Problem Solving in Abdominal Imaging

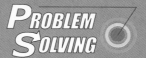
Problem Solving in Abdominal Imaging

Neal C. Dalrymple, MD
Clinical Associate Professor
The University of Texas Health Science Center, Department of Radiology
San Antonio, Texas

John R. Leyendecker, MD
Associate Professor of Radiology
Wake Forest University School of Medicine, The Bowman Gray Campus
Clinical Director—MRI
Wake Forest University Baptist Medical Center
Winston-Salem, North Carolina

Michael Oliphant, MD, FACR
Professor of Radiology
Wake Forest University School of Medicine, The Bowman Gray Campus
Winston-Salem, North Carolina

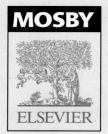

MOSBY

ELSEVIER

1600 John F. Kennedy Blvd.
Ste 1800
Philadelphia, PA 19103-2899

PROBLEM SOLVING IN ABDOMINAL IMAGING ISBN: 978-0-323-04353-3

Notice

Knowledge and best practice in this field are constantly changing. As new research and experience broaden our knowledge, changes in practice, treatment and drug therapy may become necessary or appropriate. Readers are advised to check the most current information provided (i) on procedures featured or (ii) by the manufacturer of each product to be administered, to verify the recommended dose or formula, the method and duration of administration, and contraindications. It is the responsibility of the practitioner, relying on their own experience and knowledge of the patient, to make diagnoses, to determine dosages and the best treatment for each individual patient, and to take all appropriate safety precautions. To the fullest extent of the law, neither the Publisher nor the authors assume any liability for any injury and/or damage to persons or property arising out of or related to any use of the material contained in this book.

The Publisher

Library of Congress Cataloging-in-Publication Data
Dalrymple, Neal C.
 Problem solving in abdominal imaging with CD-ROM / Neal C. Dalrymple,
John R. Leyendecker, Michael Oliphant. -- 1st ed.
  p. ; cm. -- (Problem solving in radiology series)
 ISBN 978-0-323-04353-3
 1. Abdomen--Imaging--Handbooks, manuals, etc. I. Leyendecker, John R. II. Oliphant, Michael, 1941- III. Title. IV. Series: Problem solving in radiology.
 [DNLM: 1. Radiography, Abdominal--methods. 2. Diagnostic Imaging--methods. WI 900 D151p 2010]
 RC944.D35 2010
 617.5'507572--dc22

                    2008049004

Acquisitions Editor: Rebecca Gaertner
Editorial Assistant: Elizabeth Hart
Project Manager: David Saltzberg
Design Director: Steve Stave
Marketing Manager: Nancy Ciliberti

Printed in China

Last digit is the print number: 9 8 7 6 5 4 3 2 1

To my wife, Monika, and to my daughter, Alexandra, for their steadfast patience, love, and support

NCD

To Mary, Michael, and Bridget for their love and support

JRL

To Phyllis—All my love always

MO

Contributors

Matthew Blurton, MD
Radiology Department
Singleton Associates, PA
Houston, Texas
22: Percutaneous Biopsy and Drainage

Samir A. Chhaya, MD
Assistant Professor of Radiology
Musculoskeletal Radiology Section
The University of Texas Health Science Center
   at San Antonio
San Antonio, Texas
26: Survival Guide to Bone Findings in the Abdomen and Pelvis

David Childs, MD
Assistant Professor of Radiology
Abdominal Imaging Section
Wake Forest University School of Medicine
Winston-Salem, North Carolina
21: Female Reproductive System

Paige Clark, MD
Assistant Professor
Department of Radiology
Wake Forest University School of Medicine
Winston-Salem, North Carolina
4: Positron Emission Tomography

Monika Dalrymple, MD
Staff Radiologist
South Texas Radiology Group
San Antonio, Texas
25: Survival Guide to Findings in the Lower Chest

Neal C. Dalrymple, MD
Associate Professor of Radiology
The University of Texas Health Science Center
   at San Antonio
San Antonio, Texas
1: Ultrasound; 2: Multidetector Computed Tomography; 5: A Multidimensional Approach to Abdominal Imaging; 7: Computed Tomography Incidentalomas; 8: Imaging Evaluation of Acute Abdominal Pain; 9: Imaging Evaluation of Trauma; 17: Adrenal Glands; 18: Kidneys; 19: Ureters, Bladder, and Urethra; 20: Male Reproductive System; 21: Female Reproductive System; 25: Survival Guide to Findings in the Lower Chest; 26: Survival Guide to Bone Findings in the Abdomen and Pelvis

Andrew Deibler, MD
Resident, Diagnostic Radiology
Department of Radiology
Wake Forest University School of Medicine
Winston-Salem, North Carolina
11: Common Inherited and Metabolic Disorders

David J. DiSantis, MD, MS
Associate Professor
Department of Radiology
Wake Forest University School of Medicine
Winston-Salem, North Carolina
16: Gastrointestinal Tract

Constanza J. Gutierrez, MD
Assistant Professor of Radiology
Cardiothoracic Radiology Section
The University of Texas Health Science Center
   at San Antonio
San Antonio, Texas
25: Survival Guide to Findings in the Lower Chest

Adam J. Jung, MD
Resident, Diagnostic Radiology
Graduate Student in Radiological Sciences
The University of Texas Health Science Center
  at San Antonio
San Antonio, Texas
20: Male Reproductive System

John R. Leyendecker, MD
Associate Professor of Radiology
Department of Radiology
Wake Forest University School of Medicine
Winston-Salem, North Carolina
*3: Magnetic Resonance Imaging; 6: Localization and Spread of
Disease; 7: Computed Tomography Incidentalomas; 8: Imaging
Evaluation of Acute Abdominal Pain; 10: A Brief Guide to Cancer
Imaging; 11: Common Inherited and Metabolic Disorders; 12:
Liver; 13: Gallbladder and Bile Ducts; 14: Pancreas; 15: Spleen;
16: Gastrointestinal Tract; 22: Percutaneous Biopsy and Drainage;
23: Lesion Composition; 24: Atlas of Basic Surgical Procedures*

Michael Oliphant, MD, FACR
Professor of Radiology
Wake Forest University School of Medicine
Winston-Salem, North Carolina
*6: Localization and Spread of Disease; 8: Imaging Evaluation
of Acute Abdominal Pain; 9: Imaging Evaluation of Trauma;
10: A Brief Guide to Cancer Imaging; 14: Pancreas; 16: Gastrointestinal Tract*

Phil Ralls, MD
Professor, Department of Radiology
Keck School of Medicine
University of Southern California
Los Angeles, California
1: Ultrasound

Hisham Tchelepi, MD
Instructor of Radiology
Department of Radiology
Keck School of Medicine
University of Southern California
Los Angeles, California
*1: Ultrasound; 13: Gallbladder and Bile Ducts;
23: Lesion Composition*

Anthony I. Zarka, MD
Staff Radiologist
Wilford Hall Medical Center
Lackland Air Force Base, Texas
20: Male Reproductive System

Foreword

The field of abdominal imaging is quite broad, having implications for a variety of imaging specialists. This is primarily because of the abdomen's central location within the body, because it is a frequent focus of emergent conditions, and because it includes several different organs and their associated disease processes. Ideally, all radiologists who are responsible for the interpretation of images in the abdomen and pelvis should acquire subspecialty training in abdominal imaging. This notion, of course, is neither practical nor realistic. Alternatively, one can attempt to acquire some level of expertise from continuing medical educational endeavors, such as attending meetings or viewing on-line content. While these formats are indeed informative, they may not be well suited to one's particular pace, area of interest, or clinical need. This book provides an excellent solution to this problem, particularly in the way that the material is presented.

In a way, this publication is like a "fellowship in a book." Having said that, it might be prudent to ask, "What exactly does one receive from fellowship subspecialty training?" First, a fellowship allows the individual to concentrate or focus his or her efforts on a specific group of anatomic and disease processes. Second, a fellowship allows the individual to become familiar with the design and implementation of imaging protocols, particularly in CT, MRI, and PET. Third, a fellowship gives the individual ample opportunities to develop diagnostic algorithms relative to a multi-modality organ-oriented approach. Fourth, a fellowship exposes the individual to a high volume and wide variety of cases, thereby allowing his or her diagnostic skills to mature. Maturity yields diagnoses that are more specific with superior handling of tough and challenging cases. Lastly, a fellowship may provide expertise in certain interventional techniques.

How will this book help one approximate fellowship training in abdominal imaging? While it won't give you experience performing interventional procedures, it will definitely provide a handy resource that focuses on the anatomy and disease processes in the abdomen and pelvis, familiarize you with the issues related to protocol design, aid in the development of multi-modality organ-oriented diagnostic algorithms, and expose you to a large variety of interesting and challenging cases. If the end result is a mature diagnostician, then the intended purpose of the book can be considered sound.

The editors of this book, Drs. John Leyendecker, Neal Dalrymple, and Michael Oliphant, are noted experts in the field of abdominal imaging and are well suited to teaching the principles emphasized in this new and exciting book. On a personal note, I am particularly honored and delighted to have been invited to write the Foreword for this book, as John Leyendecker and I worked together years ago when he was a resident in Diagnostic Radiology at Emory University. It was obvious to me and the other faculty back then that John was a unique and special radiologist, destined to make a difference in our specialty. His work ethic and attention to detail are attributes that have made him an outstanding editor of the material presented in this exceptional book.

Rendon C. Nelson, MD
Reed and Martha Rice Distinguished Professor of Radiology
Division of Abdominal Imaging
Duke University

Preface

The field of abdominal imaging has grown beyond the ability of most practitioners to maintain expertise in all of the relevant modalities, anatomic concepts, and disease processes. This expansion in knowledge has created two distinct needs. One is for concise, readily accessible information relevant to the daily practice of abdominal imaging. The other is for an effective approach to the problems that can be encountered at various steps in the imaging management of a patient. These steps include selection of an appropriate imaging modality to investigate a patient's symptoms, physical findings, and laboratory abnormalities. Imaging findings must be actively sought and accurately interpreted to yield a diagnosis or list of possible diagnoses. If the diagnosis remains in doubt after initial imaging, one must determine whether additional imaging or intervention is appropriate. Even after a diagnosis is revealed, it is important to seek additional relevant imaging findings that might impact patient management or prognosis. This volume in the Problem Solving series was created to assist and guide the imager through these steps.

This is not simply a book of radiologic differential diagnoses. Initial chapters summarize key aspects of relevant imaging modalities, including ultrasound, multidetector computed tomography, magnetic resonance imaging, and positron emission tomography. We go beyond image acquisition with a section on problem-solving applications of three-dimensional techniques and other forms of image processing. Subsequent chapters describe our approach to common clinical scenarios and disease processes such as pain, trauma, and cancer. Common "incidentalomas" are addressed, and organ-specific chapters lead the reader from imaging findings to diagnosis. When discussing pathologic processes and disease entities, the various imaging modalities are often discussed together in an attempt to encourage cross-modality thinking; this mirrors typical general practice; encourages correlative interpretation; and acknowledges that human anatomy, physiology, and pathology are constant regardless of imaging technique.

Traditionalists might not approve of our approach of mixing modalities while deviating from the standard organizational framework that has served imaging textbooks for decades. Admittedly, the type of organization we employ may take some getting used to. However, we firmly believe that to remain vital to modern medicine imagers need to evolve from pattern recognition and rote memorization toward a more insightful approach to the imaging of disease processes. The best radiologists see beyond the images to visualize a patient with a disease that has a distinct composition, biological behavior, and pattern of spread that determine the imaging findings and clinical presentation. Such radiologists are not just playing a high-tech game of seek-and-find; they are true problem solvers who are also likely to be valued consultants.

There is no question that we have undertaken an ambitious task in attempting to combine multiple abdominal imaging modalities, clinical scenarios, and organ systems in a single, readable text. To accomplish this, we could not possibly include an in-depth discussion of every known pathologic condition of the abdomen and pelvis. Instead, we chose to focus on topics that commonly vex practicing radiologists, such as characterizing and managing cystic pancreatic lesions, what to do with an incidental adrenal nodule, and how to best approach an abdominal abscess. Throughout this book, we try to help the reader separate clinically insignificant findings from life-threatening abnormalities and, ultimately, to render more definitive and comprehensive interpretations. Whenever possible, we consolidate key concepts into tables or illustrations and highlight important points as "pearls" or "pitfalls." We have also tried to produce the type of book we would want by our sides every day but can still read at night.

To some extent, this book is a reflection of our own individual struggles experienced during the daily practice and teaching of abdominal imaging. As such, it is important to acknowledge that there are often multiple, equally valid ways to evaluate a patient's symptoms or further assess an abnormal finding. Our recommendations should serve only as a starting point to be modified as appropriate in light of one's individual practice environment, weighing of conflicting opinions, and subsequent advances in knowledge and technology. While the variable and dynamic nature of abdominal imaging presents obvious challenges to anyone attempting to write a timely and practical treatise on the field, we believe that the very same complexity creates a need for a text such as this. We hope readers agree.

Acknowledgments

Thanks to John Leyendecker for inviting me to work with him to create this book. I could not have asked for a better partner. Thanks also to Mike Oliphant, whose insights helped me to see familiar structures in an entirely new way. I am grateful to those who taught me over the years (too many of my professors, colleagues, residents, and technologists to name!) for challenging me to learn more every day. I appreciate the patience shown to me by my support staff at the University of Texas Health Science Center, especially Gladys, Edie, and Lissette, as I juggled this project with my other responsibilities. Most of all, I am fortunate that my wife, Monika, not only worked hard to maintain a "normal" family life through the countless nights and weekends during which I worked on this book, but also, as a radiologist herself, provided me with invaluable feedback on text and figures when asked (regardless of the hour).

NCD

I would like to acknowledge my Abdominal Imaging friends and colleagues at Wake Forest University for their direct and indirect contributions to this work: Ray Dyer, for whom I have tremendous respect despite his love of eponyms, for his dedication to mentoring and for his constant vigilance for interesting cases, many of which are featured in this book; Ron Zagoria, our section head, for maintaining a challenging, productive, and fun academic environment at a time when many institutions have given up trying; David DiSantis, who, through his knowledge of gastrointestinal radiology more than compensates for his use of "junk rubber"; Hisham Tchelepi, the best sonologist I know, for his advice on all things ultrasound, for never being afraid to change his mind or mine, and for always hitting a forehand smash, even when he shouldn't.

I would also like to thank the editors at Elsevier, who stood by us and encouraged us every step of the way, even when it seemed this day would never come.

JRL

Contents

Advanced Modalities as Problem-Solving Tools

CHAPTER 1.

Ultrasound

Hisham Tchelepi, Neal C. Dalrymple, and Phil Ralls

Ultrasound is an interactive modality that integrates the art of the physical examination with modern high-resolution imaging technology. In some ways the evolutionary offspring of the stethoscope, ultrasound is a handheld diagnostic tool that is only as powerful as the experience and expertise of its user.

Ultrasound is often the first-line modality for imaging patients suspected of having abdominal or pelvic disease. It provides comprehensive anatomic detail for many abdominal and pelvic organs, yet remains less costly than the other cross-sectional imaging modalities, making it widely available. Because sonography also lacks the risks associated with ionizing radiation and iodinated contrast media, little disadvantage exists to imaging patients with ultrasound.

In recent years, significant advances have been made in the field of sonography. Current systems make use of sophisticated technology to produce high-resolution images incorporating anatomy and pathology. Applications such as color and power Doppler, tissue harmonic imaging, and speckle reduction imaging have helped to revolutionize the role of sonography as a problem solver in medical imaging. The ready availability and standard use of real-time imaging is unique to ultrasound among cross-sectional imaging modalities. Contrast-enhanced sonography is emerging in the twenty-first century as an imaging modality that will likely play an important role in the management and follow-up of disease progression in patients with cancer.

Of course, sonography does have some limitations. The patient's body habitus often determines the image quality and visibility that can be achieved. Beyond size, the location of a lesion or anatomic structure is critical because sonography is unable to visualize structures that lie deep to bone or air. Perhaps the most critical limitation is that the diagnostic yield is highly dependent on the skill of the individual performing the examination.

■ GENERAL PRINCIPLES OF ULTRASOUND TECHNIQUE

Ultrasound scanners use the piezoelectric effect to transform electricity into acoustic energy. The transducer serves to generate and transmit energy into the body, as well as to receive acoustic energy as it returns after being altered by tissues. Some of the many factors that influence image quality are listed in Box 1-1.

Contact

Although the variable acoustic conductivity of tissues is the cornerstone of its utility, poor conductivity through air and particularly through abrupt air/soft-tissue interfaces is of particular concern where the ultrasound transducer contacts the skin. A low-impedance gel is used to bridge the gap between the transducer and skin, providing enough texture to conform to contours of the skin and transducer while fluid enough to act as a lubricant, minimizing patient discomfort during manipulation.

Window

Contact at the skin surface is only the first obstacle from the transducer to the anatomic structures of interest. Skin, fat, lung, bowel, and bone can intervene and reflect or attenuate acoustic energy. It is usually desirable to use a structure with low acoustic impedance as a "window" to the structures to be examined. For example, the transducer is often placed between ribs but overlying the liver to visualize the gallbladder because bowel loops can obscure a more direct approach. The liver is often used as a window into the pancreas and right kidney as well. If gastric air obscures the pancreas, this can be improved by asking the patient to drink water. The spleen often provides a window to the left kidney, although variable location of the spleen makes this unreliable. A distended bladder is commonly used as a window for transabdominal sonography of the gynecologic organs. Because some of these organs may move when the patient moves, repositioning the patient may be useful when faced with difficulty finding a satisfactory window.

Transducer Array

Several basic types of transducers are available, and advantages and disadvantages are associated with each. These include sector scanners, curved arrays, linear arrays, and phased arrays.

Sector Scanner

Sector scanners are the earliest type of transducer, and they utilize a single piezoelectric crystal. Because the source is a single point of oscillation, it results in a cone-shaped beam (Fig. 1-1). Sector scanners usually have a fixed range and are not in common use today.

Curved Array

Curved array transducers have become the mainstay for most abdominal and pelvic applications. The convex surface results in a mildly diverging beam, optimizing anatomic coverage from a given window (Fig. 1-2). The smooth convexity also provides for patient comfort as the transducer is moved along the skin surface. Endocavitary transducers rely on small, curved arrays with high frequency to provide high-resolution images of the pelvic organs.

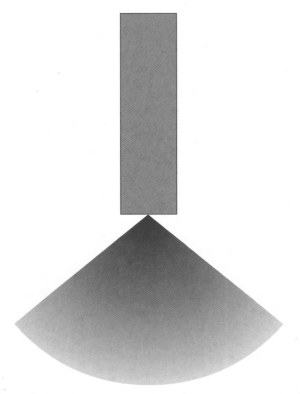

Figure 1-1 Footprint and field of view for sector scanner. Phased array transducers usually have a similar appearance, but the beam can be steered, increasing utility.

Figure 1-2 Footprint and field of view for curved array transducer.

Linear Array

Using a flat footprint and high-frequency element, linear arrays have become the preferred transducer for most vascular applications, as well as for the evaluation of superficial small parts (testicles, thyroid). Parallel waves result in a rectangular field of view and provide for minimal distortion of anatomic structures (Fig. 1-3).

Phased Array

Phased array transducers orchestrate multiple elements activated in sequence to create a beam that can be steered electronically. Phased array transducers usually provide a cone-shaped field of view that appears similar to a sector scanner (see Fig. 1-1) but are more versatile because the beam can be steered from side to side. A small footprint makes these transducers useful when only a small sonographic window is available (e.g., intercostal approach, neonatal heads, postsurgical patients with wounds/bandages).

Transducer Frequency

Frequency selection is a key element that affects image quality. High-frequency transducers offer high-resolution imaging of superficial structures but are more susceptible to beam attenuation than low-frequency transducers. Low-frequency transducers provide better penetration, so they are useful for examining deep structures and large patients, but at a cost of lower image resolution. Thus a balance exists between the desired resolution and tissue

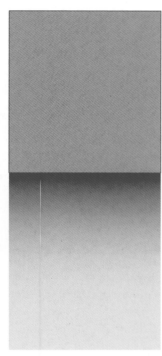

Figure 1-3 Linear array transducer.

interaction between the radiologist and sonographer, rescanning patients with different transducers when necessary, will help achieve consistent image quality within an ultrasound department.

Gain

Many think of the two-dimensional gain on the ultrasound machine simply as controlling the brightness of the ultrasound image. Adjusting the gain does not alter the intensity of the ultrasound beam; rather, it increases the sensitivity for receiving the incident acoustic information, similar to turning up the volume on a radio. Decreasing the gain results in a dark image, increasing it results in a bright image. Optimal image contrast is found somewhere in between.

Because the tissues along the depth of a given field of view attenuate acoustic waves to a variable extent, a single gain setting cannot optimize image quality throughout the field of view. Time gain compensation is used to adjust gain settings according to depth to optimize gain throughout the image (Fig. 1-4).

Focal Zone

The focal zone describes the distance from the transducer at which the beam is optimized for spatial resolution. In general, the focal zone should be adjusted to the depth of the object being examined (Fig. 1-5). Many

penetration required to reach the object in question. In general, optimal image quality is achieved when using the highest frequency transducer that provides sufficient penetration. If that sounds subjective, it is! Frequent

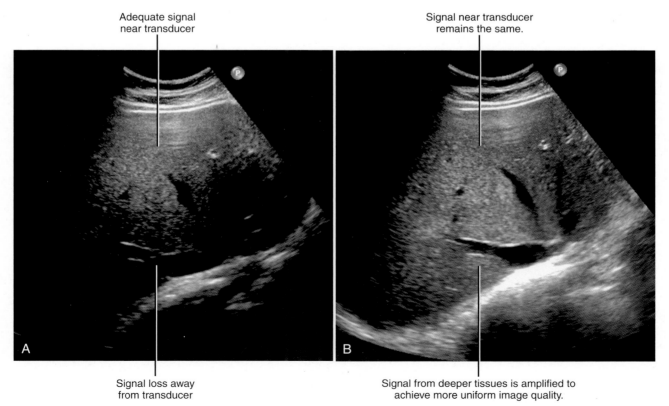

Adequate signal near transducer

Signal near transducer remains the same.

Signal loss away from transducer

Signal from deeper tissues is amplified to achieve more uniform image quality.

Figure 1-4 Effects of using time gain compensation (TGC) shown by using flat TGC settings (**A**), then by using TGC to amplify signal from deeper tissues (**B**).

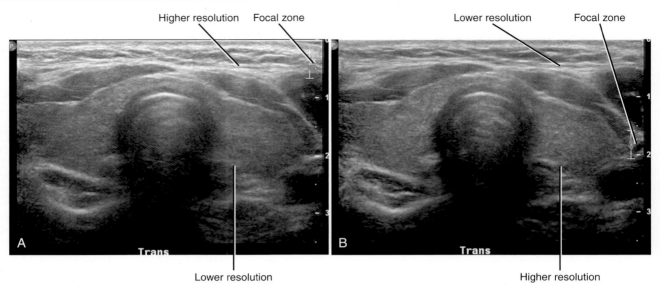

Figure 1-5 Impact of adjusting the focal zone shown with two images of the same location in the thyroid gland with the focal zone near (**A**), then away (**B**) from the transducer.

transducers now provide multiple focal zones, allowing for more uniform image quality.

Harmonic Imaging

Although acoustic signal is transmitted at a specific frequency, the interaction of the beam with different tissues generates harmonic waves that resonate at frequencies that are double, triple, or quadruple the transmitted frequency. Because the types of tissue interfaces that generate most types of artifact do not produce harmonic waves, integrating harmonic information with the primary frequency improves the ratio of signal to noise (Fig. 1-6). Tissue harmonic imaging is particularly helpful with large body habitus or "noisy" tissues such as an echogenic liver.

■ COMMON ARTIFACTS

English dictionaries define the word *artifact* to mean something created by humans, whereas medical dictionaries define it as something that results from technique. In fact, every sonographic image is a human creation born of technical innovation. Perhaps the more

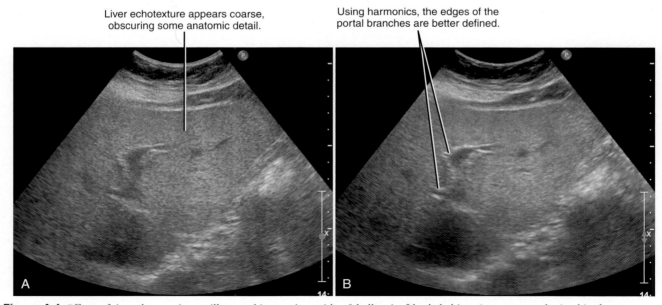

Figure 1-6 Effects of tissue harmonics are illustrated in a patient with a "challenging" body habitus. Images were obtained in the same location of the liver without (**A**) and then with (**B**) tissue harmonics.

common radiologic use of the word describes the *unintended* production of an image because of technical factors. This parsing of words may seem trivial, but despite the often negative connotation associated with the word *artifact* in the field of imaging, artifacts are sometimes a key diagnostic finding in sonography. Because the presence and recognition of an artifact can lead to diagnosis and the lack or recognition may lead to misdiagnosis, a basic understanding of the most common artifacts is critical to the effective use of sonography.

Acoustic Shadowing

Acoustic shadowing results when tissues absorb or reflect the incident ultrasound beam. Because there is no signal representing the tissues distal to that point, the image is replaced with a dark band along the projected course of the beam (Fig. 1-7). Shadowing is commonly seen with urinary or biliary calculi.

Calcium deposits and their interface with soft tissues can reflect and/or absorb ultrasound waves effectively. This has two main impacts on the ultrasound image: (1) a highly echogenic appearance at the near margin of the calcified object, and (2) a loss of signal beyond that object. The presence and type of posterior acoustic shadowing produced is related to the size and surface morphology of a structure. In the case of small calcium deposits, color Doppler can be used to increase conspicuity of tissue reflectivity in the form of the color comet tail artifact (CCTA), also called *twinkle artifact* (see Fig. 23-37 on CD-ROM).

Shadowing often results in a uniform dark stripe distal to the object, but this is not always the case. Although the authors prefer to avoid the term *dirty shadowing,* it is sometimes used in the literature to describe less uniform absorption, usually at soft-tissue interfaces or from gas (see Fig. 1-7). Although this has been reported to be helpful to identify structures or processes including lung, bowel, pneumobilia, and portal venous gas, caution must be applied. The sign is neither sensitive nor specific because there can be overlap with the more traditional shadowing.

Reverberation

Reverberation occurs when acoustic energy "bounces" between two or more adjacent highly reflective surfaces. The result is a series of bands perpendicular to the beam, each representing a different delay in the return of energy to the transducer (Fig. 1-8). The effect is more pronounced when these surfaces are in the near field and in the center of the field of view. Reverberation artifact can be mistaken for sludge within the gallbladder, although examining the gallbladder from a different angle should eliminate the artifact. Reverberation is useful in creating the "comet tail" artifact characteristic of adenomyomatosis of the gallbladder wall. Color Doppler can be used to accentuate the reverberation effects of adenomyomatosis. The result is another form of CCTA (twinkle artifact) (Fig. 1-9).

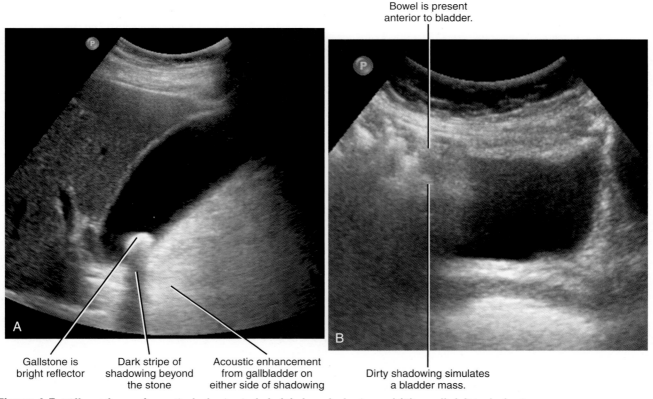

Bowel is present
anterior to bladder.

A

B

Gallstone is
bright reflector

Dark stripe of
shadowing beyond
the stone

Acoustic enhancement
from gallbladder on
either side of shadowing

Dirty shadowing simulates
a bladder mass.

Figure 1-7 Different forms of acoustic shadowing include (**A**) clean shadowing and (**B**) so-called dirty shadowing.

Anterior peritoneum is a bright
reflector near the transducer.

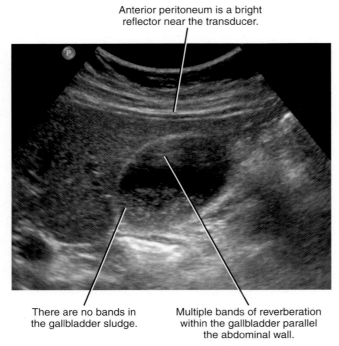

There are no bands in
the gallbladder sludge.

Multiple bands of reverberation
within the gallbladder parallel
the abdominal wall.

Figure 1-8 Reverberation artifact in the gallbladder.

Side Lobe

Side lobes are the result of nonuniformity of the ultrasound beam at the periphery of the transducer. Although most of the beam is concentrated in the intended field of imaging, additional waves extend toward the periphery, out of the field of view. These "side lobes" typically account for only a minute component of the overall ultrasound energy, and only a small portion of it actually reflects back into the field of view most of the time. However, if those sound waves encounter an effective reflector and return to the field of view, they produce bands that are parallel to the primary incident beam. This is often seen as an apparent septation extending from the side of the gallbladder, the urinary bladder, or a simple cyst (Fig. 1-10). Unlike true septations, these bands will disappear or change with adjustment of the scan angle or focal zone.

Refraction Artifact

Much like light entering water, the ultrasound beam bends when it encounters tissues that conduct sound at widely disparate velocities. As a result, an object may appear to be in a place other than where it actually is. Usually only part of the beam bends, causing an object to appear duplicated. This can result in the "now you see it, now you don't" phenomenon, where there appear to be two cysts in the liver on first inspection, but only one is seen later.

Mirror Image

Also known as multipath artifact, mirror image artifact is the result of the ultrasound beam "bouncing" off two strong specular reflectors before returning to the transducer. This is analogous to a billiard ball shot near a

Small areas of comet tail artifact

Twinkle artifact represents color
Doppler enhancement of
the comet tail artifact.

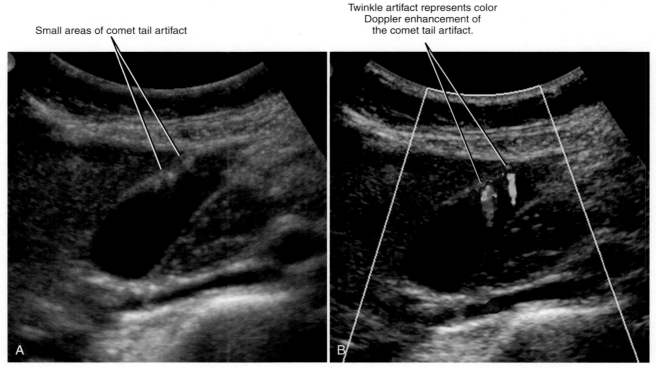

Figure 1-9 Comet tail (**A**) and color comet tail artifact or twinkle (**B**) artifacts in adenomyomatosis of the gallbladder.

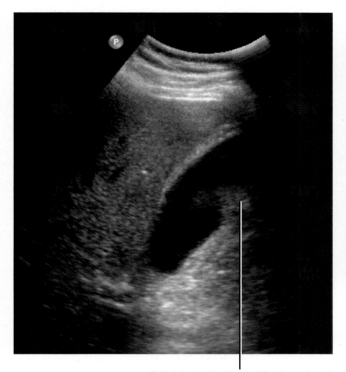

Side lobe artifact looks like linear band
of sludge or a mass but did not persist
when scanning from different angles.

Figure 1-10 Ultrasound image of the gallbladder shows side lobe artifact caused by adjacent bowel.

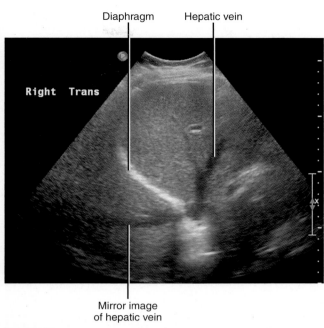

Diaphragm   Hepatic vein

Right Trans

Mirror image
of hepatic vein

Figure 1-11 Transverse ultrasound image of the right hepatic lobe shows mirror image artifact of liver beyond the diaphragm.

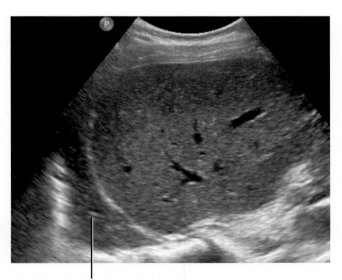

Markings within consolidated lung
do not mirror vascular structures
within the liver.

Figure 1-12 Right lower lobe pneumonia first identified by ultrasound in a patient with right upper quadrant pain. The diagnosis was confirmed by chest radiograph.

corner striking two cushions before returning to the shooter. Because the travel between the reflectors is not acknowledged by the ultrasound system, the result is duplication of the near-field image beyond the reflector. This occurs most commonly when the ultrasound beam reflects off two points of the diaphragm, resulting in projection of the liver into the thorax (Fig. 1-11). If structures do not precisely mirror the near field, consider alternative explanations for the image appearance (Fig. 1-12).

Acoustic Enhancement

Acoustic enhancement refers to a zone of increased signal (usually a bright stripe) seen deep to a structure with low acoustic impedance. This is most commonly seen deep to the gallbladder, urinary bladder, simple cysts, or large blood vessels (Fig. 1-13). Acoustic enhancement is usually omitted from lists of ultrasound artifacts, perhaps because of its utility in characterizing cystic structures. Nonetheless, acoustic enhancement is merely an unintended technical phenomenon, and although it is often useful, it can also lead to errant diagnosis if unrecognized. For example, ascites in the hepatorenal space can make the kidney appear echogenic, prompting an inaccurate diagnosis of diffuse renal parenchymal disease (Fig. 1-14).

■ ULTRASOUND OF THE UPPER ABDOMEN

Ultrasound of the Liver

The liver is best imaged with the patient in the supine and left lateral decubitus positions, starting with 3- to 7-MHz curved array transducers. In most cases, harmonic imaging improves image quality in the liver. A subcostal acoustic window should be attempted first,

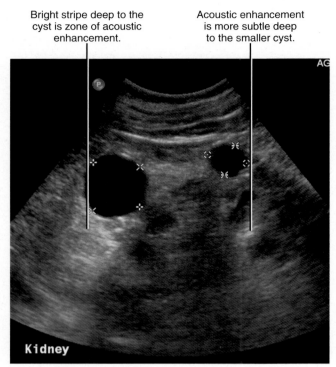

Bright stripe deep to the cyst is zone of acoustic enhancement.

Acoustic enhancement is more subtle deep to the smaller cyst.

Kidney

Figure 1-13 Ultrasound image of the right kidney shows two renal cysts causing acoustic enhancement.

supplemented with intercostal scanning as necessary. The liver surface (usually the ventral left lobe) should be evaluated for nodularity with a near-field, optimized, 5- to 12-MHz linear array transducer. It is easier to appreciate subtle nodularity during real-time examination or on video clips than on hard-copy images. Furthermore, surface characteristics are easier to appreciate when ascites is present (Fig. 1-15) Angling the transducer so that it is not perpendicular to the liver surface may falsely simulate nodularity.

Routine color flow imaging is useful in patients with suspected liver disease. Optimal color flow and spectral Doppler sonography of the liver generally require relatively low-frequency (2-3 MHz) scanning and good acoustic access. Spectral Doppler sonography can help distinguish arterial from venous flow and detect abnormal hemodynamics within vessels.

Viral Hepatitis

No specific sonographic findings are found in acute hepatitis. The most common sonographic finding in hepatitis is probably hepatomegaly, although this is easily overlooked. The so-called starry sky pattern, increased periportal echoes coupled with decreased parenchymal echogenicity, is relatively insensitive for the detection of acute viral hepatitis. In one series, the starry sky liver pattern was found in only 19 of 791 patients with viral hepatitis. In the same study, there was no difference in sonographic findings between a control group and patients with acute viral hepatitis. Marked gallbladder wall thickening is sometimes present in patients with acute hepatitis (Fig. 1-16).

Hepatomegaly and heterogeneously increased echogenicity are common in chronic hepatitis and are related to the amount of fatty infiltration and fibrosis present. The liver surface is smooth, unless cirrhosis is also present. In chronic active hepatitis, enlarged arteries are noted on color Doppler sonography because of increased arterial flow. This may cause a "double-channel"

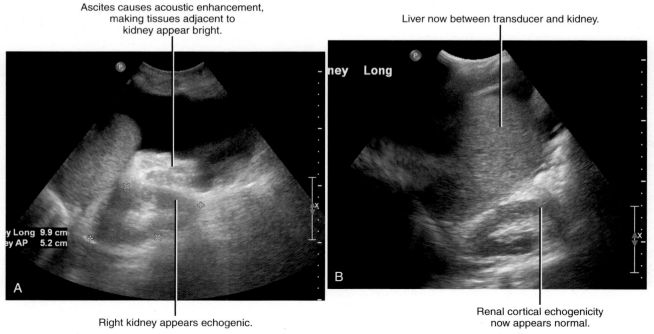

Ascites causes acoustic enhancement, making tissues adjacent to kidney appear bright.

Liver now between transducer and kidney.

Right kidney appears echogenic.

Renal cortical echogenicity now appears normal.

Figure 1-14 Two images from the same ultrasound examination, first using ascites as a window to the right kidney (**A**), then using the right lobe of the liver as a window (**B**).

Nodular surface
of the liver

Ascites improves delineation
of the liver surface.

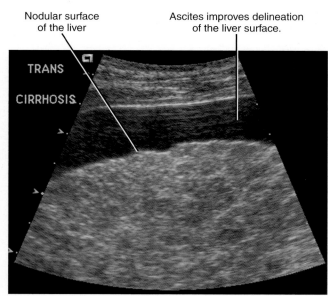

Figure 1-15 Sonographic demonstration of surface nodularity in a patient with cirrhosis.

Thick gallbladder wall

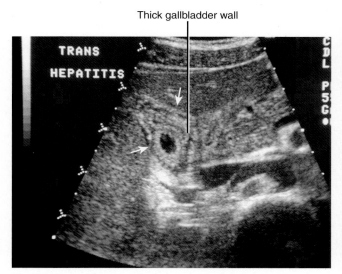

Figure 1-16 Thickening of the gallbladder wall in acute viral hepatitis.

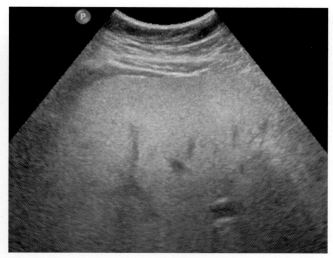

Figure 1-17 Diffuse fatty infiltration of the liver. The liver is diffusely echogenic, and the portal radicals are not apparent.

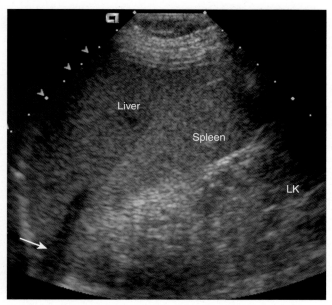

Liver

Spleen

LK

Figure 1-18 Relative echogenicity of the liver, spleen, and left kidney *(LK)* in a healthy patient.

sign on grayscale images that can be confused with biliary dilatation. Lymph nodes are often detected in the hepatoduodenal ligament.

Steatohepatitis

Severe fatty infiltration of the liver often results in hepatomegaly and diffusely increased echogenicity (Fig. 1-17). Acoustic penetration may be decreased, resulting in indistinctness of blood vessels and the diaphragm. Hepatic echogenicity is usually equal to or greater than that of the renal cortex. Although subjective assessment of the renal cortex and liver parenchyma echogenicity is useful in severe fatty infiltration, this approach is error prone and insensitive. Although unproven, we prefer to use the relative echogenicity of the kidneys compared with the spleen and liver (Fig. 1-18). The normal spleen is slightly more

echogenic than the normal liver. Therefore, if the difference in echogenicity between the liver and right kidney is greater than the difference between the spleen and left kidney, the liver parenchyma has abnormally increased echogenicity. This approach assumes, of course, that the echogenicity of the kidneys is equal bilaterally.

Fat deposition and sparing are not always uniform, with focal (Fig. 1-19) and regional (Fig. 1-20) differences possible within the liver. Patterns of fat deposition and sparing are discussed in more detail in Chapter 12.

Cirrhosis

Cirrhosis is the end stage of chronic hepatocellular injury, characterized by bridging fibrosis and regeneration. The most common sonographic findings in cirrhosis are listed in Table 1-1. Unfortunately, many of these signs

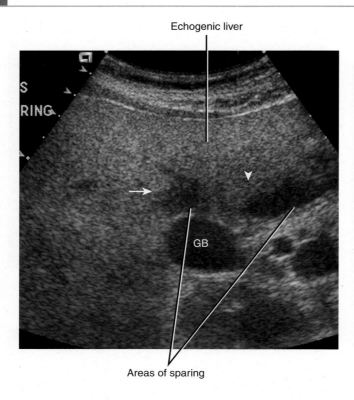

Echogenic liver

GB

Areas of sparing

Figure 1-19 Typical focal sparing adjacent to the gallbladder *(GB)* and in the dorsal left lobe in an otherwise diffusely fatty infiltrated liver.

are insensitive and insufficiently specific for cirrhosis to be diagnosed reliably with sonography. Furthermore, the extent of sonographic changes is not a reliable predictor of disease severity. Nevertheless, evaluation of the liver surface with a high-resolution linear array transducer is useful because surface nodularity may be the only sonographic sign of cirrhosis (Fig. 1-21). Be aware that metastases to the liver can also result in a nodular liver contour, and this nodularity may be the only indication of metastatic disease in patients with a known primary malignancy (Fig. 1-22).

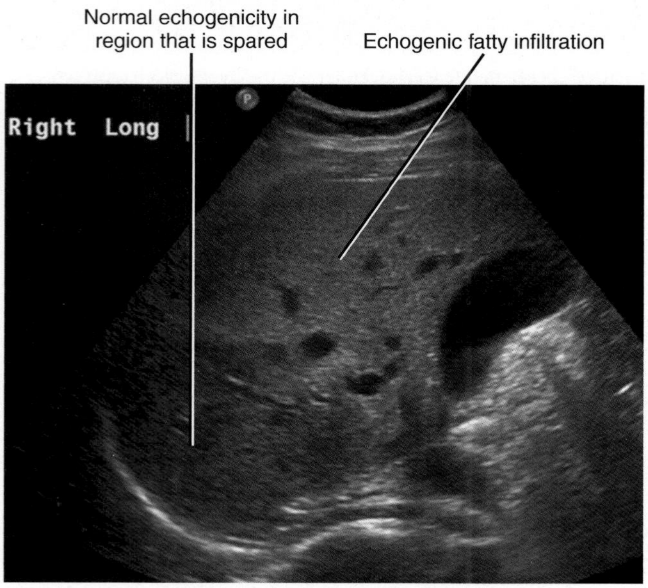

Normal echogenicity in region that is spared

Echogenic fatty infiltration

Right Long

Figure 1-20 Regional sparing of the posterior right lobe of the liver.

Color Doppler sonography can show portal vein flow reversal or portosystemic collaterals, suggesting the diagnosis of portal hypertension (Fig. 1-26). Because considerable variation exists in the size of the portal vein with changes in respiration and patient position, absolute portal vein diameter is not a reliable predictor of portal hypertension. In fact, a lack of respiratory variation (an increase in portal vein diameter during inspiration and a decrease during expiration) can indicate portal hypertension. Other portal flow abnormalities include bidirectional flow and, rarely, nearly static blood flow. Be aware that transient portal flow reversal also occurs in some clinical conditions not related to liver disease such as tricuspid regurgitation and heart failure (Fig. 1-27).

Table 1-1   Sonographic Findings of Cirrhosis

Finding	Comments
Nodular liver surface	More specific than sensitive; however, also consider metastatic disease if patient has known primary malignancy
Echogenic liver	Nonspecific, commonly seen with fatty infiltration
Flow reversal in portal vein	Specific finding, although transient reversal occasionally seen with cardiac disease
Collateral venous flow	Specific finding when present (Fig. 1-23)
Enlarged hepatic arteries (Fig. 1-24)	Also seen with portal vein thrombosis and arteriovenous shunting
Narrowing of the hepatic veins and intrahepatic IVC	Dampens transmission of cardiac waveform (see Fig. 1-25)

IVC, Inferior vena cava.

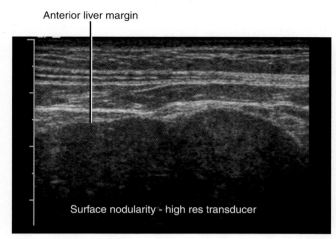

Anterior liver margin

Surface nodularity - high res transducer

Figure 1-21 Demonstration of nodular liver contour using high-resolution linear transducer. The nodular contour can be seen even in the absence of ascites.

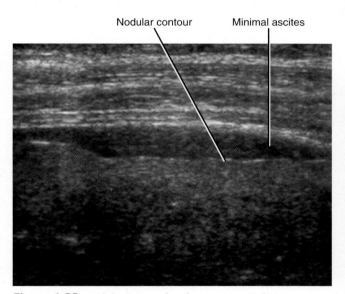

Nodular contour   *Minimal ascites*

Figure 1-22 Nodular liver surface from metastatic disease.

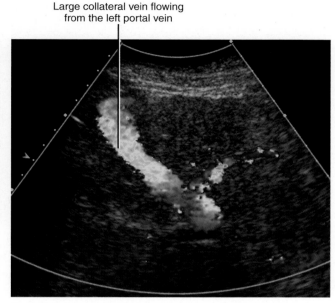

Large collateral vein flowing from the left portal vein

Figure 1-23 Demonstration of a paraumbilical vein using color Doppler imaging.

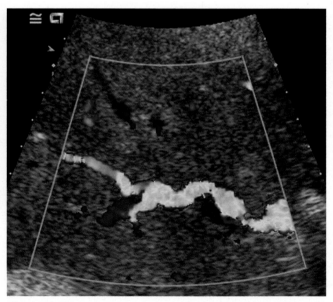

Figure 1-24 Tortuous and enlarged hepatic artery in cirrhosis.

Sonography also plays an important role in the evaluation and follow-up of patients with known liver cirrhosis. Although focal fatty infiltration, regenerating nodules, and other benign lesions can occur in a cirrhotic liver, any sonographically detected mass within a cirrhotic liver should be considered suspicious for hepatocellular carcinoma (HCC) and referred for additional diagnostic evaluation.

Focal Liver Lesions

Sonography excels at the detection and characterization of cystic lesions in the liver. These cystic lesions can be easily classified based on their sonographic features as simple or complex. Simple cysts are usually well-defined, echo-free, round or oval lesions with thin walls and enhanced through transmission. Thin septations are a frequent finding in simple hepatic cysts. Thicker septations or mural nodules are generally a sign of a cystic neoplasm such as biliary cystadenoma or cystic metastases.

The sonographic appearance of hydatid disease in the liver can range from simple cystic to complex, demonstrating calcifications, mural nodules, and the so-called water lily sign. The latter finding represents separation of the endocyst layer of the hydatid cyst. When a hydatid cyst has dense egg-shell calcification, the shadowing produced from the reflected echoes may simulate a granuloma or be confused with other solid lesions (Fig. 1-28).

In the United States, 85% of HCCs occur in patients with cirrhosis or precirrhotic conditions. Small HCCs (<5 cm) are often hypoechoic. With further progression, lesions become more numerous and heterogeneous, and often develop a hypoechoic peripheral rim (Fig. 1-29). Advanced HCC is often multifocal, making

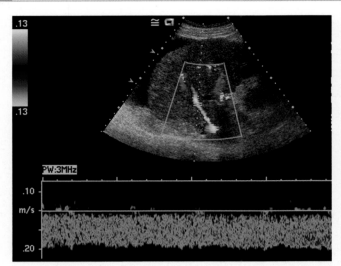

Figure 1-25 Narrowing of the hepatic veins in cirrhosis. Note loss of the triphasic waveform shown by spectral Doppler imaging.

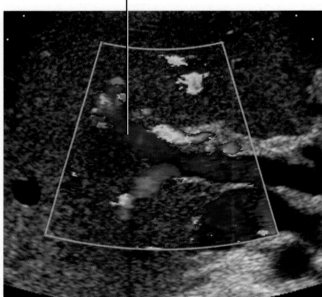

Flow is reversed (away from the liver) in the right, left, and main portal veins

Figure 1-26 Reversal of flow in the portal vein demonstrated by color Doppler imaging. The color scale (not shown) was set so that flow toward the transducer is red and flow away from the transducer is blue.

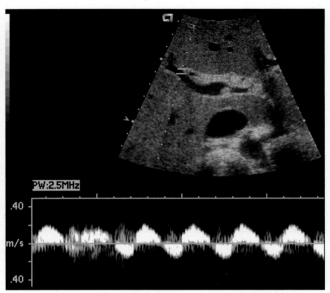

Figure 1-27 Spectral Doppler imaging shows a biphasic waveform in portal vein in patient with tricuspid regurgitation.

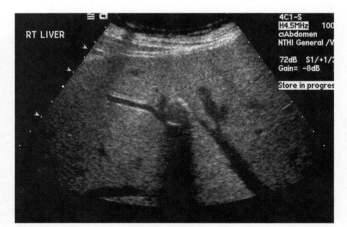

Figure 1-28 Calcified hydatid cyst in the liver.

it difficult to distinguish from metastatic disease. Echogenic nodules are fairly common in multifocal HCC (Fig. 1-30). Fatty metamorphosis of HCC also causes increased echogenicity and can result in confusion with hemangioma. A mass associated with invasion of the portal or hepatic veins should suggest the diagnosis of HCC (Fig. 1-31), although other liver tumors occasionally invade venous structures. About three-fourths of HCCs have identifiable internal color flow, a feature present in only one-third of metastases.

Because patients presenting with right upper quadrant pain, fever, and leukocytosis usually undergo an ultrasound as the initial imaging examination, liver abscesses are frequently identified with ultrasound. The sonographic appearance of liver abscess is quite variable. Abscesses are usually round or oval and hypoechoic with irregular margins (Fig. 1-32). The abscesses can be homogeneous or inhomogeneous. They may also simulate solid masses, and acoustic enhancement is frequently absent. Often, the internal contents of a liver abscess can be seen to move during real-time sonography, distinguishing it from a solid tumor.

The presence of echogenic fine foci within the abscess usually indicates microbubbles (Fig. 1-33). Microbubbles can also simulate the appearance of blood flow within some abscesses on color Doppler. Large, confluent pockets of gas within an abscess can be confused with bowel gas, particularly in right lobe abscesses close to the diaphragm.

Mass is predominantly
hypoechoic.

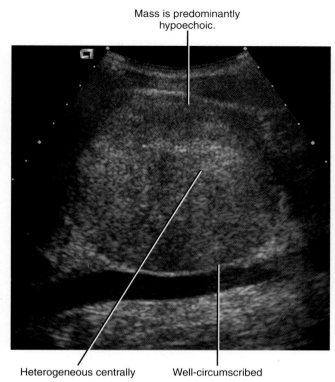

Heterogeneous centrally   Well-circumscribed

Figure 1-29 Hepatocellular carcinoma identified as a large heterogeneous mass by ultrasound.

Wall of portal vein   Blood flow within
tumor thrombus

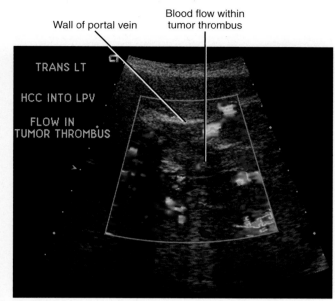

Figure 1-31 Color Doppler imaging shows arterial flow within tumor thrombus in the portal vein of a patient with hepatocellular carcinoma.

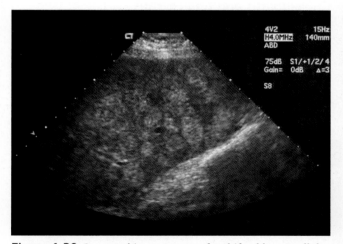

Figure 1-30 Sonographic appearance of multifocal hepatocellular carcinoma as multiple echogenic masses.

Needle advanced into lesion   Oval, hypoechoic lesion
yields infected fluid.   appears solid.

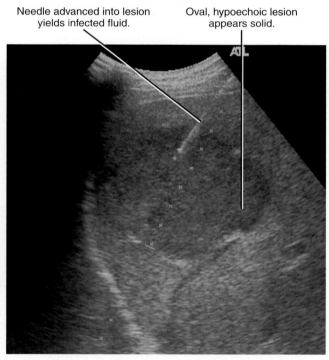

Figure 1-32 Ultrasound image of liver abscess obtained during drainage procedure.

Cavernous hemangiomas are usually well-defined, echogenic lesions that blend with the normal liver without distinctive halos and have enhanced through transmission. Larger hemangiomas frequently diverge from this pattern, with mixed echogenicity or even hypoechoic lesions (Fig. 1-34). A thin, echogenic rim surrounded by normal liver should suggest that the lesion is a hemangioma. Color Doppler sonography with high sensitivity reveals some internal flow in about half of hemangiomas. This finding is more common in larger lesions. Although it appears that advancing ultrasound technology now allows detection of blood flow within an increasing number of hemangiomas, lesions that exhibit

increased flow on color Doppler sonography should still be evaluated further using computed tomography (CT), magnetic resonance imaging (MRI), or blood pool scintigraphy.

Other focal lesions that can be seen in the liver include focal nodular hyperplasia (FNH) and hepatic adenoma. The sonographic features of both FNH and hepatic adenoma are variable. There is a tendency for FNH

Gas   Fluid

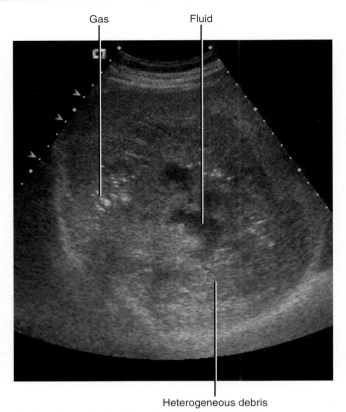

Heterogeneous debris

Figure 1-33 Ultrasound image of a liver abscess shows a variety of findings commonly seen in abscess, including fluid, debris, and gas.

to be more homogeneous than adenoma. FNH often has mildly increased echogenicity compared with normal parenchyma, whereas hepatic adenomas are usually hypoechoic and more heterogeneous. On color Doppler-flow imaging, FNH usually has markedly increased flow, sometimes with characteristic spoke-wheel pattern (Fig. 1-35).

Intraoperative Ultrasound of the Liver

The portability of ultrasound allows it to be used to provide guidance during surgery. The ultrasound transducer can be placed using a sterile cover within an open surgical incision to provide direct access to an organ or blood vessel. The main indications for intraoperative sonography include lesion localization and evaluation of blood flow within a vessel.

Sonographic localization of a lesion is performed when an organ-sparing procedure is planned, such as partial resection or tissue ablation. Intraoperative sonography is particularly useful for deep lesions when there are no surface features to allow the surgeon to identify the mass. The surgeon performing partial hepatectomy can better design the plane of resection by directly visualizing the relations among the liver surface, the mass(es), and relevant vascular structures.

Ultrasound of the Gallbladder

Cholelithiasis and Cholecystitis

Ultrasound is the imaging modality of choice for the evaluation of patients with right upper quadrant pain. Beyond cholelithiasis and cholecystitis, ultrasound is capable of diagnosing gallbladder carcinoma, gallbladder

Round echogenic lesion in the right hepatic lobe

Larger hemangioma is more heterogeneous. Note that there is no flow on color Doppler.

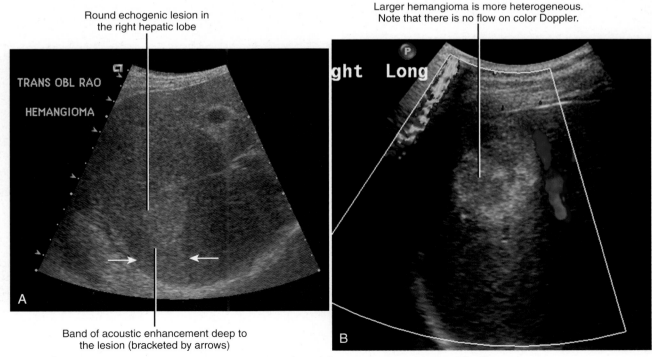

Band of acoustic enhancement deep to the lesion (bracketed by arrows)

Figure 1-34 Sonographic features in one small **(A)** and one large **(B)** cavernous hemangioma of the liver.

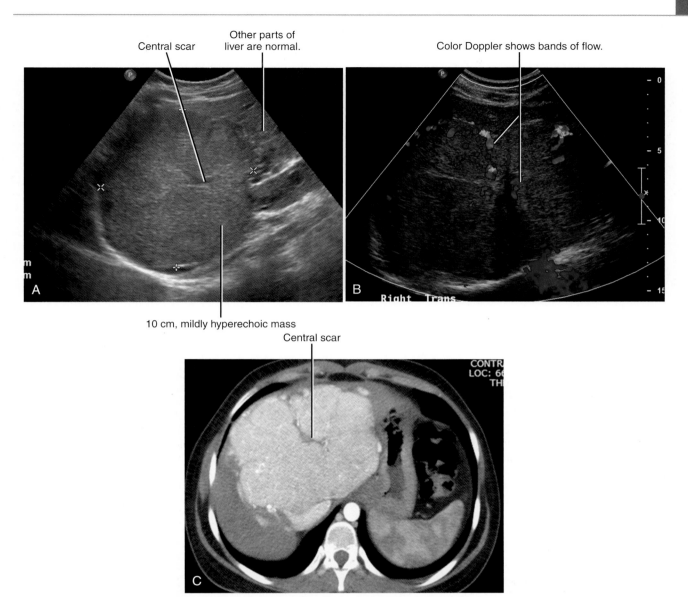

Figure 1-35 Grayscale (**A**) and color Doppler (**B**) ultrasound images of the liver in a proven case of focal nodular hyperplasia. Computed tomography was performed subsequently (**C**). (Courtesy Michael Freckleton, M.D.)

polyps, and adenomyomatosis, although these entities are usually found incidentally while searching for gallstones.

Most gallstones can be readily identified within the fundus of the gallbladder. However, stones within the gallbladder neck or the cystic duct may be overlooked (Fig. 1-36). It is therefore critical that each gallbladder examination include specific evaluation of the gallbladder neck and the cystic duct.

Pearl: Including specific evaluation of the gallbladder neck and cystic duct will improve the sensitivity and specificity of ultrasound for gallstones.

The typical sonographic features of gallstones include an echogenic focus that produces acoustic shadowing. Small stones do not reliably produce acoustic shadowing and can simulate polyps. In such cases, repositioning the patient can help distinguish mobile stones from fixed polyps. Keep in mind, however, that stones can be

adherent to the gallbladder wall; therefore, failure to move is not a specific sign for polyps.

Sludge within the gallbladder generally indicates poor gallbladder emptying. When present, gallbladder sludge should be reported because there has been considerable literature investigating the role of sludge as a potential cause of acute pancreatitis due to a "microlithiasis phenomenon."

Thickening of the gallbladder wall is a nonspecific finding that is associated with many diagnoses, ranging from acute and chronic cholecystitis to gallbladder carcinoma. Thus, thickening of the gallbladder wall alone should not be the basis of a specific diagnosis.

Pitfall: Thickening of the gallbladder wall is a nonspecific finding that is associated with many diagnoses. Thus, thickening of the gallbladder wall alone should not be the basis of a specific diagnosis.

Gallstone in neck of gallbladder
near cystic duct

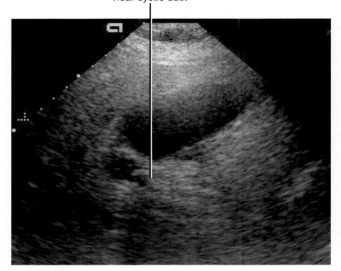

Figure 1-36 Gallstone that was difficult to detect with ultrasonography. No stone was detected on an ultrasound examination performed 1 day before this one. Examination was repeated after positive nuclear medicine scan. The stone was confirmed at cholecystectomy.

Patients with acute cholecystitis usually present with fever, right upper quadrant pain, and leukocytosis. In such patients, ultrasound demonstration of gallstones within a distended gallbladder accompanied by either gallbladder wall thickening (>3 mm) or a positive sonographic Murphy sign allows diagnosis of acute cholecystitis with relative confidence (Fig. 1-37). The sonographic Murphy sign is focal, reproducible tenderness when the transducer is used to apply pressure directly over the gallbladder and must be performed correctly to achieve an accurate diagnosis. Although specificity of the sonographic Murphy sign was originally described to be 92%, other studies have found specificity as low as 35%, likely because of incorrect performance.

Pearl: Because proper application of the sonographic Murphy sign is a critical element to diagnosis of acute cholecystitis, it is worth taking time to rescan patients when possible and to educate ultrasound technologists to be certain it is performed correctly.

Biliary scintigraphy should be performed in the 20% of patients when clinical suspicion of cholecystitis persists despite the lack of an ultrasound diagnosis. Acalculous cholecystitis comprises 5% to 10% of patients with acute cholecystitis and occurs for a variety of reasons including severe illness and hyperalimentation. Diagnosis is difficult in many cases. In the appropriate clinical setting, gallbladder wall thickening with a positive sonographic Murphy sign is suggestive of acute acalculous cholecystitis.

Gangrenous cholecystitis has a more severe prognosis than typical acute cholecystitis and is associated with a greater risk for perforation. In addition to perforation, sonographic signs of gangrenous cholecystitis include gallbladder wall striations (hypoechoic bands of edema) and intraluminal membranes (sloughed mucosa) (Fig. 1-38). These intramural membranes should not be confused with normal gallbladder folds.

Gallbladder perforation with pericholecystic abscess can result in sepsis and morbidity when the diagnosis of cholecystis is delayed (Fig. 1-39). Pericholecystic abscesses are complex fluid collections contiguous with

Thickened GB wall
with wall striation   Gallstone

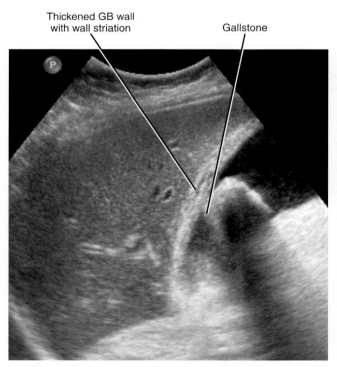

Figure 1-37 Ultrasound findings of acute cholecystitis. A sonographic Murphy sign was also present. *GB,* Gallbladder.

Sloughed mucosa results
in membranes within   Hypoechoic bands of fluid
gallbladder lumen.   in gallbladder wall

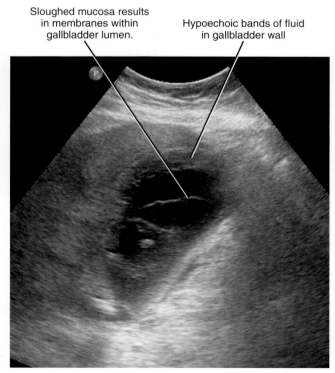

Figure 1-38 Sonographic findings in gangrenous cholecystitis.

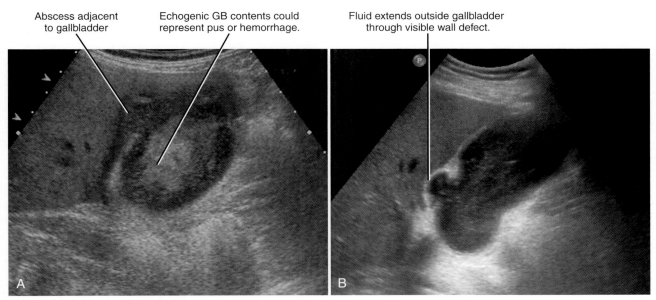

Abscess adjacent to gallbladder

Echogenic GB contents could represent pus or hemorrhage.

Fluid extends outside gallbladder through visible wall defect.

Figure 1-39 Ultrasound images from two separate patients with perforation of the gallbladder *(GB)*. **A,** Perforation is suspected due to complex fluid adjacent to the GB. **B,** In a different patient, a site of perforation is identified with fluid extending beyond a defect in the GB wall.

the gallbladder, and often the echogenic submucosa is interrupted. Echogenic, inflamed fat may be noted adjacent to the abscess, correlating with fat stranding seen on CT.

Gallbladder Masses

Polyps are the most common gallbladder mass and are commonly identified by ultrasound (Fig. 1-40). These polyps are usually identified incidentally during ultrasound examination of the right upper quadrant. They are usually of no clinical concern until the size reaches 10 mm or greater. Because polyps larger than 10 mm have an increased risk for malignant transformation and carcinoma, cholecystectomy is usually performed.

Carcinoma of the gallbladder usually presents with advanced disease. In such cases, there is replacement of the gallbladder by a mass that infiltrates into the nearby liver and lymph-node involvement (Fig. 1-41). Because of the aggressiveness of the disease, bile duct invasion is a common occurrence.

When gallbladder cancer is detected early by ultrasound, it is usually found incidentally during right upper quadrant ultrasound examination. Small gallbladder cancers can be missed by ultrasound in the presence of large and multiple stones. The sonographic findings of gallbladder carcinoma confined to its lumen range from polypoid masses to focal or irregular thickening of the gallbladder wall. Color Doppler imaging may demonstrate increased flow within the mass, which is a helpful sign when present. However, because flow can be absent

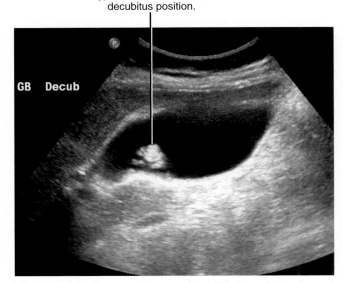

Polyp does not move despite decubitus position.

GB   Decub

Figure 1-40 Ultrasound image of the gallbladder *(GB)* performed with patient in the left lateral decubitus *(decub)* position shows a gallbladder polyp.

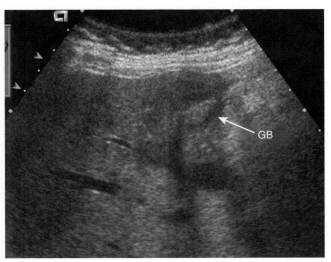

GB

Figure 1-41 Advanced gallbladder carcinoma by ultrasound. Although the region of the gallbladder *(GB)* is identified, it is difficult to define margins of the gallbladder because of liver invasion.

in malignant masses, the absence of flow on color Doppler sonography does not exclude cancer (Fig. 1-42).

Pitfall: Flow can be absent on color Doppler sonography of gallbladder cancer. Therefore, a lack of flow does not exclude the diagnosis.

Adenomyomatosis

Adenomyomatosis is a benign disease process of the gallbladder that can cause diffuse or focal wall thickening. In some cases, adenomyomatosis can cause masslike and bizarre, irregular wall thickening simulating carcinoma. A characteristic finding on ultrasound is the so-called comet tail artifact caused by reverberation from crystals trapped within hypertrophied Rokitansky–Aschoff sinuses. As mentioned earlier, twinkle artifact is the color Doppler representation of comet tail artifact from adenomyomatosis (see Fig. 1-9).

Ultrasound of the Bile Ducts

Ultrasound is commonly performed to exclude biliary obstruction as a possible explanation for abnormal liver function tests. The extrahepatic segment of the common bile duct (CBD) can usually be identified in the porta hepatis and should be measured in the region where the right hepatic artery crosses the portal vein (Fig. 1-43). Controversy exists over the reference range for CBD diameter, in particular, over the theory that the reference range increases with age and after cholecystectomy (see Normal Imaging Appearance of the Biliary System section in Chapter 13). Many authors use 5 mm as the upper limit of normal for the CBD and recommend further evaluation with laboratory tests, magnetic resonance cholangiopancreatography, and/or endoscopic retrograde cholangiopancreatography (ERCP) for a larger duct size.

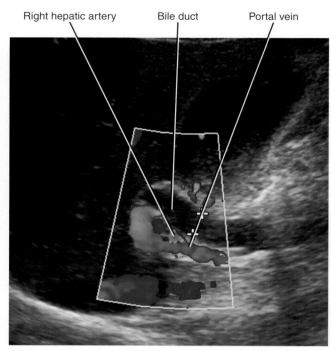

Right hepatic artery   Bile duct   Portal vein

Figure 1-43 Preferred location for measuring the common bile duct diameter by ultrasonography. In this case, the duct is dilated and contains sludge, which is also present in the gallbladder.

Others allow for an additional 1 mm per decade of life over 60 years and up to 10 mm in patients who have undergone cholecystectomy. What can be said with confidence is that clinical context is an important consideration when CBD enlargement is an isolated finding and there is no evidence of intrahepatic duct dilatation.

The right and left hepatic ducts may be considered dilated when they exceed 2 mm in diameter (Fig. 1-44).

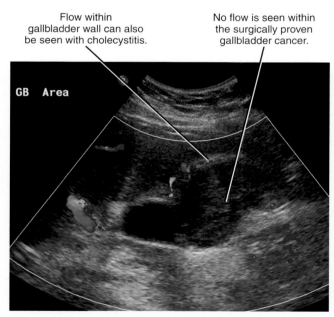

Flow within gallbladder wall can also be seen with cholecystitis.   No flow is seen within the surgically proven gallbladder cancer.

GB   Area

Figure 1-42 Absence of flow within proven gallbladder (*GB*) carcinoma on color Doppler sonography. The sonographic appearance is similar to sludge.

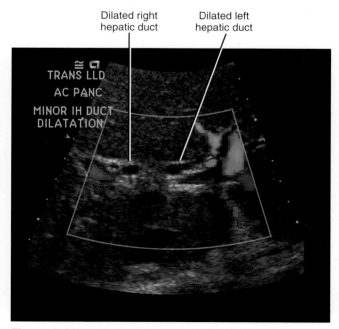

Dilated right hepatic duct   Dilated left hepatic duct

TRANS LLD
AC PANC
MINOR IH DUCT DILATATION

Figure 1-44 Mildly dilated intrahepatic bile ducts in a patient with pancreatic carcinoma.

Therefore, the region of the bile duct confluence should always be specifically examined in patients with clinical evidence of biliary obstruction. Color Doppler sonography is often helpful in distinguishing between vascular structures and dilated intrahepatic bile ducts.

Choledocholithiasis

Choledocholithiasis is the most common cause of bile duct dilatation in patients with gallstones. Approximately 85% of obstructing bile duct stones are found in the distal duct near the head of the pancreas. This region of the duct is often difficult to visualize with ultrasound. Visualization of the distal duct can be improved by placing the patient in the left lateral decubitus position so that the gallbladder provides an acoustic window to the bile duct (Fig. 1-45).

CDB stones appear as intraductal echogenic foci with acoustic shadowing (Fig. 1-46). Potential mimics include air in the bile duct, extrabiliary calcification, or surgical clips. Stones in normal-size ducts can be identified but are more difficult to detect than stones in dilated ducts. Small intrahepatic ductal stones such as those seen in patients with cystic fibrosis are difficult to identify, particularly when significant biliary dilatation is absent.

Cholangitis

Ultrasound plays a limited role in the diagnosis of cholangitis. Ultrasound can identify wall thickening in the bile ducts, although normal studies can occur. Causes of bile duct wall thickening include acute cholangitis, parasitic disease, human immunodeficiency virus, and other cholangiopathies, as well as primary and secondary malignancy (Fig. 1-47). In some cases, the thickened echogenic wall of the CBD results in a narrowed bile duct lumen that can be confused with a normal duct.

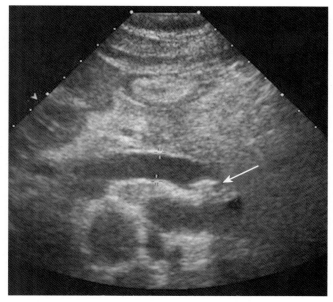

Figure 1-46 Ultrasound appearance of choledocholithiasis. The echogenic stone in the distal common bile duct is indicated by the *white arrow.*

Recurrent pyogenic cholangitis (previously known as Oriental cholangiohepatitis) is characterized by recurrent bacterial cholangitis promoted by strictures and primary bile duct stones that can occur in any part of the biliary tree. Massively dilated ducts (>2 cm) with sludge and large stones are common.

Cholangiocarcinoma

Sonography can diagnose cholangiocarcinoma in patients with jaundice. The versatility of infinite imaging planes with ultrasound can be an advantage over CT in

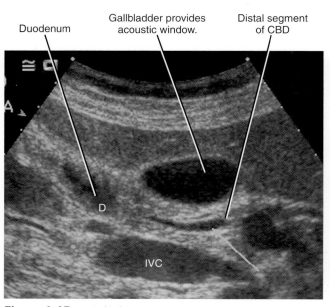

Figure 1-45 Use of left lateral decubitus position to visualize distal common bile duct (CBD). *IVC,* Inferior vena cava.

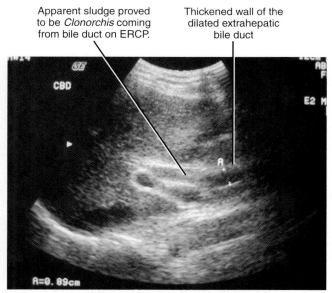

Figure 1-47 Wall thickening in the bile duct caused by infection with *Clonorchis sinensis. ERCP,* Endoscopic retrograde cholangiopancreatography.

defining the relation between tumor and adjacent structures. Assessment for resectability is best performed before stenting the ducts, which can cause an inflammatory reaction, simulating tumor. Stents also make it difficult to visualize the intraductal extent of the mass. In challenging cases when a determination cannot be made regarding resectability even after multiple imaging studies are performed, intraoperative ultrasound can be used in a final attempt to stage the disease and guide resection.

Congenital Bile Duct Abnormalities

Choledochal cysts are readily identified with ultrasound. Some choledochal cysts contain stones and, if large enough, may simulate a gallbladder with stones (Fig. 1-48). This pitfall may be avoided by tracing the CBD carefully above and distal to the focal area of ductal dilatation, making sure to identify the gallbladder as separate from the duct in the plane of the interlobar fissure.

Ultrasound of the Pancreas

Acute Pancreatitis

Sonography is often performed in patients with acute pancreatitis to identify gallstones, biliary obstruction, or both. If stones are identified, ERCP with sphincterotomy may be performed.

Evaluation of the pancreas itself is sometimes limited in patients with pancreatitis. Dilated, gas-filled bowel loops are often interposed between the transducer and the pancreas. Sometimes this limitation can be overcome by using compression and repositioning the patient (decubitus or semi-upright).

The sonographic appearances of acute pancreatitis can be divided into three major groups: (1) pancreatic abnormalities, (2) peripancreatic abnormalities, and (3) miscellaneous associated abdominal findings.

Although the thickness of the pancreas varies widely, published measurement for the thickness of the body of the normal pancreas in 261 adults was 10.1 ± 3.8 mm with a range of 4 to 23 mm. A maximum anteroposterior diameter of 23 mm at the body of the pancreas, measured at the level of the superior mesenteric artery in the transverse plane, represents the upper limit of normal. A measurement of more than 23 mm is considered abnormal (Fig. 1-49).

The echogenicity of the gland is compared with that of the liver. A normal-appearing pancreas has echogenicity similar or greater than that of the liver. The normal pancreas is of relatively homogeneous echogenicity. The gland is considered abnormal if there is a heterogeneous echo pattern or focal hypoechoic areas. Masslike changes are occasionally encountered in acute pancreatitis and are almost always hypoechoic (Fig. 1-50). Inflammatory masses can be difficult to distinguish from solid tumors, although the presence of associated peripancreatic and extrapancreatic imaging findings can help establish the diagnosis of acute pancreatitis.

The most common peripancreatic features seen in patients with acute pancreatitis are findings of extraperitoneal inflammation and fluid collections. These changes can be seen in the pararenal and perirenal spaces (Fig. 1-51). When the pancreas is adequately visualized, inflammation can be seen ventral to the pancreas, along the transverse mesocolon, and less commonly in the omental fat. Perivascular inflammation can be seen as hypoechoic or anechoic linear strands around the splenic and superior mesenteric veins (Fig. 1-52).

Acute pancreatitis sometimes results in thrombosis of the portal vein or splenic vein. The diagnosis can be established with grayscale and color Doppler sonography.

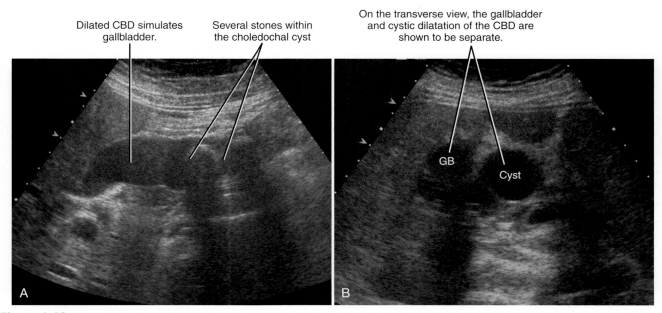

Figure 1-48 Large type I choledochal cyst with stones, an appearance that may be confused with cholelithiasis. **A,** Longitudinal view of the duct and **(B)** transverse view with the duct and gallbladder *(GB)* seen separately. CBD, common bile duct.

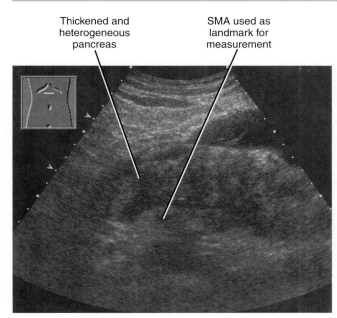

Thickened and heterogeneous pancreas

SMA used as landmark for measurement

Figure 1-49 Enlargement of the pancreatic body in acute pancreatitis. *SMA,* Superior mesenteric artery.

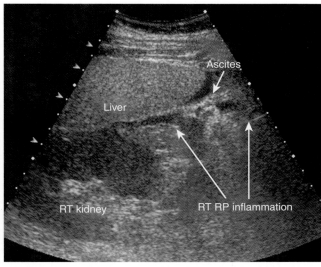

Ascites

Liver

RT kidney

RT RP inflammation

Figure 1-51 Ultrasound image of the right upper quadrant in a patient with acute pancreatitis showing retroperitoneal *(RP)* extension of fluid and inflammation. *RT,* Right.

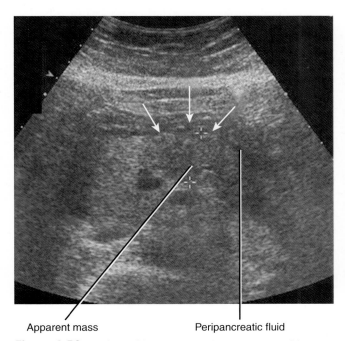

Apparent mass

Peripancreatic fluid

Figure 1-50 Focal masslike appearance in acute pancreatitis.

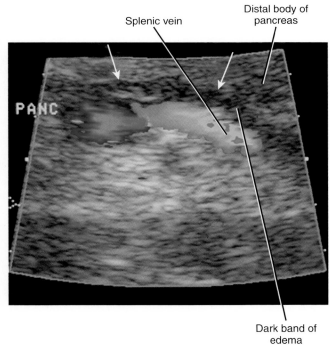

Splenic vein

Distal body of pancreas

PANC

Dark band of edema

Figure 1-52 Perivascular edema in a patient with acute pancreatitis.

Isolated splenic vein thrombosis usually results in short gastric varices with reversed flow in the coronary vein (Fig. 1-53). Extensive thrombosis of the portal vein will result in cavernous transformation, which can be seen with color Doppler sonography (Fig. 1-54). Varices of the gallbladder wall can occur in the presence of portal vein thrombosis.

Another vascular complication of pancreatitis is the formation of arterial pseudoaneurysms that are at risk for hemorrhage (Fig. 1-55). These can be identified using color Doppler, and once identified, are usually treated by transcatheter embolization. Follow-up ultrasound

examination can then be performed to detect residual or recurrent flow within the pseudoaneurysms.

Chronic Pancreatitis
Ultrasound findings of chronic pancreatitis include pancreatic duct dilatation with or without stones, volume redistribution, and atrophy of the gland (Fig. 1-56). Focal changes can be indistinguishable from cancer, and the "double duct" sign can be present in the absence of malignancy. In some instances, pancreatic biopsy (often performed with endoscopic ultrasound guidance) may be the only option to exclude malignancy.

Liver   Varices

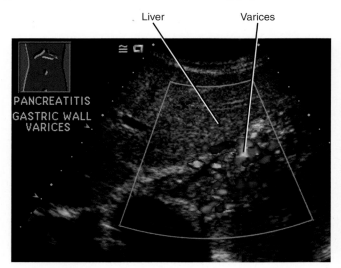

Figure 1-53 Short gastric varices in a patient with portal vein thrombosis.

Multidirectional flow is present
within tortuous vessels in
the expected location
of the portal vein.

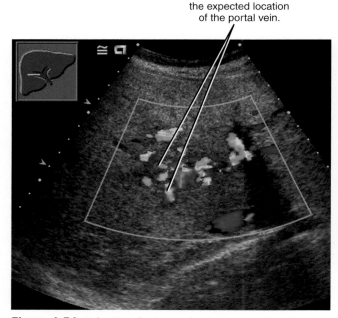

Figure 1-54 Color Doppler image showing cavernous transformation of the portal vein.

Pseudoaneurysm

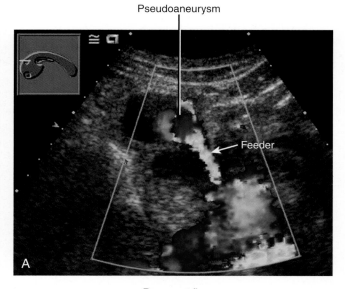

Feeder

A

Recurrent flow

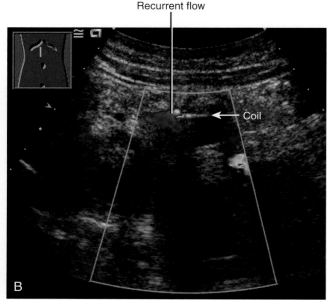

Coil

B

Figure 1-55 Pseudoaneurysm of the gastroduodenal artery (GDA) in a patient with acute pancreatitis (**A**). Follow-up postembolization image (**B**) shows recurrence of flow within the pseudoaneurysm.

Pancreatic Neoplasms

Contrast-enhanced CT is the mainstay for diagnosis and staging of pancreatic neoplasms. However, pancreatic neoplasms can be identified during the sonographic evaluation of patients with obstructive jaundice or upper abdominal pain. In experienced hands, ultrasound is superior to CT for characterization of the internal architecture of cystic masses. However, satisfactory visualization of the pancreas often requires repositioning of the patient, oral water intake to displace gas within the stomach, and considerable persistence.

Sonographically, pancreatic carcinoma is typically a hypoechoic mass that alters the morphology of the gland, although pancreatic carcinoma is occasionally heterogeneous or echogenic (Fig. 1-57). Scattered calcifications or cystic areas are present in about 5% of patients. Secondary findings of carcinoma include ductal dilation (biliary and pancreatic), vascular and extraglandular invasion, and metastatic disease. Pseudocysts, related to obstruction of a pancreatic duct, have been reported in as many as 11% of patients with pancreatic cancer.

Intraoperative ultrasound of the pancreas is the most sensitive imaging study for some types of pancreatic masses. Sonography can be used for intraoperative tumor localization when a mass is suspected but not

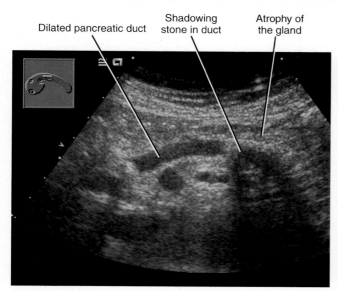

Dilated pancreatic duct   Shadowing stone in duct   Atrophy of the gland

Figure 1-56 Ultrasound findings in chronic pancreatitis.

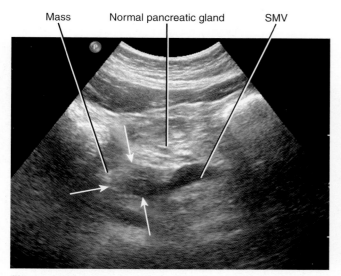

Mass   Normal pancreatic gland   SMV

Figure 1-57 Pancreatic adenocarcinoma on ultrasound performed for abdominal pain with jaundice. Images show a hypoechoic mass in the head of the pancreas. *SMV*, Superior mesenteric vein.

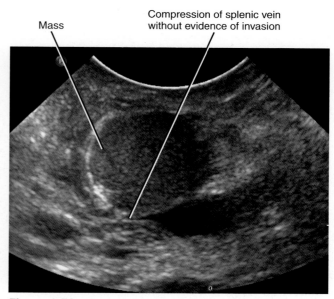

Mass   Compression of splenic vein without evidence of invasion

Figure 1-58 Intraoperative ultrasound of pancreatic mass. Placing the transducer directly on the mass facilitates high-resolution images but also eliminates the anatomic landmarks used in transabdominal scanning.

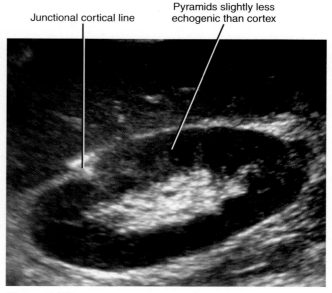

Junctional cortical line   Pyramids slightly less echogenic than cortex

Figure 1-59 Normal sonographic appearance of the kidney.

well demonstrated with other imaging. Detailed images of the mass and adjacent blood vessels provide additional intraoperative information regarding resectability (Fig. 1-58).

■ RENAL ULTRASOUND

In the normal kidney, the renal cortex is hypoechoic or isoechoic to the adjacent normal liver. Renal pyramidal echogenicity is less than that of the cortex (Fig. 1-59). In the presence of renal disease, this corticomedullary differentiation can become either lost or accentuated (Fig. 1-60). A hypertrophied column of Bertin and junctional cortical line are anatomic variants that can

be mistaken for a mass. These are discussed in greater detail in the section on pseudolesions of the kidney in Chapter 18.

Renal Cysts

Ultrasound excels at the characterization of cystic renal lesions and is commonly used to evaluate suspected cysts found incidentally with CT. Simple cysts have characteristic features. They are well-defined, anechoic round

Pyramids

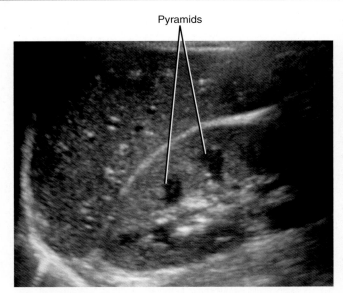

Figure 1-60 Echogenic renal cortex accentuates contrast between the cortex and medullary pyramids.

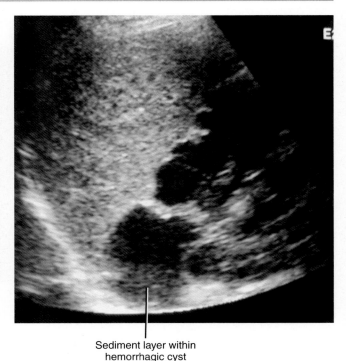

Sediment layer within hemorrhagic cyst

Figure 1-61 Longitudinal view of the right kidney in a patient with autosomal dominant polycystic kidney disease shows kidney to be enlarged and replaced with cysts of variable sizes, some of which contain hemorrhage.

or oval structures that produce posterior acoustic enhancement (see Fig. 1-13). The wall of a simple cyst can be slightly irregular but should not be thick. A few thin septa are also accepted as part of a simple renal cyst, provided no other concerning features are present.

A broad spectrum of renal cystic disease exists; this is discussed in more detail in Chapter 18. In summary, these include simple sporadic cysts, acquired cysts of dialysis, syndromic cysts, cystic dysplasia, and cystic renal cell carcinoma (RCC).

In most cases, the main goal of sonography is to determine whether a given renal lesion is cystic or solid. Because renal carcinoma can occasionally be nearly entirely cystic, each renal cyst merits close scrutiny. Mural nodules, thick septa, or irregular wall thickening are findings associated with renal carcinoma. Occasionally, the tumor can be purely cystic, with increased flow within a thickened wall on color Doppler imaging as the only hint of malignancy.

Autosomal dominant polycystic kidney disease (ADPKD) has a characteristic sonographic appearance of enlarged kidneys with multiple cysts of variable sizes. Ultrasound can detect hemorrhage within cysts of ADPKD, seen as internal echoes that often form a sediment layer (Fig. 1-61). Dystrophic calcifications are commonly seen as echogenic foci within cyst walls.

Hydronephrosis

Ultrasound is commonly used to evaluate patients with renal failure. Often, the duration of renal failure is unknown to the clinician, and ultrasound is used to determine whether hydronephrosis is present. Ultrasound is also used to look for signs of obstruction in young or pregnant patients with flank pain and suspected ureterolithiasis. Alternatively, hydronephrosis caused by

ureteral encasement or bladder outlet obstruction may be the first sign of a pelvic malignancy (Fig. 1-62).

Although diffuse enlargement of the pelvicaliceal system is not difficult to identify, be aware that renal sinus cysts and ADPKD can mimic hydronephrosis (see Hydronephrosis and Its Mimics section in Chapter 18). Continuity between adjacent fluid-filled structures is present with hydronephrosis but absent in cases of renal cystic disease.

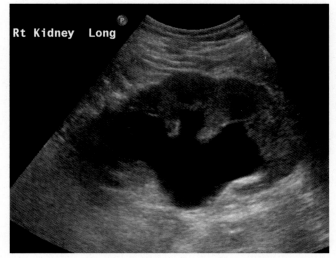

Rt Kidney Long

Figure 1-62 Renal ultrasound in a man who presented to the emergency department with renal failure. Bilateral hydronephrosis was found and subsequently shown to be the result of prostate cancer, leading to bladder outlet obstruction.

Color Doppler sonography can be used to identify the flow of urine from each ureter into the bladder. These "ureteral jets" are identified by finding the mildly protuberant part of the lower posterior bladder wall that signifies each ureteral orifice, then looking for intermittent linear bursts of flow (Fig. 1-63). Examination of ureteral jets has become a standard component of the renal ultrasound examination. Absence of both jets in the absence of hydronephrosis is usually of no clinical significance. However, absence of one ureteral jet or significant asymmetry is usually abnormal, particularly if accompanied by hydronephrosis.

Diffuse Renal Parenchymal Disease

Considerable overlap exists between the sonographic appearances of various types of acute and chronic diffuse renal parenchymal disease. Ultrasound can be of utility in identifying various patterns of disease, such as increased or decreased renal size, hyperechoic or hypoechoic renal echotexture, unilateral or bilateral disease, and smooth or irregular contours.

End-stage renal disease has characteristic sonographic features. Typical findings include bilateral echogenic kidneys that are small (Fig. 1-64). Patients with diabetes mellitus with clinically documented renal failure often have normal to increased kidney size with normal or subtly increased echogenicity. It is also important to remember that increased echogenicity does not necessarily indicate chronic disease, although decreased renal size usually does.

Although it is useful to use the liver for comparison to assess the echogenicity of the right kidney, remember that the liver can also have abnormal echogenicity; that is, an echogenic kidney can appear slightly hypoechoic compared with a fatty or cirrhotic liver. Alternatively, a

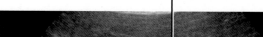
Calcification with calyceal diverticulum

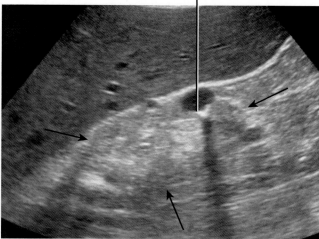

Figure 1-64 Small echogenic kidney *(arrows)* by ultrasound in a patient with chronic renal parenchymal disease.

normal kidney might appear slightly echogenic compared with the liver in the presence of abdominal ascites (see Fig. 1-14). It is helpful to include enough hepatic parenchyma in images of the right kidney to allow the interpreter to determine whether the liver is appropriate for comparison in each case.

Renal Infection

Uncomplicated urinary tract infections usually do not require imaging. In most cases of acute pyelonephritis, the kidney appears sonographically normal. If baseline imaging is available, edema may make the affected kidney appear relatively more rounded at the poles. Focally severe pyelonephritis manifests as an area of increased echogenicity with diminished or absent flow with color Doppler imaging (Fig. 1-65). This finding results from cortical edema, which also causes compression of the renal sinus. When collecting system dilatation is present in a patient with acute pyelonephritis, urothelial thickening can be demonstrated (Fig. 1-66).

Occasionally, pyelonephritis progresses to renal abscess. Small abscesses are usually hypoechoic and can be confined to the renal cortex or extend to the perinephric space (Fig. 1-67). Large abscesses can be confused with cysts, although the presence of internal echoes usually prevents their classification as simple.

A perinephric abscess may be the only abnormal sonographic finding in a patient with pyelonephritis. To help identify a subtle perinephric abscess, supplemented optimized color or power Doppler images of the kidney cortex will demonstrate the abscess as an abnormal hypoechoic area between the colorized kidney cortex and the normal echogenic perinephric fat (Fig. 1-68). Although this appearance is not specific for abscess because perinephric hematoma can have a similar appearance, the diagnosis of abscess can be made confidently in the appropriate clinical setting.

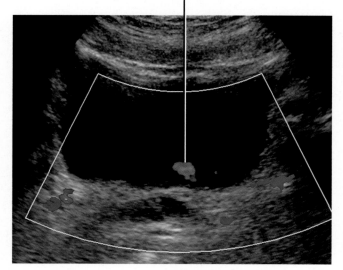
Color shows urine moving away from trigone and toward US transducer.

Figure 1-63 Color Doppler image of the bladder shows a left ureteral jet. The right ureteral jet was identified separately (not shown). *US,* Ultrasound.

Region of increased
echogenicity in the
superior pole

Corresponding region
of decreased color flow

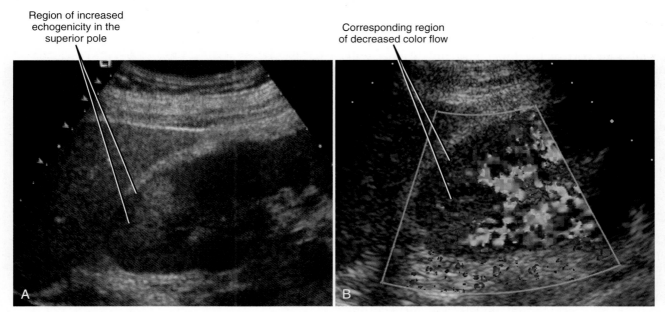

Figure 1-65 Appearance of acute bacterial pyelonephritis on grayscale (**A**) and color Doppler (**B**) ultrasound.

Thick wall of
the renal pelvis

Thin rim of extra
luminal fluid in
renal sinus

Cortical echogenicity
is mildly increased
diffusely.

Hypoechoic region
indicates area of
abscess formation.

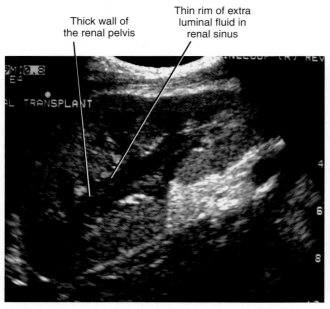

Figure 1-66 Ultrasound of an infected transplanted kidney shows diffuse urothelial thickening in the renal pelvis. This finding can also be seen with rejection.

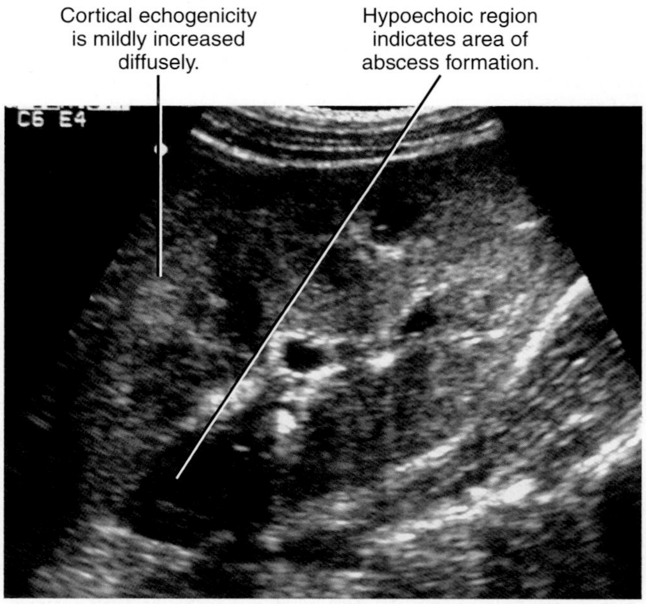

Figure 1-67 Ultrasound of the right kidney in a patient with a small renal abscess.

Renal Masses

For a detailed discussion of renal masses, see Chapter 18. This section summarizes important sonographic features of commonly encountered renal masses.

Angiomyolipoma (AML) is a benign kidney tumor containing varying amounts of fatty tissue, smooth muscle and blood vessels. The typical sonographic appearance of an AML is a well-defined echogenic mass within the renal cortex (Fig. 1-69). Exophytic AMLs can blend with perirenal fat and are easily overlooked. Rarely, if the adipose component of the AML is relatively small, the mass can appear hypoechoic and indistinguishable from RCC. If an echogenic mass has a hypoechoic halo, RCC is more likely than AML. Because some overlap exists between even typical AML and RCC on ultrasound, most advocate confirming the diagnosis of AML with CT or MRI, although some literature shows many radiologists do not recommend additional studies for suspected AMLs of 1 cm or smaller.

Pearl: If an echogenic mass has a hypoechoic halo, RCC is more likely than AML.

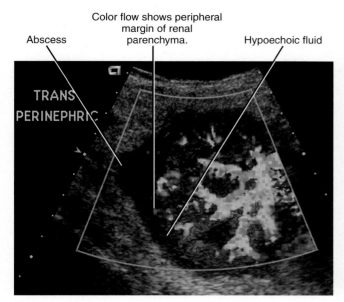

Abscess · Color flow shows peripheral margin of renal parenchyma. · Hypoechoic fluid

Figure 1-68 Use of color Doppler imaging to improve conspicuity of a perirenal abscess.

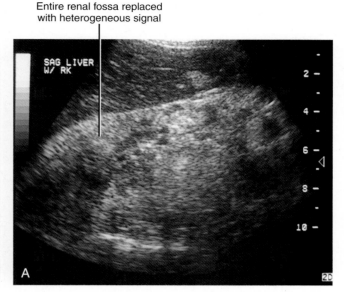

Entire renal fossa replaced with heterogeneous signal

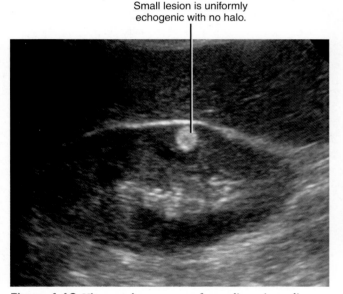

Small lesion is uniformly echogenic with no halo.

Figure 1-69 Ultrasound appearance of sporadic angiomyolipoma. Fat attenuation was confirmed by computed tomography.

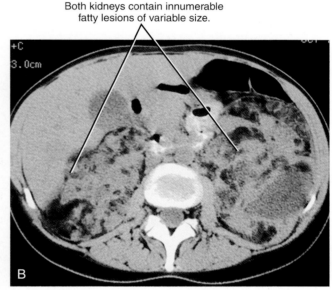

Both kidneys contain innumerable fatty lesions of variable size.

Figure 1-70 Ultrasound (**A**) and computed tomography (CT) (**B**) of a patient with tuberous sclerosis (TS) shows how difficult it can be to identify discrete renal lesions by ultrasound in TS. In this case, CT was more useful for assessing and following the renal masses.

Most discussions of AML describe the characteristics of isolated, sporadic masses. AMLs associated with tuberous sclerosis are a much more heterogeneous population of tumors. Rather than appearing as discrete masses, multiple masses of variable size and composition can replace much of the renal parenchyma. This often results in a bizarre appearance on ultrasound (Fig. 1-70).

Despite significant advances in ultrasound technology, the sensitivity of sonography for small asymptomatic RCC remains limited. When RCC is identified by ultrasound, it can be solid or cystic (Fig. 1-71). Although solid masses without evidence of fat content are always suspicious for malignancy, cystic lesions become more suspicious with increasing complexity (number and thickness of septations, mural nodularity) and increased vascularity on color Doppler sonography.

The echogenicity of solid RCC is variable, ranging from hypoechoic (10%) to relatively isoechoic (86%) and echogenic (4%). Large exophytic renal masses can be missed by sonography (Fig. 1-72), although awareness of this phenomenon and inclusion of parasagittal images improve detection. Each renal ultrasound examination should demonstrate defined margins of the upper and lower poles of each kidney with the surrounding organs and tissues. If these are not apparent, seek additional images.

Pitfall: Large exophytic renal masses can be missed by sonography, particularly if parasagittal images are not

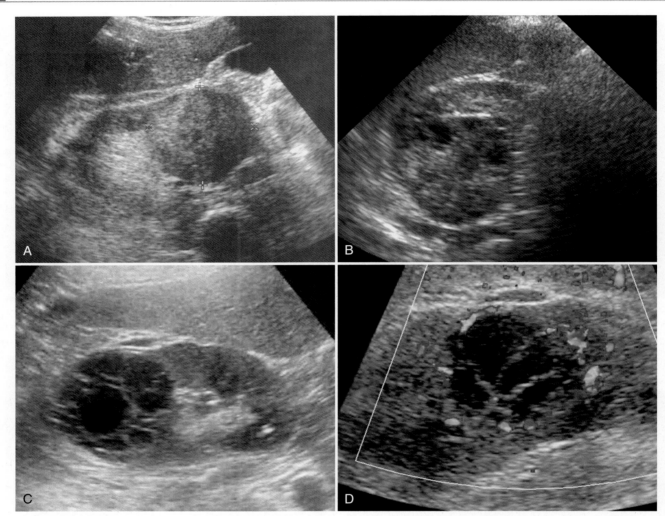

Figure 1-71 Variable appearance of renal cell carcinoma by ultrasound. Solid (**A**), predominantly solid with some cystic areas (**B**), and predominantly cystic (**C**) lesions are shown. **D,** Color Doppler evaluation of the cystic lesion shows flow within the septa.

obtained and all margins of the kidney are not visualized.

Intraoperative sonography facilitates partial nephrectomy for renal mass by helping to localize lesions that are not visible from the kidney surface, and to identify proximity of the mass to major vessels and the renal sinus (Fig. 1-73). Because there is no subcutaneous tissue between the transducer and the kidney, intraoperative images can be somewhat disorienting at times. If the mass is not identified at first, consider changing the image depth.

Pearl: Because most sonography is performed through the subcutaneous tissues, placing the transducer placed directly on the organ of interest can be disorienting. In some cases, a relatively small lesion may fill nearly the entire field of view. It is useful to inspect any available preoperative imaging before any intraoperative scan. Changing depth settings can provide additional perspective as well.

■ ULTRASOUND IMAGING OF THE PELVIS

Ultrasound is usually the initial modality for evaluation of the reproductive organs of both sexes. In fact, it is often the only modality used in a variety of common conditions. Because of this, ultrasound findings for many pelvic disorders are discussed at length in Chapters 20 and 21. Included in this chapter is a summary of the common applications of ultrasound in the pelvis.

Transvaginal Ultrasound of the Female Pelvis

Uterine Applications
Transvaginal scanning provides high-resolution images of the uterus. With the transducer only millimeters from the uterus, ultrasound provides excellent detail of the

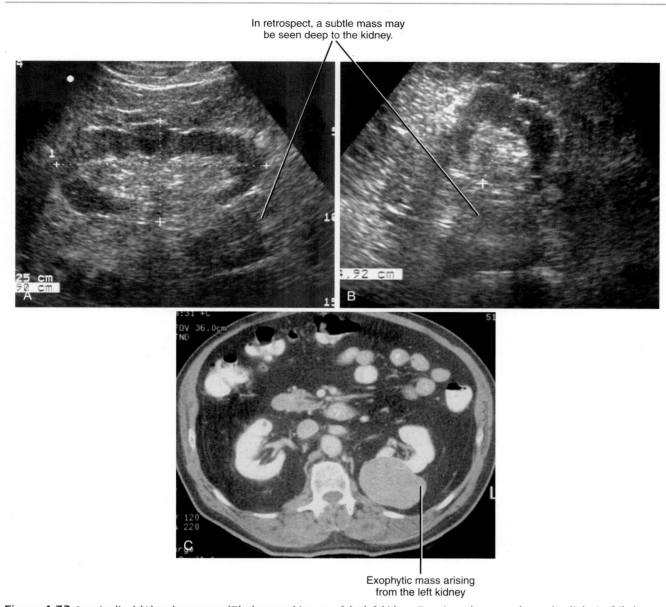

In retrospect, a subtle mass may
be seen deep to the kidney.

Exophytic mass arising
from the left kidney

Figure 1-72 Longitudinal (**A**) and transverse (**B**) ultrasound images of the left kidney. Experienced sonographer and radiologist failed to identify a mass. When computed tomography (**C**) was performed for an indeterminate lesion on the right side, an exophytic left renal mass was identified.

endometrium and myometrium (Fig. 1-74). Hormonal influences on the endometrium result in a variable appearance throughout each menstrual cycle with alternating phases of proliferative and secretory endometrium. Transabdominal scanning remains useful by providing perspective regarding orientation of the pelvic organs, particularly if a large mass is present.

Pelvic pain is the most common indication for pelvic sonography in young women. Ultrasound allows identification and characterization of leiomyomas, common benign tumors of smooth muscle. Sonographic appearance of leiomyomas is variable, but sonography allows diagnosis of complications such as torsion of a pedunculated leiomyoma or hemorrhagic degeneration. Sonographic findings can also suggest

the presence of adenomyosis, although MRI may be required to confirm the diagnosis.

Abnormal uterine bleeding is a common indication for pelvic sonography for perimenopausal and postmenopausal women. The endometrium stripe becomes atrophic after menopause, resulting in thinning of the endometrial stripe on sonography. Among asymptomatic postmenopausal women, the normal endometrial stripe is 8 mm or less. If a woman reports abnormal uterine bleeding, however, an endometrial stripe measurement of greater than 5 mm should prompt further investigation with sonohysterography or endometrial biopsy. A variety of diffuse and focal abnormalities of the endometrial stripe exist that signal the need for further investigation as well.

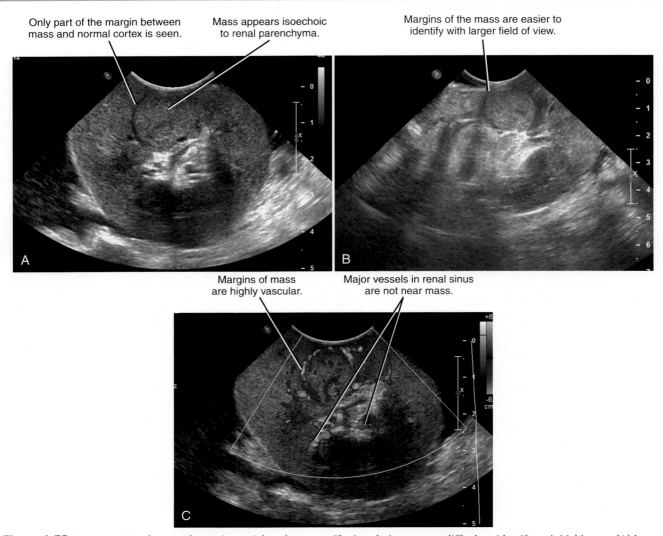

Figure 1-73 Intraoperative ultrasound to assist partial nephrectomy. The isoechoic mass was difficult to identify on initial images (**A**) but more apparent with increased field of view (**B**). Color Doppler was used to localize central vessels (**C**).

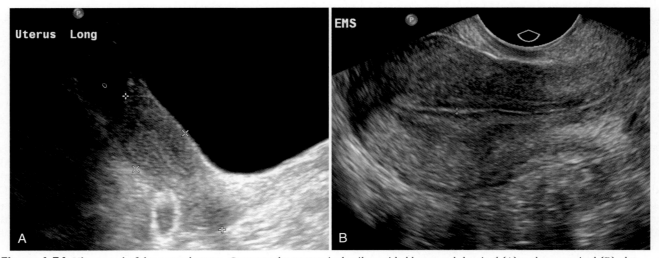

Figure 1-74 Ultrasound of the normal uterus. Compare the anatomic detail provided by transabdominal (**A**) and transvaginal (**B**) ultrasound images of the uterus during a single examination.

Adnexal Applications

Despite variable location of the ovaries, they can be identified with transvaginal sonography in nearly all premenopausal women (Fig. 1-75). Because of atrophy, the ovaries can be more challenging to identify after menopause but are still identified in the majority of women.

The normal ovary contains multiple small follicles, typically ranging from 1.0 to 2.5 cm. Most consider a cystic structure in the ovary that exceeds 2.5 cm in diameter to be a cyst, and most of these are functional cysts that will become smaller over time. Cysts that become large, rupture, torse, or hemorrhage cause acute pelvic pain, a palpable adnexal mass, or both. Ovarian cysts and related complications are both the most common cause of acute pelvic pain in young women and better characterized by transvaginal sonography than by CT. Thus, most acute-care settings use sonography as the initial imaging modality to evaluate premenopausal women with acute lower abdominal pain.

First-Trimester Pregnancy

Obstetrical imaging is not included in this textbook, but evaluation of early pregnancy is a key component in the investigation of pelvic pain or vaginal bleeding in premenopausal women. Sonography detects intrauterine pregnancy as early as 5 weeks gestation, making concurrent ectopic pregnancy an unlikely explanation for pelvic pain (Fig. 1-76). Absence of an intrauterine gestation, accompanied by appropriate correlation with levels of serum β-human chorionic gonadotropin, may be the only sonographic finding in ectopic pregnancy. Peritoneal fluid and adnexal mass are positive findings to support the diagnosis of ectopic pregnancy. Additional diagnostic considerations in early pregnancy include gestational trophoblastic disease and fetal demise. Early identification of multiple gestations allows the expecting parents to start saving money for diapers.

Testicular Ultrasound

Testicular Mass

In contrast with the ovaries, the testicles are usually as easy to find on physical examination as with sonography. Superficial location facilitates high-resolution images of the testis, and evaluation with color and spectral Doppler imaging can always be performed.

Ultrasound of the scrotum is often requested to evaluate a palpable abnormality. Because extratesticular malignancies in the scrotum usually become case reports and virtually all testicular masses can be identified by ultrasound, the absence of a testicular mass on sonography excludes malignancy with confidence. Common diagnoses made during sonographic evaluation of a palpable abnormality include epididymal cyst, varicocele, and hydrocele (Fig. 1-77). Before concluding that a sonographic abnormality accounts for the physical examination finding, it is helpful to correlate directly by palpating the testicle and placing the transducer directly over the nodule in question.

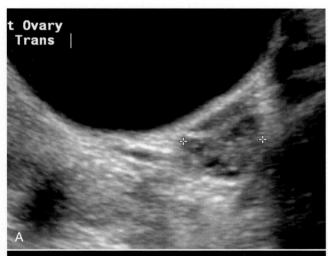

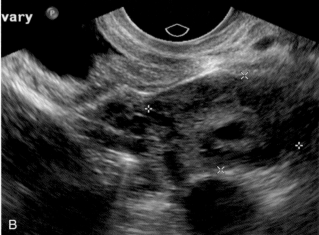

Figure 1-75 Ultrasound of the normal ovary. Compare transabdominal (**A**) and transvaginal (**B**) images of the same left ovary.

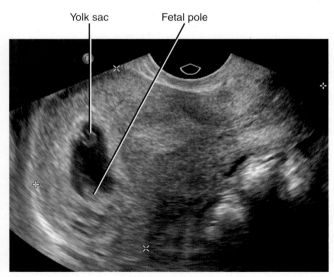

Figure 1-76 Sagittal transvaginal ultrasonographic image demonstrates an early intrauterine gestation (estimated at 6 weeks, 4 days by menstrual cycle).

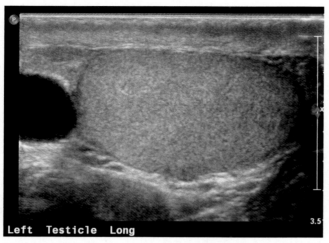

Figure 1-77 Ultrasound performed for palpable abnormality on physical examination. There is no testicular mass. A cyst is present in the epididymis, which correlated with the physical examination finding.

Acute Scrotum

Increased blood flow is seen in the epididymis and testis when they are infected; enlargement and decreased flow are usually identified in the event of testicular torsion. Epididymitis is the most common diagnosis among men evaluated for acute scrotal pain. However, excluding testicular torsion is essential because irreversible damage occurs within hours of the onset of torsion.

Pearl: Whenever ultrasound is performed for acute scrotal pain, a transverse scan of both testes with color Doppler imaging should be performed to compare vascularity. A discrepancy between the two sides raises concern for infection or torsion.

■ DOPPLER ULTRASOUND AS A PROBLEM SOLVER

One of the strengths of ultrasound as a problem-solving modality is the real-time blood flow evaluation made possible by a variety of Doppler techniques. Because no contrast media is required, prolonged interrogation can be performed from a variety of angles, and serial examinations can be performed without risk to the patient.

The Doppler principle forms the basis of Doppler imaging. Sound reflected from blood cells moving within vessels undergoes frequency shifts that are dependent on the direction and velocity of blood flow. Flow velocity and direction can be quantified based on the relative magnitude of the frequency shift and angle of insonation.

Spectral Doppler (also called *pulsed-wave Doppler*) ultrasound is performed by placing a sampling cursor over a specific vessel. The range of flow velocities within the sampling gate is displayed as a graph, with flow toward the transducer specified as positive and flow away as negative. Positive flow is usually displayed above the baseline, but this can be inverted, so it is always important to note how these are positioned on the scale. Because of mathematical constraints of the

Doppler equation, it is important to keep the sampling angle less than 60 degrees to maintain accuracy. Because blood cells travel at a range of velocities within the blood vessels, some degree of spectral broadening is expected. When blood flow is complex or disordered, as occurs near vascular stenoses, considerable spectral broadening results. Alterations in the shape of the spectral tracing (waveform) can also signal abnormal hemodynamics.

Color Doppler is the most commonly used form of sonographic flow analysis. A color scale is always provided on the image, specifying the color of flow toward and away from the transducer. Velocity is displayed as color intensity along the spectrum of the color scale. Be aware that adjustments to the velocity scale, wall filter, or color gain can make it appear that there is no flow within a normal vessel.

Power Doppler appears similar to color Doppler ultrasound in that it maps color flow using a color scale. At first glance, the main difference is that power Doppler ultrasound uses only a single color to map blood flow. Although there are technical reasons for the difference that are beyond this discussion, the result is that power Doppler provides no information regarding flow direction or velocity, but it is more sensitive to slower flow than color Doppler and is less angle dependent.

Duplex ultrasound describes the display of two different ultrasound modes simultaneously. Spectral Doppler is almost always used in a duplex mode, using grayscale images to identify vessels and spectral Doppler to sample blood flow.

Renal Artery Stenosis

Doppler sonography is a valuable tool to screen patients with hypertension for renal arterial stenosis (RAS). It has evolved into a technique that is not only appropriate for primary diagnosis but also for posttherapeutic surveillance.

The reported sensitivity and specificity of Doppler sonography in the evaluation of RAS vary considerably. Likewise, criteria used to diagnose RAS vary from one investigator to another. The degree of stenosis required to produce RAS-related hypertension has been variously reported from 50% to 70%.

Currently, two basic Doppler techniques are available to study RAS. The first approach is direct Doppler of the renal arteries. Sampling near the origin of the renal arteries may appear ideal for this purpose. However, the technique is difficult in many cases and often limited by body habitus, anatomic variants in the origin of the renal arteries, and the presence of multiple renal arteries in one or both kidneys. Measurements using this technique (peak systolic velocity [PSV] and renal artery/aorta peak velocity ratio [RAR]) are more accurate than those obtained from intrarenal arteries (acceleration indices). The main criteria for diagnosing RAS with direct renal artery Doppler are: (1) a renal-aortic ratio greater than 3.5, and (2) PSV greater than 180 to 200 cm/sec (Fig. 1-78). Color Doppler ultrasound is an important part of the study because it is used to ensure

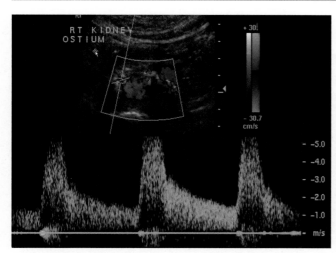

Figure 1-78 Spectral Doppler demonstration of severe renal arterial stenosis (RAS) with peak systolic velocity in the main renal artery exceeding 500 cm/sec.

waveform in segmental renal arteries (the early systolic compliance peak/reflective-wave complex [ESP]) is adequate to suggest the diagnosis of RAS, and that this method was better than other calculation methods such as PSV or acceleration time (Fig. 1-79). Loss of the ESP is the first step in development of a tardus parvus waveform. With a reported sensitivity of 95% and specificity of 97%, many sonologists use this criterion in practice.

A more pronounced aberration of the shape of the Doppler waveform in RAS is the so-called tardus-parvus waveform. This appearance results from the slow rise to PSV distal to the site of stenosis. Identification of the tardus-parvus waveform is highly suggestive of RAS (Fig. 1-80).

placement of the sample volume over the site of a high-velocity jet, if present.

The second technique used is Doppler of the intrarenal arteries. This technique may be less sensitive than direct evaluation of the main renal arteries but is often more practical because it is technically easier and more reliable. Direct Doppler techniques are commonly combined with intrarenal measurements to improve diagnostic confidence. Investigators have evaluated many intrarenal Doppler parameters for the diagnosis of RAS. These include acceleration time, acceleration index, resistive index (RI), and pulsatility index (summarized in Table 1-2). The best Doppler signals for evaluation come from the large segmental or interlobar arteries as they course directly toward the transducer. In this location, signals are the strongest and most reproducible.

Before attempting a Doppler study for renal artery stenosis, the operator must optimize the Doppler settings to avoid false-positive and -negative outcomes. Acceleration index of less than 3 m/sec^2 is considered abnormal. Use of the acceleration time is less sensitive than other techniques and may be misleading. In many vascular laboratories, measuring acceleration time is not a common practice.

An abnormally shaped intrarenal artery waveform may indicate RAS. Stavros showed that a loss of the sharp peak that normally precedes the curved part of the

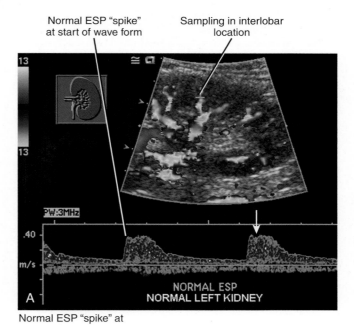

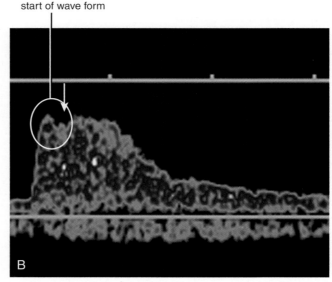

Figure 1-79 Normal spectral Doppler appearance of interlobar artery within the kidney (**A**). A magnified view of the waveform (**B**) better shows the normal early systolic compliance peak (ESP).

Table 1-2   Guide to Intrarenal Doppler Parameters

Parameter	Description
Acceleration time	Time interval between the start of systole and peak systole
Acceleration index	Ratio of acceleration time to peak systolic velocity
Pulsatility index	(PSV − EDV)/mean velocity
Resistive index	(PSV − EDV)/PSV

EDV, End-diastolic velocity; *PSV*, peak systolic velocity.

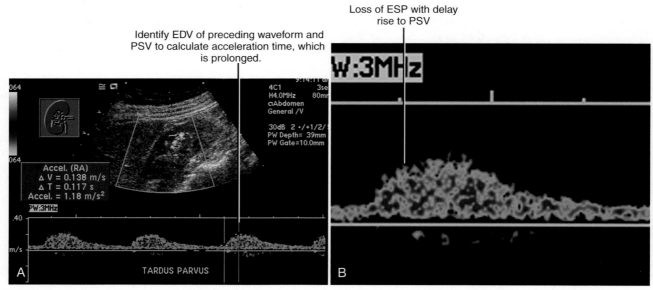

Figure 1-80 **A,** Tardus-parvus waveform in an interlobular artery in renal arterial stenosis (RAS). **B,** Enlarged view of the waveform. Compare this waveform with the one shown in Figure 1-79. *EDV,* End-diastolic velocity; *ESP,* early systolic compliance peak; *PSV,* peak systolic velocity.

Early studies attempted to use measurements of intrarenal vascular resistance such as RI to detect RAS. These measurements were proved to be inaccurate because they are influenced by other factors such as underlying intrinsic kidney disease, obstruction, patient age, and compliance of the arteries under study. More recent studies show the RI may play a role in evaluating efficacy after intravascular stent placement. Furthermore, evidence has been reported that RI measurements can predict whether patients with RAS will benefit from stent placement. An RI value of more than 0.8 makes a treatment effect highly unlikely.

Transjugular Intrahepatic Portosystemic Shunt

Doppler sonography is the preferred surveillance modality after transjugular intrahepatic portosystemic stent shunt (TIPS) creation for the treatment of portal hypertension. Preprocedure evaluation can also be helpful to verify patency of the portal and hepatic veins. Post-TIPS sonographic follow-up is performed in the first 24 hours to confirm appropriate shunt function and to establish a baseline. Subsequent follow-up examinations are performed at regular intervals to allow early detection of shunt malfunction. Low-frequency Doppler imaging (e.g., 2 MHz) is generally best for imaging patients with TIPS. Recommended techniques include color and spectral Doppler imaging to determine direction and velocity of flow in the stent, main portal vein, and branches of the portal and hepatic vein. Grayscale imaging is important to detect and quantify ascites, and screen for hepatocellular carcinoma.

Many factors influence intrastent velocity, including respiration. Considerable decrease in flow velocity can occur during inspiration compared with quiet respiration.

Pearl: Coaching the patient to maintain quiet, smooth respiration will enhance the accuracy of TIPS evaluation with ultrasound.

TIPS stenosis occurs most commonly near the hepatic venous end and can result in either increased or decreased flow velocity within the stent. As yet, no consistently accurate Doppler criteria exist for TIPS malfunction in the literature. Most of the authors use a velocity range of 90 to 200 cm/sec in the mid and distal (HV side) stent as normal (Fig. 1-81). Velocities outside this range suggest shunt malfunction (Fig. 1-82). Other

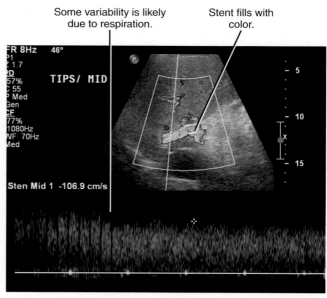

Figure 1-81 Normal color and spectral Doppler evaluation of transjugular intrahepatic portosystemic stent shunt (TIPS) stent.

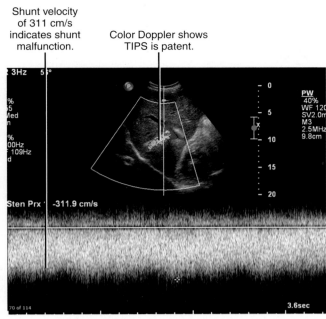

Shunt velocity of 311 cm/s indicates shunt malfunction.

Color Doppler shows TIPS is patent.

Figure 1-82 Spectral Doppler diagnosis of transjugular intrahepatic portosystemic stent shunt (TIPS) malfunction with markedly increased intrastent velocity. An increased pressure gradient was confirmed at revision.

Table 1-3   Doppler Ultrasound Findings of Transjugular Intrahepatic Portosystemic Shunt Malfunction

Finding	Comments
Absent or reversed flow within shunt	Very accurate
High-velocity flow within the shunt	200 cm/sec* vs. 250 cm/sec
Low-velocity flow within the shunt	90 cm/sec* vs. 50 cm/sec
Velocity difference within the stent (spatial gradient)	>50 cm/sec*
Change in peak velocity since prior examination (temporal change, higher or lower)	>50 cm/sec*
Decreased peak velocity of main portal vein	<30 cm/sec*
Main portal vein peak velocity decrease from baseline	>33%
Inversion of flow to pre-TIPS direction within intrahepatic portal veins	Usual post-TIPS flow in these veins is toward the stent

*Indicates parameters used by most of the authors.
TIPS, Transjugular intrahepatic portosystemic shunt.

published velocity thresholds within the stent include a lower limit of 50 cm/sec and upper limit of 250 cm/sec (these parameters are more specific but less sensitive for malfunction) (Table 1-3). Velocity measurements in the proximal portion (portal venous side) of the stent must be approached with caution because readings can be quite variable. Reversal of flow in the main portal vein is specific for shunt dysfunction.

With color Doppler, flow should be detectable throughout the stent. Flow is often turbulent in stents that are functioning well. Intrastent velocity parameters are fairly sensitive for stent dysfunction, but occasional false-positive results will result in venography.

Pitfall: The only highly specific sign for thrombosed shunt is complete or near-complete absence of color flow. In most cases, abnormal velocities must be reevaluated with venography.

Recently, many centers have begun to use stents covered with polytetrafluoroethylene (PTFE) for TIPS creation. Initial results indicate that these stents are less prone to thrombosis and stenosis when compared with conventional uncovered or "bare" stents. It has been also suggested that these stents last longer and even improve the overall survival in patients with cirrhosis. However, the PTFE causes significant shadowing immediately after covered stent placement, creating a blind spot for sonography that could be misinterpreted as a shunt malfunction (Fig. 1-83). Whereas shunt patency and direction of flow can be verified in the portal and hepatic veins, covered stents can be evaluated only 48 hours or more after TIPS creation (some advocate 7-14 days unless there is clinical suspicion of shunt malfunction).

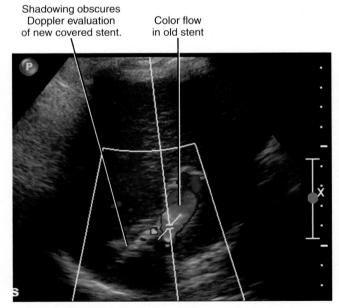

Shadowing obscures Doppler evaluation of new covered stent.

Color flow in old stent

Figure 1-83 Ultrasound evaluation of covered stent placed just 1 day before the examination as part of a revision. Color Doppler imaging can visualize flow within the original proximal stent but not the more distal covered stent.

Suggested Readings

Akan H, Arik N, Saglam S et al: Evaluation of the patients with renovascular hypertension after percutaneous revascularization by Doppler ultrasonography, *Eur J Radiol* 46:124-129, 2003.
Benito A: Doppler ultrasound for TIPS: does it work? Abdom Imaging 29:45-52, 2004.

Campbell SC: Slow flow or no flow? Color and power Doppler US pitfalls in the abdomen and pelvis, *RadioGraphics* 24:497-506, 2004.

Charboneau JW, Hattery RR, Ernst EC 3rd et al: Spectrum of sonographic findings in 125 renal masses other than benign simple cyst, *Am J Roentgenol* 140:87-94, 1983.

Desser TS, Jeffrey RB Jr, Lane MJ, Ralls PW: Tissue harmonic imaging: utility in abdominal and pelvic sonography, *J Clin Ultrasound* 27(3):135-142, 1999.

Dodd GD: Detection of transjugular intrahepatic portosystemic shunt dysfunction: value of duplex Doppler sonography, *Am J Roentgenol* 164:1119-1124, 1995.

Finstad TA, Tchelepi H, Ralls PW: Sonography of acute pancreatitis: prevalence of findings a pictorial essay, *Ultrasound Q* 21(2):95-104; quiz 150, 153-154, 2005.

Giorgio A: Ultrasound evaluation of uncomplicated and complicated acute viral hepatitis, *J Clin Ultrasound* 14:675-679, 1986.

Giorgio A, Amoroso P, Lettieri G et al: Cirrhosis: value of caudate to right lobe ratio in diagnosis with US, *Radiology* 161:443-445, 1986.

Gupta P: Fibrolamellar carcinoma: an unusual clinico-radiological presentation. *Eur J Radiol* 32:119-123, 1999.

Huang J: Imaging artifacts of medical instruments in ultrasound-guided interventions, *J Ultrasound Med* 26:1303-1322, 2007.

Ikeda AK, Korobkin M, Platt JF et al: Small echogenic renal masses: how often is computed tomography used to confirm the sonographic suspicion of angiomyolipoma? *Urology* 46:311-315, 1995.

Jungst C: Gallstone disease: microlithiasis and sludge, *Best Pract Res Clin Gastroenterol* 20:1053-1062, 2006.

Laing FC: US analysis of adnexal masses: the art of making the correct diagnosis, *Radiology* 191:21-22, 1994.

Laing FC, Kurtz AB: The importance of ultrasonic side-lobe artifacts, *Radiology* 145:763-768, 1982.

Lake D, Guimaraes M, Ackerman S et al: Comparative results of Doppler sonography after TIPS using covered and bare stents, *Am J Roentgenol* 186:1138-1143, 2006.

Maizlin ZV, Gottlieb P, Corat-Simon Y et al: Various appearances of multiple angiomyolipomas in the same kidney in a patient without tuberous sclerosis, *J Ultrasound Med* 21:211-213, 2002.

McGahan JP, Gerscovich E: Intraoperative and interventional ultrasound, *Curr Opin Radiol* 2(2):213-222, 1990.

McLarney JK, Rucker PT, Bender GN et al: From the Archives of the AFIP: fibrolamellar carcinoma of the liver: radiologic-pathologic correlation, *Radiographics* 19:453-471, 1999.

Middleton WD, Teefey SA, Darcy MD: Doppler evaluation of transjugular intrahepatic portosystemic shunts, *Ultrasound Q* 19(2):56-70, 2003.

Miralles M, Cairols M, Cotillas J et al: Value of Doppler parameters in the diagnosis of renal artery stenosis, *J Vasc Surg* 23:428-435, 1996.

Nino-Murcia M, Jeffrey RB Jr: Imaging the patient with right upper quadrant pain, *Semin Roentgenol* 36(2):81-91, 2000.

Puylaert JBCM: Ultrasonography of the acute abdomen: gastrointestinal conditions, *Radiol Clin North Am* 41:1227-vii, 2003.

Ralls PW: Inflammatory disease of the liver, *Clin Liver Dis* 6(1):203-225, 2002.

Rubens DJ: Doppler artifacts and pitfalls, *Radiol Clin North Am* 44:805-835, 2006.

Rubin JM: Clean and dirty shadowing at US: a reappraisal, *Radiology* 181:231-236, 1991.

Rubin JM: Power Doppler US: a potentially useful alternative to mean frequency-based color Doppler US, *Radiology* 190:853-856, 1994.

Rubin JM, Adler RS, Bude RO et al: Clean and dirty shadowing at US: a reappraisal, *Radiology* 181:231-236, 1991.

Sandler MA: Ultrasound case of the day. Duplication artifact (mirror image artifact), *RadioGraphics* 7:1025-1028, 1987.

Sharafuddin MJA, Raboi CA, Abu-Yousef M et al: Renal artery stenosis: duplex US after angioplasty and stent placement, *Radiology* 220:168-173, 2001.

Siegel CL, Middleton WD, Teefey SA et al: Angiomyolipoma and renal cell carcinoma: US differentiation, *Radiology* 198:789-793, 1996.

Stavros AT, Parker SH, Yakes WF et al: Segmental stenosis of the renal artery: pattern recognition of tardus and parvus abnormalities with duplex sonography, *Radiology* 184:487-492, 1992.

Williams GJ, Macaskill P, Chan SF et al: Comparative accuracy of renal duplex sonographic parameters in the diagnosis of renal artery stenosis: paired and unpaired analysis, *Am J Roentgenol* 188:798-811, 2007.

Zizka J, Elias P, Krajina A et al: Value of Doppler sonography in revealing transjugular intrahepatic portosystemic shunt malfunction: a 5-year experience in 216 patients, *Am J Roentgenol* 175:141-148, 2000.

CHAPTER 2

Multidetector Computed Tomography

Neal C. Dalrymple

Computed tomography (CT) is one of the cornerstones of abdominal imaging in the United States. Rapid assessment of multiple organ systems has made CT popular among radiologists and clinicians alike. The introduction of single-detector helical computed tomography (SDCT) in 1989 was the first step in a transition from viewing CT as a series of sequential axial sections to perceiving each examination as a volumetric acquisition of anatomic data. Technical innovations in multidetector computed tomography (MDCT) have accelerated this transition. Collecting multiple channels of data with MDCT has allowed simultaneous improvements in spatial resolution and volume coverage within the finite constraints of a single breath hold or contrast bolus.

■ BASIC PRINCIPLES OF COMPUTED TOMOGRAPHIC TECHNIQUE

Every clinical CT examination requires a number of steps from patient preparation to image transfer. Although the radiologist may not routinely participate in or witness each step, the processes of patient preparation, scan acquisition, data reconstruction, postprocessing, and image transfer must be considered when designing scan protocols.

Preparation

CT examinations of most regions of the body require little patient preparation. CT examinations of the abdomen and pelvis often require additional preparation, particularly for evaluation of the intestinal tract. Oral contrast media is often administered several hours before the examination to improve detection of bowel abnormalities. For CT colonography, a thorough bowel preparation is required including a cathartic accompanied by a clear liquid diet or fecal tagging agent to minimize confusion between polyps and fecal material. Patients are usually asked to refrain from other oral intake for several hours before intravenous (IV) contrast injection to minimize nausea and decrease the risk for aspiration.

Scan Acquisition

Scan acquisition is a critical step for every CT examination. Even the most sophisticated protocols performed on state-of-the-art scanners yield unsatisfactory images if the patient moves or if tube current is insufficient. Despite the rapid acquisition times of the newest scanners, breath holding is still necessary to avoid motion artifact for abdominal acquisitions. Experienced CT technologists are aware of the benefits of coaching patients through this step. The impact of poor breath-hold instructions may not be readily apparent to all technologists; therefore, if a radiologist notices frequent problems with breathing-related motion, informing the technologists may help to improve scan quality considerably. If it is unclear whether a CT abnormality is due to patient motion, multiplanar reformations (MPRs) can be useful (Fig. 2-1).

Pearl: MPRs can help to confirm that an abnormality seen on axial images is, in fact, the result of motion artifact. If MPRs are performed, look for a step off at the margin of organs and at the skin surface.

Detector configuration and radiographic technique parameters are specified for each scan acquisition and cannot be altered retrospectively. Fortunately, each generation of new scanner seems to make the "lower resolution" choices better than the "higher resolution" data on older scanners. Selecting a wide collimation setting to decrease the time required for a breath hold or to increase the amount of volume coverage during a contrast injection does not necessarily lead to "poor" long-axis resolution, although it does determine the finite restraints of reconstructed section thickness.

The characteristics of the radiation that passes through the patient during CT may be altered by modifying two parameters: tube current and tube potential. Tube current describes the quantity of photons emitted and is specified in milliamperes per second (mAs). Increasing tube current results in a decrease in image noise (Fig. 2-2) but also increases radiation dose to the patient in a linear fashion (a doubling of tube current results in twice as much radiation). Tube potential describes the energy of each photon emitted and is quantified in kilovolt potential (kVp). Increases in tube potential also decrease image noise and improve low-contrast resolution (ability to

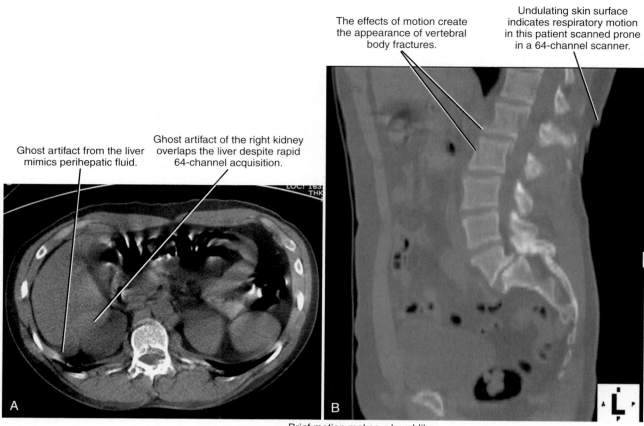

Ghost artifact from the liver mimics perihepatic fluid.

Ghost artifact of the right kidney overlaps the liver despite rapid 64-channel acquisition.

The effects of motion create the appearance of vertebral body fractures.

Undulating skin surface indicates respiratory motion in this patient scanned prone in a 64-channel scanner.

Brief motion makes a band-like step off in the kidney, liver and spleen on this coronal reformation from a 16-channel scanner.

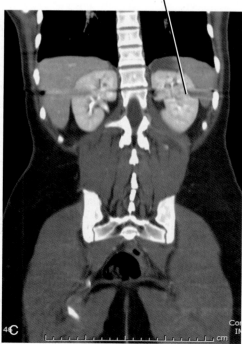

Figure 2-1 Axial computed tomographic image (**A**) and sagittal reformation (**B**) of data acquired on a 64-channel scanner, and coronal reformation (**C**) of data acquired on a 16-channel scanner show respiratory motion artifact.

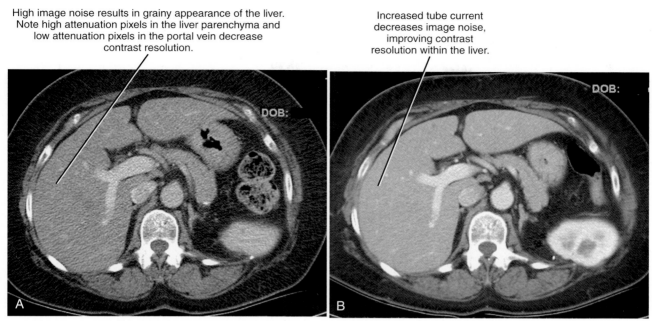

High image noise results in grainy appearance of the liver. Note high attenuation pixels in the liver parenchyma and low attenuation pixels in the portal vein decrease contrast resolution.

Increased tube current decreases image noise, improving contrast resolution within the liver.

Figure 2-2 Axial computed tomographic image (**A**) in a patient scanned initially with tube current set to 100 mA. For follow-up examination (**B**), tube current was set to 398 mA with marked decrease in image noise.

detect subtle differences in soft-tissue density) (Fig. 2-3). Unlike tube current, increases in tube potential result in an exponential increase in radiation dose.

Data Reconstruction

Data reconstruction is the process of converting the projection data generated during scan acquisition into axial sections for display. This process was relatively straightforward with step-and-shoot axial CT, because attenuation values were calculated to fill a specified matrix within a section that was determined by table position and collimator setting. Data reconstruction is more complicated with helical CT because no complete axial sections are obtained during acquisition, and interpolation algorithms are necessary to create axial sections from volumetric helical data.

Section Thickness and Section Increment

With SDCT, section thickness is determined by beam collimation and thus cannot be altered retrospectively (as with axial CT acquisition). However, because interpolation algorithms generate axial sections at arbitrary locations along the helix, the increment (also called *interval*) between sections can be adjusted retrospectively with SDCT. If the increment has a smaller value than the section thickness, the sections are considered to be overlapped. Overlapping images may be used to avoid segments of "skipped" tissue that could occur with increased pitch (increasing table speed to "stretch" out the helix, covering more volume per gantry rotation). Overlapping can also be used to improve the longitudinal resolution and smoothness of multiplanar and three-dimensional (3D) images created from axial CT sections (Fig. 2-4). These interpolation algorithms become increasingly

complex with MDCT because axial sections are reconstructed at arbitrary intervals along multiple helices. Because MDCT data are partitioned into small components, axial sections of variable thickness may be reconstructed for a given scan acquisition. Restrictions on reconstructed section thickness and increment on axial CT, SDCT, and MDCT are summarized in Table 2-1.

Initial or *primary data reconstruction* refers to the first set of axial images reconstructed from a given scan acquisition. The parameters of this reconstruction are specified on the scanner console before scan acquisition. Additional data reconstruction may be performed with a different algorithm or kernel to optimize evaluation of soft tissue, lung, or bone (Figs 2-5 and 2-6). Alternatively, data using a small section thickness and overlapping interval may be used to improve longitudinal resolution of small vessels or the margins of a mass. Data reconstruction performed subsequent to the initial reconstruction is usually called *secondary data reconstruction*. Most scanners now include the option to prescribe multiple sets of reconstructed sections that are generated automatically after the initial data reconstruction.

Sometimes the need for more than one set of reconstructed data is not anticipated or specified in the protocol. Additional data reconstruction prescribed after completion of the examination is referred to as *retrospective data reconstruction*. The ability to perform thin section data reconstruction retrospectively accounts for the versatility of newer MDCT scanners but relies on access to the projection data or "raw data" available only on the scanner. Because these data are not archived, no additional data reconstruction can be performed once it is deleted. On early MDCT scanners, the window of opportunity for data reconstruction was often only hours or a few days. As the tremendous utility of retrospective data reconstruction has become recognized (and the

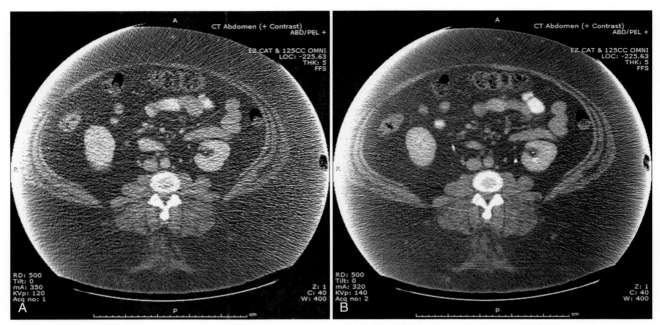

Figure 2-3 Images from a computed tomographic urogram showing effect of tube potential on image quality. Tube potential was increased from 120 **(A)** to 140 kVp **(B)** between the nephrographic and excretory phases. Note a decrease in image noise despite a slight decrease in tube current from 350 **(A)** to 320 mA **(B)**.

price of memory has decreased), vendors have been prolonging the time raw data is preserved.

Trade-offs are to be made when selecting section thickness. Although the thin sections available with MDCT have expanded multiplanar and 3D capabilities, thin sections are not always desirable. A balance exists between spatial resolution and low-contrast resolution. Decreasing section thickness necessarily increases image noise, decreasing low-contrast resolution. It is possible to decrease thin section noise by increasing tube

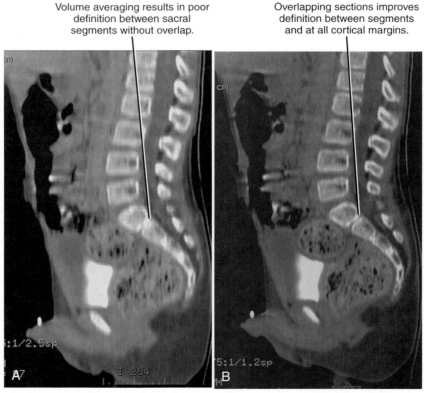

Volume averaging results in poor definition between sacral segments without overlap.

Overlapping sections improves definition between segments and at all cortical margins.

Figure 2-4 Sagittal reformations performed with computed tomographic data reconstructed using section thickness and increment of 2.5 mm **(A)**, then using section thickness of 2.5 mm and overlapping increment of 1.25 mm **(B)**.

Table 2-1 Availability of Retrospective Data Reconstruction on Different Computed Tomographic Scanner Platforms

CT Platform	Section Thickness	Increment
Axial CT	Fixed	Fixed
SDCT	Fixed	Variable
MDCT	Variable	Variable

CT, Computed tomography.

Soft tissue algorithm optimizes contrast resolution in the liver.

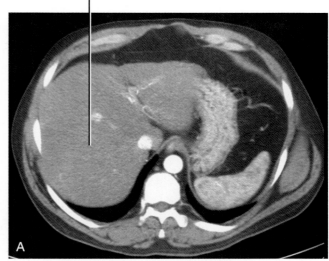

Lung markings appear smooth on images reconstructed using soft tissue algorithm.

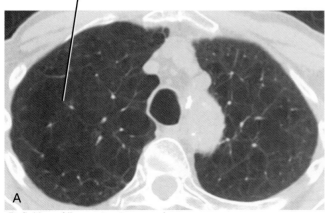

Definition of linear structures such as lung markings improved with edge-defining lung algorithm.

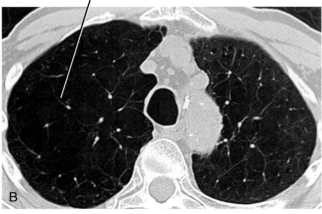

Figure 2-5 Unenhanced axial computed tomographic images through the lungs without (A) and with (B) lung algorithm demonstrate impact of reconstruction algorithm on image quality.

Use of a lung algorithm sharpens definition of linear structures such as small vessels with a mild increase in image noise.

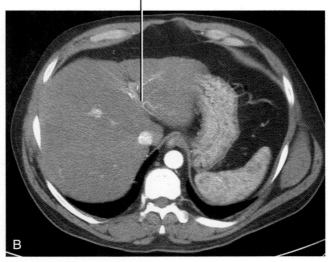

Figure 2-6 Enhanced axial computed tomographic images reconstructed with soft-tissue algorithm (A) and lung algorithm (B) demonstrate impact of reconstruction algorithm on image quality.

current, but this results in a greater radiation dose to the patient. Thin sections also worsen beam hardening and helical artifacts (Fig. 2-7).

Postprocessing

MDCT makes available thin section data that may be used to create exquisitely detailed multiplanar and 3D images. Unlike MRI, which is capable of acquiring coronal or sagittal images directly, multidimensional CT images always require the use of software to convert axial section data. In the past, most postprocessing was performed by technologists on highly specialized 3D workstations. Although this still occurs today, networked 3D systems are now available that help to integrate 3D review of CT examinations into the primary interpretation session. This is discussed in greater detail in Chapter 5.

Image Transfer

Transferring CT images to picture archiving and communication system (PACS) for viewing seems such an obvious step it might not deserve mention. However, MDCT can create examinations with hundreds or thousands of

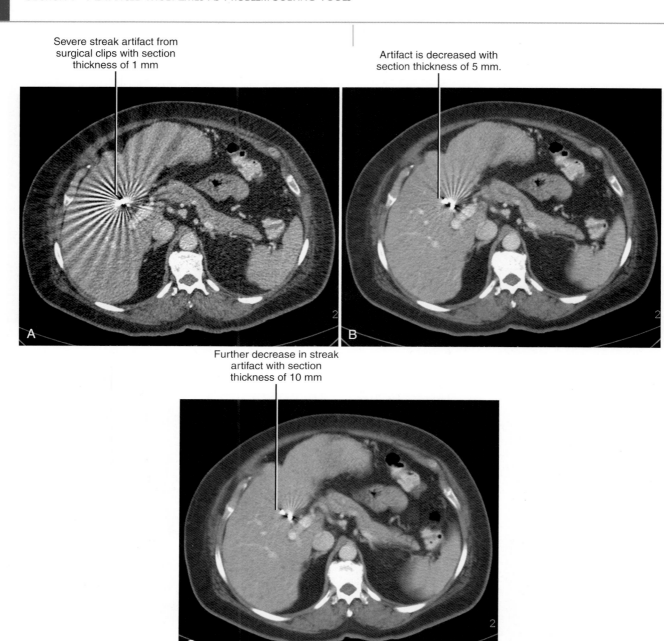

Severe streak artifact from surgical clips with section thickness of 1 mm

Artifact is decreased with section thickness of 5 mm.

Further decrease in streak artifact with section thickness of 10 mm

Figure 2-7 Impact of reconstructed section thickness on image artifact. A single scan acquisition reconstructed with section thickness of (**A**) 1, (**B**) 5, and (**C**) 10 mm.

images, and transferring all of those images may not be desirable. Radiologists may choose to transfer only axial sections of traditional thickness (2-5 mm) for primary axial review to PACS, whereas channeling the entire thin-section data set separately to a 3D workstation or 3D network server. In this workflow model, postprocessed 3D and multiplanar images are eventually sent to join the original axial examination in the PACS. Others may choose to reconstruct thin-section data primarily, performing all interpretation on thin data either on PACS or with a 3D system. This limits redundancy of data, although the thin section images may appear noisy if not postprocessed.

■ TYPES OF MULTIDETECTOR COMPUTED TOMOGRAPHIC SCANNERS

Rapid development in CT technology has produced considerable variety among the types of MDCT scanners in use today. Not surprisingly, some of the terminology used to describe scanners can be misleading. Even the term *single detector* is not entirely accurate when describing SDCT. In truth, SDCT scanners typically have a single row containing hundreds of detectors exposed to a fan beam as it rotates around the patient in the axial plane. If the patient is stationary during exposure, scan

‌

acquisition is considered to be "axial." If the patient is advancing continuously during exposure, scan acquisition is "helical."

Development of MDCT involved converting from a single row of detectors (imagine a single hula hoop) to multiple rows of detectors (imagine multiple hula hoops). Each detector row exposed provides a separate channel of data that can be used to reconstruct axial sections. When a scanner is described as "4-slice," "16-slice," or "64-slice," the number describes the maximum number of data channels available for acquisition. For example, a 64-slice scanner can acquire 40 mm of data per rotation, allowing reconstruction of up to 64 axial sections each with a thickness of 0.625 mm or, if selected, 8 axial sections each with a thickness of 5 mm. In comparison, data from a 16-slice scanner acquiring 10 mm of data per rotation may be used to generate sixteen 0.625-mm sections or two 5-mm sections per rotation. For this reason, it may be less confusing to refer to scanners as "16-channel" or "64-channel" scanners.

It is necessary to know the number of data channels available and the selectable values for section thickness during data reconstruction to design effective scan protocols with MDCT. Combined, these two variables are described as the "detector configuration," as illustrated in Fig. 2-8. For example, a 16-channel scanner may be set to obtain 16 channels of data each with a section thickness of 1.25 mm or 16 channels of data each with a section thickness of 0.625 mm. In this example, available detector configurations would include 16 × 1.25 mm and 16 × 0.625 mm.

Multiplying the number of data channels by the section thickness yields the width of beam collimation used to acquire the scan (e.g., 16 × 1.25 mm = 20 mm or 64 × 0.625 mm = 40 mm). Beam collimation is an important variable to consider when designing protocols because it is the combination of beam collimation, gantry rotation time, and table speed that determines the length of scan coverage that can be acquired within a given period. For example, a CT examination of the abdomen and pelvis using a 4-channel scanner that can

be performed in a single 25-second breath hold using a 4 × 5-mm configuration may require two similar breath holds within the 4 × 2.5-mm configuration.

Pearl: When using a scanner with 16 or fewer channels, selecting a detector configuration using the largest collimation practical for the application at hand will minimize the radiation dose to the patient.

◾ USE OF INTRAVENOUS AND ENTERIC CONTRAST MEDIA FOR MULTIDETECTOR COMPUTED TOMOGRAPHY

Intravenous Contrast Media

Use of IV contrast media is a crucial component of most CT examinations of the abdomen and pelvis. IV contrast media increase tissue attenuation through: (1) vascular opacification, (2) tissue enhancement, and (3) urinary excretion. Therefore IV contrast media can be used to create images of the vasculature (CT angiography), to improve the conspicuity of abnormalities of the abdominal organs, or to assess the urinary tract (CT urography).

In the case of CT angiography, IV contrast media facilitate the creation of detailed 3D images of the blood vessels and improve the detection of vascular extravasation, thrombosis, and embolism. Relatively long scan times on single-channel scanners result in progression through multiple phases of vascular and parenchymal enhancement during scan acquisition. This limits the utility of single-channel scanners for vascular imaging, although it does simplify protocols. The short acquisition times of modern multichannel scanners permit imaging of discrete phases of enhancement, forcing the radiologist to make choices regarding scan delays and contrast injection profiles. For example, an examination performed early in the peak of arterial enhancement provides excellent vascular detail but little information about the veins or enhancement of solid organs (Fig. 2-9). Rapid injections of short duration are also useful for CT arteriography but

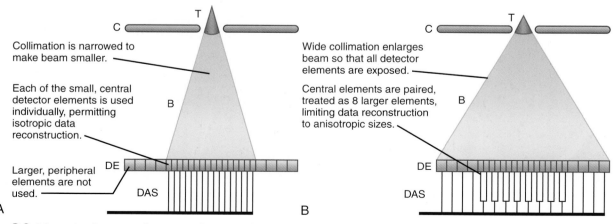

Figure 2-8 Schematic of common detector configurations for 16-channel scanners shows relation between detector configuration and the geometric constraints of the data obtained. Narrow **(A)** and wide **(B)** collimation settings are illustrated. *B,* x-ray beam; *C,* collimator; *DAS,* data acquisition system; *DE,* detector elements; *T,* x-ray tube. (Reprinted from Dalrymple NC, Prasad SR, Freckleton MW et al: Informatics in Radiology (InfoRAD): introduction to the language of three-dimensional imaging with multidetector CT, *Radiographics* 25:1409-1428, 2005, by permission.)

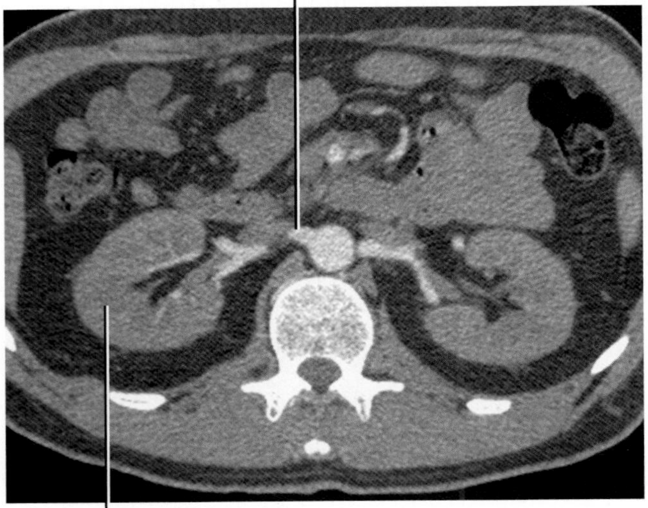

Good opacification of
aorta and renal arteries

Renal parenchyma is
not yet opacified.

Figure 2-9 Axial computed tomographic (CT) image acquired early in the arterial phase of contrast enhancement performed for CT angiography examination.

quality can be improved by using contrast media with a high concentration of iodine.

Most often, IV contrast media are used to improve the conspicuity of abnormalities. In some cases, conspicuity is increased because the abnormality enhances to a lesser degree than surrounding structures. Renal cysts are a common example of this phenomenon. In other cases, the increased conspicuity results from increased vascular perfusion (as with hypervascular liver metastases) or extracellular contrast media accumulation (as with desmoplastic tumors) relative to background tissues. In addition to increasing lesion conspicuity, IV contrast media can improve the specificity of CT for focal lesions. For example, with the aid of IV contrast media, cysts, hemangiomas, and solid neoplasms of the liver can be accurately distinguished from one another. For characterizing abnormalities of the abdomen and pelvis, the enhancement pattern (e.g., diffuse, nodular, etc.) and the timing of enhancement (e.g., arterial, portal, equilibrium, delayed) must be taken into account. The degree to which contrast is retained within a lesion is also a relevant feature that aids in characterization.

Bolus Tracking

Precise timing of scan initiation during or after injection of contrast media may be achieved by using bolus tracking. Bolus tracking monitors the attenuation within a vessel or target organ on repeated axial sections. When the attenuation within the region of interest (ROI) reaches a selected threshold, scan acquisition begins, usually after an additional delay of several seconds while the table moves into position (Fig. 2-10). This

may result in minimal arterial opacification during the portal venous phase (PVP). A slower rate of injection may be used to achieve some residual arterial opacification during the PVP. Because automated vessel segmentation used in most 3D workstations is more effective with uniform, dense vascular opacification, CT angiography image

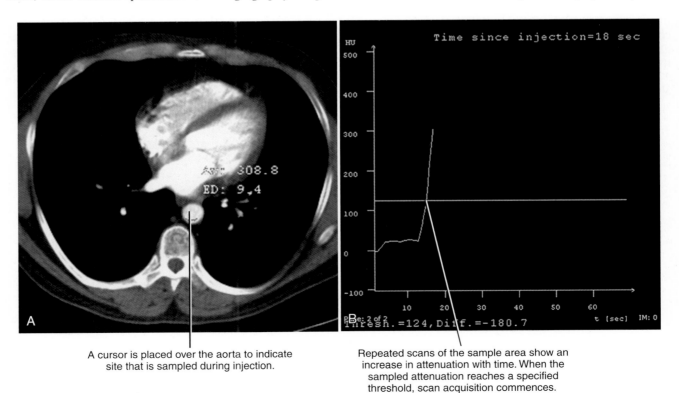

A cursor is placed over the aorta to indicate
site that is sampled during injection.

Repeated scans of the sample area show an
increase in attenuation with time. When the
sampled attenuation reaches a specified
threshold, scan acquisition commences.

Figure 2-10 Demonstration of use of bolus tracking to trigger initiation of scan acquisition.

technique allows consistent scan quality in the face of variable cardiac output and patient size. Acquisition can be started within several seconds of arterial enhancement for CT angiography or after a prescribed delay such as 10 seconds after aortic enhancement for arterial imaging of the liver. Because unopacified blood within vessels typically measures approximately 30 Hounsfield units (HU) and peak arterial opacification can result in attenuation measurements of 250 to 350 HU, a wide range of trigger thresholds may be selected.

Combining the precision of bolus tracking with dual injection using a saline "push" allows excellent vascular opacification using relatively small amounts of contrast media. However, the degree of parenchymal opacification of the liver, spleen, pancreas, and kidneys is affected not only by the rate of injection and scan delay, but also by the total amount of iodine injected. Therefore solid organ imaging requires administration of a sufficient quantity of injected contrast medium.

Enteric Contrast Media

CT evaluation of gastrointestinal structures may be improved considerably with the addition of enteric contrast media. Traditionally, patients have been asked to drink a dilute barium solution or iodine-based water-soluble solution 90 minutes to 2 hours before the CT examination. If the patient is unable to drink, the contrast media can be administered through a nasogastric tube. Colonic opacification can be achieved by prolonging prep time or by administering additional contrast through a rectal tube. If bowel perforation is considered in the clinical differential diagnosis, water-soluble contrast should be substituted for barium.

Contrast media that results in high attenuation within the bowel lumen is referred to as *positive enteric contrast.* Abnormalities well demonstrated with positive enteric contrast include low-attenuation filling defects, bowel wall thickening, and bowel perforation (Figs. 2-11, 2-12, and 2-13, respectively).

Negative enteric contrast consists of water or another low-attenuation liquid. This is usually administered in conjunction with rapid injection of IV contrast to assess enhancement of the bowel wall and adjacent structures. Negative contrast may improve visualization of such structures as the ampulla of Vater (Fig. 2-14). In the setting of inflammatory bowel disease, negative oral contrast medium improves visualization of wall enhancement within thickened segments of bowel (Fig. 2-15). Negative contrast improves visualization of bowel segments during CT angiography without compromising 3D images by obscuring vascular structures with high-attenuation enteric agents. Some advocate the use of negative contrast agents routinely with MDCT because the presence of positive contrast could hinder 3D applications to evaluate unexpected abnormalities (Fig. 2-16).

Recently, a *weakly positive oral contrast* medium has been introduced. This consists of dilute barium (0.1% solution) combined with an agent that causes bowel distention. Weakly positive, bowel-distensing, oral contrast media may be used for dedicated evaluation of the stomach or small intestine. Although slightly denser

Linear low attenuation filling defect appears conspicuous against high attenuation enteric contrast material. A toothpick within a Meckel's diverticulum was found at surgery.

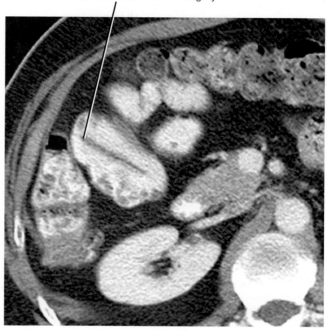

Figure 2-11 Computed tomographic examination of the abdomen demonstrating the utility of positive oral contrast media for evaluation of abdominal pain.

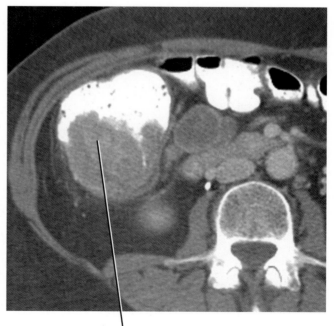

Large filling defect in posterior cecum confirmed to be cecal carcinoma at surgery.

Figure 2-12 Computed tomographic examination of the abdomen demonstrating the utility of positive oral contrast media for evaluation of abdominal pain.

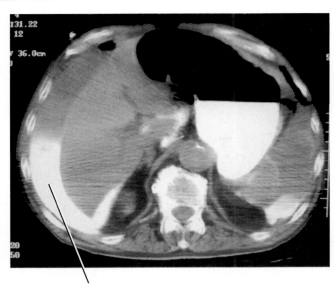

High attenuation contrast media
indicates perihepatic fluid from
a perforation of the GI tract.

Figure 2-13 Computed tomography of the abdomen performed with water-soluble positive oral contrast media for the evaluation of abdominal pain. Perforated duodenal ulcer was found at surgery. GI, gastrointestinal.

Combination of negative oral contrast media with
intravenous contrast enhancement allows
visualization of major papilla against
low attenuation background.

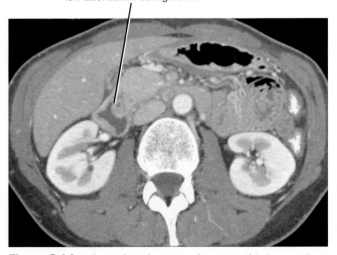

Figure 2-14 Enhanced axial computed tomographic image using water as negative oral contrast media in combination with intravenous contrast media.

than water, bowel wall and mucosal detail can be visualized when combined with rapid injection of IV contrast media in a manner similar to negative contrast media but with improved bowel distention (Fig. 2-17). Whereas traditional positive oral contrast media contain enough barium to attenuate emission during positron emission tomography/CT (resulting in artifactually decreased activity), weakly positive oral contrast media result in less attenuation, improving bowel visualization.

Low attenuation contrast media within small
bowel lumen optimizes visualization
of mucosal enhancement.

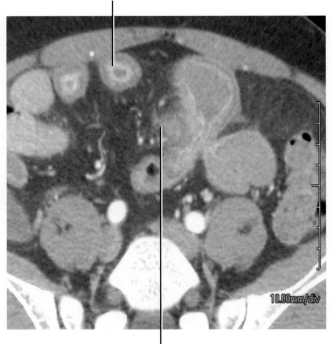

Extra-luminal inflammatory changes are
still easily distinguished from
fluid within bowel lumen.

Figure 2-15 Axial enhanced computed tomographic scan in a patient with Crohn disease scanned using negative oral contrast.

Rectal administration of contrast media may be beneficial in some circumstances. Colonic opacification through a rectal tube is much faster than antegrade filling of the colon via oral administration. Rectal administration also improves colonic distention, improving detection of small colonic perforations and fistulae. Some surgeons prefer the use of rectal contrast for patients with suspected appendicitis because this allows the patient to remain NPO (nothing by mouth) in the event surgery is required. Because most of the indications for rectal contrast involve suspected perforation or at least potential surgical disease, water-soluble contrast is usually used. Rectal contrast media for CT evaluation can be administered through a small, soft tube without a retention balloon. It is important to note that rectal contrast administration will distend the colon and possibly the distal small bowel, potentially masking the caliber transition used to identify bowel obstruction. On the other hand, rectal contrast administration can be useful for distinguishing between fixed luminal narrowings and collapsed colon segments.

■ ATTENUATION VALUES

The data acquired by CT is a grayscale representation of the variable attenuation of the x-ray beam by tissues of differing densities. Although this is used predominantly to define normal and abnormal anatomic detail by

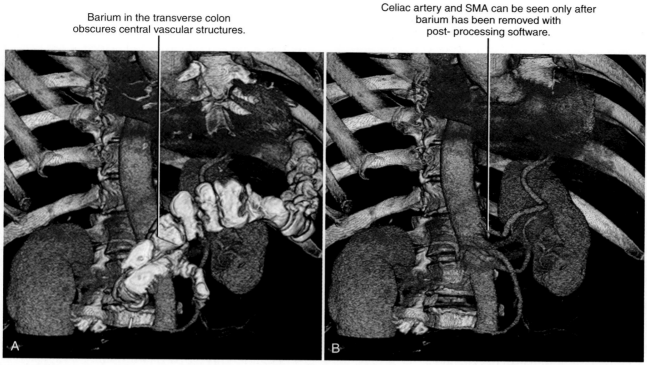

Barium in the transverse colon obscures central vascular structures.

Celiac artery and SMA can be seen only after barium has been removed with post- processing software.

Figure 2-16 Three-dimensional volume rendering of abdominal aorta performed after positive oral contrast administration shows how positive contrast agents can interfere with visualization of other high-attenuation structures. **A,** Barium in the colon obscures vascular structures on original rendering. **B,** Manually removing the barium "uncovers" the structures of interest. *SMA,* Superior mesenteric artery.

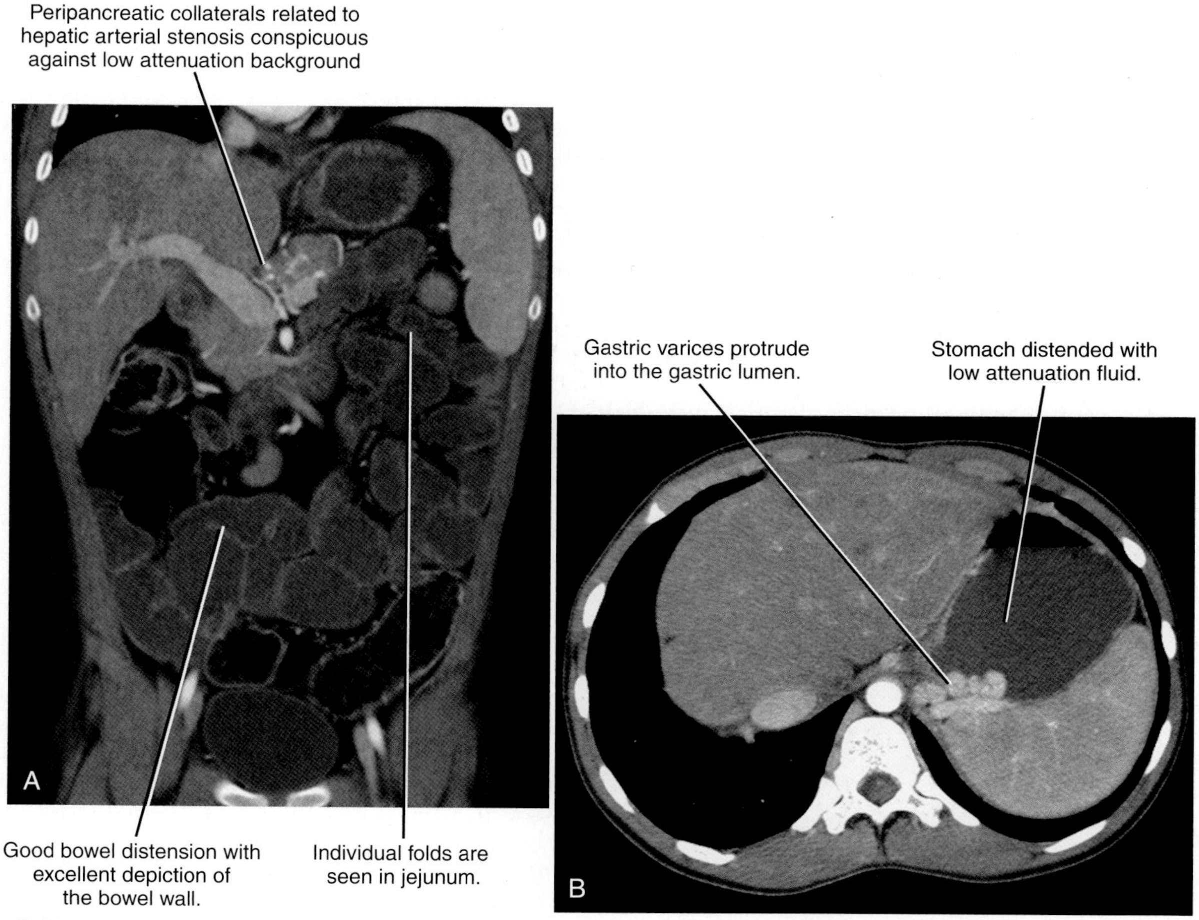

Peripancreatic collaterals related to hepatic arterial stenosis conspicuous against low attenuation background

Gastric varices protrude into the gastric lumen.

Stomach distended with low attenuation fluid.

Good bowel distension with excellent depiction of the bowel wall.

Individual folds are seen in jejunum.

Figure 2-17 Computed tomographic examinations performed in two separate patients (**A, B**) using weakly positive, distensing, oral contrast media demonstrate excellent conspicuity of high-attenuation structures.

differentiating among soft tissue, air, fluid, bone, and contrast media (Table 2-2), there are circumstances in which the quantitative values of acquired data are useful. The attenuation value of a ROI reported in Hounsfield units is the most frequently used quantitative measurement. Although the mean attenuation value within a user-defined ROI is most often used to ascertain whether a given lesion is composed of fluid or soft tissue, attenuation may be used in a variety of circumstances. Sequential attenuation measurements of a given lesion before and after the administration of IV contrast media is used to search for evidence of lesion enhancement. The attenuation of fluid collections may be used to discriminate between water/serous fluid and collections that contain blood. Fluid attenuation within an adrenal lesion more commonly indicates the averaging of intracellular lipid and soft tissue of an adenoma than an adrenal cyst. Pixel mapping displays the value of each pixel within an ROI and has been used to add specificity to the characterization of adrenal lesions when at least 10% of included pixels measure 10 HU or less. Because acquired values may vary according to scan technique or when artifacts are present, it is important to optimize general scan technique and to consider scan parameters such as tube current and tube potential used in the literature if quantitative evaluation is anticipated.

■ RADIATION DOSE WITH MULTIDETECTOR COMPUTED TOMOGRAPHY

A full discussion of the implications of radiation dose to the patient and methods for estimation of the effective dose from a given examination are beyond the scope of this textbook. However, some general principles merit consideration during the routine performance of CT examinations.

Automated Modulation of Tube Current

Most MDCT scanners with 16 or more channels include some type of automated program that adjusts tube current. These programs use ionizing radiation efficiently by adjusting tube current to achieve similar signal-to-noise

Table 2-2 Approximate Computed Tomographic Attenuation Values for Different Tissue Types

Tissue Type	Attenuation Value (HU)
Air	−2000 to −200
Fat	−190 to −30
Water	0 to 20
Soft tissue	20 to 60
Hemorrhage	45 to 80
Intravenous contrast media	50 to 350
Calcium	130 to 2500

characteristics among different areas of the body. In other words, tube current is decreased when exposing less dense regions (such as the lungs) and increased when exposing regions of higher density (such as the pelvis or shoulders). This type of tube current adjustment along the length of the body is called *z-axis current modulation*. Because supine patients are usually "thicker" from side to side than front to back, some systems also adjust tube current throughout a given rotation, to achieve uniform photon flux. Adjustment in tube current within a given gantry revolution is called *angular current modulation*.

Automated exposure control programs differ considerably among vendors, and it is important to become familiar with their use. For example, if no maximum limit is specified and the default low-noise setting is not adjusted on some platforms, default settings may result in a radiation dose to the patient that is greater than expected. Some systems allow selection of a "noise index" that will usually result in a predictable level of image noise. This allows selection of high noise settings when loss of low tissue contrast is unlikely to affect diagnostic accuracy (Fig. 2-18).

MDCT scanners offer multiple choices for gantry rotation rate. Increasing the rate of rotation decreases acquisition time or allows a larger volume of tissue to be covered per unit time. This is particularly useful for cardiac imaging when temporal resolution is critical. Although rapid rates of gantry rotation allow large-volume coverage for CT angiography, scanners with 16 or more channels can cover large areas without necessitating increases in gantry rotation. This is important because increases in gantry rotation rate require a compensatory increase in tube current to avoid increases in image noise. Greater levels of image noise may be acceptable in CT angiography where there is high inherent contrast between brightly enhanced vessels and low-density surrounding soft tissues. However, solid organ imaging requires optimization of soft-tissue contrast resolution. Because automated current modulation may not be able to increase tube current enough to compensate for the most rapid rates of gantry rotation, slower rates (between 0.7 and 1.0 second per rotation) are typically more desirable when imaging the abdomen and pelvis (Fig. 2-19).

Collimation

With SDCT, narrowing collimation generally results in an increase in radiation dose to the patient. Narrow beam collimation has a similar effect with MDCT. Narrow collimation results in less efficient use of the incident beam, including unused or "wasted" exposure at the margins of the exposed array (Fig. 2-20). In addition, because narrow collimation is usually used to achieve thin sections, tube current is often increased to balance the increase in noise encountered with thin CT sections. These effects are particularly pronounced with the 4- to 16-channel platforms. Most platforms with more than 16 channels achieve changes in available section thickness with either a smaller effect or no effect on size of the incident beam. Therefore relative changes in patient radiation dose become less significant when

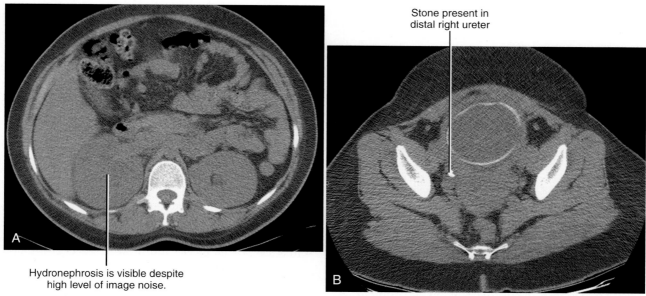

Stone present in
distal right ureter

Hydronephrosis is visible despite
high level of image noise.

Figure 2-18 Computed tomography performed through the abdomen (**A**) and the pelvis (**B**) with deliberately increased noise index (to decrease radiation dose) in pregnant patient with right flank pain.

switching between thin and thick section modes on higher channel platforms.

Multiphase Examinations

The speed of acquisition and increasing tube capacity with modern CT scanners makes dynamic imaging of multiple phases tempting. Multiphase imaging provides valuable information about many types of hepatic, renal, and

pancreatic lesions. Initial nonenhanced images provide a baseline to measure lesion enhancement, essential for differentiating a high-attenuation cyst from a homogeneously enhancing mass. Innumerable articles describe the utility of noncontrast, arterial, portal venous, corticomedullary, nephrographic, and delayed excretory phase images for different purposes. However, because each phase of acquisition contributes to the radiation dose, the ALARA (as low as reasonably achievable) principle requires careful attention to the clinical utility of each phase.

Tube current is insufficient to compensate for
rapid gantry rotation. High image noise
decreases conspicuity of liver lesion.

Slower gantry rotation allows sufficient tube
current to decrease image noise, making
regions of increased or decreased
enhancement more conspicuous.

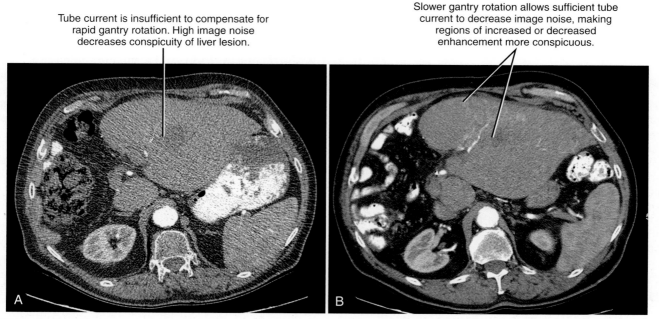

Figure 2-19 Axial enhanced computed tomographic image of the liver in a patient with metastases from colon cancer performed with automated current modulation and variable gantry rotation of 0.5 (**A**) and 0.8 second (**B**). Because the noise index was fixed, image quality would be expected to be similar on both images. However, the tube current could not be raised sufficiently to compensate for the increased gantry rotation speed. As a result, diagnostic information is compromised in (**A**).

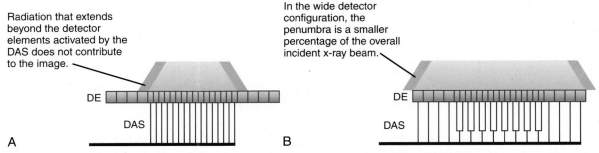

Figure 2-20 Illustration of 16-channel scanner with penumbra of "extra" or "wasted" radiation shown in red at the margins of the incident x-ray beam (yellow) with the collimator in the narrow (**A**) and wide (**B**) settings. *DAS*, Data acquisition system; *DE*, detector elements. (Reprinted from Dalrymple NC, Prasad SR, El-Merhi FM et al: Price of isotropy in multidetector CT, *RadioGraphics* 27:49-62, 2007, by permission.)

Imaging the Obese Patient

When imaging the abdomen or pelvis of an obese patient, increases in exposure parameters are sometimes necessary to ensure adequate image quality. Image noise can be reduced by increasing either tube potential or current, and increases in both are often used by CT technologists. However, technologists sometimes overlook the effect of exposure time on image noise. When a maximum value for tube current has already been selected, additional exposure may be achieved by slowing the rate of gantry rotation. For example, selecting a tube current of 400 mA and gantry rotation time of 0.8 second per rotation results in 400 mA × 0.8 second = 320 mAs. Slowing the rate of gantry rotation to 1.0 second per rotation would result in 400 mA × 1.0 second = 400 mAs or a 25% increase in photons available for imaging.

Pearl: It may be helpful to preprogram a protocol designed for obese patients for each common type of examination. This ensures that a low rate of gantry rotation and high tube current and potential are selected.

■ PROTOCOLS AND TIPS

The varying characteristics of available MDCT scanners and diverse preferences of radiologists make it challenging to offer detailed scan protocols. Tube current settings, in particular, vary considerably between scanner platforms and are not included in the protocols that follow. However, we can discuss general principles to consider when tailoring common CT protocols and provide a few individual protocols tailored to common abdominal and pelvic indications. Each protocol will likely require additional adjustments to accommodate specific equipment and practice environments.

Breath Hold

Respiratory motion can compromise scan quality with even the most rapid scan acquisitions currently available (see Fig. 2-1). A patient's respiratory status, mental status, age, or language abilities can affect compliance with breath-hold commands. If respiratory motion is a recurring problem, it may be useful to address the issue with the CT technologists, emphasizing the benefits of coaching patients to comply with instructions. In some cases, the short scan delay programmed after bolus tracking of IV contrast media injection may not give patients adequate time to complete inspiration before the scan is initiated. If this is the case, adding a few additional seconds to the triggering delay may reduce motion artifact with minimal impact on contrast timing.

Narrow Collimation

Narrow beam collimation describes exposing only the central small detector elements, allowing the smallest possible reconstructed section thickness for a given MDCT scanner platform.

Wide Collimation

With wide beam collimation, the entire detector array is exposed, and smaller elements are paired to provide "thicker" data. The smallest available section thickness is greater than 1 mm, but this allows faster coverage and generally results in a lower radiation dose to the patient.

Examples of narrow and wide collimation are provided in Table 2-3. Similar settings are available for most scanners with slight variations according to vendor.

Scan Delay

The short scan times possible with MDCT permit dynamic scanning but also make it easy to improperly time exposures. Following are some general principles for achieving satisfactory images:

■ *Unenhanced phase:* Scan without contrast injection, either as an unenhanced study or as a precontrast baseline for dynamic examination. Unenhanced images are essential when calcifications are a key

Table 2-3 Detector Configuration by Scanner Platform

Scanner Platform	Narrow Settings	Wide Settings
4-Channel	4 × 1.0 mm 4 × 1.25 mm	4 × 2.5 mm 4 × 3.75 mm 4 × 5.0 mm
16-Channel	16 × 0.5 mm 16 × 0.625 mm 16 × 0.75 mm	16 × 1.0 mm 16 × 1.25 mm 16 × 1.5 mm
40-Channel	40 × 0.625 mm	40 × 1.25 mm
64-Channel	64 × 0.5 mm 64 × 0.6 mm 64 × 0.625 mm	64 × 1.0 mm 64 × 1.25 mm

element of the diagnosis (e.g., stones in the urinary tract) or when the enhanced attenuation value has particular significance (e.g., adrenal mass or renal cyst). Some of the more common indications for unenhanced scanning are listed in Box 2-1. Because radiographic technique has an impact on attenuation measurements, use kilovolt potential and milliamperes per second values similar to the enhanced series if a change in attenuation will affect diagnosis.

■ *Arterial phase:* To obtain an arterial phase scan, we recommend using bolus tracking. We often place the cursor in the abdominal aorta near the celiac artery for liver, kidney, and abdominal aorta studies. For vascular studies, we generally recommend an attenuation peak of 150 HU and minimal start delay (it always takes some time to stop taking the tracking images, reposition the table to start the clinical scan, and instruct the patient to hold his or her breath). For parenchymal studies (liver, kidneys, pancreas), an additional 5-second delay provides improved parenchymal opacification. If bolus tracking is not available, consider using a 25-second delay for arterial phase studies and a 30-second delay for solid organ imaging.

BOX 2-1 Indications for Unenhanced Computed Tomography of the Abdomen, Pelvis, or Both

- Suspected urinary calculus
- Possible adrenal adenoma
- Detection of calcifications or high-attenuation foreign bodies
- Baseline attenuation measurement before contrast administration
- Evaluation for intramural hemorrhage in abdominal aortic aneurysm
- Patient-related contraindication to contrast media (e.g., prior contrast reaction, renal compromise, recent contrast injection, poor venous access)

■ *Portal venous phase (PVP):* Many centers use standard delay scanning in the PVP. Typical scan delays for the PVP according to the scanner platform are as follows:

4-channel	60 seconds
16-channel	70 seconds
40- to 64-channel	80 seconds

■ *Nephrographic phase (NP):* The NP is useful for detecting renal masses. The NP occurs slightly later than the PVP. A 100-second delay is usually satisfactory for the NP, although some individuals prefer to wait 120 seconds to include the early excretory phase.

■ *Delayed excretory phase:* The delayed excretory phase is used primarily for CT urography. Many versions of CT urography exist in the literature. Dispersion of contrast material within the collecting systems and distention of the ureters can be augmented by the administration of IV saline, a diuretic, or both.

Sample Protocols

The following abbreviations are used to describe the phase of scan delay in the sample protocols presented in Tables 2-4 through 2-10:

UP – unenhanced phase
AP – arterial phase
PVP – portal venous phase
NP – nephrographic phase
DEP – delayed excretory phase

Table 2-4 Routine Abdominal-Pelvic Survey

Indications	Pain, oncologic survey, trauma, suspected intraabdominal infection
Preparation	Clear liquids 12 hours prior, nothing by mouth 4 hours prior
Oral contrast	Positive agent 2 hours prior
Intravenous contrast	Yes
Injection rate	3 ml/sec
Scan delay	Portal venous phase
Collimation	Wide
Thickness	5 mm
Increment	5 mm
Pitch	1-1.5
Rotation time	0.7-1.0 second
Voltage	120 kVp
Filter	Standard
Additional data reconstruction	Per request

Table 2-5 Liver Mass Protocol

Indications	Characterize focal liver lesions, screen for hepatocellular carcinoma
Preparation	Clear liquids 12 hours prior, nothing by mouth 4 hours prior
Oral contrast	None or negative agent
Intravenous contrast	Yes
Injection rate	4 ml/sec
Scan delay	Unenhanced phase, arterial phase, portal venous phase Add 3- to 5-minute delay for suspected hemangioma Add 10-minute delay for suspected cholangiocarcinoma
Collimation	Wide for unenhanced phase and portal venous phase Narrow for arterial phase
Thickness	5 mm
Increment	5 mm
Pitch	1-1.5
Rotation time	0.7-1.0 second
Voltage	140 kVp
Filter	Standard
Additional data reconstruction	Routine arterial phase 1 mm overlapped

Table 2-6 Pancreatic Mass Protocol

Indications	Detect and characterize focal pancreatic lesions
Preparation	Clear liquids 12 hours prior, nothing by mouth 4 hours prior
Oral contrast	Negative agent
Intravenous contrast	Yes
Injection rate	4-5 ml/sec
Scan delay	Unenhanced, arterial phase, portal venous phase
Collimation	Wide for unenhanced phase Narrow for arterial phase and portal venous phase
Thickness	2.5 mm
Increment	2.5 mm
Pitch	1-1.5
Rotation time	0.7-1.0 second
Voltage	140 kVp
Filter	Standard
Additional data reconstruction	Routine arterial phase and portal venous phase 1 mm overlapped

Table 2-7 Renal Mass Protocol

Indications	Characterize focal renal lesions, hematuria (unless computed tomographic urography performed)
Preparation	Clear liquids 12 hours prior, nothing by mouth 4 hours prior
Oral contrast	None or negative agent
Intravenous contrast	Yes
Injection rate	4 ml/sec
Scan delay	Unenhanced, arterial phase, nephrographic phase
Collimation	Wide for unenhanced and portal venous phase Narrow for arterial phase
Thickness	2.5 mm
Increment	2.5 mm
Pitch	1-1.5
Rotation time	0.7-1.0 second
Voltage	120 kVp
Filter	Standard
Additional data reconstruction	Routine arterial phase 1 mm overlapped Routine nephrographic phase 1 mm overlapped
Comments	Computed tomographic urography can be performed with above protocol by adding delayed excretory phase images in narrow collimation setting Reconstruct 0.6 mm overlapped

Table 2-8 Abdominal Computed Tomographic Angiography

Indications	Characterize abdominal aortic aneurysm; suspected renal, aortoiliac, or mesenteric arterial disease; follow-up aortic aneurysm repair
Preparation	Clear liquids 12 hours prior, nothing by mouth 4 hours prior
Oral contrast	None or negative agent
Intravenous contrast	Yes
Injection rate	4-5 ml/sec
Scan delay	Arterial phase
Collimation	Narrow
Thickness	2.5 mm
Increment	2.5 mm
Pitch	1-1.5
Rotation time	0.5-0.8 second
Voltage	140 kVp
Filter	Standard
Additional data reconstruction	Routine arterial phase and portal venous phase 1 mm overlapped

Table 2-9   Flank Pain Protocol

Indications	Suspected ureteral stone May be used for suspected appendicitis
Preparation	None
Oral contrast	None
Intravenous contrast	None
Injection rate	Not applicable
Scan delay	Not applicable
Collimation	Wide
Thickness	3 mm or less
Increment	Contiguous
Pitch	1.5
Rotation time	0.6-0.8 second
Voltage	120 kVp
Filter	Standard
Additional data reconstruction	As requested
Comments	Consider scanning with patient in the prone position to discriminate stones within the uterovesical junction from those within the bladder

Table 2-10   Computed Tomographic Colonography

Indications	Failed colonoscopy Colon cancer screening
Preparation	Dry colon cleansing prep, fecal tagging agent if available
Enteric contrast	Air or CO_2 via rectal tube
Intravenous contrast	None
Injection rate	Not applicable
Scan delay	Not applicable
Collimation	Wide for 16-channel (dose reduction) Narrow for 4-, 40-, 64-channel
Thickness	3 mm or less
Increment	Contiguous
Pitch	1.5
Rotation time	0.6-0.8 second
Voltage	120
Filter	Edge enhancing
Additional data reconstruction	Thinnest overlapping sections available for workstation interpretation
Comments	Scan patient in both supine and prone positions

Suggested Readings

Brink JA, Heiken JP, Balfe DM et al: decreased spatial resolution in vivo due to broadening of section-sensitivity profile, *Radiology* 185:469-474, 1992.

Cody DD MD, Davros W, Silverman PM: Principles of multislice computed tomographic technology. In Silverman PM, editors: *Multislice computed tomography: principles, practice, and clinical protocols*, Philadelphia, 2002, Lippincott Williams & Wilkins.

Dalrymple NC, Prasad SR, Freckleton MW et al: Informatics in Radiology (InfoRAD): Introduction to the language of three-dimensional imaging with multidetector CT, *Radiographics* 25:1409-1428, 2005.

Dalrymple NC, Prasad SR, El-Merhi FM et al: Price of isotropy in multidetector CT, *RadioGraphics* 27:49-62, 2007.

Hsieh J: A general approach to the reconstruction of x-ray helical computed tomography, *Med Phys* 23:221-229, 1996.

Hu H: Multi-slice helical CT: scan and reconstruction, *Med Phys* 26:5-18, 1999.

Hu H, He HD, Foley WD, Fox SH: Four multidetector-row helical CT: image quality and volume coverage speed, *Radiology* 215:55-62, 2000.

Kalender WA, Polacin A: Physical performance characteristics of spiral CT scanning, *Med Phys* 18:910-915, 1991.

Kalender WA, Polacin A, Suss C: A comparison of conventional and spiral CT: an experimental study on the detection of spherical lesions. [erratum appears in J Comput Assist Tomogr 1994 Jul-Aug;18(4):671], *J Comput Assist Tomogr* 18:167-176, 1994.

Kalra MK, Maher MM, Toth TL et al: Strategies for CT radiation dose optimization, *Radiology* 230:619-628, 2004.

Mahesh M: The AAPM/RSNA physics tutorial for residents: search for isotropic resolution in CT from conventional through multiple-row detector, *Radiographics* 22:949-962, 2002.

McCollough CH, Zink FE: Performance evaluation of a multi-slice CT system, *Med Phys* 26:2223-2230, 1999.

Ney DR, Fishman EK, Magid D et al: Three-dimensional volumetric display of CT data: effect of scan parameters upon image quality, *J Comput Assist Tomogr* 15:875-885, 1991.

Polacin A, Kalender WA, Marchal G: Evaluation of section sensitivity profiles and image noise in spiral CT, *Radiology* 185:29-35, 1992.

Rankin SC: Spiral CT: vascular applications, *Eur J Radiol* 28:18-29, 1998.

Rubin GD, Napel S, Leung AN: Volumetric analysis of volumetric data: achieving a paradigm shift, *Radiology* 200:312-317, 1996.

Rubin GD: Multislice imaging for three-dimensional examinations. In Silverman PM, editor: *Multislice helical tomography: A practical approach to clinical protocols*, Philadelphia, 2002, Lippincott Williams & Wilkins.

Rubin GD: 3-D imaging with MDCT, *Eur J Radiol* 45(suppl 1):S37-S41, 2003.

Rydberg J, Liang Y, Teague SD: Fundamentals of multichannel CT, *Radiol Clin North Am* 41:465-474, 2003.

Saini S: Multi-detector row CT: principles and practice for abdominal applications, *Radiology* 233:323-327, 2004.

CHAPTER 3

Magnetic Resonance Imaging

John R. Leyendecker

The problem-solving role of MRI stems from its exceptional ability to differentiate between different types of tissue and to detect subtle degrees of enhancement after intravenous (IV) contrast administration. Thus, MRI provides a high level of specificity for many disease processes without compromising sensitivity for most abnormalities. The role of MRI as a problem-solving modality will likely continue to expand as new techniques and applications continue to be developed.

■ ESSENCE OF MAGNETIC RESONANCE IMAGING

In conventional MRI, we measure the response of hydrogen protons to radiofrequency (RF) pulses. Hydrogen protons placed in a static magnetic field (the magnetic resonance scanner magnet) precess at their Larmor frequency, which is determined by the strength of the magnetic field. Because hydrogen protons are spinning charged particles, each proton is itself like a small magnet. A large population of hydrogen protons (as in the body) will be associated with a net magnetization vector that is aligned along the static magnetic field. This is referred to as longitudinal magnetization. The trick to MRI is to convert this longitudinal magnetization into transverse magnetization (aligned perpendicular to the static magnetic field) through the use of an RF pulse. Transverse magnetization is essentially a rotating magnetic field that induces a current in the receiver coil. This current represents the signal from which images are eventually made.

Spatial localization is accomplished in MRI through the use of magnetic gradients. Specialized coils within the scanner are used to create magnetic fields that vary with distance and allow signal to be localized within the body through clever gradient manipulations and mathematics. Image contrast in MRI can be created through several mechanisms. The most commonly applied properties of tissue used to create image contrast are the T1 and T2 relaxation times. The T1 relaxation time is a measure of how quickly a tissue recovers its initial longitudinal magnetization after an RF pulse. T2 relaxation time is a measure of how quickly a tissue loses transverse magnetization created by an RF pulse (after correcting for magnetic field imperfections). Over the years, additional means of generating image contrast have been developed, including the use of IV contrast agents, making MRI a powerful tool for tissue characterization.

■ MAGNETIC RESONANCE IMAGING TOOLBOX

Although many imagers liken the MRI scanner to a black box, I like to think of the MRI scanner as a toolbox full of useful tools for localizing and characterizing lesions of the abdomen and pelvis. The most frequently used tools include T1- and T2-weighted imaging, fat suppression, chemical shift imaging, and contrast-enhanced (CE) imaging. Additional tools used considerably less often include spectroscopy and diffusion-weighted imaging (DWI). A discussion of these techniques follows.

T1-Weighted Imaging

T1-weighted images emphasize differences in the T1 relaxation times of different types of tissue. The repetition time (TR) is kept relatively short to maximize differences in T1 relaxation, and the echo time (TE) is kept relatively short to minimize differences in T2 relaxation. T1-weighted imaging plays an important role in the characterization of certain substances and tissue types in the abdomen and pelvis. In particular, only a few substances and tissues have sufficiently short T1 relaxation times to appear as bright on T1-weighted images. These include fat (Fig. 3-1), hemorrhage (Fig. 3-2), melanin (Fig. 3-3), and proteinaceous fluid. Some gallstones, some cirrhotic nodules, and RF ablation sites may also appear bright on T1-weighted images. Paramagnetic contrast agents, including the gadolinium chelates, shorten the T1 relaxation times of tissues. This causes enhancing organs, blood vessels, and abnormalities such as tumors or inflammatory processes to increase in signal intensity on T1-weighted scans. Solid organs generally appear as intermediate signal intensity on T1-weighted images, with the normal pancreas appearing slightly hyperintense and the normal spleen slightly hypointense compared with the normal liver.

Fat enveloping the left renal hilum is
bright on this T1-weighted image

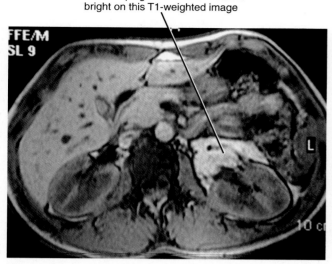

Figure 3-1 Axial T1-weighted, gradient-echo, magnetic resonance image through the liver and kidneys.

Hemorrhage is bright on
this T1-weighted image

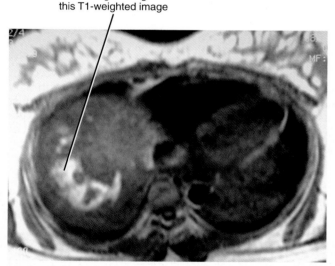

Figure 3-2 Axial T1-weighted, gradient-echo image through the dome of the liver in a patient with subcapsular hematoma.

Changes in these relative signal intensities may be a sign of abnormality. Because fat has a short T1 relaxation time relative to other tissues, organ outlines are clearly depicted on T1-weighted images performed without fat suppression.

T2-Weighted Imaging

T2-weighted images emphasize differences in the T2 relaxation times of different tissues. By combining a relatively long TR with a relatively long TE, differences in T1 relaxation times between tissues are minimized and differences in the T2 relaxation times are emphasized. T2-weighted imaging is important both for lesion

Melanoma metastasis is bright
on this T1-weighted image

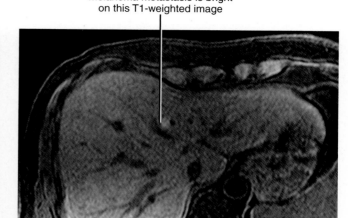

Figure 3-3 Axial fat-suppressed, T1-weighted, gradient-echo image through the liver in a patient with metastatic melanoma.

detection and characterization, as well as anatomic delineation in the abdomen and pelvis. Certain tissues or substances are highly conspicuous on T2-weighted images. These include simple fluid, myxoid stroma, and mucin (Fig. 3-4). Uncomplicated bile, urine, gastrointestinal fluid, and pancreatic fluid are also bright on T2-weighted images. Therefore, T2-weighted images are useful for imaging the biliary tree, pancreatic duct, and urinary tract. A variety of lesions are bright on T2-weighted images, including simple cysts (Fig. 3-5),

Mucinous material is bright on this T2-weighted
image, making it indistinguishable
from simple fluid

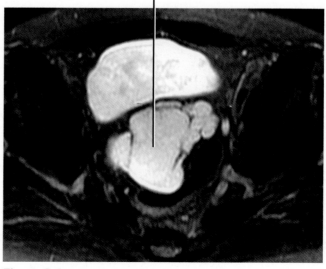

Figure 3-4 Axial fat-suppressed, T2-weighted, fast spin-echo image in a patient with peritoneal spread of mucinous adenocarcinoma of appendix.

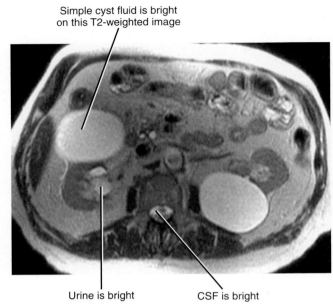

Simple cyst fluid is bright on this T2-weighted image

Urine is bright

CSF is bright

Figure 3-5 Axial T2-weighted, single-shot, fast spin-echo image through the kidneys in a patient with bilateral simple renal cysts. *CSF,* Cerebrospinal fluid.

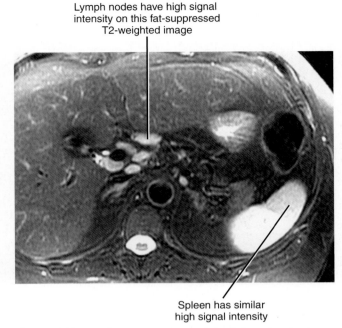

Lymph nodes have high signal intensity on this fat-suppressed T2-weighted image

Spleen has similar high signal intensity

Figure 3-7 Axial fat-suppressed, T2-weighted, fast spin-echo image through the porta hepatis in a patient with hepatitis C infection and hepatoduodenal ligament adenopathy.

hemangiomas (Fig. 3-6), cystic or necrotic neoplasms, mucinous and myxoid tumors, and peripheral nerve sheath tumors such as schwannomas and neurofibromas. Certain anatomic structures are inherently bright on T2-weighted images, such as the spleen, lymph nodes (Fig. 3-7), and testes. Zonal anatomy of the prostate and uterus can best be appreciated on T2-weighted images (Figs. 3-8 and 3-9).

Fat Suppression

Fat suppression is one of the most frequently utilized options in abdominal and pelvic MRI. Two primary reasons exist to use fat-suppression techniques. The first is to eliminate signal from background fat to improve the conspicuity of anatomic structures and enhancement with paramagnetic contrast agents. This is the reason

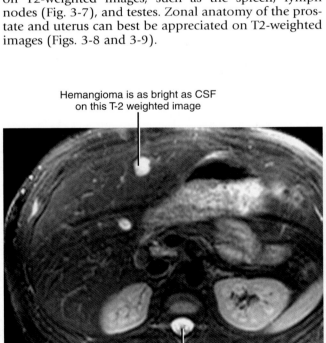

Hemangioma is as bright as CSF on this T-2 weighted image

CSF

Figure 3-6 Axial fat-suppressed, T2-weighted, fast spin-echo image through the liver and kidneys in a patient with small hepatic hemangioma. *CSF,* Cerebrospinal fluid.

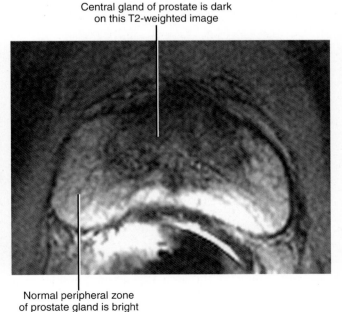

Central gland of prostate is dark on this T2-weighted image

Normal peripheral zone of prostate gland is bright

Figure 3-8 Axial T2-weighted, magnetic resonance image performed with endorectal coil in a patient with normal prostate gland.

most gadolinium-enhanced, T1-weighted sequences include fat suppression. The other primary reason for using fat suppression is to characterize an anatomic structure or abnormality, such as a tumor, by demonstrating or excluding the presence of fat (Fig. 3-10). Therefore, fat suppression is an important technique for helping to confirm such diagnoses as lipoma, myelolipoma, angiomyolipoma, and cystic teratoma. Several methods of fat suppression currently are in common use, and most of these methods take advantage of the different resonant frequencies or T1 relaxation times of fat and water protons. The advantages and disadvantages of the various fat-suppression techniques are listed in Table 3-1. Frequency-selective fat saturation is the most prevalent form of fat suppression used for the abdomen and pelvis. This technique uses a frequency-selective RF excitation pulse (at the precessional frequency of fat) and a spoiler gradient (eliminates phase coherence of fat protons) to null signal from fat. The technique of short tau inversion recovery (STIR) is an inversion recovery technique that relies on the difference in T1 relaxation times between fat and other tissues. STIR is preferred when the imaging volume is far from isocenter or when orthopedic hardware is present. Therefore, STIR has its greatest utility for musculoskeletal imaging. STIR should not be used for T1-weighted imaging after administration of paramagnetic contrast agents. This is because the T1 relaxation time of enhancing tissues may be sufficiently close to that of fat, resulting in suppression of signal from enhancing tissues. Spectral presaturation inversion recovery (SPIR) is a specialized form of fat

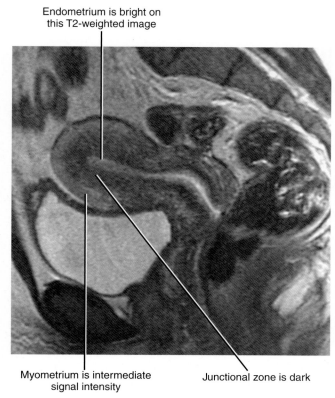

Endometrium is bright on this T2-weighted image

Myometrium is intermediate signal intensity

Junctional zone is dark

Figure 3-9 Sagittal T2-weighted, fast spin-echo image through the uterus demonstrates normal zonal anatomy.

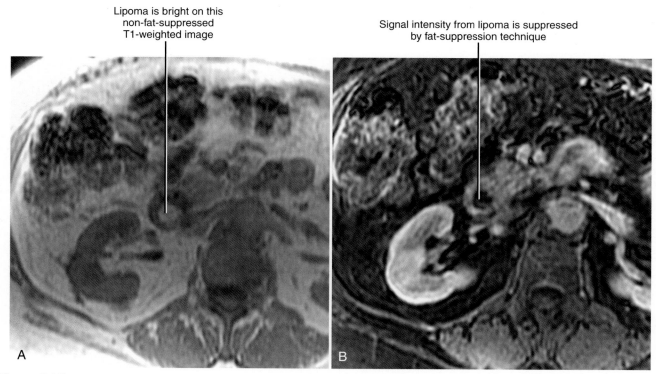

Lipoma is bright on this non-fat-suppressed T1-weighted image

Signal intensity from lipoma is suppressed by fat-suppression technique

A

B

Figure 3-10 **A,** Axial T1-weighted, gradient-echo image in a patient with duodenal lipoma. **B,** Axial fat-suppressed, T1-weighted, gradient-echo image in same patient as in **A** shows suppression of signal in lipoma with use of fat suppression.

Table 3-1 Methods of Fat Suppression

Method	Advantages	Disadvantages
Chemically selective fat saturation	Widely available	Requires homogeneous field May increase scan time
Short tau inversion recovery	Effective even with heterogeneous field	May increase scan time May suppress blood products and gadolinium
Spectral presaturation inversion recovery	Works well with gadolinium	May increase scan time Requires homogeneous field
Water excitation	Minimal effect on scan time	Not as widely available
Dixon method	Generates in- and opposed-phase and water-only and fat-only images	Only recently available

suppression that combines elements of standard fat saturation and STIR, and has clinical utility similar to fat saturation. One advantage of SPIR over STIR is that the former technique can be used successfully for T1-weighted imaging after gadolinium chelate administration. Dixon techniques are now available that provide in-phase, opposed-phase, fat-only, and water-only images from a single acquisition. Water excitation techniques are not available on all scanners but will likely increase in popularity given their effectiveness.

Chemical Shift Imaging

Chemical shift imaging is a powerful tool for the detection of intracellular lipid (also called *microscopic lipid* or *intracytoplasmic lipid*) and lesion characterization in the abdomen and pelvis. Fat and water can be conceptualized as containing two distinct populations of protons, each with its own net magnetization vector. These vectors rotate in the transverse plane at slightly different frequencies, causing the magnetization vectors of fat and water protons to periodically become out of phase. If a tissue voxel containing similar amounts of fat and water protons is imaged at a time when the fat and water transverse magnetization vectors are approximately 180 degrees out of phase, the vectors cancel out, resulting in a reduced signal. By comparing such out-of-phase images with images obtained when fat and water protons are precessing in phase, the presence of intracellular lipid can be confirmed. However, the signal intensity of voxels containing mostly fat or mostly water will not be significantly altered by chemical shift imaging. Chemical shift imaging is effective at detecting fatty infiltration of solid organs such as the liver (Fig. 3-11) and pancreas, or for detecting intracellular lipid in tumors such as adrenal adenoma, hepatic adenoma, hepatocellular carcinoma, and renal cell carcinoma (Fig. 3-12). Tiny amounts of macroscopic fat in tumors such as angiomyolipoma (Fig. 3-13) or cystic teratoma can be detected using this technique. In such cases, tiny foci of fat will appear as small rings of low signal intensity representing the border voxels between fat and water-containing tissues.

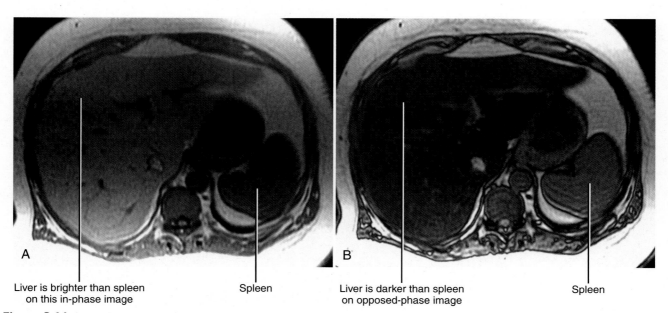

A, Liver is brighter than spleen on this in-phase image — Spleen

B, Liver is darker than spleen on opposed-phase image — Spleen

Figure 3-11 **A,** Axial T1-weighted, in-phase, gradient-echo image of a patient with hepatic steatosis. **B,** Opposed-phase, gradient-echo of the same patient with hepatic steatosis, demonstrating signal loss in the liver.

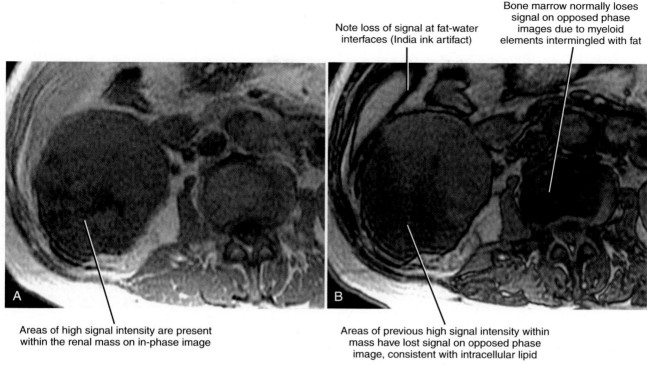

Note loss of signal at fat-water interfaces (India ink artifact)

Bone marrow normally loses signal on opposed phase images due to myeloid elements intermingled with fat

Areas of high signal intensity are present within the renal mass on in-phase image

Areas of previous high signal intensity within mass have lost signal on opposed phase image, consistent with intracellular lipid

Figure 3-12 **A,** Axial T1-weighted, in-phase, gradient-echo image of a patient with clear cell carcinoma of the right kidney. **B,** Opposed-phase, gradient-echo image of the same patient with clear cell carcinoma of the kidney shows area of signal loss caused by intracytoplasmic lipid.

Spectroscopy

Until recently, proton magnetic resonance spectroscopy (MRS) has been limited to structures that are not prone to gross physiologic motion such as the brain, breast, and prostate gland. MRS may be used to localize

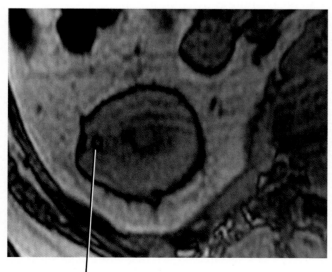

Ring of low signal intensity within right kidney suggests presence of small focus of macroscopic fat

Figure 3-13 Axial T1-weighted, opposed-phase, gradient-echo image in a patient with small angiomyolipoma.

adenocarcinoma of the prostate by demonstrating alterations in the normal ratio of choline (a substance found to be increased in many tumors) to citrate (a substance found in healthy prostate tissue). That is, prostate cancer will demonstrate a reduction in citrate and a relative increase of choline compared with normal healthy prostate tissue. This alteration in relative metabolite abundance can be detected with spectroscopy (Fig. 3-14). Because the metabolic peak of creatine overlaps with that of choline, a ratio of choline and creatine to citrate is usually obtained when performing spectroscopy at 1.5 Tesla. Provided one has access to necessary software, one can perform spectroscopy for multiple voxels distributed over the prostate gland like a grid. These data can then be displayed in a number of formats including individual spectral traces or a color-coded map. Because of the software expense, limited collective clinical experience, and relatively low spatial resolution of prostate spectroscopy at 1.5 Tesla, this technique is not currently widely performed.

Over time, interest in spectroscopy of other abdominal and pelvic organs has increased. Areas that have been interrogated with MRS include the liver, pancreas, kidneys, and uterus and ovaries. It is hoped that such investigations will eventually lead to improved methods of diagnosing or quantifying hepatic steatosis and fibrosis, distinguishing inflammation from tumor, and characterizing focal abnormalities of the abdomen and pelvis. The improved signal-to-noise ratio (SNR) and spectral resolution inherent in 3-Tesla scanners may enhance the abdominal and pelvic applications of

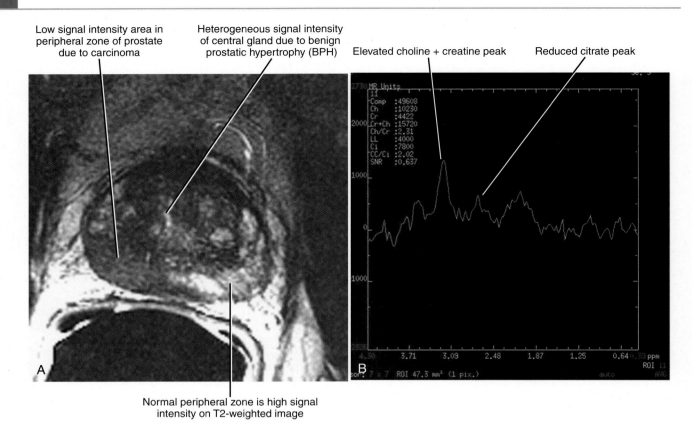

Low signal intensity area in peripheral zone of prostate due to carcinoma

Heterogeneous signal intensity of central gland due to benign prostatic hypertrophy (BPH)

Elevated choline + creatine peak

Reduced citrate peak

Normal peripheral zone is high signal intensity on T2-weighted image

Figure 3-14 A, Axial T2-weighted magnetic resonance (MR) image of prostate performed with endorectal coil in a patient with prostate carcinoma. **B,** MR spectrum from region of carcinoma in the same patient.

spectroscopy, although this potential advantage of higher field strength will apply only if 3-Tesla software and coil technology manage to keep pace with that available for 1.5-Tesla scanners. Currently, much work is yet to be done to validate and disseminate MRS applications for the abdomen and pelvis.

Diffusion-Weighted Imaging

In the setting of MRI, diffusion refers to the microscopic motion of water molecules/protons. Focal changes in water proton diffusion, or diffusivity, within an organ may signal an alteration in tissue cellularity, permeability, or organization indicative of disease. This altered diffusivity can be detected with DWI. It is beyond the scope of this text to give a detailed description of the various pulse sequences designed to measure diffusion. However, the basic principle that allows diffusion of water protons to be measured is easily understood. Spins moving in the presence of a magnetic field gradient will accumulate phase based on the direction and rate of their motion. A group of water protons moving randomly in the presence of a magnetic field gradient will experience random phase shifts that ultimately result in signal attenuation. As diffusion of water molecules increases within a tissue, the signal produced by the tissue becomes further attenuated. Pulse sequences can be designed that

measure and display diffusion effects through the brief application of strong magnetic field gradients. Areas within organs or tissues that have restricted diffusion will be relatively less affected by the application of these gradients and produce relatively more signal than areas of unrestricted diffusion.

The "b value" is a user-defined parameter that determines the strength of the diffusion gradients. For abdominal and pelvic MRI, most investigators have used b values in the range of 50 to 1,000. At lower b values, sensitivity increases. At greater b values, only lesions with severely restricted diffusion will remain bright, potentially offering some improvement in specificity. A typical DWI study will include measurements at several b values.

DWI has proved most useful for the early detection of ischemic infarction in the brain. Several applications of DWI in the abdomen and pelvis have also been investigated, with the ultimate goal of determining the apparent diffusion coefficient values for normal and diseased organs, as well as for a variety of focal lesions. It is hoped that such work will lead to new tools for distinguishing normal from diseased organs (e.g., detection and staging of cirrhosis) and benign from malignant lesions. Early results suggest that DWI may improve sensitivity for detection of malignant lesions in the liver and elsewhere, although specificity remains a problem. It is possible that DWI will become a standard part of abdominal imaging protocols in the near future (Fig. 3-15).

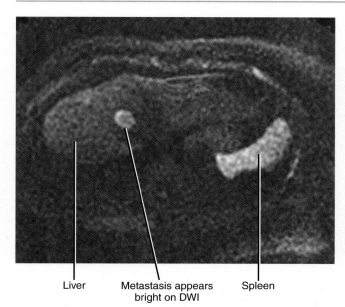

Liver   Metastasis appears   Spleen
         bright on DWI

Figure 3-15 Axial diffusion-weighted image (b value = 500) through the liver dome in a patient with metastatic breast carcinoma. The entire liver was imaged in two 14-second breath holds. *DWI,* Diffusion-weighted imaging.

■ CONTRAST AGENTS

A variety of IV and enteric MR contrast agents are commercially available. These contrast agents can be divided into positive and negative contrast agents. Positive agents are those that increase the signal intensity of a target organ or lumen. Negative contrast agents decrease the signal intensity of the same. Whether an agent has a positive or negative effect on the target organ or lumen may depend on the pulse sequence used. For example, water is a positive enteric contrast agent on a T2-weighted scan and a negative contrast agent on a T1-weighted scan. A positive IV contrast agent such as gadolinium chelate is often combined with a negative enteric agent to improve the conspicuity of enhancement.

Intravenous Agents

Currently, gadolinium chelates constitute the main group of IV paramagnetic contrast agents in widespread use for abdominal and pelvic MRI. Gadolinium chelates shorten the T1 relaxation time of tissues, rendering enhancing tissues bright on T1-weighted images. As extracellular agents, the gadolinium chelates have a similar biodistribution in the body to iodinated CT contrast agents. Like CT contrast agents, gadolinium chelates are suitable for bolus injection. They are predominately eliminated via renal excretion, although some newer agents also have a component of biliary elimination. Although free gadolinium is toxic, the commercially available chelated forms have favorable safety profiles at approved doses in patients with normal renal function. Relatively recently, the use of gadolinium chelates in patients on dialysis or with severely

compromised renal function has been linked to a potentially severe and debilitating condition known as nephrogenic systemic fibrosis. Knowledge and recommendations regarding the use of gadolinium-based contrast media in the setting of renal insufficiency were rapidly evolving at the time of this writing. Therefore, readers are encouraged to familiarize themselves with the latest information and guidelines regarding the use of gadolinium-based contrast media in patients with renal insufficiency.

IV gadolinium chelates have a variety of uses in the abdomen and pelvis. First-pass vascular imaging allows creation of exquisite MR angiograms. Rapid multiphase (dynamic) imaging of abdominal organs allows assessment of tissue perfusion and differentiation of lesions based on enhancement characteristics (Fig. 3-16). Delayed images may be helpful in further characterizing focal abnormalities, and images obtained during the renal excretory stage may be used to evaluate the urinary tract. Box 3-1 provides a list of potential indications for use of IV gadolinium chelates for abdominal and pelvic MRI.

Some newer gadolinium-based contrast agents can be classified as hepatobiliary agents in that some percentage of the agent is taken up by hepatocytes and excreted in the bile. At least two such agents, gadobenate dimeglumine (Gd-BOPTA) and gadoxetate disodium (Gd-EOB-DTPA), are approved for clinical use in the United States and elsewhere at the time of this writing, although only Gd-EOB-DTPA is approved in the U.S. for liver imaging at the time of this writing. One advantage of these agents is that they can be administered as an IV bolus at rates necessary to image discrete vascular phases. This was not possible with mangafodipir, an alternative manganese-based hepatobiliary agent. Only about 3% to 5% of Gd-BOPTA is taken up by hepatocytes and eliminated in bile, while up to half of the administered dose of Gd-EOB-DTPA is eliminated in the bile of patients with normal renal function. Both Gd-BOPTA and Gd-EOB-DTPA demonstrate higher relaxivity than other agents in human plasma. Because of this high relaxivity, the approved dose of Gd-EOB-DTPA is 0.025 mmol/kg body weight rather than the 0.1 mmol/kg body weight dose approved for other gadolinium-based contrast agents. Hepatobiliary contrast agents may be beneficial in distinguishing between focal nodular hyperplasia (FNH), a relatively common benign hepatic lesion, and nonhepatocellular lesions such as metastases. Because FNH contains functioning hepatocytes, it typically retains Gd-BOPTA and Gd-EOB-DTPA to a similar or greater degree than normal liver during the hepatobiliary phase of imaging (at approximately 20 minutes for Gd-EOB-DTPA and approximately 1 to 3 hours for Gd-BOPTA (Fig. 3-17). Lesions that do not contain functioning hepatocytes, such as metastases, typically become hypointense to normal liver parenchyma during the hepatobiliary phase.

One final IV contrast agent deserves mention for its role in problem solving. Superparamagnetic iron oxide particles, or ferumoxides, are taken up by the reticuloendothelial system and act as a negative contrast agent. One commercially available preparation of this contrast agent is used to decrease the signal intensity of

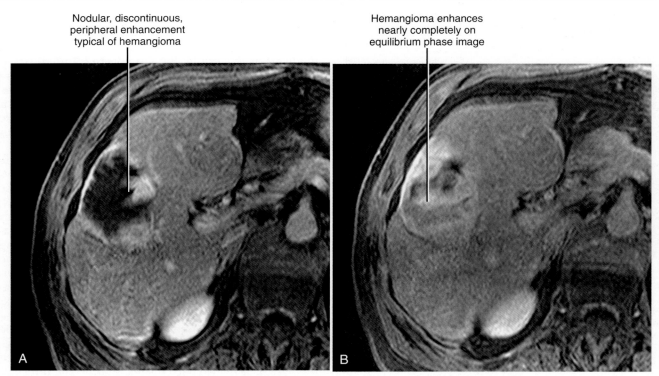

Figure 3-16 A, Portal-phase, axial, fat-suppressed, T1-weighted, gradient-echo image performed after intravenous gadolinium chelate administration through the liver in a patient with hepatic hemangioma demonstrates typical enhancement pattern. **B,** Equilibrium-phase image in the same patient as in **A** shows typical progressive enhancement.

the liver on T2- or T2*-weighted images, potentially making hepatic lesions more conspicuous with these sequences (Fig. 3-18). This may be advantageous when screening for hepatocellular carcinoma or planning liver resection in the setting of hepatic metastases. Liver lesions containing sufficient numbers of functioning Kupffer cells will also take up ferumoxides, making ferumoxides potentially useful for the characterization of lesions such as FNH. The commercially available form of ferumoxides is typically administered as a slow IV infusion (over approximately 30 minutes) through a filter rather than as a rapid bolus. This potentially creates logistical problems that, combined with early reports of unique adverse reactions, have limited widespread clinical use of this agent. In our experience, however, adverse reactions are uncommon when this agent is administered according to manufacturer guidelines.

Oral Contrast Agents

A variety of oral MR contrast agents have been proposed and evaluated, although most are seldom used clinically. Water remains the least expensive and easiest to administer oral contrast agent, although bowel absorption limits the utility of water to the stomach and proximal small bowel. A commercially available superparamagnetic iron oxide preparation (ferumoxsil) may be helpful to diminish the signal intensity of the luminal contents of the entire bowel. This agent acts as a negative contrast agent on both T1- and T2-weighted images. Dilute barium is another readily available and effective negative (on T1-weighted images) oral contrast agent.

In general, positive oral contrast agents are effective at demonstrating intraluminal abnormalities of the gastrointestinal tract. Positive oral contrast agents may degrade overall image quality when significant bowel peristalsis is present unless rapid imaging sequences are used. Negative oral contrast agents may help eliminate some motion artifact caused by bowel peristalsis and are useful in eliminating bright intraluminal signal that may interfere with magnetic resonance angiography (MRA) or magnetic resonance urography (MRU) reconstructions. Negative agents also may be helpful when assessing enhancement of the bowel wall after IV gadolinium chelate administration in patients with inflammatory bowel disease.

BOX 3-1   Potential Indications for the Use of Intravenous Magnetic Resonance Contrast Agents in the Abdomen and Pelvis

Characterization of abnormalities detected with other sequences or imaging modalities
Detection of primary neoplasms and metastatic disease
Staging of malignant neoplasms
Evaluation of inflammatory diseases
Assessment of organ or tumor perfusion and viability
Depiction and assessment of arteries and veins
Depiction and assessment of the urinary tract

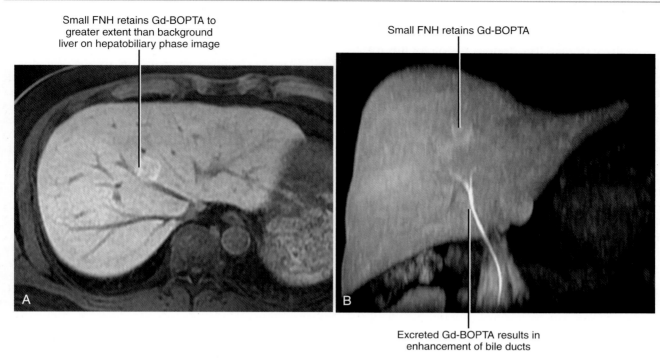

Small FNH retains Gd-BOPTA to greater extent than background liver on hepatobiliary phase image

Small FNH retains Gd-BOPTA

Excreted Gd-BOPTA results in enhancement of bile ducts

Figure 3-17 **A,** Axial fat-suppressed, T1-weighted, gradient-echo image performed several hours (hepatobiliary phase) after intravenous administration of gadobenate dimeglumine (Gd-BOPTA) in a patient with small focal nodular hyperplasia (FNH). **B,** Coronal maximum intensity projection image of liver during hepatobiliary phase in the same patient.

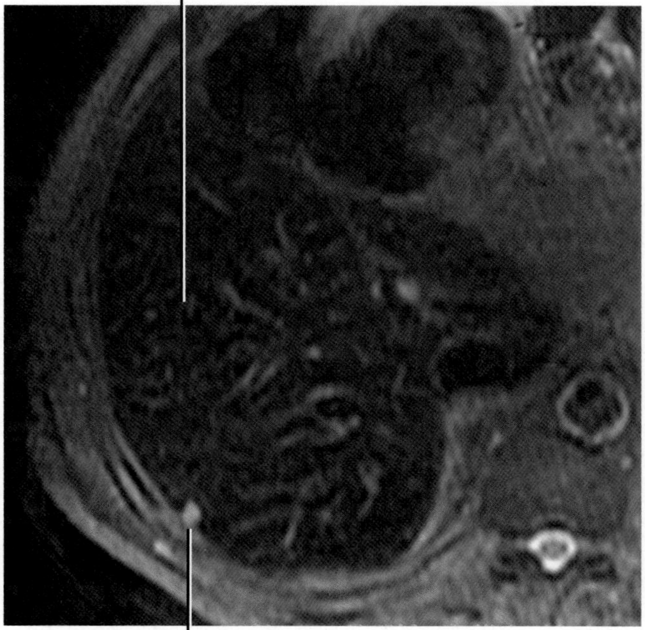

Low signal intensity liver after ferumoxides administration

Small lesion is very conspicuous against background of dark liver

Figure 3-18 Axial T2-weighted image through liver performed after intravenous administration of ferumoxides.

■ PROTOCOLS

Basic Components

The majority of abdominal and nonmusculoskeletal pelvic MRI examinations in the United States are performed to further evaluate abnormalities detected with an initial imaging modality such as CT or sonography. Protocols must be optimized not only to detect lesions, but they also must provide specificity superior to that of the initial imaging modality. Effective MRI protocols include a variety of pulse sequences, each with a different image contrast mechanism to aid in distinguishing different tissue types. At least one CE sequence is often included to augment information obtained from standard noncontrast sequences.

At a minimum, most abdominal and pelvic MRI protocols include a scout- or survey-type sequence, a T1-weighted sequence, a T2-weighted sequence, and an IV CE sequence. The initial survey sequence primarily serves to provide the technologist with anatomic information in multiple planes on which to plan subsequent imaging sequences. Because this localizing scan often consists of a free breathing sequence that produces images of marginal diagnostic utility, many protocols include an additional breath-held localizer utilizing either a single-shot FSE/turbo spin echo (TSE) or a steady state free precession-type sequence performed in the coronal plane. These latter sequences provide superior image quality to most standard gradient-echo scout sequences and provide a diagnostically useful anatomic overview of the abdomen and pelvis. Notably, many scanner manufacturers now offer a single-shot FSE/TSE or a steady state free precession-type sequence as a multiplanar localizer.

For T1-weighted imaging, many MR imagers prefer gradient-echo rather than spin-echo sequences, particularly in the abdomen. The primary reason for this preference is the ability to image large anatomic regions such as the liver during a single breath hold using gradient-echo sequences. In addition, gradient-echo imaging allows for the acquisition of in-phase and opposed-phase images that are important for detection of intracellular lipid. When possible, it is more time efficient to perform in-phase and opposed-phase imaging as a single dual-echo sequence. This option allows both in-phase and opposed-phase images to be created from a single acquisition. Not only does this eliminate the time necessary to repeat the sequence, it allows signal intensity measurements to be directly compared between the in-phase and opposed-phase images without having to correct for differences in transmitter and receiver gain.

T2-weighted imaging may be performed using one of a variety of pulse sequences. These include conventional spin echo, FSE/TSE, or GRASE. Conventional spin-echo sequences have largely been abandoned by most practices because of long scan times. GRASE is a gradient-echo/spin-echo hybrid that is relatively time efficient and capable of providing similar image contrast to FSE/TSE. FSE/TSE sequences can be performed during free breathing (in which case multiple signal averages are used to eliminate respiratory motion artifact), with respiratory triggering, or during breath holding. Each of these methods has advantages and drawbacks, and ultimately one must choose some compromise between the SNR, scan time, and scan resolution. T2-weighted

imaging is often performed with fat suppression to improve lesion conspicuity and improve detection of edema and fluid (Fig. 3-19).

Clinical experience supports the use of IV gadolinium chelates for many abdominal and pelvic MR protocols. Gadolinium chelates improve lesion detection in solid organs such as the liver and are critical to characterizing many abnormalities detected with other sequences. Because MRI exposes the patient to no ionizing radiation, no additional risk is associated with multiphase imaging. Therefore precontrast, arterial, portal venous, and equilibrium phase images are often routinely obtained, particularly when imaging the liver, kidneys, and pancreas. Timing of the acquisition after contrast administration is variable depending on the rate of contrast injection, circulation time, sequence acquisition time, and k-space trajectory (e.g., sequential, centric, elliptical centric, etc.). When in doubt as to when to begin acquiring data after contrast injection, a timing bolus may be beneficial. Alternatively, some form of automated bolus detection software or real-time monitoring may be used. Imaging after gadolinium chelate administration typically is accomplished with a T1-weighted gradient-echo sequence optimized so that the entire organ of interest can be imaged during a single breath hold. Fat suppression is beneficial when imaging after administration of IV gadolinium chelates, making enhancing structures and abnormalities more conspicuous.

For most abdominal and pelvic imaging, a phased array surface coil is recommended because of a significant

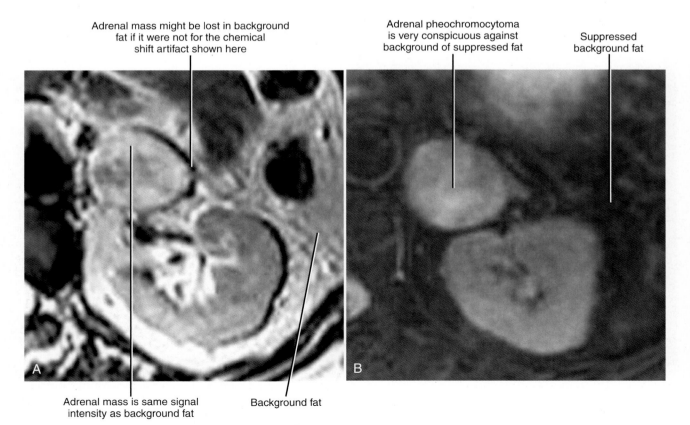

Figure 3-19 A, Axial T2-weighted image performed without fat suppression through left adrenal gland in a patient with pheochromocytoma. B, Axial T2-weighted image performed with fat suppression through the left adrenal gland in a different patient with pheochromocytoma.

improvement in SNR compared with the main body coil (built into the scanner). Use of an appropriate phased array surface coil also allows the use of parallel imaging techniques, which dramatically reduce scan times at the expense of a modest reduction in SNR.

Specific Protocols

This section provides some protocols capable of addressing the most commonly encountered indications for abdominal and pelvic MRI (Tables 3-2 through 3-9). These are based on a 1.5-Tesla scanner, and minor modifications may be necessary to accommodate other field strengths. There are seemingly endless combinations of sequence and protocol modifications possible with MRI, and a complete discussion of every permutation is well beyond the scope of this textbook. The interested imager is encouraged to experiment with variations on standard protocols to the extent practical, keeping in mind that each protocol or sequence alteration may result in a compromise of study time, SNR, or other indicator of image quality. Ultimately, one must always keep in mind the goal of producing diagnostic images in a reasonable period with the least amount of patient discomfort and risk.

Protocol Abbreviations
b-FFE – balanced fast field echo
FAME – fast acquisition with multiphase Efgre3D
FIESTA – fast imaging employing steady state acquisition
FSE – fast spin echo
HASTE – half-Fournier single-shot turbo spin echo
LAVA – liver acquisition volume acceleration
THRIVE – T1W high-resolution isotropic volume examination
TrueFISP – fast imaging with steady state precession

Sequences
1. Half-Fourier single-shot echo train spin echo (e.g., ssFSE, ssTSE, HASTE)
2. Echo train spin echo (e.g., FSE, TSE)
3. Conventional spin echo (e.g., SE)
4. Gradient-echo/spin-echo hybrid (GRASE)
5. Two-dimensional gradient echo (spoiled gradient-echo recalled acquisition [SPGR], fast low-angle shot [FLASH], FFE)
6. Three-dimensional interpolated gradient echo (FAME, LAVA, VIBE, THRIVE)
7. Two-dimensional steady state free precession (FIESTA, trueFISP, b-FFE)
8. Thick-slab, breath-hold, heavily T2-weighted (T2W), echo train spin echo (FSE, TSE)
9. Three-dimensional, respiratory-triggered, heavily T2W, echo train spin echo (FSE, TSE)

■ SPECIALIZED TECHNIQUES

Several specific MRI techniques are worthy of additional comment. These include MRA, magnetic resonance cholangiopancreatography (MRCP), and MRU.

Table 3-2   Liver Magnetic Resonance Protocol

Scan Description	Sequences	Comments
Three-plane localizer	1, 5, or 7	
COR BH survey	1 or 7	
AX BH I/O phase T1W	5	Dual echo if possible
AX FS T2W	2, 3, or 4	RT or BH
AX BH multiphase CE T1W	5 or 6	Includes precontrast, FS if possible
AX BH delayed CE T1W	5 or 6	Optional, FS if possible
MRCP	8 or 9	Optional

AX, Axial; *BH*, breath hold; *CE*, contrast enhanced; *COR*, coronal; *FS*, fat suppressed; *I/O*, in and opposed; *MRCP*, magnetic resonance cholangiopancreatography; *RT*, respiratory triggered; *T1W*, T1 weighted; *T2W*, T2 weighted.

Table 3-3   Pancreas Magnetic Resonance Protocol

Scan Description	Sequences	Comments
Three-plane localizer	1, 5, or 7	
COR BH survey	1 or 7	
AX BH I/O phase T1W	5	Dual echo if possible
AX FS T2W	2, 3, or 4	RT or BH
AX FS T1W	2, 3, 5, or 6	Optional
AX BH multiphase CE T1W	5 or 6	Includes precontrast, FS if possible
COR or OBL MRCP	8 or 9	Optional

AX, Axial; *BH*, breath hold; *CE*, contrast enhanced; *COR*, coronal; *FS*, fat suppressed; *I/O*, in and opposed; *MRCP*, magnetic resonance cholangiopancreatography; *OBL*, oblique; *RT*, respiratory triggered; *T1W*, T1 weighted; *T2W*, T2 weighted.

Table 3-4   Kidney Magnetic Resonance Protocol

Scan Description	Sequences	Comments
Three-plane localizer	1, 5, or 7	
COR BH survey	1 or 7	
AX BH I/O phase T1W	5	Dual echo if possible
AX FS T2W	2, 3, or 4	RT or BH
COR BH static MRU	8	Optional, precontrast
AX BH multiphase CE T1W	5 or 6	Includes precontrast, FS if possible
AX BH T2W	1	Optional
COR BH delayed CE T1W	5 or 6	Optional, FS if possible

Static magnetic resonance urography *(MRU)* is essentially the same as magnetic resonance cholangiopancreatography but centered over the kidneys, ureters, and bladder. The delayed coronal contrast-enhanced *(CE)* T1-weighted *(T1W)* scan can serve as a CE MRU by hydrating the patient and administering a low dose of furosemide if necessary.
AX, Axial; *BH*, breath hold; *COR*, coronal; *FS*, fat suppressed; *I/O*, in and opposed; *RT*, respiratory triggered; *T2W*, T2 weighted.

Table 3-5   Adrenal Magnetic Resonance Protocol

Scan Description	Sequences	Comments
Three-plane localizer	1, 5, or 7	
COR BH survey	1 or 7	
AX BH I/O phase T1W	5	Dual echo if possible
COR BH I/O phase T1W	5	Optional
AX FS T2W	2, 3, or 4	RT or BH
AX BH multiphase CE T1W	5 or 6	Optional Includes precontrast FS if possible

AX, Axial; BH, breath hold; CE, contrast enhanced; COR, coronal; FS, fat suppressed; I/O, in and opposed; RT, respiratory triggered; T1W, T1 weighted; T2W, T2 weighted.

Table 3-6   Female Pelvis Magnetic Resonance Protocol: Uterus

Scan Description	Sequences	Comments
Three-plane localizer	1, 5, or 7	
COR survey	1	Optional
AX T1W	2, 3, or 5	
AX FS T1W	2, 3, 5, or 6	
AX T2W	1, 2, 3, or 4	FS optional
SAG OBL T2W	1, 2, 3, or 4	SAG relative to uterus
COR OBL T2W	1, 2, 3, or 4	COR relative to uterus
Multiphase CE T1W	5 or 6	Optional, SAG or AX relative to uterus Includes precontrast FS if possible
AX delayed CE T1W	2, 3, 5 or 6	Optional, FS if possible

Sagittal (SAG) and coronal (COR) scans are planned along the long axis of the uterus rather than relative to the pelvis. This provides a more accurate assessment of uterine morphology and endometrial abnormalities. Contrast-enhanced (CE) imaging is usually not necessary for evaluation of Müllerian anomalies. The plane for multiphase CE images should be one that best demonstrates the endometrial abnormality in question and the underlying myometrium. If study is done for uterine fibroids before embolization, multiphase imaging performed in the coronal plane may be used to provide vascular anatomic information.
AX, Axial; FS, fat suppressed; OBL, oblique; T1W, T1 weighted; T2W, T2 weighted.

Magnetic Resonance Angiography

A variety of MRA techniques have been proved effective for the evaluation of the arteries and veins of the abdomen and pelvis. These techniques may be divided into dark blood techniques and bright blood techniques. Dark blood techniques rely on the use of saturation bands or inversion prepulses to null the signal of flowing blood. Dark blood MRA is particularly useful for the evaluation of tumor thrombus in large vessels such as the renal vein and inferior vena cava (IVC) (Fig. 3-20). Bright blood techniques may be further divided into non-CE and CE methods. Noncontrast bright blood

Table 3-7   Female Pelvis Magnetic Resonance Protocol: Adnexa

Scan Description	Sequences	Comments
Three-plane localizer	1, 5, or 7	
COR survey	1	Optional
AX T1W	2, 3, or 5	Consider in/opposed phase
AX FS T1W	2, 3, 5, or 6	
AX T2W	2, 3, or 4	FS optional
SAG OBL T2W	1, 2, 3, or 4	Optional SAG relative to uterus
AX multiphase CE T1W	5 or 6	Includes precontrast, FS if possible
AX delayed CE T1W	2, 3, 5, or 6	Optional, FS if possible

Gradient-echo T1-weighted (T1W) imaging may be performed using in- and opposed-phase echo times to demonstrate small amounts of intralesional fat. Sagittal (SAG) T2-weighted (T2W) images are obtained relative to the uterine axes to allow assessment of the endometrium and junctional zone.
AX, Axial; CE, contrast enhanced; COR, coronal; FS, fat suppressed; OBL, oblique.

Table 3-8   Male Pelvis Magnetic Resonance Protocol: Generic

Scan Description	Sequences	Comments
Three-plane localizer	1, 5, or 7	
COR survey	1	Optional
AX T1W	2, 3, or 5	
AX FS T1W	2, 3, 5, or 6	Optional
AX T2W	2, 3, or 4	FS optional
AX multiphase CE T1W	5 or 6	Includes precontrast, FS if possible
AX delayed CE T1W	2, 3, 5, or 6	Optional, FS if possible

AX, Axial; CE, contrast enhanced; COR, coronal; FS, fat suppressed; T1W, T1 weighted; T2W, T2 weighted.

Table 3-9   Male Pelvis Magnetic Resonance Protocol: Prostate

Scan Description	Sequences	Comments
Three-plane localizer	1, 5, or 7	
SAG localizer	1	
AX T1W	2, 3, or 5	Small FOV
AX T2W	2 or 3	Small FOV
SAG T2W	2 or 3	Optional
COR T2W	2 or 3	Optional
AX BH multiphase CE T1W	5 or 6	Optional Includes precontrast, FS if possible Small FOV

Endorectal coil provides significant improvement in signal-to-noise ratio.
Multiple signal averages may be necessary given small field of view (FOV). Typical FOVs range from 12 to 16 cm for endorectal prostate magnetic resonance imaging.
AX, Axial; BH, breath hold; CE, contrast enhanced; COR, coronal; FS, fat suppressed; SAG, sagittal; T1W, T1 weighted; T2W, T2 weighted.

Sharp interface between tumor and blood

Dark blood in patent portion of IVC

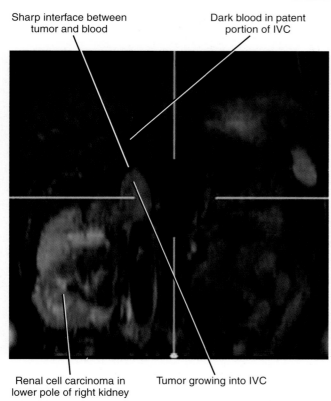

Renal cell carcinoma in lower pole of right kidney

Tumor growing into IVC

Figure 3-20 Coronal reformation of T2-weighted dark blood images in a patient with renal cell carcinoma of the right kidney invading the inferior vena cava (IVC).

Background tissues are suppressed by repeated RF pulses (RF saturation)

IVC

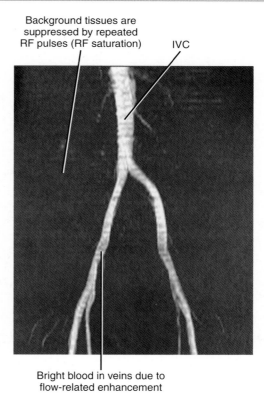

Bright blood in veins due to flow-related enhancement

Figure 3-21 Coronal maximum intensity projection image of a normal time-of-flight venogram of the lower inferior vena cava (IVC) and pelvic veins. Images originally acquired axially. *RF,* Radiofrequency.

sequences include time-of-flight (TOF), phase contrast, and steady state free precession. Although these techniques have largely been replaced by CE MRA for routine applications, they remain useful for limited applications. TOF MRA provides a relatively simple method of performing venography that is useful in patients with limited IV access (Fig. 3-21). The data obtained with phase-contrast MRA is inherently quantitative and may be used to determine flow direction and velocity. Steady state free precession techniques are extremely fast and motion resistant, providing a robust method of quickly assessing vascular anatomy (Fig. 3-22).

CE MRA techniques have rapidly emerged as the dominant method of imaging the abdominal and pelvic vasculature with MRI. Also referred to as three-dimensional (3D) gadolinium-enhanced MRA, the typical CE MRA uses a 3D gradient-echo sequence applied after the IV injection of a gadolinium chelate. Gadolinium contrast agents shorten the T1 relaxation time of blood, resulting in bright blood on the images (Fig. 3-23). CE MRA has proved useful for the evaluation of vascular stenoses, thromboses, dissections, aneurysms, and malformations, as well as the delineation of complex vascular anatomy. The typical CE MRA sequence closely resembles newer fat-suppressed volumetric MRI techniques (VIBE, FAME, LAVA, THRIVE) used to image the solid organs. Provided adequate through-plane resolution is obtained, these latter methods of imaging the abdomen

Middle hepatic vein   IVC   CSF   Aorta

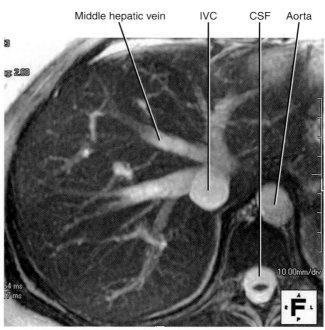

Figure 3-22 Axial maximum intensity projection image of hepatic veins acquired using steady state free precession technique (FIESTA). *CSF,* Cerebrospinal fluid; *IVC,* inferior vena cava.

Right kidney   Aortic aneurysm

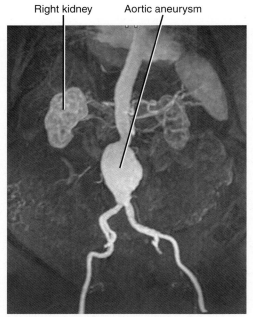

Figure 3-23 Coronal maximum intensity projection image of three-dimensional gadolinium-enhanced magnetic resonance angiography (MRA) of the abdominal aorta in a patient with aortic aneurysm. Images originally acquired in the coronal plane.

and pelvis may also provide MRA-like images when appropriately postprocessed.

Magnetic Resonance Cholangiopancreatography

MRCP has dramatically enhanced our ability to noninvasively evaluate the biliary and pancreatic ducts. MRCP may be divided into two categories: static and CE MRCP. Static MRCP utilizes heavily T2-weighted techniques to image fluid within ducts. CE MRCP techniques utilize a T1-weighted sequence to image paramagnetic contrast agents with some element of biliary excretion. CE MRCP has the potential to provide information about bile duct patency and integrity. Box 3-2 lists some clinical indications for performing MRCP.

Static MRCP images may be obtained in a variety of ways. The most familiar technique involves obtaining one or more thick-slab (typically 4 cm or thicker) acquisitions using a long echo train heavily T2-weighted sequence during a single breath hold. This type of sequence uses a long TE that results in attenuation of signal from most soft tissues, creating a clear depiction of fluid-containing structures (Fig. 3-24, *A*). This technique is not specific for the biliary and pancreatic ducts, so fluid within the bowel, urinary tract, and peritoneal cavity will also be demonstrated. Therefore care must be taken to position the imaging volume only over the structures of interest to provide the optimal views. Most often, multiple oblique coronal thick slabs are positioned in a radial manner around the common bile duct to provide multiple projections of the ducts. This is

necessary because the data are acquired as a single slice and cannot be manipulated in the same manner as volumetric data. When intrahepatic biliary ductal abnormalities are suspected, it may be helpful to perform a similar radial acquisition in the oblique axial plane (see Fig. 3-24, *B*). Because each projection takes only a few seconds to perform, this technique may be applied in multiple planes or projections with only minimal time investment. One disadvantage of the thick-slab technique is that overlapping structures may obscure findings or anatomy if the optimal projection is not obtained. For this reason, it is commonplace to supplement these images with thin-slice T2-weighted images obtained in multiple (most commonly axial and coronal) planes. These thin-section images may be obtained during breath holding using a half-Fourier single-shot echo train spin-echo technique such as HASTE, ssFSE, or ssTSE. Alternatively, a respiratory-triggered, heavily T2-weighted, echo train spin-echo sequence can be performed with extremely thin sections, although such sequences typically take several minutes to complete. One advantage of the latter technique is the ability to create detailed 3D models that can be manipulated in a variety of ways to demonstrate relevant anatomy or disease (Fig. 3-25).

A thick-slab MRCP sequence can be repeated multiple times over the same volume of interest and played as a cine loop. Care must be taken to allow sufficient time between acquisitions to avoid saturation effects. This technique may be helpful in demonstrating the dynamic appearance of the ampulla and documenting that the ampullary segment of the bile duct is patent. Some clinical sites have begun to administer secretin in conjunction with MRCP to aid in the evaluation of pancreatic exocrine function. The amount of pancreatic juice excreted into the duodenum can be quantified based on signal intensity within a volume of interest and is a reflection of the pancreatic exocrine reserve in patients with chronic pancreatitis.

CE MRCP requires the IV administration of a paramagnetic contrast agent that has at least some biliary excretion of the paramagnetic component. In the past, a manganese-based contrast agent, mangafodipir, served this purpose well but was removed from the market and

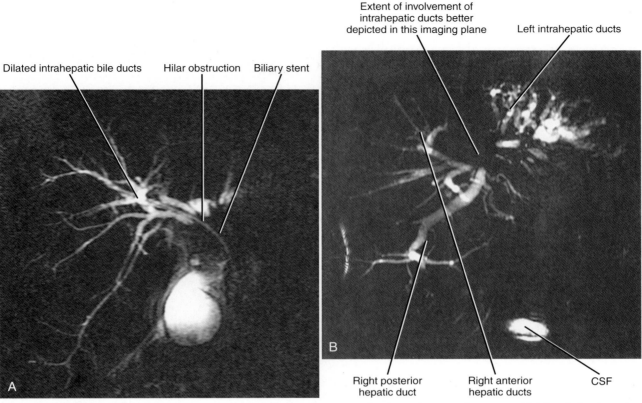

Figure 3-24 **A,** Coronal thick-slab magnetic resonance cholangiopancreatographic (MRCP) image of a patient with hilar cholangiocarcinoma. Total acquisition time for this image was approximately 2 seconds. **B,** Thick-slab MRCP performed in oblique axial plane in the same patient to better demonstrate involvement of secondary biliary radicals. *CSF,* Cerebrospinal fluid.

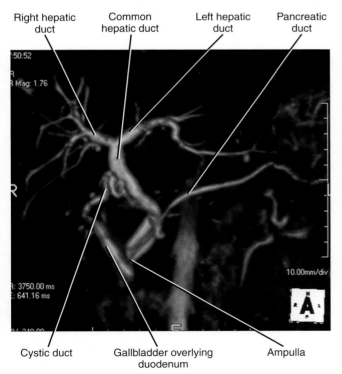

Figure 3-25 Three-dimensional, volume-rendered, magnetic resonance cholangiopancreatographic image created from thin-section respiratory-triggered images that required several minutes to complete.

was not available in the United States at the time of this writing. Gadolinium-based hepatobiliary agents such as Gd-BOPTA and Gd-EOB-DTPA could potentially fill this void, although little has been published regarding their efficacy in this regard (see Fig. 3-17, *B*). Imaging of hepatobiliary contrast agents may be accomplished with the same fat-suppressed, 3D, gradient-echo sequences used for multiphase liver imaging or MRA. In the past, CE MRCP with manganese-based mangafodipir was particularly useful for demonstrating intrahepatic biliary ductal anatomy in patients with nondistended bile ducts and the evaluation of suspected bile leaks. It is likely that CE MRCP will increase in popularity as more contrast agents with sufficient hepatobiliary activity become commercially available.

Magnetic Resonance Urography

MRU is not currently a widely applied technique of MRI, but given its favorable safety profile, use of existing sequences and software, and preliminary success, MRU may one day experience growth similar to that enjoyed by MRA and MRCP. The basic sequences used to produce MRU images do not differ significantly from many used for MRA and MRCP. Static MRU is essentially identical to static MRCP, as both techniques attempt to image fluid within a tubular structure using heavily T2-weighted sequences. MRU can be performed in any plane. As with MRCP, static MRU is most successful when the target structures are fluid filled and well distended (Fig. 3-26). Poorly distended ureters in a dehydrated patient are extremely difficult to display with static MRU. Static MRU is highly accurate for determining the level of urinary tract obstruction.

Excretory MRU involves imaging the urinary tract during the excretory phase after administration of a gadolinium chelate (Fig. 3-27). Imaging is generally performed with a 3D gradient-echo sequence. The use of fat suppression improves visualization of the ureters. Excretory MRU obviously requires a moderate degree of renal function and is usually enhanced through the use of hydration and low-dose furosemide. In addition to distending the ureters, these latter accompaniments serve to prevent signal loss caused by the T2* effects of concentrated gadolinium within the collecting systems.

MRU is best performed in conjunction with additional sequences designed to evaluate the solid organs and soft tissues to take complete advantage of the diagnostic capability of MRI. Because a wide variety of alternative imaging techniques exist for evaluation of the urinary tract, MRU is often reserved for patients who have a contraindication to iodinated contrast, and for whom noncontrast CT and ultrasound have been unrevealing or

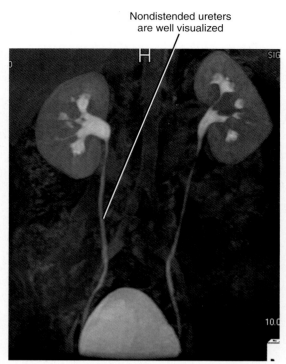

Nondistended ureters are well visualized

Figure 3-27 Coronal maximum intensity projection of excretory urogram facilitated by administration of low-dose intravenous furosemide and hydration in a patient without urinary tract obstruction.

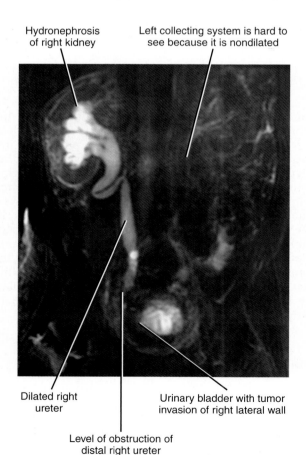

Hydronephrosis of right kidney

Left collecting system is hard to see because it is nondilated

Dilated right ureter

Urinary bladder with tumor invasion of right lateral wall

Level of obstruction of distal right ureter

Figure 3-26 Coronal static magnetic resonance urogram in a patient with right distal ureteral obstruction caused by metastatic prostate cancer (pelvic lymph-node metastasis). (From Leyendecker JR, Barnes CE, Zagoria RJ. MR urography: techniques and clinical applications. *Radiographics* 28: 23-46, 2008, with permission.)

nondiagnostic. MRU has the additional benefit of not exposing patients to ionizing radiation, and this factor alone may result in some increased interest in this technique.

■ ARTIFACTS AND PITFALLS

When an abnormality is detected on an MRI examination of the abdomen and pelvis, it is essential to consider the possibility that the finding in question represents an artifact of imaging. As discussed in this section, a number of artifacts exist that may closely mimic disease and lead to errant management if not recognized. Most interpretive pitfalls can be overcome through meticulous attention to all sequences obtained. Such review is necessary because each sequence of a carefully crafted abdominal or pelvic MRI protocol serves a unique purpose, and not all lesions will be clearly evident on all sequences.

Artifacts and Pitfalls That Simulate Masses

Wraparound artifact may mimic masses within the abdomen or pelvis when anatomic structures (e.g., an arm) or other objects (e.g., IV tubing) positioned outside the field of view are wrapped into an image. Such structures may become superimposed on organs such as the liver and simulate a tumor. When IV tubing filled with gadolinium wraps into the image, it may simulate an aberrant vessel or drainage catheter (Fig. 3-28).

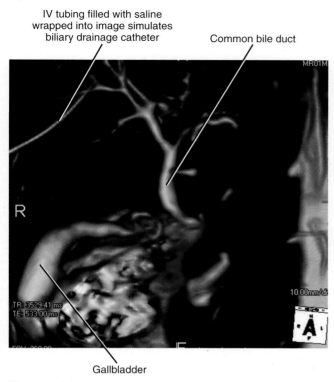

IV tubing filled with saline
wrapped into image simulates
biliary drainage catheter

Common bile duct

R

Gallbladder

Figure 3-28 Volume-rendered reconstruction of thin-section magnetic resonance cholangiopancreatographic images in a patient with peripheral IV demonstrating wraparound artifact.

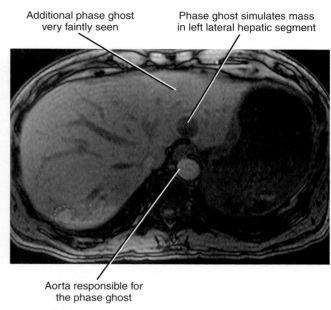

Additional phase ghost
very faintly seen

Phase ghost simulates mass
in left lateral hepatic segment

Aorta responsible for
the phase ghost

Figure 3-29 Axial fat-suppressed, T1-weighted, gradient-echo image through the liver demonstrating pulsation artifact.

Because wraparound is automatically suppressed in the frequency encoding direction, wraparound artifact typically manifests along the phase-encoding direction. To eliminate this artifact, one can increase the field of view or apply an option available on most scanners known as phase oversampling, although this latter option may considerably increase scan time for some sequences.

Pulsation artifact results from motion-induced phase errors related to pulsatile blood flow and, like wraparound artifact, manifests along the phase-encoding axis. This is a common artifact that may be difficult to completely suppress on every sequence. Pulsatile flow within a vessel causes faint images of the responsible vessel to occur in both directions along the phase-encoding axis. These "ghosts," as they are sometimes called, may be confused with mass lesions, most commonly of the liver and spine (Fig. 3-29). The key to uncovering the true nature of this artifact is recognizing the multiplicity of the abnormality at regular intervals in a straight line along the phase-encoding axis. The use of saturation bands above and below the imaging volume may reduce the effects of vascular ghosts.

Flow artifacts are commonly seen within fluid-containing structures imaged with single-shot echo train spin-echo sequences such as ssFSE, ssTSE, and HASTE. These low signal intensity artifacts are commonly encountered in pleural effusions, ascites, the common bile duct, and the urinary bladder. Even some large renal cysts may demonstrate signal loss resulting from the bulk movement of fluid. Such flow artifacts may appear masslike and simulate mural nodules, pleural or

peritoneal implants, or bladder masses (Fig. 3-30). Thin-section axial images created with long echo train FSE sequences may demonstrate artifact simulating a filling defect within the common bile duct because of the through-plane motion of bile (Fig. 3-31). This artifact is easily mistaken for a common bile duct stone by the unsuspecting radiologist. This pitfall may be avoided

Urinary bladder

Flow artifact caused by ureteral
jet resembles bladder mass

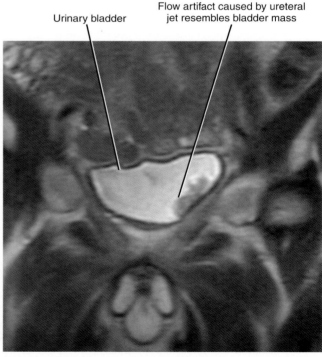

Figure 3-30 Coronal single-shot fast spin-echo image through the urinary bladder demonstrates flow artifact (ureteral jet) simulating bladder wall mass.

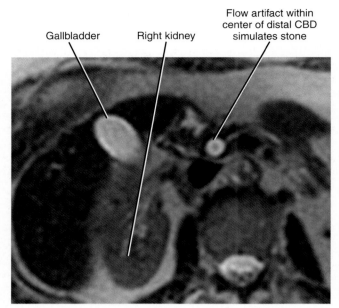

Gallbladder   Right kidney   Flow artifact within center of distal CBD simulates stone

Figure 3-31 Axial single-shot fast spin-echo image through distal common bile duct (CBD) demonstrates flow artifact centrally within the duct.

by making it a practice to confirm any suspected filling defect in the common bile duct identified on axial images with the corresponding coronal images.

Artifacts and Pitfalls That Simulate Stenoses, Thromboses, and Occlusions

Many unenhanced MRA sequences are prone to flow-related artifacts that manifest as areas of signal loss that may be confused with intravascular thrombus. Such artifacts are common at sites of complex flow such as venous confluences, or in regions of vascular stenoses or aneurysms. When an area of intravascular signal loss is seen on a non-CE MRA sequence such as TOF, one should attempt to confirm the abnormality on an alternate sequence or by administering IV contrast material before concluding that thrombus is present. Non-CE MRA techniques are also prone to saturation of in-plane flow. Blood flowing parallel to the imaging plane of an unenhanced MRA sequence may be subjected to the same repeated RF pulses that suppress the background tissues. As a result, there may be sufficient signal loss within a vessel to create the impression of absent flow (i.e., thrombosis or occlusion). A similar impression may be created by retrograde flow on an unenhanced TOF MRA sequence that utilizes a saturation band to selectively eliminate arterial or venous flow.

Slow flow may be misinterpreted as absent flow when the flow velocity is below the threshold of the imaging technique. This latter problem may be successfully overcome with CE imaging, provided a sufficiently long imaging delay is used after contrast administration. On T2-weighted images of the abdomen, flow within blood vessels usually manifests as a signal void. Although

absence of this signal void may be a manifestation of thrombosis, vessels that contain slowly moving blood or spend sufficient time within the imaging plane may appear as high signal intensity even when patent.

Some artifacts occur with both IV CE and unenhanced MRA sequences. Susceptibility artifact associated with metallic objects may extend to adjacent vessels, simulating stenosis or occlusion (Fig. 3-32). Metallic intravascular stents and IVC filters produce variable artifact depending on the material (Figs. 3-33 and 3-34). Artifact associated with nitinol and tantalum may be mild, but stainless-steel stents are associated with considerably more artifact. When intravascular signal loss is not accompanied by the presence of vascular collaterals, one should always verify the absence of an intravascular device before proclaiming the vessel occluded. Occasionally, extrinsic compression of a vessel by normal anatomic structures may simulate a fixed stenosis. This is a common problem where the right common iliac artery crosses the left common iliac vein. A similar artifact is also frequently encountered on MRCP images where the right hepatic artery crosses the common hepatic bile duct, simulating a stricture or stone (Fig. 3-35).

One final artifact that may simulate vascular thrombosis is caused by mixing of IV contrast material with unopacified blood, as commonly occurs in the IVC at the renal vein confluence during the portal venous phase of CE imaging. Fortunately, most of us are familiar with this artifact, as it occurs commonly with CE CT. This artifact can usually be disregarded if the vessel in question enhances homogeneously on equilibrium-phase images.

Artifacts and Pitfalls That Simulate Enhancement

When a phase misregistration ghost resulting from pulsatile vascular flow appears as high signal intensity on a CE image, it may be mistaken for an enhancing lesion, particularly if it appears of low signal intensity on precontrast images. Fat and fat-suppression techniques may be responsible for a number of pitfalls in the category of pseudoenhancement. When non–fat-suppressed, T1-weighted images are performed before contrast, and fat-suppressed T1-weighted images are performed after IV gadolinium chelate administration, lesions that have a short T1 relaxation time may appear to enhance relative to background, particularly if the abnormality in question was previously surrounded by fat. Signal intensity measurements of the lesion in question or the use of subtraction will resolve this problem, provided the precontrast and postcontrast sequences are otherwise identical (Fig. 3-36). Opposed-phase imaging may create a similar impression when in-phase T1-weighted imaging is performed before contrast but opposed-phase imaging is performed after gadolinium chelate administration in a patient with a fatty liver. Loss of signal intensity in the fatty liver on the opposed-phase sequence may unmask focal lesions or make them more conspicuous (Fig. 3-37). Geographic areas of fatty sparing may cause a similar problem. This pitfall is easy to

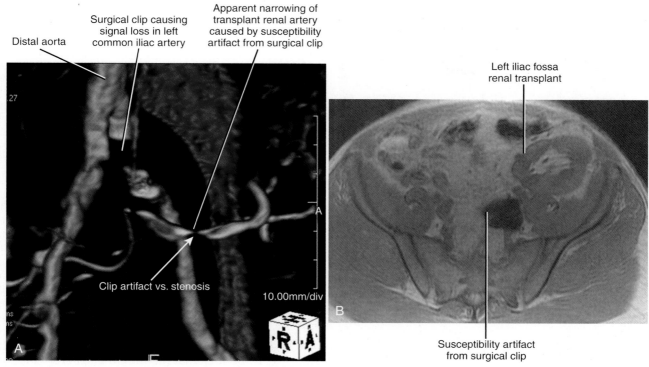

Figure 3-32 **A,** Volume-rendered gadolinium-enhanced magnetic resonance angiogram (MRA) in a patient with left iliac fossa renal transplant and surgical clip simulating stenosis of transplant artery. **B,** Axial T1-weighted, gradient-echo image through level of renal transplant in the same patient shows large amount of susceptibility artifact from surgical clips. Numerous clips were present in the pelvis and responsible for signal loss and pseudostenosis seen on MRA reconstructions.

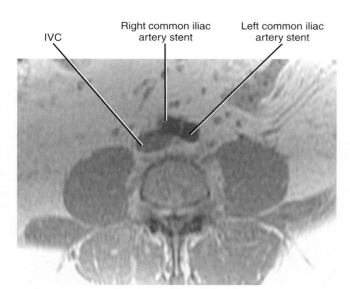

Figure 3-33 Axial T1-weighted, gradient-echo image at the level of aortic bifurcation in a patient with bilateral common iliac stents. *IVC,* Inferior vena cava.

avoid by consulting the in- and opposed-phase images performed before contrast.

When sufficient magnetic field heterogeneity is present, frequency selective fat saturation techniques may fail to suppress fat in a portion of an image. This failure of fat suppression may be misinterpreted as enhancement due to inflammation on fat suppressed postcontrast images.

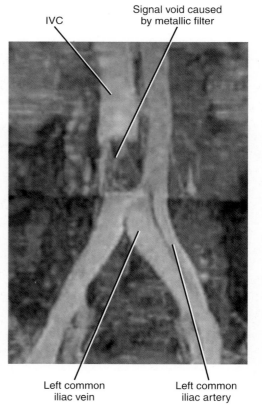

Figure 3-34 Coronal maximum intensity projection reconstruction of contrast-enhanced, T1-weighted, gradient-echo images in a patient with inferior vena cava (IVC) filter.

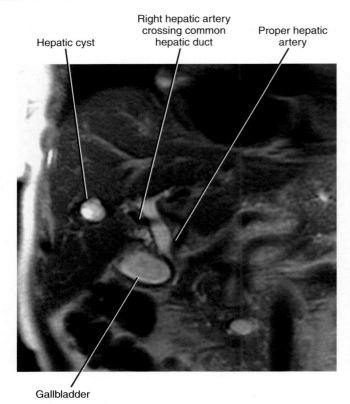

Figure 3-35 Coronal T2-weighted, single-shot, fast spin-echo image through the common bile duct demonstrates the right hepatic artery crossing the common hepatic duct.

While the use of subtraction may avoid the pitfall of pseudoenhancement, subtraction may also be a source of this pitfall. Subtraction works by subtracting the precontrast data set from a data set performed after IV contrast administration using identical scanning parameters. If precontrast and postcontrast data sets are not obtained during the same breath hold, respiratory misregistration may occur between data sets, simulating enhancement (Fig. 3-38).

Artifacts and Pitfalls That Obscure Disease

Of the artifacts and pitfalls encountered on a daily basis on a busy MRI service, those that obscure disease are the most concerning, because the interpreter may be entirely unaware that an abnormality exists. Perhaps the most common problem encountered when imaging the abdomen with MRI is respiratory motion. Respiratory motion results in obscuration of disease by reducing the apparent signal intensity of lesions and producing obscuring ghosts along the phase-encoding direction (Fig. 3-39). Several strategies may be used to reduce or eliminate the effects of respiratory motion. Breath-hold imaging is the preferred method of respiratory motion suppression but may not be an option for some patients. Scanning quickly using a single-shot echo train spin-echo or steady state free precession technique will often produce images free of respiratory artifact even when obtained during free breathing. However, some compromises made to reduce scan time may also reduce the contrast-to-noise ratio between lesions and

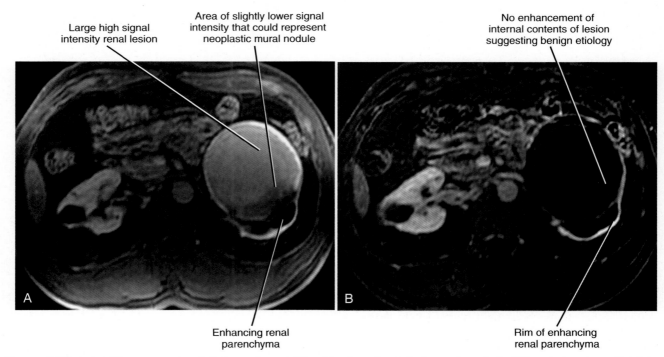

Figure 3-36 A, Axial fat-suppressed, gadolinium-enhanced, T1-weighted, gradient-echo image through the kidneys in a patient with a large hemorrhagic cyst of left kidney. B, Image created by subtracting the precontrast data set from the postcontrast data set in the same patient.

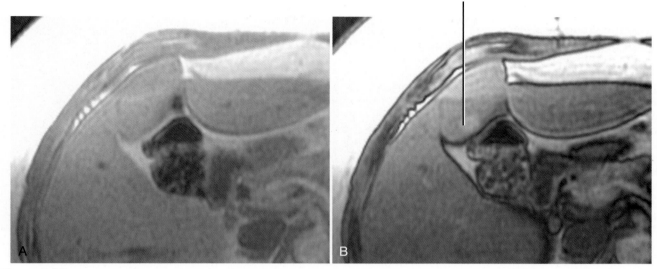

Lesion is now brighter than background liver due to relative signal loss of fatty liver on opposed-phase image. This could be confused with enhancement of the lesion

Figure 3-37 **A,** Axial unenhanced, in-phase, gradient-echo image through the liver in a patient with hepatic steatosis in segment IVb shows no focal abnormality in liver. **B,** Axial unenhanced, opposed-phase, gradient-echo image through the liver of the same patient shows lesion in segment IVb. Lesion is now visible because of signal loss in adjacent fatty parenchyma.

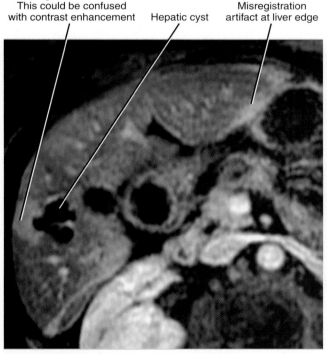

Misregistration artifact. This could be confused with contrast enhancement

Hepatic cyst

Misregistration artifact at liver edge

Figure 3-38 Subtraction image of a patient with hepatic cysts demonstrates a misregistration artifact because the postcontrast data set was obtained in a different degree of inspiration than the precontrast data set.

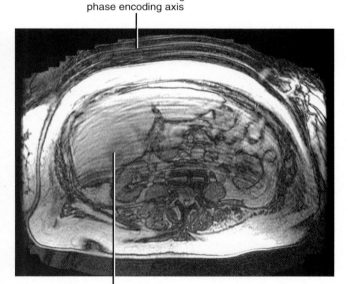

Multiple ghosts of anterior abdominal wall along phase encoding axis

Respiratory ghosts partially obscure lesion in liver

Figure 3-39 Axial T1-weighted, gradient-echo image demonstrates severe respiratory artifact.

background tissues. Respiratory triggering or navigator pulses are helpful for T2-weighted sequences when breathing is regular, although this option may add significantly to acquisition times. Respiratory compensation may reduce the effects of respiratory motion on

spin-echo T1-weighted images without a significant time penalty, although this option tends to be only partially successful. Because the signal intensity of a motion artifact is related to the signal intensity of the structure causing it, respiratory ghost artifacts can be reduced by applying a saturation band over the anterior abdominal fat. Unfortunately, this may not be an option for some pulse sequences. Peristalsis is another cause of motion-related artifacts that may be reduced by having patients fast for several hours before imaging or through the use of antiperistaltic agents such as glucagon.

Certain obscuring artifacts are intrinsic to the patient and not easily corrected. For example, certain types of metallic implanted objects are associated with considerable susceptibility artifact but are not easily removed (Fig. 3-40). In addition to the susceptibility artifact created by metallic implanted devices, metallic objects may cause local failure of frequency-selective fat-suppression techniques. A focal area of nonsuppressed fat on an otherwise fat-suppressed sequence could be misinterpreted as high signal intensity edema or inflammation on a T2-weighted sequence if the offending metallic device lies outside the field of view (Fig. 3-41). This is often the situation with MRI scans of the abdomen in a patient with a metallic hip prosthesis. Occasionally, soft-tissue structures of interest will be suppressed instead of fat when using a frequency-selective form of fat suppression in a patient with an intrinsic metallic object.

Wraparound artifact may also obscure disease. This occurs when the portion of the body wrapping into the image overlays an area of abnormality. Fortunately, this problem may be overcome by increasing the field of view in the phase-encoding direction or use of the phase oversampling option. The use of sensitivity-encoding (SENSE) parallel imaging techniques (array spatial sensitvity encoding technique [ASSET]) to shorten acquisition times has resulted in a common artifact that may obscure abnormalities if not corrected. These parallel imaging techniques essentially work by purposely creating wraparound in the phase-encoding direction and then "unwrapping" the image using sensitivity data obtained for the individual phased array coil elements during an initial calibration scan. If too small a field of view is initially chosen in the phase-encoding direction or if the calibration scan is improperly performed, one will see a faint residue of the wraparound artifact on the

images (Fig. 3-42). If the field of view is much too small, a bright line will appear in the center of the image. These artifacts may be eliminated or reduced by expanding the field of view or repeating the calibration scan, ensuring that patient position and respiration are consistent.

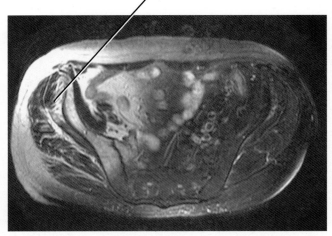

Local failure of fat suppression caused by metallic hip prosthesis could be confused with soft tissue edema. Using STIR to suppress the fat would eliminate this problem

Figure 3-41 Axial T2-weighted, fast-spin echo image through upper pelvis in a patient with right hip prosthesis. Chemically selective fat saturation was applied. *STIR,* Short tau inversion recovery.

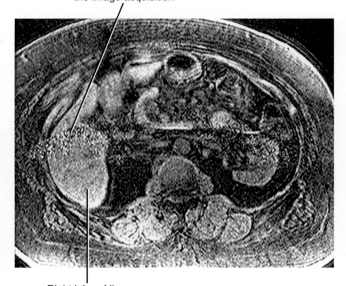

Parallel imaging artifact. This can be improved by increasing the field-of-view and by recalibrating while ensuring that patient breath holds are consistent between the calibration scan and the image acquisition

Right lobe of liver

Figure 3-42 Axial fat-suppressed, T1-weighted, gradient-echo image through the abdomen obtained using parallel imaging technique.

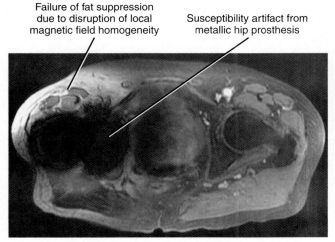

Failure of fat suppression due to disruption of local magnetic field homogeneity

Susceptibility artifact from metallic hip prosthesis

Figure 3-40 Axial fat-suppressed, T1-weighted, gradient-echo image in a patient with right hip prosthesis.

3-Tesla Artifacts

As more radiologists transition to 3-Tesla imaging, a new host of artifacts and pitfalls will emerge, whereas others will become more noticeable. For example, susceptibility and chemical shift artifacts are more apparent on higher field strength systems. T1 relaxation times are increased at higher field strength, potentially resulting in loss of image contrast on T1-weighted images. It is also important to be aware that on 3-Tesla MRI systems, the in- and opposed-phase echo times differ from those at 1.5 Tesla. Not only are the times different, but the order in which the in- and opposed-phase echoes are collected may be reversed on dual-phase acquisitions. At 1.5 Tesla, the opposed-phase echo is usually measured first, followed by the in-phase echo. At 3 Tesla, the in-phase echo may be collected first on some scanners (even though an opposed-phase occurs sooner), resulting in a longer TE for the opposed-phase echo. At first glance, this may not appear to present much of a problem. However, consider that at 1.5 Tesla, fatty infiltration of the liver or intracellular lipid in abdominal masses will "drop out" on opposed-phase images, whereas hemosiderosis will do so on in-phase images because of the longer TE. At 3 Tesla, both intracellular lipid and iron will demonstrate signal loss on opposed-phase images, potentially limiting the usefulness of this valuable sign for distinguishing iron from fat. This problem may be easily overcome by performing in- and opposed-phase imaging as separate acquisitions rather than as a single dual-phase acquisition. Implementation of this solution does result in an increase in overall imaging time.

"Standing waves" and circulating currents created within the body can produce large areas of signal loss on some images performed at 3 Tesla. These effects can be exacerbated by the presence of ascites. Vendor-designed "RF cushions" may help reduce these effects.

Suggested Readings

Balci NC, Semelka RC: Contrast agents for MR imaging of the liver, *Radiol Clin North Am* 43:887-898, 2005.

Blandino A, Gaeta M, Minutoli F et al: MR urography of the ureter, *AJR Am J Roentgenol* 179:1307-1314, 2002.

Broome DR, Girguis MS, Baron PW et al: Gadodiamide-associated nephrogenic systemic fibrosis: why radiologists should be concerned, *AJR Am J Roentgenol* 188:586-592, 2007.

Coakley FV, Qayyum A, Kurhanewicz J: Magnetic resonance imaging and spectroscopic imaging of prostate cancer, *J Urol* 170:S69-S75, 2003.

Delfaut EM, Beltran J, Johnson G et al: Fat suppression in MR imaging: techniques and pitfalls, *RadioGraphics* 19:373-382, 1999.

Ersoy H, Rybicki FJ: Biochemical safety profiles of gadolinium-based extracellular contrast agents and nephrogenic systemic fibrosis, *J Magn Reson Imaging* 26:1190-1197, 2007.

Giovagnoni A, Fabbri A, Maccioni F: Oral contrast agents in MRI of the gastrointestinal tract, *Abdom Imaging* 27:367-375, 2002.

Glockner JF: MR angiography interpretation: techniques and pitfalls, *Magn Reson Clin N Am* 13:23-40, 2005.

Grobner T: Gadolinium—a specific trigger for the development of nephrogenic fibrosing dermopathy and nephrogenic systemic fibrosis? *Nephrol Dial Transplant* 21:1104-1108, 2006.

Hood MN, Ho VB, Smirniotopoulos JG et al: Chemical shift: the artifact and clinical tool revisited, *RadioGraphics* 19:357-371, 1999.

Ichikawa T, Haradome H, Hachiya J et al: Diffusion-weighted MR imaging with single-shot echo-planar imaging in the upper abdomen: preliminary clinical experience in 61 patients, *Abdom Imaging* 24:456-461, 1999.

Irie H, Honda H, Kuroiwa T et al: Pitfalls in MR cholangiopancreatographic interpretation, *RadioGraphics* 21:23-37, 2001.

Keogan MT, Edelman RR: Technologic advances in abdominal MR imaging, *Radiology* 220:310-320, 2001.

Koyama T, Tamai K, Togashi K: Current status of body MR imaging: fast MR imaging and diffusion-weighted imaging, *Int J Clin Oncol* 11:278-285, 2006.

Laissy JP, Trillaud H, Douek P: MR angiography: noninvasive imaging of the abdomen, *Abdom Imaging* 27:488-506, 2002.

Lin S-P, Brown JJ: MR contrast agents: physical and pharmacologic basics, *J Magn Reson Imaging* 25:884-899, 2007.

Merkle EM, Dale BM, Paulson EK: Abdominal MR imaging at 3T, *Magn Reson Imaging Clin N Am* 14:17-26, 2006.

Mirowitz SA: Diagnostic pitfalls and artifacts in abdominal MR imaging: a review, *Radiology* 208:577-589, 1998.

Motohara T, Semelka RC, Bader TR: MR cholangiopancreatography, *Radiol Clin North Am* 41:89-96, 2003.

Nitz WR, Reimer P: Contrast mechanisms in MR imaging, *Eur Radiol* 9:1032-1046, 1999.

Nitz WR: Fast and ultrafast non-echo-planar MR imaging techniques, *Eur Radiol* 12:2866-2882, 2002.

Nolte-Ernsting CC, Staatz G, Tacke J et al: MR urography today, *Abdom Imaging* 28:191-209, 2003.

Rofsky NM, Lee VS, Laub G et al: Abdominal MR imaging with a volumetric interpolated breath-hold examination, *Radiology* 212:876-884, 1999.

Semelka RC, Balci NC, Op de Beeck B et al: Evaluation of a 10-minute comprehensive MR imaging examination of the upper abdomen, *Radiology* 211:189-195, 1999.

Van Hoe L, Mermuys K, Vanhoenacker P: MRCP pitfalls, *Abdom Imaging* 29:360-387, 2004.

CHAPTER 4

Positron Emission Tomography

Paige Clark

Positron emission tomography (PET) provides information about molecular processes that cannot be obtained with conventional cross-sectional imaging techniques such as ultrasound, computed tomography (CT), and magnetic resonance imaging (MRI). Such information about cellular metabolism provides an additional method for detecting disease, accurately characterizing tissues, and determining tumor activity. When combined with anatomic imaging using a hybrid technique such as PET/CT, metabolic data can be combined with anatomic localization to create a powerful problem-solving tool.

■ THE ESSENCE OF PET AND PET/CT

With 18F-fluoro-2-deoxy-D-glucose (FDG) PET, a radio-active glucose analogue is trapped in cells hypermetabolic because of malignant transformation, infection, or inflammation. Positrons emitted as the 18F-FDG decays encounter electrons in the body and annihilate, releasing two 511 keV gamma emissions that travel 180 degrees apart. Crystals arranged in a ring around the patient detect these photons, which are localized through tomographic reconstruction algorithms.

Due to photon attenuation by different body tissues (e.g., gamma rays travel more effectively through lung tissue than liver tissue), attenuation maps are necessary. These are created by using transmission scans or CT scans. Attenuation correction with CT allows quick attenuation mapping, shortening the attenuation correction scan by about 25 minutes. PET/CT scanners offer other advantages over PET-only scanners, including more accurate anatomic localization (compared to side-by-side PET and CT comparison) and lack of need for complex image fusion software.

As mentioned earlier, the radiopharmaceutical 18F-FDG is taken up by metabolically active cells regardless of the underlying reason for the increased metabolic activity. Therefore there is much room for improvement in the specificity of PET for various types of tissues and disease processes. In efforts to improve specificity, several alternative positron-emitting radiopharmaceuticals are under development. As a measure of protein synthesis in tumors, amino acid imaging with PET radiopharmaceuticals incorporating methionine and tyrosine have been studied in rectal and ovarian carcinoma. Nucleoside imaging as a measure of cellular proliferation is also being evaluated for such tumors as those involved in esophageal cancer, colon cancer, and lymphoma.

■ PROBLEM-SOLVING APPLICATIONS OF PET AND PET/CT

In the literature, 18F-FDG PET has been shown to provide incremental clinical value over anatomical imaging in three main clinical scenarios: (1) lesion detection; (2) lesion characterization; and (3) directing cancer therapy. A summary of some current indications for PET imaging are listed in Box 4-1. We will now consider these applications in more detail.

Lesion Detection

In patients with known malignant tumor, PET/CT may be beneficial in the detection of metastases, particularly those distant from the primary tumor. In a study of colon cancer patients by Cohade and colleagues, 30% more lesions were detected by PET/CT than by CT alone. In this same study, the accuracy of tumor staging increased from 78% to 89% with PET/CT. Similar results were reported in a review by Subhas and colleagues on the use of PET in patients with cervical and endometrial cancer. These authors showed greater than 95% sensitivity and 76% specificity in detecting disease recurrence. Schiepers and colleagues reported sensitivities of 82% to 99% and specificities of approximately 99% for initial staging and posttherapy evaluation of non-Hodgkin lymphoma. In addition to detecting distant metastases in patients with newly diagnosed malignant tumors, PET and PET/CT are useful for detecting metastases in patients with rising tumor markers despite negative anatomic imaging (Figs. 4-1 and 4-2). Unfortunately, very small (<6 mm) lesions such as peritoneal implants often are not evident on PET despite increased metabolism.

When considering the use of PET to detect malignant lesions in the abdomen and pelvis, the avidity of 18F-FDG for various malignancies should be considered.

BOX 4-1   Potential Problem-Solving Uses for PET in the Abdomen and Pelvis

Direct biopsy
Characterization of lymph nodes
Direct exploratory oncologic surgery
Detection of occult lesions in patients with negative contrast-enhanced CT and rising serum tumor markers
Evaluation of posttherapy residual tumor (i.e., after surgery or thermal ablation)
Evaluation of response to systemic cancer therapy
Detection of lytic bone metastases (e.g., renal cell carcinoma)
Evaluation of fever of unknown origin (FUO)
Evaluation of suspected infected prosthesis

The most common abdominal and pelvic tumors known to be strongly positive on 18F-FDG PET in the majority of cases are listed in Box 4-2.

Abdominal malignancies commonly regarded as showing no or little hypermetabolic activity on 18F-FDG PET include mucinous adenocarcinoma, well-differentiated hepatocellular carcinoma, and well-differentiated prostate cancer (Fig. 4-3). Testicular cancer shows variable 18F-FDG uptake. While high-grade lymphomas usually are hypermetabolic, low-grade lymphoma may be difficult to detect with PET/CT. Up to half of all renal cell carcinomas are not 18F-FDG avid (Fig. 4-4). 18F-FDG PET for renal cell carcinoma presents additional challenges even when the tumor is hypermetabolic. Renal cell carcinoma may be isointense to surrounding renal parenchyma on PET images, and renal excretion of 18F-FDG can obscure primary renal lesions adjacent to the renal collecting system. Despite these limitations, PET may be occasionally useful for finding distant metastatic deposits from renal cell carcinoma. In particular, 18F-FDG PET seems to be very sensitive for early detection of lytic bone metastases when compared with plain film, CT or bone scan. For tumors with variable avidity for 18F-FDG, if PET/CT shows hypermetabolic activity in lesions with anatomic correlates, then the study may be a reliable indicator of extent of disease.

The utility of 18F-FDG PET is not limited to the detection of malignant neoplasms. The highly sensitive nature of PET imaging may be exploited for the evaluation of patients with fever of unknown origin, vasculitis, arthroplasty infections, and inflammatory disorders such as sarcoidosis (Fig. 4-5). Because PET and PET/CT are emerging technologies, not all potential applications are reimbursed by insurers. As with any imaging modality, incidental findings are common on PET and PET/CT scans (Figs. 4-6 and 4-7). Normal physiologic FDG uptake (e.g., bowel, brown fat) is also common and must be distinguished from pathologic FDG activity.

Lesion Characterization

Incidental lesions, such as pulmonary nodules or adrenal masses, are commonly encountered on CT or MRI examinations. Often such a study is not optimized for the unsuspected lesion, resulting in the unsatisfying

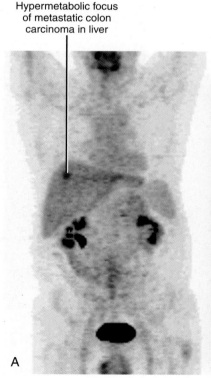

Hypermetabolic focus
of metastatic colon
carcinoma in liver

Hypermetabolic focus
(colon carcinoma metastasis)
localizes to liver dome

A

B

Figure 4-1 **A,** Coronal MIP reconstruction of PET data from a patient with rising CEA after surgery for colon cancer and negative contrast-enhanced CT. **B,** Coronal PET/CT image in the same patient as in **A.**

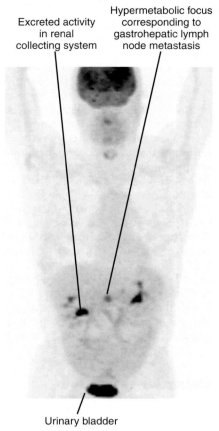

Excreted activity in renal collecting system

Hypermetabolic focus corresponding to gastrohepatic lymph node metastasis

Urinary bladder

Figure 4-2 Coronal PET image in a patient with gastrohepatic lymph node metastasis after surgery for colon cancer with rising CEA. No enlarged lymph nodes were visible on contrast-enhanced CT.

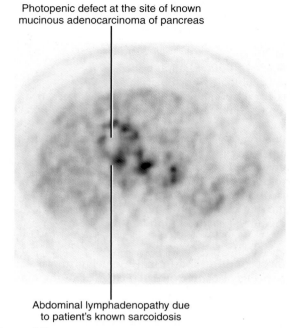

Photopenic defect at the site of known mucinous adenocarcinoma of pancreas

Abdominal lymphadenopathy due to patient's known sarcoidosis

Figure 4-3 Axial PET image at the level of the pancreatic head in a patient with a mucinous adenocarcinoma of the pancreas. Mucin-producing tumors can show variable uptake on PET, limiting sensitivity of this modality for these lesions.

designation of indeterminate abnormality. 18F-FDG PET can effectively characterize many indeterminate abdominal and pelvic abnormalities. In the case of lung and adrenal nodules incidentally discovered on a CT scan, if there is high index of suspicion for malignant neoplasm, a PET/CT can be performed to characterize the lung and adrenal lesions and provide information regarding possible nodal and bone metastases. If the lung and adrenal lesions measure at least one centimeter in diameter and are metabolically inactive, these lesions are very unlikely to represent metastatic disease.

BOX 4-2 Tumors of the Abdomen and Pelvis with High 18F-FDG Avidity

High-grade lymphoma
Colorectal cancer
Cholangiocarcinoma
Pheochromocytoma
Poorly differentiated hepatocellular carcinoma
Ovarian cancer
Cervical cancer
Endometrial cancer
Metastatic melanoma
Lung, breast, esophageal, and gastric cancer metastases

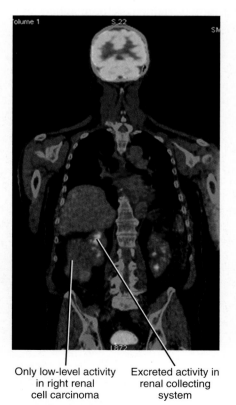

Only low-level activity in right renal cell carcinoma

Excreted activity in renal collecting system

Figure 4-4 Coronal fused PET/CT image in a patient with large right renal cell carcinoma that is not particularly FDG avid.

Extensive uptake in
abdominal lymph nodes

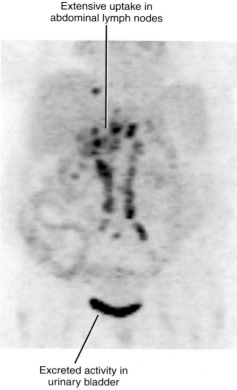

Excreted activity in
urinary bladder

Figure 4-5 Coronal PET image in a patient with sarcoidosis (same patient as in Fig. 4-3).

Hepatic metastasis
from colon cancer

Excreted activity in
renal collecting
system

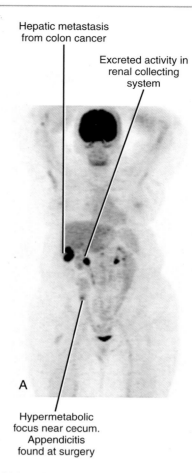

A

Hypermetabolic
focus near cecum.
Appendicitis
found at surgery

Abnormally thickened appendix
with mild stranding in adjacent fat

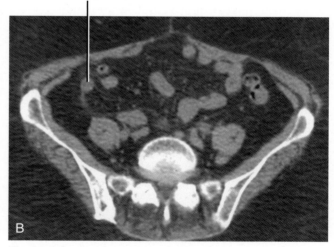

B

Figure 4-6 **A,** Coronal PET image of a patient with metastatic colon cancer being evaluated for possible hepatic resection of solitary hepatic lesion. The patient also had early appendicitis accounting for increased metabolic activity near the cecum. **B,** Axial CT image of the same patient as in A shows thickened appendix with fat stranding corresponding to increased activity on PET scan and appendicitis at surgery.

If either lesion is metabolically active in the setting of additional hypermetabolic foci, the likelihood of metastatic disease is very high. In this manner, PET/CT may obviate further anatomic imaging in addition to bone scan.

For indeterminate adrenal lesions detected incidentally on anatomic imaging studies, hypermetabolic adrenal activity on PET is highly specific for malignancy. To determine if an adrenal lesion is hypermetabolic, most PET readers compare adrenal activity with hepatic activity. If the adrenal lesion is more metabolically active than liver, it is most likely malignant. If the adrenal lesion shows similar or less activity than liver, it is indeterminate or benign by PET criteria. Comparison of functional PET data with findings on anatomic imaging can usually yield a satisfactory clinical answer.

Despite less-than-perfect specificity, PET can be beneficial in attempting to distinguish between benign and malignant lymph nodes. Anatomic imaging requires lymph nodes to reach a certain size (often 8-10 mm) before they are considered abnormal. PET can often detect hypermetabolic activity in smaller lymph nodes involved with metastatic disease. However, PET is not 100% sensitive or specific for lymph node metastases, even in the setting of a tumor known to be FDG avid. Tiny metastatic deposits may be missed, and lymph nodes in close proximity to a hypermetabolic tumor (such as gastric cancer) may be eclipsed by the primary tumor's activity. In addition, not all enlarged lymph

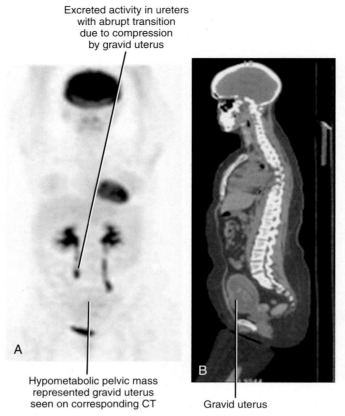

Excreted activity in ureters
with abrupt transition
due to compression
by gravid uterus

A

Hypometabolic pelvic mass
represented gravid uterus
seen on corresponding CT

B

Gravid uterus

Figure 4-7 **A,** Coronal PET image shows a hypometabolic pelvic mass *(arrow)* with concomitant urinary stasis due to unexpected intrauterine pregnancy. **B,** Sagittal reformation of the same patient as in **A** showing unexpected intrauterine pregnancy accounting for findings on PET portion of exam.

nodes with increased FDG uptake are indicative of nodal metastases. A hypermetabolic lymph node that manifests benign imaging characteristics (e.g., well-defined fatty hilum) may be reactive. As with anatomic imaging, coexistent malignant neoplasm and infection or inflammation is problematic and may necessitate biopsy or follow-up imaging to fully characterize suspicious lymph nodes.

PET may also be useful in lymphoma patients with mild or no splenic enlargement on anatomic imaging. In this setting, splenic involvement is evidenced by focal or diffusely increased splenic activity on PET. As with the adrenal gland, splenic activity is compared with the liver: If activity is greater in the spleen than in the liver, malignant involvement is presumed.

Anatomic imaging findings after cancer treatment are often ambiguous or nonspecific. Decreased activity in a tumor site post-therapy suggest response or, if performed immediately after therapy, tumor stunning (Fig. 4-8). When combined with anatomic imaging, PET may be useful for distinguishing between tumor recurrence and expected posttreatment changes such as scarring. Examples of such utility include distinguishing between scarring and pelvic tumor recurrence after colorectal cancer resection and differentiating between post-radiofrequency ablation changes within the liver and residual tumor. In each case, residual hypermetabolic activity that does not decrease over time

or that is new since a prior exam suggests viable residual or recurrent tumor (Figs. 4-9 and 4-10).

When findings on anatomic and PET imaging are not definitive, biopsy-proven disease elsewhere greatly increases the specificity of PET/CT for additional lesions in the same patient. Clinical history and anatomic imaging findings of concomitant granulomatous, infectious, or degenerative bone disease similarly aid interpretation of PET/CT, decreasing false positive interpretations. Therefore the importance of clinical and anatomic imaging correlation cannot be overemphasized.

Directing Therapy

For select malignant tumors, PET/CT has become critical to patient management prior to, during, and after therapeutic intervention. For example, for patients with many types of lymphoma, PET has been shown to be accurate for pretherapy staging, evaluating response to therapy, and detecting relapse. In the case of endometrial cancer, PET has been shown to be highly sensitive and specific for detection of tumor recurrence. In the setting of a suspected isolated colorectal cancer metastasis to the liver, PET can exclude additional hepatic lesions or detect distant metastases outside the liver that may preclude resection of the hepatic disease. With a

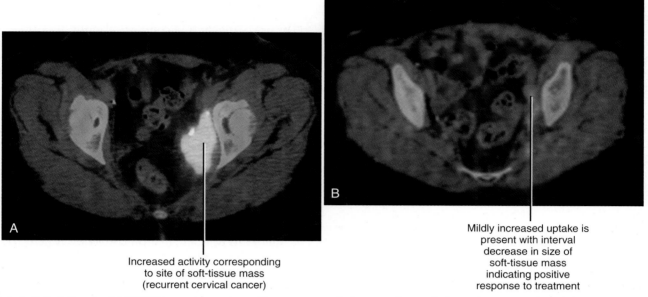

Increased activity corresponding
to site of soft-tissue mass
(recurrent cervical cancer)

Mildly increased uptake is
present with interval
decrease in size of
soft-tissue mass
indicating positive
response to treatment

Figure 4-8 A, Fused axial PET/CT image in a patient with recurrent cervical cancer after surgical resection. **B,** Fused axial PET/CT image in same patient as in **A** obtained after a course of therapy for recurrent cervical cancer shows diminished activity and smaller soft-tissue mass consistent with therapeutic response.

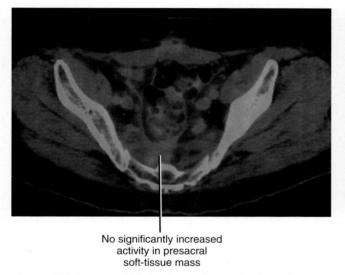

No significantly increased
activity in presacral
soft-tissue mass

Figure 4-9 Fused axial PET/CT in a patient with colorectal cancer performed after resection shows residual presacral soft-tissue mass without increased FDG activity, denoting benignity.

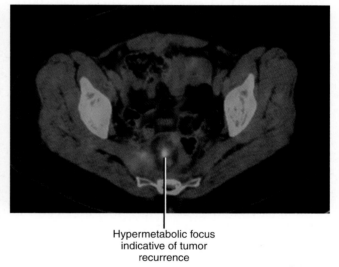

Hypermetabolic focus
indicative of tumor
recurrence

Figure 4-10 Fused axial PET/CT shows presacral focus of increased activity after surgery for colorectal cancer suspicious for tumor recurrence.

reported sensitivity for the detection of colorectal liver metastases exceeding 90%, PET may spare patients with multicentric disease major surgery. As previously alluded to, PET may also aid in distinguishing recurrent colorectal cancer from benign postoperative scarring. Of course, one cannot expect PET or PET/CT to provide all the answers regarding tumor extent and activity in all patients. If PET/CT shows equivocal lesions in the abdomen and pelvis, an exploratory laparotomy may be indicated, particularly if patient management would be significantly different depending on the nature of the lesions.

■ PROTOCOLS

Patient Preparation and Instructions

Due to physiologic handling of 18F-FDG, appropriate patient preparation is imperative prior to PET imaging. Patients fast at least 4 hrs prior to 18F-FDG injection to reduce postprandial insulin levels which, if too high, can cause high muscle uptake. This can lead to false negative PET findings, especially for small lesions. In addition, blood glucose levels are checked on every patient prior to 18F-FDG injection. At our center, a blood glucose level of less than 150 mg/dl is preferred.

Patients with blood glucose levels greater than 200 mg/dl can be scanned, with the understanding that the study may be less than optimal. Diabetic patients are instructed to eat breakfast and take insulin as they normally would on the day of the PET scan. Diabetic patients with blood glucose levels greater than 200 mg/dl are rescheduled when possible. Assistance from the patient's endocrinologist or primary caregiver is enlisted to bring the blood glucose under better control before the next PET appointment.

Because clothing and metallic objects can cause artifacts, we recommend patients change into a gown and remove jewelry prior to PET imaging. During the 45 to 60 minutes after 18-F-FDG injection and prior to PET scan, patients are instructed to sit quietly without talking, chewing, or writing. Any of these activities can cause increased physiologic uptake of 18F-FDG in the laryngeal muscles, muscles of mastication, and forearm/hand muscles, respectively. Patients are asked to void just prior to scanning to decrease excreted 18F-FDG activity in the urinary bladder.

CT Considerations

With hybrid PET/CT scanners, CT attenuation correction provides a quicker attenuation scan (~30 seconds) when compared to transmission scans (~25 minutes) on PET-only scanners. In addition, CT provides valuable anatomic correlation. CT protocol parameters that need to be considered specifically for PET/CT include patient positioning, respiration, starting point, slice thickness, tube current and energy, and IV or oral contrast.

When possible, patients are positioned with arms over their heads for both CT and PET acquisitions. This is particularly important to reduce scatter from the arms on CT and to increase sensitivity for axillary lesions (e.g., lymphoma). If patients are unable to keep their arms overhead for the entire exam, the arms are positioned in the most optimal secondary position based on region of interest of the exam. For example, with pelvic malignancy, the arms may be best positioned crossed over the upper abdomen or chest.

Respiratory motion causes artifacts and misregistration between PET and CT images. Due to the long acquisition time of PET, this scan is obtained during quiet breathing. While breath-hold protocols produce optimal lung images on CT, respiratory misregistration can cause artifacts in the lower lung fields and upper abdominal organs. Therefore, most centers perform CT during quiet breathing as well.

CT images are typically obtained from the top of the skull to mid-thigh. CT settings for PET/CT vary between institutions, but typical settings might include 0.8 second per revolution gantry speed, 6:1 pitch, 22.5 mm/sec table speed, and 140 kVp and 80 mA tube settings. If CT scans are only used for attenuation correction and low-quality anatomic localization, the tube settings may be set lower. On the other hand, if diagnostic-quality CT is desired, these tube settings may be set higher. Adjustment of these parameters for patient

weight may also be necessary. Slice thicknesses in the 2.5-mm to 5-mm range are commonly used.

The use of oral and IV contrast currently also varies by institution. In the abdomen and pelvis, dilute oral contrast prior to PET/CT can be extremely useful in differentiating masses from normal bowel. A low-density barium solution that is glucose free can be an effective oral CT contrast that causes little artifact on PET. If barium is present in the gut and thought to cause an attenuation correction artifact, this suspicion can be confirmed on non–attenuation-corrected images. IV contrast can be especially useful in correlating PET findings with anatomic imaging. CT-based attenuation correction of PET can be affected by intravenous contrast in the vasculature, causing artifactual regions of increased activity. It is therefore recommended that attenuation correction be performed using a low-radiation-dose noncontrast CT. Alternatively, if attenuation correction is performed from a contrast-enhanced CT, increased activity corresponding to vasculature can be expected by the reader. If the increased activity is truly an artifact, evaluation of non–attenuation-corrected images will show background activity in the same region overlying the vasculature.

PET Considerations

In general, the dose of 18F-FDG administered for PET imaging is 10-15 mCi injected intravenously. The amount of 18F-FDG administered to the patient will affect radiation dose to patient, scan time, and count statistics. Sites interested in high patient throughput usually use higher 18F-FDG doses and shorter scan times. PET images are obtained starting from mid-thighs to reduce the amount of excreted 18F-FDG in the bladder. A whole-body scan can be completed in 7 bed positions. (Each bed position covers approximately 15 cm at the time of this writing.) Images can be obtained in two-dimensional (2D) or three-dimensional (3D) mode. Images in 3D mode are obtained without septa in front of the detector crystal, which leads to increased sensitivity but also increased image noise. Images in 2D mode are obtained with septa in front of the crystal, take longer than 3D mode for equivalent count statistics, and have less noise.

Image Processing and Display

CT data are acquired and reconstructed into images with a 512 × 512 matrix and 50-cm field of view. CT data are applied to the PET scan using attenuation mapping algorithms. PET data are reconstructed using iterative methods on a 128 × 128 matrix and 50-cm field of view. Once processed, the images are displayed on a two-monitor workstation. Workstation users can set up display characteristics per personal preference. Images available on a typical workstation include both PET and CT in axial, sagittal, and coronal views. Maximum intensity projection (MIP) PET images, CT scout images, and fused PET/CT images are also typically available. Windowing of both PET and CT images can be performed separately. Preset windows for brain, lung, soft tissue, and bone are common. On PET, standardized uptake values (SUVs) can be set according to various parameters, such as grams, kilograms, mCi, or MBq. Attenuation measurements (HU) can also be performed on CT.

Physician Review

At the completion of the PET study, a physician often reviews the PET and CT images for artifacts and findings that may benefit from re-imaging. For example, a patient with ovarian cancer may need to have the pelvis re-imaged if a significant amount of urine activity is present in the bladder at the time of imaging. Occasionally, catheterization with instillation of normal saline may benefit interpretation of the pelvic images. If no re-imaging is required, the patient is discharged.

■ INTERPRETATION

Interpretation of PET/CT involves interpreting the PET images, CT images, and combined PET/CT data. 18F-FDG is a metabolic agent that has a different biodistribution than the extracellular contrast agents used for CT. One mistake that new PET/CT readers (particularly anatomic imagers) make is to read the CT first and then correlate the CT findings with PET data. If the PET data set is not evaluated completely, important findings may escape detection. It is likewise important that an individual interpreting PET/CT be appropriately trained in the interpretation of CT images. In highly subspecialized imaging departments, consensus interpretations between nuclear medicine experts and diagnostic radiologists may be helpful.

One effective method for reading PET/CT involves first evaluating the 3D maximum intensity projection (MIP) PET image. This allows a quick and sensitive whole-body overview of findings that will need to be characterized further. Often, this view gives a quick impression of tumor stage, directing attention to specific lesions. Higher-stage disease may not require close scrutiny of each individual lesion (e.g., diffuse lymphoma). Bone lesions are particularly conspicuous on the MIP view. It is important to note, however, that a glance at the MIP view does not obviate a more detailed review of the source data in most cases. As axial interpretation is comfortable and familiar for most readers, axial PET, axial CT, and fused axial PET/CT image interpretation is standard.

Windowing the PET intensity on a workstation can cause great variations in qualitative interpretation of PET. To increase sensitivity, it can be beneficial to over-intensify the PET images at first. This may quickly draw attention to subtle findings. However, reading the entire PET in an over-intensified window can lead to wasted time spent on spurious lesions. For example, normal hepatic heterogeneity on PET can be misconstrued as hepatic metastases if over-intensified. On the other hand, reading the PET images in an under-intensified state can lead to decreased sensitivity for lesions.

■ LIMITATIONS, ARTIFACTS, AND PITFALLS

Physiologic distribution of 18F-FDG in the abdomen and pelvis is commonly evident in the liver, spleen, bone marrow, genitalia, bowel, and urinary tract. Urinary tract activity can be dealt with in a variety of ways, including voiding, bladder catheterization, intravenous hydration, or diuretic administration. Ureteral activity may be confused with retroperitoneal lymphadenopathy, although the latter process typically appears more nodular and medially positioned. It is not unusual for ureteral activity to accumulate where the ureters cross the iliac arteries. Excretory bladder activity can obscure adjacent hypermetabolic lesions of the pelvis. Bowel activity is less predictable and may be influenced in part by bacterial concentration. The tubular appearance of bowel activity distinguishes it from most pathologic conditions. Intense localized uptake is not typical of bowel and should prompt a search of anatomic images for a corresponding mass (Figs. 4-11 and 4-12). Mildly increased activity can be present in the cecum due to normal lymphoid tissue. The liver normally has a mottled appearance on PET that should not be mistaken for diffuse metastatic disease. Unfortunately, this heterogeneity may mask small malignant lesions. In the pelvis, hypermetabolic activity can be present in the normal secretory-phase endometrium of premenopausal women, follicular phase of normal ovaries, and follicular

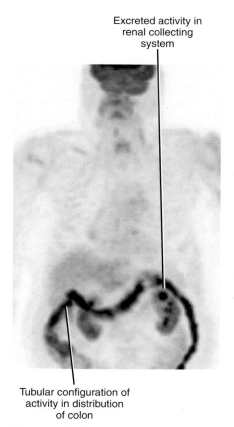

Excreted activity in
renal collecting
system

Tubular configuration of
activity in distribution
of colon

Figure 4-11 Coronal PET image shows physiologic activity in the colon and renal collecting systems.

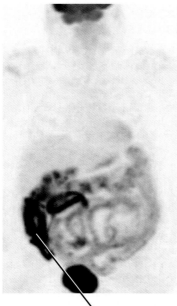

Focally increased activity in region
of right colon. Compare with colon
activity seen in Fig. 4.11

Figure 4-12 Coronal PET image shows increased pericolonic activity in the right abdomen due to lymphoma.

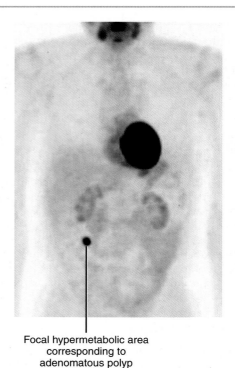

Focal hypermetabolic area
corresponding to
adenomatous polyp

Figure 4-13 Coronal PET image in a patient with adenomatous polyp of right colon.

ovarian cysts. Brown fat deposits in the neck, thorax, and abdomen can take up 18F-FDG. Retrocrural brown fat that has taken up 18F-FDG can mimic adrenal metastases. A large amount of brown fat can decrease the sensitivity and specificity of PET findings. Particularly in the case of lymphoma staging, repeating the PET after warming the patient from 45 minutes prior to 18F-FDG injection until completion of the scan can decrease brown fat activity.

Many nonmalignant pathologic changes in abdominal and pelvic organs such as ulceration, inflammation, infection, and hyperplasia can show hypermetabolic activity on PET/CT. In the colon, hyperplastic polyps, adenomatous polyps, inflammatory bowel disease, and diverticulitis all may show hypermetabolic activity (Fig. 4-13). When focal, such uptake may be confused with cancer. Mesenteric adenitis and appendicitis also may result in 18F-FDG uptake. Mildly increased activity in the stomach is common and may indicate gastritis. Pancreatitis and pancreatic cancer may be indistinguishable with PET imaging. Sacral fractures, uterine fibroids, and abscesses are additional nonmalignant entities that can show hypermetabolic activity on PET. Correlative anatomic imaging (CT, MR, or US) and careful attention to clinical details (e.g., tumor marker levels, recent surgery, biopsy, trauma, infection, or radiation therapy) are essential for distinguishing benign from malignant 18F-FDG uptake in the abdomen and pelvis.

Inflammation related to radiation therapy, biopsy, or surgical incision may result in mildly increased FDG uptake for months after treatment. Unlike residual or recurrent tumor, however, posttreatment inflammatory changes should gradually diminish or remain stable over time.

On PET, spuriously increased or decreased activity can be caused by attenuation correction errors. Common etiologies for attenuation correction errors include patient or respiratory motion between the PET acquisition and CT acquisition and dense intravenous or enteric contrast material. Review of non–attenuation-corrected PET images confirms the presence or absence of attenuation correction artifacts. Misregistration of PET and CT images may be inherent in the PET/CT hardware and should be evaluated upon acceptance testing.

Suggested Readings

Antoch G, Freudenberg LS, Beyer T, et al. To enhance or not to enhance? 18F-FDG and CT contrast agents in dual-modality 18F-FDG PET/CT. *J Nucl Med* 45:S56-S65, 2004.

Bingham JB. Where can FDG-PET contribute most to anatomical imaging problems? *Br J Radiol* 75:S39-S52, 2002.

Cohade C, Osman M, Leal J, et al. Direct comparison of (18)F-FDG PET and PET/CT in patients with colorectal carcinoma. *J Nucl Med* 44(Nov):1797-803, 2003.

Groves AM, Kayani I, Dickson JC, et al. Oral contrast medium in PET/CT: should you or shouldn't you? *Eur J Nucl Med Mol Imaging* 32:1160-1166, 2005.

Maher MM, Kalra MK, Singh A, et al. "Hot" spots in hybrid positron emission tomography/computed tomography scanning of the abdomen: protocols, indications, interpretation, responsibilities, and reimbursements. *Curr Probl Diagn Radiol* 35:35-54, 2006.

Schiepers C, Filmont JE, Czernin J. PET for staging of Hodgkin's disease and non-Hodgkin's lymphoma. *Eur J Nucl Med Mol Imaging* 30:S82-88, 2003.

Subhas N, Patel PV, Pannu HK, et al. Imaging pelvic malignancies with in-line FDG PET-CT: case examples and common pitfalls of FDG PET. *Radiographics* 25:1031-1043, 2005.

Wahl RL. Why nearly all PET of abdominal and pelvic cancers will be performed as PET/CT. *J Nucl Med* 45:S82-S95, 2004.

Zhuang H, Yu JQ, Alavi A. Applications of fluorodeoxyglucose-PET imaging in the detection of infection and inflammation and other benign disorders. *Radiol Clin North Am* 43:121-134, 2005.

CHAPTER 5

A Multidimensional Approach to Abdominal Imaging

Neal C. Dalrymple

Through development of computed tomography (CT), Geoffrey Hounsfield and Allen Cormack left a truly remarkable legacy. Part of their legacy, however, is that after CT scanners became available for clinical use in the early 1970s, many physicians began to think about human anatomy in axial sections. Previously, understanding of anatomy was learned through cadaveric and then surgical dissection, as well as physical examination. Atlases of cross-sectional anatomy were designed to act as a "translation" of sectional anatomy to the three dimensions of human anatomy and disease. Ultrasound, of course, permits sections to be obtained in virtually any plane as long as there is access or a "window" to peer through. However, the presence of intestinal gas and bone, as well as variable operator dependence, secured a significant role for CT for imaging the abdomen and pelvis despite being restricted to axial sections.

The development of magnetic resonance imaging (MRI) introduced physicians to the benefits of obtaining large data-rich sections of anatomic detail that were not limited to the axial imaging plane. Clearly, spinal imaging with MRI illustrated the advantages for some organ systems of obtaining images along the long plane or z-axis of the patient. Even with MRI, however, nonaxial imaging remained arbitrary, depending on acquisition within a prescribed imaging plane that could not be altered once the examination was complete. Although useful for predictable anatomic structures such as the spine, bones, joints, and some blood vessels, even the dimensional versatility of MRI might not image the relation between diseased and anatomic structures that are not identified during scan acquisition.

Dramatic technical improvements in CT and magnetic resonance (MR) technology now permit the acquisition of data that provide the substrate for subsequent postprocessing. Availability of this "volumetric" data allows a sort of virtual dissection at the discretion of the interpreting physician. Although conventional planes of imaging are still provided, robust data sets allow the radiologist to manipulate the imaging plane, and even the data processing algorithm, long after the patient has left the department. Thus, an initially unsuspected mass can be interrogated in multiple planes, defining relations that can help guide therapeutic decisions. Although integration of three-dimensional (3D) processing software into picture archiving and communication

systems (PACSs) is improving radiologist access to these programs during image interpretation, most image postprocessing is still performed by CT and MR technologists under the supervision of a radiologist. However, just as the captain of a ship must first learn to sail, effective use of 3D imaging techniques requires the radiologist to have an understanding of the basic principles underlying data processing techniques.

■ PIXELS AND VOXELS

Just as a masterpiece by Seurat is composed of hundreds of small independent points of color, each CT, MR, or ultrasound image is composed of hundreds of small squares that vary from black to white along a spectrum of gray. Together, these squares or *pixels* combine to comprise images that represent anatomic structures. The number of pixels used to compose each image is defined as the matrix size. For most CT examinations today, each image consists of 512 pixels in both the x- and y-planes, described as a matrix of 512×512 and yielding 262,144 pixels per image. (Remember this the next time you complain that your PACS is too slow!) The size of each pixel can be calculated easily by dividing the scan field of view (FOV) by 512. For example, for an acquisition using a 36-cm FOV, each square pixel measures 360 mm divided by 512, or 0.7 mm.

If the depth of each data component used to construct an image is considered, the square pixel is transformed into a 3D cuboid called a *voxel*. The depth or z-axis dimension of the voxel is defined by the value of the reconstructed section thickness. Until recently, virtually all CT and MR acquisitions yielded reconstructed voxels that were much thicker than the pixel size, usually by several fold. With the introduction of multidetector CT scanners (MDCT), particularly with 16 or more data channels, voxels can now be achieved routinely that are cubic in shape. Voxels with similar length in all three planes are called *isotropic*. Voxels that are not cube shaped are *anisotropic* (Fig. 5-1).

Voxel geometry has limited significance if axial sections alone comprise the total utilization of CT data. Because the voxel length in the z-axis is determined by reconstructed section thickness, voxel geometry does determine the degree of volume averaging that occurs

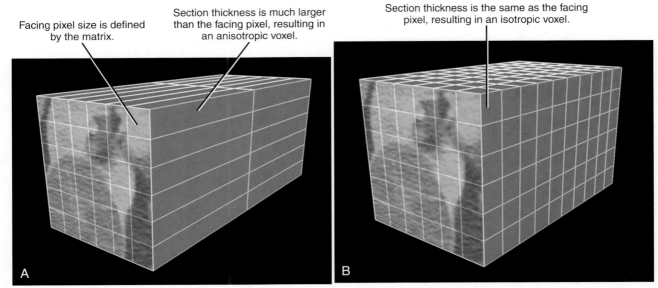

Facing pixel size is defined by the matrix.

Section thickness is much larger than the facing pixel, resulting in an anisotropic voxel.

Section thickness is the same as the facing pixel, resulting in an isotropic voxel.

Figure 5-1 **A,** Anisotropic and **(B)** isotropic voxels. Axial computed tomographic section of a renal cyst superimposed over voxels represents facing pixels of an axial image with the other surfaces showing the overall dimensions of each voxel. Image is not to scale. (Modified from Dalrymple NC, Prasad SR, Freckleton MW, Chintapalli KN: Informatics in radiology (infoRAD): introduction to the language of three-dimensional imaging with multidetector CT, *Radiographics* 25:1409-1428, 2005, by permission.)

(affecting image noise) but has minimal other impact on axial imaging. Such geometry, however, is one of the most crucial elements to successful application of nonaxial image processing. In general, these imaging applications may be divided into three main types: multiplanar reformations (MPRs), slab projections, and volume rendering.

■ MULTIPLANAR REFORMATIONS

As mentioned earlier, each axial section that comprises a CT or MR examination is created by calculating attenuation or signal values for each of its component voxels. An MPR is created by using a computer to create a new nonaxial imaging plane through the voxels of a "stacked" set of reconstructed sections. With CT, the reconstructed sections are always axial, so axial sections are stacked and a nonaxial imaging plane one voxel in thickness is defined within that volume (Fig. 5-2). With MR, the original scan data can be in any acquisition-defined imaging plane.

Choosing an Imaging Plane for Multiplanar Reformation

The additional perspective available with MPRs may be beneficial in two distinct ways: (1) improved lesion detection, and (2) lesion characterization. Lesion detection is improved when the structure does not lend itself to thorough evaluation in the axial plane. For example, because compressive deformity of vertebral bodies may be difficult to detect on axial sections, sagittal reformations can improve detection of spine fractures on routine abdominal CT scans (Fig. 5-3). Coronal and sagittal

Sagittal section created by selecting a paper-thin plane through a stack of axial sections.

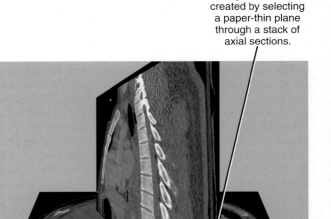

Figure 5-2 Graphic representation of how multiplanar reformations are formed. (Modified from Dalrymple NC, Prasad SR, Freckleton MW, Chintapalli KN: Informatics in radiology (infoRAD): introduction to the language of three-dimensional imaging with multidetector CT, *Radiographics* 25:1409-1428, 2005, by permission.)

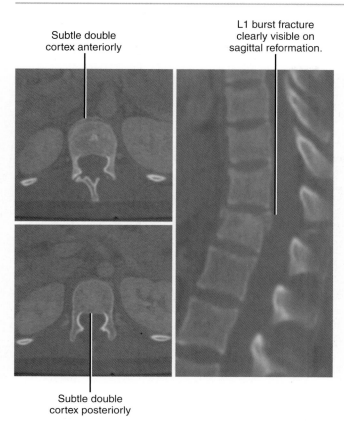

Subtle double cortex anteriorly

L1 burst fracture clearly visible on sagittal reformation.

Subtle double cortex posteriorly

Figure 5-3 Axial and sagittal computed tomographic (CT) images of a patient with an L1 burst fracture. The fracture is visible on the axial images but could be mistaken for degenerative change. Cortical disruption and loss of vertebral body height are much more conspicuous on the sagittal reformation.

MPRs are helpful for the diaphragm and the hips. In most cases, the imaging plane is flat, similar to a pane of glass inserted into the volume of data.

MPRs may facilitate lesion characterization by helping to identify the origin of a lesion or its shape. In some cases, MPRs are useful to characterize a specific lesion such as a suprarenal mass of uncertain origin. In other cases, the change in perspective may provide insight into the shape of a lesion, either providing a diagnosis or directing more specific investigation (Fig. 5-4). MPRs are also useful in lesion detection, such as locating an appendix not readily apparent on axial sections. Because the potential benefit of MPRs rests on an improved alignment between the orientation of the organ in question and the selected imaging plane, arbitrary imaging planes may not be the optimal choice. Oblique planes are those that are off-axis from standard axial, coronal, and sagittal planes. One of the most commonly prescribed oblique planes is a coronal oblique view of the abdominal aorta (Fig. 5-5). In certain cases, it is helpful to manipulate the imaging plane in real time to clarify issues raised during the interpretive session.

For focused evaluation of a curvilinear structure such as a blood vessel, an imaging plane may be defined that follows that one particular structure. This is a curved planar reformation (CPR), and the resulting image transforms a curved length of vessel, ureter, or intestine into a straight segment (Fig. 5-6). Because all other structures in the image are distorted by the curved imaging plane, CPR is useful only to investigate the structure used to define its imaging plane. Similar to MPRs, CPRs are a single voxel in depth.

■ PROJECTION TECHNIQUES

Although MPRs can provide perspective tailored to the anatomic structure or clinical question at hand, thickening the MPR into a slab of data that is two or more voxels in thickness opens the door to additional possibilities that further enhance the diagnostic value of the data (Fig. 5-7). The imaging algorithms become more complex using slabs, because utilizing the "depth" of a slab requires extrapolating a line of sight from the viewer's eye through the slab, intersecting all voxels within the slab along that specific path. If the image is rotated, the line of sight intersects different combinations of voxels as the incident angle changes. Because the line of projection determines the appearance of the resulting image, these are called *projection techniques.*

The main benefit of thickening an MPR into a slab projection is that it incorporates multiple voxels along the line of sight to determine the displayed value. This allows the user to select from among different mathematical algorithms to determine how the collection of voxel values will be processed (Fig. 5-8). Each of these types of projection processing techniques is discussed briefly in the following sections.

Maximum Intensity Projection

Maximum intensity projection (MIP) is perhaps the most well-known type of projection technique and one of the most commonly used. When MIP is used, of all the voxels intersected by a particular line of sight, only the one with the greatest value is represented in the image. This technique is effective at demonstrating continuous segments of high-attenuation or high-signal structures such as arteries opacified with intravascular contrast media or ureters filled with excreted contrast media (Fig. 5-9). Note that because high-intensity voxels are emphasized and low-attenuation voxels are ignored or deemphasized, evaluation of soft-tissue structures may be limited (Fig. 5-10), and small filling defects within a high-intensity lumen may be obscured (Fig. 5-11).

MIP first gained popularity using data from magnetic resonance angiography (MRA) but has become increasingly popular for CT applications as well. The number of images required to visualize the full length of a structure depends on the orientation and thickness of the slab, as well as how straight or tortuous the structure in question is. As with all projection techniques, the thickness and orientation of the slab are selected by the operator, and thus are likely to be of greater utility with a knowledgeable user.

Soft tissue mass identified between
the bladder and rectum

Sagittal MPR shows the mass conforms to the bladder and colon.
This unusual configuration and the patient's age and history
raised suspicion for splenosis.

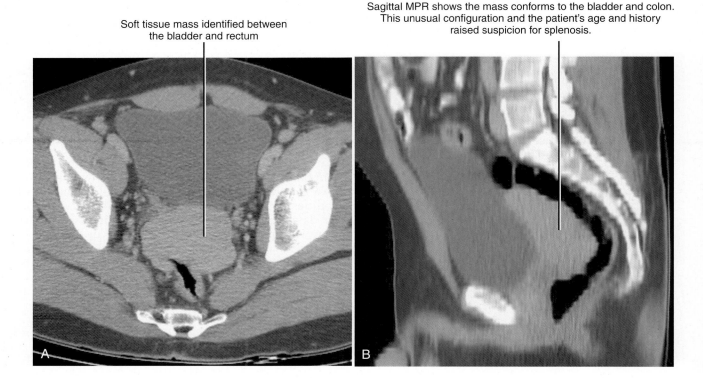

Sagittal SPECT image from damaged RBC
study confirms the mass is splenic tissue.

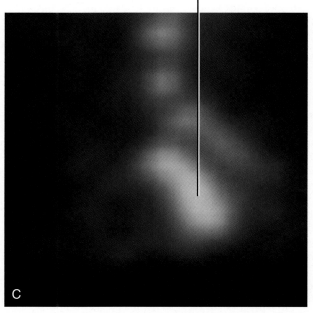

Figure 5-4 Thirty-three-year-old man with abdominal pain. Images of the upper abdomen showed a history of left nephrectomy and splenectomy for prior trauma. Pelvic malignancy was suspected on the axial images (**A**) initially, but sagittal reformations (**B**) prompted a technetium 99m (Tc-99m)–labeled heat-damaged red blood cell (RBC) study (**C**) that led to the correct diagnosis of trauma-related splenosis. *MPR*, Multiplanar reformation; *SPECT*, single-photon emission computed tomography.

Average Intensity Projection and Ray Sum

Average intensity projection (AIP) applies a different algorithm than the slab technique used by MIP. When AIP is applied to a slab, the average value of the voxels intersected by the ray of projection is used to construct the image (see Fig. 5-8). The result is an image quality similar in appearance to traditional axial sections used for CT interpretation. Similar to the way that increasing section thickness is an effective method for decreasing

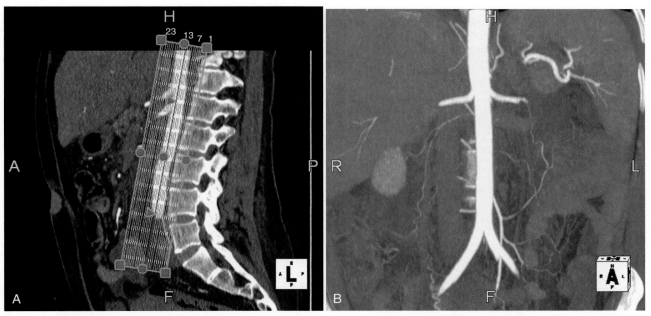

Figure 5-5 Prescribing coronal oblique images of the abdominal aorta. **A,** A sagittal image through the abdominal aorta is used to select the optimal oblique plane for the aorta. **B,** The coronal oblique maximum intensity projection image includes the entire abdominal aorta and its major branches.

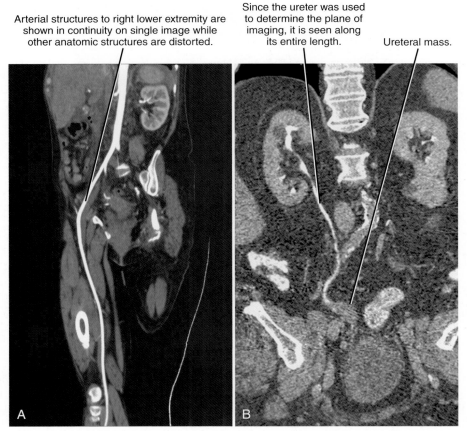

Arterial structures to right lower extremity are shown in continuity on single image while other anatomic structures are distorted.

Since the ureter was used to determine the plane of imaging, it is seen along its entire length.

Ureteral mass.

Figure 5-6 Two examples of curved planar reformations (CPRs). **A,** CPR of the abdominal aorta and contiguous arterial system to level of popliteal artery. **B,** CPR of the right ureter in a patient with urothelial carcinoma of the ureter.

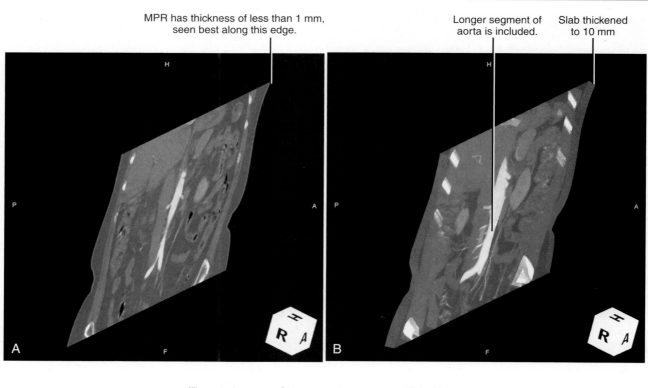

MPR has thickness of less than 1 mm, seen best along this edge.

Longer segment of aorta is included.

Slab thickened to 10 mm

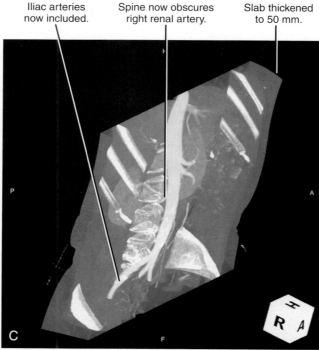

Iliac arteries now included.

Spine now obscures right renal artery.

Slab thickened to 50 mm.

Figure 5-7 A-C, Thickening a coronal multiplanar reformation (MPR) into a slab allows application of projection techniques (maximum intensity projection in this example). This image was rotated off-axis to allow visualization of the edge of the slab.

image noise, AIP uses thickening of the slab to decrease the noise that is otherwise present in many MPR images. A relatively thin AIP is less likely than MIP to obscure small filling defects within a segment of artery or ureter. However, a shorter segment of each artery or ureter is included in each image (see Figs. 5-9 and 5-10), decreasing the sense of continuity on the image.

Ray sum uses a different algorithm to achieve an appearance similar to AIP. As the name implies, when ray sum is applied, the sum of values within each

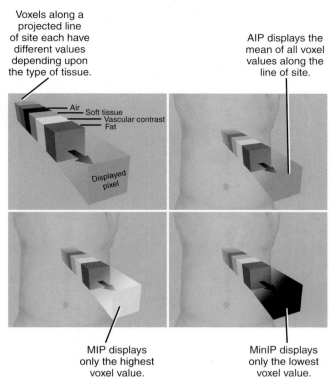

Voxels along a projected line of site each have different values depending upon the type of tissue.

AIP displays the mean of all voxel values along the line of site.

Air
Soft tissue
Vascular contrast
Fat

Displayed pixel

MIP displays only the highest voxel value.

MinIP displays only the lowest voxel value.

Figure 5-8 Graphic representation of projection techniques. *AIP*, Average intensity projection; *MinIP*, minimum intensity projection; *MIP*, maximum intensity projection. (Modified from Dalrymple NC, Prasad SR, Freckleton MW, Chintapalli KN: Informatics in radiology (infoRAD): introduction to the language of three-dimensional imaging with multidetector CT, *Radiographics* 25:1409-1428, 2005, by permission.)

voxel along a given ray of projection is used to construct the image. Although the mean is not obtained as in AIP, each voxel in the row defined by the line of sight influences the ultimate value; therefore, the overall result is similar and in most cases indistinguishable from AIP.

Minimum Intensity Projection

Minimum intensity projection (MinIP) is, in effect, the opposite of MIP. When MinIP is applied, of the voxels intersected by the ray of projection through a slab, only the lowest value along each ray is used to contrast the image (see Fig. 5-8). This technique emphasizes low-attenuation structures and is used most commonly for air-filled structures such as airways or regions of air trapping within the lung, although it is occasionally useful to evaluate fat or fluid within a high-attenuation object. The utility of MinIP can be illustrated by comparing the effects of MinIP with MIP and AIP techniques on the appearance of a segment of bowel with pneumatosis (Fig. 5-12). Because abnormal air can usually be detected on axial source images, MinIP is not usually necessary. However, it can be applied to increase sensitivity for small amounts of air when suspected or to further characterize indeterminate low-attenuation foci.

■ VOLUME RENDERING

Volume rendering was first developed to improve animation for entertainment. By entering 3D data into a computer and designing algorithms to render the data

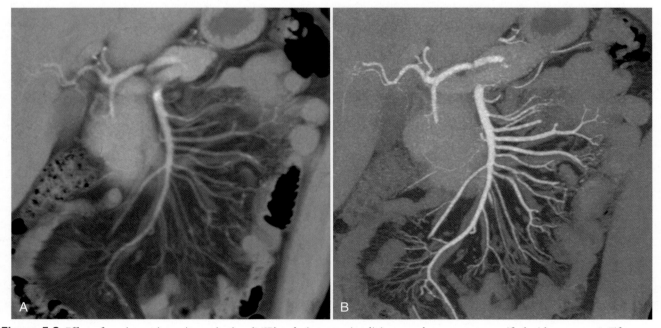

Figure 5-9 Effect of maximum intensity projection (MIP) technique on visualizing vascular structures opacified with contrast. **A,** Fifteen-millimeter slab image using ray sum. **B,** Same 15-mm slab using MIP displays greater detail of superior mesenteric artery and its branches.

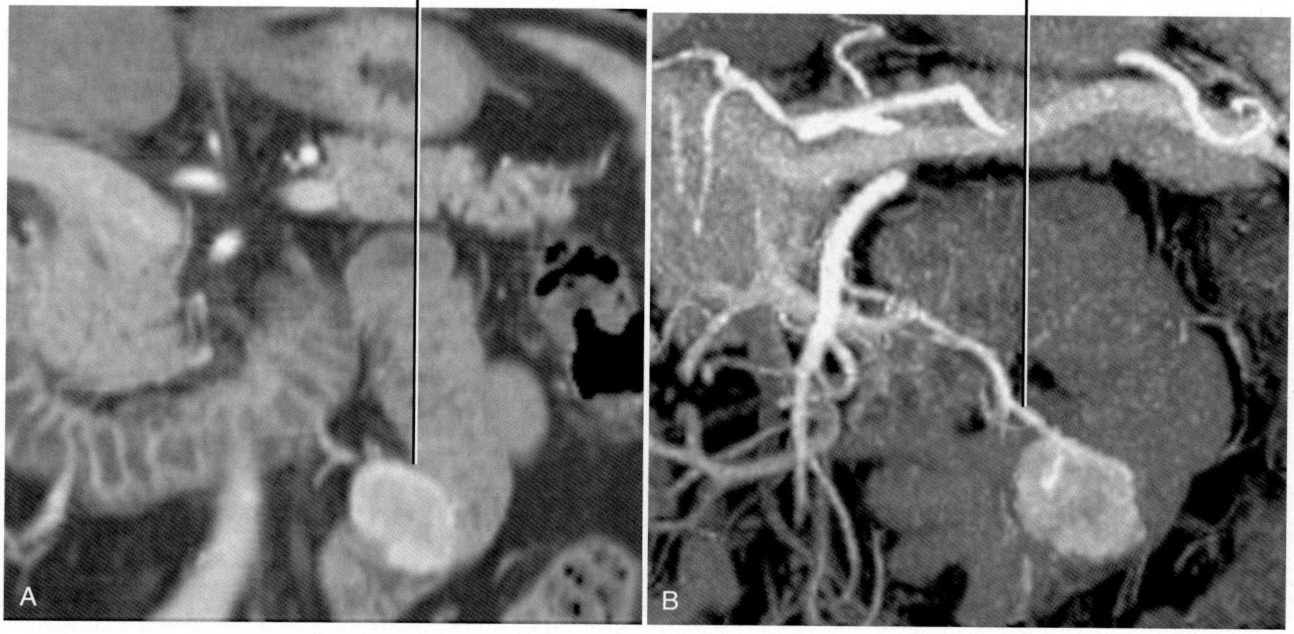

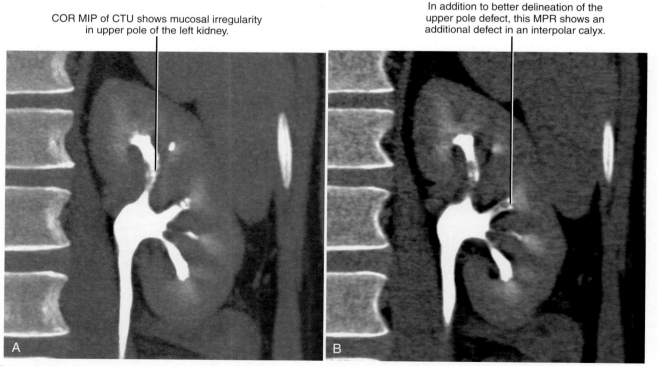

Coronal AIP image shows enhancing soft tissue mass arising from wall of the proximal jejunum. Notice mucosal folds are visible.

MIP image shows vessels supplying the mass to its origin from the SMA. However, bowel wall detail is no longer visible.

Figure 5-10 Coronal computed tomographic images of jejunal mass surgically proven to be gastrointestinal stromal tumor. **A,** Average intensity projection and **(B)** maximum intensity projection (MIP). *AIP,* Average intensity projection; *SMA,* superior mesenteric artery.

COR MIP of CTU shows mucosal irregularity in upper pole of the left kidney.

In addition to better delineation of the upper pole defect, this MPR shows an additional defect in an interpolar calyx.

Figure 5-11 "Blooming" of maximum intensity projection *(MIP)* image obscures filling defects. Coronal *(COR)* MIP **(A)** and multiplanar reformation *(MPR)* **(B)** images from excretory phase of computed tomographic urogram *(CTU).*

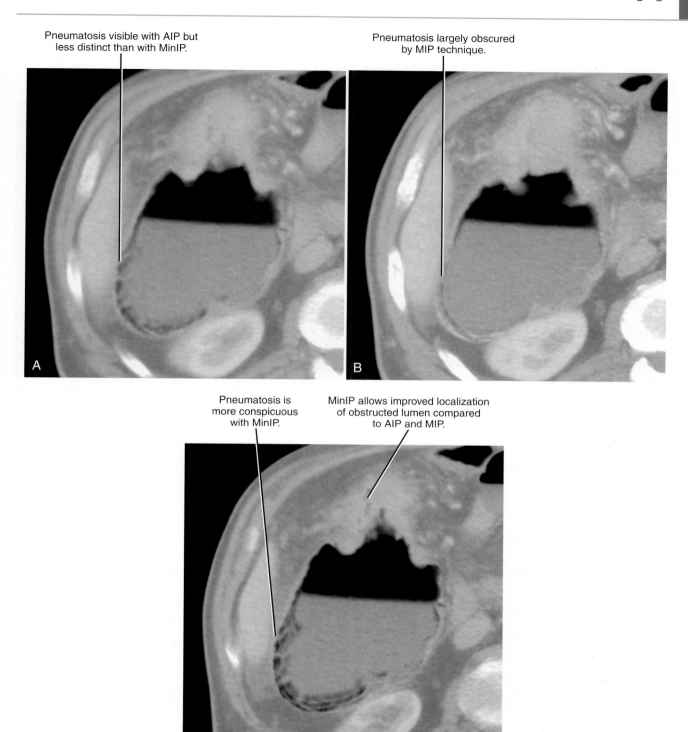

Pneumatosis visible with AIP but less distinct than with MinIP.

Pneumatosis largely obscured by MIP technique.

Pneumatosis is more conspicuous with MinIP.

MinIP allows improved localization of obstructed lumen compared to AIP and MIP.

Figure 5-12 Axial sections of a patient with colonic pneumatosis caused by malignant obstruction displayed in **(A)** average intensity projection *(AIP)*, **(B)** maximum intensity projection *(MIP)*, and **(C)** minimum intensity projection *(MinIP)*.

so that the computer recognized and treated data as 3D objects, lifelike spatial relations, motion, and shading could be accomplished, and computer animation was born. The first volume-rendered animated short film was released in 1984, and tremendous computing power was required to generate only 4 minutes of film. Several years later, medical image data were entered into the

Pixar computers used to create the evolving computer-generated animation, and medical volume rendering was born.

Although the technique appeared promising, the sophisticated computers required for rendering were not widely available, limiting access to rendering technology. In just over a decade, however, computers have advanced to the point that volume rendering can be performed on a home personal computer.

Early attempts had already been made at 3D imaging; the most common by the early 1990s was shaded surface display (SSD). However, the SSD technique had limited potential because only surface-defining data were included in the binary application, yielding an image reflecting only the outer shell of a structure (Fig. 5-13). After the outer surface of a structure has been defined, no other information can be added or subtracted.

Volume rendering revolutionized 3D imaging by including all data within a data set to generate an image (Fig. 5-14). Segmentation profiles are applied to categorize tissues according to their attenuation (air, water, soft tissue, contrast, bone). Combining variable attenuation value ranges to a variable number of tissue settings provides a virtually unlimited number of color/opacity schemes that may be utilized. These are available on commercial 3D systems as templates that provide rapid adjustments to achieve images useful for the desired task (e.g., analysis of vessels, the colon, or the airways), although images may be refined further with user-defined adjustments.

Tissue segmentation can also be used to isolate portions of the image that are of particular interest. For example, automated programs can be used to either remove bone or to add only the contrast-opacified vessels of interest (Fig. 5-15).

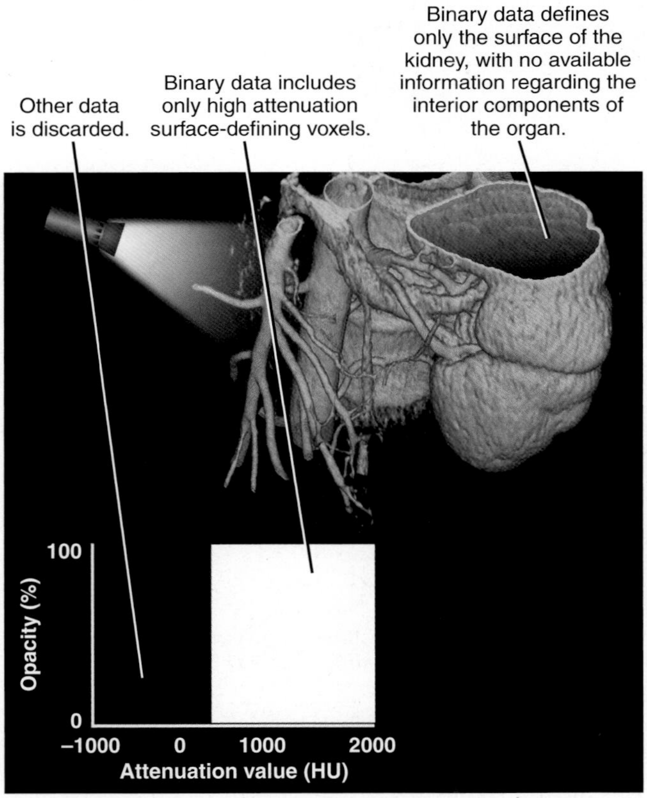

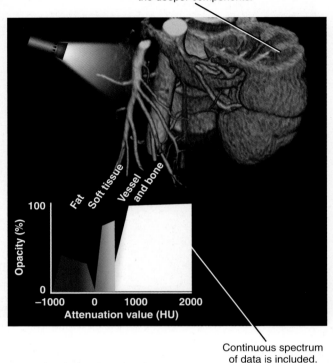

Complete spectrum of data means that even when image settings are adjusted to display the surface of the organ, data is available to permit virtual dissection of the deeper components.

Continuous spectrum of data is included.

Figure 5-14 Volume rendering of the left kidney and central abdominal blood vessels. (Modified from Dalrymple NC, Prasad SR, Freckleton MW, Chintapalli KN: Informatics in radiology (infoRAD): introduction to the language of three-dimensional imaging with multidetector CT, *Radiographics* 25:1409-1428, 2005, by permission.)

Binary data defines only the surface of the kidney, with no available information regarding the interior components of the organ.

Binary data includes only high attenuation surface-defining voxels.

Other data is discarded.

Figure 5-13 Shaded surface display of the left kidney and central abdominal blood vessels. (Modified from Dalrymple NC, Prasad SR, Freckleton MW, Chintapalli KN: Informatics in radiology (infoRAD): introduction to the language of three-dimensional imaging with multidetector CT, *Radiographics* 25:1409-1428, 2005, by permission.)

Although volume rendering is usually used to provide perspective to abnormalities seen initially on 2D images, volume rendering can also be used to improve lesion detection or characterization. Because of its ability to define the boundary between air and the wall of a distended colon, polypoid lesions are often more conspicuous on virtual colonoscopic images than on 2D images. Because of the sensitivity of volume rendering to subtle differences in attenuation, differences in organ or lesion perfusion may be more conspicuous on volume rendering than on axial or multiplanar 2D images (Figs. 5-16 and 5-17).

Orthographic volume rendering is the most common type of rendering used in medical imaging. An orthographic rendering is similar to a statue on display in a museum (Fig. 5-18). The image can be rotated in space, or made larger or smaller, without distortion of the anatomic perspective.

Perspective volume rendering uses distortion of the image to simulate the appearance of fiberoptic endoscopy (Fig. 5-19). Virtual colonoscopy, virtual cystoscopy, and virtual bronchoscopy create images similar to the appearance of the respective anatomy through an endoscope or bronchoscope. The main purpose for simulation is to enhance the intuitive nature of

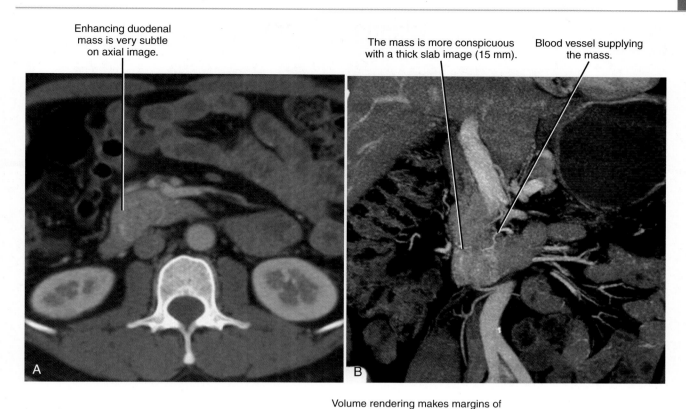

Enhancing duodenal
mass is very subtle
on axial image.

The mass is more conspicuous
with a thick slab image (15 mm).

Blood vessel supplying
the mass.

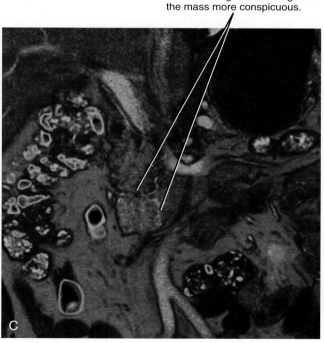

Volume rendering makes margins of
the mass more conspicuous.

Figure 5-17 Lesion conspicuity demonstrated on axial reconstruction (**A**), coronal maximum intensity projection (MIP) image (**B**), and slab volume rendering (**C**) of a duodenal carcinoma.

distinguish bowel strictures from normal peristalsis, or detect tethered loops of bowel indicating intraabdominal adhesions. Persistently dilated bowel can be demonstrated proximal to strictures with these techniques (Fig. 5-23).

Temporal Evaluation of Physiologic Stress

Some conditions simply cannot be detected reliably using typical cross-sectional imaging techniques. Abdominal hernias are perhaps the most commonly

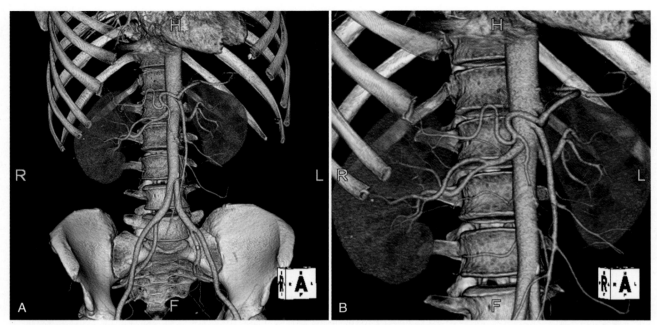

Figure 5-18 Orthographic volume rendering of abdominal-pelvic computed tomographic angiogram. Full view **(A)** and close-up **(B)** views result in different viewing angles and degrees of magnification without distortion of the object.

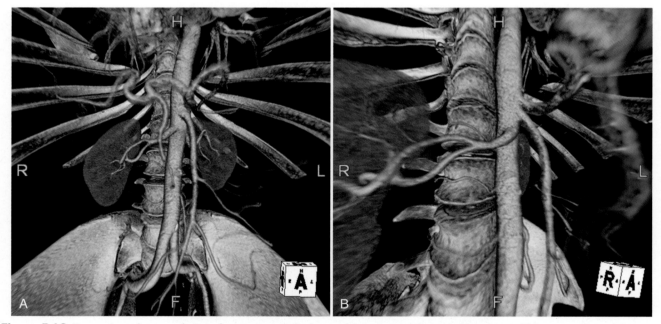

Figure 5-19 Perspective volume rendering of same computed tomographic angiogram shown in Figure 5-18. Objects near the periphery are distorted less near the center of view to simulate fiberoptic endoscopy/laparoscopy. This results in different types of distortion on far **(A)** and close-up **(B)** views.

encountered example. Although thin-section MDCT examinations allow identification of most of the fascial defects that allow herniation of abdominal contents, the size of the defect and its usual contents may be underestimated in the supine position at rest. When evaluating a known or suspected abdominal wall hernia with CT, performing acquisitions with Valsalva

maneuver may improve characterization of hernia size and contents (Fig. 5-24).

Evaluation of the female pelvic floor for laxity has been challenging over the years. Fluoroscopic evaluation requires opacification of the bladder, rectum, and small intestine to allow identification of cysto-cele, rectocele, and enterocele. Real-time fluoroscopic

In the arterial phase, there is a small amount of peripheral nodular enhancement.

Contrast enhancement fills toward the center in the portal venous phase.

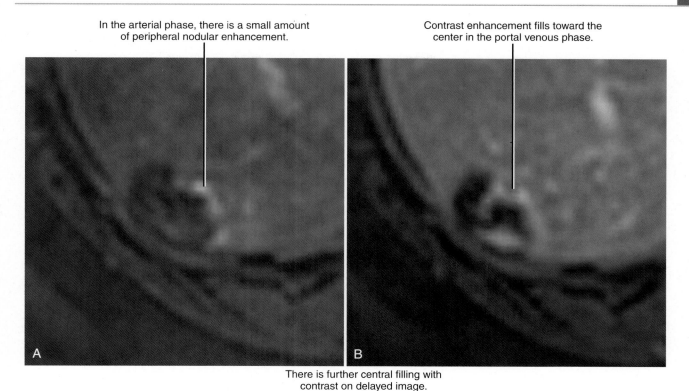

There is further central filling with contrast on delayed image.

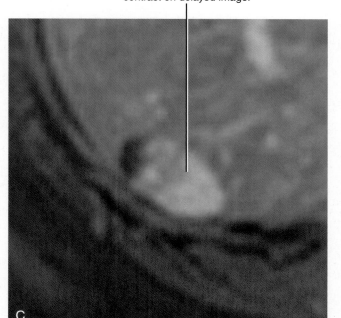

Figure 5-20 Dynamic contrast-enhanced magnetic resonance image of a cavernous hemangioma of the liver in the arterial (**A**), portal venous (**B**), and delayed (**C**) phases of enhancement.

examination provides high temporal resolution but requires an experienced operator to identify abnormal changes in the relations between opacified viscera and osseous landmarks of the pelvis. Rapid MR acquisition in the sagittal plane at rest and during stress provides additional detailed information regarding the soft-tissue structures of the pelvis and perineum (Fig. 5-25).

■ SPECIFIC THREE-DIMENSIONAL APPLICATIONS

Computed Tomographic and Magnetic Resonance Angiography

Noninvasive vascular imaging has replaced diagnostic catheter-directed angiography for many clinical applications. This is the result of simultaneous evolutions in

Oval structures within the renal sinus of both kidneys are of uncertain significance in the early excretory phase of enhancement.

Dense opacification during the arterial phase shows these structures to be bilateral renal AVMs.

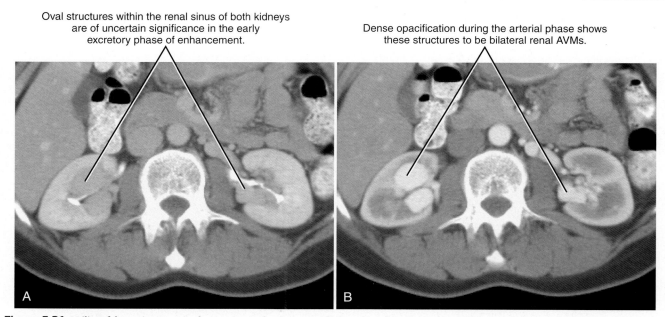

Figure 5-21 Utility of dynamic contrast enhancement in the diagnosis of bilateral renal arteriovenous malformations *(AVMs)*. **(A)** Excretory phase and **(B)** arterial phase images from multiphase enhanced computed tomography examination demonstrate the transient nature of vascular enhancement.

Columnization of urine above small ureteral stone

Mild hydronephrosis

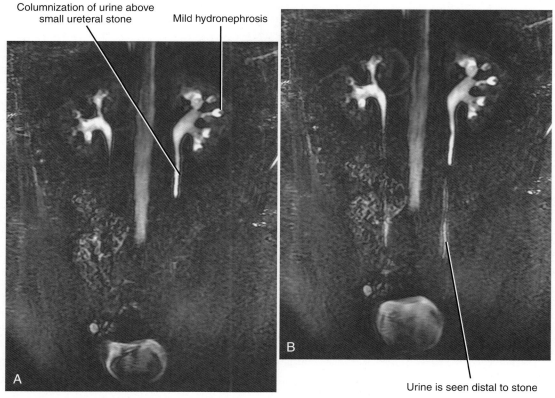

Urine is seen distal to stone

Figure 5-22 Two successive coronal T2-weighted magnetic resonance urogram images **(A, B)** of a patient with a small left ureteral calculus demonstrating columnization of urine within the left proximal ureter. A small amount of urine can be seen distal to the stone **(B)**, excluding complete obstruction. (From Leyendecker JR, Childs DD: Kidneys and MR urography. Magn Reson Imaging Clin N Am 2007 Aug;15(3):373-382, vii, by permission.)

scanner technology allowing rapid scan acquisition (optimizing use of a given contrast bolus and minimizing patient motion) and in 3D image processing software. There is no doubt that large anatomic regions can now be imaged with excellent spatial resolution. However, computed tomographic angiographic (CTA) and MRA examinations can generate thousands of images. Image processing has the potential of decreasing image interpretation time whereas also improving diagnostic accuracy.

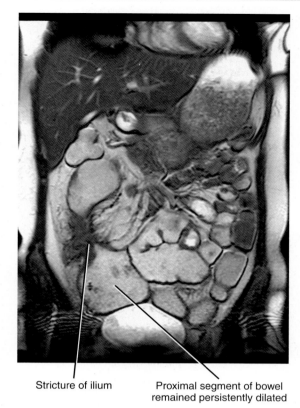

Stricture of ilium   Proximal segment of bowel
                            remained persistently dilated

Figure 5-23 Coronal steady state free precession image of a patient with Crohn disease demonstrating a small bowel stricture in the right lower quadrant. Twenty-five individual images of this area were performed in succession (approximately 1 frame/sec). However, the narrowing and the proximal bowel distention remained unchanged.

MPRs offer several advantages over axial images. Because few vessels are seen in-plane on axial images, coronal, sagittal, and oblique MPR images allow visualization of longer segments of most vascular structures in the abdomen and pelvis. Because sections are typically less than 1 mm for CTA, only minimal volume averaging occurs, and calcified plaque is thus unlikely to obscure the residual lumen of a high-grade stenosis (Fig. 5-26).

The advantages of MPR can be enhanced by tailoring the image plane to specific vessels. Many vendors offer vessel analysis packages that ask the operator to place a cursor in several defined regions to generate a predictable CPR of a vessel. This allows in-depth interrogation of that vessel and often includes automated features to allow comparison with an orthogonal view. This provides an image axial to the vessel itself (Fig. 5-27). Although the validity of measuring stenoses using most of these packages is not scientifically proved, they do provide perspective that enhances the multiplanar evaluation of the vessel.

One potential disadvantage of MPR is that the image noise inherent in thin sections may make intermediate density lesions difficult to identify by CT, particularly if the contrast bolus is suboptimal. Image noise can be improved by using a thin-slab AIP or raysum image, although these techniques introduce volume averaging, which can affect plaque evaluation.

MIP allows visualization of long vascular segments without requiring designation of a curved imaging plane. This is particularly useful in MRA because most of the nonvascular structures are of low signal intensity, allowing long vascular segments to be displayed without interference from calcium or bone. Remember that, even with a good-quality, thick-slab MIP, orthogonal views are necessary because stenoses can be obscured in a single imaging plane (Fig. 5-28).

Because calcium typically has a greater attenuation value than vascular contrast media, it will be displayed in preference to vessel lumen on MIP images created from CT data. Thus, with CTA, the spine can obscure the abdominal aorta on a thick-slab MIP image despite excellent contrast bolus timing (Fig. 5-29). Likewise, MIP can allow the calcium of a high-grade lesion to obscure the lumen entirely (see Fig. 5-26). This does not eliminate the utility of MIP in the interpretation of CTA, provided MPR or original axial views are consulted.

Volume rendering provides the most exciting and realistic appearing images of CTA and MRA acquisitions, but these images are usually less useful than MPR or MIP images when attempting to characterize a particular stenosis. In fact, caution must be used when attempting to characterize a stenosis with volume rendering because volume rendering settings can affect the appearance significantly (Fig. 5-30). Three-dimensional volume-rendered images can be useful in planning a surgical or transcatheter intervention; however, MPR or projection views provide more accurate information regarding the degree of stenosis or length of vessel involved.

Computed Tomographic and Magnetic Resonance Urography

CT and MR urography bring the advantages of cross-sectional imaging to the evaluation of the urinary tract. Although T2-weighted images can provide evaluation of the urinary tract without contrast media, contrast-enhanced images are an important component of both MR and CT urography. With both techniques, signal-to-noise ratio between excreted contrast media and adjacent soft tissues proves to be advantageous to many image-processing techniques. MIP is commonly used to allow visualization of long segments of the ureter. Areas of apparent ureteral stenosis or mass can then be further evaluated using corresponding axial or MPR images (Fig. 5-31).

Despite the many advantages of CT, limiting evaluation to a single imaging plane can be problematic. Small renal masses that enhance similar to renal cortex can be overlooked when located at the superior or inferior pole. Although polar masses are better seen on sagittal and coronal images (Fig. 5-32), anterior and posterior masses are not seen well on coronal images. Lesion detection is improved only when orthogonal planes are viewed in each case.

Early concerns about CT urography focused on its ability to detect collecting system abnormalities such as papillary necrosis or longitudinal abnormalities of the ureter.

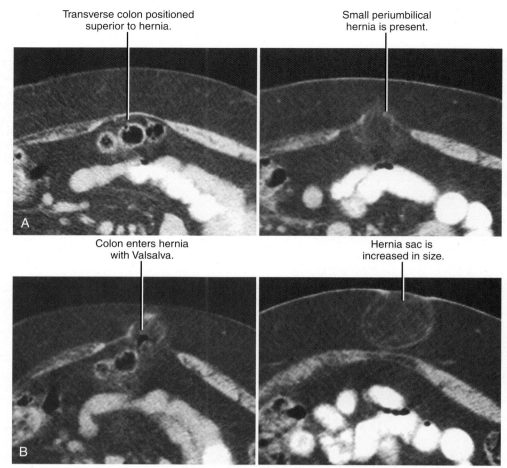

Transverse colon positioned superior to hernia.

Small periumbilical hernia is present.

Colon enters hernia with Valsalva.

Hernia sac is increased in size.

Figure 5-24 Computed tomography of periumbilical region performed first without **(A)** and then with **(B)** Valsalva maneuver shows the impact of physiologic stress on imaging findings.

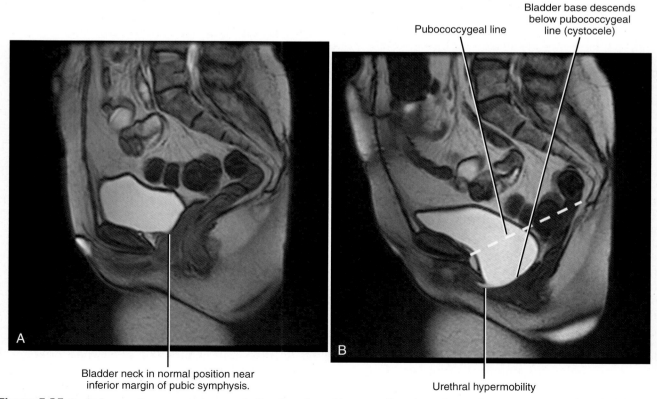

Pubococcygeal line

Bladder base descends below pubococcygeal line (cystocele)

Bladder neck in normal position near inferior margin of pubic symphysis.

Urethral hypermobility

Figure 5-25 Sagittal magnetic resonance images of a female patient with stress urinary incontinence. Images were acquired at rest **(A)** and during Valsalva maneuver **(B)**. A total of 25 images were performed in less than 30 seconds during straining.

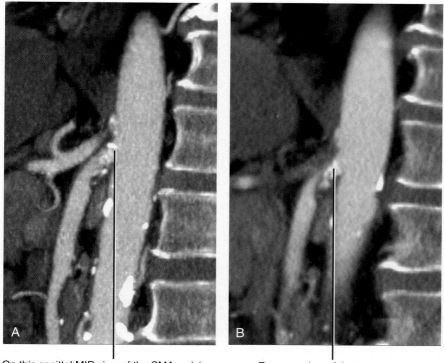

On this sagittal MIP view of the SMA, calcium appears to nearly occlude the origin.

Ray sum view of the same area shows no visible patent lumen.

Sagittal MPR view shows a thin patent lumen.

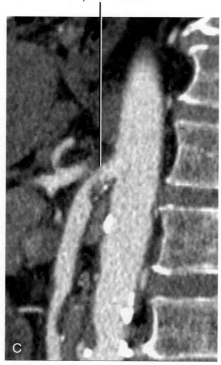

Figure 5-26 Comparison of 5-mm-thick slab maximum intensity projection *(MIP)* **(A)** and ray sum **(B)** to multiplanar reformation *(MPR)* **(C)** of same sagittal section from computed tomographic angiogram shows impact of these techniques on evaluation of plaque at the origin of the superior mesenteric artery *(SMA)*.

CPR shows blue
line indicating level
of orthogonal axial
evaluation at level of
plaque in proximal SMA.

Orthogonal section
automatically
calculates
diameter at level
of stenosis.

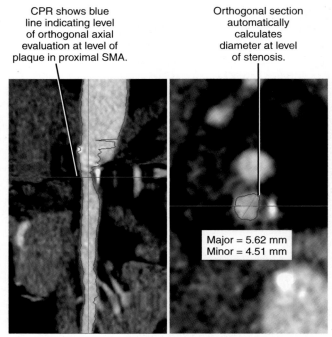

Major = 5.62 mm
Minor = 4.51 mm

Figure 5-27 Vessel analysis package applied to same case as Figure 5-26 demonstrates automated generation of orthogonal sections based on curved planar reformation *(CPR)*. *SMA,* Superior mesenteric artery.

In most cases, long-axis (usually coronal) MIP or AIP images show these abnormalities well. Despite lower spatial resolution compared with plain radiography, the improved contrast resolution of CT often shows small urothelial lesions, papillary necrosis, and medullary sponge kidney with greater conspicuity than conventional urography (Fig. 5-33).

Although images are acquired at fewer points in time than with conventional urography, temporally spaced acquisitions are an essential component of CT urography. Dynamic patterns of enhancement aid in the characterization of renal lesions, and changes in the urinary tract over time are useful in characterizing lesions such as calyceal diverticula and renal sinus cysts (Fig. 5-34).

Whether image postprocessing is performed by a technologist or a radiologist, it is important to remember that basic principles of image review remain similar to review of traditional axial sections. Although this may not seem to require particular mention, it is tempting to accept postprocessed images "as is" and to overlook the potential benefits of further manipulation of window and level settings on the PACS. With CT urography, it is of particular importance to use window and level settings similar to bone windows when looking at detailed structures of the urinary tract in the excretory phase (Fig. 5-35). Although soft-tissue windows provide information regarding the renal parenchyma and adjacent organs, calyceal detail may be obscured.

Computed Tomographic Colonography

Computed tomographic colonography (CTC) offers several advantages over fiberoptic endoscopy in screening patients for colon cancer. It is less invasive, requiring only insufflation of the colon with air through a rectal tube. Because no sedation is required, there is minimal

Coronal image shows irregular
plaque but no focal stenosis

Sagittal image in same location shows plaque pedunculated
from posterior wall of common iliac artery.

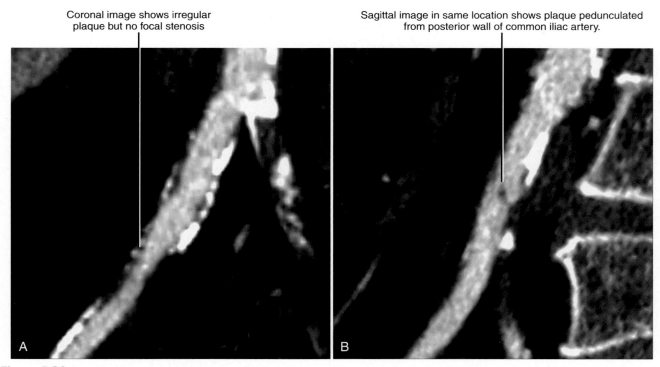

Figure 5-28 Coronal (**A**) and sagittal (**B**) images from computed tomographic angiography of the iliac arteries demonstrate the utility of viewing orthogonal images.

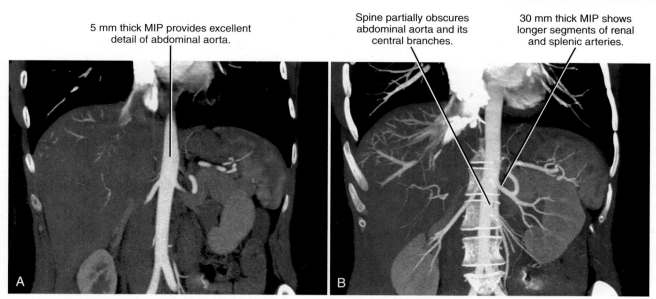

5 mm thick MIP provides excellent detail of abdominal aorta.

Spine partially obscures abdominal aorta and its central branches.

30 mm thick MIP shows longer segments of renal and splenic arteries.

Figure 5-29 Obscuration of the abdominal aorta by the spine when using thick-slab technique with computed tomographic angiography. Thin **(A)** and thick **(B)** slabs are provided for comparison. *MIP,* Maximum intensity projection.

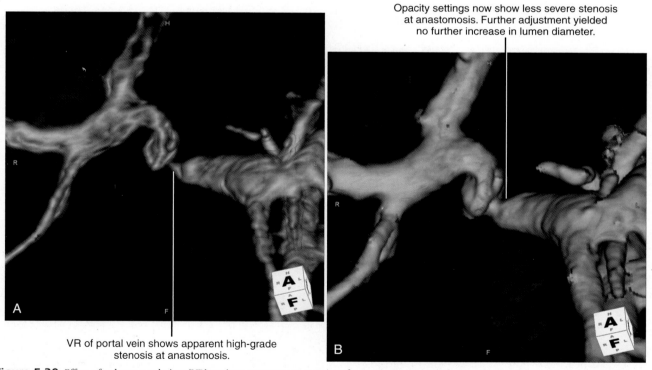

Opacity settings now show less severe stenosis at anastomosis. Further adjustment yielded no further increase in lumen diameter.

VR of portal vein shows apparent high-grade stenosis at anastomosis.

Figure 5-30 Effect of volume-rendering *(VR)* settings on apparent severity of stenosis on computed tomography of the portal vein on a liver transplant patient with suspected portal vein stenosis. The same data viewed with different opacity settings in **A** and **B** result in a marked difference in the appearance of stenosis. Multiplanar reformations confirmed only mild stenosis at the anastomosis (not shown).

time spent setting up the procedure, and no recovery time is required. Provided an adequate colon preparation is performed, CTC reliably identifies polyps and other colon masses, allowing for effective cancer screening in patients who are at low risk for development of colon cancer. CTC also provides an alternative method for evaluating the proximal colon when conventional colonoscopy is incomplete. Because of limited sensitivity of CTC for flat lesions and a greater prevalence of such lesions in high-risk patients, fiberoptic examination is preferred in this patient population.

The key to successful CTC is an adequate interface between air and the colon wall. With proper insufflation, polyps protrude from the wall into the air-filled

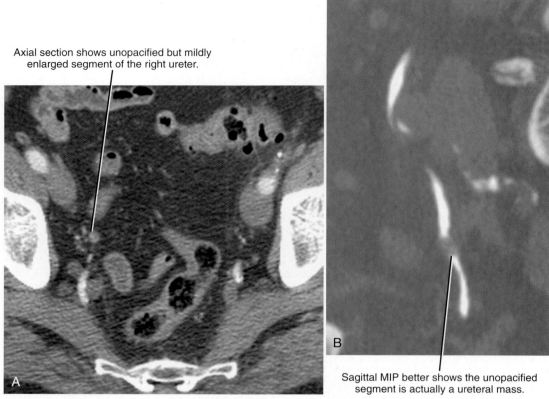

Axial section shows unopacified but mildly enlarged segment of the right ureter.

B

Sagittal MIP better shows the unopacified segment is actually a ureteral mass.

A

Figure 5-31 Multiplanar evaluation of the ureter. Axial source image **(A)** and coronal maximum intensity projection *(MIP)* image **(B)** of a mass in the right ureter. This was proved to be urothelial carcinoma.

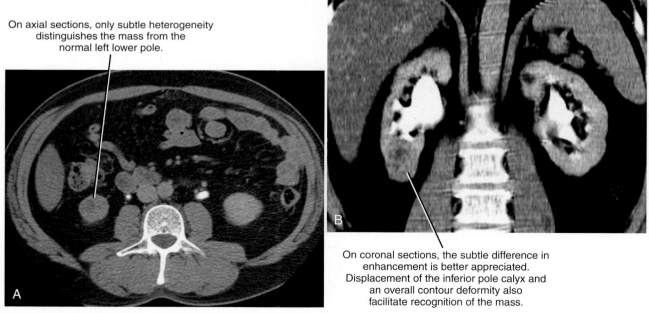

On axial sections, only subtle heterogeneity distinguishes the mass from the normal left lower pole.

B

On coronal sections, the subtle difference in enhancement is better appreciated. Displacement of the inferior pole calyx and an overall contour deformity also facilitate recognition of the mass.

A

Figure 5-32 Improved detection of polar renal masses using orthogonal imaging planes. Axial **(A)** and coronal **(B)** images from a computed tomographic urogram each show renal cell carcinoma in the inferior pole of the right kidney.

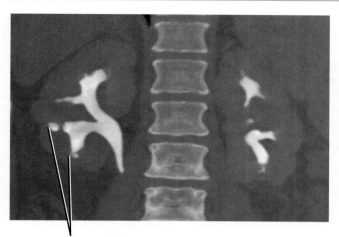

Collections of contrast in
the renal papillae are
readily identified on
MIP images.

Figure 5-33 Detection of papillary necrosis on computed tomographic urography. *MIP,* Maximum intensity projection.

lumen (Fig. 5-36). Because most polyps are relatively small and might be overlooked on soft-tissue settings, use of window and level settings closer to those used for lung or bone improves sensitivity. Because polyps may lay flat against the colon wall when dependent, scan acquisition is performed with the patient in the supine and prone positions. Repositioning the patient also

helps to distinguish retained fecal material from mucosal lesions, because fecal material often dramatically changes position between acquisitions (Fig. 5-37). Caution must be applied, however, because pedunculated polyps can change position although the stalk remains attached.

Most diagnoses can be made by reviewing images in a 2D mode, with supine and prone acquisitions displayed synchronously side by side. Certainly, review of 2D source and multiplanar images are a key step to identifying abnormalities deep to the mucosa (Figs. 5-38 and 5-39). Two-dimensional image review also provides an opportunity to diagnose extracolonic findings. In some cases of CTC performed after failed fiberoptic colonoscopy, the 2D images provide an explanation for the failed procedure, such as the presence of colon in a ventral or inguinal hernia (Fig. 5-40).

Effective interpretation of CTC requires effective integration of multiple types of 3D techniques (Fig. 5-41). MPRs provide a good overview of colonic anatomy, 2D evaluation of the colonic wall including mucosal surface and wall thickness, as well as inspection of extracolonic structures. The endoluminal view provided by perspective volume rendering encourages a detailed inspection of the mucosal surface for polyps. An air-highlighted orthographic volume rendering of the insufflated colon facilitates localization during endoluminal survey. Orthographic volume renderings with various forms of automated dissection allow 3D manipulation of specific findings, often helpful in characterizing specific lesions (Fig. 5-42).

Fluid in the renal sinus has the
appearance of hydronephrosis.

Unopacified fluid can be
diagnosed as renal sinus
cysts with confidence.

Components of the renal collecting
system are opacified with
excreted contrast.

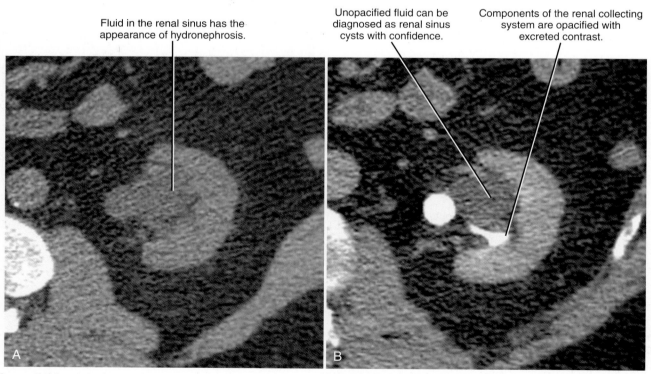

Figure 5-34 Enhancement of the urinary tract defines the presence of renal sinus cysts. Images shown in the precontrast **(A)** and excretory **(B)** phases.

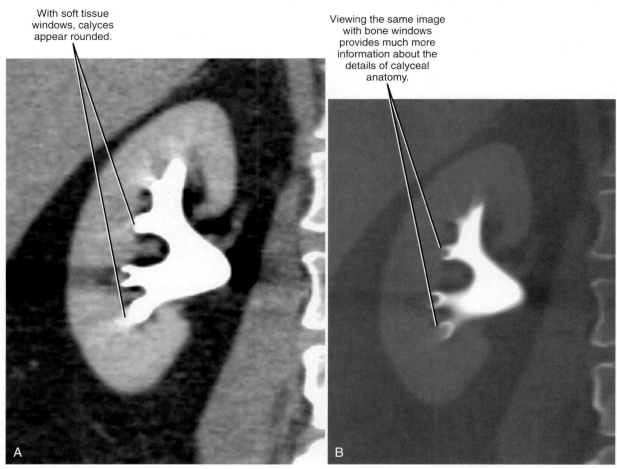

With soft tissue windows, calyces appear rounded.

Viewing the same image with bone windows provides much more information about the details of calyceal anatomy.

A

B

Figure 5-35 Importance of adjusting window and level settings on postprocessed images. Coronal maximum intensity projection (MIP) image of computed tomographic urography in excretory phase displayed with soft-tissue **(A)** and bone **(B)** windows.

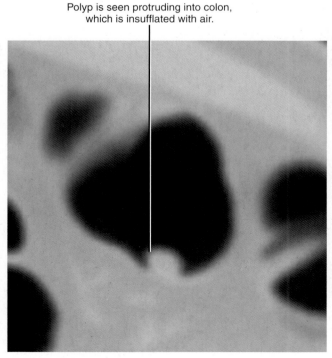

Polyp is seen protruding into colon, which is insufflated with air.

Figure 5-36 Appearance of polyp on two-dimensional images from computed tomographic colonography.

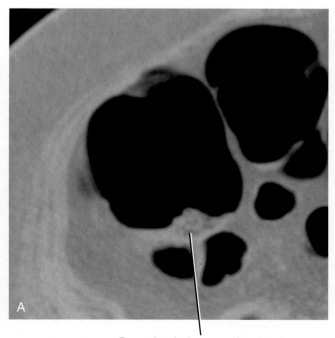

A

Dependent lesion on supine views. Mottled appearance suggests feces.

Figure 5-37 Role of patient repositioning in identifying retained fecal material. Axial images from computed tomographic colonography examination with patient supine **(A)** *(cont'd)*

Lesion moves to opposite side on prone
view, confirming retained fecal material.

Axial section shows nodule
of soft tissue attenuation
within a diverticulum

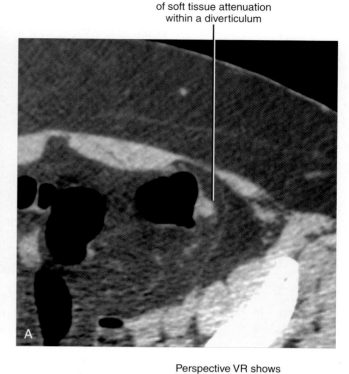

Figure 5-37, cont'd. and prone (**B**).

Coronal image of the
sigmoid colon shows an
annular lesion with wall
thickening.

Breath hold scan
misregistration due to
single detector CT
acquisition.

Perspective VR shows
air-filled diverticulum.

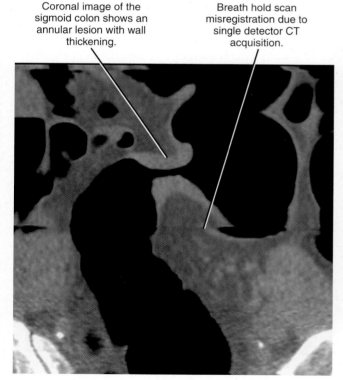

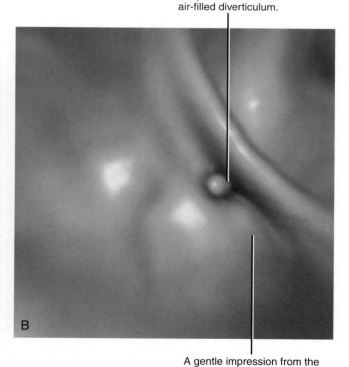

A gentle impression from the
mass-filled diverticulum could
easily be overlooked.

Figure 5-38 Two-dimensional images of computed tomographic
(CT) colonography allow the reader to identify wall thickening in a
collapsed segment, indicating a mass is present. Colon carcinoma
was confirmed at colonoscopy.

Figure 5-39 Material within diverticulum on two-dimensional
source images (**A**) and perspective volume rendering *(VR)* (**B**). Although this proved ultimately to be fecal material, a mass could
have a similar appearance.

Sigmoid colon within left
inguinal hernia

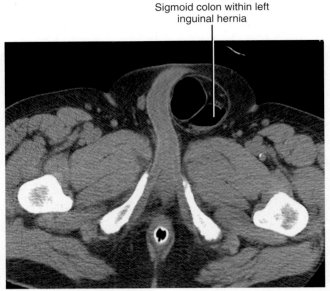

Figure 5-40 Axial image from computed tomographic colonography examination performed for incomplete colonoscopy because of "tortuous sigmoid colon." Two-dimensional review demonstrates a segment of sigmoid colon within a left inguinal hernia, accounting for failed colonoscopy. This finding was not apparent on the endoluminal view.

Coronal MPR of ascending colon
provides overview of the region.

Endoluminal view provides detailed
survey of the interior surface
of the colon.

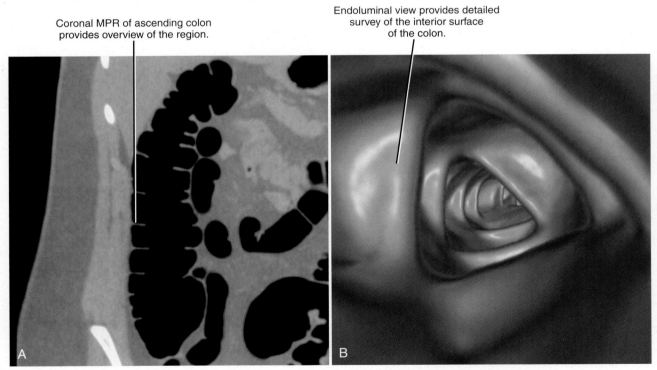

Figure 5-41 Coordinated review of multiplanar reformation *(MPR)* **(A)**, perspective volume rendering (VR) **(B)**,   *(cont'd)*

Orthographic VR of the insufflated colon allows the reader to localize specific findings.

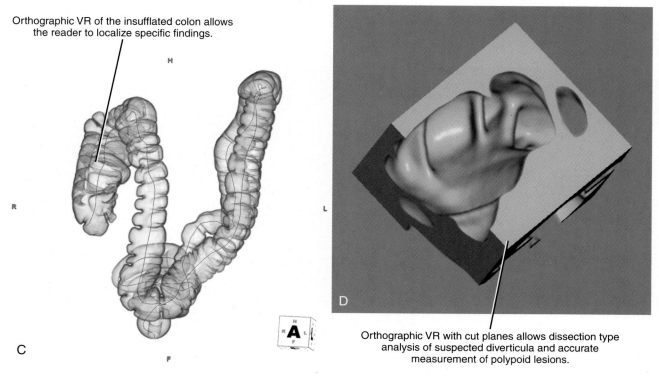

C

D

Orthographic VR with cut planes allows dissection type analysis of suspected diverticula and accurate measurement of polypoid lesions.

Orthographic VR "dissection view" is similar to curved planar reformation by making a curved object appear straight. This provides an additional review of the colonic surface without the distortion associated with perspective rendering.

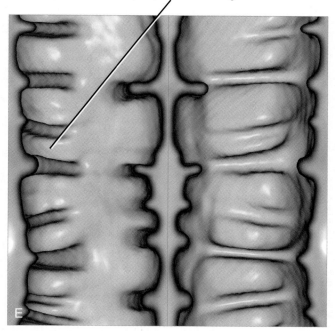

E

Figure 5-41, cont'd. and various forms of orthographic VR **(C-E)** facilitate effective use of computed tomographic colonography.

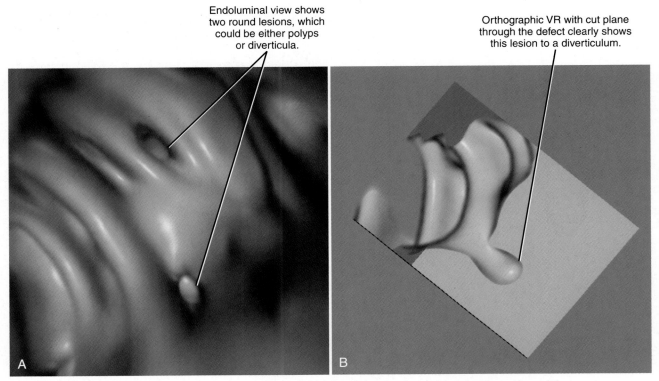

Endoluminal view shows two round lesions, which could be either polyps or diverticula.

Orthographic VR with cut plane through the defect clearly shows this lesion to a diverticulum.

Figure 5-42 Colonic diverticulum on perspective volume rendering *(VR)* **(A)** and orthographic VR with cut planes **(B)**.

Suggested Readings

Calhoun PS, Kuszyk BS, Heath DG et al: Three-dimensional volume rendering of spiral CT data: theory and method, *Radiographics* 19:745-764, 1999.

Dalrymple NC, Prasad SR, El-Merhi FM, Chintapalli KN: The price of isotropy in multidetector CT, *Radiographics* 27:49-62, 2007.

Dalrymple NC, Prasad SR, Freckleton MW et al: Informatics in radiology (infoRAD): introduction to the language of three-dimensional imaging with multidetector CT, *Radiographics* 25:1409-1428, 2005.

Fishman EK, Drebin RA, Hruban et al: Three-dimensional reconstruction of the human body, *AJR Am J Roentgenol* 150:1419-1420, 1988.

Fishman EK, Drebin B, Magid D et al: Volumetric rendering techniques: applications for three-dimensional imaging of the hip, *Radiology* 163:737-738, 1987.

Fishman EK, Magid D, Ney DR et al: Three-dimensional imaging and display of musculoskeletal anatomy, *J Comput Assist Tomogr* 12:465-467, 1988.

Heath DG, Soyer PA, Kuszyk BS et al: Three-dimensional spiral CT during arterial portography: comparison of three rendering techniques, *Radiographics* 15:1001-1011, 1995.

Hu H, He HD, Foley WD et al: Four multidetector-row helical CT: image quality and volume coverage speed, *Radiology* 215:55-62, 2000.

Jaffe TA, Martin LC, Miller CM et al: Abdominal pain: coronal reformations from isotropic voxels with 16-section CT-reader lesion detection and interpretation time, *Radiology* 242:175-181, 2007.

Kalender WA, Polacin A: Physical performance characteristics of spiral CT scanning, *Med Phys* 18:910-915, 1991.

Kim JK, Kim JH, Bae SJ et al: CT angiography for evaluation of living renal donors: comparison of four reconstruction methods, *Am J Roentgenol* 183:471-477, 2004.

Kuszyk BS, Heath DG, Bliss DF et al: Skeletal 3-D CT: advantages of volume rendering over surface rendering, *Skeletal Radiol* 25:207-214, 1996.

Leyendecker JR, Barnes CE, Zagoria RJ: Urography: techniques and clinical applications. *Radiographics* 28:23-46, 2008.

Leyendecker JR, Childs DD: Kidneys and MR urography, *Magn Reson Imaging Clin N Am* 15:373-382, vii, 2007.

Mahesh M: The AAPM/RSNA Physics Tutorial for Residents: search for isotropic resolution in CT from conventional through multiple-row detector, *Radiographics* 22:949-962, 2002.

Napel S, Marks MP, Rubin GD et al: CT angiography with spiral CT and maximum intensity projection, *Radiology* 185:607-610, 1992.

Ney DR, Fishman EK, Magid D et al: Three-dimensional volumetric display of CT data: effect of scan parameters upon image quality, *J Comput Assist Tomogr* 15:875-885, 1991.

Raman R, Napel S, Beaulieu CF et al: Automated generation of curved planar reformations from volume data: method and evaluation, *Radiology* 223: 275-280, 2002.

Raman R, Napel S, Rubin GD: Curved-slab maximum intensity projection: method and evaluation, *Radiology* 229:255-260, 2003.

Rankin SC: Spiral CT: vascular applications, *Eur J Radiol* 28:18-29, 1998.

Rubin GD: 3-D imaging with MDCT, *Eur J Radiol* 45(suppl 1):S37-S41, 2003.

Rubin GD, Beaulieu CF, Argiro V et al: Perspective volume rendering of CT and MR images: applications for endoscopic imaging, *Radiology* 199:321-330, 1996.

Rubin GD, Dake MD, Napel S et al: Spiral CT of renal artery stenosis: comparison of three-dimensional rendering techniques, *Radiology* 190:181-189, 1994.

Rubin GD, Napel S, Leung AN: Volumetric analysis of volumetric data: achieving a paradigm shift, *Radiology* 200:312-317, 1996.

Rubin GD, Silverman SG: Helical (spiral) CT of the retroperitoneum, *Radiol Clin North Am* 33:903-932, 1995.

Rydberg J, Liang Y, Teague SD: Fundamentals of multichannel CT, *Radiol Clin North Am* 41:465-474, 2003.

Saini S: Multi-detector row CT: principles and practice for abdominal applications, *Radiology* 233:323-327, 2004.

Sommer FG, Olcott EW, Ch'en I et al: Volume rendering of CT data: applications to the genitourinary tract [erratum appears in Am J Roentgenol 1997 Aug;169(2):602], *Am J Roentgenol* 168:1223-1226, 1997.

Udupa JK: Three-dimensional visualization and analysis methodologies: a current perspective, *Radiographics* 19:783-806, 1999.

van Ooijen PM, van Geuns RJ, Rensing BJ et al: Noninvasive coronary imaging using electron beam CT: surface rendering versus volume rendering, *Am J Roentgenol* 180:223-226, 2003.

Vining DJ, Zagoria RJ, Liu K et al: CT cystoscopy: an innovation in bladder imaging, *Am J Roentgenol* 166:409-410, 1996.

PROBLEM SOLVING: DISEASE CATEGORIES

CHAPTER 6

Localization and Spread of Disease

Michael Oliphant and John R. Leyendecker

Imaging to investigate problems of the abdomen and pelvis is often focused to a specific organ or body system. This can be problematic because diseases are often not confined to a specific organ, and pathologic processes can present distant from their origins. A thorough approach to abdominal and pelvic disease processes necessitates a basic understanding of how disease is contained and spread within the abdomen and pelvis. Such knowledge allows one to diagnose disease distant from its site of origin and predict the primary site of abnormality. This chapter considers how diseases are spread throughout the abdomen and pelvis, and examines relevant anatomic relations, the classic concepts of intraperitoneal and extraperitoneal, and the unifying concept of the subperitoneal space.

■ PERITONEUM

The peritoneum is defined by a continuous serous membrane that divides the coelomic cavity into the peritoneal cavity and the subperitoneal space (Fig. 6-1). The peritoneal lining develops from a splitting of the lateral mesoderm. The somatic mesoderm (parietal peritoneum) lines the body wall, and the splanchnic mesoderm (visceral peritoneum) covers the abdominal viscera and forms the abdominal mesenteries. The peritoneal cavity is a potential space that is outside the peritoneal lining and contains the suspended abdominal viscera. The space beneath the parietal peritoneum, containing a variable amount of areolar tissue, is the extraperitoneum. Early in embryonic life, the extraperitoneal space extends into the mesenteries and forms the subperitoneal space. The mesenteries provide avenues for the blood vessels, lymphatics, and nerves of the abdominal viscera to course to and from the extraperitoneum. The single subperitoneal space lies beneath the peritoneal lining and contains both the extraperitoneal space and the network of interconnecting mesenteries of the abdomen and pelvis.

■ MESENTERIES AND LIGAMENTS OF THE ABDOMEN AND PELVIS

Ventral and Dorsal Mesenteries

The primitive mesentery is divided by the primitive gut into the ventral and dorsal mesenteries. The ventral mesentery regresses except for the portion that is associated

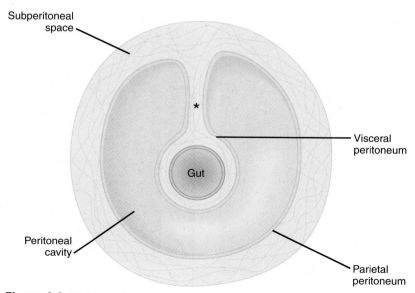

Figure 6-1 Divisions of the peritoneum.

with the foregut (ventral mesogastrium). The rapid growth of the liver within the ventral mesentery divides this mesentery into the lesser omentum (gastrohepatic ligament) and falciform ligament. The visceral peritoneum forms the liver capsule as it encases the liver, except for the surface embedded within the septum transversum (the bare area). Here, the peritoneum is reflected as the coronary ligament. The reflections of the coronary ligament again oppose each other as they attach to the parietal peritoneum anteriorly as the falciform ligament and laterally as the triangular ligaments. The falciform ligament extends from fissure for the ligamentum venosum to the anterior abdominal wall (Fig. 6-2). The falciform ligament provides a potential conduit for transmission of inflammation or hemorrhage from remote organs such as the pancreas (via the gastrohepatic ligament) to the anterior abdominal wall.

The dorsal mesentery extends in continuity from the intraabdominal portion of the esophagus to the rectum. This mesentery, in addition to giving support to the gut, serves as a conduit for the blood vessels, lymphatics, and nerves of the body organs. The spleen and dorsal portion of the pancreas appear by the fifth gestational week between the folds of the dorsal mesogastrium, which contains the splenic artery and vein, accompanying nerves, and lymphatics. The mesentery of the pancreas fuses with the posterior parietal peritoneum, leaving the spleen suspended by the splenorenal ligament and gastrosplenic ligament (Fig. 6-3). This is followed by posterior fusion of the splenorenal ligament. Inflammation or neoplasm may extend between the stomach and spleen via the gastrosplenic ligament. It is important to recognize that the pancreas is positioned beneath the posterior parietal peritoneum. The pancreas is centrally located within the subperitoneal space and in continuity with the abdominal organs via their mesenteric attachments. Neoplasms and inflammation can spread from the pancreas directly to the spleen via the

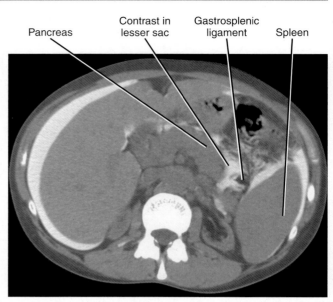

Figure 6-3 Axial computed tomographic image after administration of peritoneal contrast material.

splenorenal ligament, to the colon via the transverse mesocolon, to the liver via the hepatoduodenal ligament, and into the small bowel mesentery along the superior mesenteric vessels (Fig. 6-4). It is important to remember that the derivatives of the dorsal and ventral mesenteries remain in continuity after development, and that the individual named mesenteries are identified by their contained vessels (Tables 6-1 and 6-2).

Pearl: Neoplasms and inflammation can spread from the pancreas directly to the spleen via the splenorenal ligament, to the colon via the transverse mesocolon, to the liver via the hepatoduodenal ligament, and into the small bowel mesentery along the superior mesenteric vessels.

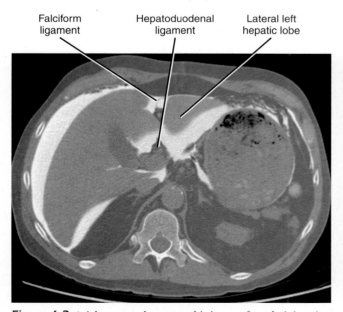

Figure 6-2 Axial computed tomographic image after administration of peritoneal contrast material.

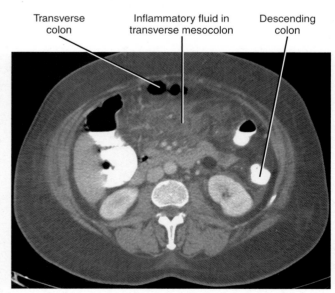

Figure 6-4 Axial enhanced computed tomographic scan through the abdomen in a patient with acute pancreatitis demonstrates spread of inflammation to the transverse mesocolon.

Table 6-1   Ventral Mesentery Derivatives

Name	Landmarks
Gastrohepatic ligament	Left gastric vessels, right gastric vessels
Hepatoduodenal ligament	Portal vein, hepatic artery, bile duct
Falciform ligament	Ligamentum teres

Table 6-2   Dorsal Mesentery Derivatives

Name	Landmarks
Gastrosplenic ligament	Short gastric vessels, left gastroepiploic vessels
Splenorenal ligament	Splenic artery and vein
Gastrocolic ligament	Right and left gastroepiploic vessels, gastrocolic trunk
Transverse mesocolon	Middle colic vessels
Greater omentum	Epiploic vessels

Gastrohepatic and Hepatoduodenal Ligaments

The ventral mesogastrium is one mesentery in continuity as it attaches the foregut to the ventral abdominal wall. Its derivatives include the lesser omentum and the falciform ligament. The lesser omentum (gastrohepatic ligament) extends from the liver to the stomach. More specifically, this ligament extends from the fissure for the ligamentum venosum and porta hepatis to the lesser curvature of the stomach (Fig. 6-5). The gastrohepatic ligament contains the left and right gastric arteries, coronary vein, and left gastric lymph nodes. The gastrohepatic ligament provides a pathway for bidirectional spread of disease between the stomach and the

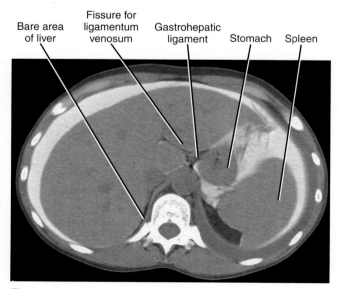

Figure 6-5 Axial computed tomographic image after administration of peritoneal contrast material.

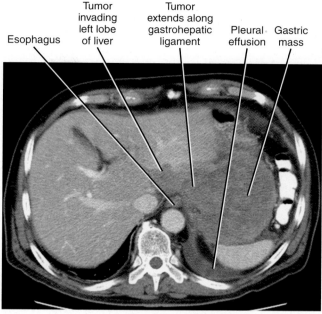

Figure 6-6 Axial enhanced computed tomographic scan in a patient with non-Hodgkin's lymphoma extending from the stomach to the left hepatic lobe via the gastrohepatic ligament.

left hepatic lobe (Fig. 6-6). The free margin of the lesser omentum (hepatoduodenal ligament) attaches to the duodenum ventrally and contains the portal vein, hepatic artery, and common bile duct.

Pearl: The gastrohepatic ligament provides a pathway for bidirectional spread of disease between the stomach and the left hepatic lobe.

Ligamentous Support of the Colon and Small Bowel

The transverse mesocolon is derived from the dorsal mesocolon and is in continuity with the root of the small-bowel mesentery (Fig. 6-7). The phrenicocolic ligament is the left lateral extension of the root of the transverse mesocolon, and the duodenocolic ligament is the right lateral extension. The posterior reflections of the small intestine mesentery extend from the region below the transverse mesocolon in the left upper abdomen to the right lower abdomen, providing continuity between the left upper and right lower abdomen (Fig. 6-8). The dorsal mesocolon undergoes extensive posterior fusion after reentry to the abdominal cavity during development. The ascending and descending portions of the dorsal mesocolon lie in their lateral positions and fuse with the parietal peritoneum, as does the mesorectum. For imaging purposes, the ascending and descending colon and rectum are considered extraperitoneal structures. The appendix cecum, transverse mesocolon, and sigmoid mesocolon persist (Fig. 6-9). Therefore, the transverse and sigmoid portions of the colon are considered to be intraperitoneal. However, it is important to realize that the entire mesentery of the colon and rectum remains in continuity regardless of fused portions.

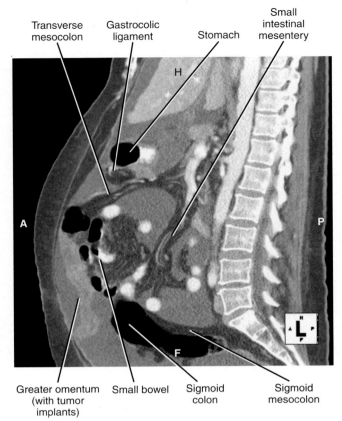

Figure 6-7 Sagittal enhanced computed tomographic image of a patient with peritoneal carcinomatosis and ascites demonstrating continuity of the mesenteries of the abdomen.

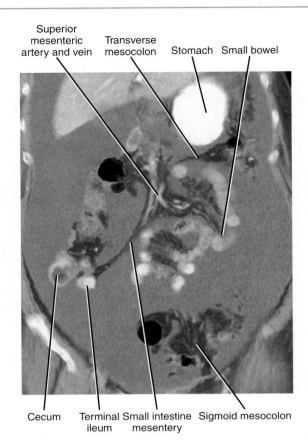

Figure 6-8 Coronal reformation of enhanced computed tomographic scan of a patient with ascites caused by peritoneal carcinomatosis.

Pelvic Ligaments

Of the numerous supporting ligaments of the pelvis, the broad ligament is the most relevant for disease spread and containment. The broad ligament forms from a mesenchymal shelf within the pelvis and bridges the lateral pelvic walls (Table 6-3). The visceral peritoneum encases the broad ligament, uterus, and adnexa. Specialized portions of the broad ligament form the mesovarium and mesosalpinx superiorly, and the cardinal ligament inferiorly. The broad ligament contains the blood vessels, lymphatics, and nerves of the uterus and adnexa. Thus, the subperitoneal space extends into the pelvis as the broad ligament (analogous to the mesenteries of the abdomen) and interconnects the female pelvic organs with the abdomen.

■ EXTRAPERITONEAL SPACES

Spread and containment of extraperitoneal disease is related to the anatomy of the extraperitoneal spaces. The localization of a process within an extraperitoneal compartment also allows for development of a differential diagnosis related to organs within that space. The three classic extraperitoneal spaces are demarcated by fascial planes that divide the extraperitoneum into compartments with specific contents and

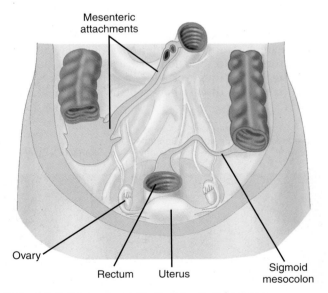

Figure 6-9 Pelvic mesenteric attachments and recesses.

Table 6-3   Pelvic Ligaments

Name	Landmarks
Broad ligaments	Uterine vessels, fallopian tubes, ovaries, uterus
Round ligaments	Inguinal canals

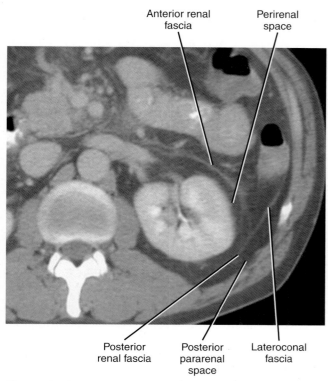

Anterior renal fascia — Perirenal space

Posterior renal fascia — Posterior pararenal space — Lateroconal fascia

Figure 6-10 Axial enhanced computed tomographic scan through left kidney in a patient with acute pancreatitis demonstrates classic retroperitoneal anatomy.

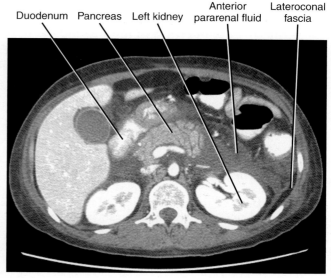

Duodenum   Pancreas   Left kidney   Anterior pararenal fluid   Lateroconal fascia

Figure 6-11 Axial enhanced computed tomographic scan in a patient with acute pancreatitis and anterior pararenal fluid.

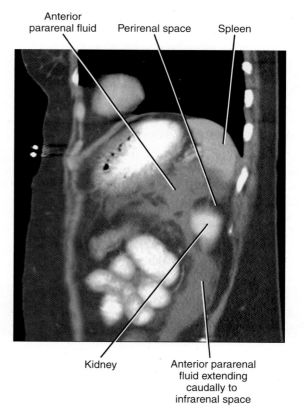

Anterior pararenal fluid   Perirenal space   Spleen

Kidney   Anterior pararenal fluid extending caudally to infrarenal space

Figure 6-12 Sagittal computed tomographic reformation to left of midline in a patient with acute necrotizing pancreatitis.

relations. The anterior and posterior renal fascias (collectively known as Gerota's fascia, although the posterior renal fascia was first described by Zuckerkandl) segment the extraperitoneum into the anterior pararenal, posterior pararenal, and perirenal spaces (Fig. 6-10). The anterior and posterior pararenal spaces combine below the iliac crest and continue inferiorly as the extraperitoneal space of the pelvis, providing anatomic continuity.

Anterior Pararenal Space

The anterior pararenal space lies between the posterior parietal peritoneum and the anterior renal fascia (Figs. 6-11 and 6-12). This space contains the pancreas, extraperitoneal portion of the duodenum, and the ascending and descending colon. Its cephalad extent is the bare area of the liver (on the right) and its caudad extent is the level of the iliac fossae. The anterior pararenal space is continuous as the subperitoneal space of the mesenteries of the upper abdomen, transverse mesocolon, and small bowel. In this manner, disease processes may spread bidirectionally between the organs of the upper abdomen, pancreas, small bowel, and colon. The anterior pararenal space is constrained laterally by the lateroconal fascia formed by fusion of the layers of the anterior and posterior renal fascia. Anatomically, the anterior pararenal space is compartmentalized into colonic and pancreaticoduodenal compartments by fusion of the primitive mesenteries. This process of fusion results in creation of the retropancreaticoduodenal and retromesenteric interfascial planes that can serve as conduits for spread of fluid within the extraperitoneum.

Perirenal Space

The perirenal space lies between the anterior and posterior renal fascia. Pathologic processes or fluid collections occurring within the right or left perirenal space most often do not cross the midline, as the renal fascias fuse with the connective tissue surrounding the aorta and inferior vena cava. The caudad extent of the perirenal space is at the iliac crest where the fascial layers are poorly fused and blend with the periureteric connective tissue. Controversy exists as to the anatomic patency of the inferior perirenal space. In practice, however, perirenal fluid collections are usually confined to the perirenal space (Fig. 6-13). If there is deficiency in the cephalad extent of the anterior renal fascia, the superior perirenal space may be open. In such a case, abnormalities of the perirenal space can extend cephalad with the anterior pararenal space to the level of the bare area of the liver.

Posterior Pararenal Space

The posterior pararenal space is located between the posterior renal fascia and the transversalis fascia, and continues cephalad to beneath the diaphragm, caudad to the iliac crest, and lateral to form the properitoneal fat stripe. This space contains no organs and does not cross the midline, as the posterior renal fascia fuses with the fascia of the psoas and quadratus lumborum muscles.

Bare Area of the Liver

The bare area of the liver is formed by the peritoneal reflection over the posterior portion of the liver embedded in the diaphragm. The bare area is delineated by the falciform ligament (anterior), the coronary ligament (central), and the right and left triangular ligaments

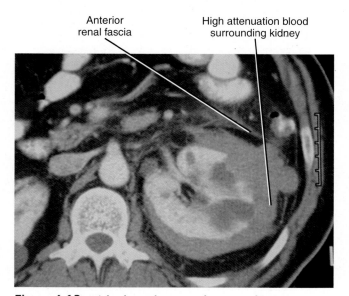

Anterior renal fascia

High attenuation blood surrounding kidney

Figure 6-13 Axial enhanced computed tomographic scan in a patient with perirenal hematoma.

(lateral). It is the cephalad extent of the right anterior pararenal space. Occasionally, the perirenal space is open superiorly and in continuity with the anterior pararenal space in the region of the bare area of the liver. Right pararenal or perirenal hematoma, infection, or neoplasm may extend superiorly to the bare area of the liver, and hematoma from hepatic injury may enter the pararenal or perirenal space via the same pathway. Abscesses can also arise from the liver and extend into the bare area. The bare area of the liver is difficult to visualize on cross-sectional imaging modalities in the absence of peritoneal fluid. However, in patients with sufficient ascites, the bare area is identified as the area along the posterior surface of the liver adjacent to the diaphragm that is spared by the fluid (see Fig. 6-5).

■ UNIFYING CONCEPT OF THE SUBPERITONEAL SPACE

Several problems arise with the traditional approach to the peritoneum and extraperitoneum (e.g., explaining disease spread involving several classic compartments). These problems can be resolved by viewing the abdomen and pelvis as one space, the subperitoneal space. The subperitoneal space is defined as the anatomic continuum deep to the peritoneum that covers the coelomic cavity and organs extending in continuity to form a network of interconnecting peritoneal folds known as the ligaments and mesenteries of the abdomen and pelvis.

Viewed this way, the organs suspended by mesenteries in the peritoneal cavity are really an extension of the extraperitoneal space. The extraperitoneum and the mesenteries and ligaments form a continuous interconnecting network as demonstrated by their embryonic development and imaged by their vascular and lymphatic contents. Visualization of the abdomen and pelvis as a continuum provides a concept not only to explain confinement of disease but pathways for spread. The subperitoneal space provides a conduit for spread of fluid, air, inflammation, and tumor from the thorax to the pelvis. Hematogenous, lymphatic, and perineural dissemination of disease may all be considered forms of subperitoneal spread because these structures all travel within the subperitoneal space. Examples of subperitoneal spread of disease between the various visceral organs are listed in Table 6-4.

■ PERITONEAL COMPARTMENTS AND RECESSES

Spread of disease within the peritoneal cavity is determined in large part by the constraints imposed by the peritoneal attachments and the dynamics of fluid flow within the peritoneal cavity. The peritoneal compartments and recesses are potential spaces within the abdominal cavity formed by the posterior and anterior parietal attachments of the membranes and ligaments discussed earlier.

Table 6-4   Subperitoneal Spread of Disease via the Ligaments and Mesenteries

Disease Spreads Between:	Spread of Disease Occurs Via The:
Pancreas and anterior abdominal wall	Gastrohepatic and falciform ligaments
Pancreas and transverse colon	Transverse mesocolon
Pancreas and spleen	Splenorenal ligament
Pancreas and liver	Hepatoduodenal ligament
Pancreas and small bowel	Small intestinal mesentery
Stomach and spleen	Gastrosplenic ligament
Stomach and transverse colon	Gastrocolic ligament
Stomach and liver	Gastrohepatic ligament
Duodenum and colon (hepatic flexure)	Duodenocolic ligament
Uterus and pelvic sidewall	Broad ligament

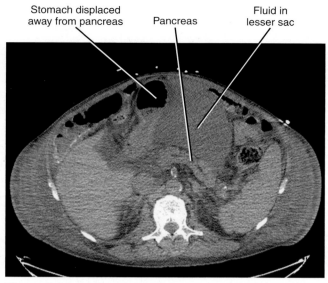

Stomach displaced away from pancreas   Pancreas   Fluid in lesser sac

Figure 6-14 Axial unenhanced computed tomographic image in a patient with lesser sac fluid collection.

Dorsal Peritoneal Recesses

The root of the transverse mesocolon is the central dorsal attachment that divides the abdominal cavity into the supramesocolic and inframesocolic compartments (see Fig. 6-7). The attachment of the root of the small intestinal mesentery divides the inframesocolic compartment into the right and left inframesocolic recesses (see Fig. 6-8). The lateral extensions of the inframesocolic recesses are the paracolic gutters. The left paracolic gutter is in continuity with the pelvis above the root of the sigmoid mesocolon but is not in continuity with the supramesocolic recess because it is interrupted by the phrenicocolic ligament. The right paracolic gutter is larger than the left and extends from the pelvis to the right subhepatic recess. The posterior extent of this recess is Morison's pouch. Morison's pouch extends medially as the recess between the hepatoduodenal ligament and the inferior vena cava to the epiploic foramen (of Winslow). The right subhepatic recess continues lateral to the liver, around the coronary and triangular ligament, and superiorly to the right subphrenic recess. The falciform ligament separates the right and left subphrenic recesses. The left subphrenic recess is divided into the gastrohepatic recess and gastrosplenic recess.

The lesser sac is located on the left, behind the stomach and gastrohepatic ligament (lesser omentum), and anterior to the posterior peritoneal reflection overlying the pancreas. The lesser sac communicates with the remainder of the peritoneal cavity only via the epiploic foramen (foramen of Winslow). The lesser sac is confined caudally by the transverse colon, transverse mesocolon, and gastrocolic ligament; left laterally by the gastrosplenic ligament, splenorenal ligament, and the spleen; and right laterally by the duodenum and hepatoduodenal ligament. These boundaries separate the lesser sac from the left subphrenic recess and the left posterior peritoneal recesses. Fluid accumulated in the lesser sac typically displaces the stomach away from the pancreas, although extraperitoneal peripancreatic fluid may do the same (Fig. 6-14).

The dorsal peritoneal recess of the pelvis is located between the urinary bladder and rectum (rectovesical recess). Women have further division of this space by the uterus, forming the vesicouterine recess (pouch of Douglas). The dorsal and ventral recesses are connected laterally by the paravesical recesses of the pelvis.

Ventral Peritoneal Recesses

Ventral peritoneal recesses are defined by the umbilical ligaments. The median umbilical ligament extends from the apex of the urinary bladder to the umbilicus and contains the urachus. The medial umbilical ligaments course anterior and medial from the internal iliac arteries to the umbilicus and contain the obliterated umbilical arteries. The lateral umbilical ligaments contain the inferior epigastric arteries and veins, and lie medial to the inguinal canal.

The supravesical fossa is the recess between the medial umbilical ligaments. The medial inguinal recesses are between the medial and lateral umbilical ligaments, and the lateral inguinal recesses are lateral to the lateral umbilical ligaments. The ventral peritoneal recesses are illustrated in Figure 6-15.

■ FLUID DYNAMICS WITHIN THE PERITONEAL SPACE

Intraperitoneal spread of disease is influenced by the patterns of ascitic flow dictated by the anatomy of the peritoneal attachments and recesses, as well as regional variations in intraperitoneal pressures. The normal 100 ml of peritoneal fluid is formed and absorbed by passive exchange over the entire peritoneal lining. Gastrointestinal peristalsis facilitates lateral flow of peritoneal fluid, whereas caudad flow results from gravity. Cephalad flow is facilitated by respiration and the creation of

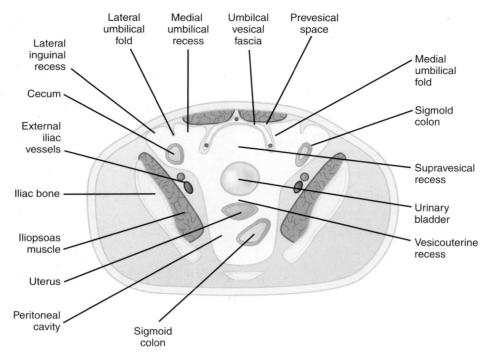

Figure 6-15 Pelvic peritoneal recesses.

negative subdiaphragmatic pressure. On the right, fluid ascends up the right paracolic gutter to Morison's pouch, a frequent site of infection or tumor implantation (Fig. 6-16). From this location, fluid tracks into the right subphrenic recess. Cephalad flow of ascites is constrained on the left by the phrenicocolic ligament. This explains why the propagation of pelvic infection to the subphrenic recess tends to occur more commonly on the right. Left subphrenic collections are more likely to result from regional surgery (e.g., splenectomy or gastric surgery). The falciform ligament tends to restrict spread of subphrenic infection across the midline.

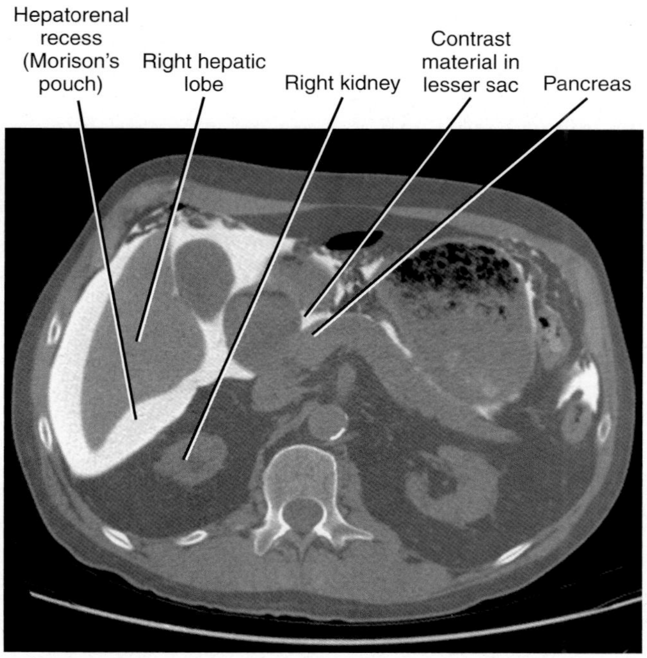

Fluid accumulates in regions of stasis within the peritoneal cavity. These potential pooling spots are created by the intraabdominal ligaments and their posterior attachments. The typical locations of stasis are the dorsal peritoneal recesses of the pelvis, the small intestinal mesentery attachment in the right lower quadrant, the superior sigmoid mesocolon, and the right paracolic gutter. It is in these locations that one is most likely to encounter accumulations of fluid, hemorrhage, pus, or tumor seeding (Fig. 6-17). This is evidenced by the frequent appearance of pelvic abscesses and peritoneal metastatic implants in the pouch of Douglas, which represents the most dependent part of the peritoneal cavity in both the upright and supine positions. The lower end of the small bowel mesentery also represents a frequent site for peritoneal seeding.

There are potential peritoneal recesses where fluid does not initially flow (e.g., between the folds of the small intestine mesentery or into the lesser sac). Lesser sac fluid collections are more likely to arise from perforation of the posterior walls of the intraabdominal esophagus, stomach, or duodenum directly into the lesser sac than from spread of fluid or infection through the epiploic foramen. Pancreatitis may also result in lesser sac fluid accumulation, although peripancreatic fluid within the subperitoneal space may mimic lesser sac fluid.

Pearl: Lesser sac fluid collections more commonly originate from the border-forming organs of the lesser sac than from spread through the epiploic foramen.

Figure 6-16 Axial computed tomographic image after administration of peritoneal contrast material.

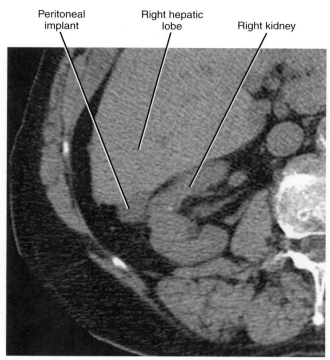

Figure 6-17 Axial unenhanced computed tomographic scan in a patient with metastatic mucinous adenocarcinoma of the appendix.

The frequent involvement of the greater omentum with peritoneal metastases reflects the role of this structure in the lymphatic absorption of peritoneal fluid. Omental metastases may occur in great numbers, creating a confluent neoplastic mantle referred to as *omental cake* (Figs. 6-7 and 6-18). Fluid is also cleared

through lymphatic vessels in the diaphragmatic portion of the peritoneum to the lymphatics within the anterior mediastinum.

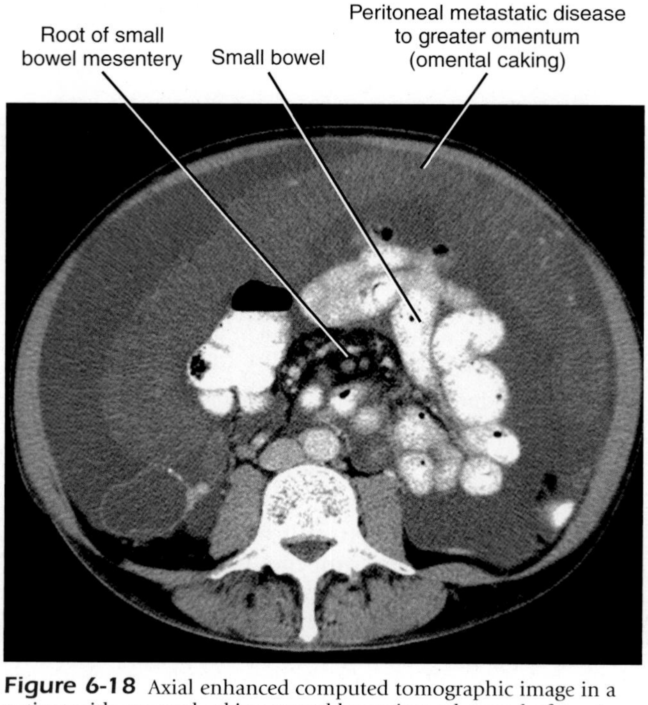

■ ORIGIN OF ABNORMAL GAS COLLECTIONS

Gas is free to move throughout the intraperitoneal recesses and subperitoneal spaces unless impeded by the normal ligaments, peritoneal reflections, and fascia. Therefore, determining the origin of an abnormal gas collection within the abdomen and pelvis may be a challenge. However, certain clues may be helpful in at least narrowing the list of possibilities.

Gas is more constrained within the extraperitoneum than in the peritoneal cavity. Therefore, extraperitoneal gas is more likely than peritoneal gas to remain on the side of origin. Although extraperitoneal gas from many locations can spread bilaterally, this occurs most commonly in the pelvis. Gas may be presumed to originate from the gastrointestinal tract when there is evidence of disruption or discontinuity of bowel wall, abnormal mural thickening, perienteric inflammation, evidence of foreign body or penetrating trauma, or leakage of enteric contrast material present (Fig. 6-19). A large volume of peritoneal gas is more likely the result of gastroduodenal perforation than more distal bowel perforation unless the patient has had bowel obstruction or recent endoscopy. The "sentinel bubble" sign represents a small locule of gas in the recess adjacent to the duodenal bulb (Fig. 6-20). When present, one should suspect a perforated duodenal or pyloric channel ulcer. Gas within the lesser sac usually arises from one of its border-defining organs such as the stomach, duodenum, or less often, the transverse

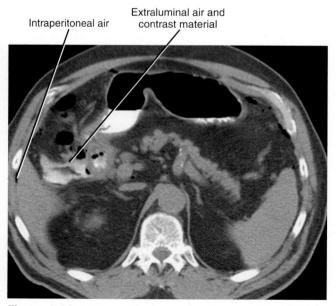

Figure 6-18 Axial enhanced computed tomographic image in a patient with omental caking caused by peritoneal spread of ovarian carcinoma.

Figure 6-19 Axial unenhanced computed tomographic scan in a patient who sustained perforation of the duodenum during endoscopy. Intraperitoneal gas and enteric contrast material are seen in the region of the duodenocolic ligament.

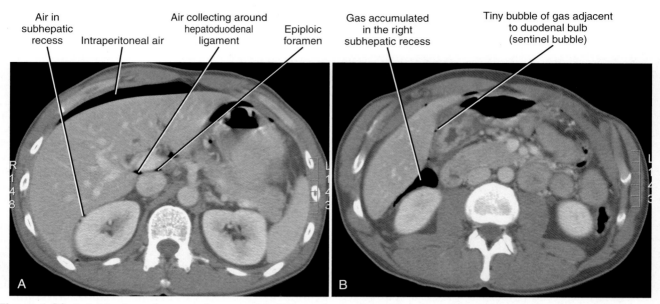

Air in subhepatic recess | Intraperitoneal air | Air collecting around hepatoduodenal ligament | Epiploic foramen | Gas accumulated in the right subhepatic recess | Tiny bubble of gas adjacent to duodenal bulb (sentinel bubble)

Figure 6-20 **A,** Axial enhanced computed tomographic (CT) scan in a patient with perforated duodenal ulcer. **B,** More caudal image in the same patient.

colon. Table 6-5 provides some clues to localizing gastrointestinal sources of abnormal gas collections based on the location of the extraluminal gas.

Pearl: Extraperitoneal gas is more likely than peritoneal gas to remain on the side of origin and near the site of origin.

Not all abnormal gas collections within the abdomen and pelvis originate from the gastrointestinal tract. Other sources of pneumoperitoneum include peritoneal dialysis, recent abdominal surgery, thoracic abnormalities, and the female genital tract (Fig. 6-21).

Table 6-5   Gastrointestinal Origins of Abnormal Gas Collections

Location of Air	Sources to Consider
Lesser sac	Posterior stomach, duodenum, lower esophagus, transverse colon
Fissure for the ligamentum teres	Stomach, duodenal bulb
Recess adjacent to duodenal bulb	Duodenal bulb or pyloric channel
Mesenteric folds	Colon or small bowel
Extraperitoneum	Extraperitoneal portions of the duodenum, ascending colon, descending colon, sigmoid colon, rectum
Right anterior pararenal space	Duodenum, ascending colon
Left anterior pararenal space	Descending colon, sigmoid colon
Perirenal space	Kidney, renal collecting system
Bilateral extraperitoneum	Rectum
Intraperitoneal and extraperitoneal	Extraperitoneal source (usually sigmoid diverticular disease)

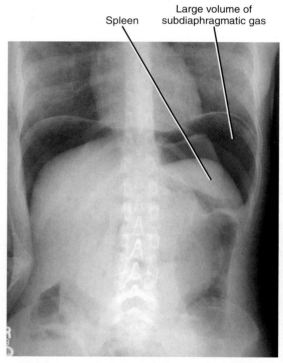

Spleen | Large volume of subdiaphragmatic gas

Figure 6-21 Upright abdominal radiograph demonstrates a large volume of free intraperitoneal air caused by vaginal fornical laceration.

Extraperitoneal gas may result from infections, surgical procedures, and pneumomediastinum (Fig. 6-22).

Gas within the biliary system (pneumobilia) most commonly originates from the duodenum and usually results from procedures such as ERCP, biliary stent placement, sphincterotomy, or biliary-enteric anastomosis (Fig. 6-23). Other causes include nonsurgical biliary-enteric fistula or infection with a gas-forming organism.

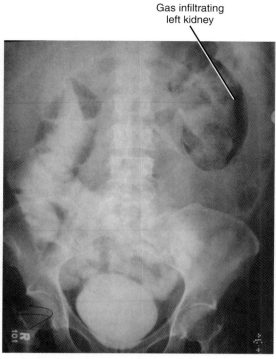

Gas infiltrating
left kidney

Figure 6-22 Abdominal radiograph performed after a computed tomographic (CT) scan demonstrates an abnormal gas collection outlining the left kidney in a patient with emphysematous pyelonephritis.

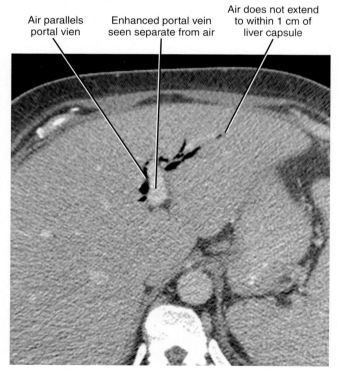

Air parallels   Enhanced portal vein   Air does not extend
portal vien   seen separate from air   to within 1 cm of
                                                   liver capsule

Figure 6-23 Axial enhanced computed tomographic scan in a patient with biliary enteric anastomosis demonstrates typical appearance of pneumobilia.

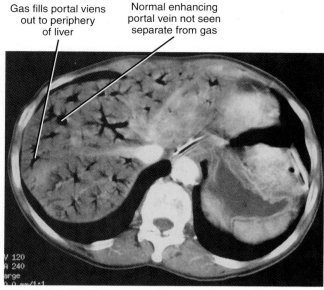

Gas fills portal viens   Normal enhancing
out to periphery   portal vein not seen
of liver   separate from gas

Figure 6-24 Extensive portal venous gas in a patient with bowel necrosis.

Gas within the portal vein usually originates from the gastrointestinal tract. When small amounts of gas are present within the portal vein, it can often be distinguished from pneumobilia by its tendency to appear in a peripheral location within the liver on radiographs and CT scans (Fig. 6-24). Gas within mesenteric veins follows the course of these veins and tends to occur on the mesenteric rather than antimesenteric side of the bowel. Causes to consider when portal venous gas is identified include intestinal ischemia, inflammatory bowel conditions, bowel distention, blunt trauma, and infection. In some patients, the cause is never identified.

Pearl: When small amounts of gas are present within the portal vein, it can often be distinguished from pneumobilia by its tendency to appear in a peripheral location within the liver on radiographs and CT scans.

■ LOCALIZING FLUID COLLECTIONS

The location of a fluid collection may be a clue to its origin. This section describes how one can localize fluid to a specific compartment or space and mentions some of the more common causes of fluid collections by location.

Pleural versus Subphrenic Fluid

The distinction between pleural fluid and peritoneal fluid has important diagnostic and therapeutic implications. Free-flowing pleural fluid layers dependently along the chest wall on decubitus films. With ultrasound, pleural fluid is generally hypoechoic with variable amounts of echogenic debris depending on fluid content. Compressed lung parenchyma is often seen moving within pleural fluid with real-time sonography. On CT and MRI studies, pleural fluid collects posterior to the crus of the diaphragm and tends to displace the crus away from the spine ("displaced crus" sign) (Fig. 6-25). In contrast, intraabdominal fluid collects anterolateral to the crus. Because the bare area of the liver restricts the movement of peritoneal fluid, fluid crossing this right posteromedial area tends to be pleural. When an empyema is present, thickening of the visceral and parietal pleura results in the "split pleura" sign. This sign may also be seen with neoplastic and inflammatory processes that thicken the pleura. Multiplanar reconstructions of volumetric data may be helpful in identifying the relation of a fluid collection to the diaphragm.

Pleural fluid may result from a wide variety of infectious, neoplastic, and inflammatory processes of the thorax or abdomen, but intrathoracic processes rarely cause subphrenic fluid to accumulate. Isolated right-sided subphrenic collections are often bilomas, particularly after liver surgery (Fig. 6-26). Isolated left-sided subphrenic collections are often of pancreatic origin and commonly coexist with left-sided pleural effusions.

Lesser Sac Fluid

The lesser sac has two recesses. The left gastric artery is the landmark that divides the lesser sac into a small medial component (superior recess) and a larger lateral component (inferior recess) (Fig. 6-27). Fluid in the superior recess collects to the right of the left gastric artery, behind the stomach, and is bordered by segments I (caudate) and IV (medial left) of the liver. Inferior recess fluid collects to the left of the left gastric artery, behind the stomach, and is bordered laterally by the spleen and gastrosplenic ligament. Although a small amount of lesser sac fluid can be

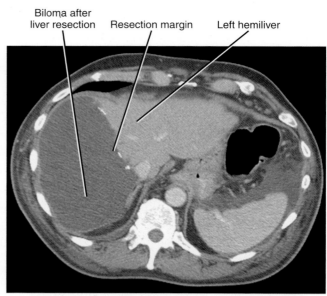

Figure 6-26 Axial enhanced computed tomography after right hepatectomy for cholangiocarcinoma demonstrates large right upper quadrant fluid collection subsequently shown to represent biloma.

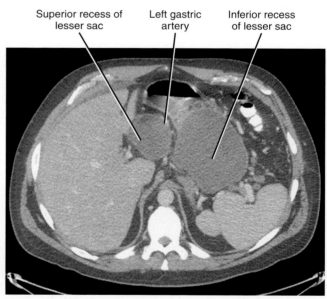

Figure 6-27 Axial enhanced computed tomographic scan of a patient with lesser sac fluid collection.

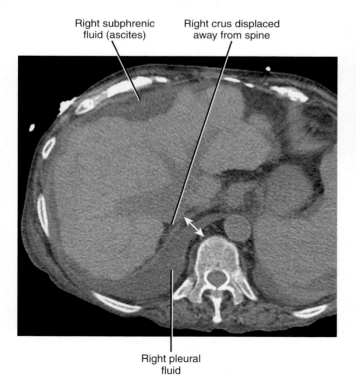

Figure 6-25 Axial unenhanced computed tomographic scan of a patient with cirrhosis, ascites, and pleural effusions.

seen with ascites, fluid collecting predominately in the lesser sac is typically secondary to a disease process of one of its border-defining organs (e.g., stomach, duodenum, spleen, pancreas) or peritoneal lining (Fig. 6-28). Fluid within the lesser sac may occasionally be seen extending between leaves of the greater omentum.

Interloop Fluid

Fluid within the peritoneal cavity may accumulate between mesenteric folds. Generally, this does not occur to any great degree until fluid has accumulated in more

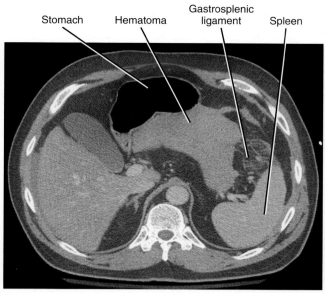

Stomach   Hematoma   Gastrosplenic ligament   Spleen

Figure 6-28 Axial enhanced computed tomography of a patient with hematoma of the inferior recess of the lesser sac caused by small splenic laceration.

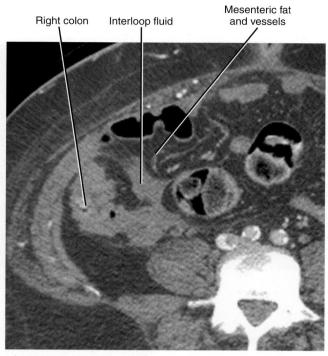

Right colon   Interloop fluid   Mesenteric fat and vessels

Figure 6-30 Axial enhanced computed tomographic scan demonstrates stellate appearance of interloop fluid.

dependent recesses of the peritoneal cavity. Fluid within the subperitoneal space of the mesentery must be distinguished from interloop fluid. Because the mesenteric vessels run within the subperitoneal space, fluid (such as blood) and other processes (such as inflammation) within this space tend to surround the vessels and obscure the fat (Fig. 6-29). On the other hand, interloop fluid does not surround the vessels, preserves the fat, and often has a stellate or triangular appearance as it collects between the mesenteric leaves (Fig. 6-30).

Pearl: Interloop fluid does not surround the vessels, preserves the fat, and often has a stellate or triangular appearance.

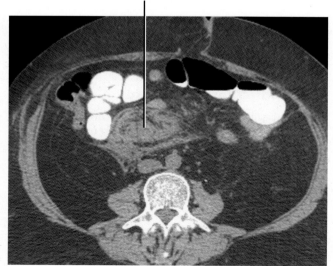

Blood in small bowel mesentery obscures vessels and fat

Figure 6-29 Axial unenhanced computed tomography in a patient with acute hemorrhage into the small bowel mesentery from pseudoaneurysm of a small mesenteric artery branch.

Peritoneal Pelvic Fluid

Fluid within the pelvic peritoneal recesses may arise from within the pelvis or from distant sites such as the liver. The rectouterine pouch (between the rectum and uterus in women) and rectovesical pouch (between the rectum and bladder in men) represent the most dependent aspects of the peritoneal cavity. Fluid accumulation in these regions is extremely common regardless of cause or site of origin. The pelvic peritoneal recesses are also divided by the urinary bladder into supravesical and paravesical recesses, and ventrally by the umbilical ligaments.

Anterior Pararenal Fluid

Fluid accumulating between the posterior peritoneal lining and the anterior renal fascia occupies the anterior pararenal space. Such fluid may originate from the duodenum (e.g., perforated ulcer), ascending or descending colon (e.g., diverticulitis), and most commonly, the pancreas (e.g., pancreatitis). Fluid may extend within the anterior pararenal space to the bare area of the liver, to the interconnecting mesenteries (e.g., gastrohepatic ligament, gastrosplenic ligament, small bowel mesentery, transverse mesocolon), or to the pelvis (Fig. 6-31). Fluid in the anterior pararenal space may originate from distant organs and spread via the mesenteries to the anterior pararenal space.

Posterior Pararenal Fluid

Fluid within the posterior pararenal space accumulates behind the posterior renal fascia. This is the most common space for idiopathic retroperitoneal bleed and is a

Inflammation and fluid
surround pancreatic tail

Inflammatory fluid extends from pancreas
caudally in infrarenal space

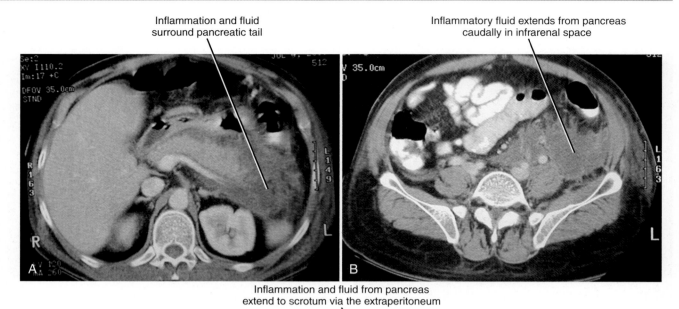

Inflammation and fluid from pancreas
extend to scrotum via the extraperitoneum

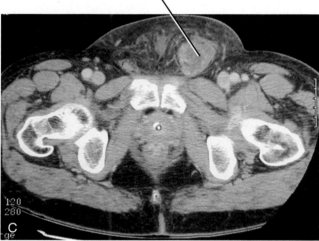

Figure 6-31 **A,** Axial enhanced computed tomographic (CT) scan in a patient with acute pancreatitis shows inflammatory fluid in the left anterior pararenal space. **B,** Axial enhanced CT scan in same patient shows caudal extension of extraperitoneal inflammatory fluid from acute pancreatitis. **C,** Axial enhanced CT scan in same patient shows spread of inflammation and fluid from acute pancreatitis as far as the left scrotum.

common site of extension of abdominal aortic aneurysm rupture (Fig. 6-32). Fluid originating from inflammatory processes of the duodenum, pancreas, and ascending and descending colon can track within the planes of the posterior renal fascia (retrorenal plane).

Interfascial Fluid

Hemorrhage and inflammation may spread throughout the extraperitoneum via interfascial planes alluded to earlier. These planes are formed by fusion of the primitive mesenteries during embryologic development. Fluid or blood from aortic rupture, pancreatitis, or colonic processes may be seen dissecting into the retromesenteric and retrorenal interfascial planes. The spread of pancreatitis into the retrorenal plane (visualized as fusion of the lateral conal fascia and the anterior renal fascia) is commonly seen with imaging (Fig. 6-33).

Blood from aortic rupture often extends into the psoas space or retrorenal (posterior) interfascial plane.

Perinephric/Perirenal Fluid

Perinephric fluid collects within the confines of the renal fascia that enclose the kidneys, adrenal glands, and renal hilar structures. Fluid can appear compartmentalized within the perirenal space by perirenal septations. Perirenal fluid often results from renal infection, hemorrhage, or urine leakage (urinoma) (see Fig. 6-13).

Mesenteric Subperitoneal Fluid

Fluid may accumulate within the subperitoneal spaces of the abdominal mesenteries. For example, inflammatory fluid from pancreatitis may dissect into the transverse

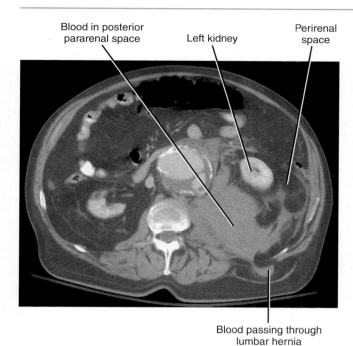

Blood in posterior pararenal space   Left kidney   Perirenal space

Blood passing through lumbar hernia

Figure 6-32 Enhanced computed tomographic (CT) scan of a patient with ruptured abdominal aortic aneurysm.

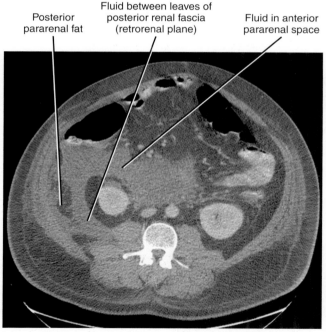

Posterior pararenal fat   Fluid between leaves of posterior renal fascia (retrorenal plane)   Fluid in anterior pararenal space

Figure 6-33 Axial enhanced computed tomographic scan of a patient with acute pancreatitis and inflammatory fluid dissecting into retrorenal plane.

mesocolon, hepatoduodenal ligament, and other interconnecting ligaments and mesenteries of the abdomen. These spaces are best identified by tracing the vessels that they normally transmit. Traumatic injury to the vessels that normally run within these mesenteries may result in hematoma formation in the involved mesentery.

Prevesical Fluid

Often referred to as the "space of Retzius," this retropubic extraperitoneal space is located between the transversalis fascia (deep to the rectus abdominus muscles) and the fascia covering the obliterated umbilical arteries and urachus (umbilicovesical fascia). Large volumes of fluid (most commonly blood or urine) may accumulate within this space. The limitations of this space imposed by the attachments of the umbilicovesical fascia create a characteristic "molar tooth" appearance (Figs. 6-34 and 6-35).

Pearl: Fluid within the prevesical space often has a characteristic "molar tooth" appearance.

■ ORIGIN OF MASSES

Determining the organ or compartment of origin has important implications for the differential diagnosis of a mass. For example, a fatty tumor arising from the kidney or adrenal gland is almost certainly benign. However, a fatty tumor arising from the perirenal or pararenal space is concerning for liposarcoma. A large mass arising from the uterus has a markedly different differential diagnosis from a large mass arising from the ovary.

Small masses arising from within an organ do not present a dilemma in terms of localization, provided they are entirely surrounded by parenchyma. It is important to distinguish serosal implants to the surface of an organ such as the liver from hematogenous metastases to the parenchyma, because hematogenous metastases may be resectable, whereas the presence of serosal implants implies unresectability (Figs. 6-36 and 6-37). Sometimes this distinction is not possible with imaging.

Large masses that compress and displace surrounding structures present a challenge. The first determination that one might make in such a setting is whether the mass is intraperitoneal or extraperitoneal. Clues to the extraperitoneal origin of a mass include anterior displacement of a kidney, adrenal gland, pancreas, ureter, or extraperitoneal segment of bowel (e.g., transverse duodenum, ascending colon) and anterior displacement or encasement of extraperitoneal vessels such as the inferior vena cava, aorta, renal arteries, and iliac vessels (Fig. 6-38).

Because tumors often derive their blood supply from the vessels normally feeding the organ of origin, blood supply to the tumor is a clue to its origin. Identifying the blood supply is particularly helpful in distinguishing between uterine masses and ovarian masses. Ovarian masses are typically supplied and drained by the gonadal vessels (Fig. 6-39). Therefore, if the gonadal vessels can be followed directly to a pelvic mass, it is likely of ovarian origin. On the other hand, subserosal uterine fibroids are more often supplied by the uterine arteries (Fig. 6-40). Identifying vessels extending between the normal myometrium and a pelvic mass confirms its uterine origin (bridging vascular sign) (Fig. 6-41).

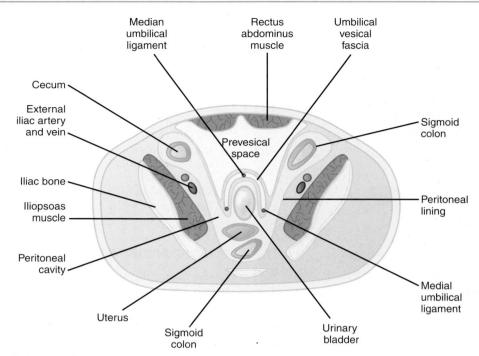

Figure 6-34 Expanded prevesical space.

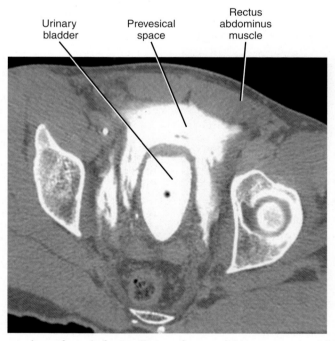

Figure 6-35 Axial computed tomography performed after instillation of water-soluble contrast material into bladder in a patient with pelvic trauma and extraperitoneal bladder rupture demonstrates contrast accumulation in the prevesical space.

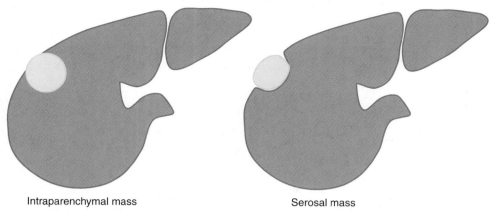

Intraparenchymal mass   Serosal mass

Figure 6-36 Distinguishing between a parenchymal mass and serosal implant (peritoneal metastasis).

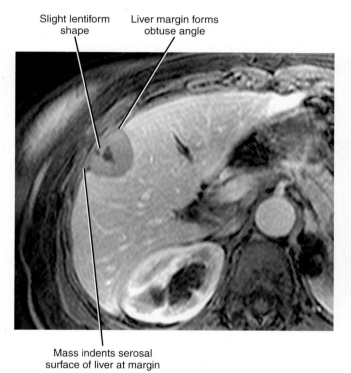

Slight lentiform shape   Liver margin forms obtuse angle

Mass indents serosal surface of liver at margin

Figure 6-37 Axial contrast-enhanced magnetic resonance imaging in a patient with perihepatic serosal implant from a metastatic gastrointestinal stromal tumor. Such serosal masses may closely mimic parenchymal tumors.

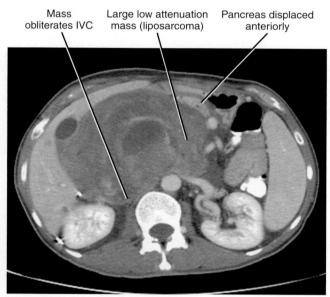

Mass obliterates IVC   Large low attenuation mass (liposarcoma)   Pancreas displaced anteriorly

Figure 6-38 Axial enhanced computed tomographic scan of a patient with large liposarcoma. Anterior displacement of the pancreas confirms that mass arises from extraperitoneum. *IVC,* Inferior vena cava.

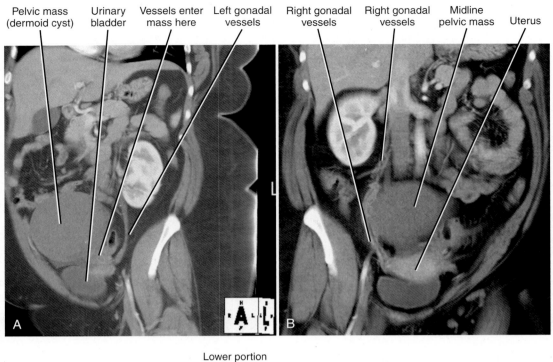

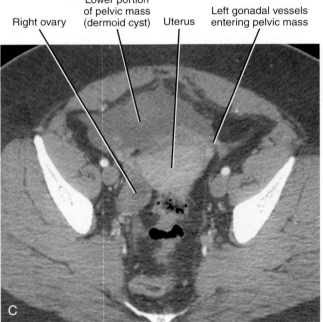

Figure 6-39 **A,** Oblique sagittal reconstruction of enhanced computed tomography (CT) shows left gonadal vessels supplying a large pelvic dermoid cyst. **B,** Coronal reconstruction of enhanced CT in the same patient shows right gonadal vessels bypassing midline pelvic mass (dermoid cyst). **C,** Axial enhanced CT scan in the same patient shows a normal right ovary separate from the pelvic mass (dermoid cyst). A normal left ovary could not be located separate from mass.

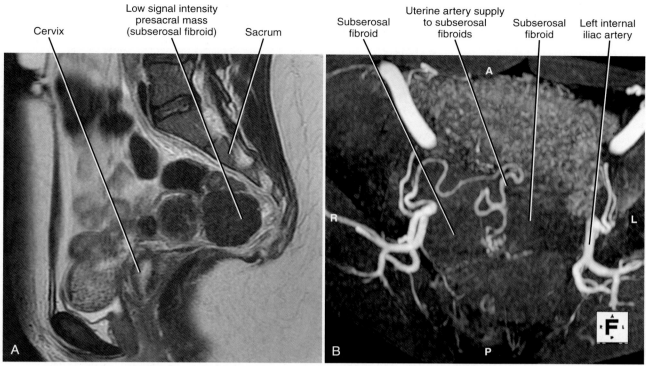

Figure 6-40 A, Sagittal T2-weighted magnetic resonance image (MRI) of the pelvis in a woman with subserosal uterine fibroids. B, Oblique axial maximum intensity projection (MIP) image from contrast-enhanced MRI of the pelvis in same patient. Note the uterine artery supply.

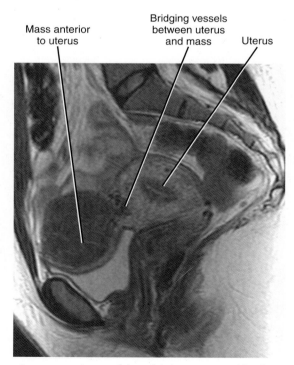

Figure 6-41 Sagittal T2-weighted magnetic resonance image of the pelvis in a woman with a large subserosal fibroid demonstrating the bridging vascular sign, confirming uterine origin of the mass.

Pearl: *If the gonadal vessels can be followed directly to a pelvic mass, it is likely of ovarian origin.*

Occasionally, the organ of origin may be implied by the presence of the "beak sign" or "claw sign." This sign is present when a crescent or beak of normal parenchyma is seen extending from the organ of origin around the margin of a mass (Fig. 6-42). Organ of origin may also be implied when a parenchymal defect is present within an organ along the interface between a mass and its organ of origin (Fig. 6-43). When the organ of origin cannot be determined directly, it can occasionally be inferred by excluding other possibilities. For example, the presence of a normal adrenal gland clearly separate from a suprarenal mass excludes the adrenal gland as a potential site of origin (Fig. 6-44). Therefore, a directed search should always be performed for all organs that are normally present in the general vicinity of an abnormality. When an organ that is normally present cannot be identified in the vicinity of a mass (phantom organ sign), that organ becomes a potential site of origin for the mass. The presence of an intact fat plane on CT or MRI between a mass and an adjacent organ is a useful indicator that the mass originates outside that organ. It should be mentioned that invasion or obliteration of an organ by a malignant tumor can mimic a primary neoplasm originating from that organ. Signs that are helpful in determining the organ of origin for a mass are listed in Box 6-1.

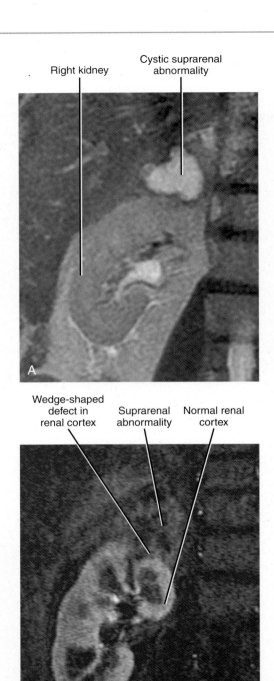

Figure 6-43 **A,** Coronal T2-weighted magnetic resonance image shows suprarenal lesion initially thought to represent a cystic adrenal mass. **B,** Coronal gadolinium-enhanced T1-weighted image of the right kidney (corticomedullary phase) in the same patient shows a wedge-shaped area of cortical interruption that implies renal origin of the mass (perinephric abscess).

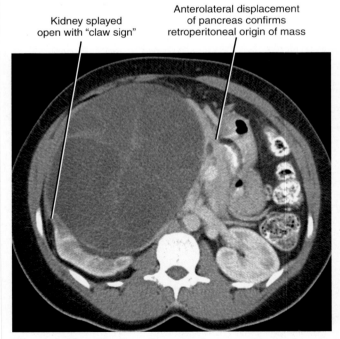

Figure 6-42 Axial enhanced computed tomographic scan in a patient with a large multilocular cystic nephroma. Renal origin of mass suggested by "claw sign."

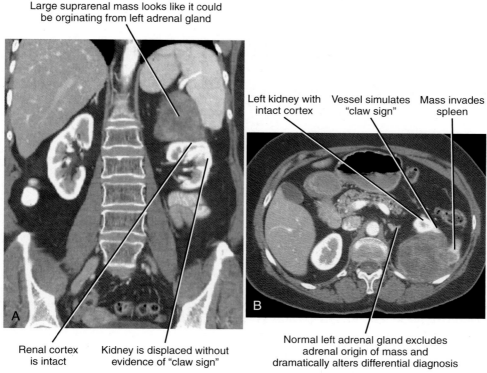

Large suprarenal mass looks like it could be orginating from left adrenal gland

Left kidney with intact cortex

Vessel simulates "claw sign"

Mass invades spleen

A

B

Renal cortex is intact

Kidney is displaced without evidence of "claw sign"

Normal left adrenal gland excludes adrenal origin of mass and dramatically alters differential diagnosis

Figure 6-44 A, Coronal reformation of enhanced axial computed tomographic (CT) scan in a patient with suprarenal myxoid liposarcoma. **B,** Axial enhanced CT image in the same patient shows normal left adrenal gland, excluding adrenal origin of mass.

BOX 6-1   Signs That a Mass Originates from a Particular Organ

Beak/claw sign present
Mass shares same blood supply as organ
Vessels extend between mass and organ (bridging vascular sign)
Lack of intact fat plane between mass and organ
Mass contiguous with parenchymal defect in organ
Normal organ not visible (phantom organ sign)

Suggested Readings

Arenas AP, Sanchez LV, Albillos JM et al: Direct dissemination of pathologic abdominal processes through perihepatic ligaments: identification with CT, *Radiographics* 14:515-528, 1994.

Coakley FV, Hricak H: Imaging of peritoneal and mesenteric disease: key concepts for the clinical radiologist, *Clin Radiol* 54:563-574, 1999.

DeMeo JH, Fulcher AS, Austin RF Jr: Anatomic CT demonstration of the peritoneal spaces, ligaments, and mesenteries: normal and pathologic processes, *Radiographics* 15:755-770, 1995.

Furukawa A, Sakoda M, Yamasaki M et al: Gastrointestinal tract perforation: CT diagnosis of presence, site, and cause, *Abdom Imaging* 30:524-534, 2005.

Hashimoto M, Okane K, Hirano H et al: Pictorial review: subperitoneal spaces of the broad ligament and sigmoid mesocolon—imaging findings, *Clin Radiol* 53:875-881, 1998.

Kim S, Kim TU, Lee JW et al: The perihepatic space: comprehensive anatomy and CT features of pathologic conditions, *Radiographics* 27:129-143, 2007.

Mastromatteo JF, Mindell HJ, Mastromatteo MF et al: Communications of the pelvic extraperitoneal spaces and their relation to the abdominal extraperitoneal spaces: helical CT cadaver study with pelvic extraperitoneal injections, *Radiology* 202:523-530, 1997.

Nishino M, Hayakawa K, Minami M et al: Primary extraperitoneal neoplasms: CT and MR imaging findings with anatomic and pathologic diagnostic clues, *RadioGraphics* 23:45-57, 2003.

Okino Y, Kiyosue H, Mori H et al: Root of the small-bowel mesentery: correlative anatomy and CT features of pathologic conditions, *Radiographics* 21:1475-1490, 2001.

Oliphant M, Berne AS: Computed tomography of the subperitoneal space: demonstration of direct spread of intraabdominal disease, *J Comput Assist Tomogr* 6:1127-1137, 1982.

Oliphant M, Berne AS, Meyers MA: The subperitoneal space: normal and pathologic anatomy, In Myers MA, editor: *Dynamic radiology of the abdomen*, ed 5, New York, 2000, Springer.

Saksouk FA, Johnson SC: Recognition of the ovaries and ovarian origin of pelvic masses with CT, *RadioGraphics* 24:S133-S146, 2004.

CHAPTER 7

Computed Tomography Incidentalomas

John R. Leyendecker and Neal C. Dalrymple

The discovery of small, incidental, asymptomatic lesions during the routine review of computed tomographic (CT) images is a common and often frustrating occurrence in routine clinical practice. Such lesions are often referred to as indeterminate, nonspecific, or "too small to characterize." Because most busy radiologists cannot devote more than a brief moment to determining the significance and subsequent evaluation of such lesions, this section is dedicated to "incidentalomas." We do not advocate a single approach to small incidental lesions because recommendations remain in flux. Each individual radiologist must determine the degree of uncertainty he or she is willing to tolerate, taking into consideration patient anxiety and prognosis, the personality and typical practices of the referring physician, and the number of malpractice attorneys preying on the local medical community. Regardless, one should always use common sense. If a lesion has a small chance of being malignant, recommending further costly or potentially morbid tests is of no immediate benefit to a patient with significant comorbidities of an acutely life-limiting nature. Likewise, incidental lesions should not be viewed as an opportunity for revenue building through the recommendation of frequent follow-up imaging studies. In contrast, with the increasing availability of minimally invasive therapies for malignant tumors, early detection and diagnosis of incidental malignant neoplasms has taken on new imperative.

■ LIVER

When faced with a small, nonspecific liver lesion, it is helpful to determine whether the patient has risk factors for a malignant hepatic tumor (primary or secondary). Most patients in this category can be identified by asking if they have a history of chronic liver disease (e.g., viral hepatitis, cirrhosis, hemochromatosis, primary sclerosing cholangitis) or known extrahepatic primary malignancy. The definition of a liver lesion that is "too small to characterize" varies in the literature but typically includes lesions smaller than 2 cm in greatest dimension. With the widespread use of thin-section multidetector CT, the size criteria for "too small to characterize" has diminished. Common causes of "too small to characterize" liver lesions include hepatic cysts, hemangiomas, and bile duct hamartomas.

Patients with No Known Cancer or Chronic Liver Disease

In the absence of risk factors such as cancer or chronic liver disease, the likelihood that a small, incidental, indeterminate liver lesion is malignant is extremely low, regardless of the age of the patient or number of lesions. Therefore, we do not automatically recommend additional evaluation of incidental nonspecific lesions smaller than 1 cm in diameter in patients without risk factors for malignant disease, provided no other compelling indications exist. Examples of lesions that might require additional evaluation include multiple lesions in an immunocompromised patient or a lesion that shows evidence of growth.

Large lesions detected incidentally in asymptomatic healthy individuals have a greater chance for being malignant than small lesions. In a study of 107 asymptomatic patients with hepatic lesions incidentally discovered with a variety of imaging techniques, Liu and colleagues found that 58% of lesions were malignant. On multivariate analysis, male sex, age older than 50 years, and tumor size greater than 4 cm were predictive of malignant disease.

Ultrasound may be a reasonable initial step to evaluate a low-attenuation liver lesion in an accessible location in an average-size patient. Lesions less than 5 mm are unlikely to be detected with ultrasound. However, up to two thirds of lesions larger than 5 mm detected with CT can be located by ultrasound, provided the CT scan is used to direct the search. Targeted ultrasound is much more likely to succeed for a lesion in a favorable location (e.g., not the dome of the liver) and in a person of average body habitus. If ultrasound reveals a simple cyst, no further evaluation is necessary. Targeted ultrasound of an indeterminate hepatic lesion may also help to determine whether sonographically guided biopsy is an option.

Magnetic resonance imaging (MRI) has the highest sensitivity and specificity of available hepatic imaging techniques but is typically reserved for the evaluation of patients with risk factors for malignant tumor or infection. MRI is capable of distinguishing between benign and malignant lesions in the majority of cases referred for a small indeterminate lesion discovered with CT. However, MRI is costly and should be reserved for cases when further characterization of a lesion is likely to affect patient management. Such situations include oncology patients for whom hepatic resection or an alternate chemotherapy regimen is contemplated.

Nuclear medicine techniques are rarely helpful in the evaluation of small, incidentally discovered hepatic lesions because of limited spatial resolution.

Patients with Known Extrahepatic Cancer

Even in patients with known primary malignancy, a small incidental lesion discovered with CT is more likely benign than malignant (Fig. 7-1). In patients with known primary cancer, a lesion considered "too small to characterize" by CT has a greater than 80% chance of being benign according to most studies. The actual number can be expected to vary with the population studied, the criteria used to define small or "too small to characterize," the imaging technique, and the interpreting individual. Patients with breast cancer with one or more small (≤15 mm) hypoattenuating lesions on a baseline contrast-enhanced CT scan without other evidence of hepatic metastases are no more likely to experience development of subsequent hepatic metastases than patients with no such lesions. In another study of patients with breast cancer, too small to characterize lesions represented benign findings in more than 90% of women. Patterson and researchers studied the MRI evaluation of "too small to characterize" liver lesions discovered with CT in patients with breast cancer and found that only 5% of such

lesions were shown to represent metastases. In a study of hepatic lesions 15 mm or smaller in patients with gastric and colorectal cancer, almost 80% were benign. In that study, if patients with larger coexistent liver metastases were excluded, small hypoattenuating lesions were metastases in only approximately 2% of patients.

In some respects, it is not surprising that small incidental lesions discovered with CT are likely benign. After all, benign hepatic lesions are extremely common, and tiny, low-attenuation, simple cysts are likely to be more conspicuous against a background of enhancing liver than equally sized enhancing metastatic lesions.

A brief analysis of lesion features can sometimes help identify worrisome lesions, although no imaging features are entirely specific. Benign lesions tend to be lower in attenuation and have more discrete margins than malignant lesions, whereas target enhancement (low-attenuation border surrounding a lower attenuation center) is suggestive of metastatic disease. For patients with extrahepatic tumors, one may also take into account the stage and imaging characteristics of the primary tumor when analyzing a small focal hepatic lesion. For example, patients with known extrahepatic metastases are more likely to have liver metastases than patients with carcinoma in situ.

Pearl: Even in patients with known extrahepatic malignant neoplasm, most liver lesions too small to characterize with CT are benign. In such cases, ultrasound or MRI can be helpful for further characterization.

Multiple small low-attenuation lesions scattered throughout the liver

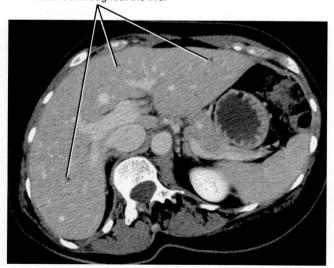

Figure 7-1 Enhanced axial computed tomographic image through the abdomen of a patient with colorectal carcinoma and multiple low-attenuation liver lesions. Given the small size and number of lesions, a diagnosis of biliary hamartomas was suggested and subsequently confirmed at the time of colectomy.

Patients with Chronic Liver Disease

Patients with chronic viral hepatitis or cirrhosis are at increased risk for development of hepatocellular carcinoma. Unfortunately, patients with chronic liver disease are also likely to be plagued by small, incidental, arterially enhancing lesions on dynamic, multiphase, contrast-enhanced imaging. The cause of such lesions varies and may include arterial-portal shunt, regenerative nodule, or benign neoplasm (e.g., hemangioma or focal nodular hyperplasia–like lesions). Fortunately, small (<2 cm), arterially enhancing nodules not visible on other phases of enhancement are more likely to be benign than malignant in the setting of chronic liver disease, although it may be difficult to distinguish benign nodules from hepatocellular carcinoma based on imaging criteria alone. Therefore, patients with chronic liver disease who have small arterially enhancing nodules on dynamic, multiphase, contrast-enhanced CT (or MRI) are usually followed with CT or MRI at approximately 6-month intervals. Small, arterially enhancing lesions that demonstrate intralesional washout of contrast material during the portal venous phase, a nodule-within-nodule appearance, rim enhancement, or evidence of a pseudocapsule on portal phase images should be considered malignant until proved otherwise.

Pearl: Liver lesions smaller than 2 cm seen only on arterial phase enhanced CT or MR images are more likely benign than malignant. Worrisome features include portal phase washout, interval growth, pseudocapsule, nodule-within-nodule appearance, and rim enhancement.

■ PANCREAS

Pancreatic lesions are less likely to be discovered incidentally than liver lesions, although this gap is narrowing with the widespread availability and frequent utilization of multidetector CT and MRI. Incidentally discovered solid lesions of the pancreas usually require further evaluation and intervention because many such lesions will subsequently be shown to represent adenocarcinoma or neuroendocrine tumor. Given that little controversy surrounds the management of incidentally discovered solid pancreatic masses, this is not discussed here in further detail.

Incidental asymptomatic cystic lesions are a more common occurrence. Zhang and colleagues found a prevalence rate of pancreatic cystic lesions of 19.6% in a population of 1444 patients studied with single-shot fast spin-echo MR. In general, cystic lesions are less likely to be malignant than solid lesions. Asymptomatic pancreatic cysts had a 14% chance of being malignant in one study by Goh and researchers, which included cysts of any size. Distinguishing between different types of cystic pancreatic lesions is critical to patient management. For example, a simple pancreatic cyst can be managed nonsurgically, whereas mucinous cystic neoplasm is resected when possible. Lesions of serous (microcystic) cystadenoma are benign and left alone when asymptomatic.

When faced with an incidentally discovered pancreatic cystic lesion, many factors should be considered when determining subsequent management. Patient age and surgical risk, lesion size and location, and imaging characteristics of the lesion all contribute to decisions about subsequent patient management. In general, large size, thick septations, large locules, enhancing nodules, or biliary or pancreatic duct dilatation are concerning features. If a lesion is readily accessible to interrogation with endoscopic ultrasound (EUS), aspiration and cyst fluid analysis can be helpful in management decisions. The presence or level of mucin, amylase, carcinoembryonic antigen, CA-19-9, prostaglandin E_2, and malignant cytology have all been investigated as potential discriminators between surgical and nonsurgical cystic lesions of the pancreas with variable results.

The appearance of certain cystic pancreatic lesions can be suggestive of a specific diagnosis. This is true for some serous/microcystic adenomas and intraductal papillary mucinous neoplasms. Unfortunately, most cystic pancreatic lesions lack a specific appearance, and even experienced abdominal imagers have trouble accurately characterizing cystic pancreatic masses, even when convinced of a specific diagnosis. In Visser and colleagues' study, expert reviewers accurately characterized fewer than 50% of cystic pancreatic lesions with CT or MRI despite a high level of confidence in many of the cases. Another disturbing finding of this study was that 2 of 13 unilocular thin-walled cysts smaller than 4 cm were subsequently proved malignant; an additional 3 such lesions were premalignant mucinous cystadenomas.

Few would argue with resecting a nonspecific 4-cm cystic lesion of the pancreas, particularly if suspicious features such as solid components are present. Smaller (<2 to 3 cm), simple-appearing cystic lesions present more of a dilemma. Many centers consider serial imaging follow-up to be a reasonable alternative for small, asymptomatic, simple-appearing cystic lesions of the pancreas. Handrich and colleagues managed patients with simple-appearing pancreatic cysts of 2 cm or smaller discovered on ultrasound or CT with imaging (minimum follow-up of 5 years), review of clinic notes (minimum follow-up 8 years), or questionnaire (minimum follow-up of 8 years). These authors concluded that small (≤2 cm), incidentally discovered, simple-appearing pancreatic cystic lesions can be observed safely, with further evaluation or invasive management reserved for lesions that grow beyond 2 cm. Some groups have advocated 3 cm be used as a cutoff for serial observation provided no suspicious features are present, while others have concluded that cyst aspiration is a more reliable indicator of the need for surgery than cyst size.

For simple-appearing cystic lesions of the pancreas smaller than 1 cm, a follow-up interval of 6 months is probably reasonable. For cystic lesions between 1 and 3 cm in size, we believe that EUS with cyst aspiration should be considered. Magnetic resonance cholangiopancreatography can occasionally be helpful to demonstrate communication with the pancreatic duct (supporting a diagnosis of intraductal papillary mucinous tumor in a patient without a history of pancreatitis) or evidence of complicating features such as mural nodules. In most cases, however, a cystic lesion that is indeterminate by CT will remain indeterminate despite MRI. For lesions between 1 and 2 to 3 cm without concerning features at EUS, a 6-month follow-up interval could be considered. Surgical intervention should be considered for lesions that demonstrate interval growth (Fig. 7-2).

A unilocular cyst in the setting of pancreatitis is suggestive of, but not diagnostic for, a pseudocyst. Even in patients with prior pancreatitis, cystic lesions should be followed to ensure resolution. For asymptomatic cystic lesions larger than 2 to 3 cm that occur in a patient without a history of pancreatitis, or for lesions that are not typical of microcystic (serous) cystadenoma, surgical resection should be considered for reasonably fit patients.

Management recommendations for patients with asymptomatic, incidentally discovered cystic lesions of the pancreas are in a state of evolution and vary by

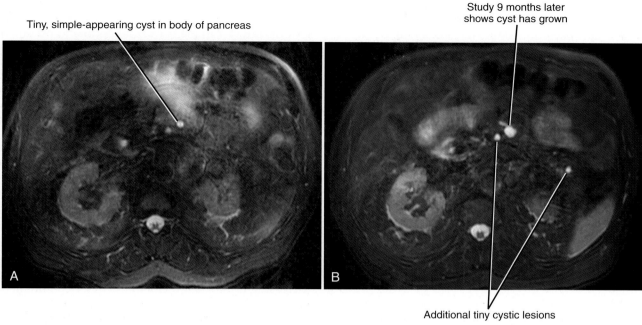

Figure 7-2 Enlarging pancreatic cysts. **A,** Axial T2-weighted magnetic resonance image through the pancreas of a man with an incidentally discovered 1-cm cystic lesion of the pancreas. **B,** T2-weighted image obtained 9 months after (**A**) demonstrates interval growth. The patient was referred to a pancreatic surgeon for further management.

institution. Therefore, refer to the Suggested Readings for more detailed discussions of this topic. Figure 7-3 presents one algorithm for the management of incidentally discovered pancreatic cysts, although this represents just one potential approach and should not be considered an established protocol to which to rigidly adhere.

Pearl: Intervention should be considered for any incidentally discovered cystic pancreatic lesion that demonstrates enhancing septa, nodules, size greater than 2 to 3 cm, or interval growth unless clinical and imaging features are highly suggestive of serous cystadenoma or pancreatic pseudocyst.

■ KIDNEY

The incidental discovery of a renal lesion on a CT examination performed for other reasons is a common occurrence. It is helpful to divide incidental lesions of the kidney into low-attenuation lesions (usually benign) and enhancing masses (usually malignant).

Low-Attenuation Lesions of the Kidney

Low-attenuation lesions, often called *hypodensities,* are by far the most commonly encountered lesion in the kidney. This is largely due to the high incidence of renal

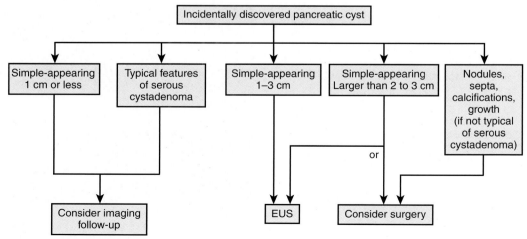

Figure 7-3 Algorithm for the management of incidentally discovered pancreatic cysts. *EUS,* Endoscopic ultrasound.

cysts in the general population. Although unusual in children and young adults, one third of people older than 60 years have at least one renal cyst (Table 7-1). In all likelihood, the renal cysts in our senior citizens grew from "renal hypodensities that are too small to characterize" over years or even decades.

Many incidentally detected renal lesions can be characterized definitively as simple cysts on the initial examination. However, the CT criteria used to characterize renal cysts are most effective when applied to lesions 2 cm or greater in diameter. Although increased use of thin sections and dynamic imaging with multidetector CT has likely improved our ability to apply the Bosniak classification system to lesions just smaller than 2 cm, it remains difficult to diagnose many of these lesions with confidence. Before relegating the lesion to the "too small to characterize" status, look closely for any positive signs that increase the likelihood of malignancy. On occasion, enhancement or wall irregularity can be seen even in very small lesions.

Keep in mind that any reference to low-attenuation lesion in the kidney assumes that intravenous contrast has been administered. Because even highly vascular renal lesions can appear lower in attenuation than unenhanced renal parenchyma on CT, any focal renal lesion detected on unenhanced CT (e.g., renal stone protocol) merits further evaluation.

It is difficult to devise a one-size-fits-all algorithm to deal with small, low-attenuation lesions of the kidney. In patients with no known malignancy or predisposition to renal malignancy (von Hippel–Lindau disease or other hereditary syndromes), lesions that measure 5 mm or less can probably be ignored because the yield with additional imaging and surveillance is extremely low. For lesions larger than 1 cm in diameter in patients of modest size, ultrasound is a reasonable next step because many renal cysts can be characterized definitively with lower risk, less discomfort, and at a lower cost than with dynamic contrast-enhanced CT or MRI.

When ultrasound is not definitive, several options are available. Depending on the age of the patient, concurrent disease, and the patient's and referring physician's level of comfort with a wait-and-see approach, many small lesions can be observed with imaging. If further imaging is desired by any of the involved parties (including the radiologist), it is reasonable to start with a multiphase renal CT for lesions 2 cm or greater. Because smaller lesions are

likely to remain indeterminate on dedicated renal CT, MRI is the preferred imaging modality for small renal lesions. MR technique is less susceptible to pseudoenhancement, and many benign lesions have specific signal characteristics, allowing definitive characterization in the majority of cases.

Lesions that remain indeterminate with MRI are likely either benign or slow-growing neoplasms. An initial follow-up is recommended at 6 months with subsequent annual surveillance. The authors recommend that follow-up be performed with whichever imaging modality (CT or MR) provided best images of that particular lesion in the initial diagnostic evaluation.

Enhancing Lesions of the Kidney

Detection of any internal enhancement within a renal lesion is usually a sign of malignancy. However, with increased utilization of cross-sectional imaging, the increasing number of incidentally detected enhancing renal masses has resulted in a larger percentage of surgically removed renal tumors that prove to be benign (Fig. 7-4). In Vasudevan's series that reviewed 70 cases of incidentally detected renal masses, each less than 5 cm in diameter and characterized as "renal cell carcinoma" by the radiologist, 33% were, in fact, benign lesions. Another series by Frank found a rate of benign lesions of 46% in lesions smaller than 1 cm but only 6% in those lesions greater than 7 cm. This last finding is consistent with older literature reporting a 5% to 7% rate of benign lesions at nephrectomy,

Enhancing renal mass

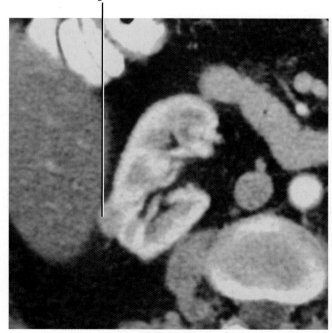

Figure 7-4 Enhanced computed tomographic image of the right kidney demonstrates an enhancing renal lesion reported (appropriately) as highly suspicious for malignancy. Partial nephrectomy was performed, yielding a pathological diagnosis of angiomyolipoma. Even in retrospect, no fat could be detected within the lesion.

Table 7-1 Incidence of Renal Cysts by Age of Patient

Age (yr)	Incidence Rate of Renal Cysts
<30	4%
30-39	15%
40-49	22%
50-59	23%
>60	33%

because until recently, imaging detected only larger tumors. The most commonly reported benign lesions are oncocytoma, angiomyolipoma, papillary adenoma, and metanephric adenoma.

The main impact of this discovery is increasing discussion of the role of biopsy in the management of small renal masses. Current image-guided needle biopsy techniques have a low complication rate, with rate of hemorrhage as low as 1% in some series. Despite isolated reports of tumor seeding in the biopsy track, it has not been reported as a significant factor despite an increasing number of renal mass biopsies in recent years. Even some cases of reported tumor seeding may be inaccurate, because recent evidence reports that percutaneous procedures in the kidney may result in benign nodular changes along the needle track.

■ ADRENAL GLAND

In most cases of clinically significant adrenal disease, the diagnosis is made in the context of a collection of clinical symptoms, laboratory findings, and often a history of primary malignancy elsewhere. More often, however, an unsuspected adrenal mass is detected when CT is performed for unrelated reasons. These incidentally detected and clinically inapparent adrenal masses are among the most common incidental masses encountered in abdominal imaging. These adrenal incidentalomas are present in as many as 3% of middle aged adults and up to 10% in the elderly.

On identifying an adrenal mass, the first step is to search for any of the characteristics that might provide a specific diagnosis (fluid or fat content suggests a benign lesion; large internally calcified or necrotic-appearing lesions suggest malignancy). If a definitive diagnosis cannot be made, consideration must be given to patient age and history, as well as size of the lesion. Because of the increasing prevalence of adrenal nodules with increasing patient age, some advocate more aggressive investigation of medium-size adrenal masses (3-4 cm) for patients younger than 50. An endocrine evaluation is often performed, searching for signs of increased production of cortisol.

Because size of the mass, patient age, and the presence or absence of a known malignancy all impact the likelihood that a given adrenal mass is malignant, it is impossible to develop a one-size-fits-all algorithm for the management of the incidental adrenal mass. However, if one starts with the most invasive options (adrenalectomy and biopsy) and works back, an algorithm begins to emerge.

When Is Adrenalectomy Performed?

Adrenalectomy is generally reserved for hyperfunctioning adrenal masses and adrenal masses with a high probability of being a primary malignancy. These include an isolated adrenal mass 6 cm or greater in size because there is high likelihood of adrenal cortical carcinoma. Biopsy can help confirm the diagnosis before surgery in some cases but is not performed as often for primary tumors as it is for suspected metastatic disease. Because biopsy of pheochromocytoma is associated with a risk for hypertensive crisis, adrenalectomy is often performed without a preceding biopsy as long as there is no evidence of metastases to the liver, lungs, or other organs.

When Is Biopsy of an Adrenal Mass Indicated?

The most common indication for adrenal biopsy is an adrenal mass that remains indeterminate after noninvasive imaging in a patient with known cancer (usually lung cancer) for whom the presence of an adrenal metastasis would alter therapy. Recent developments in the use of positron emission tomography (PET) and PET-CT have helped some confirm the diagnosis of metastatic disease noninvasively and have thus resulted in a decline in the number of biopsies performed at some centers. Nonetheless, a number of masses remain that cannot be completely characterized by CT, MRI, and PET, and for whom definitive diagnosis has important therapeutic implications. In those cases, imaging-guided biopsy may be performed, usually under CT guidance. A relatively small risk for pneumothorax and hemorrhage exists.

When Is Surveillance Imaging Appropriate?

In patients without a history of malignancy, most small (<2 cm) incidentally detected adrenal masses are benign. If laboratory evaluation does not show evidence of a hyperfunctioning adrenal adenoma and the lesion remains indeterminate after MRI and/or washout CT of the adrenal gland, serial imaging examination may be performed to detect growth of the nodule or document stability. Similar surveillance can be applied to slightly larger masses if they remain indeterminate after washout CT or chemical shift MR, or both, and are shown to have low activity by PET. If the mass increases in size on subsequent examinations, biopsy or excision should be considered.

Imaging surveillance can be performed using either noncontrast-enhanced CT or MRI. Noncontrast-enhanced CT is less expensive and usually more available, but it does expose the patient to additional ionizing radiation. Because size is the main parameter being followed, low-dose protocols may be used. Surveillance by MR is somewhat more expensive but does not expose the patient to ionizing radiation. Figure 7-5 proposes an algorithm for managing incidental adrenal masses detected on CT in patients who have no preexisting history of malignancy.

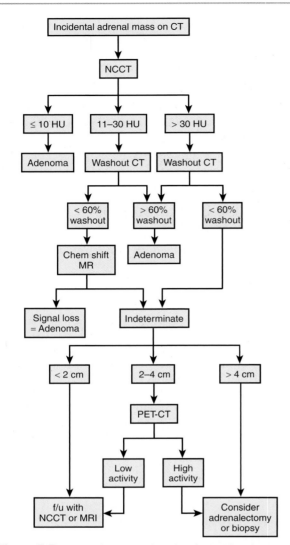

Figure 7-5 Proposed imaging algorithm for incidental mass when there is no history of malignancy or positive history of extra-adrenal malignancy without known activity on positron emission tomography (PET). Note that if the patient has a history of extra-adrenal malignancy that is known to have increased activity on PET, it is reasonable to proceed directly to PET computed tomography (CT) after identification of an adrenal mass. *MR*, Magnetic resonance; *NCCT*, noncontrast-enhanced computed tomography.

Suggested Readings

Allen PJ, Brennan MF: The management of cystic lesions of the pancreas, *Adv Surg* 41:211-228, 2007.

Allen PJ, D'Angelica M, Gonen M et al: A selective approach to the resection of cystic lesions of the pancreas: results from 539 consecutive patients, *Ann Surg* 244:572-582, 2006.

Blake MA: Distinguishing benign from malignant adrenal masses: multi-detector row CT protocol with 10-minute delay, *Radiology* 238:578-585, 2006.

Byrnes V, Shi H, Kiryu S et al: The clinical outcome of small (<20 mm) arterially enhancing nodules on MRI in the cirrhotic liver, *Am J Gastroenterol* 102:1654-1659, 2007.

Curry NS: Small renal masses (lesions smaller than 3 cm): imaging evaluation and management, *AJR Am J Roentgenol* 164:355-362, 1995.

Eberhardt S, Choi P, Bach A et al: Utility of sonography for small hepatic lesions found on computed tomography in patients with cancer, *J Ultrasound Med* 22:335-343, 2003.

Elsayes K, Leyendecker J, Menias C et al: MRI characterization of 124 CT-indeterminate focal hepatic lesions: evaluation of clinical utility, *HPB (Oxford)* 9:208-215, 2007.

Frank I, Blute ML, Cheville JC, et al. Solid renal tumors: An analysis of pathological features related to tumor size, *J Urol* 170:2217-2220, 2003.

Goh BK, Tan YM, Cheow PC et al: Cystic lesions of the pancreas: an appraisal of an aggressive resectional policy adopted at a single institution during 15 years, *Am J Surg* 192:148-154, 2006.

Handrich SJ, Hough DM, Fletcher JG et al: The natural history of the incidentally discovered small simple pancreatic cyst: long-term follow-up and clinical implications, *AJR Am J Roentgenol* 184:20-23, 2005.

Holland AE, Hecht EM, Hahn WY et al: Importance of small (< or = 20-mm) enhancing nodules seen only during the hepatic arterial phase at MR imaging of the cirrhotic liver: evaluation and comparison with whole explanted liver, *Radiology* 237:938-944, 2005.

Jang H-J, Lim HK, Lee WJ et al: Small hypoattenuating lesions in the liver on single-phase helical CT in preoperative patients with gastric and colorectal cancer: prevalence, significance, and differentiating features, *J Comput Assist Tomogr* 26:718-724, 2002.

Jones EC, Chezmar JL, Nelson RC et al: The frequency and significance of small (less than or equal to 15 mm) hepatic lesions detected by CT, *AJR Am J Roentgenol* 158:535-539, 1992.

Khalid A, Brugge W: ACG practice guidelines for the diagnosis and management of neoplastic pancreatic cysts, *Am J Gastroenterol* 102:2339-2349, 2007.

Khalil H, Patterson SA, Panicek DM: Hepatic lesions deemed too small to characterize at CT: prevalence and importance in women with breast cancer, *Radiology* 235:872-878, 2005.

Korobkin M: Differentiation of adrenal adenomas from nonadenomas using CT attenuation values, *AJR Am J Roentgenol* 166:531-536, 1996.

Krakora GA, Coakley F, Williams G et al: Small hypoattenuating hepatic lesions at contrast-enhanced CT: prognostic importance in patients with breast cancer, *Radiology* 233:667-673, 2004.

Kutikov A: Incidence of benign pathologic findings at partial nephrectomy for solitary renal mass presumed to be renal cell carcinoma on preoperative imaging, *Urology* 68:737-740, 2006.

Lee CJ, Scheiman J, Anderson MA, et al: Risk of malignancy in resected cystic tumors of the pancreas < or = 3 cm in size: is it safe to observe asymptomatic patients? A multi-institutional report, *J Gastrointest Surg* 12:234-242, 2008.

Liu CH, Fan ST, Lo CM, et al: Hepatic resection for incidentaloma, *J Gastrointest Surg* 8:785-793, 2004.

Lokken RP: Inflammatory nodules mimic applicator track seeding after percutaneous ablation of renal tumors, *AJR Am J Roentgenol* 189:845-848, 2007.

McNicholas MM: An imaging algorithm for the differential diagnosis of adrenal adenomas and metastases, *AJR Am J Roentgenol* 165:1453-1459, 1995.

Megibow AJ, Lombardo FP, Guarise A et al: Cystic pancreatic masses: cross-sectional imaging observations and serial follow-up, *Abdom Imaging* 26:640-647, 2001.

Moparty B, Brugge WR: Approach to pancreatic cystic lesions, *Curr Gastroenterol Rep* 9:130-135, 2007.

Mueller GC, Hussain HK, Carlos RC et al: Effectiveness of MR imaging in characterizing small hepatic lesions: routine versus expert interpretation, *AJR Am J Roentgenol* 180:673-680, 2003.

O'Malley ME, Takayama Y, Sherman M: Outcome of small (10-20 mm) arterial phase-enhancing nodules seen on triphasic liver CT in patients with cirrhosis or chronic liver disease, *Am J Gastroenterol* 100:1523-1528, 2005.

Park BK: Comparison of delayed enhanced CT and chemical shift MR for evaluating hyperattenuating incidental adrenal masses, *Radiology* 243:760-765, 2007.

Patterson SA, Khalil HI, Panicek DM: MRI evaluation of small hepatic lesions in women with breast cancer, *AJR Am J Roentgenol* 187:307-312, 2007.

Robinson PJ, Arnold P, Wilson D: Small "indeterminate" lesions on CT of the liver: a follow-up study of stability, *Br J Radiol* 76:866-874, 2003.

Rofsky NM: MR imaging in the evaluation of small (< or = 3.0 cm) renal masses, *Magn Reson Imaging Clin N Am* 5:67-81, 1997.

Sahani DV, Kadavigere R, Saokar et al: Cystic pancreatic lesions: a simple imaging-based classification system for guiding management, *Radiographics* 25:1471-1484, 2005.

Sahdev A: The indeterminate adrenal mass in patients with cancer, *Cancer Imaging* 7(spec no A):S100-S109, 2007.

Schwartz LH, Gandras EJ, Colangelo SM et al: Prevalence and importance of small hepatic lesions found at CT in patients with cancer, *Radiology* 210:71-74, 1999.

Silverman SG: Hyperattenuating renal masses: etiologies, pathogenesis, and imaging evaluation, *Radiographics* 27:1131-1143, 2007.

Silverman SG, Gan YU, Mortele KJ et al: Renal masses in the adult patient: the role of percutaneous biopsy, *Radiology* 240:6-22, 2006.

Somani BK: Image-guided biopsy-diagnosed renal cell carcinoma: critical appraisal of technique and long-term follow-up, *Eur Urol* 51:1289-1296, 2007.

Song JH: The incidental indeterminate adrenal mass on CT (> 10 H) in patients without cancer: is further imaging necessary? Follow-up of 321 consecutive indeterminate adrenal masses, *AJR Am J Roentgenol* 189:1119-1123, 2007.

Spinelli KS, Fromwiller TE, Daniel RA et al: Cystic pancreatic neoplasms: observe or operate, *Ann Surg* 239:651-657, 2004.

Vasudevan A: Incidental renal tumours: the frequency of benign lesions and the role of preoperative core biopsy, *BJU Int* 97:946-949, 2006.

Visser BC, Yeh BM, Qayyum A et al: Characterization of cystic pancreatic masses: relative accuracy of CT and MRI, *AJR Am J Roentgenol* 189:648-656, 2007.

Walsh RM, Vogt DP, Henderson JM et al: Natural history of indeterminate pancreatic cysts, *Surgery* 138:665-671, 2005.

Zagoria RJ: Imaging of small renal masses: a medical success story, *AJR Am J Roentgenol* 175:945-955, 2000.

Zhang XM, Mitchell DG, Dohke M et al: Pancreatic cysts: depiction on single-shot fast spin-echo MR images, *Radiology* 223:547-553, 2002.

CHAPTER 8

Imaging Evaluation of Acute Abdominal Pain

Neal C. Dalrymple, Michael Oliphant, and John R. Leyendecker

■ ACUTE ABDOMINAL PAIN: A DIAGNOSTIC DILEMMA

Acute abdominal pain is a common clinical syndrome and a diagnostic dilemma for clinicians. For centuries, physicians relied on obtaining a history of illness that elicited characteristic clinical symptoms. This history, combined with careful elicitation of physical examination findings, allowed physicians to discriminate among many potential disease processes. Unfortunately, historical, physical examination, and laboratory data are often nonspecific and inconclusive, spurring a shift in the diagnostic approach to patients with abdominal pain toward imaging. As with physical examination, image interpretation is facilitated by familiarity with the relevant anatomic structures and common diagnoses to be considered in patients presenting with specific pain syndromes (Table 8-1).

Keep in mind that significant overlap exists between the diseases listed in Table 8-1 and their clinical presentations. A confusing influence in the diagnosis of abdominal pain is related to the overlapping innervation of the abdominal organs. For example, there exists considerable overlapping innervation of the stomach (T5-7), biliary tract (T6-8), and pancreas (T5-9). Therefore, a gastric process can be difficult to differentiate from biliary colic or pancreatitis based on location of pain alone. Overlapping innervation of structures such as the colon (T10-L1), small bowel (T8-10), and kidney (T10-L1) can obscure the precise origin of pain elsewhere in the abdomen as well. Also, remember that abdominal organs do not always reside in their expected locations. For example, the cecum and appendix have a notorious propensity to extend to locations beyond the right lower quadrant, and patients with situs anomalies or bowel malrotation are not uncommon. Finally, disease processes often present remote from their organ of origin. Inflammation and tumor can spread via the subperitoneal space within the ligaments and mesenteries of the abdomen and pelvis or via the peritoneal space. Knowledge of these pathways of disease spread as discussed in Chapter 6 can greatly facilitate image interpretation and explain apparent discrepancies between the clinical presentation and the actual diagnosis.

Pitfall: Overlapping innervation, developmental anatomic variations, and potential mobility of the abdominal organs combined with complex pathways of disease spread can result in apparent discrepancies between a patient's clinical presentation and the actual diagnosis. The astute radiologist understands these complexities and applies imaging to provide a cohesive explanation for the patient's symptoms.

The role of laboratory data in narrowing a differential diagnosis should not be underestimated. At a minimum, a radiologist interpreting an imaging study of a patient with acute abdominal pain should be familiar with the patient's blood cell counts, liver function tests, amylase and lipase levels, and urinalysis if they are available.

Not all imaging modalities are equally capable of demonstrating the structures and disease processes listed in Table 8-1. For example, computed tomography (CT) would be an inappropriate first test to perform in a patient presenting with scrotal pain, whereas transabdominal ultrasound would be a poor choice for excluding peptic ulcer disease. Therefore, when imaging is deemed necessary for further evaluation of a patient's pain, the first decision to make involves the choice of imaging modality. A carefully optimized protocol must be selected and combined with appropriate patient preparation to maximize the effectiveness of the chosen modality.

■ COMPUTED TOMOGRAPHY: THE WORKHORSE OF THE EMERGENCY DEPARTMENT

Why Computed Tomography Rules the Emergency Department

Despite the wide variety of available imaging options, CT has been adopted as the modality of choice for the evaluation of patients presenting with acute abdominal pain not clearly localized to the right upper quadrant or pelvis (in females of child-bearing age). The use of plain radiographs in the acute setting has come under criticism, mainly because of low sensitivity of conventional radiography for most common causes of abdominal pain. Some studies recommend use of unenhanced CT of the abdomen and pelvis rather than abdominal radiography, arguing that plain films rarely provide a specific diagnosis. CT is much more likely than plain radiographs to show a specific cause of abdominal pain and

Table 8-1   Causes of Acute Abdominal Pain Based on Location of Symptoms

Location of Pain	Relevant Structures and Common Diagnoses to Consider
Right upper quadrant	Cardiopulmonary: pneumonia, pulmonary embolism, acute myocardial infarction Gallbladder: cholelithiasis, acute cholecystitis, torsion Liver: abscess, tumor, hepatitis, hemorrhage, hepatic necrosis Bile ducts: obstruction, choledocholithiasis, cholangitis, bile leak, hemobilia from biopsy or other trauma Hepatic flexure: diverticulitis, colitis, tumor, obstruction, epiploic appendagitis Duodenum: peptic ulcer, perforation, duodenitis, obstruction Omentum: segmental omental infarction Peritoneum: perihepatitis (Fitz–Hugh–Curtis syndrome)
Left upper quadrant	Cardiopulmonary: pneumonia, pulmonary embolism, acute myocardial infarction Stomach: peptic ulcer, gastritis, tumor, obstruction Spleen: infarction, hemorrhage, tumor Pancreas: acute pancreatitis, pancreatic cancer Splenic flexure: diverticulitis, colitis, tumor, obstruction, ischemia Peritoneum: abscess
Midepigastric	Esophagus: esophagitis, reflux disease, dysmotility, tumor, impaction Stomach: peptic ulcer, gastritis, tumor, obstruction, volvulus Duodenum: peptic ulcer, perforation, duodenitis, obstruction Pancreas: pancreatitis, pancreatic cancer Abdominal wall: ventral hernia Aorta: aneurysm (with or without rupture)
Right lower quadrant	Appendix: appendicitis Ileum: Crohn disease, infectious enteritis, Meckel diverticulitis Colon: colitis, diverticulitis, epiploic appendagitis, perforated tumor, perforated foreign body, ischemia Adnexa: cyst, endometriosis, torsion, tuboovarian abscess, ectopic pregnancy Abdominal wall: hernia
Left lower quadrant	Colon: diverticulitis, perforated tumor, perforated foreign body, colitis, ischemia Adnexa: cyst, endometriosis, torsion, tuboovarian abscess, ectopic pregnancy Abdominal wall: hernia
Generalized	Bowel: obstruction (neoplastic, inflammatory, or volvulus), ileus, ischemia, perforation, inflammation Peritoneum: peritonitis, pneumoperitoneum Aorta: aneurysm (with or without rupture)
Flank and back	Kidney and ureters: ureterolithiasis, pyelonephritis/abscess, embolism/infarction, venous thrombosis, cyst rupture, hemorrhage, nephritis Adrenal gland: hemorrhage Appendix: appendicitis (retrocecal) Aorta: aneurysm (with or without rupture), dissection Musculoskeletal: trauma, infection, hemorrhage, neoplasm, disc herniation, spinal stenosis
Pelvis and groin	Adnexa: cyst, endometriosis, torsion, tuboovarian abscess, ectopic pregnancy Uterus: endometritis, obstruction, rupture Rectosigmoid colon: colitis/proctitis, ischemia, diverticulitis, foreign body Small bowel: inflammation Appendix: appendicitis Bladder and ureters: bladder outlet obstruction, ureteral calculus, cystitis Lymph nodes: lymphadenitis Abdominal wall: hernia Peritoneum: abscess
Scrotal or inguinal	Testis: torsion, orchitis, abscess, hematoma Epididymis: epididymitis Bowel and peritoneum: hernia

can be useful in distinguishing between those processes that require urgent surgical intervention and those suitable for conservative management. Several studies have shown that routine evaluation of the abdomen and pelvis with CT in the emergency setting decreases both the number of hospital admissions and the length of stay in the emergency department.

Although ultrasound is routinely performed for the evaluation of right upper quadrant and pelvic pain, CT has many advantages over sonography for the evaluation of patients with other types of pain. CT can be performed in a matter of seconds on a modern scanner, allowing surgical triage to be accomplished with utmost efficiency. CT is less limited by patient body habitus, and displays all organ systems and many disease processes with near equal clarity. Finally, CT image quality is far less operator dependent than sonography.

One final advantage of CT is its exquisite ability to demonstrate the full extent of a disease process that spans multiple abdominal organ systems or abdominal compartments. No other modality has the ability of CT to fully document the spread of diseases via the peritoneal cavity or abdominal mesenteries and ligaments. This avoids the potential diagnostic pitfall created by diseases presenting remote from their organs of origin.

Computed Tomography Protocol Considerations for Acute Abdominal Pain

Because of the overlapping innervation of abdominal and pelvic organs and the possibility of a disease process presenting remote from the organ of origin, the entire abdomen and pelvis should be included on a CT examination performed for evaluation of acute abdominal pain. Although CT performed without the addition of enteric and intravenous contrast media can provide valuable diagnostic information, the appropriate use of these agents often improves sensitivity and defines disease to better advantage. For this reason, most survey examinations of the abdomen and pelvis for acute pain are performed using both intravenous and enteric (typically oral) contrast. The portal venous phase of enhancement is preferred in most situations. The CT examination can be modified to accommodate specific patient conditions, such as renal insufficiency, contrast sensitivity, or compromised hemodynamic status.

Traditional positive oral contrast (high attenuation) is useful for distinguishing bowel from other structures and for demonstrating perforation of the gastrointestinal tract. Negative oral contrast (low attenuation) accompanied by injection of intravenous contrast media can be useful for demonstrating inflammation and other enhancing lesions of the bowel wall (Fig. 8-1). When urgency dictates, examinations can be performed without enteric contrast media.

Helpful Computed Tomographic Findings in the Acute Abdomen

Because of the all-inclusive survey provided by CT and the overlapping clinical presentations that can cloud the origins of abdominal pain, radiologists must be facile with interpreting CT scans of the abdomen and pelvis. This skill requires a systematic approach and knowledge of findings that aid in disease localization. A number of signs have been proved effective in localizing the source of acute abdominal pain (Box 8-1).

Focal Fat Stranding or Fascial Thickening

Fat stranding adjacent to a bowel loop or solid organ is often a key CT finding indicating the origin of pain. Stranding is seen as linear or hazy increased attenuation within a region of fat, usually caused by fluid or inflammatory cells infiltrating the tissues (Fig. 8-2) and often accompanied by thickening of nearby fascial planes. Stranding is most useful when it is localized because

---

BOX 8-1   Computed Tomographic Signs That Localize or Characterize Disease in the Acute Abdomen

Focal fat stranding or fascial thickening
Segmental bowel dilatation
Segmental bowel wall thickening
Extraluminal gas collections
Focal fluid collections
Altered contrast enhancement
Distortion of bowel/vessels
Displacement of structures
Soft-tissue mass
Regional lymphadenopathy
Asymmetry of paired organs (kidneys, testes, ovaries, adrenals)

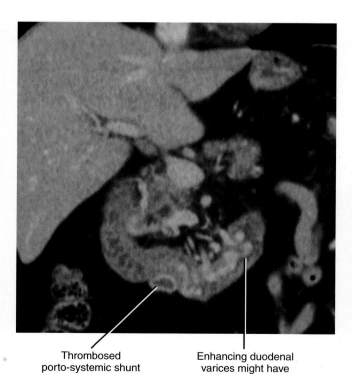

Thrombosed porto-systemic shunt

Enhancing duodenal varices might have been obscured by barium

Figure 8-1 Coronal reformation of computed tomography performed with intravenous and negative oral contrast demonstrates varices within the fourth part of the duodenum. The scan was performed to evaluate abdominal pain and occult gastrointestinal bleeding in a patient with prior placement of a portosystemic shunt that was found to be thrombosed on this examination.

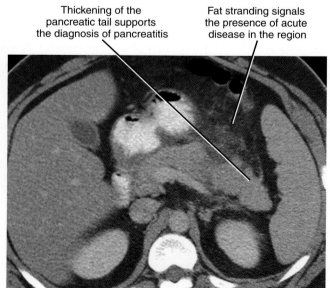

Thickening of the pancreatic tail supports the diagnosis of pancreatitis

Fat stranding signals the presence of acute disease in the region

Figure 8-2 Axial image from a contrast-enhanced computed tomographic scan of the upper abdomen demonstrates fat stranding anterior to the pancreas in a patient with acute pancreatitis.

generalized stranding is nonspecific and can be seen with any systemic cause of edema (e.g., congestive heart failure or hypoproteinemia). Focal fat stranding can signal a focus of acute disease and should always prompt focused inspection of the adjacent structures.

Disproportionate fat stranding refers to focal stranding adjacent to bowel associated with minimal or absent bowel wall thickening. Its presence suggests entities that typically result in a greater degree of inflammation in the adjacent mesentery than in the bowel wall itself. The presence or absence of disproportionate fat stranding is one method used to differentiate colonic diverticulitis from colon cancer, because diverticulitis tends to result in a greater degree of pericolic inflammation relative to the degree of bowel wall thickening (Fig. 8-3). Disease processes associated with disproportionate fat stranding are listed in Table 8-2.

Table 8-2   Disease Processes Associated with Disproportionate Fat Stranding

Diagnosis	Clinical Discriminators	Imaging Discriminators
Appendicitis	Right lower quadrant pain, nausea, fever, leukocytosis	Periappendiceal inflammation
Diverticulitis	Left lower quadrant pain, fever, leukocytosis	Pericolonic inflammation, adjacent diverticulum
Epiploic appendagitis	Nausea and fever are rare	Fatty pericolonic mass with dense rim and central high-attenuation focus
Omental infarction	Right-sided greater than left-sided pain Nausea and fever are rare	Triangular or ovoid fatty/heterogeneous lesion deep to right anterior abdominal wall

Degree of fat stranding and thickening of fascia exceed the degree of wall thickening in diverticulitis

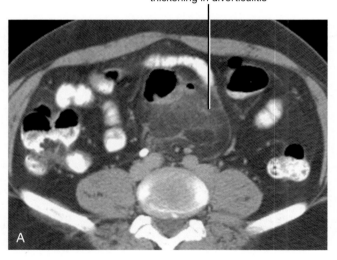

Severe wall thickening with minimal fat stranding is typical of cancer

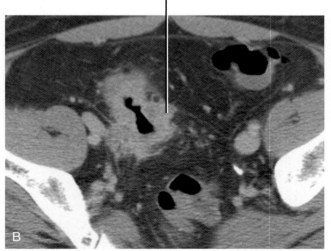

Figure 8-3 Axial computed tomographic images from two patients demonstrate how the presence of disproportionate fat stranding can help to differentiate between **(A)** diverticulitis and **(B)** colon cancer.

Mesenteric fat stranding can result from a broad variety of inflammatory and neoplastic disease processes; therefore, it is important to consider this finding in the context of clinical presentation and other imaging findings (Fig. 8-4). The most common causes of mesenteric fat stranding are listed in Box 8-2.

Sclerosing mesenteritis is an uncommon primary inflammatory disorder of the mesentery. An elusive disease that can be difficult to diagnose and to treat, sclerosing mesenteritis has been known by many names, including mesenteric panniculitis, retractile mesenteritis, fibrosing mesenteritis, mesenteric lipodystrophy, and mesenteric Weber–Christian disease. The most common CT finding is fat stranding in the mesentery, a nonspecific finding sometimes referred to as a "misty" mesentery (Fig. 8-5). Additional findings of sclerosing mesenteritis may include: (1) a "fat halo," or ring of low attenuation surrounding mesenteric vessels within a region of mesenteric fat stranding; (2) a dense pseudocapsule surrounding the area of involved fat; and (3) small soft-tissue nodules within the affected region of mesentery.

The most common malignant neoplasms to involve the mesenteries are lymphoma and carcinoid tumor, although other tumors, such as adenocarcinoma, can also extend into the mesenteries or incite a local desmoplastic reaction. Neoplastic disease of the mesentery rarely presents as acute abdominal pain.

Perinephric stranding is commonly seen in healthy individuals, but when asymmetric, should prompt a search for a cause. Some causes to consider include obstructive urinary calculus, pyelonephritis, inflammatory nephritides, renal infarction, and renal vein thrombosis.

Segmental Bowel Dilatation
Bowel becomes distended when the intestinal tract is obstructed or when there is a decrease in normal bowel motility. In the case of obstruction, the proximal gastrointestinal tract distends, unless partially decompressed by vomiting or nasogastric tube suction. In cases of decompressed obstruction, bowel distention may be limited to the immediately proximal segment.

Swirled appearance of
the omental vessels

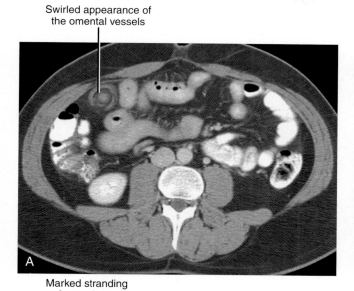

Marked stranding
from edema

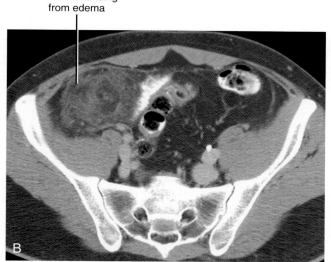

Figure 8-4 Axial images from contrast-enhanced computed to-mography of the **(A)** abdomen and **(B)** pelvis demonstrate fat stranding because of omental torsion. Stranding extended into the right inguinal canal where the omentum was tethered by a hernia.

BOX 8-2   Causes of Localized Mesenteric Fat Stranding

Inflammation
Lymphoma
Sclerosing mesenteritis
Portal hypertension
Mesenteric contusion/hematoma
Carcinoid tumor
Vascular thrombosis or embolism
Intestinal volvulus or other closed-loop obstruction
Intestinal lymphangiectasia

Adynamic or paralytic ileus is often associated with a generalized decrease in bowel motility, resulting in relatively uniform distention of the small intestine and colon. However, a focal area of inflammation in the peritoneal cavity can result in segmentally decreased motility

Regional mesenteric
fat stranding with
well-defined margins   Perivascular sparing

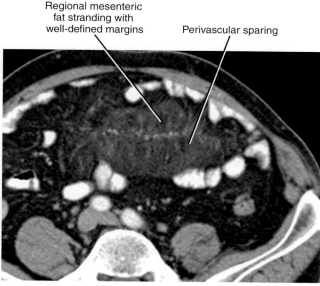

Figure 8-5 Axial image from contrast-enhanced computed tomography (CT) in a patient with upper abdominal pain demonstrates a well-defined region of hazy fat stranding within the mesentery. In the absence of other evidence of disease, a diagnosis of sclerosing mesenteritis was made, and the findings were followed by CT. (Courtesy Srinivasa R. Prasad, M.D.)

in bowel loops immediately adjacent to the acute process. This accounts for the "sentinel loop" sign associated with intraabdominal inflammation (Fig. 8-6) and can be a clue to the nature and location of the underlying disease process.

Segmental Bowel Wall Thickening
Distinguishing between normal and abnormal bowel wall thickness is one of the greatest challenges in abdominal imaging. Even the combination of a diligent

Dilated loop of
proximal jejunum   Fat stranding extends
anteriorly from anterior
pararenal space

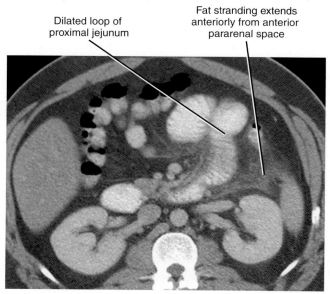

Figure 8-6 Axial image from contrast-enhanced computed tomographic scan performed in a patient with pancreatitis demonstrates focal dilatation of a jejunal loop adjacent to mesenteric stranding. This is comparable with the sentinel loop sign described on plain radiographs.

technologist and compliant patient rarely results in uniform bowel distention throughout the gastrointestinal tract. Because some bowel loops are likely to be incompletely distended during the examination, it is common to mistakenly describe a collapsed bowel segment as "thickened." Of course, if one becomes accustomed to ignoring apparently thickened loops of bowel, critical diagnoses can be missed.

If a bowel loop appears thickened, it is useful to look for a segment of that loop that contains air. Because air rises to the most nondependent portion of the lumen and produces some degree of luminal distension, the presence of air underlying apparent bowel wall thickening suggests that the loop in question is truly abnormal.

Be cautious about calling wall thickening in the jejunum on CT examinations. The normal jejunum contains many more redundant folds than ileum. The CT correlate of redundant folds in the jejunum is a thicker appearance of the bowel wall (Fig. 8-7). As stated earlier, looking for areas of nondependent air between folds may help distinguish normal from thickened jejunum.

Whereas thickening of the entire cecum can be seen with colitis or colon cancer, focal thickening of the cecal apex near the base of the appendix is often seen with acute appendicitis. Sometimes called the *cecal arrow* sign, wall thickening at the junction of the cecum and appendix causes the lumen of the cecum to point toward the appendix, supporting the diagnosis of acute appendicitis (Fig. 8-8).

Table 8-3 lists the disease processes most commonly associated with segmental thickening of the bowel wall on CT, as well as some parameters that can be used to refine the differential diagnosis.

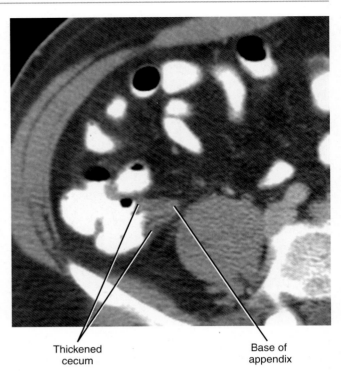

Thickened cecum

Base of appendix

Figure 8-8 Cecal arrow sign in acute appendicitis. Axial computed tomographic image demonstrates focal thickening of the cecum at its junction with an inflamed appendix. The high-attenuation enteric contrast within the cecum tapers to "point" toward the appendix.

Table 8-3   Diseases Associated with Segmental Bowel Wall Thickening

Diagnosis	Imaging Discriminators
Appendicitis	Thickening of appendix and adjacent cecal apex Appendicolith Interruption in enhancing appendiceal wall Periappendiceal fat stranding or fluid
Crohn disease	Thickened segment of distal ileum Skip lesions Fistulas and interloop abscesses
Colonic diverticulitis	Fat stranding usually more severe than wall thickening Eccentric wall thickening Adjacent diverticulosis
Gastritis	Thickening of gastric wall Usually more severe in the antrum
Malignancy	Bowel wall thickening more severe than fat stranding Eccentric wall thickening Loss of wall stratification on enhanced images Pericolonic lymphadenopathy
Meckel's diverticulitis	Blind ending loop from ileum, not from cecum

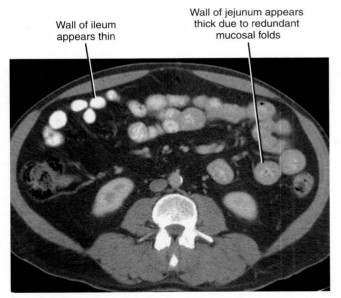

Wall of ileum appears thin

Wall of jejunum appears thick due to redundant mucosal folds

Figure 8-7 Axial image from contrast-enhanced computed tomographic examination performed in an asymptomatic patient to follow a small liver lesion demonstrates the differences in appearance between normal jejunum and ileum. Note the redundant folds of the normal jejunum results in a thickened appearance when compared with the ileum.

Extraluminal Gas

PNEUMOPERITONEUM

The interpretation of CT examinations performed for acute abdominal pain should always include a directed search for peritoneal gas. Gas usually rises to the most nondependent recesses of the peritoneal cavity; therefore, a focused survey along the anterior peritoneal surface can increase sensitivity. During the search, it is helpful to use window and level settings that allow differentiation between fat and gas. The peritoneal space extends into the fissures for the ligamentum teres and ligamentum venosum, so include those locations in the search pattern. When gas is present in these fissures, duodenal or distal stomach perforation is often the source (Fig. 8-9). The most common causes of pneumoperitoneum are listed in Table 8-4.

Notably, many causes of pneumoperitoneum do not require emergent therapy. The most common among these is postoperative pneumoperitoneum. Gas in the peritoneal cavity can be a normal finding up to 10 days after surgery. This can be confounding in a postoperative patient with acute abdominal pain or signs of infection. Postoperative peritoneal gas is typically seen in trace amounts after the first few days and should decrease in quantity on successive examinations. An increase in gas over time raises concern for complications.

Pitfall: Although pneumoperitoneum can persist for up to 10 days after abdominal surgery, increasing gas can be a sign of infection, breakdown of a bowel anastomosis, or perforated postoperative stress ulcer. If a patient is imaged repeatedly for suspected complications, pay close attention to the quantity and distribution of gas.

Iatrogenic pneumoperitoneum can also occur when air is inadvertently injected into a peritoneal dialysis catheter. As with postoperative pneumoperitoneum, the presence of a dialysis catheter does not prove that gas in the peritoneal space is an insignificant finding in the patient with acute abdominal pain. Pneumoperitoneum is also occasionally seen when a percutaneous gastrostomy tube is present. Retrograde passage of air through the female genital tract has been reported in association with

Table 8-4   Causes of Pneumoperitoneum

Surgical Causes (90%)*	Nonsurgical Causes (10%)
Bowel perforation Penetrating injury	Recent laparotomy Transabdominal peritoneal or enteric catheter Mechanical ventilation Pulmonary disease Spontaneous bacterial peritonitis Pneumatosis cystoides intestinalis Scleroderma Retrograde passage through female genital system

*Requirement for urgent, often surgical, therapy.

sexual activity and pelvic examination, as well as with activities such as horseback riding and water skiing.

PNEUMORETROPERITONEUM
Extraperitoneal gas is usually the result of bowel perforation or infection. Because gas is more restricted within the extraperitoneal compartments than within the peritoneal cavity, the location of gas within the retroperitoneum is often more useful for identifying the source. In general, by determining whether the gas is within the anterior pararenal space, the perirenal space, or posterior pararenal space, and noting whether it is unilateral or bilateral, the differential diagnosis can be narrowed considerably. The most likely causes for retroperitoneal gas within each space are outlined in Table 8-5.

INTRAMURAL GAS COLLECTIONS
Pneumatosis intestinalis describes gas in the wall of the alimentary tract. Because the gas is confined between the mucosal and serosal layers, pneumatosis does not move freely through the abdomen and is usually confined to one region of the intestinal tract. On plain film, pneumatosis appears as a combination of curvilinear and mottled gas, and can easily be confused with fecal

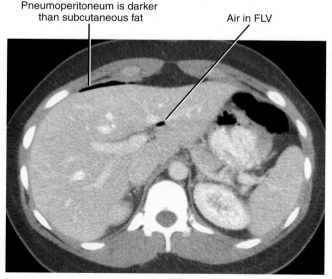

Pneumoperitoneum is darker than subcutaneous fat

Air in FLV

Figure 8-9 Axial image from contrast-enhanced computed tomographic scan demonstrates pneumoperitoneum in the fissure for the ligamentum venosum (FVL) and anterior to the liver. A perforated duodenal ulcer was found at surgery. Note that the window/level settings are set to make air darker than fat.

Table 8-5   Correlation between Location of Extraperitoneal Gas and Its Source

Compartment	Side	Likely Source
Anterior pararenal	Right	Perforation of descending duodenum (e.g., duodenal ulcer or recent ERCP) (Fig. 8-10)
	Left	Perforation of descending or sigmoid colon (e.g., diverticulitis)
	Bilateral	Sigmoid or rectal perforation (Fig. 8-11) Complicated pancreatitis
Perirenal	Right or left	Renal infection
Posterior pararenal	Left	Perforated sigmoid diverticulitis
	Bilateral	Rectal perforation (traumatic) Supradiaphragmatic origin (pneumomediastinum)

Air in right anterior
pararenal space

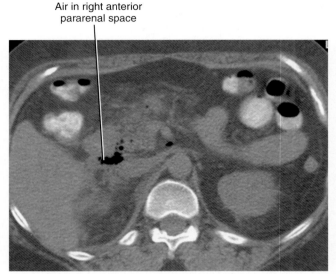

Figure 8-10 Axial image from noncontrast-enhanced computed tomographic examination performed after difficult endoscopic retrograde cholangiopancreatogram demonstrates air in the right anterior pararenal space. The patient recovered with conservative management.

Right anterior
pararenal space

Left anterior
pararenal space

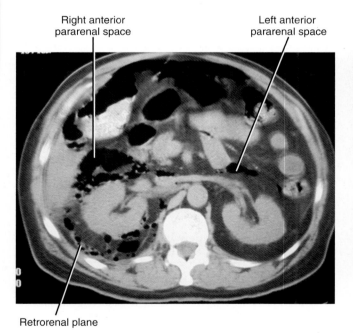

Retrorenal plane

Figure 8-11 Axial computed tomographic image at the level of the kidneys demonstrates air in the anterior pararenal space bilaterally in patient with perforated sigmoid diverticulitis. On the right side, air also enters the perirenal space and retrorenal plane (between the layers of the posterior renal fascia).

material (Fig. 8-12). Although the curvilinear shape of the gas collections are better appreciated by CT, differentiation from fecal material can still be challenging. Because the mucosal and serosal layers can be thin when distended, pneumatosis can be difficult to detect when located adjacent to gas within the bowel lumen. However, when fluid is present adjacent to intramural gas, the gas is much more conspicuous.

Mottled and curvilinear collections
of gas in colonic wall

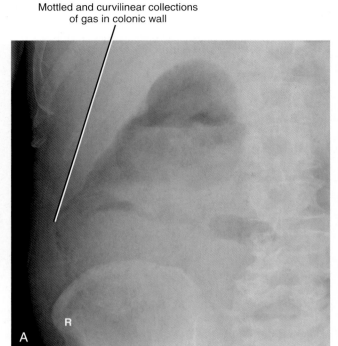

A   R

Obstructing colon cancer

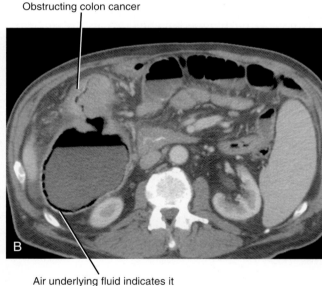

B

Air underlying fluid indicates it
is within colonic wall

Figure 8-12 Pneumatosis of the colon demonstrated by (**A**) abnormal radiograph and by (**B**) computed tomographic scan in a patient with an obstructing cancer of the hepatic flexure.

Most of the many causes of intestinal pneumatosis are listed in Table 8-6. Pneumatosis is often seen in association with acute gastrointestinal disease processes such as bowel ischemia, bowel obstruction, and severe bowel infections. When seen in the presence of bowel ischemia, it is associated with reported mortality rates of 50% to 75%. However, pneumatosis is also associated with chronic disease processes such as obstructive pulmonary disease, Whipple disease, and scleroderma. Iatrogenic pneumatosis can result from endoscopy with or without biopsy, barium enema, or bowel surgery,

Table 8-6   Causes of Intestinal Pneumatosis

Causes that Usually Require Urgent Therapy	Causes that Usually Do Not Require Therapy
Bowel ischemia	Mechanical ventilation
Severe bowel infections	Chronic obstructive pulmonary
Bowel obstruction	disease
Trauma	Recent endoscopy
	Barium enema
	Recent bowel surgery
	Whipple disease
	Scleroderma
	Systemic lupus erythematosus
	Idiopathic

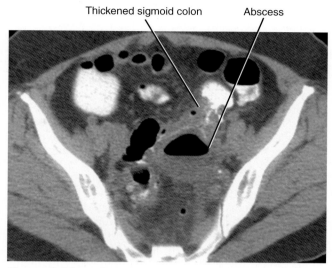

Thickened sigmoid colon   Abscess

Figure 8-14 Axial image of the pelvis from computed tomographic scan performed with oral contrast demonstrates an air–fluid level within a peridiverticular abscess.

particularly if a bowel anastomosis is performed. Occasionally, idiopathic pneumatosis is seen as an unsuspected finding in patients without acute abdominal symptoms. When pneumatosis is present, always look at the mesenteric vessels and liver for evidence of portal venous gas (Fig. 8-13).

As with the bowel, gas can also collect within the walls of other structures such as the gallbladder (emphysematous cholecystitis) and the urinary bladder (emphysematous cystitis). These entities are almost always infectious in nature and particularly common in individuals with diabetes. Gas within the vagina (vaginitis emphysematosa) is an uncommon but clinically benign entity characterized by gas-filled mucosal cysts. Although vaginitis emphysematosa can be associated with organisms such as *Trichomonas vaginalis,* it does not represent a life-threatening gas-producing infection.

OTHER GAS COLLECTIONS

A contained collection of extraluminal gas near bowel is a common sign of perforation with or without abscess formation. Abscesses contain infected material with variable proportions of fluid, debris, and gas (Fig. 8-14). Common causes of abscess include bowel perforation, superinfected postoperative

fluid, hematogenous dissemination of bacteria, pyelonephritis, or anastomotic leak. Because the bowel also contains differing proportions of gas, fluid, and semisolid material, it is sometimes mistaken for an abscess. A key feature that distinguishes an abscess from bowel is discontinuity or eccentric location with respect to the alimentary tract. When an abscess is identified near a bowel loop without evidence of diverticula or inflammatory bowel disease, be certain to look for a foreign body such as a fish bone.

Gelatin bioabsorbable sponge (Gelfoam) and oxidized cellulose (Surgicel) used for intraoperative hemostasis can result in an appearance similar to abscess on CT. Clues to the presence of these materials on CT include a history of recent surgery, linear organization of small gas bubbles (best seen on bone windows), stable

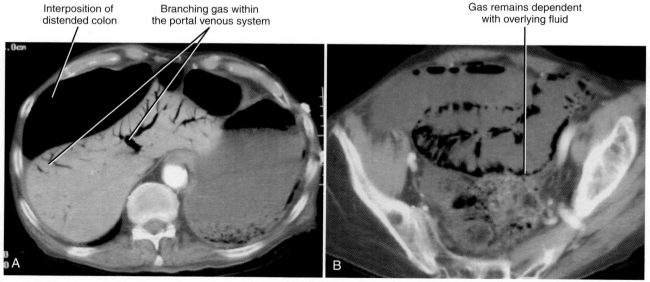

Interposition of distended colon   Branching gas within the portal venous system   Gas remains dependent with overlying fluid

Figure 8-13 Axial images from computed tomographic examination performed for development of abdominal distention after resuscitation from recent cardiac arrest demonstrate **(A)** extensive portal venous gas in association with **(B)** colonic pneumatosis.

appearance of the gas on sequential examinations, and unusual shape of the collection. Because most postoperative abscesses contain at least some fluid, a predominantly mottled gas appearance and the absence of an air–fluid level favor hemostatic material (Fig. 8-15). This general rule does not work in reverse, however; because the material may be surrounded by hematoma, the presence of fluid does not necessarily indicate abscess. Note that this material can occasionally become superinfected, but because it is semisolid and typically in an area of recent hemorrhage, catheter drainage is not usually performed.

Hospitalized patients often have gas in the urinary bladder from bladder catheterization. However, gas within the urinary tract can also be a sign of urinary tract infection (UTI) or enterovesical fistula. Biliary gas is commonly present in patients who have had prior sphincterotomy, biliary stent placement, or choledochoenteric anastomosis, but it can signify acute cholangitis in an acutely ill patient with right upper quadrant pain.

Focal Fluid Collections

Under normal circumstances, fluid in the abdominal pelvic cavity is contained within the hollow viscera of the gastrointestinal, biliary, and urinary tracts. Women of reproductive age often have small amounts of "physiologic" fluid in the pelvis as a result of the rupture of follicular cysts. However, larger amounts of peritoneal fluid in women and more than trace amounts of peritoneal fluid in the male patient must be viewed with suspicion.

Fluid collecting adjacent to thickened or inflamed bowel often indicates bowel perforation with or without abscess formation. For example, although acute appendicitis and diverticulitis without perforation can result in inflammation of the adjacent fat, a nonlinear fluid collection near a thickened appendix or inflamed diverticulum increases the likelihood of perforation (Fig. 8-16).

A similar principle can be applied to perirenal collections. Urinary obstruction often results in stranding of

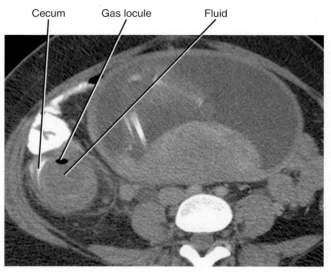

Cecum   Gas locule   Fluid

Figure 8-16 Focal fluid collection as a sign of perforation in appendicitis. Axial image of the pelvis from computed tomography performed to evaluate right lower quadrant pain at 32 weeks of gestation demonstrates a rounded fluid collection compressing the cecum. The appendix was thickened on other images (not shown). Percutaneous catheter drainage was performed initially, followed by cesarean section and appendectomy, which confirmed the diagnosis of perforated appendicitis.

the perinephric fat, appearing as thin linear and curvilinear areas of fluid attenuation within otherwise low-density fat. If the areas of fluid attenuation become wider or rounded in the setting of urinary obstruction, forniceal rupture should be suspected (Fig. 8-17).

The presence of fluid in the lesser sac presents a limited differential diagnosis, particularly if there is little or no fluid in the rest of the peritoneal cavity. The most likely causes of fluid in the lesser sac include processes that affect the pancreas, stomach or gastroesophageal junction (Fig. 8-18), duodenum, or spleen.

As mentioned earlier, the pelvis is the most common site for physiologic fluid to accumulate. In addition,

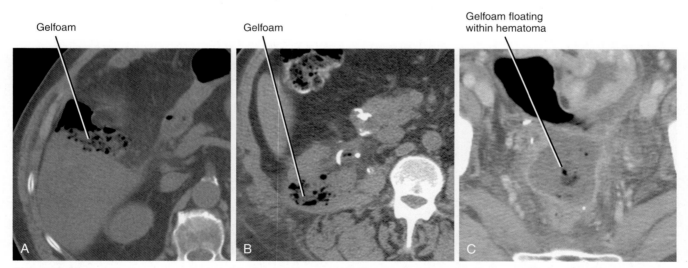

Gelfoam   Gelfoam   Gelfoam floating within hematoma

A   B   C

Figure 8-15 Variable appearance of gelatin bioabsorbable sponge (Gelfoam) on axial computed tomographic images of three separate patients. **A,** Mottled gas in gallbladder fossa. **B,** Mottled gas in partial nephrectomy defect. **C,** Low-attenuation material surrounded by hematoma after hysterectomy. Because the material is used to stop bleeding, it is often located in places at high risk for delayed bleeding.

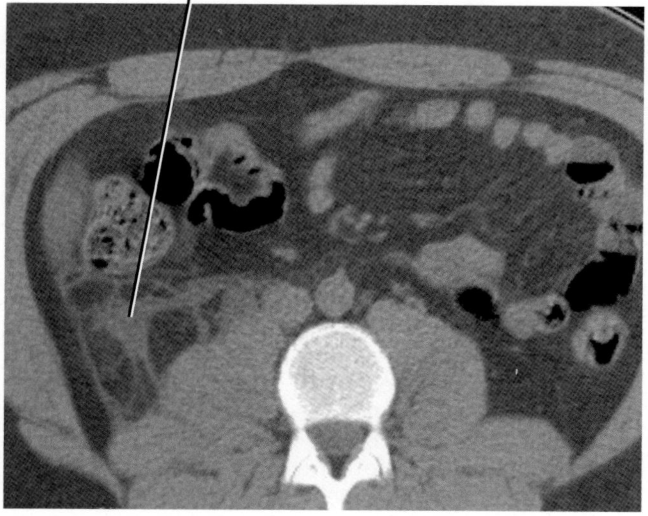

Fluid bands are too wide
for simple stranding

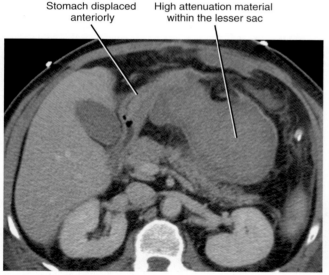

Figure 8-17 Axial image just inferior to the right kidney from noncontrast-enhanced computed tomographic examination demonstrates wide, polygonal bands of perinephric fluid indicating forniceal rupture. A small distal ureteral calculus and hydronephrosis were also identified (not shown).

Stomach displaced   High attenuation material
anteriorly   within the lesser sac

Figure 8-18 Axial image from contrast-enhanced computed tomographic scan performed after difficult repair of a tear at the gastroesophageal junction demonstrates high-attenuation material in the lesser sac. Percutaneous aspiration confirmed hematoma.

peritoneal fluid from inflammatory or malignant disease processes originating anywhere within the peritoneal space often accumulates first within the pelvis because of its dependent location. Primary pelvic processes that result in focal pelvic fluid collections include pelvic inflammatory disease (PID), endometriosis, ovarian cancer, bladder injury, and pelvic surgery.

Extraperitoneal fluid is commonly identified in patients with acute abdominal pain. Knowledge of the compartments and fascial planes of the extraperitoneum

provides a tool for identifying the causative factors of extraperitoneal fluid collections.

The anterior pararenal space contains the pancreas, the ascending and descending colon, and the extraperitoneal portion of the duodenum. Therefore, fluid in the anterior pararenal space is likely to originate from these structures. Although the anterior pararenal space is continuous across the midline, fluid collections from the duodenum and colon are often confined to the side of origin. Bilateral anterior pararenal fluid collections usually are of pancreatic origin (Fig. 8-19).

Pearl: When fluid in the anterior pararenal space is bilateral, it is most often the result of acute pancreatitis.

The perirenal space contains the kidneys and adrenal glands, and is divided into right and left because the anterior renal fascia fuses with the fascia surrounding the abdominal aorta and inferior vena cava. Despite this compartmentalization, fluid under pressure within the perirenal space can occasionally cross to the contralateral side (Fig. 8-20). The perirenal space extends caudally to the upper pelvis, where it communicates with the anterior pararenal space. Despite these potential avenues of communication, the majority of perirenal fluid collections remain confined to the perirenal space.

The posterior pararenal space contains no organs and is primarily filled with adipose tissue. Infection within this space can extend from the psoas compartment or result from penetrating trauma. Interestingly, idiopathic extraperitoneal hemorrhage is most frequent in the posterior pararenal space, left greater than right.

An additional potential space exists between the two layers of the posterior renal fascia, sometimes called the *retrorenal plane*. Fluid collections in this potential space most often arise from pancreatitis (Fig. 8-21) and are in continuity with the anterior pararenal space (see Fig. 6-33).

Fluid in right APS   Thickened duodenum   Fluid in left APS

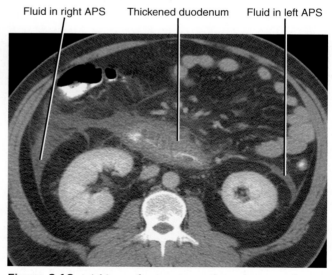

Figure 8-19 Axial image from contrast-enhanced computed tomographic scan in a patient with acute pancreatitis demonstrates fluid in the anterior pararenal space *(APS)* bilaterally. The transverse duodenum (also located within the APS) is markedly thickened.

Fluid in right APS

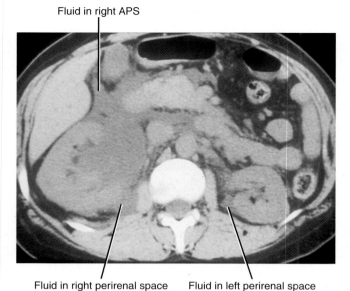

Fluid in right perirenal space   Fluid in left perirenal space

Figure 8-20 Axial image from noncontrast-enhanced computed tomography demonstrates a large amount of fluid in the left renal sinus and perirenal space. A ureteral calculus was present in the distal ureter (not shown). In this case of severe forniceal rupture, urine extends into the anterior pararenal space *(APS)* with a small amount of fluid crossing the midline to the left perirenal space.

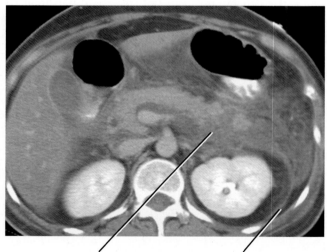

Region of pancreatic necrosis   Fluid in retrorenal plane

Figure 8-21 Axial image from contrast-enhanced computed tomographic examination performed in evaluation of necrotizing pancreatitis demonstrates fluid dissecting between the superficial and deep layers of the posterior renal fascia (retrorenal plane). Regions of pancreatic parenchyma that do not enhance indicate necrosis.

Extraperitoneal hemorrhage is usually the result of ruptured aortic aneurysm, trauma, hemorrhagic tumor, or a bleeding disorder. The significance of periaortic fluid depends largely on the clinical setting. In the presence of an abdominal aortic aneurysm (AAA), high-density periaortic fluid implies leak or rupture. If an aortic repair has already been performed, low-attenuation fluid in the vicinity of the repair can be a sign of infection in a patient with leukocytosis and fever, especially when a gas locule

is present. Periaortic fluid collections are uncommon after endograft repair of aortic aneurysm.

Table 8-7 correlates each extraperitoneal space with acute disease processes that are most often responsible for fluid accumulating within that space.

Altered Contrast Enhancement

INCREASED ENHANCEMENT

An area of increased contrast enhancement can be a key finding when interpreting a CT examination of the abdomen and pelvis in a patient with acute pain. The hyperemia and increased capillary permeability often associated with tissue injury often results in increased delivery of intravenous contrast media to the affected structure. For example, increased bowel wall enhancement is commonly seen in active stages of Crohn disease but can also be seen with nonocclusive mesenteric ischemia (caused by increased capillary permeability) and appendicitis (Fig. 8-22). If peritoneal fluid is present, it may be possible to detect increased peritoneal enhancement in patients with inflammatory or neoplastic disease of the peritoneum (Fig. 8-23). A rim of increased enhancement around a fluid collection is usually a sound indicator of an abscess or pseudocyst.

Other forms of inflammatory disease can cause hyperenhancement in the setting of acute abdominal pain. For example, severe acute cholecystitis is often associated with increased enhancement of the adjacent liver on early phase images. Of course, many neoplastic processes also demonstrate enhancement above that of the background organ after intravenous contrast administration.

DECREASED CONTRAST ENHANCEMENT

Focal areas of decreased contrast enhancement are also key to diagnosing patients with acute abdominal pain. Decreased delivery of contrast material to all or part of an organ can be caused by obstructed inflow (as in the case of arterial occlusion), increased interstitial pressure (as in the case of urinary tract obstruction), or obstructed outflow (as in the case of venous occlusion).

Table 8-7   Acute Disease Processes Most Likely to Account for Fluid in Each Extraperitoneal Space

Space	Disease Processes
Anterior pararenal space	Pancreatitis Extraperitoneal duodenal ulcer or injury (right side) Colonic diverticulitis (left or both sides) Ruptured abdominal aortic aneurysm
Perirenal space	Ureteral stone with forniceal rupture Pyelonephritis Renal injury
Between layers of posterior renal fascia (retrorenal plane)	Pancreatitis
Posterior pararenal space	Trauma Extension of psoas or renal abscess Idiopathic hemorrhage

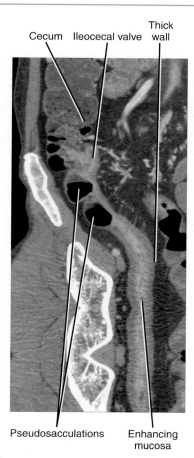

Cecum   Ileocecal valve   Thick wall

Pseudosacculations   Enhancing mucosa

Figure 8-22 Curved planar reformation of terminal ileum from computed tomographic (CT) examination performed with intravenous contrast and negative oral contrast for CT enterography. Mucosal enhancement and diffuse wall thickening exist within the ileal segment, as well as focal areas of pseudosacculation. Endoscopy confirmed a diagnosis of Crohn disease.

Decreased enhancement can also result from infiltration of an organ by inflammatory or neoplastic cells (as in the case of infection or lymphoma).

Parenchymal infarction caused by embolic disease most often affects the kidneys and spleen because of the limited collateral arterial blood flow available within these organs and high volume of perfusion. Infarcts are typically wedge shaped, defining the vascular distribution of an end arteriole. It is common to see a rim of persistent or increased enhancement overlying areas of infarction because of the presence of capsular vessels (Fig. 8-24; see also Fig. 9-23).

Acute venous obstruction reduces early enhancement of organs such as the kidney but can actually increase enhancement of organs such as the liver because of hepatic autoregulatory mechanisms. Decreased enhancement of the intestinal wall is an important sign of bowel necrosis and perforated appendix.

Whenever an enhanced CT scan is performed on a patient with acute pancreatitis, one should assess the degree of pancreatic enhancement because significant pancreatic necrosis portends a complicated course (Fig. 8-25).

DISTORTION OF BOWEL/VESSELS

Distortion of normal anatomic structures can be an important finding when searching for a cause of acute pain. Within a solid organ such as the liver, displacement and distortion of vascular structures can signal the presence of mass lesions including malignant tumor or abscess. Distortion (twisting) of mesenteric vessels may be an important sign of volvulus (Fig. 8-26).

Kinking or unusual angulation of bowel loops can be a sign of peritoneal adhesions or desmoplastic response to a neoplasm (Fig. 8-27). Crohn disease can cause a significant increase in the amount of mesenteric fat adjacent to affected bowel loops, most

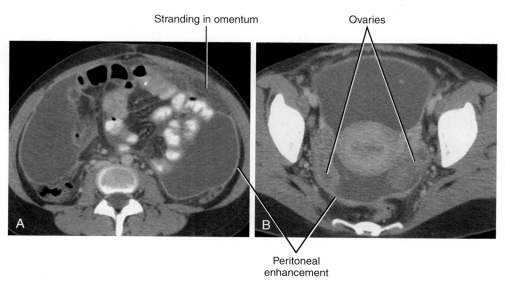

Stranding in omentum   Ovaries

Peritoneal enhancement

Figure 8-23 Axial images from contrast-enhanced computed tomographic (CT) examination performed in a 25-year-old woman with abdominal pain and distention. Images of the **(A)** abdomen and **(B)** pelvis demonstrate ascites with diffuse peritoneal enhancement, infiltration of the omentum, and enlargement of the ovaries. Initially presumed to be ovarian carcinoma, the diagnosis ultimately proved to be tuberculous peritonitis.

Geographic zone
of low attenuation

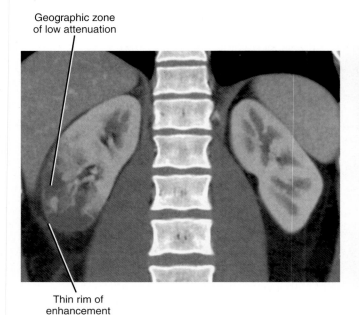

Thin rim of
enhancement

Figure 8-24 Coronal reformation from contrast-enhanced computed tomography performed for severe right flank pain demonstrates a region of decreased perfusion to the inferior pole of the right kidney consistent with infarction. Note the rim of enhancement surrounding the region of infarction.

Necrotic tissue   Enhancing tissue

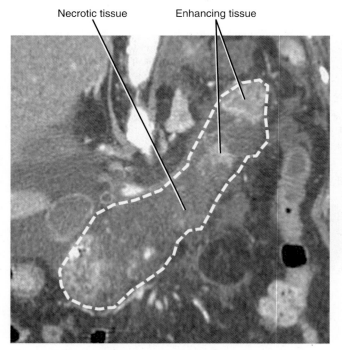

Figure 8-25 Curved planar reformation of the pancreas (outlined) from contrast-enhanced computed tomographic examination performed to evaluate patient with necrotizing pancreatitis. Only approximately 20% of the gland enhances.

Dilated small bowel   Whirling vessels

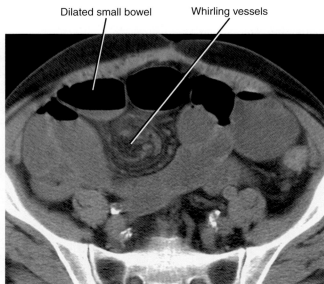

Figure 8-26 Axial image from noncontrast-enhanced computed tomography performed for acute abdominal pain and distention demonstrates "whirling" of mesenteric vessels and dilated small bowel loops. Small bowel volvulus was confirmed at laparotomy.

Mass   Tethering

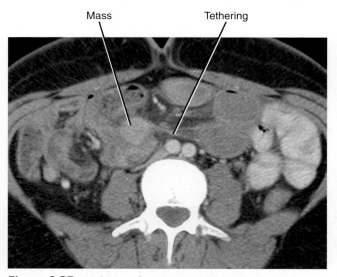

Figure 8-27 Axial image from contrast-enhanced computed tomographic examination performed for right-sided abdominal pain demonstrates tethering of small-bowel loops. While looking for the cause of tethering, an enhancing mass was identified, subsequently proved to be carcinoid tumor.

commonly in the right lower quadrant surrounding the terminal ileum. The increased amount of fat separates the ileum from other loops. Unusually "good" visualization of the terminal ileum as a structure separated from other bowel loops by a layer of fat

should prompt consideration of inflammatory bowel disease (Fig. 8-28).

SOFT-TISSUE MASS

A focal area of masslike soft-tissue density is often a key finding indicating the source of a patient's pain. Benign or malignant masses can stretch an organ's capsule or compress adjacent structures to cause pain. Extraperitoneal masses such as lymphoma, metastases, or sarcomas

More fat here than elsewhere
in abdomen

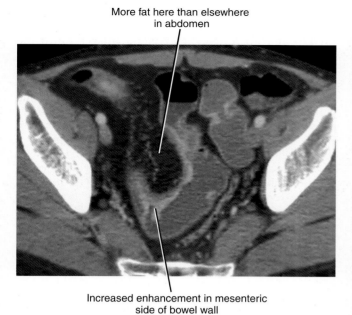

Increased enhancement in mesenteric
side of bowel wall

Figure 8-28 Axial image from contrast-enhanced computed tomographic scan in a patient with Crohn disease demonstrates fatty hypertrophy in the right lower quadrant. Also, note mucosal enhancement is more pronounced along the mesenteric wall of the ileum, a common finding in the disease.

Enhancing mass within the mesentery

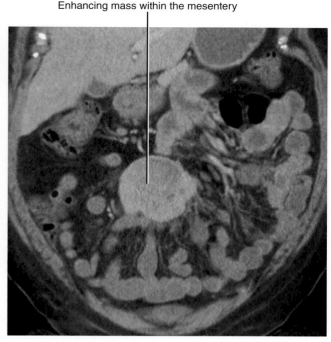

Figure 8-29 Coronal reformation from contrast-enhanced computed tomographic examination performed to evaluate a patient with abdominal pain demonstrates a large soft-tissue mass within the mesentery. Percutaneous biopsy proved this to be a carcinoid tumor.

can displace the kidneys or vascular structures, causing pain that is sometimes difficult to localize clinically. Lymphoma and carcinoid tumor are the most common malignancies to form soft-tissue masses within the mesentery (Fig. 8-29).

It may be difficult to differentiate areas of soft-tissue mass from hematoma, particularly in the patient with acute pain. Contrast enhancement is helpful in making this distinction because hematomas do not enhance unless actively bleeding. Active hemorrhage is typically visible on enhanced CT as a well-defined perivascular focus of intense enhancement that becomes progressively larger and more ill-defined on subsequent phases of imaging.

REGIONAL LYMPHADENOPATHY

Regional lymphadenopathy in the abdomen or pelvis can signal the presence of neoplastic or inflammatory disease. In some cases, the lymph nodes are a secondary finding (colon cancer, inflammatory disorders), whereas in other cases, the lymph nodes represent the primary abnormality (lymphoma). In either case, the presence of abnormally large or numerous lymph nodes should prompt a careful inspection of that region.

Mesenteric adenitis is a syndrome of regional lymphadenopathy in the right lower quadrant associated with pain, diagnosed more commonly in children but also seen in young adults. It is likely the result of mild infectious enteritis, although enlarged lymph nodes are usually the only imaging finding. Primary mesenteric adenitis should be considered only when there is no identifiable other cause of inflammation in the region.

Although criteria for diagnosing mesenteric adenitis vary, we suggest the diagnosis if the site of pain corresponds with a group of three or more enlarged mesenteric lymph nodes in the right lower quadrant, provided other causes of pain have been excluded (Fig. 8-30). Because ileocolic lymph nodes are often found incidentally, and because many neoplastic and inflammatory disease processes are associated with mesenteric lymphadenopathy, it is important to seek out additional imaging findings and clinical information before making the diagnosis of mesenteric adenitis.

Although many malignant tumors can spread to lymph nodes in the retroperitoneum and mesentery, lymphoma is the most commonly encountered process causing abdominal lymphadenopathy. However, lymphoma rarely presents as acute abdominal pain. When it does, the pain is usually due to mass effect.

ASYMMETRY OF PAIRED ORGANS

Even a novice at CT interpretation quickly learns to use paired anatomic structures to their advantage. Asymmetry in size, attenuation, or contrast enhancement is useful in detecting disease in the adrenal glands, kidneys, ureters, and ovaries. Of course, the organ involved and the particular characteristic of the asymmetric finding generates a different differential in each case, but noting the asymmetry is often the first step in diagnosis. With sonography, similar comparison is used to detect altered echotexture or vascularity of the testes. Although some degree of asymmetry is normal in virtually every paired organ system, and abnormalities can be bilateral and symmetric, asymmetry should at least warrant further scrutiny.

Enlarged lymph nodes

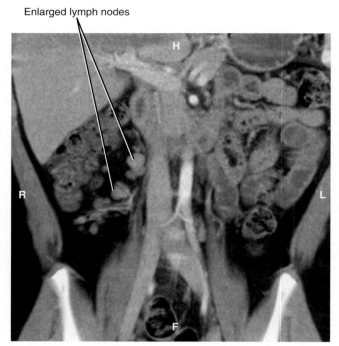

Figure 8-30 Coronal reformation from contrast-enhanced computed tomographic examination performed in evaluation of right lower quadrant pain demonstrates multiple enlarged lymph nodes along the ileocolic vessels. A diagnosis of mesenteric adenitis was made in the absence of other findings and with clinical correlation confirming the location of pain.

■ UPPER ABDOMINAL PAIN

Many physicians begin the imaging evaluation of patients with upper abdominal pain with ultrasound, particularly when the pain is localized to the right upper quadrant. Subsequent decisions regarding further imaging are based on a combination of ultrasound findings and clinical information. The astute radiologist will also think outside the abdomen, considering diagnoses such as rib fracture, pneumonia, or shingles when evaluating the patient with upper abdominal pain.

Start with Ultrasound

Because gallbladder and biliary disease are among the most common causes of acute pain in the upper abdomen, ultrasound is usually the first-line imaging examination. Cost and risk to the patient also compare favorably with CT; therefore, there is little to lose by starting with sonography. Even in patients with a clinical diagnosis of pancreatitis, ultrasound is helpful in excluding gallstones as the causative agent. The upper abdominal sonogram includes evaluation of the liver, gallbladder, bile ducts, pancreas, spleen, and kidneys. The "right upper quadrant (RUQ) sonogram" omits the spleen and left kidney to save time when symptoms are on the right side. If, however, an abnormality is encountered in the liver or kidney, converting a limited RUQ sonogram to a complete abdominal sonogram can provide additional valuable information.

Acute cholecystitis can be diagnosed with ultrasound in the appropriate clinical setting when gallstones are present and accompanied by either thickening of the gallbladder wall or a sonographic Murphy sign. Pericholecystic fluid or striation of the wall is sometimes present on grayscale images. Proper technique can minimize false-positive results. For an accurate measurement, the gallbladder wall nearest the transducer should be measured in the anteroposterior dimension on a transverse image of the gallbladder. Side-to-side measurement of the gallbladder wall is more prone to error.

With regard to the sonographic Murphy sign, communication with the patient is crucial. It is important not to "lead the witness" by placing the transducer over the gallbladder while asking if that is where it hurts. If placing the transducer over the gallbladder evokes guarding, try to "provoke" a pain response in multiple regions of the abdomen, noting where the pain seems to be maximal. It is sometimes helpful to ask the patient to place a single finger over the point of maximal pain and then scan that area to determine whether the patient is pointing to the gallbladder. Whenever cholelithiasis is diagnosed in a patient with acute abdominal pain, a search should be conducted for evidence of choledocholithiasis.

Hepatobiliary scintigraphy is useful when there is persistent clinical suspicion of acute cholecystitis despite a negative ultrasound examination. The physiologic information from scintigraphy allows for diagnosis of acute cholecystitis with or without gallstones. Rarely, acute cholecystitis is identified by CT after a negative ultrasound examination, usually when there is a small stone in the cystic duct and no significant thickening of the gallbladder wall.

Other common causes of upper abdominal pain that can be diagnosed with ultrasound include pancreatitis, choledocholithiasis, and urinary obstruction. Less common diagnoses include malignant neoplasm, liver abscess, and ascending cholangitis (Fig. 8-31).

Upper Abdominal Diagnoses Likely to Require Computed Tomography or Magnetic Resonance

When complicated cholecystitis is suspected based on sonographic findings, CT can be helpful for confirming the presence of gallbladder wall gas, perforation, or abscess formation (Fig. 8-32). Ultrasound findings in the gallbladder that should prompt further evaluation by CT include hyperechoic, shadowing foci in the wall (air), nonlinear pericholecystic or intrahepatic fluid (abscess), shadowing without distinct visualization of a soft-tissue wall (porcelain gallbladder), or unusual shape or orientation of the gallbladder (gallbladder torsion). Magnetic resonance cholangiopancreatography (MRCP) can be helpful in confirming the latter diagnosis (see Fig. 13-15).

Once ultrasound has been performed to exclude gallstones in a patient with clinical evidence of acute pancreatitis, CT is often performed to assess disease severity and detect complications. In some cases, ultrasound fails to

Echogenic gas in the biliary tree

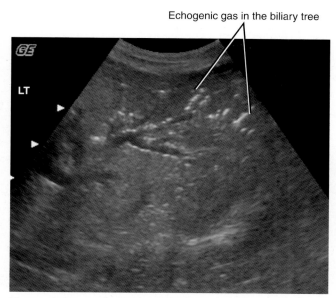

Figure 8-31 Transverse ultrasound image of the left hepatic lobe in a patient with ascending cholangitis demonstrates linear echogenic structures in the nondependent regions. The clinical diagnosis, absence of flow-type movement, and lack of pneumatosis on computed tomography indicated pneumobilia rather than portal venous gas. Symptoms resolved with antibiotic therapy.

Abscess   GB lumen

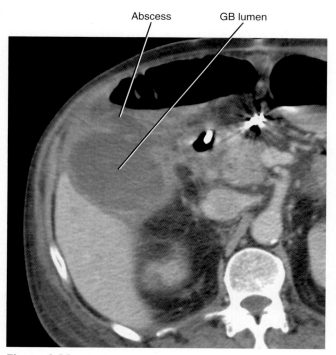

Figure 8-32 Axial image from contrast-enhanced computed tomographic scan of the upper abdomen demonstrates gallbladder (GB) perforation that was not identified by ultrasound. Medial gallbladder perforation near the bowel is more likely to be missed by ultrasound than is lateral perforation (compare with Fig. 1-39).

identify any cause for acute abdominal pain. In such cases, an alternate imaging modality can be helpful. CT can provide information regarding bowel wall thickening and identify extraluminal gas in cases of intestinal perforation (Fig. 8-33). MRI can identify stones within the common

bile duct that are not identified with sonography (Fig. 8-34). MRCP is often performed to determine the need for therapeutic endoscopic retrograde cholangiopancreatogram. Finally, endoscopic techniques are often helpful for diagnosis of gastrointestinal and biliary disorders with the added benefit of being potentially therapeutic.

Low attenuation thickening of gastric wall

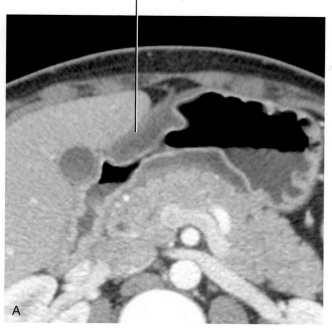

A

Gas adjacent
to gallbladder

Pneumoperitoneum

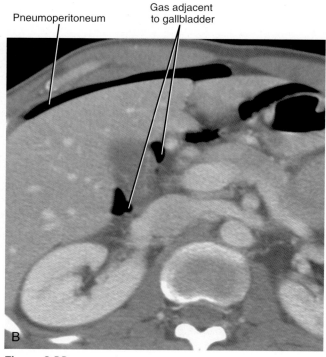

B

Figure 8-33 Images of the upper abdomen from contrast-enhanced computed tomographic examinations in different patients demonstrating some of the causes of upper abdominal pain that could be missed by a cursory right upper quadrant ultrasound. Cases shown include (**A**) axial image demonstrating gastritis, (**B**) axial image demonstrating perforated duodenal ulcer,

Continued

Thickening of colonic wall

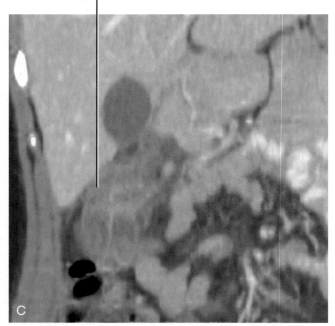

Figure 8-33, cont'd and (C) coronal reformation demonstrating colitis in the hepatic flexure.

Dilated common bile duct   Stone in distal bile duct

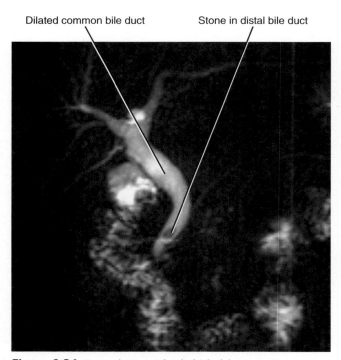

Figure 8-34 Coronal, T2-weighted, thick-slab, magnetic resonance cholangiopancreatography image demonstrates a stone in the distal common bile duct, retained after cholecystectomy. Duct dilatation was evident by ultrasound, but no stone was visualized.

Table 8-8   Causes of Upper Abdominal Pain for Which Ultrasound May Be Inadequate for Diagnosis

Ultrasound Often Negative or Nonspecific*	Ultrasound Findings Often Prompt Further Imaging
Peptic ulcer disease	Choledocholithiasis
Gastritis, duodenitis	Emphysematous cholecystitis
Transverse colitis	Gallbladder torsion
Pyelonephritis	Upper abdominal abscess
Splenic infarction	Acute pancreatitis
Epiploic appendigitis	Malignant neoplasm
Omental infarction	
Pulmonary disease	
Myocardial infarction	
Herpes zoster	

*Many of the entities on this list have been diagnosed with ultrasound by an expert sonographer at some point. However, we believe this table represents the typical experience in a typical radiology practice.

Spleen with normal perfusion   Infarcted segment   Enhancing rim

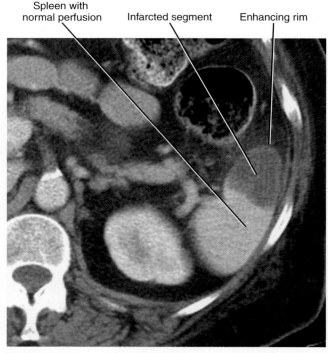

Figure 8-35 Axial image from contrast-enhanced computed tomographic scan performed for evaluation of left upper quadrant pain demonstrates a region of hypoperfusion to the spleen consistent with an infarct. Note the faint rim of enhancement surrounding the region of infarction.

Table 8-8 summarizes disease processes that cause upper abdominal pain that commonly result in a negative or inconclusive ultrasound examination. Note that although less common, acute upper abdominal pain is sometimes localized to the left side. In addition to atypical presentation of cardiac pain, diagnoses to consider in such cases include splenic infarction, pancreatitis, or masses involving the pancreatic tail, gastritis, and diverticulitis/colitis at the splenic flexure (Fig. 8-35). In most of these cases, diagnosis is made by CT rather than by ultrasound.

■ LOWER ABDOMINAL PAIN

Most cases of lower abdominal pain originate in the appendix, colon, ileum, reproductive system or bladder. Since the differential diagnosis varies significantly with the side of the pain, our discussion is divided into right and left lower quadrant pain.

Right Lower Quadrant Pain

Although the differential diagnosis for right lower quadrant pain is lengthy, the workup can begin with a short list of potential diagnoses. In women of reproductive age, a pelvic examination and serum beta human chorionic gonadotropic hormone (β-HCG) should be performed before making decisions regarding imaging. If physical examination does not exclude gynecologic origin, pelvic ultrasound should be considered. Once the above tests are negative, other diagnoses can be pursued.

The next order of business is usually to exclude appendicitis. Acute appendicitis is the most common cause of acute abdominal pain requiring surgery in the Western world. Interestingly, it is much less common in developing countries, and although the appendix has been described anatomically for centuries, inflammation of the appendix was not described until the nineteenth century.

The appendix is a long diverticulum arising from the cecum. It averages 10 cm in length, but can be as long as 20 cm. The appendix originates from the tip of the cecum, typically from the inferomedial wall, although this is variable. If the lumen of the appendix becomes obstructed by impacted fecal material (fecalith), lymphoid hyperplasia, parasites, or even foreign bodies, the obstructed lumen becomes inflamed and, eventually, ischemic from distention. Untreated acute appendicitis can progress to perforation with clinical outcome ranging from chronic abscess formation to death.

CT is usually the imaging modality of choice for evaluating adult patients with right lower quadrant pain not of gynecologic origin. Ultrasound is often used for children with suspected acute appendicitis, but larger body habitus and longer list of potential diagnoses decrease its utility in the adult population. CT provides adequate visualization of the appendix in most cases and clearly depicts complications of acute appendicitis.

Finding the Appendix

The appendix must first be identified to confirm or exclude the diagnosis of appendicitis by CT. It is usually found as a small, blind-ending, tubular structure arising from the cecum. The location of the tip of the appendix is variable and can be found as far cephalad as the gallbladder fossa or caudad within a right inguinal hernia (Fig. 8-36). Fortunately, the origin of the appendix is more predictable. The appendix usually originates from the medial wall of the cecum approximately 3 cm inferior to the ileocecal valve. If the cecum has an atypical orientation, the base of the appendix will still arise from the same wall that has the ileocecal valve. Thus, if the appendix is not readily apparent by CT, it is often useful to first identify the ileocecal valve. If the cecum is positioned horizontally, the appendix can course superiorly or inferiorly from the cecum. In problem cases, coronal or sagittal images can be useful. It is important to note when the appendix is in a retrocecal extraperitoneal location (17% are retrocecal, and half of these are extraperitoneal). Extraperitoneal appendicitis presents with atypical signs and symptoms, and alters the surgical approach.

Pearl: Use the ileocecal valve to locate the appendix because they often both arise from the same wall of the cecum.

Pitfall: Extraperitoneal appendicitis presents with atypical signs and symptoms, and alters the surgical approach.

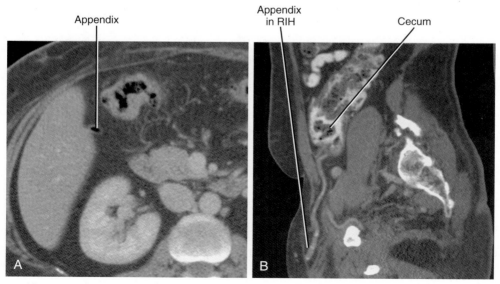

Figure 8-36 Unusual locations of the appendix in two separate patients. **A,** Axial computed tomographic (CT) image demonstrates the appendix in the right upper quadrant near the gallbladder fossa. **B,** Sagittal reformation from CT scan in a different patient demonstrates the appendix within a right inguinal hernia *(RIH).*

Computed Tomographic Findings in Acute Appendicitis

Because acute appendicitis is caused by obstruction of the lumen, the inflamed appendix is usually distended. Some studies correlate an appendiceal diameter of greater than 6 mm with appendicitis, although such numbers should be applied with caution. Distended with air, a normal appendix can have a luminal diameter greater than 6 mm; therefore, numeric criteria should be applied only to a fluid-filled appendix. Appendiceal diameter should be interpreted in the context of clinical presentation and ancillary findings to maintain specificity.

Ancillary signs are useful to the diagnosis of acute appendicitis. The inflamed appendiceal wall is typically thickened, and this inflammation usually causes some stranding in the adjacent fat. In "tip appendicitis," only the end of the appendix is affected, and soft-tissue stranding around the tip may be the main finding. A calcified fecalith, though a classic radiologic sign, is only variably present. Although a fecalith is reported to be present in 11% to 52% of acutely inflamed appendices under pathologic evaluation, fewer are calcified and visible with CT. In addition, calcified fecaliths can be seen in asymptomatic patients, limiting the specificity of this finding. Also, not all densities are fecaliths, and both lower quadrants are common sites for ingested foreign bodies to become imbedded (Fig. 8-37).

Acute appendicitis is a continuum of disease, ranging from acute focal appendicitis to perforative appendicitis (Table 8-9). Because conservative management is sometimes used for mild cases of acute focal appendicitis, and percutaneous drainage may be used in the initial treatment of periappendiceal abscess in perforative appendicitis, precise description of the extent of disease can help guide the surgeon in making therapeutic decisions.

Although periappendiceal stranding is a common finding in acute suppurative appendicitis (Fig. 8-38), a loculated fluid collection adjacent to the appendix usually indicates perforation, particularly if contained by an enhancing rim (Fig. 8-39). In the absence of loculated fluid, one should look for interruption of the enhancing appendiceal wall as a sign of ischemia and gangrenous appendicitis, which can lead to perforation (Fig. 8-40). Perforation can also be suggested when localized gas collections are noted adjacent to the appendix. Pneumoperitoneum can result from perforation but is uncommon.

Table 8-9   Categorizing Acute Appendicitis with Computed Tomography

Type	Imaging Findings
Acute focal	Distension, wall thickening, and enhancement are main findings Minimal fat stranding
Acute suppurative	Marked periappendiceal inflammation May be phlegmonous Wall enhancement still *increased*
Gangrenous	Venous thrombosis causes wall ischemia, leading to marked thickening with *decreased enhancement*
Perforative	Discontinuity of the appendiceal wall Discrete fluid or air collections Fecalith in peritoneum

Well-defined "calcification"

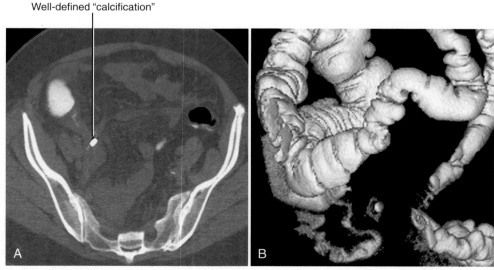

Figure 8-37 Foreign body mimics appendicolith. **A,** Axial image from computed tomography performed with oral but no intravenous contrast demonstrates a high-attenuation object in the right lower quadrant. **B,** Because of the unnaturally well-defined margins, volume rendering was performed for further characterization, demonstrating an iron tablet inadvertently taken by this elderly patient while it was still within the foil blister pack. At surgery, the packet was found to have eroded through the bowel wall.

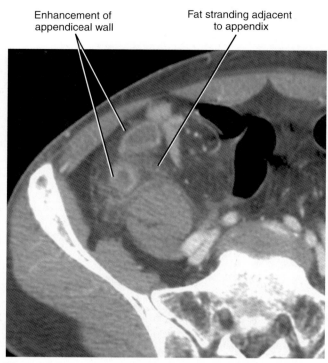

Enhancement of appendiceal wall

Fat stranding adjacent to appendix

Figure 8-38 Acute suppurative appendicitis. Axial image from contrast-enhanced computed tomography demonstrates a distended, fluid-filled appendix with increased enhancement of the appendiceal wall and marked periappendiceal fat stranding. Despite the inflammatory changes, no discrete fluid collections were present.

Appendicitis versus Crohn Disease

Crohn disease can present with clinical findings identical to acute appendicitis, but most treating physicians will avoid surgery in patients with Crohn disease if at all possible. The CT appearance of Crohn disease is variable, but findings in the right lower quadrant typically include thickening of the distal ileum and stranding of the adjacent fat. Thus, Crohn disease and appendicitis can usually be differentiated by following the thickened loop. If it is a blind-ending loop that joins the cecum, the diagnosis is appendicitis. If the loop is in continuity with small bowel and meets the ileocecal valve, Crohn disease is likely, although other forms of ileitis must be considered clinically. Identifying a normal appendix confirms localization of disease to the small bowel (Fig. 8-41).

When inflammatory changes are severe, the appendix and small bowel may both appear thickened (Fig. 8-42). The more thickened loop is usually the point of origin, and inflammatory changes are often centered on it. This method usually works, but because the appendix is occasionally directly involved with Crohn disease, some diagnoses are still left to the pathologist (Fig. 8-43).

In addition to increased wall enhancement discussed in the previous section on CT findings, increased vascularity in Crohn disease often results in enlarged mesenteric vessels surrounded by mesenteric fat (Fig. 8-44). This appearance has been described as the "comb sign" and usually indicates Crohn disease.

Appendicitis versus Meckel's Diverticulitis

Imaging differentiation between appendicitis and Meckel's diverticulitis may be considered more for style than substance, because surgery is indicated for both processes. Nonetheless, to preserve your reputation, be sure to trace an abnormal appendix to its origin at the cecum. In the uncommon event that an inflamed, blind-ending structure arises from the distal ileum instead, the appropriate diagnosis is Meckel's diverticulitis (Fig. 8-45). Imaging findings are otherwise similar to appendicitis. Note that a Meckel's diverticulum arises from the antimesenteric side of the bowel and is often larger than the normal appendix. Retained enteric material may occasionally cause pain without inflammation (Fig. 8-46).

Appendicitis versus Pelvic Inflammatory Disease (PID)

Although the presentation is often different, some potential overlap exists between PID and appendicitis clinically. In many cases of PID, hydrosalpinx is present and visible on imaging studies. The finding of hydrosalpinx with adjacent inflammatory fluid and a normal appendix elsewhere is consistent with PID (Fig. 8-47). If the appendix is adjacent to the adnexa, apply a principle similar to the one mentioned earlier for Crohn disease; the more abnormal structure is usually the point of origin. In some cases, surveillance or exploratory laparoscopy is necessary for diagnosis. Table 8-10 summarizes clinical and imaging findings that are useful for discriminating among different causes of right lower quadrant abdominal pain.

Left Lower Quadrant Pain

Although right lower quadrant pain is a more common presentation in young adults, older adults are more likely to present with left lower quadrant pain. Timely diagnosis of the cause of left lower quadrant pain allows initiation of therapy at an early stage of disease. Diverticulitis is a key example. Although many older patients with clinical suspicion of diverticulitis are treated empirically, the diagnosis of diverticulitis might be overlooked in younger patients without the aid of imaging. Identification of subtle pericolonic fat stranding can help clinicians diagnose and treat diverticulitis before surgical intervention or percutaneous drainage is required (Fig. 8-48).

When peridiverticular inflammation is severe, not only is fat stranding more pronounced, but there is often thickening of the adjacent colon. In some cases, colonic wall thickening is so severe that it mimics colon cancer. With diverticulitis, the degree of fat stranding usually exceeds the degree of wall thickening (see Fig. 8-3). The opposite can be said of colon cancer. However, because overlap exists between the two, follow-up imaging or colonoscopy is recommended in most cases of diverticulitis in which colonic wall thickening is identified by CT (Fig. 8-49). Table 8-11 lists some of the more common causes of left lower quadrant pain.

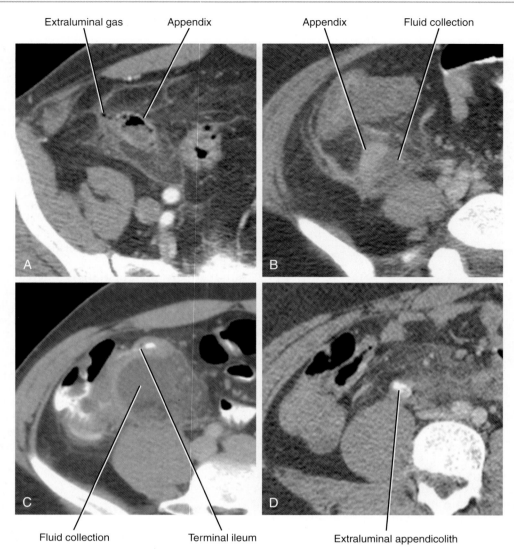

Figure 8-39 Axial computed tomographic images from four different patients demonstrate a spectrum of findings in acute perforative appendicitis. **A.** Trace air adjacent to appendix. **B,** Small amount of extraluminal fluid. **C,** Large fluid collection with secondary effects on the cecum and ileum. **D,** Extraluminal appendicolith.

■ PELVIC PAIN

We use the term *pelvic pain* to describe pain confined to or originating from the most inferior portions of the torso in the region of the bladder, rectum, prostate, and female reproductive organs. Because the differential diagnosis for pelvic pain differs considerably between male and female patients, these will be discussed separately.

Female Pelvic Pain

Pain in the female pelvis usually originates in the gynecologic organs. Some entities (e.g., uterine contractions of menstruation or small endometrial implants) are usually occult on medical imaging. Some causes of pelvic pain in women that can be reliably imaged are described later and listed in Table 8-12. Endovaginal ultrasound is typically the first (and often only) imaging examination used for women with acute pelvic pain.

Ovarian Cysts

Ovarian cysts are best diagnosed with sonography but often visible on CT images. Determining the clinical relevance of an ovarian cyst may be difficult. Endovaginal sonography offers the opportunity to correlate symptoms with anatomic structures. Similar to eliciting the sonographic Murphy sign for acute cholecystitis, asking questions during the examination can help confirm that an ovarian cyst correlates with the site of the patient's pain. Rupture of a functional cyst or follicle can cause severe pain. In such cases, ultrasound can identify the presence of a collapsed cyst in the presence of free pelvic fluid. However, the diagnosis of ruptured ovarian cyst should be rendered only after life-threatening causes of abdominal pain have been excluded.

Retrocecal appendix

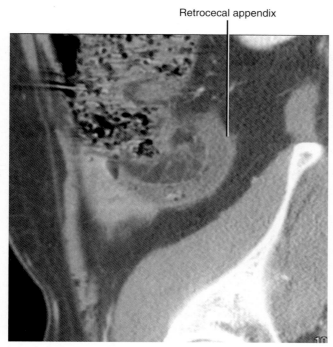

Normal appendix

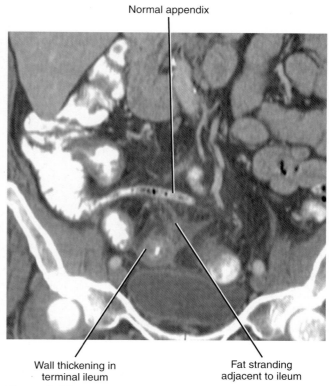

Wall thickening in terminal ileum

Fat stranding adjacent to ileum

Figure 8-40 Sagittal reformation from computed tomographic examination demonstrates a distended, fluid-filled appendix with stranding of the periappendiceal fat but poor enhancement of the wall of the appendix (despite excellent enhancement in the portal venous phase elsewhere on the examination). Acute gangrenous appendicitis was found at surgery.

Figure 8-41 Coronal reformation of computed tomographic examination performed for right lower quadrant pain demonstrates marked thickening of a loop of distal ileum adjacent to a normal appendix. The diagnosis of Crohn disease was confirmed based on clinical and endoscopic findings.

Diffuse thickening of the appendix

Secondary focal thickening of ileum

Secondary thickening of the appendix

Terminal ileum thickened by Crohn disease

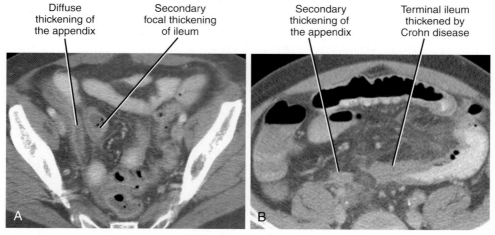

Figure 8-42 Thickening of "bystander" bowel loops on axial computed tomographic images from two different patients. **A,** Acute appendicitis causes thickening of an adjacent loop of ileum. **B,** Crohn disease causes thickening of the appendix. In both cases, the loop of primary pathology appears to be more severely affected than the bystander.

Appendix   Terminal ileum

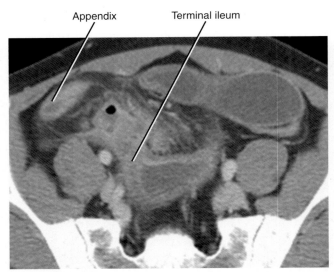

Figure 8-43 Axial image from contrast-enhanced computed tomographic examination demonstrates wall thickening involving both the appendix and the terminal ileum. Which one is responsible? Surgery proved Crohn disease of the appendix and the distal ileum.

Inflamed Meckel diverticulum

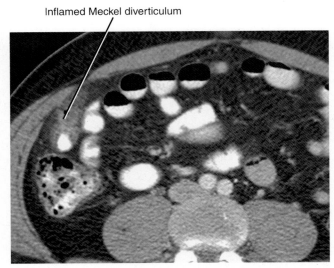

Figure 8-45 Axial image from contrast-enhanced computed tomographic examination performed for right lower quadrant pain demonstrates an inflamed, blind-ending loop in the right lower quadrant. The appendix was identified separately and appeared normal (not shown). Meckel's diverticulitis was confirmed at surgery.

Hypertrophy of
mesenteric fat

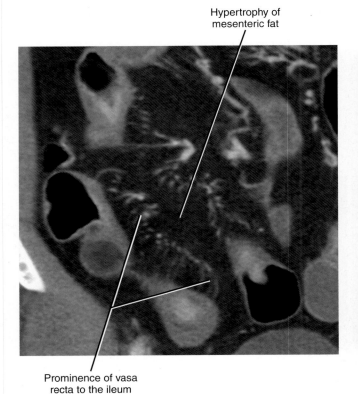

Prominence of vasa
recta to the ileum

Figure 8-44 "Comb sign" and fat proliferation in Crohn disease. Coronal reformation from enhanced axial computed tomographic examination in a patient with Crohn disease shows engorged vessels within hypertrophied mesenteric fat.

Toothpick

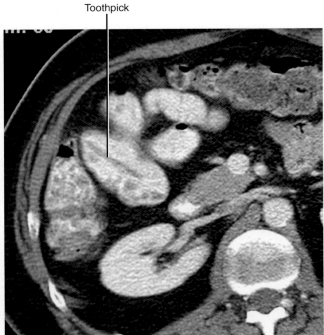

Figure 8-46 Axial image from contrast-enhanced computed tomographic examination performed in evaluation of recurring right lower quadrant pain. In addition to a normal appendix (not shown), a blind loop was identified originating from the small bowel and containing a linear filling defect. At surgery, a Meckel diverticulum was removed and found to contain a broken piece of toothpick.

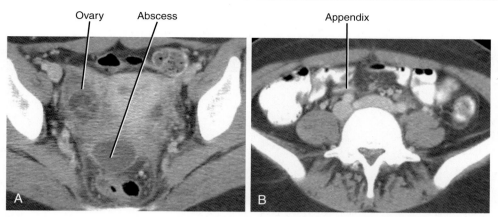

Ovary   Abscess   Appendix

Figure 8-47 Two axial images from computed tomographic examination performed to evaluate abdominal pain in a 17-year-old girl. **A,** An abscess is identified in the cul-de-sac with inflammation in the right adnexa. **B,** Identification of the normal appendix facilitated making the correct diagnosis of tuboovarian abscess rather than perforated appendicitis.

Table 8-10   Differentiating Causes of Right Lower Quadrant Abdominal Pain with Computed Tomography

Diagnosis	Clinical Discriminators	Imaging Discriminators
Acute appendicitis	Anorexia, fever, leukocytosis	Thickened, fluid-filled appendix Appendicolith Periappendiceal fat stranding
Mesenteric lymphadenitis	Anorexia and leukocytosis less likely	Normal appendix Three or more enlarged mesenteric lymph nodes
Ovarian torsion	Adnexal tenderness	Enlarged ovary Abnormal position of ovary Adnexal fat stranding
Pelvic inflammatory disease	Cervical motion tenderness	Dilated fallopian tube Normal appendix
Crohn disease	Diarrhea	Small or large intestinal wall thickening Mesenteric vascular engorgement ("comb sign") Increased mesenteric fat
Cecal diverticulitis	Similar to appendicitis	Fat stranding > wall thickening Normal appendix Inflammation centered on cecal diverticulum
Cecal carcinoma	Older patients Mild pain (unless perforated)	Wall thickening > fat stranding
Meckel's diverticulitis	Presents similar to appendicitis in adults	Normal appendix Pseudoappendix connects with ileum
Epiploic appendagitis	No fever or leukocytosis	Fat surrounded by stranding and rim Central dot of high attenuation
Mucocele of the appendix	Older patients Mild pain	Dilatation more pronounced than stranding May have wall calcification
Infectious ileitis/colitis	Diarrhea Cramping	Diffuse thickening of bowel segment(s)
Inguinal or spigelian hernia	Lump or bulge in left lower quadrant (often lacking with spigelian hernia)	Fat or bowel in inguinal canal or posterior to external oblique aponeurosis

Subtle fat stranding

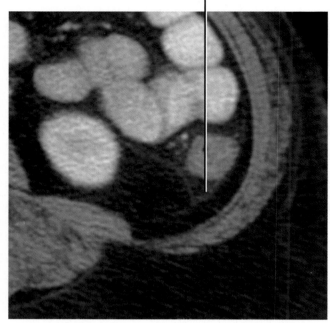

Figure 8-48 Computed tomographic (CT) findings in early diverticulitis. Axial image from contrast-enhanced CT scan shows subtle stranding of the adjacent fat and thickening of lateral conal fascia compared with other regions on the scan. Focal tenderness corresponded precisely to this location on physical examination. The responsible diverticulum was visible on an adjacent image (not shown).

Table 8-11   Differentiating Causes of Left Lower Quadrant Pain with Imaging

Diagnosis	Clinical Discriminators	Imaging Discriminators
Diverticulitis	Older patients Change in bowel habits Left lower quadrant tenderness Fever, leukocytosis may be present	Disproportionate fat stranding Thickened colon wall Colonic diverticulosis
Ovarian cyst	Female patient Midportion of menstrual cycle	Ovarian cyst on side of pain Pelvic fluid associated with rupture Internal echoes if hemorrhagic cyst
Ovarian torsion	Abrupt onset Nausea Adnexal tenderness	Enlarged ovary with peripheral follicles Abnormal position of ovary Pelvic fluid Decreased flow on color Doppler imaging
Inflammatory or ischemic colitis	Loose stools Hematochezia	Smooth segment of bowel wall thickening
Epiploic appendagitis	Fever unusual No leukocytosis	Disproportionate fat stranding Fat surrounded by stranding and rim Central dot of high attenuation
Colon cancer	Blood in stool Gradual onset	Focal, irregular thickening of colon wall Lymphadenopathy in sigmoid mesocolon
Inguinal or spigelian hernia	Lump or bulge in left lower quadrant (often lacking with spigelian hernia)	Fat or bowel in inguinal canal or posterior to external oblique aponeurosis

Masslike but eccentric thickening of sigmoid colon   Wall thickening has resolved

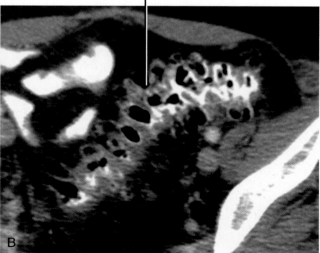

Figure 8-49 Follow-up for resolution of diverticulitis. **A,** Axial image from contrast-enhanced computed tomographic (CT) examination obtained during clinical episode of diverticulitis demonstrates masslike thickening of the sigmoid colon. **B,** Axial image from repeat CT examination performed several months later demonstrates complete resolution of colonic wall thickening.

Table 8-12   Common Causes of Pelvic Pain in Women

Diagnosis	Clinical Discriminators	Imaging Discriminators
Ovarian cyst	Cyclic pain, enlarged ovary on physical examination	Adnexal cyst Simple pelvic fluid
Ectopic pregnancy	Increased serum beta human chorionic gonadotropic hormone level Vaginal bleeding	No intrauterine gestation Pseudogestational sac Complex pelvic fluid Extrauterine gestation or decidual reaction
Pelvic inflammatory disease	Cervical motion tenderness Vaginal discharge	Hydrosalpinx, often bilateral
Ovarian torsion	Sudden onset	Enlarged ovary in unusual location Blood flow often diminished Twisted adnexal vessels
Endometriosis	Cyclic pelvic pain	May see blood-filled paraovarian cysts Pelvic adhesions
Uterine leiomyoma	Enlarged uterus on physical examination	Uterine mass visible with degeneration or torsion
Uterine rupture	Recent Cesarian section or vaginal delivery after prior Cesarian section	Disruption of anterior uterine wall
Migration of IUD	IUD placement in past	IUD outside endometrial cavity
Cystitis	Voiding symptoms Hematuria, pyuria	Air in lumen or bladder mucosa Bladder wall thickening

IUD, Intrauterine device.

Ectopic Pregnancy

Ectopic pregnancy is a potentially life-threatening cause of pelvic pain. Any woman of child-bearing age with acute pelvic pain should be tested for the presence of β-HCG, because the presence or absence of this hormone is a critical piece of diagnostic data. Patients with suspected ectopic pregnancy should undergo endovaginal ultrasound. Although identification of a fetal heartbeat outside the uterus provides a conclusive imaging diagnosis of ectopic pregnancy, this is found in only a minority of cases. Much more often, the diagnosis is made when a hypervascular heterogeneous (often hyperechoic) mass is seen in the adnexa in the absence of intrauterine pregnancy (Fig. 8-50). Complex pelvic fluid and a pseudogestational sac are important ancillary findings. When ultrasound findings are inconclusive, as is often the case with very early gestations, close follow-up with serial serum β-HCG levels and ultrasound can be helpful.

Pelvic Inflammatory Disease

PID is a continuum of ascending infection from cervicitis to endometritis to salpingitis to peritonitis. Complications include hydrosalpinx, tuboovarian abscess (TOA), and Fitz–Hugh–Curtis syndrome. Ultrasound findings of hydrosalpinx, free pelvic fluid, and adnexal tenderness usually indicate PID. If the diagnosis remains in doubt in a woman with right lower quadrant pain, visualization of a normal appendix improves diagnostic certainty. A delay in diagnosis of PID can result in formation of TOA. With TOA, inflammatory changes can be severe enough to cause secondary effects on the appendix. A combination of physical examination findings (site of greatest tenderness) and extent of appendiceal involvement facilitate a correct diagnosis.

It can sometimes be difficult to differentiate sigmoid diverticulitis from PID (Fig. 8-51). Unlike with appendicitis, however, both PID and diverticulitis often respond to nonoperative treatment.

Ovarian Torsion

The diagnosis of ovarian torsion can be problematic because symptoms and physical findings are nonspecific. Fortunately, an accurate diagnosis can usually be made with ultrasound.

Whether torsion is the result of an underlying adnexal mass (usually a cyst or teratoma) or redundant mesovarium, a torsed ovary is almost always enlarged on ultrasound. Multiple peripheral follicles may be visible in the affected ovary ("string of pearls" sign), and fluid is often present in the cul-de-sac (Fig. 8-52). Doppler ultrasound may demonstrate absent flow to the ovary. However, arterial flow is present in 54% and venous flow is present in 33% of patients with surgically proven ovarian torsion. High-resistance arterial flow or diminished blood flow compared with the contralateral side also suggests the diagnosis. Other helpful signs are twisted adnexal vessels and an unusual or abnormal position of the ovary (e.g., anterior to the uterus).

Pearl: Torsion should be considered when a woman has pelvic pain and an enlarged ovary that contains multiple peripheral follicles, has diminished or absent blood flow, or occupies an unusual position.

Pitfall: The presence of flow within an ovary on Doppler sonography does not exclude torsion.

Because the clinical presentation of ovarian torsion can mimic acute appendicitis, patients are often initially imaged with CT. CT findings of ovarian torsion include an enlarged ovary and free fluid (Figs. 8-53 and 8-54). A twisted appearance of the vascular pedicle has been reported. Images performed after administration of intravenous contrast media can show diminished or absent enhancement of the ovary. As with ultrasound, the ovary may lie in an unusual position. If all of these findings are present, diagnosis is usually certain enough for surgical therapy. If the diagnosis remains in doubt, ultrasound can be performed for further confirmation.

Uterine Fibroids

Uterine fibroids (leiomyomata) are discussed in detail in Chapter 21. Some discussion is relevant here because they are a common cause of chronic, intermittent pelvic

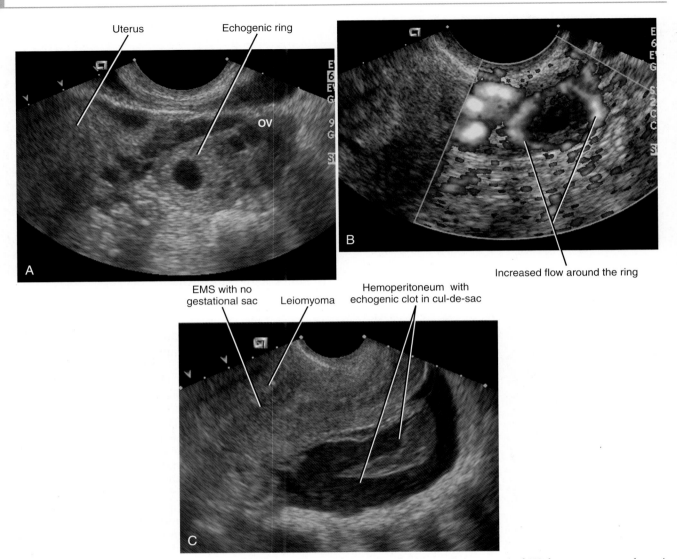

Figure 8-50 Ectopic pregnancy on ultrasound (US). **A,** Transverse image of the left adnexa using transvaginal US demonstrates an echogenic ring between the uterus and left ovary *(OV)*. **B,** Power Doppler image of the adnexal ring shows peripheral hypervascularity with no central flow. **C,** Sagittal midline image in the same patient demonstrates hemoperitoneum in the cul-de-sac. The endometrial stripe *(EMS)* is displaced by a leiomyoma, but no intrauterine gestation was identified.

pain but can occasionally cause acute abdominal pain of sufficient severity to require urgent imaging. Complications of uterine fibroids that can present acutely include torsion of a pedunculated subserosal fibroid or hemorrhagic degeneration of a fibroid. If torsion goes untreated and progresses to detachment from the uterus, a "parasitic" fibroid results.

Ultrasound is the preferred modality for evaluating the uterus and is usually performed if fibroids are the suspected cause of pain. A twisting of the vascular pedicle to a fibroid can be seen in some cases of torsion, with no perfusion or peripheral flow visible in the mass.

On contrast-enhanced CT, fibroid torsion appears as an exophytic mass connected to the uterus by a pedicle, often with peripheral hyperemia that is presumed to be due to venous congestion. Simple pelvic fluid and adjacent fat stranding are often present. On both CT and ultrasound images, torsion of a pedunculated fibroid can resemble ovarian torsion. Therefore, the presence of two normal ovaries should be documented before excluding ovarian torsion. If not conspicuous, the normal ovaries can often be located by following the gonadal vessels into the pelvis.

Intrauterine Device Migration
An intrauterine device provides contraception requiring minimal patient compliance. In most cases, it is safe and effective. In rare instances, the devices become imbedded in the myometrium of the uterine wall or even pass completely through the wall into the peritoneal cavity (Fig. 8-55).

Urinary Tract Infection (UTI)
Pelvic pain associated with UTI is usually accompanied by urgency to void and dysuria, although there are exceptions. Urinalysis is typically included in the workup

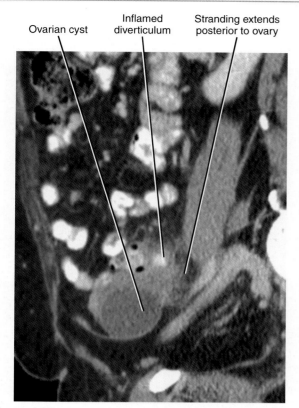

Ovarian cyst   Inflamed diverticulum   Stranding extends posterior to ovary

Figure 8-51 Diverticulitis affecting the adnexa. Sagittal reformation of contrast-enhanced computed tomographic examination demonstrates thickening of the sigmoid colon immediately adjacent to the superior margin of the left ovary with fat stranding that extends to the ovary. Incidental note is made of an ovarian cyst.

of abdominal or pelvic pain, so imaging does not usually play a role. On occasion, however, the radiologist may be the first to encounter evidence of infection. Air in the bladder is usually the result of catheterization but can signal the presence of a UTI. In more severe cases, particularly in individuals with diabetes, air can be seen within the bladder mucosa (emphysematous cystitis) (Fig. 8-56).

Interstitial cystitis is an idiopathic bladder disorder that is probably immune mediated. It is more common in women, and symptoms mimic UTI, although cultures remain negative. In severe cases, bladder wall thickening can be seen with cross-sectional imaging (see Chapter 19, Figure 19-62).

Pain in the Male Pelvis

Pelvic pain is much less common in men than in women. Furthermore, the main cause of male-specific pelvic pain, prostatitis, is usually diagnosed and treated without imaging. On occasions when imaging is performed, findings are often normal or nonspecific unless an abscess is present. Because prostatic pain is rarely confused with other types of lower abdominal pain (provided a physical examination is performed), this is discussed in Chapter 22.

■ FLANK PAIN

Flank pain is located more laterally than pain typically described as abdominal and usually involves one side. The primary diagnostic consideration in a patient with acute flank pain is a ureteral calculus. Other disease processes that occur in the extraperitoneum can mimic ureteral colic, including pyelonephritis, pancreatitis, rupture of an AAA, or diseases that involve extraperitoneal segments of the gastrointestinal tract (duodenum and portions of the colon). The term *renal colic* is often used to describe this type of pain, but its use without a diagnosis can draw attention away from potential nonurinary causes.

Noncontrast-enhanced CT (NCCT) is the preferred study for evaluating most patients believed to have a ureteral stone. Because neither intravenous nor enteric contrast is necessary, the examination does not interfere with performance of subsequent studies. Because many other diseases that cause flank pain can also be identified using NCCT, emergency physicians around the country have embraced the technique.

Thin sections available with MDCT facilitate following the ureter in continuity. Sections 2.5 to 5 mm in thickness are commonly used. Some institutions choose to scan patients in the prone position for suspected renal colic so that a calculus in the bladder can be distinguished from one lodged at the uterovesical junction (UVJ) (Fig. 8-57).

Interpretation of Noncontrast-Enhanced Computed Tomography for Urinary Stones

A systematic approach to the interpretation of NCCT will improve accuracy for diagnosing ureteral stone disease. The basic steps are outlined in Box 8-3.

Signs of Urinary Obstruction

Although NCCT provides less physiologic information than intravenous urography, obstruction can still be discerned from secondary signs (Table 8-13).

Pitfall: Extrarenal pelvis and renal sinus (peripelvic) cysts can mimic hydronephrosis. In the case of extrarenal pelvis without obstruction, the calyces will be normal. To confirm the presence of renal sinus cysts, consider obtaining images in the excretory phase after intravenous contrast administration.

Phleboliths

Most false-positive diagnoses of ureteral calculi result from phleboliths in the vicinity of the ureters. Following the ureter in continuity is the most accurate method of establishing that a calcification lies within the ureter. Unfortunately, this can be difficult or impossible in patients with a paucity of extraperitoneal fat or who have orthopedic hardware in the spine, hips, or pelvis. When the ureters cannot be confidently followed along their entire extents, additional steps can be taken to avoid misdiagnosis.

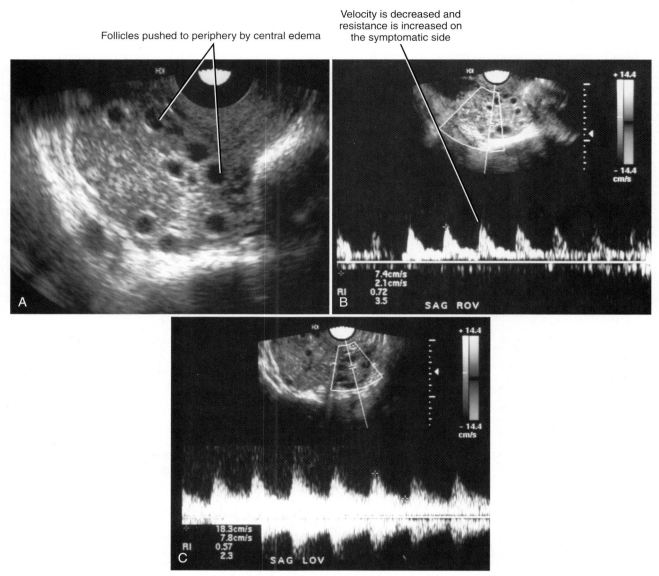

Figure 8-52 Ovarian torsion with asymmetric blood flow on transvaginal ultrasound. **A,** Grayscale image demonstrates an enlarged right ovary (6.9 × 4.9 cm) with the "string of pearls" sign. **B,** Spectral Doppler evaluation of the right ovary demonstrates flow is present, but with decreased peak systolic velocity (7 cm/sec) compared with the **(C)** left ovary (18 cm/sec). Right ovarian torsion was confirmed at surgery.

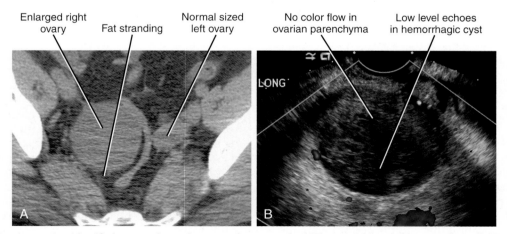

Figure 8-53 Ovarian torsion identified on unenhanced computed tomography (CT). **A,** Axial image from unenhanced CT performed for right-sided abdominal pain demonstrates an enlarged right ovary with subtle stranding of the adjacent fat. **B,** Longitudinal transvaginal ultrasound image of the right ovary with color Doppler demonstrates a region with low-level echoes typical of a hemorrhagic cyst but no demonstrable flow within the crescent of solid ovarian parenchyma. Ovarian torsion with a hemorrhagic ovarian cyst was confirmed at surgery.

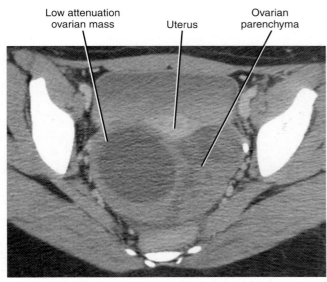

Figure 8-54   Ovarian torsion on contrast-enhanced computed tomography (CT). Axial image from contrast-enhanced CT examination performed for acute lower abdominal pain demonstrates a markedly enlarged ovary posterior to the uterus. A low-attenuation mass was presumed to be a cyst. A normal right ovary was present on more superior images (not shown). Surgery confirmed infarction of the left ovary caused by torsion. The low-attenuation ovarian mass was found to be an ovarian adenofibroma (benign fibrous tumor).

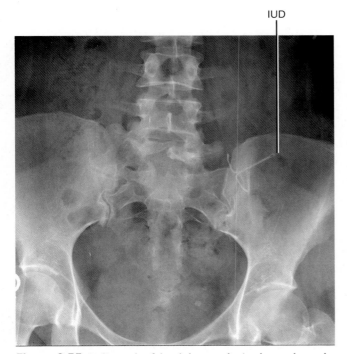

Figure 8-55   Radiograph of the abdomen obtained to evaluate abdominal pain shows a T-shaped intrauterine device in the left lower quadrant. The device is well away from the expected location of the uterus.

To better characterize calcifications above the pelvic brim, identify the gonadal veins. Anatomy of the gonadal veins is relatively predictable. Just as following the ureter allows confident classification of a calcification as ureteral in location, following the gonadal veins will confirm whether a calcification is a phlebolith. The right gonadal

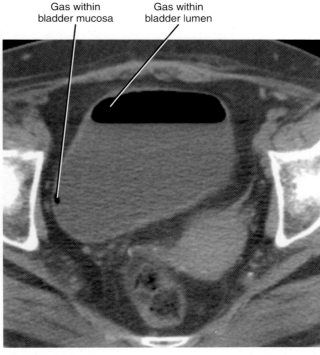

Figure 8-56   Bladder infection demonstrated by computed tomography (CT). Axial image of the pelvis from contrast-enhanced CT performed for abdominal pain in a 62-year-old woman with diabetes demonstrates gas within the lumen and mucosa of the bladder. The patient had not been catheterized and subsequent urinalysis demonstrated pyuria. Mucosal gas indicates emphysematous cystitis.

vein usually enters the inferior vena cava at approximately the 10- to 11-o'clock position near the lower pole of the kidney and can usually be followed retrograde into the pelvis. The vein crosses over the ureter from medial to lateral above the bony pelvis. The left gonadal vein enters the left renal vein but otherwise follows a similar course. Correctly identifying both gonadal veins early in the process of interpreting a stone protocol CT scan can avoid confusion later.

To better characterize calcifications in the pelvis, follow the ureters back from the UVJ. The ureters exit from the posterior wall of the bladder, typically at an angle of approximately 45 degrees (see Chapter 19, Figure 19-5). By following the ureters retrograde from their bladder insertions, ureteral calculi can often be distinguished from pelvic phleboliths (Fig. 8-61).

If these steps fail, look for the presence or absence of a soft-tissue rim around the calcification (Fig. 8-62). The presence of a rim of soft tissue surrounding a calcification indicates it is likely within the ureter. This *rim sign* is most useful for small calculi because larger stones stretch the ureteral wall and obliterate the soft-tissue rim. The *comet tail sign* (also called the *comet sign* or the *tail sign*) describes linear soft tissue extending from a pelvic calcification. The soft tissue is a vein, and the finding indicates that the calcification is a phlebolith.

Human Immunodeficiency Virus and Stone Disease

Protease inhibitor medications used to treat human immunodeficiency virus (HIV) infection have been associated with the formation of urinary precipitates of the

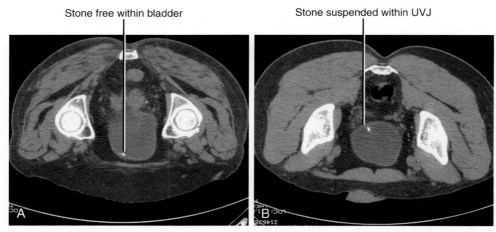

Figure 8-57 Utility of prone scanning for urinary stones. **A,** Axial image from computed tomographic (CT) examination obtained with the patient prone demonstrates a stone that has passed into the bladder dependent along the anterior bladder wall. **B,** Axial image from CT scan of a different patient also in the prone position demonstrates a stone that remains suspended within the uterovesical junction (often not visible around the stone).

BOX 8-3   Steps for Interpretation of Noncontrast-Enhanced Computed Tomography for Urinary Stones

1. Look for renal and perirenal asymmetry (size, density).
2. Look for hydroureteronephrosis.
3. Inspect the entire course of both ureters for stones and transitions.
   a. Use of bone windows is useful for detecting stones adjacent to stents (Fig. 8-58).
   b. Identify each gonadal vein near the kidneys to avoid confusion with the ureter.
   c. Follow distal ureters back from the ureterovesical junction if necessary.
4. Look for stones or other abnormal densities in the kidneys, bladder, and urethra.
5. Consider nonurologic causes of flank pain.

Table 8-13   Secondary Signs of Urinary Obstruction on Noncontrast-Enhanced Computed Tomography

Sign	Comments
Hydronephrosis	Renal pelvis can be misleading. Look for rounding of the collecting system structures at either pole of the kidney (Fig. 8-59).
Asymmetric fat stranding	Symmetric fat stranding is common. Look for subtle asymmetry adjacent to each renal pole. Stranding should be linear. Rounded or crescentic collections suggest calyceal rupture.
Ureteral dilatation	Follow the complete course of the ureter to avoid confusion with the gonadal vein. Compare with the other side to look for asymmetry.
Pale kidney sign	The renal parenchymal edema caused by urinary obstruction often decreases the attenuation of the affected kidney by 5 HU or more. This is sometimes useful for differentiating between a passed stone and pyelonephritis (Fig. 8-60).
Unilateral absence of the white pyramid	When protein in the renal tubules makes the pyramids appear dense, it does so bilaterally. When it is present in only one kidney, the pyramids of the other kidney are probably diluted because of obstruction.

excreted portion of the medication. The resulting clay-like proteinaceous substance is usually not dense enough to be seen on NCCT. The diagnosis of a protease inhibitor "stone" should be suspected when a person with HIV has secondary CT findings of ureteral obstruction without identifiable calcification. The main competing diagnostic possibility is pyelonephritis.

Diagnoses to Consider When Stone Disease Is Absent

Despite evidence of increasing use of NCCT for flank pain, no evidence has been reported of a similar increase in the incidence of urinary stone disease. As a result, the percentage of examinations demonstrating ureteral stones has declined, whereas the list of alternate diagnoses established with NCCT has grown. Box 8-4 includes some of the most commonly encountered alternate diagnoses together with helpful clinical and imaging findings.

■ GENERALIZED ABDOMINAL PAIN

Sometimes abdominal pain cannot be localized to a particular quadrant of the abdomen. Unfortunately, generalized abdominal pain can be the presenting symptom for a vast spectrum of diseases that range from minor to life-threatening. Table 8-14 presents an abbreviated list of some of the more common causes of generalized acute abdominal pain. As a result of the nonspecific nature of generalized abdominal pain and the long list of possible causes, CT plays a dominant role in managing these patients.

A single high attenuation structure is
visible and presumed to be the stent

Stone   Stent

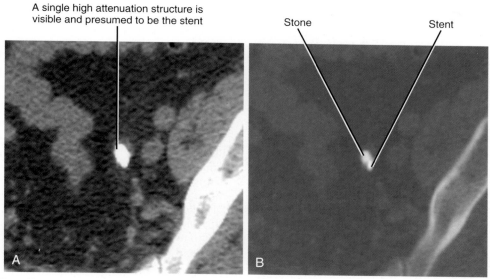

Figure 8-58 Utility of bone windows for identifying ureteral calculi adjacent to ureteral stent. **A,** Axial image from noncontrast-enhanced computed tomographic scan viewed in soft-tissue windows demonstrates a single high-attenuation object within the ureter, presumed to be the stent. **B,** When the same axial image is viewed with bone windows, a ureteral stone can be identified adjacent to the stent.

Dilated ureter   Hydronephrosis   Asymmetric fat
stranding

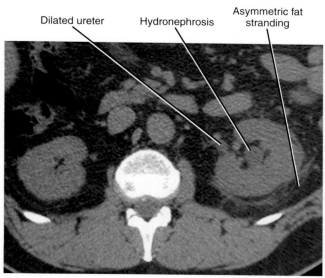

Figure 8-59 Axial image from noncontrast-enhanced computed tomographic examination performed for suspected ureterolithiasis demonstrates secondary signs of urinary obstruction. A small calculus was present at the left uterovesical junction (not shown).

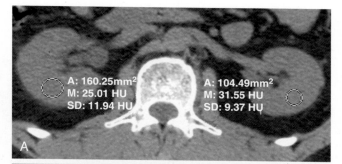

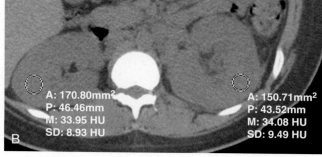

Figure 8-60 Pale kidney sign. **A,** Attenuation measurements of the renal parenchyma on noncontrast-enhanced computed tomographic images from a patient with a right ureteral stone demonstrate lower attenuation in the obstructed kidney (25 vs. 31 HU). **B,** When a similar measurement is made in a patient with left pyelonephritis, no significant attenuation difference exists between the kidneys. *M,* Mean attenuation; *SD,* standard deviation.

Most of the causes listed in Table 8-14 are readily diagnosed on CT when they are severe enough to result in generalized pain. Several of the disease processes listed can also cause localized pain and have been discussed in preceding sections of this chapter. Bowel ischemia is worthy of a specific discussion in the context of problem solving because it is often difficult to diagnose but is associated with a high rate of mortality. Although diagnosis of ruptured AAA is less problematic, given the urgency of this condition, some of the imaging characteristics of this entity are discussed as well.

Ischemic Bowel

Bowel ischemia results from decreased intestinal perfusion. Although many disease processes lead to bowel ischemia, they may be categorized into three major types: acute mesenteric ischemia, chronic mesenteric ischemia, and nonocclusive (hypoperfusion) mesenteric ischemia.

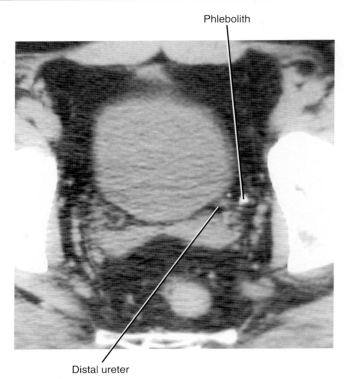

Phlebolith

Distal ureter

Figure 8-61 Identification of the uterovesical junction (UVJ) used to characterize a pelvic calcification. Axial image from noncontrast-enhanced computed tomographic examination demonstrates a calcification that is separate from the UVJ, indicating that it is a phlebolith. Note also the absence of a soft-tissue rim around the calcification.

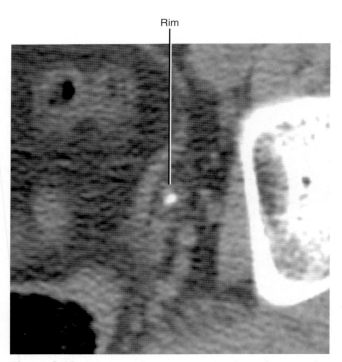

Rim

Figure 8-62 Axial image from noncontrast-enhanced computed tomographic examination demonstrates a soft-tissue rim around a calcification, indicating that the calcification is located within the ureter. The rim is the thickened wall of the ureter and is seen more commonly with small stones.

BOX 8-4 Alternate Diagnoses to Look for on Noncontrast-Enhanced Computed Tomography Performed for Suspected Stone Disease

Noncalculous ureteral obstruction
Pyelonephritis
Renal vein thrombosis
Perinephric hemorrhage
Adrenal hemorrhage
Ovarian cyst/torsion
PID
Pancreatitis
Cholecystitis
Appendicitis
Diverticulitis
Epiploic appendagitis
Spontaneous retroperitoneal hemorrhage
Ruptured abdominal aortic aneurysm (AAA)

These entities are described in detail in the organ-specific sections of this book.

Acute Mesenteric Ischemia

Acute mesenteric ischemia describes an abrupt loss of perfusion to a segment of bowel and is most commonly the result of embolic disease (50%), although there are a variety of causes (Table 8-15). The small intestine has limited peripheral collateral blood supply; therefore, acute occlusion of the superior mesenteric artery or its branches can become rapidly fatal, with a mortality rate of at least 80% without early intervention.

Before widespread availability of computed tomographic angiography (CTA) and magnetic resonance angiography (MRA), conventional angiography was the mainstay of imaging patients with suspected acute mesenteric ischemia. Angiography does offer the potential advantage of access for percutaneous intervention such as thrombolysis or suction embolectomy at the time of diagnosis, although most patients will require emergent surgery.

CTA using MDCT offers the advantage of effective and rapid diagnosis of mesenteric vascular disease with additional ability to detect other causes of acute abdominal pain. Because most emboli lodge within the main trunk of the superior mesenteric artery at the level of the first arterial division within 3 cm of the aorta, emboli are often visible even when the scan is acquired in the portal venous phase. If mesenteric ischemia is the primary diagnostic concern, however, detection of more distal emboli can be optimized by scanning during the arterial phase. Because small, peripheral branches of the bowel are opacified later than central arteries, a slightly longer scan delay than typically used for renal arteries will improve the quality of CTA (Fig. 8-63). Standard delays of 35 to 40 seconds are usually sufficient. It is often useful to repeat the scan in the portal venous phase to evaluate for mesenteric venous thrombosis.

Table 8-14   Causes of Generalized Abdominal Pain

Intestinal	Adynamic ileus Bowel perforation Bowel obstruction Bowel ischemia Foreign body Inflammatory bowel disease (infectious, idiopathic) Gastroenteritis Volvulus
Pancreatic	Pancreatitis (chronic, acute) Pancreatic neoplasm
Genitourinary	Bladder outlet obstruction Massive uterine fibroids
Peritoneal	Peritonitis (infectious, biliary) Endometriosis Abscess Pneumoperitoneum (nonintestinal origin)
Vascular	Abdominal aortic aneurysm Vasculitis Mesenteric/portal venous thrombosis Hemorrhage
Lymphatic	Mesenteric lymphadenitis Lymphoma
Mesenteric	Omental infarction Sclerosing mesenteritis

These entities are described in detail in the organ-specific sections of this book.

Table 8-15   Causes of Acute Mesenteric Ischemia

Category	Comments
Arterial embolus	Caused by blood clot, plaque, or cholesterol
Arterial thrombosis	Gradual progressive stenosis leads to sudden occlusion
Venous thrombosis	Related to portal hypertension, pancreatitis, tumor, or hypercoagulable state
Nonocclusive	Low-flow state associated with cardiac dysfunction, hypotension, and dehydration
Arterial dissection	Primary mesenteric or caused by aortic dissection
Vasculitis	Often involves small arteries beyond resolution of ultrasound, computed tomography, and magnetic resonance imaging
Iatrogenic	Intraaortic balloon pump

Chronic Mesenteric Ischemia

Chronic mesenteric ischemia describes a rare outcome of stenosing atherosclerotic disease. Because atherosclerosis is a systemic disease, all three mesenteric vessels are usually involved to some extent in these patients. The classic presentation of chronic mesenteric ischemia is a gradual onset of recurring postprandial abdominal pain, typically 10 to 15 minutes after eating. Although the pain is most often periumbilical or epigastric, the pain is variable depending on the segment of bowel affected. The cause of pain is thought to be analogous to

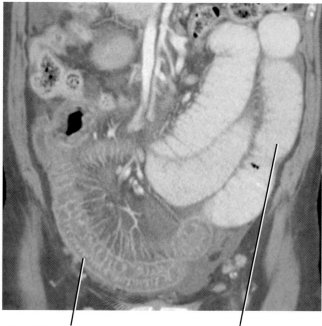

Wall thickening with serosal and mucosal enhancement

Small bowel loops proximal to the affected segment are dilated

Figure 8-63 Coronal maximum intensity projection image from mesenteric multidetector computed tomographic angiogram using a 40-second scan delay. Excellent opacification of even small vessels excludes embolic disease, whereas patent venous branches exclude thrombosis. A diagnosis of vasculitis-related bowel ischemia was presumed in this patient with systemic lupus erythematosus. Symptoms resolved with high-dose steroid therapy.

stress-induced cardiac angina, with sufficient flow through the stenotic vessel to supply resting viscera but no capacity to accommodate augmented flow when the metabolic demands increase. For this reason, the clinical symptoms of chronic mesenteric ischemia are sometimes called *mesenteric angina*. Because there are many potential proximal collateral pathways in the mesenteric arterial system, development of symptoms usually requires significant disease in at least two of the three mesenteric arteries. Because nausea and vomiting frequently accompany mesenteric angina, patients develop an aversion to food, and by the time patients seek treatment, they often report significant weight loss.

Imaging plays an important role in the diagnosis of chronic mesenteric ischemia. In the past, catheter angiography was usually required to establish the diagnosis, although CTA and MRA techniques have significantly reduced its role. Most clinically significant atheromatous plaques are at vessel origins or proximal branch points, rendering the higher spatial resolution of catheter angiography moot for most cases of chronic intestinal ischemia. With proper technique, stenoses in such locations can be effectively characterized with cross-sectional imaging (see Figs. 5-26 and 5-27).

Hypoperfusion-Related Intestinal Ischemia

Ischemic colitis is the most common cause of colitis in the elderly. Patients often present with bloody diarrhea, and the rectum is spared on imaging studies. Decreased perfusion to the bowel can result from any cause of systemic hypotension or decreased cardiac output. Most of the colon is relatively protected from regional hypoperfusion, because collateral flow is available through the marginal artery of Drummond and the arc of Riolan. There are, however, three watershed areas where the collateral cascade is often insufficient. These are the ileocecal region, the splenic flexure, and the rectosigmoid region (Fig. 8-64). Although colitis in these areas should prompt consideration of an ischemic cause, ischemic colitis often extends beyond these watersheds. Ischemic colitis more often involves the left colon than the right.

> **Pearl:** *When evidence of colitis (e.g., wall thickening) is identified in any of the three watershed areas of the colon, ischemic colitis should be considered.*

Abdominal Aortic Aneurysm (AAA)

Identification of an AAA on an imaging study is relatively simple. Far more important is the radiologist's role in identifying signs of AAA rupture or instability that warrant immediate intervention. These signs are listed in Table 8-16.

The most common sign of aortic rupture is the presence of extraperitoneal hematoma near an aortic aneurysm, an indication for emergent surgery. Hemorrhage can extend into the anterior pararenal space, perirenal spaces, and even the peritoneal space (Fig. 8-65).

Table 8-16   Computed Tomographic Signs of Aortic Rupture and Impending Rupture

Signs of Rupture	Signs of Impending Rupture
Extraperitoneal hematoma	Increasing aneurysm size
Draped aorta sign	Focal contour bulge
Discontinuity of aortic wall	"Hyperdense crescent" sign
Extravasation of intravenous contrast media	

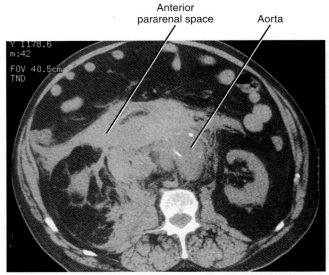

Figure 8-65 Retroperitoneal hemorrhage from ruptured abdominal aortic aneurysm. Axial image from noncontrast-enhanced computed tomographic examination for suspected ureteral stone demonstrates extensive hemorrhage into the anterior pararenal spaces, along the right psoas muscle and into the right perirenal space.

The draped aorta sign describes an apparent contour abnormality of the posterior wall of the aorta as it conforms to the contour of the adjacent vertebral body. The actual deformity represents a pseudoaneurysm with contained hematoma extending posterior and to the left. Discontinuity of the aortic wall and extravasation of intravenous contrast are additional signs of ruptured AAA.

Aortic rupture can remain contained by the fascia within the extraperitoneum. In such cases, the hematoma can have fluid attenuation. It is important to maintain a high level of suspicion regarding any extraperitoneal fluid collection in the presence of AAA because attempted catheter drainage could be disastrous (see Fig. 22-1).

Identifying signs of impending AAA rupture allows urgent intervention with a lower rate of morbidity and mortality. Signs of impending rupture include increasing size of the aneurysm, focal bulges in contour, and the presence of a hyperdense crescent within the aneurysm wall on unenhanced CT images (Fig. 8-66).

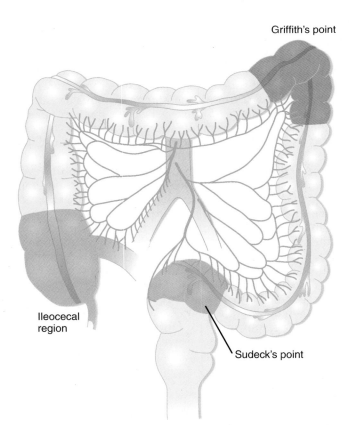

Figure 8-64 Illustration demonstrating the regions of watershed perfusion in the colon. These are the areas most susceptible to ischemic colitis.

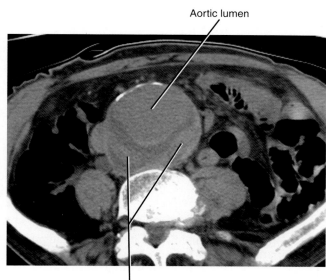

Aortic lumen

Hyperdense crescent

Figure 8-66 Signs of impending rupture of abdominal aortic aneurysm. Unenhanced axial computed tomographic image (performed prone for suspected ureteral stone!) demonstrates a high-attenuation crescent within the wall of the aorta. Acute hemorrhage into the aortic wall also creates a contour bulge adjacent to the spine ("draping" of the aorta).

Suggested Readings

Ahn SH, Mayo-Smith WW, Murphy BL et al: Acute nontraumatic abdominal pain in adult patients: abdominal radiography compared with CT evaluation, *Radiology* 225:159-164, 2002.

Albayram F, Hamper UM: Ovarian and adnexal torsion: spectrum of sonographic findings with pathologic correlation, *J Ultrasound Med* 20:1083-1089, 2001.

Bennett GL, Slywotzky CM, Giovanniello G: Gynecologic causes of acute pelvic pain: spectrum of CT findings, *Radiographics* 22:785-801, 2002.

Boridy IC, Nikolaidis P, Kawashima A et al: Ureterolithiasis: value of the tail sign in differentiating phleboliths from ureteral calculi at nonenhanced helical CT, *Radiology* 211:619-621, 1999.

Brown DF, Fischer RH, Novelline RA et al: The role of abdominal computed tomography scanning in patients with non-traumatic abdominal symptoms, *Eur J Emerg Med* 9:330-333, 2002.

Byun JY, Ha HK, Yu SY et al: CT features of systemic lupus erythematosus in patients with acute abdominal pain: emphasis on ischemic bowel disease, *Radiology* 211:203-209, 1999.

Dalrymple NC, Verga M, Anderson KR et al: The value of unenhanced helical computerized tomography in the management of acute flank pain, *J Urol* 159:735-740, 1998.

Del Campo L, Arribas I, Valbuena M et al: Spiral CT findings in active and remission phases in patients with Crohn disease, *J Comput Assist Tomogr* 25:792-797, 2001.

Hanbidge AE, Buckler PM, O'Malley ME et al: From the RSNA refresher courses: imaging evaluation for acute pain in the right upper quadrant, *Radiographics* 24:1117-1135, 2004.

Hernandez JA, Swischuk LE, Angel CA et al: Imaging of acute appendicitis: US as the primary imaging modality, *Pediatr Radiol* 35:392-395, 2005.

Kalish GM, Patel MD, Gunn ML et al: Computed tomographic and magnetic resonance features of gynecologic abnormalities in women presenting with acute or chronic abdominal pain, *Ultrasound Q* 23:167-175, 2007.

Langer JE, Cornud F: Inflammatory disorders of the prostate and the distal genital tract, *Radiol Clin North Am* 44:665-677, vii, 2006.

Lucey BC, Stuhlfaut JW, Soto JA: Mesenteric lymph nodes seen at imaging: causes and significance, *Radiographics* 25:351-365, 2005.

Macari M, Hines J, Balthazar E et al: Mesenteric adenitis: CT diagnosis of primary versus secondary causes, incidence, and clinical significance in pediatric and adult patients, *AJR Am J Roentgenol* 178:853-858, 2002.

MacKersie AB, Lane MJ, Gerhardt RT et al: Nontraumatic acute abdominal pain: unenhanced helical CT compared with three-view acute abdominal series, *Radiology* 237:114-122, 2005.

Madura MJ, Craig RM, Shields TW: Unusual causes of spontaneous pneumo-peritoneum, *Surg Gynecol Obstet* 154:417-420, 1982.

Meyers MA, McGuire PV: Spiral CT demonstration of hypervascularity in Crohn disease: "vascular jejunization of the ileum" or the "comb sign," *Abdom Imaging* 20:327-332, 1995.

Mindell HJ, Mastromatteo JF, Dickey KW et al: Anatomic communications between the three retroperitoneal spaces: determination by CT-guided injections of contrast material in cadavers, *Am J Roentgenol* 164:1173-1178, 1995.

Mularski RA, Sippel JM, Osborne ML: Pneumoperitoneum: a review of non-surgical causes, *Crit Care Med* 28:2638-2644, 2000.

Pereira JM, Sirlin CB, Pinto PS et al: Disproportionate fat stranding: a helpful CT sign in patients with acute abdominal pain, *Radiographics* 24:703-715, 2004.

Pinto Leite N, Pereira JM, Cunha R et al: CT evaluation of appendicitis and its complications: imaging techniques and key diagnostic findings, *Am J Roentgenol* 185:406-417, 2005.

Rakita D, Newatia A, Hines JJ et al: Spectrum of CT findings in rupture and impending rupture of abdominal aortic aneurysms, *Radiographics* 27:497-507, 2007.

Rao PM, Rhea JT, Novelline RA: CT diagnosis of mesenteric adenitis, *Radiology* 202:145-149, 1997.

Raptopoulos V, Katsou G, Rosen MP et al: Acute appendicitis: effect of increased use of CT on selecting patients earlier, *Radiology* 226:521-526, 2003.

Raptopoulos V, Kleinman PK, Marks S Jr et al: Renal fascial pathway: posterior extension of pancreatic effusions within the anterior pararenal space, *Radiology* 158:367-374, 1986.

Rosen MP, Sands DZ, Longmaid HE 3rd et al: Impact of abdominal CT on the management of patients presenting to the emergency department with acute abdominal pain, *AJR Am J Roentgenol* 174:1391-1396, 2000.

Roth C, Tello R, Sutherland K et al: Prediction rule for etiology of vague abdominal pain in the emergency room: utility for imaging triage, *Invest Radiol* 37:552-556, 2002.

Roy C, Bierry G, El Ghali S et al: Acute torsion of uterine leiomyoma: CT features, *Abdom Imaging* 30:120-123, 2005.

Sandrasegaran K, Lall C, Rajesh A et al: Distinguishing gelatin bioabsorbable sponge and postoperative abdominal abscess on CT, *AJR Am J Roentgenol* 184:475-480, 2005.

Seo BK, Ha HK, Kim AY et al: Segmental misty mesentery: analysis of CT features and primary causes, *Radiology* 226:86-94, 2003.

Shadinger LL, Andreotti RF, Kurian RL: Preoperative sonographic and clinical characteristics as predictors of ovarian torsion, *J Ultrasound Med* 27:7-13, 2008.

Smith RC, Dalrymple NC, Neitlich J: Noncontrast helical CT in the evaluation of acute flank pain, *Abdom Imaging* 23:10-16, 1998.

CHAPTER 9

Imaging Evaluation of Trauma

Neal C. Dalrymple and Michael Oliphant

■ ROLE OF IMAGING IN TRAUMA

Imaging plays an important role in the early evaluation of trauma patients. Current trauma management protocols use imaging more liberally than in the past in an effort to detect injuries that might otherwise be overlooked because of distracting pain or inaccurate historical information. Knowledge regarding patterns of injury in the abdomen and pelvis helps the radiologist detect subtle injuries or associated injuries that might be missed.

It is important to keep the role of imaging in the trauma setting in perspective. The diagnostic acumen of the trauma physician remains the most important factor in directing therapy. Patients with hypotension following severe blunt or penetrating injury often go directly to surgery. In such cases, the time required for imaging may cause unacceptable delay of life-saving therapy. When imaging is used, it must be interpreted within its clinical context to avoid errant interpretation leading to unnecessary intervention. When a trauma-related finding is present on imaging, management options include observation, surgery, and transcatheter intervention. Injuries that require emergent therapy must be immediately identified and accurately communicated to the trauma team.

Ultrasound and Computed Tomography

Despite earlier literature that implied competition between computed tomography (CT) and ultrasound in the trauma setting, the two have evolved as complementary imaging tools. CT has emerged as the cornerstone of trauma imaging of the abdomen and pelvis because of high sensitivity for injuries of the solid and hollow organs, fractures of the spine and pelvis, hemorrhage, and extraluminal gas.

Ultrasound, in contrast, can be used in the trauma room while members of the trauma team continue to assess and support the patient. Focused abdominal sonogram for trauma (FAST) has largely replaced diagnostic peritoneal lavage by providing a rapid noninvasive method for identifying hemoperitoneum. Box 9-1 shows the search pattern for FAST examination. Up to 40% of patients with injuries to the abdominal viscera are taken to the operating room immediately after sonographic determination of hemoperitoneum, and injuries are diagnosed during laparotomy rather than with CT.

A key limitation of the FAST examination is that nearly one in three injuries to the liver or spleen do not result in hemoperitoneum and are more likely to be identified on CT. Understanding the relative strengths and weakness of imaging modalities is an important step in creating effective trauma protocols. Table 9-1 summarizes the advantages and disadvantages of ultrasound and CT.

Blunt versus Penetrating Trauma

Until recently, CT played a limited role in the initial management of patients with penetrating injury to the abdomen and pelvis because most such patients received emergent surgery. Early in its history, CT had only limited sensitivity for detecting bowel injury. Therefore, CT was reserved for those patients in whom the depth of injury remained in question.

As advancements in multidetector computed tomography (MDCT) technology have improved sensitivity for bowel injury, the number of CT examinations performed for penetrating injuries has increased. Pneumoperitoneum, focal bowel wall thickening, isolated bowel dilatation, and mesenteric hematoma are CT findings that suggest bowel injury. Rarely, the site of discontinuity within the bowel wall can be seen. Some centers administer water-soluble enteric contrast media via a nasogastric tube in the trauma room, improving sensitivity for injuries to the stomach and proximal small bowel. Patients with hemodynamic compromise are still likely to be taken directly to surgery without any imaging beyond FAST ultrasound.

BOX 9-1   FAST Search Pattern

Pericardium
Right subphrenic space above the liver
Hepatorenal space
Left subphrenic space above the spleen
Perisplenic space at the inferior margin of the spleen
Peritoneal recesses of the pelvis

Table 9-1   Comparison of Ultrasound and Computed Tomography in Trauma Imaging

Imaging Type	Advantages	Disadvantages
Ultrasound	• Does not require patient transport	• Operator dependent
	• Other procedures can be performed simultaneously	• Requires sonographic window
	• No radiation or contrast media	• Limited in obese patients
	• Can be repeated	• May miss injuries without associated hemoperitoneum
Computed tomography	• Accurate characterization of solid organ injuries	• Requires contrast media
	• Sensitive for extraperitoneal injuries	• Ionizing radiation
	• Less operator dependent	• Requires patient transport and transfer to scanner

Imaging is routinely performed for blunt force trauma. Injury in blunt force trauma is the result of direct crush injury, sheer forces, or burst injury from an abrupt increase in intraluminal pressure. The most common source of blunt force trauma that requires imaging is motor vehicle collision. Victims of severe blunt force trauma with hemodynamic compromise may still require immediate surgical exploration, but occasionally even unstable patients require imaging if the site of injury is not apparent by physical examination. Imaging surveys often include CT examinations of the head, cervical spine, chest, abdomen, and pelvis.

The American Association for the Surgery of Trauma (AAST) provides a scoring system that categorizes the severity of solid organ injury based on imaging findings. Familiarity with that system allows the radiologist to report specific imaging findings that may affect the surgeon's classification of a particular injury.

■ KEY COMPUTED TOMOGRAPHIC FINDINGS IN THE TRAUMA PATIENT

Lacerations

As with most disease processes, the key radiographic findings in trauma include both direct and indirect findings. Most direct CT findings are relatively straightforward but can be subtle at times. Low-attenuation parenchymal defects indicating laceration of a solid organ are perhaps the most common direct sign on enhanced CT images. The location of the laceration should be noted, with particular attention to involvement of the capsule of the organ in addition to any other vital structures such as blood vessels, bile ducts, or urinary collecting system. In addition, the approximate length of the laceration

should be noted, particularly if it results in complete or near-complete transection of the organ involved.

Contrast Extravasation

Active contrast extravasation (ACE) describes the presence of vascular contrast media outside the vascular space and is a direct sign of hemorrhage. Attenuation of extravasated contrast medium is as high as in major arterial structures nearby and is often located within or adjacent to a parenchymal laceration (Fig. 9-1). When ACE is present, transcatheter or surgical intervention is often required to stop the hemorrhage. Before the significance of ACE was known, some patients were managed with observation that included prolonged replacement of blood products and fluids. In this scenario, the patient can become coagulopathic by the time the intervention is performed, increasing risk of the procedure and potentially decreasing its efficacy. ACE is now considered to be a risk factor independent of other AAST criteria.

Pearl: ACE is a sign that urgent transcatheter or surgical intervention may be necessary to prevent prolonged hemorrhage.

Leakage of excreted contrast material from the urinary tract is a highly specific sign of urinary tract injury. It is seen most often with injuries to the intrarenal collecting system and bladder, and only rarely with ureteral injuries. Because urine will be opacified only in the excretory phase, delayed (>2-3 minutes) CT images are helpful in confirming the diagnosis (Fig. 9-2).

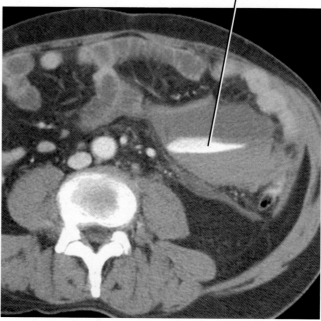

Contrast pooling within the mesenteric hematoma has attenuation similar to the aorta

Figure 9-1 Axial image from a contrast-enhanced computed tomographic scan demonstrates active contrast extravasation in the jejunal mesentery after blunt force trauma.

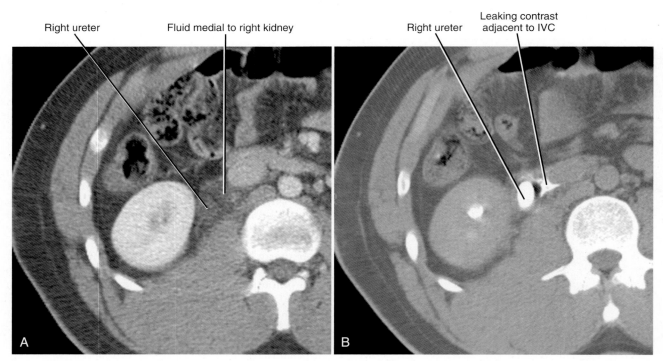

Right ureter   Fluid medial to right kidney   Right ureter   Leaking contrast adjacent to IVC

Figure 9-2 Importance of delayed images for urinary trauma. **A,** Axial image from initial contrast-enhanced computed tomographic examination performed after a motor vehicle collision demonstrates minimal fluid adjacent the right ureter. **B,** The scan was repeated 20 minutes later at the radiologist's request, demonstrating excreted contrast leaking into the periureteral tissues. *IVC,* Inferior vena cava.

Some centers administer enteric contrast as part of the CT trauma evaluation in an attempt to increase sensitivity for gastrointestinal injury (Fig. 9-3). Because this technique can delay imaging (up to an hour for complete small-bowel opacification) and carries some increased risk for aspiration during surgery, many institutions no longer routinely use enteric contrast media in trauma patients.

Extraluminal Fluid and Air

Extraluminal fluid and air are important indirect signs of injury. It is critical to characterize the precise location of fluid and air in the abdomen because pathways of intraperitoneal and extraperitoneal spread are usually predictable and help direct the search for the site of injury (see Chapter 6).

Large amounts of hemoperitoneum are often associated with injuries to the spleen or liver. Fluid in the lesser sac is usually associated with injury to the structures that form its borders (i.e., spleen, stomach, or pancreas) (Fig. 9-4). When extraperitoneal fluid or hemorrhage is present, look for injuries to the urinary tract, pancreas, and vessels such as the aorta and its major branches. Fluid within the mesentery and between bowel loops is better seen with CT than with ultrasound. When mesenteric injury is present, also look for evidence of bowel injury such as wall thickening, absent mural enhancement, or extraluminal gas. Remember to adjust window/level settings to make fat appear gray to facilitate detection of pneumoperitoneum (Fig. 9-5).

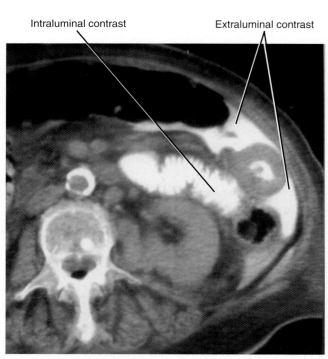

Intraluminal contrast   Extraluminal contrast

Figure 9-3 Axial computed tomographic image demonstrates extravasated enteric contrast caused by blunt force injury to the bowel during motor vehicle collision. A jejunal perforation was confirmed at surgery.

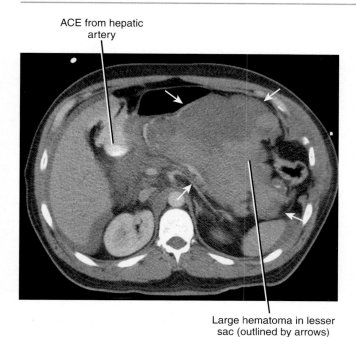

ACE from hepatic artery

Large hematoma in lesser sac (outlined by arrows)

Figure 9-4 Axial image from contrast-enhanced computed tomography performed after a motor vehicle collision demonstrates hematoma in the lesser sac as the result of active hemorrhage from the hepatic artery. *ACE,* Active contrast extravasation.

Pearl: *Increase your sensitivity for detecting extraluminal fluid with CT by including a directed search for fluid using the FAST pattern. Increase your sensitivity for detection of extraluminal air by reviewing the entire scan with bone or lung windows.*
Pitfall: *Window/level settings that make fat appear nearly black decrease the conspicuity of pneumoperitoneum. Adjusting settings to make the fat appear gray will facilitate detection of small amounts of extraluminal gas.*

Signs of Hemodynamic Compromise

Aside from ACE, other CT findings indicate life-threatening hemorrhage. The most common are flattening of the inferior vena cava (IVC) and increased enhancement of the bowel, kidneys, and adrenal glands. Box 9-2 lists key findings of hemodynamic compromise. Figure 9-6 shows some of these findings.

■ HEPATIC TRAUMA

The liver is the largest solid organ in the abdominal cavity, and its relatively brittle parenchyma makes it susceptible to laceration and fracture from the compressive and shear forces of blunt abdominal trauma. The size of the

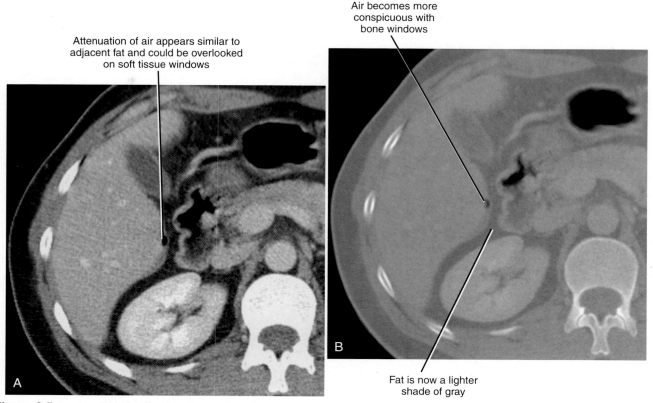

Attenuation of air appears similar to adjacent fat and could be overlooked on soft tissue windows

Air becomes more conspicuous with bone windows

Fat is now a lighter shade of gray

Figure 9-5 Impact of window/level settings on detecting pneumoperitoneum. **A,** Axial image from computed tomographic scan viewed in soft-tissue windows demonstrates a small pneumoperitoneum in the upper abdomen after a motor vehicle collision. **B,** Viewing the same image using bone windows increases conspicuity of the air.

BOX 9-2   CT Findings of Hemodynamic Compromise

Flattening of the IVC
Small aortic diameter
Low-attenuation halo around the IVC or pancreas
Shock bowel: wall thickening with increased enhancement
Increased enhancement of the kidneys, adrenal glands, and pancreas
Decreased enhancement of the spleen or liver

liver also makes it the most commonly injured solid organ from penetrating injury. Although the posterior segment of the right hepatic lobe and the interlobar region are most commonly injured, injuries can occur anywhere in the liver. Therapeutic options most commonly used to treat liver injury include transcatheter embolization, hepatotomy with vessel ligation, segmentectomy, and lobectomy. Despite these options, the mortality rate from liver injuries remains near 10%.

Types of Injury to the Liver

Injuries to the liver are classified into several types, listed in Box 9-3. The most common injuries are *lacerations*, which are parenchyma tears that extend to the

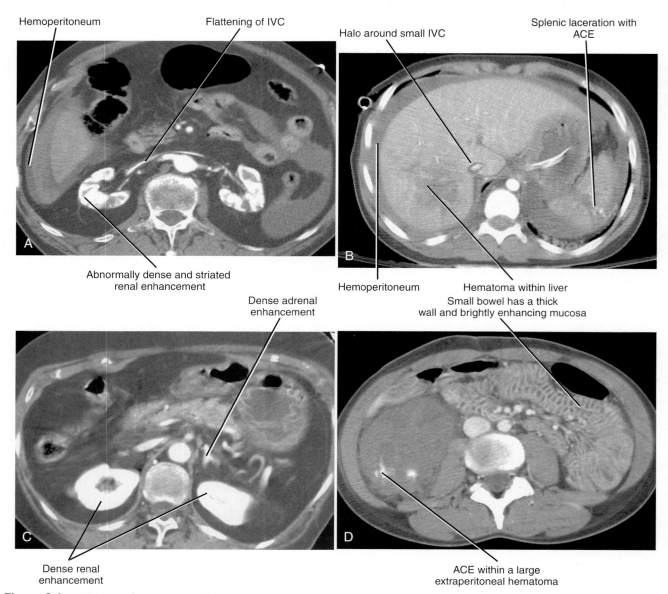

Figure 9-6 Axial images from contrast-enhanced computed tomographic examinations in four different patients demonstrate findings of hemodynamic compromise. **A,** Hemoperitoneum with flattening of the inferior vena cava (*IVC*). **B,** Halo of low attenuation around the IVC. **C,** Bright enhancement of the kidneys and adrenal glands. **D,** Shock bowel appearance. *ACE,* Active contrast extravasation.

BOX 9-3   Types of Hepatic Injury

Laceration
Parenchymal hematoma
Subcapsular hematoma
Biloma
Vascular injury
Hepatic avulsion

liver surface. On contrast-enhanced CT, most lacerations appear as linear or curvilinear hypoattenuating defects. Characterization of a laceration should include its location and any important structures (particularly vascular structures) involved. A superficial laceration is sometimes called a *capsular tear* (Fig. 9-7). A laceration that continues from one liver surface to another (full thickness) is called a *fracture*.

Hematomas are nonlinear (often lentiform or round) collections of blood within the liver parenchyma (Fig. 9-8). *Subcapsular hematomas* occur between the liver capsule and the hepatic parenchyma, and are often curvilinear or lentiform.

Portosystemic shunting, arteriovenous fistula, ACE, and infarction near areas of laceration are all signs of vascular injury. ACE can be seen within any type of hepatic hematoma, and should be noted and reported immediately because prompt transcatheter or surgical intervention can be lifesaving. Infarction occurs with transection of arterial and portal venous structures but should not occur with

Parenchymal hematoma

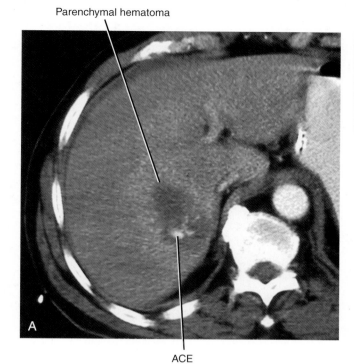

ACE

Pressure of the confined
hematoma compresses the liver

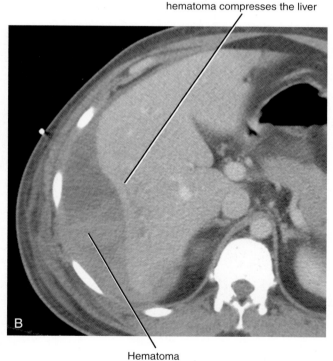

Hematoma

Figure 9-8 Axial images from contrast-enhanced computed tomographic scans of two different patients with liver hematomas. **A,** Parenchymal hematoma with active contrast extravasation *(ACE).* **B,** Subcapsular hematoma.

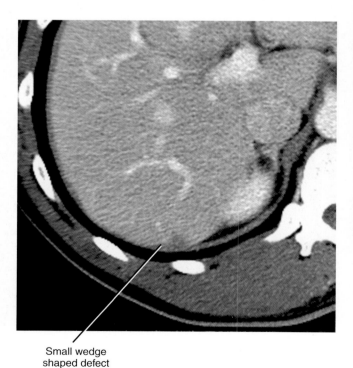

Small wedge
shaped defect

Figure 9-7 Axial image from contrast-enhanced computed tomography performed after a motor vehicle collision demonstrates a small peripheral laceration extending to the capsule of the liver, commonly called a *capsular tear.*

hepatic venous injury alone. Vascular avulsions or sheer injuries can occur within the porta hepatis (hepatic artery, portal vein, or both) (Fig. 9-9), or at either the superior or inferior margin of the hepatic attachment of the inferior vena cava (Fig. 9-10). Subtle laceration to the central

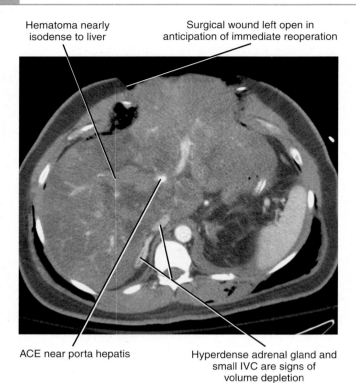

Hematoma nearly isodense to liver

Surgical wound left open in anticipation of immediate reoperation

ACE near porta hepatis

Hyperdense adrenal gland and small IVC are signs of volume depletion

Figure 9-9 Pedestrian struck by motor vehicle. Immediate exploratory laparotomy was unsuccessful at controlling liver hemorrhage. Postsurgery contrast-enhanced computed tomographic scan demonstrates active contrast extravasation *(ACE)* in the left hepatic lobe. Angiography confirmed active hemorrhage from a branch of left hepatic artery. Transcatheter embolization was successful at achieving hemostasis. *IVC,* Inferior vena cava.

hepatic veins can result in dramatic blood loss if exacerbated during manipulation by an unsuspecting surgeon (Fig. 9-11).

Pearl: Warning the surgeon of injury to the large central hepatic veins can help prevent rapid, unexpected intraoperative hemorrhage caused by manipulation of the liver.

Grading Hepatic Trauma

Trauma surgeons use the classification system adopted by the AAST to stratify liver injuries. Table 9-2 summarizes the AAST classification. In most centers, the radiologist is not expected to provide the precise grading for the injury. However, knowledge of the classification system paired with precise observation of the relevant findings facilitates effective patient management. In most cases, the key imaging findings used for the AAST classification can be distilled to the short list included in Table 9-3.

Pitfalls in Imaging Hepatic Trauma

Intravenous contrast media is essential for detecting lacerations of the solid organs. Timing of image acquisition is also important. Imaging the liver before the portal venous phase causes the hepatic veins to appear as low-attenuation linear structures that can be mistaken for or obscure a laceration.

Hepatic fissures can also mimic laceration. Similarly, a laceration in the expected location of a normal fissure

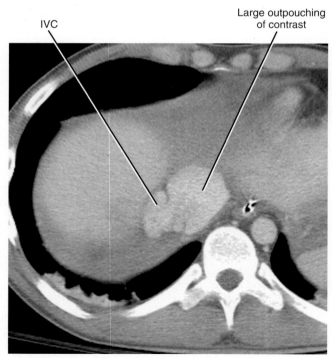

IVC

Large outpouching of contrast

Figure 9-10 Axial image of the liver dome from contrast-enhanced computed tomographic scan demonstrates a venous pseudoaneurysm at the superior margin of the intrahepatic inferior vena cava *(IVC)*. At surgery, a partial hepatic avulsion from the IVC was repaired successfully.

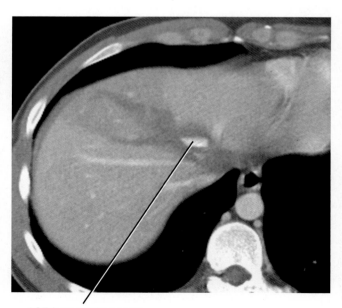

ACE from middle hepatic vein near convergence of hepatic veins

Figure 9-11 Axial image from contrast-enhanced computed tomographic scan demonstrates active contrast extravasation *(ACE)* from the middle hepatic vein. Note near-complete interlobar fracture of the liver.

Table 9-2   American Association for the Surgery of Trauma Classification of Hepatic Trauma

Grade	Laceration	Hematoma	Vascular
I	Capsular tear < 1 cm deep	Subcapsular hematoma < 10% surface area	None
II	1-3 cm deep <10 cm long	Subcapsular hematoma: 10%-50% surface area Intraparenchymal hematoma < 10 cm	None
III	Parenchymal laceration more than 3 cm deep	Subcapsular hematoma > 50% surface area, expanding or ruptured (regardless of size) Parenchymal hematoma > 10 cm or expanding	None
IV	Involves 25-75% of hepatic lobe or 1-3 Couinaud segments within a single lobe	Not determining factor	None
V	Involves > 75% of a hepatic lobe or > 3 Couinaud segments within a single lobe	Not determining factor	Juxtahepatic venous injuries

Continued

Table 9-2 American Association for the Surgery of Trauma Classification of Hepatic Trauma—cont'd

Grade	Laceration	Hematoma	Vascular
VI	Not determining factor	Not determining factor	Hepatic avulsion

The presence of multiple injuries increases grade by one up to grade III.

Table 9-3 Key Imaging Findings in Hepatic Trauma

Finding	Significance
Presence of active contrast extravasation	Likely to require embolization or surgery
Laceration to a central hepatic vein	Risk for severe hemorrhage when liver is moved during surgery
Central collection of low-attenuation fluid (rare)	Possible bile leak; consider endoscopic retrograde cholangiopancreatogram or scintigraphy when stable
Regions of hepatic infarction (rare)	Vascular injury is present, increased risk for further hemorrhage

can be overlooked. Multiplanar reformations are useful when differentiating between fissures and lacerations (Fig. 9-12). Aggressive volume resuscitation can affect the appearance of the liver on contrast-enhanced CT images, with periportal edema resulting in a halo of low attenuation around portal branches (Fig. 9-13).

■ SPLENIC TRAUMA

The spleen is the most commonly injured abdominal organ. A soft and relatively mobile but highly vascular organ, the spleen is quite susceptible to injury from blunt force trauma. In addition to motor vehicle collisions, the spleen is commonly injured in fights, falls, and athletic activities.

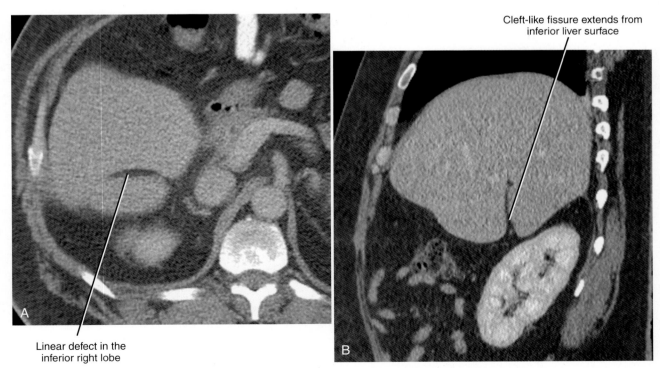

Cleft-like fissure extends from inferior liver surface

Linear defect in the inferior right lobe

Figure 9-12 Accessory fissure in right hepatic lobe mimics liver laceration. **A,** Axial image from contrast-enhanced computed tomographic (CT) scan demonstrates a linear low-attenuation defect in the right hepatic lobe, but fat attenuation and absence of perihepatic fluid suggest that this is not a laceration. **B,** Sagittal reformation of the CT scan demonstrates an anatomic (nontraumatic) cleft.

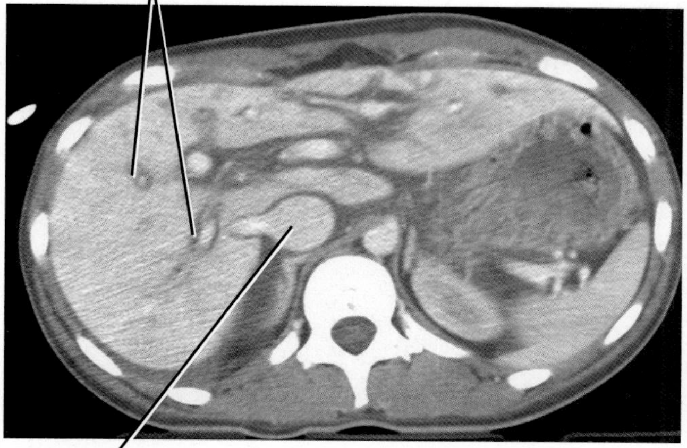

Low attenuation fluid tracks
along portal venous branches

IVC is distended

Figure 9-13 Axial image from contrast-enhanced computed tomographic scan after aggressive volume resuscitation demonstrates extensive periportal edema. Distention of the inferior vena cava (IVC) suggests volume overload.

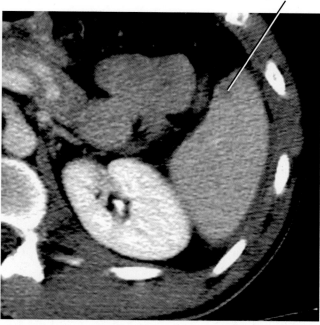

Capsular tear

Figure 9-14 Axial image of the spleen from contrast-enhanced computed tomographic scan performed after a motor vehicle collision demonstrates a small, superficial defect in the anterior aspect of the spleen.

With increasing understanding of postsplenectomy sepsis, nonoperative management of splenic injury has become increasingly emphasized in recent years. Because the risk for death from sepsis in patients who have undergone splenectomy is approximately 10 times that in the general population, efforts are made to preserve functioning splenic tissue whenever possible. Currently, at least 70% of patients with splenic injury who are hemodynamically stable are treated without surgery. Because delayed hemorrhage can be life threatening, patients with splenic injuries are often observed in an inpatient setting for at least 72 hours.

Types of Injury to the Spleen

As with the liver, most splenic injuries can be described as lacerations, hematomas, or vascular injuries. Small, superficial lacerations are commonly called *capsular tears* (Fig. 9-14). Hematomas contained by the splenic capsule are called *subcapsular hematomas* (Fig. 9-15). Although sometimes difficult to differentiate from areas of parenchymal hematoma, regions of devitalized spleen signify vascular injury (Fig. 9-16). ACE indicates severe vascular injury with active hemorrhage and usually requires immediate surgical or transcatheter intervention.

Grading Splenic Trauma

Table 9-4 provides the AAST system for grading splenic injury. As already discussed for the liver, it is useful to be familiar with the AAST system of classification for splenic injuries, but the key imaging findings to be reported can be abbreviated to a simpler list (Table 9-5). In general, the presence of active or expanding hemorrhage, extensive

hemorrhage into the peritoneum (Fig. 9-17), or central vascular injury are the key imaging findings that the trauma surgeon combines with clinical data to determine appropriate management.

Pitfalls in Imaging Splenic Trauma

The heterogeneous vascular lymphatic tissue of the spleen results in a mosaic-appearing enhancement pattern during early arterial enhancement (Fig. 9-18). Thus, splenic injuries are less conspicuous on images obtained during the arterial phase of enhancement. A scan delay of at least 70 seconds with MDCT scanners should ensure uniform splenic enhancement and optimize detection of lacerations.

The lobulated contour of the spleen sometimes results in clefts that may be difficult to differentiate from small capsular tears (see Fig. 15-1). The absence of associated hematoma or perisplenic fluid makes laceration less likely but is not always conclusive. Coronal or sagittal reformations may aid differentiation between anatomic clefts and small lacerations.

■ RENAL TRAUMA

The kidneys are partially protected by the ribs posteriorly and soft tissues anteriorly, and their relatively fixed retroperitoneal position helps decrease sheer forces in the adult. As a result, renal injuries are less frequent than hepatic or splenic injuries. In children, the kidneys occupy a relatively large proportion of the abdomen,

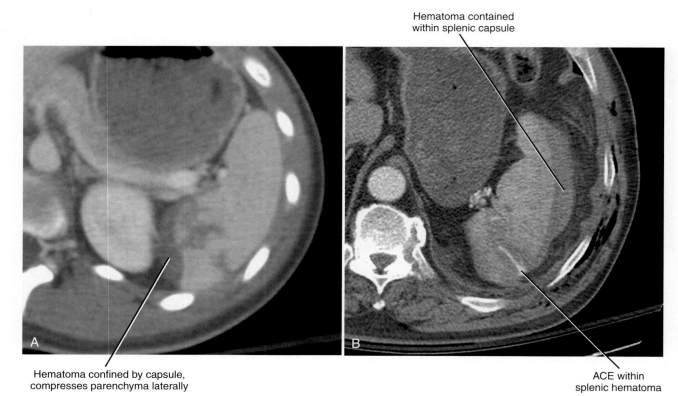

Figure 9-15 Splenic hematomas on axial contrast-enhanced computed tomographic scans of two patients. **A,** Small subcapsular hematoma along the posterior margin of the spleen. **B,** Larger subcapsular splenic hematoma in addition to active hemorrhage within a parenchymal hematoma. *ACE,* Active contrast extravasation.

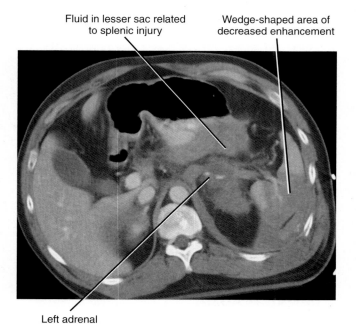

Figure 9-16 Axial image from contrast-enhanced computed tomographic scan after a motorcycle collision demonstrates a large hypoenhancing region of the spleen, indicating vascular injury. Left upper quadrant injury complex included the spleen, left adrenal gland, and left kidney (not shown). *ACE,* Active contrast extravasation.

increasing vulnerability to both blunt and penetrating injury. In addition, the elasticity of tissues in children results in increased mobility of the kidneys, increasing susceptibility to sheer forces. As a result, blunt force injuries to the renal pedicle are approximately 10 times more common in children than in adults.

Types of Injury to the Kidneys

In addition to parenchymal lacerations, hematomas, and vascular injuries, contusions are sometimes seen in renal trauma. Increased pressure from soft-tissue contusion decreases regional perfusion. Areas of contusion appear as regions of rounded or wedge-shaped low attenuation during the nephrographic phase of enhancement or can result in a diffusely abnormal nephrogram (Fig. 9-19). Contusions are less distinct than infarcts, which are much lower in attenuation than adjacent enhancing parenchyma. Contusion is also presumed to be present when hematuria occurs in the absence of imaging findings within the urinary tract.

Grading Renal Trauma

Conservative management has become the preferred method of management for most cases of renal trauma. Growing evidence supports a trial of conservative management for all but the most severe (grade V) injuries,

Table 9-4   Grading Splenic Injuries Using the American Association for the Surgery of Trauma Organ Injury Scale

Grade	Laceration	Hematoma	Vascular
I	Small laceration (capsular tear) less than 1 cm in depth	Subcapsular hematoma occupies < 10% surface area	None
II	Laceration 1-3 cm parenchymal depth and not involving a vessel	Subcapsular hematoma 10%-50% of surface area or intraparenchymal hematoma < 5 cm in diameter	None
III	>3 cm parenchymal depth or involving trabecular vessels	Subcapsular hematoma > 50% surface area or ruptured/expanding any size. Any hematoma > 5 cm	None
IV	Not determining factor	Not determining factor	Laceration of segmental or hilar vessels producing major devascularization (>25% spleen)

Continued

Table 9-4   Grading Splenic Injuries Using the American Association for the Surgery of Trauma Organ Injury Scale—cont'd

Grade	Laceration	Hematoma	Vascular
V	Shattered spleen	Not determining factor	Hilar vascular injury with devascularized spleen

Presence of multiple injuries increases grade by one up to grade III.

Table 9-5   Key Imaging Findings in Splenic Trauma

Finding	Significance
Presence of active contrast extravasation	Embolization or surgery likely to be required
Peritoneal fluid with splenic laceration	Possible hemoperitoneum from disrupted splenic capsule High risk for continued bleeding
Regions of splenic infarction	Central vascular injury is present, increased risk for continued or delayed hemorrhage

unless hemorrhage threatens hemodynamic stability. Table 9-6 presents the AAST system for grading renal trauma.

As elsewhere, ACE is the most critical finding in any renal injury and indicates a high likelihood that intervention

is necessary (Fig. 9-20). Renal collecting system injury may require surgery but can also respond to decompression with a ureteral stent or percutaneous nephrostomy catheter. Urine and blood can have a similar appearance on images obtained during the portal venous phase. Therefore, delayed images can be helpful to identify contrast material leaking from the collecting system (Figs. 9-2 and 9-21). Segmental renal infarction indicates injury to a segmental branch of the renal artery (Fig. 9-22), whereas global infarction suggests vascular pedicle injury (Fig. 9-23). Key imaging findings and their effect on management of renal trauma are shown in Table 9-7.

Congenital Anomalies in Renal Trauma

Preexisting congenital anomalies of the kidneys increase the risk for renal trauma. In the case of horseshoe kidney, compression between a lap belt and the spine is

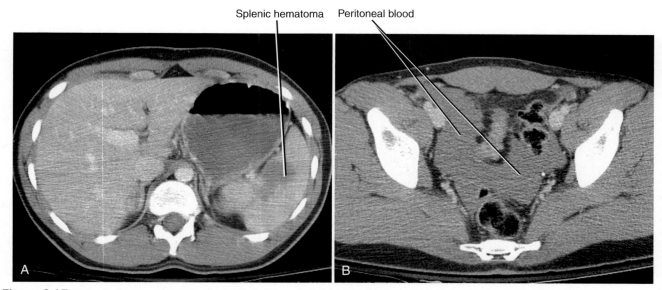

Splenic hematoma   Peritoneal blood

Figure 9-17   Extensive hemoperitoneum from splenic injury. **A,** Axial image from computed tomographic examination performed after blunt trauma demonstrates a splenic hematoma near the hilum. **B,** Axial image of the pelvis demonstrates a large amount of peritoneal blood. Exploratory laparotomy revealed isolated splenic injury.

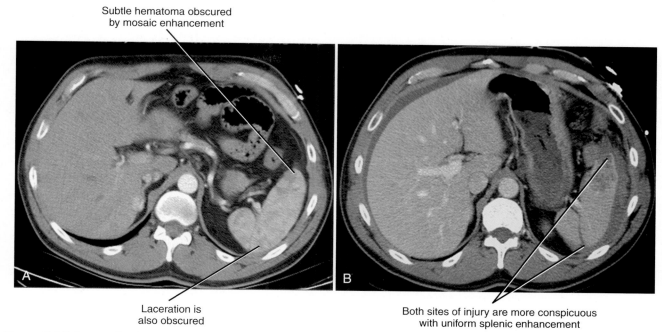

Subtle hematoma obscured
by mosaic enhancement

Laceration is
also obscured

Both sites of injury are more conspicuous
with uniform splenic enhancement

Figure 9-18 Impact of early scanning on conspicuity of splenic injury. **A,** Axial image from initial contrast-enhanced computed tomography (CT) acquired in the late arterial phase shows a mosaic pattern of splenic enhancement. No splenic injury was described. **B,** Axial image from a repeat CT scan performed in the portal venous phase to evaluate decreasing hematocrit demonstrates a conspicuous splenic laceration and new perisplenic hematoma.

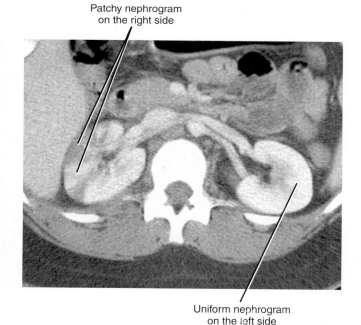

Patchy nephrogram
on the right side

Uniform nephrogram
on the left side

Figure 9-19 Axial image from contrast-enhanced computed tomographic (CT) scan after blunt force abdominal trauma demonstrates a patchy nephrogram in the right kidney typical of renal contusion. Microscopic hematuria was present. Follow-up CT performed the following day demonstrated near normalization of the nephrogram with no laceration or hematoma.

often the mechanism of renal injury. The midline segment of the kidney is not necessarily the region injured. More commonly, as that portion is "pinned" against the spine, one side or the other is torn away from it, resulting in an eccentric laceration that is usually posterior

(Fig. 9-25). A pelvic kidney or ptotic kidney situated anterior to the iliac crest is similarly vulnerable. A congenital ureteropelvic junction (UPJ) obstruction (or any other cause of hydronephrosis, for that matter) increases the chance of renal pelvic rupture, and by increasing the weight of the kidney makes it more vulnerable to deceleration injuries such as UPJ avulsion (Fig. 9-26).

Pitfalls in Imaging Renal Trauma

Extravasation of unopacified urine can mimic other traumatic abdominal fluid collections. Therefore, delayed excretory images are essential for the confident diagnosis of injuries to the renal collecting system.

■ ADRENAL TRAUMA

Trauma to the adrenal glands is relatively infrequent, and isolated injury to the adrenal glands rarely requires more than observation. The central location of the adrenal glands between the superior poles of the kidneys and the spine provide protection from blunt force trauma, a relatively fixed position minimizes effects of sheer forces, and small size decreases likelihood of injury from penetrating trauma or deceleration injury. Thus, when adrenal injury does occur, severe blunt force trauma is the most common mechanism and other organ injuries are usually present (Table 9-8). Although adrenal hemorrhage itself only rarely requires therapy such as transcatheter embolization, the severity of associated injuries carries with it a high risk for morbidity and mortality. Adrenal hemorrhage occurs more commonly on the right side in both children and

Table 9-6   Grading Renal Injuries Using the American Association for the Surgery of Trauma Organ Injury Scale

Grade	Laceration	Hematoma	Vascular
I	Hematuria with normal imaging findings Contusion without laceration	Small subcapsular hematoma	None
II	Laceration < 1 cm parenchymal depth	Nonexpanding perirenal hematoma	None
III	>1 cm parenchymal laceration without involvement of collecting system	Not determining factor	None
IV	Laceration with urinary extravasation	Not determining factor	Injury to main renal artery or vein with contained hemorrhage
V	Shattered kidney	Not determining factor	Hilar injury with devascularized kidney Ureteropelvic junction avulsion

adults, although the explanation for this remains controversial.

Types of Injury to the Adrenal Gland

The most common finding of adrenal injury at CT is hematoma replacing all or part of the gland. *Adrenal* hematoma results in round or ovoid enlargement of the gland, usually with stranding of the adjacent extraperitoneal fat (Fig. 9-27). *ACE* can occasionally be seen, and when present, embolization may be required to control hemorrhage (see Fig. 9-16).

With large hematomas, it is sometimes difficult to determine whether the source of hemorrhage is the adrenal gland, superior pole of the kidney, or even the liver (on the right side). Coronal or sagittal multiplanar reformations can be helpful in localizing the source of hemorrhage (Fig. 9-28).

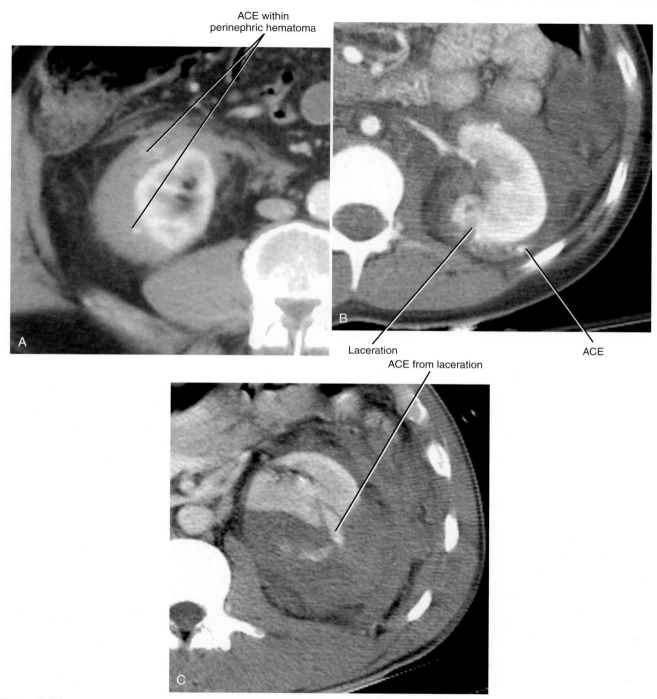

Figure 9-20 Axial computed tomographic images from three different patients demonstrate variable appearance of hemorrhage from the kidneys. **A,** Perinephric hematoma from capsular vessels with no visible renal laceration. **B,** Perinephric active contrast extravasation *(ACE)* adjacent to renal laceration. **C,** Stab wound to the left kidney with active hemorrhage from the renal laceration.

■ PANCREATIC TRAUMA

Pancreatic injuries are the least common type of solid organ injury in the abdomen and are rarely isolated. Because blunt force injury to the pancreas usually occurs as a result of direct compression, injuries to the adjacent left hepatic lobe, left adrenal gland, and spleen are commonly associated (Fig. 9-29). Penetrating injuries to the pancreas require a deep path to the center of

the abdomen; therefore, serious vascular injuries are present in approximately 75% of cases.

Unlike the other solid abdominal organs, the pancreas is linear, and its vascular supply and exocrine drainage follow a linear pattern. Thus, a 1-cm laceration in the neck of the pancreas is associated with higher morbidity than a similar laceration in the pancreatic tail. This is reflected in the AAST classification system as

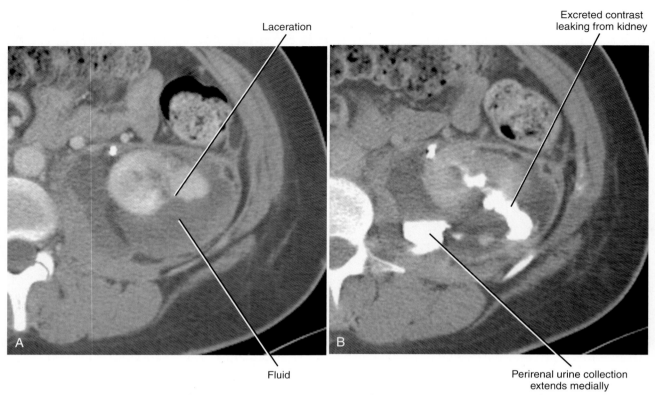

Laceration

Excreted contrast
leaking from kidney

Fluid

Perirenal urine collection
extends medially

Figure 9-21 Utility of delayed images for detecting collecting system injury. **A,** Axial image of the left kidney from a computed tomographic scan acquired in the portal venous phase demonstrates a renal laceration with fluid surrounding the kidney. **B,** Axial image from repeat scan acquired 20 minutes later clearly demonstrates contrast-opacified urine leaking into the collection.

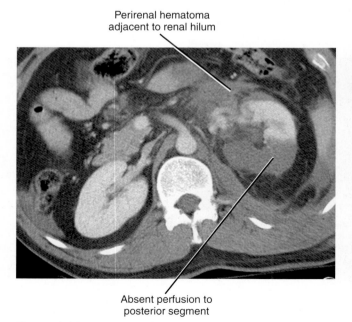

Perirenal hematoma
adjacent to renal hilum

Absent perfusion to
posterior segment

Figure 9-22 Axial image from a contrast-enhanced computed tomographic scan after a motorcycle collision demonstrates a segmental infarct of the left kidney.

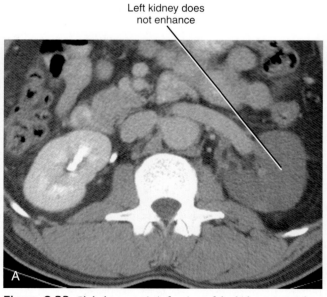

Left kidney does
not enhance

Figure 9-23 Global traumatic infarction of the kidney. **A,** Axial image from a contrast-enhanced computed tomographic scan after a motor vehicle collision demonstrates global infarction of the left kidney. Because no significant hemorrhage was present, it was managed conservatively.

Continued

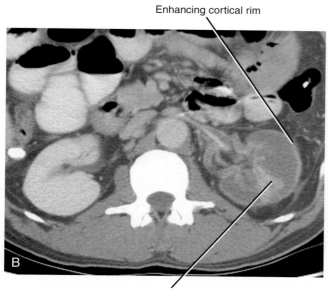

Enhancing cortical rim

Trace parenchymal enhancement

Figure 9-23, cont'd B, Axial image from follow-up examination 10 days later demonstrates rim enhancement of the infarcted kidney.

Table 9-7   Key Imaging Findings in Renal Trauma

Finding	Significance
Presence of active contrast extravasation	Embolization or surgery likely to be required
Low-attenuation fluid near kidney or deep laceration	Possible collecting system injury; delayed computed tomographic images helpful to identify extravasation of excreted contrast media
Regions of renal infarction	Vascular injury is present, increased risk for continued or delayed hemorrhage
Large subcapsular hematoma	Risk for development of Page kidney*

*The mass effect of hematoma contained by the renal capsule increases interstitial pressure within the kidney, decreasing perfusion and causing systemic hypertension through the renin-angiotensin system (Fig. 9-24).

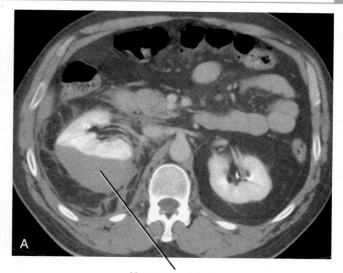

Hematoma deforms
right kidney
Hematoma surrounds and
deforms left kidney

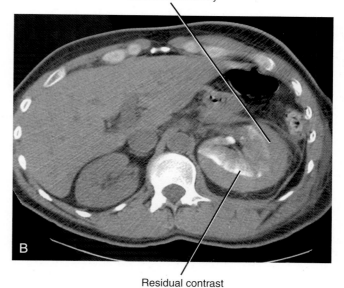

Residual contrast
in renal cortex

Figure 9-24 Subcapsular hematoma of the kidney in two patients. **A,** Axial image from contrast-enhanced computed tomography demonstrates a subcapsular hematoma compressing the right kidney with a nephrogram that is slightly increased in density. **B,** Axial image from an unenhanced computed tomographic scan performed to follow a subcapsular hematoma in a different patient demonstrates compression of the left kidney resulting in a persistent, striated nephrogram 1 day after injection.

shown in Table 9-9. Note that when applying this classification system, the location of the superior mesenteric artery is usually used to define "proximal" and "distal," with proximal injuries to the right and distal injuries to the left side of the superior mesenteric artery on axial CT images.

Pearl: Proximal pancreatic injuries are those that occur to the right side of the superior mesenteric artery and are associated with a worse prognosis.

Pitfalls in Imaging Pancreatic Trauma

Perhaps the greatest hindrance to identifying subtle pancreatic injuries is that they are uncommon, even in busy trauma centers. This is confounded by the lobulated margins of the pancreas and variable orientation of the pancreatic tail, requiring a deliberate inspection of the tail in each case.

■ TRAUMA TO THE URETER AND LOWER URINARY TRACT

Ureteral Injuries

Injuries to the ureter are uncommon. Injuries at the UPJ may result from sheer forces of blunt trauma, whereas more distal injuries are usually the result of penetrating

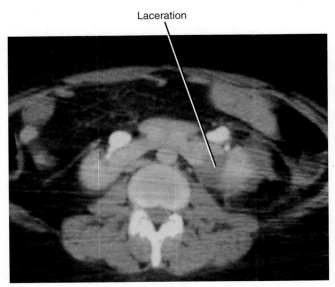

Laceration

Figure 9-25 Axial image from a contrast-enhanced computed tomographic scan after a motor vehicle collision demonstrates a laceration involving the left side of a horseshoe kidney.

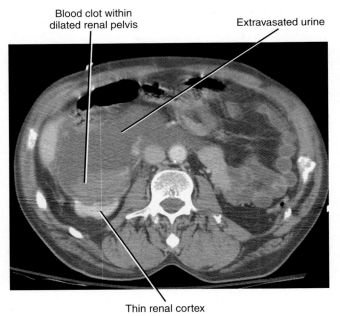

Blood clot within dilated renal pelvis

Extravasated urine

Thin renal cortex

Figure 9-26 Axial image from a contrast-enhanced computed tomographic scan after a low-speed motor vehicle collision demonstrates a large amount of retroperitoneal fluid resulting from rupture of the renal pelvis enlarged by a congenital ureteropelvic junction (UPJ) obstruction.

Table 9-8   Organs Commonly Injured with Adrenal Trauma

Right Adrenal Gland	Left Adrenal Gland
Liver	Spleen
Right kidney	Left kidney
Duodenum	Pancreatic tail
Pancreatic head	Lung
Lung	

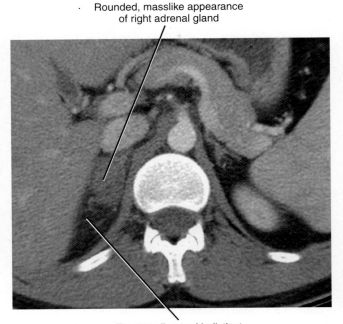

Rounded, masslike appearance of right adrenal gland

Fat stranding and indistinct margins consistent with hematoma

Figure 9-27 Axial image from a contrast-enhanced computed tomographic scan after a motor vehicle collision demonstrates enlargement of the right adrenal gland with stranding of the adjacent fat. The combination of image findings and clinical presentation is consistent with hematoma rather than adenoma.

or iatrogenic (surgical) trauma. Unlike injuries elsewhere in the urinary tract, hematuria is uncommon with ureteral injuries, because the flow of urine through the affected segment is usually disrupted and the associated hemorrhage is predominantly extraperitoneal. On CT, hematoma, soft-tissue air, or projectiles in the expected region of the ureter are usually accompanied by hydronephrosis and delayed renal enhancement and contrast excretion on the affected side (Fig. 9-32). If the patient is otherwise stable, delayed CT images or plain films can be performed to better define the region of injury (Fig. 9-33). Occasionally, retrograde urography is required.

Because deep penetrating injury is likely to cause bowel or central vascular injury that requires immediate laparotomy, ureteral injury may be first suspected in the operating room. In such cases, an intraoperative "one-shot" intravenous urogram may be performed by injecting iodinated contrast media intravenously and obtaining an abdominal urograph 5 to 10 minutes later. Ureteral injury usually results in obstruction on the affected side, with an abnormal nephrogram, hydronephrosis, and delayed excretion. Intravenous injection of methylene blue is sometimes performed so that extravasated urine can be identified visually at surgery.

Ureteral strictures can develop days after the trauma event. This usually indicates disruption of the delicate vessels that supply the ureter. The rare ureteral strictures that follow severe blunt abdominal trauma occur in the region of the UPJ. This is not surprising because the kidney is more mobile than the ureter, and sheer forces

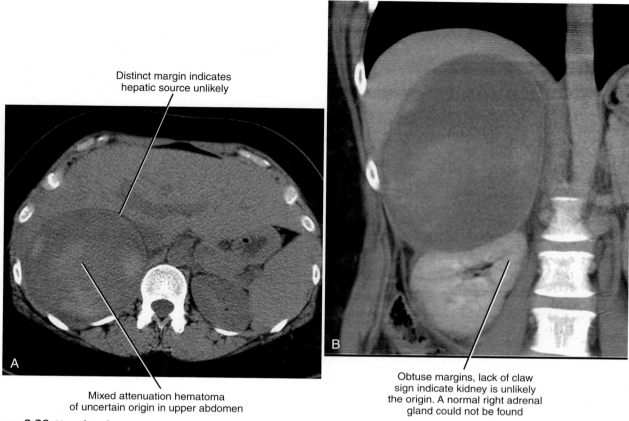

Distinct margin indicates
hepatic source unlikely

Mixed attenuation hematoma
of uncertain origin in upper abdomen

Obtuse margins, lack of claw
sign indicate kidney is unlikely
the origin. A normal right adrenal
gland could not be found

Figure 9-28 Use of a reformatted image to determine the origin of an adrenal hematoma. **A,** Axial image from an unenhanced computed tomographic scan demonstrates a large heterogeneous hematoma in the right upper quadrant that appears separated from the liver by a fat plane. **B,** Coronal reformation from the same examination demonstrates an interface with the kidney indicating extrarenal origin. The hematoma resolved on follow-up examinations.

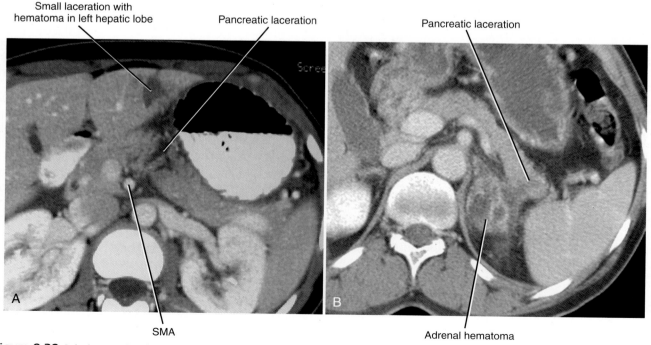

Small laceration with
hematoma in left hepatic lobe

Pancreatic laceration

Pancreatic laceration

SMA

Adrenal hematoma

Figure 9-29 Injuries associated with pancreatic trauma in different patients. **A,** Axial image from contrast-enhanced computed tomography (CT) demonstrates a pancreatic laceration associated with liver laceration after an assault. **B,** Axial image from enhanced CT in another patient demonstrates a pancreatic laceration associated with a left adrenal hematoma from a motor vehicle collision. *SMA,* Superior mesenteric artery.

Table 9-9   Grading Pancreatic Injuries Using the American Association for the Surgery of Trauma Classification

Grade	Description of Injury
I	Minor contusion or superficial laceration without duct injury
II	Major contusion or laceration without duct injury or devitalized parenchyma
III	Distal transection or parenchymal injury with duct injury (Fig. 9-30)
IV	Proximal transection or parenchymal injury involving ampulla (Fig. 9-31)
V	Massive disruption of pancreatic head

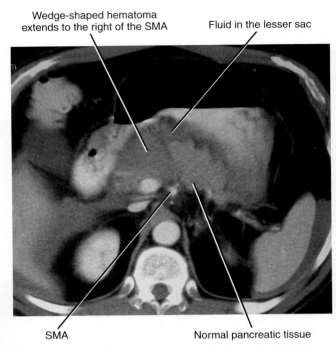

Figure 9-31 Axial image from a contrast-enhanced computed tomographic scan after blunt abdominal trauma demonstrates proximal pancreatic transection. *SMA*, Superior mesenteric artery.

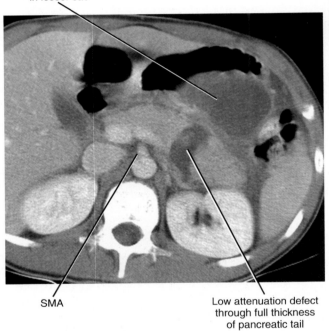

Figure 9-30 Distal pancreatic transection. Axial image from a contrast-enhanced computed tomographic scan performed several days after blunt abdominal trauma demonstrates a distal transection of the pancreas. Although the duct is not seen, the depth of laceration and developing pseudocyst indicate duct injury. *SMA*, Superior mesenteric artery.

at the UPJ are likely to tear the fine blood vessels before tearing the ureter itself. Often a hazy stranding is in the fat surrounding the ureter on the initial examination, but this is commonly overlooked because there is usually a more severe injury to the adjacent kidney (Fig. 9-34).

Bladder Injuries

Bladder injuries are usually the result of blunt trauma. Although as many as 70% of bladder injuries are associated with pelvic fractures, bone fragments are usually

not directly responsible for bladder injury. Instead, the compressive and sheer forces of blunt trauma tear tissues attached to the extraperitoneal portions of the bladder, or the abrupt increase in intravesical pressure causes the bladder dome to burst into the peritoneum. Overall, approximately 62% of bladder ruptures are extraperitoneal, 25% are intraperitoneal, and 12% are combined.

Hematuria is the most common sign of bladder injury. Because the peritoneal space reabsorbs the urine that leaks into it, intraperitoneal bladder rupture can result in a rapid increase in serum creatinine (within hours of the injury). Intraperitoneal bladder rupture usually requires surgical therapy.

Extraperitoneal bladder rupture, in contrast, is usually treated conservatively with placement of a suprapubic bladder catheter. Associated rectal injury or severe pelvic fractures can increase the risk for severe infection or fistula formation; therefore, surgical repair is often performed in such cases. In addition, untreated bladder injury may increase the risk for vesicocutaneous fistula formation when laparotomy is performed for other reasons.

Findings of Bladder Injury on Initial Trauma Computed Tomography

Evidence of bladder injury should be specifically sought when pelvic fractures or perivesical fat stranding, hematoma, or fluid are present on CT images. The presence of any of these findings associated with hematuria is an indication for CT cystography. The types of pelvic fractures most often associated with bladder rupture are

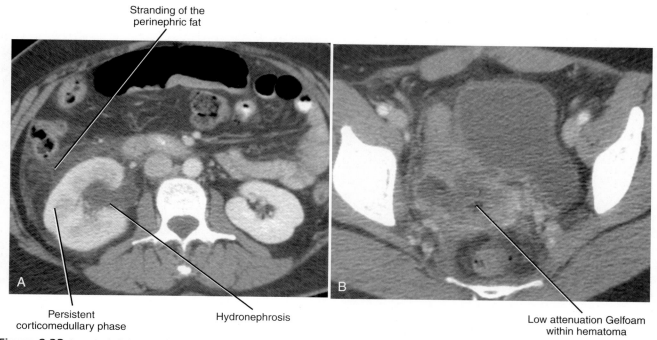

Stranding of the
perinephric fat

Low attenuation Gelfoam
within hematoma

A

B

Persistent
corticomedullary phase

Hydronephrosis

Figure 9-32 Iatrogenic injury to the distal left ureter during hysterectomy demonstrated on contrast-enhanced computed tomography. **A,** Axial image at the level of the kidneys demonstrates evidence of right ureteral obstruction. **B,** Axial image in the pelvis demonstrates hematoma and Gelfoam in the expected location of the distal right ureter.

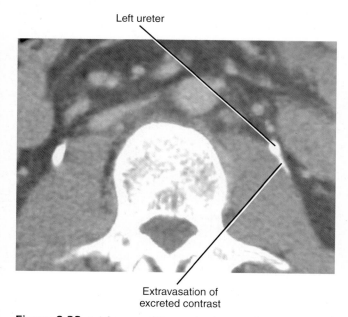

Left ureter

Extravasation of
excreted contrast

Figure 9-33 Axial image of the proximal ureters from a computed tomographic scan in the excretory phase after a motor vehicle collision demonstrates extravasation of excreted contrast adjacent to the left ureter. This was treated conservatively with a ureteral stent.

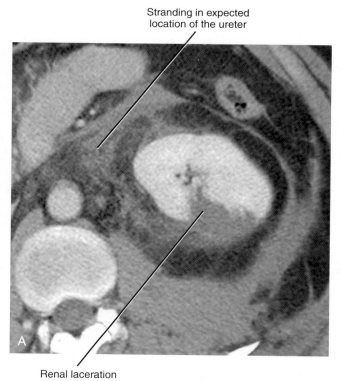

Stranding in expected
location of the ureter

A

Renal laceration

Figure 9-34 Delayed diagnosis of ureteral injury. **A,** Axial image from a contrast-enhanced computed tomographic scan after a motorcycle collision demonstrates a left renal laceration and multiple areas of soft-tissue hematoma.

included in Box 9-4. Soft-tissue changes that suggest bladder injury are often seen in the extraperitoneal tissues between the bladder and the pubic symphysis (Fig. 9-35). Low-attenuation peritoneal fluid without apparent extravesical source raises suspicion of intraperitoneal bladder rupture.

Continued

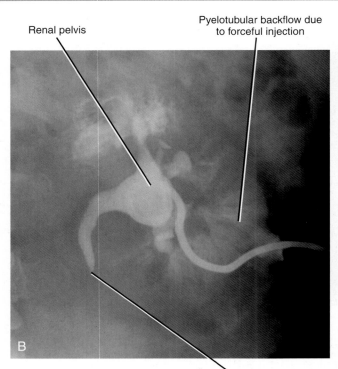

Renal pelvis

Pyelotubular backflow due to forceful injection

Stricture at approximate level of periureteral stranding.

Figure 9-34, cont'd B, Image from a nephrostogram performed approximately 1 week later demonstrates a stricture of the proximal left ureter.

BOX 9-4   Skeletal Injuries Most Often Associated with Bladder Injury

Pubic ramus fracture
Diastasis of pubic symphysis
Sacral fracture
Diastasis of sacroiliac joint

Computed Tomographic Cystography

Although an area of bladder wall disruption is sometimes identified directly on the initial CT images, more often cystography is required for diagnosis. In many trauma centers, conventional cystography has been replaced by CT cystography because small injuries can be missed with the former technique, particularly when anterior or posterior.

CT cystography is performed by instilling dilute contrast media into the bladder via a catheter before acquiring CT images. Dilution of the contrast media is necessary to prevent streak artifact that might obscure findings. One method of performing CT cystography is provided in Box 9-5, although many variations on this approach exist.

With intraperitoneal bladder rupture, CT cystography shows contrast collecting around bowel loops and in

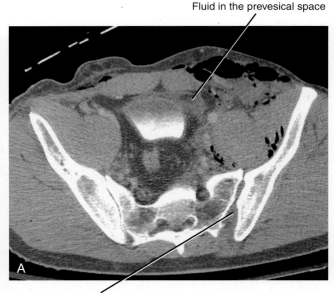

Fluid in the prevesical space

Diastasis of the SI joint

Surgical drain

Extraperitoneal extravasated contrast

Figure 9-35 Computed tomographic signs of bladder injury. **A,** Axial image from the initial contrast-enhanced computed tomographic scan in the pelvis demonstrates several signs that bladder injury is likely. **B,** Subsequent conventional cystogram demonstrates extraperitoneal bladder rupture. *SI,* Sacroiliac.

dependent recesses of the peritoneal space (Fig. 9-36). With extraperitoneal bladder rupture, contrast material disperses from the bladder in a flame-shaped configuration as it infiltrates the extraperitoneal tissues. The injury is usually in the inferior region of the bladder, near the bladder neck, trigone, or lower anterior bladder wall (Fig. 9-37). Contrast is often seen collecting around the base of the bladder or in the prevesical space of Retzius. This results in the so-called "molar tooth" pattern on

BOX 9-5   Quick Guide to Performing CT Cystography

1. Dilute contrast media (50 ml IV contrast media* in 1-L bag sterile saline).
2. Connect IV tubing to bladder catheter (cone-shaped connector).
3. Allow contrast to enter bladder under gravity pressure until it stops dripping, patient is uncomfortable, or a total of 350 ml is infused.
4. Scan pelvis from above iliac crests through pubic symphysis.

*Approximate dilution for 350 mg of iodine per ml. This can be titrated to achieve an appropriate attenuation for the available contrast media.

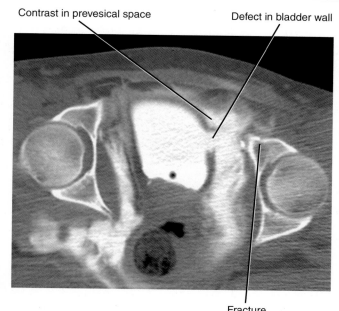

Contrast in prevesical space   Defect in bladder wall

Fracture

Figure 9-37 Extraperitoneal bladder rupture on computed tomographic (CT) cystogram. Axial image of the pelvis from a CT scan after instillation of dilute contrast material into the bladder demonstrates a large defect in the left bladder wall with extravasation of contrast into the extraperitoneal soft tissues. Also note the misalignment of the acetabula because of multiple areas of pelvic fractures and diastasis.

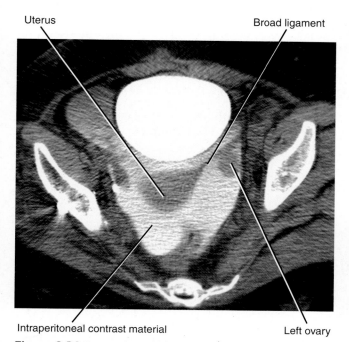

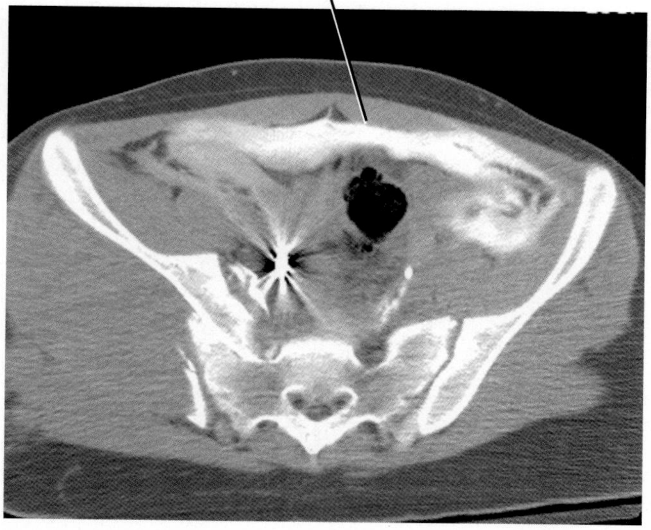

Uterus   Broad ligament

Intraperitoneal contrast material   Left ovary

Figure 9-36 Intraperitoneal bladder rupture demonstrated by computed tomographic cystography. Axial image of the pelvis performed after filling of the bladder with dilute contrast demonstrates opacified peritoneal fluid, indicating intraperitoneal bladder rupture. Optimal contrast dilution should be slightly less dense than on this image because the contrast material causes beam hardening and makes it difficult to visualize the bladder wall.

Extraperitoneal contrast makes smooth interface along the rectus sheath

Figure 9-38 Rectus sheath extension of extraperitoneal bladder rupture on computed tomographic cystography. This a more superior axial image of the same examination shown in Figure 9-37. The anterior extraperitoneal spaces must be differentiated from the ventral peritoneal recesses because a mistaken diagnosis of intraperitoneal bladder rupture can lead to unnecessary surgery.

conventional cystography and a confined anterior collection on CT cystography. If an anterior extraperitoneal tear allows urine to course along the inner margin of the rectus sheath, the resultant appearance may simulate an intraperitoneal bladder rupture on conventional cystography, although the absence of contrast material in the dependent recesses makes diagnosis by CT straightforward (Fig. 9-38).

Bladder wall contusion occurs when blunt forces or sheer injury cause hematoma within the bladder wall without disrupting it. On CT, the contused bladder wall is focally thickened but intact (Fig. 9-39). Interstitial bladder tears are usually iatrogenic incomplete disruptions of the bladder wall as the result of deep transurethral biopsy of a bladder tumor (Fig. 9-40). These are treated conservatively with bladder drainage.

ACE

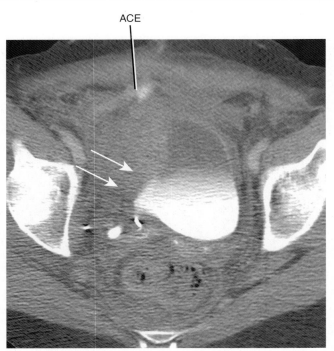

Figure 9-39 Axial image from a contrast-enhanced computed tomographic scan after a motor vehicle collision demonstrates a large right pelvic hematoma with associated thickening of the adjacent bladder wall (outer margin shown by *arrows*) indicating contusion. *ACE,* Active contrast extravasation.

■ URETHRAL INJURY

When to Suspect Urethral Injury

Injury to the male urethra occurs most often in the setting of blunt force trauma and is often associated with fractures of the pubic ramus or diastasis of the symphysis pubis. The posterior urethra is usually the site of injury. Additional mechanisms of injury include straddle injuries to the anterior urethra, iatrogenic injuries in the region of the penoscrotal junction, and penetrating injuries anywhere in the urethra.

Urethral injury is likely when there is blood at the urethral meatus, but sometimes the only clinical sign is an inability to void despite palpable bladder distension. On plain film, diastasis of the pubic symphysis should raise concern for urethral injury. CT findings commonly associated with urethral injury include fat stranding or hematoma, or both, in the region of the bulbocavernosus and obturator internus muscles, and pubic fracture/diastasis (Fig. 9-41). In such cases, retrograde urethrography (RUG) is recommended before bladder catheterization, because blind passage of a catheter can convert a partial tear to complete transection. Many partial tears can be managed with bladder drainage through a suprapubic tube, whereas most complete tears require surgical repair.

Pearl: Diastasis of or fracture near the pubic symphysis or soft-tissue injury in the region of the bulbocavernosus and obturator internus muscles should prompt performance of RUG before passage of a Foley catheter.

Thickened bladder wall is faintly visible

Contrast collects in bladder wall

Contrast moves as bladder contracts

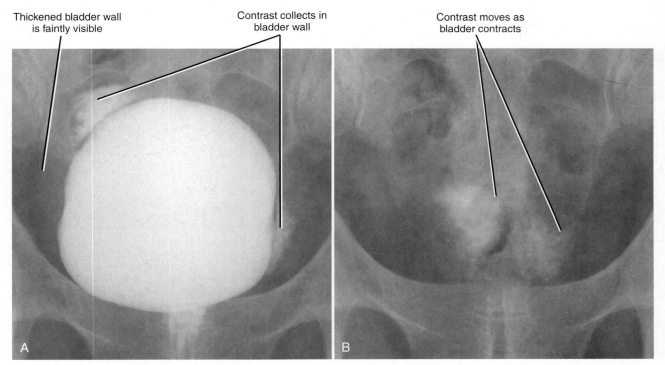

Figure 9-40 Cystogram performed after transurethral resection of bladder tumors. **A,** Two contrast collections confined to the bladder wall are consistent with interstitial bladder injury. **B,** Postvoid view shows the collections move with the bladder wall as it contracts.

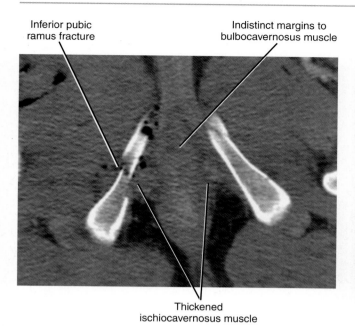

Inferior pubic ramus fracture

Indistinct margins to bulbocavernosus muscle

Thickened ischiocavernosus muscle

Figure 9-41 Computed tomographic (CT) findings associated with urethral injury. Axial image from a contrast-enhanced CT scan demonstrates hematoma in the region of ischiocavernosus and bulbocavernosus muscles.

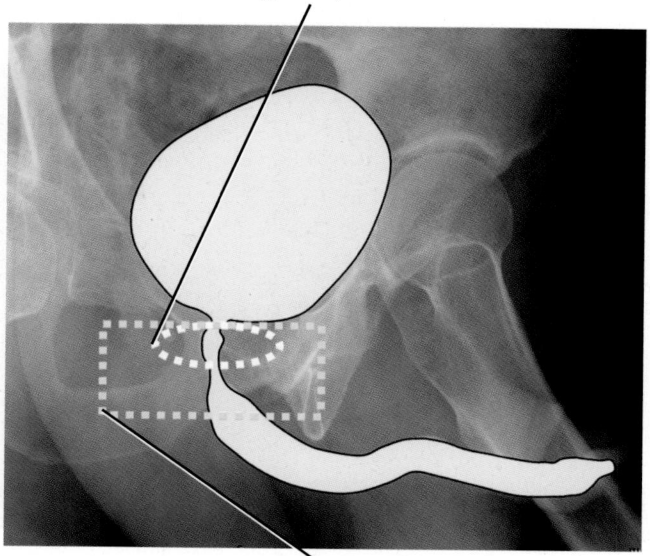

Type II injuries

Type III injuries

Figure 9-42 Illustration of a retrograde urethrogram demonstrating location of injury in type II and III urethral injuries.

Characterizing Urethral Injuries

Several systems for classifying urethral injury have been proposed. The most current system is based on anatomic and mechanical characteristics of injuries and is shown in Table 9-10. (See Chapter 19 for a detailed description of urethral anatomy and technique of RUG.) The posterior urethra (composed of the prostatic and membranous urethra) is the region most commonly injured. The main distinction of clinical importance is between type II and III injuries (Fig. 9-42). Type II injuries are uncommon, involving only the urethra above

the urogenital (UG) diaphragm. During RUG, extravasated contrast stays high in the perineum and may extend superiorly to the prevesical space. Type III injuries are more common, involving the urethra above and below the UG diaphragm. In this case, extravasated contrast material also extends inferiorly into the scrotum. When findings are equivocal on RUG images, MRI can sometimes aid in detecting and characterizing urethral injury. Examples of different types of urethral injury are shown in Figure 9-43.

Pearl: The membranous urethra (UG diaphragm) is usually located at the level of the lower half of the pubic symphysis. This can be a helpful landmark if other features of the urethra are disrupted.

Table 9-10   Classification of Urethral Injuries

Type	Description	Retrograde Urethrographic Findings
I	Stretch injury or incomplete tear	Smooth narrowing of the urethra
II	Injury above urogenital diaphragm	Contrast extravasation in perineum
III	Injury above and below urogenital diaphragm	Contrast in perineum and scrotum
IV	Injury to bladder base that may involve posterior urethra	Signs of extraperitoneal bladder rupture with contrast around posterior urethra
V	Anterior urethral injury	Contrast extravasation from bulbous or penile urethra

Adapted from Goldman SM, Sandler CM, Corriere JN et al: Blunt urethral trauma: a unified, anatomical mechanical classification, *J Urol* 157:85-89, 1997, by permission.

■ BOWEL AND MESENTERIC INJURY

Possible gastrointestinal tract injuries include wall contusion, intramural hematoma, perforation, and ischemia caused by mesenteric vascular injury. Because the small intestine fills most of the anterior abdominal cavity, it is the organ most commonly injured after penetrating injury to the anterior abdomen.

Identification of injury to the intestinal tract and its mesenteries has long been one of the great challenges in trauma imaging. Patients with signs of peritonitis are usually taken directly to laparotomy, particularly if ultrasound shows evidence of peritoneal fluid. The convoluted course and constant peristalsis of the bowel make its assessment difficult on axial CT images.

In an effort to improve detection of bowel injury, some centers administer water-soluble high-attenuation

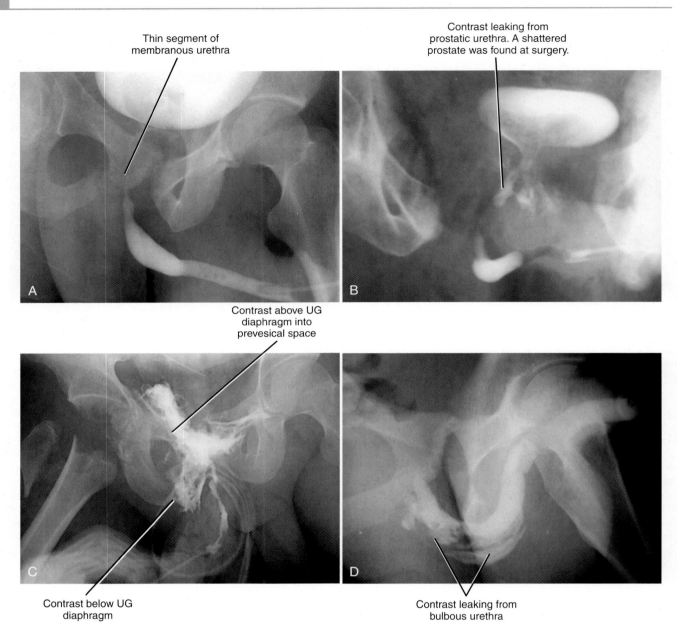

Figure 9-43 Types of urethral injuries demonstrated by retrograde urethrography. **A,** Type I stretch injury. **B,** Type II injury (above the urogenital [UG] diaphragm). **C,** Type III injury (above and below the UG diaphragm). It is difficult to exclude associated bladder injury, which would make this type IV. **D,** Type V injury (anterior urethra).

contrast media via nasogastric tube before performing CT examinations of the abdomen and pelvis for trauma. Leakage of enteric contrast media from the intestine is specific for bowel injury (see Fig. 9-3). However, this practice can delay the examination and increase the risk for aspiration.

Recent data show that MDCT without the administration of enteric contrast is a quick and sensitive technique for detection of bowel injury. On rare occasions, the precise site of bowel injury can be identified as an area of discontinuity of the bowel wall (Fig. 9-44). Additional signs of bowel injury include extraluminal gas, extraluminal fluid, alterations in bowel wall enhancement (Fig. 9-45), bowel wall thickening, and

mesenteric stranding. The most common but least specific CT sign of bowel injury is focal bowel wall thickening (Fig. 9-46). Whenever bowel injury is present, the mesentery should be inspected carefully, and vice versa.

With good MDCT technique, contrast extravasation, pseudoaneurysm, or cutoff of the mesenteric vessels can occasionally be demonstrated (Figs. 9-45 and 9-47). When fluid or blood surrounds mesenteric vessels without intervening fat, it is contained within the mesentery. Interloop fluid (between the mesenteric leaves) often has a triangular or spiculated shape and does not directly contact the vessels when sufficient mesenteric fat is present.

Skin thickening and stranding in the subcutaneous fat of the anterior abdominal wall is a sign of lap belt

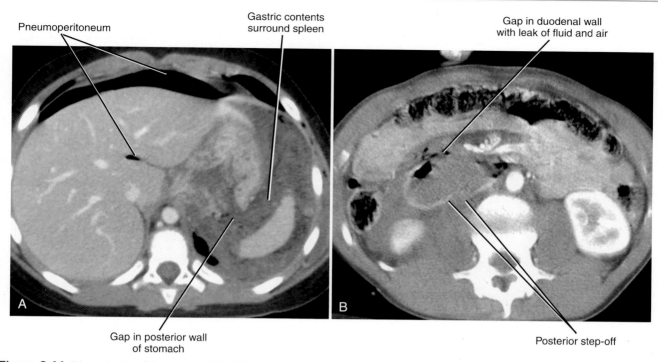

Pneumoperitoneum

Gastric contents
surround spleen

Gap in duodenal wall
with leak of fluid and air

Gap in posterior wall
of stomach

Posterior step-off

Figure 9-44 Discontinuity of the bowel wall in blunt abdominal trauma. **A,** Axial image from a contrast-enhanced computed tomographic (CT) scan demonstrates a large gastric perforation caused by a motor vehicle collision. **B,** Axial image from contrast-enhanced CT in a different patient demonstrates discontinuity of duodenal wall after an all-terrain vehicle collision.

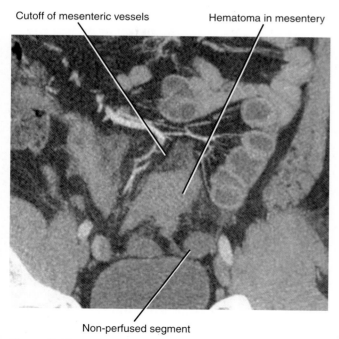

Cutoff of mesenteric vessels

Hematoma in mesentery

Non-perfused segment

Figure 9-45 Absence of wall enhancement as a sign of bowel injury. Coronal reformation from a computed tomographic scan demonstrates vessel cutoff with hematoma adjacent to the nonperfused segment of ileum. An axial image of this patient is shown in Figure 16-40.

injury (see Fig. 9-46). The presence of an abdominal wall seat belt contusion or Chance fracture of the lumbar spine, or both, carries an increased risk for bowel and mesenteric injury (see Table 9-11).

■ AORTIC INJURY

Injuries to the abdominal aorta are rarely imaged. This is likely because major injury to the abdominal aorta is extremely unusual with blunt force trauma, whereas penetrating injury to the aorta is often rapidly fatal. As a result, the possibility of injury to the abdominal aorta can be overlooked by trauma surgeons and radiologists alike, with delayed diagnosis in approximately one third of cases.

The most common mechanism of blunt force injury to the abdominal aorta is a crush injury to the aorta between a lap belt and the lumbar spine. This is more common among children, perhaps because the aorta is protected by less soft tissue than in adults. Injury affects the infrarenal abdominal aorta in 98% of reported cases.

CT findings of aortic injury can be subtle. A contour deformity may be the only finding on axial images. Because most cases involve children, the aorta is small and a paucity of retroperitoneal fat can make identification of hematoma difficult. Multiplanar images better demonstrate the contour deformity, with several reported cases presenting as circumferential hematoma (Fig. 9-48).

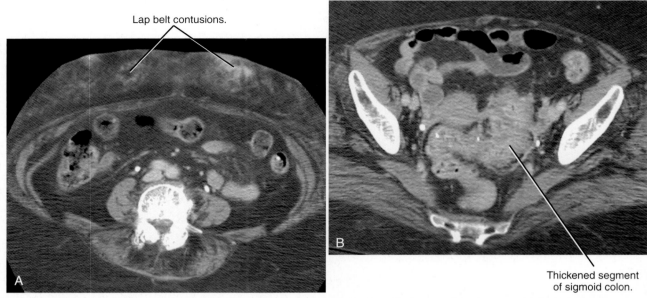

Lap belt contusions.

Thickened segment of sigmoid colon.

Figure 9-46 Lap belt injury and bowel wall thickening. **A,** Axial image from a contrast-enhanced computed tomographic scan after a motor vehicle collision demonstrates multifocal contusion in the subcutaneous fat of the anterior abdominal wall. **B,** A more inferior image demonstrates segmental wall thickening of the sigmoid colon. Surgery confirmed intramural hematoma of the sigmoid colon with a small area of perforation.

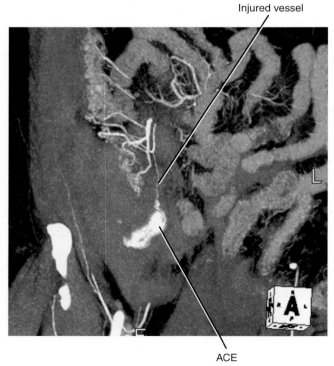

Injured vessel

ACE

Figure 9-47 Coronal oblique maximum intensity projection image of the right lower quadrant from a contrast-enhanced computed tomographic scan demonstrates active contrast extravasation (ACE) from a transected ileocolic artery.

■ SOFT TISSUE AND BONE INJURIES

Injury to the extraperitoneal soft tissues of the abdomen and pelvis are common and occasionally life threatening. The most common findings include areas of fat

Table 9-11 Findings of Bowel or Mesenteric Injury at Computed Tomography

Relative Specificity	Findings
Specific for significant injury	• Discontinuity of bowel wall • Nonenhancing bowel wall • Intraperitoneal gas • Mesenteric gas • Extravasation of enteric contrast • Mesenteric active contrast extravasation • Mesenteric vessel cutoff
Less specific for significant injury	• Focal bowel wall thickening • Mesenteric hematoma
Least specific but may indicate injury	• Mesenteric fluid • Mesenteric stranding/haziness • Abdominal wall injury • Intraperitoneal fluid without evidence of solid organ injury • Chance fracture of lumbar spine

stranding or hematoma in the subcutaneous fat, often from lap-belt injury (Figs. 9-46 and 9-49). When hemorrhage occurs deeper within the pelvis or abdominal wall, transcatheter embolization may be necessary to control bleeding (Fig. 9-50). If embolization of an abdominal wall hemorrhage is considered, it is helpful to remember that hemorrhage in the area of the rectus sheath is usually the result of injury to the inferior or superior epigastric artery, whereas more lateral abdominal wall hemorrhage is usually caused by injury to branches of the deep circumflex iliac artery.

Fractures are common in patients with intraabdominal injuries related to blunt force trauma. The presence of a fracture on CT images should prompt inspection of nearby organs and soft tissues. Likewise, the presence of

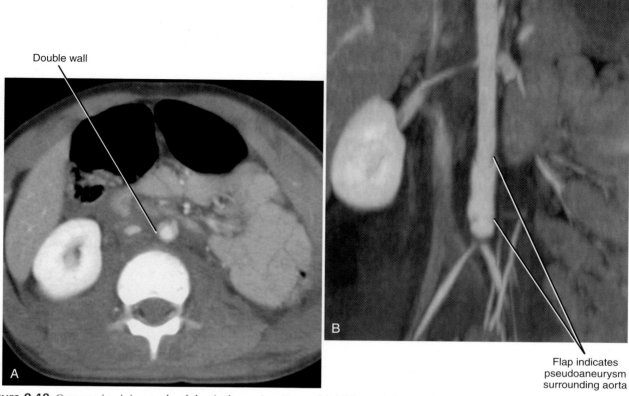

Double wall

A

B

Flap indicates
pseudoaneurysm
surrounding aorta

Figure 9-48 Compression injury to the abdominal aorta in a 7-year-old child. **A,** Axial image from a contrast-enhanced computed tomographic scan demonstrates the subtle appearance of a double wall that could be mistaken for a motion artifact. **B,** Image reformatted in the coronal plane demonstrates a stepoff in the aortic wall.

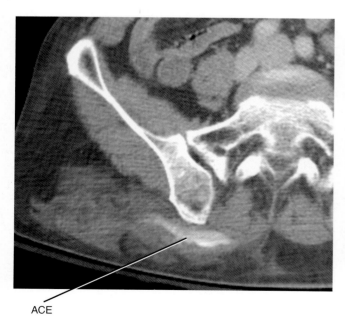

ACE

Figure 9-49 Active contrast extravasation (ACE) in the superficial soft tissues. Axial image of the pelvis from a contrast-enhanced computed tomographic scan after a motor vehicle collision demonstrates ACE in the soft tissues overlying the iliac bone. This was treated with compression and monitored by physical examination.

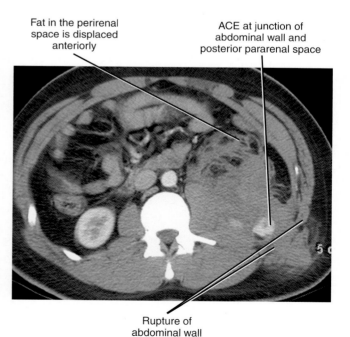

Fat in the perirenal
space is displaced
anteriorly

ACE at junction of
abdominal wall and
posterior pararenal space

Rupture of
abdominal wall

Figure 9-50 Axial image from a contrast-enhanced computed tomographic scan after a motor vehicle collision demonstrates active contrast extravasation (ACE) deep in the abdominal wall with hematoma that spans each space from the subcutaneous tissues to the perirenal space. Transcatheter embolization was performed to control hemorrhage.

an organ injury should prompt inspection of nearby bony structures. Vertebral fractures are notoriously difficult to detect on axial CT images. The presence of paraspinal hematoma or fat stranding is a clue, but often even careful inspection in the axial plane fails to detect some fractures. Therefore, we recommend including sagittal reformations of the spine for every patient imaged with abdominal and pelvic CT for trauma.

Suggested Readings

Anderson SW, Brian CL, James TR et al: 64 MDCT in multiple trauma patients: imaging manifestations and clinical implications of active extravasation, *Emerg Radiol* 14:151-159, 2007.

Brofman N, Atri M, Hanson JM et al: Evaluation of bowel and mesenteric blunt trauma with multidetector CT, *RadioGraphics* 26:1119-1131, 2006.

Burks DW, Mirvis SE, Shanmuganathan K: Acute adrenal injury after blunt abdominal trauma: CT findings, *Am J Roentgenol* 158:503-507, 1992.

Carroll PR, McAninch JW: Major bladder trauma: mechanisms of injury and a unified method of diagnosis and repair, *J Urol* 132:254-257, 1984.

Chan DP, Abujedeh HH, Cushing GL Jr et al: CT cystography with multiplanar reformation for suspected bladder rupture: experience in 234 cases, *Am J Roentgenol* 187:1296-1302, 2006.

Franklin GA, Casos SR: Current advances in the surgical approach to abdominal trauma, *Injury* 37:1143-1156, 2006.

Goldman SM, Sandler CM, Corriere JN et al: Blunt urethral trauma: a unified, anatomical mechanical classification, *J Urol* 157:85-89, 1997.

Ikeda O, Urata J, Araki Y et al: Acute adrenal hemorrhage after blunt trauma, *Abdom Imaging* 32:248-252, 2007.

Jankowski JT, Spirnak JP: Current recommendations for imaging in the management of urologic traumas, *Urol Clin North Am* 33:365-376, 2006.

Jeffrey RB, Cardoza JD, Olcott EW: Detection of active intraabdominal arterial hemorrhage: value of dynamic contrast-enhanced CT, *Am J Roentgeol* 156:725-729, 1991.

Levine CD, Gonzales RN, Wachsberg RH et al: CT findings of bowel and mesenteric injury, *J Comput Assist Tomogr* 21:974-979, 1997.

Mirvis SE, Shanmuganathan K, Erb R: Diffuse small-bowel ischemia in hypotensive adults after blunt trauma (shock bowel): CT findings and clinical significance, *Am J Roentgenol* 163:1375-1379, 1994.

Morgan DE, Nallamala LK, Kenney PJ et al: CT cystography: radiographic and clinical predictors of bladder rupture, *Am J Roentgenol* 174:89-95, 2000.

Peng MY, Parisky YR, Cornwell EE 3rd et al: CT cystography versus conventional cystography in evaluation of bladder injury, *Am J Roentgenol* 173:1269-1272, 1999.

Poletti PA, Mirvis SE, Shanmuganathan K et al: CT criteria for management of blunt liver trauma: correlation with angiographic and surgical findings, *Radiology* 216:418-427, 2000.

Rana AI, Kenney PJ, Lockhart ME et al: Adrenal gland hematomas in trauma patients, *Radiology* 230:669-675, 2004.

Roth SM, Wheeler JR, Gregory RT et al: Blunt injury of the abdominal aorta: a review, *J Trauma* 42:748-755, 1997.

Shanmuganathan K, Mirvis SE, Sover ER: Value of contrast-enhanced CT in detecting active hemorrhage in patients with blunt abdominal or pelvic trauma, *Am J Roentgenol* 161:65-69, 1993.

Shuman WP: CT of blunt abdominal trauma in adults, *Radiology* 205:297-306, 1997.

Steenburg SD, Ravenel JG: Multi-detector computed tomography findings of atypical blunt traumatic aortic injuries: a pictorial review, *Emerg Radiol* 14:143-150, 2007.

Stuhlfaut JW, Lucey BC, Varghese JC, Soto JA: Blunt abdominal trauma: utility of 5-minute delayed CT with a reduced radiation dose, *Radiology* 238:473-479, 2006.

Stuhlfaut JW, Soto JA, Lucey BC et al: Blunt abdominal trauma: performance of CT without oral contrast material, *Radiology* 233:689-694, 2004.

Tarrant AM, Ryan MF, Hamilton PA, Benjaminov O: A pictorial review of hypovolaemic shock in adults, *Br J Radiol* 81:252-257, 2008.

CHAPTER 10

A Brief Guide to Cancer Imaging

John R. Leyendecker and Michael Oliphant

Cancer imaging constitutes a significant part of the typical abdominal imaging workload of many radiology practices. Familiarity with the modes and patterns of tumor spread can improve interpretive efficiency and accuracy because malignant tumors often present distinct from their origin. Likewise, knowledge of the staging of malignant tumors helps one to convey information to the referring physician that can facilitate tumor resection or prevent unnecessary surgery in patients with advanced disease. For these reasons, this chapter is dedicated to the staging and spread of some common malignant tumors of the abdomen and pelvis.

■ MECHANISMS OF TUMOR SPREAD

The mechanisms and pathways by which malignant tumors of the abdomen and pelvis spread are determined by regional anatomy and tumor pathophysiology. Abdominal and pelvic organs are suspended in the peritoneal cavity by ligaments and mesenteries formed by the peritoneum as it reflects from the extraperitoneal surface. The abdominal ligaments and mesenteries serve as conduits through which blood vessels, nerves, and lymphatics may travel. They also may serve to facilitate tumor spread between organs or restrict tumor spread between compartments. A variety of descriptions are in common usage regarding the mechanisms of tumor spread. Tumors can spread in several ways: (1) directly from organ to organ without regard for fascial planes or anatomic compartments; (2) via the subserous connective tissue, blood vessels, or lymphatics of the abdominal mesenteries and ligaments; or (3) throughout the peritoneal cavity. Chapter 6 provides additional information regarding the spread of disease within the abdomen and pelvis.

Direct Contiguous Spread

Direct invasion by tumor can occur from the organ of origin to a contiguous organ across fascial planes. This typically occurs with locally aggressive tumors of the kidneys and pelvic organs (e.g., uterus, ovaries, prostate). Examples of this type of spread include invasion of the sigmoid colon by ovarian cancer, bladder inva-

sion by rectal cancer, and rectal invasion by prostate cancer (Figs. 10-1 and 10-2). Similarly, renal cell carcinoma may violate normal anatomic boundaries to directly invade the small bowel or colon. Direct invasion of an organ should be suspected on computed tomography (CT) or magnetic resonance imaging (MRI) when there is loss of a normal fat plane between the tumor and the secondarily involved organ.

Subperitoneal Spread

The intraperitoneal organs are suspended within the peritoneal cavity and are interconnected via a scaffolding of supporting ligaments and mesenteries. Beneath the peritoneal lining lies the subperitoneal space. This space contains connective tissue, lymphatics, and blood vessels, all of which can serve as conduits for tumor spread.

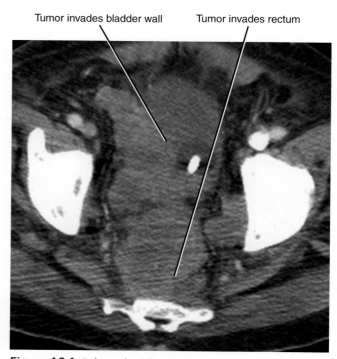

Tumor invades bladder wall   Tumor invades rectum

Figure 10-1 Enhanced axial computed tomographic scan in a patient with prostate cancer invading the bladder and rectum.

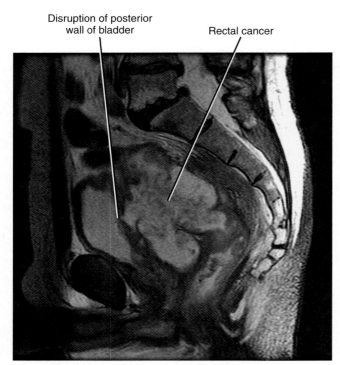

Disruption of posterior wall of bladder

Rectal cancer

Figure 10-2 Sagittal T2-weighted magnetic resonance image of the pelvis in a patient with rectal cancer that directly invades the bladder.

Subperitoneal Tumor Extension

The subperitoneal space provides a bidirectional pathway via which many tumors spread from organ to organ. This network also creates a natural communication interconnecting the extraperitoneum and the suspended intraperitoneal organs. In this manner, for example, malignant tumor may extend through the subserous connective tissues to the transverse colon via the transverse mesocolon from the pancreas or the gastrocolic ligament from

the stomach. It is important to remember that spread of tumor may occur in any direction between organs within the subperitoneal space (e.g., colon to stomach or from stomach to colon) (Figs. 10-3 to 10-5).

Pearl: The subperitoneal space of the mesenteries and ligaments of the abdomen and pelvis serves as a conduit for the bidirectional spread of tumors between organs.

Lymphatic Spread

LYMPH-NODE ANATOMY AND PATTERNS OF LYMPHATIC SPREAD OF TUMOR

Dissemination of cancer cells via the lymphatic channels to regional and distant lymph nodes constitutes a relatively common form of subperitoneal tumor spread. Knowledge of common lymph-node locations and the lymphatic drainage patterns within the abdomen and pelvis helps guide the search for lymph-node metastases in the setting of abdominal or pelvic cancer (Fig. 10-6).

In general, the lymph nodes are distributed along the blood vessels for which they are named. For example, the celiac lymph nodes are near the celiac artery, whereas the external iliac lymph nodes are distributed along the external iliac arteries (Fig. 10-7). Extraperitoneal lymph nodes along the aorta and inferior vena cava (IVC) are named in terms of their location relative to those structures (e.g., retrocaval, paraaortic, preaortic). The preaortic nodes drain the abdominal portion of the gastrointestinal tract and its derivates (e.g., liver, spleen, pancreas) supplied by the three ventral branches of the aorta: the celiac nodes drain the foregut, the superior mesenteric nodes drain the midgut (e.g., small bowel), and the inferior mesenteric nodes drain the hindgut (e.g., sigmoid colon). The paraaortic nodes drain the viscera and structures supplied by the lateral and dorsal branches of the aorta (e.g., kidneys and adrenal glands, gonads, uterus, prostate, bladder, abdominal wall, and lower extremities). A few lymph-node groups are named based on their relation to an anatomic region rather than a vessel

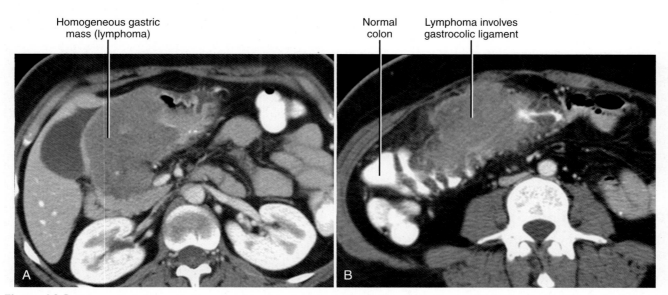

Homogeneous gastric mass (lymphoma)

Normal colon

Lymphoma involves gastrocolic ligament

Figure 10-3 Enhanced axial computed tomographic scan of a patient with malignant lymphoma of the stomach extending to the transverse colon via the gastrocolic ligament **(A, B)**.

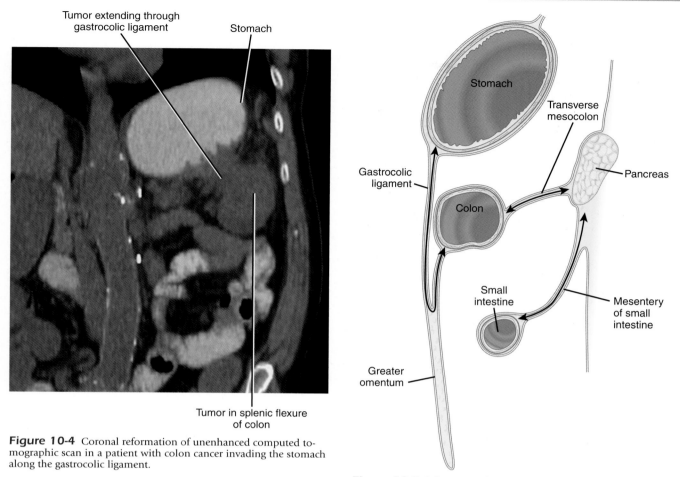

Tumor extending through gastrocolic ligament

Stomach

Tumor in splenic flexure of colon

Figure 10-4 Coronal reformation of unenhanced computed tomographic scan in a patient with colon cancer invading the stomach along the gastrocolic ligament.

Stomach

Transverse mesocolon

Gastrocolic ligament

Pancreas

Colon

Small intestine

Mesentery of small intestine

Greater omentum

Figure 10-5 Subperitoneal spread of tumor between the pancreas, stomach, and bowel.

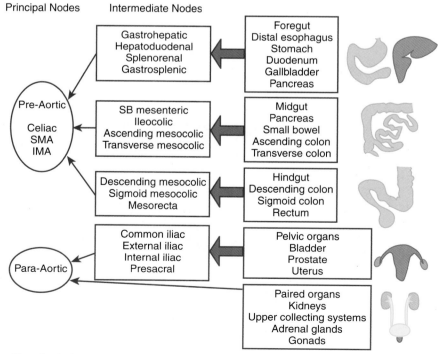

Principal Nodes   Intermediate Nodes

Gastrohepatic
Hepatoduodenal
Splenorenal
Gastrosplenic

Foregut
Distal esophagus
Stomach
Duodenum
Gallbladder
Pancreas

Pre-Aortic

Celiac
SMA
IMA

SB mesenteric
Ileocolic
Ascending mesocolic
Transverse mesocolic

Midgut
Pancreas
Small bowel
Ascending colon
Transverse colon

Descending mesocolic
Sigmoid mesocolic
Mesorecta

Hindgut
Descending colon
Sigmoid colon
Rectum

Common iliac
External iliac
Internal iliac
Presacral

Pelvic organs
Bladder
Prostate
Uterus

Para-Aortic

Paired organs
Kidneys
Upper collecting systems
Adrenal glands
Gonads

Figure 10-6 Pathways of lymphatic drainage.

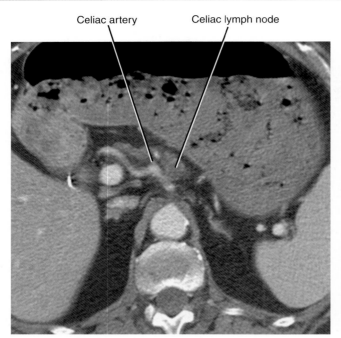

Figure 10-7 Enhanced axial computed tomographic scan shows enlarged celiac lymph node.

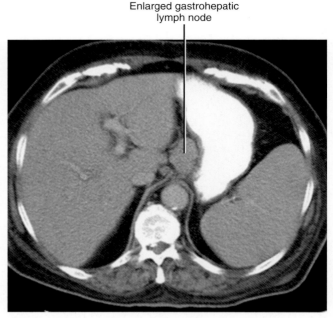

Figure 10-9 Axial enhanced computed tomographic scan shows enlarged gastrohepatic lymph node.

(e.g., retrocrural, gastrohepatic, mesorectal, presacral, inguinal) (Figs. 10-8 and 10-9). Two lymph nodes are frequently referred to by their eponyms. Virchow's node classically refers to a palpable supraclavicular lymph node (typically left) involved with metastatic disease. When an enlarged supraclavicular lymph node is present in the absence of significant chest disease, a search should be conducted for infradiaphragmatic tumor (Fig. 10-10). The node of Cloquet refers to the deepest inguinal lymph node in the femoral canal that is the first lymph node underneath the inguinal ligament (Fig. 10-11). This lymph node serves as a useful anatomic landmark. Lymph nodes central to this level are considered external iliac, whereas lymph nodes below or peripheral to this level are considered inguinal.

Lymphatic spread of tumor of the gastrointestinal tract is from primary nodes near the organ of origin to intermediate nodes within the ligaments and mesenteries, and eventually to the principle (preaortic) nodes.

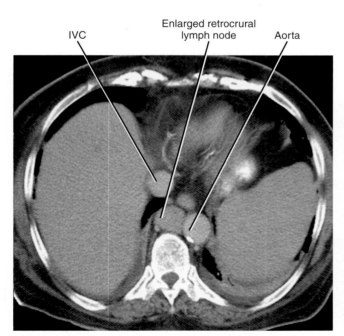

Figure 10-8 Enhanced axial computed tomographic scan shows enlarged retrocrural lymph node. *IVC,* Inferior vena cava.

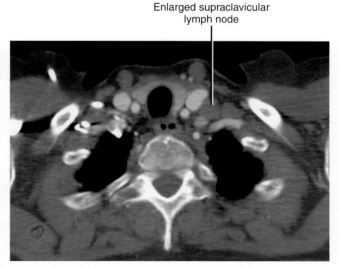

Figure 10-10 Enhanced axial computed tomographic scan in a patient with ovarian cancer with ascending lymphatic spread to a supraclavicular lymph node.

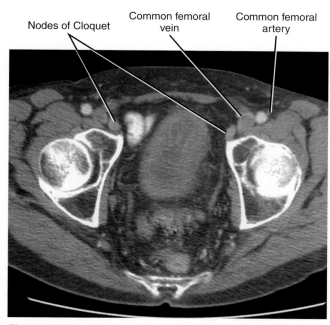

Figure 10-11 Deep inguinal lymph nodes (nodes of Cloquet).

Tumors of the kidneys, adrenal glands, gonads, uterus, prostate, bladder, abdominal wall, and lower extremities commonly spread to the paraaortic lymph nodes. Tumors arising from the pelvic organs spread to the iliac lymph nodes before reaching the paraaortic nodes, whereas testicular and ovarian neoplasms spread via their draining lymphatics traveling with the gonadal vessels to the paraaortic nodes at the level of the kidneys (Fig. 10-12). As discussed later, ovarian lymphatics also drain to the iliac chains. The lymphatic drainage of the preaortic and paraaortic lymph nodes flows to the

cisterna chyli (which is located anterior to the second lumbar vertebra and to the right of the aorta) and then cephalad within the thoracic duct to the supraclavicular region. Further information about the lymphatic spread of tumors is provided in this chapter in the sections that deal with individual tumor types.

> **Pearl:** *Malignant tumors of the gastrointestinal tract typically metastasize to mesenteric and preaortic lymph nodes, whereas tumors of the paired organs (such as the kidneys) and pelvic organs (other than the sigmoid colon and rectum) spread primarily to the paraaortic nodes.*

BENIGN VERSUS MALIGNANT LYMPH NODES

The presence or absence of lymph node metastases is one of the most important prognostic indicators for many malignant tumors. In the case of many tumors, such as colon, rectum, gallbladder, prostate, bladder, ovarian, and endometrial cancers, the stage of nodal disease parallels the stage of the primary tumor. Unfortunately, a wide range of sensitivities and specificities have been reported for CT and MRI for detecting the presence of lymph-node metastases. Suboptimal performance of cross-sectional imaging for lymph-node staging is due to both the occurrence of micrometastases that do not alter lymph-node size or morphology and the large number of benign processes that may result in lymph-node enlargement in the absence of metastatic disease. This picture is further complicated by a lack of consensus regarding what constitutes lymph-node enlargement and controversy regarding which nodal dimension should be measured (i.e., short axis, long axis, or both). Table 10-1 gives some short-axis measurements that have been suggested to distinguish normal from abnormal lymph nodes. Table 10-2 provides an easy-to-remember rough guide to lymph-node size that can be used on screening CT or MRI scans. Note that the actual measurements used

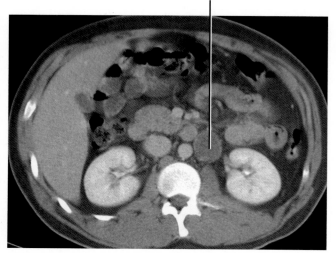

Figure 10-12 Enhanced axial computed tomographic scan in a patient with testicular cancer and metastatic disease involving a left paraaortic lymph node.

Table 10-1 Abnormal Short-Axis Lymph-Node Measurements

Site	Nodal Size (mm)
Retrocrural	6
Paracardiac	12
Gastrohepatic	8
Porta hepatis	7
Portacaval	10
Upper paraortic	9
Lower paraortic	11
Mesenteric	5
Pelvic	10
Inguinal	15

From Koh DM, Hughes M, Husband JE: Cross-sectional imaging of nodal metastases in the abdomen and pelvis, *Abdom Imaging* 31:632-643, 2006, by permission.

Table 10-2 Easy-to-Remember Approximation for Normal Lymph-Node Short Axis

<5 mm	<10 mm	<15 mm
Retrocrural	All others	Inguinal
Mesorectal		Portocaval

in individual practices may vary by several millimeters, and lymph-node size criteria are inversely correlated with sensitivity—that is, the larger the cutoff used to define an abnormal lymph node, the lower the sensitivity for detection of lymph-node metastases (although specificity increases). Clinical circumstances also play an important role in the assessment of lymph nodes. In recent years, there has been a trend toward viewing 8-mm (short-axis) lymph nodes in the internal iliac and obturator groups as metastatic in the setting of malignant pelvic neoplasm.

Table 10-3 presents some additional features that may help determine the likelihood that a lymph node is either benign or malignant. No individual feature is 100% specific for lymph-node metastasis, and for every feature of a malignant node there exists a benign mimic.

Pearl: Round, irregularly shaped, or necrotic lymph nodes are concerning for metastatic disease in the setting of known malignant tumor.

Degree of enhancement, outside its ability to identify necrosis, is not a helpful discriminator between benign and malignant nodes, although quantitative assessment of enhancement kinetics may prove useful in the future. Contrast enhancement can be helpful in distinguishing lymph nodes from vascular structures. CT density and MR signal intensity have likewise failed to reliably distinguish benign from malignant lymph nodes. Calcified lymph nodes may be seen with metastatic disease from ovarian, colon, and bladder primaries, as well as after treatment for lymphoma and seminoma. Of course, benign granulomatous disease also can produce calcified lymph nodes.

Positron emission tomographic (PET) imaging, particularly PET/CT may offer some improvement in specificity over CT and MRI alone, although sensitivity for

Table 10-3 Features of Benign and Malignant Lymph Nodes

Characteristics	Benign	Malignant
Shape	Oval	Round (Fig. 10-13)
Borders	Smooth	Irregular
Number	Few, scattered	Numerous, clustered
Fatty hilum	Present	Absent
Consistency	Homogeneous/solid	Heterogeneous/necrotic (Fig. 10-14)
Confluence	Clearly separate	Confluent/matted
Temporal stability	Stable or shrink	Grow

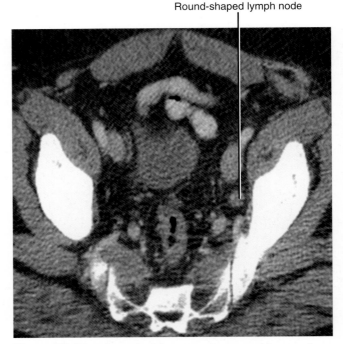

Round-shaped lymph node

Figure 10-13 Enhanced axial computed tomographic scan of a patient with prostate cancer and metastasis involving left obturator lymph node.

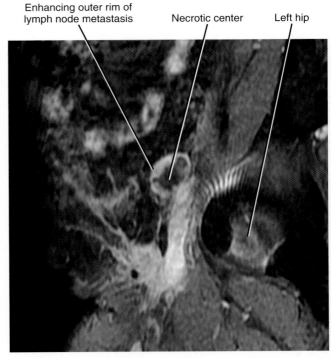

Enhancing outer rim of lymph node metastasis   Necrotic center   Left hip

Figure 10-14 Sagittal gadolinium-enhanced magnetic resonance imaging of lymph-node metastasis in a patient with vulvar cancer.

microscopic lymph-node metastases is still lacking. Fluoro-2-deoxy-D-glucose (FDG) PET imaging detects malignant lymph nodes by demonstrating increased glucose metabolism (Fig. 10-15). Therefore, PET criteria are not based on nodal morphology or size. However,

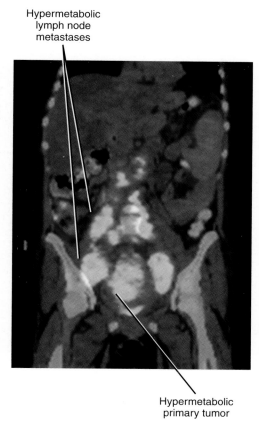

Hypermetabolic
lymph node
metastases

Hypermetabolic
primary tumor

Figure 10-15 Coronal fusion image from positron emission tomography/computed tomography in a patient with cervical cancer and bilateral hypermetabolic pelvic and paraaortic lymph-node metastases.

not all types of tumor are FDG avid. Some evidence suggests that increased FDG uptake in certain primary tumors such as gastric cancer and colorectal cancer may indicate an increased risk for lymph-node metastases, although PET may have difficulty in distinguishing between perigastric lymph nodes and a primary gastric tumor because of its poor spatial resolution.

In the near future, ultrasmall paramagnetic iron oxide particles may prove useful in distinguishing normal from metastatic lymph nodes with MRI. The appeal of these agents is based on preliminary results demonstrating their ability to show small metastatic foci in normal-size lymph nodes. However, much work remains to establish the sensitivity and specificity of such agents in large prospective trials.

One final word of caution regarding lymph-node metastases is worthy of mention. Occasionally, lymph-node metastases appear on imaging studies in the absence of a visible primary tumor. In such cases, the metastatic disease may be mistaken for a primary tumor of different origin. For example, colon cancer metastases to the lymph nodes at the root of the transverse mesocolon or left paraduodenal space may simulate a pancreatic neoplasm. By remembering the lymphatic drainage patterns discussed here, one may be able to trace the involved lymph nodes back to the true primary site of origin.

Pitfall: *Metastatic disease to the lymph nodes may sometimes mimic a primary neoplasm.*

Hematogenous Spread

Hematogenous spread of neoplasms may occur via the arteries or veins. Embolic spread occurs when malignant cells separate from the primary tumor and migrate to distant, noncontiguous sites via the blood vessels. Within the abdomen, the liver and adrenal glands are a particularly susceptible destination for hematogenous embolic metastases (Fig. 10-16; Boxes 10-1 and 10-2). Additional organs prone to hematogenous metastatic disease include the lungs and bones (Figs. 10-17 and 10-18). Visualized portions of these organs should be carefully scrutinized in every patient with known malignant tumor. Hematogenous spread to the gastrointestinal tract is uncommon but does occur. Malignant melanoma and carcinoma of the breast or lung are the most common sources of bowel metastases, with the most frequent sites of involvement being the stomach and small intestine (Fig. 10-19). Metastases to the spleen, kidneys, and pancreas are relatively uncommon but will eventually be encountered in a typical practice. Some tumors, such as malignant melanoma, have a reputation for metastasizing virtually anywhere via the hematogenous pathway. Unfortunately, a thorough scouring of the literature will ultimately reveal that virtually every malignant tumor has metastasized to virtually every organ at some time or another.

Gross contiguous extension of tumor via the lumen of a blood vessel may also occur (tumor thrombus).

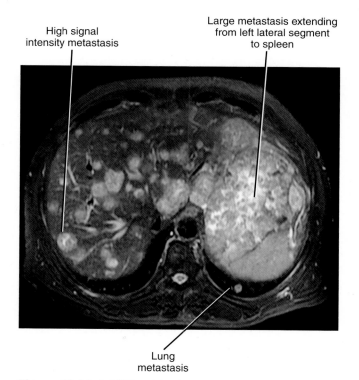

High signal
intensity metastasis

Large metastasis extending
from left lateral segment
to spleen

Lung
metastasis

Figure 10-16 Axial T2-weighted magnetic resonance image of a patient with metastatic sarcoma involving the liver and lungs.

BOX 10-1 **Common Sources of Hematogenous Liver Metastases**	
Lung	Breast
Gastrointestinal tract	Melanoma
Pancreas	Gastrointestinal stromal tumor

BOX 10-2 **Common Sources of Hematogenous Adrenal Gland Metastases**	
Lung	Thyroid
Breast	Kidney
Gastrointestinal tract	Melanoma

This latter mechanism of tumor spread is particularly common with, but not exclusive to, hepatocellular carcinoma (HCC) and renal cell carcinoma (Figs. 10-20 and 10-21).

Peritoneal Spread

Often referred to as peritoneal seeding, peritoneal spread of tumor results from neoplastic cells breaking through the peritoneal lining and entering the coelomic cavity (Fig. 10-22). Much of our understanding of

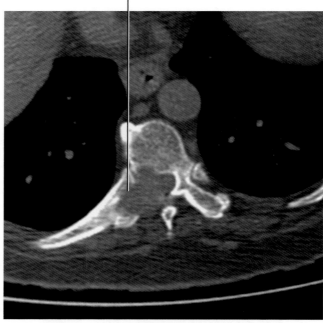

Figure 10-18 Unenhanced axial computed tomographic image through lung bases in a patient with hepatocellular carcinoma metastasis to the spine.

Destructive lesion arising from right pedicle and invading spinal canal

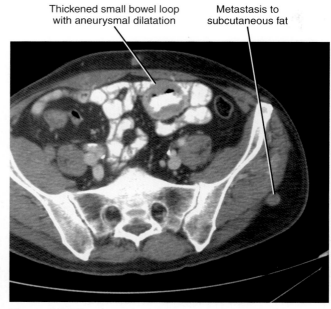

Thickened small bowel loop with aneurysmal dilatation   Metastasis to subcutaneous fat

Figure 10-19 Enhanced axial computed tomographic image through lower abdomen in a patient with metastatic melanoma to the small bowel.

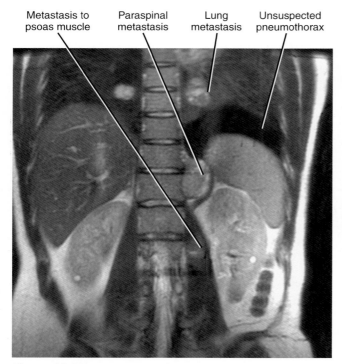

Metastasis to psoas muscle   Paraspinal metastasis   Lung metastasis   Unsuspected pneumothorax

Figure 10-17 Coronal, T2-weighted, single-shot, fast spin-echo, magnetic resonance image of a patient with metastatic sarcoma.

the intraperitoneal spread of malignant tumor can be attributed to the groundbreaking work of Dr. Morton Meyers, who demonstrated that the distribution of these malignant cells within the peritoneal cavity is dependent on the natural flow of ascites. The flow of

Cirrhotic liver | Right portal vein filled with enhancing tumor | Interface between tumor and blood pool

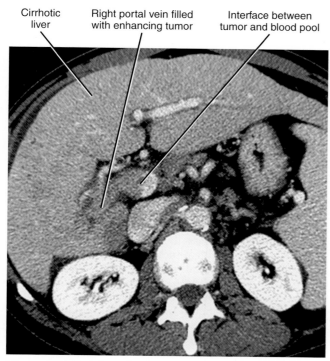

Figure 10-20 Enhanced axial computed tomographic image through liver in a patient with hepatocellular carcinoma invading portal vein.

Right kidney | Gallbladder | Tumor extending into right renal vein and IVC | Patent portion of IVC

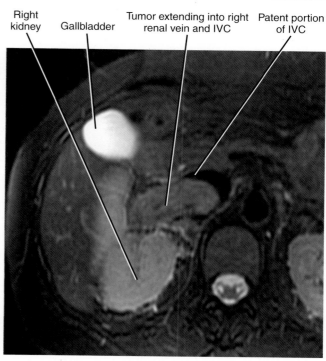

Figure 10-21 Axial T2-weighted magnetic resonance imaging through right kidney in a patient with renal cell carcinoma invading right renal vein and extending into inferior vena cava *(IVC)*.

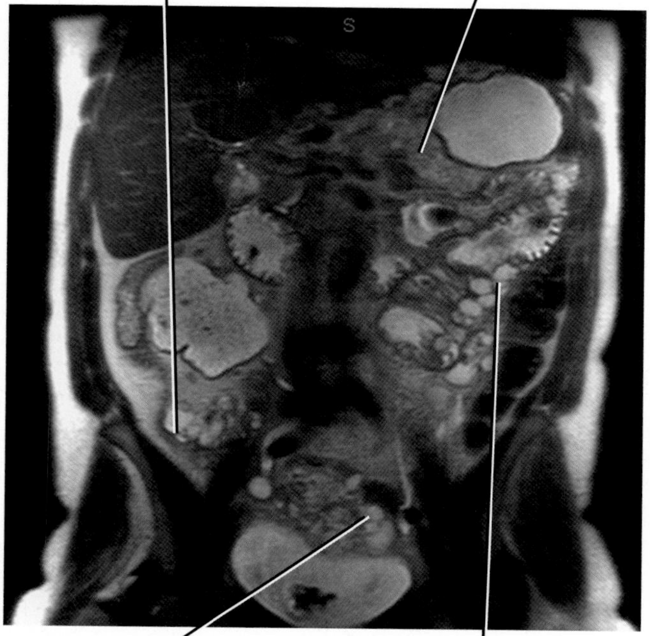

High signal intensity metastases in right lower quadrant | High signal intensity metastases around stomach

High signal intensity metastases over dome of bladder | High signal intensity metastases along left colon

Figure 10-22 Coronal T2-weighted magnetic resonance imaging through abdomen and pelvis of a patient with metastatic mucinous carcinoma of the appendix involving the peritoneum.

ascites is dependent on gravity, changes in intraabdominal pressure, and peritoneal reflections. Peritoneal reflections impose limitations on the distribution of ascitic fluid and create recesses in which static fluid accumulates. The posterior parietal attachments are particularly important anatomic barriers to the intraperitoneal spread of tumor. The pathways of fluid flowing in the peritoneal cavity are from the right supramesocolic compartment and right and left inframesocolic compartments to the pelvis. Flow from the pelvis is to the right and left paracolic gutters. Common sites of peritoneal seeding are the rectovesical or rectouterine pouch (Fig. 10-23), the right lower quadrant along the small-bowel mesentery and its insertion near the cecum, along the sigmoid mesocolon, in the posterior subhepatic recess (Morison's pouch), and along the right paracolic gutter. Peritoneal metastases are also relatively common in the perihepatic and subphrenic spaces (right greater than left because the phrenicocolic ligament impedes the cephalad flow of fluid on the left), and on the greater omental surface (Fig. 10-24). It is believed that the presence of lymphatics that absorb peritoneal fluid predisposes this latter structure to peritoneal metastatic implants.

Pearl: Malignant cells circulate within the abdomen and pelvis according to natural pressure differentials and the limitations imposed by the posterior ligamentous attachments. These cells tend to accumulate at predictable sites of fluid stasis.

Uterus   Fluid in cul-de-sac   Peritoneal metastasis

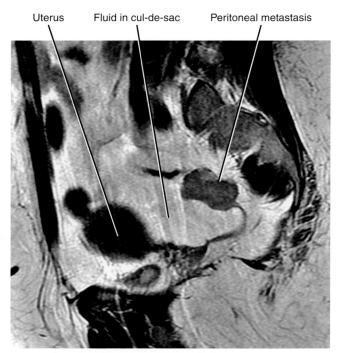

Figure 10-23 Sagittal T2-weighted magnetic resonance imaging through pelvis of a patient with endometrial cancer metastatic to the peritoneum.

Omental caking due to ovarian cancer metastases

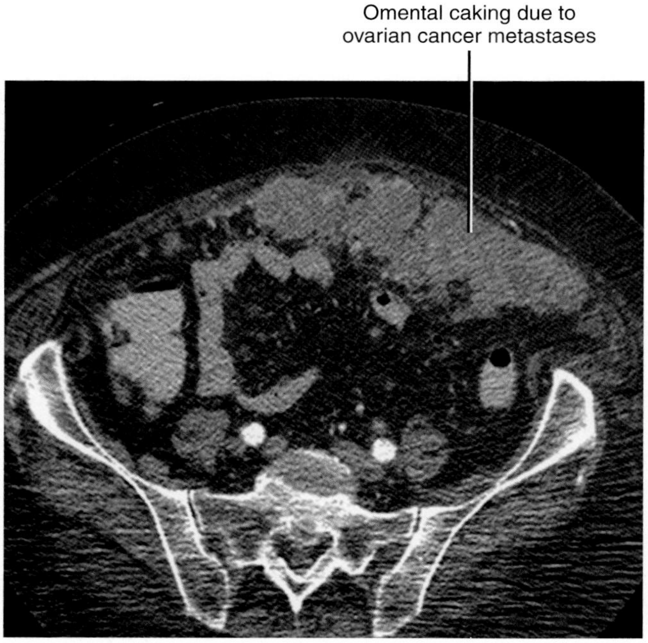

Figure 10-24 Enhanced axial computed tomographic imaging through pelvis of a patient with ovarian cancer metastatic to the greater omentum.

Box 10-3 lists some of the more common primary sites of origin of peritoneal metastases, although metastatic peritoneal implants may be seen with a variety of other tumors with lesser frequency.

BOX 10-3   Common Primary Sources of Peritoneal Metastases

Ovaries*	Colon
Appendix*	Pancreas
Stomach	Biliary tumors

*Most patients with new peritoneal metastases without previously known primary malignant neoplasm will have ovarian or appendiceal carcinoma.

Peritoneal metastases may appear on PET as diffuse uptake throughout the abdomen and pelvis, obscuring visceral outlines, or discrete, randomly distributed foci of uptake unrelated to solid organs or nodal stations (Fig. 10-25). Ascites that occurs in the setting of one of the tumors listed in Box 10-3 is concerning for (but not diagnostic of) peritoneal metastases. Visceral peritoneal metastases are suggested on CT or MRI by scalloping of organ contours (Fig. 10-26) or bowel wall thickening or distortion. The presence of enhancing areas of thickened parietal peritoneum or nodules and plaques along the parietal peritoneal surfaces also suggests intraperitoneal spread of tumor.

Other Types of Abdominal Tumor Spread

A few final conduits of tumor spread are worthy of mention. Biliary tumors (and rarely nonbiliary tumors) may extend via the bile ducts (intraductal growth pattern). Transitional cell carcinoma may

Small focus of increased metabolic activity due to perihepatic peritoneal metastasis   Liver   Second peritoneal implant

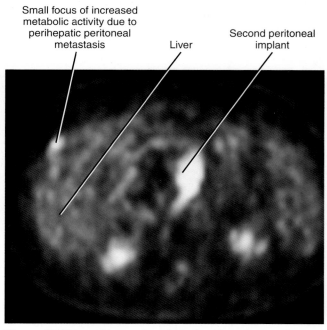

Figure 10-25 Axial image through the liver from fluoro-2-deoxy-D-glucose positron emission tomography scan of a patient with adenocarcinoma of the colon metastatic to the peritoneum.

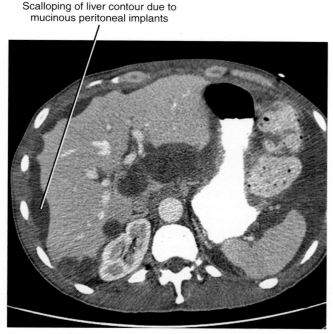

Scalloping of liver contour due to mucinous peritoneal implants

Figure 10-26 Enhanced axial computed tomographic scan through liver of a patient with mucinous adenocarcinoma of the colon metastatic to the peritoneum.

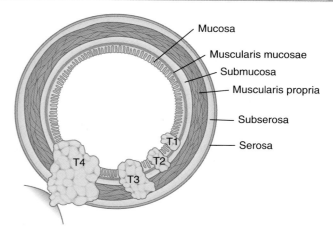

Mucosa
Muscularis mucosae
Submucosa
Muscularis propria
Subserosa
Serosa
T1
T2
T3
T4

Figure 10-27 T stage for cancer of the colon and rectum (American Joint Committee on Cancer TNM staging system).

spread via the urinary collecting system, accounting for some synchronous primary urothelial tumors. Perineural spread is a relatively common type of subperitoneal extension that is often present on pathologic specimens but rarely appreciated on imaging studies. Malignant tumor has even been known to spread between the central nervous system and the peritoneal cavity via shunt tubing.

■ INTRODUCTION TO TUMOR STAGING

Various tumor staging systems are in use throughout the world. Accurate staging is critical to determining potential treatment options and patient prognosis, and aids in standardizing clinical research trials. In the United States, the TNM staging system of the American Joint Committee on Cancer (AJCC) is in common use among pathologists, surgeons, and oncologists. The T, N, and M included in this staging system refer to <u>t</u>umor, lymph <u>n</u>ode and <u>m</u>etastasis. Figure 10-27 provides an example of T stage for cancer of the colon and rectum. This system does not take into account the degree of cellular differentiation or biological behavior of the tumor but instead relies primarily on easily determined features such as tumor size and depth of invasion. Because complete and accurate assessment of TNM stage is not possible with any imaging modality, it is most important for radiologists to be familiar with those aspects of staging with which they may be of assistance

(e.g., detection of advanced stage disease that would preclude surgical resection). Therefore, we do not include a detailed description of TNM classification for every tumor. Rather, we include the aspects of staging relevant to diagnostic imaging for those tumors most likely to be encountered on a routine basis. In most cases, we do not discuss early-stage disease (e.g., T1 and T2) that can be difficult to differentiate with cross-sectional imaging. Instead, we focus on the imaging findings of more advanced disease that can significantly alter management. For more detailed staging information, we recommend one consult the latest edition of the *AJCC Cancer Staging Manual*. The following section attempts to provide the most up-to-date information regarding staging of tumors of the abdomen and pelvis. Be aware, however, that cancer staging remains in evolution to keep pace with advances in diagnosis and treatment.

■ GUIDE TO SPECIFIC TUMORS

Hepatocellular Carcinoma

Tumor Markers

α-Fetoprotein (AFP) level is increased in 50% to 90% of patients with symptomatic HCC, but increased levels (20-400 ng/ml) may also be present in patients with hepatitis, partial hepatectomy, cirrhosis, pregnancy, and inflammatory bowel disease. A serum level exceeding 400 ng/ml (>95% positive predictive value) or a rapidly increasing level of AFP are highly suggestive of HCC. Normal levels are not unusual in patients with small tumors. For unknown reasons, AFP level is more likely to be increased in HCC patients of Asian countries compared with patients in the United States and Europe.

An assay for des-γ-carboxy prothrombin (DCP) protein induced by vitamin K abnormality (PIVKA-2) is also available for HCC. PIVKA-2 is increased in the majority of patients with HCC, although vitamin K deficiency may also cause increased levels.

Imaging Modalities

Ultrasound (US) plays a role in screening patients at risk for HCC in many practices, but once a mass is discovered, patients often proceed to contrast-enhanced CT or MRI for further evaluation. Enhanced imaging with CT and MRI should include precontrast, arterial phase, and portal venous phase images. The role of MRI in the detection and staging of HCC is likely to increase with new innovations, such as diffusion-weighted imaging, and the release of new contrast agents or novel use of existing contrast agents. CT arterial portography and delayed CT after intraarterial lipiodol injection are rarely performed in the United States for tumor detection or characterization. Many HCCs are gallium-67 avid, but nuclear scintigraphy is rarely performed for suspected HCC. FDG-PET does not currently play a significant role in the staging or management of HCC because only approximately 60% of HCCs demonstrate increased uptake of FDG.

Staging Highlights

A variety of systems are in use worldwide for the staging of HCC. This variety of staging systems reflects the difficulties encountered in attempting to provide a clinically useful staging system that accounts not only for the biological behavior of the tumor but also for the severity of the underlying liver disease. Newer methods of treatment such as chemical and thermal ablative techniques also have impacted patient prognosis and may further alter staging of this disease in the future. Because many nonsurgical treatment options are now available for HCC, imaging-based staging systems may eventually become standard.

Radiologists rarely refer to the TNM staging of HCC when interpreting cross-sectional imaging studies. The major limitations of the TNM staging system alone for HCC are that it does not take into account the degree of liver dysfunction that may be present and has limited application to unresectable patients and nonsurgical interventions. However, the TNM system has been studied and analyzed extensively, and has been through multiple revisions. Other staging systems in use around the world include the Barcelona Clinic Liver Cancer (BCLC), Cancer of the Liver Italian Program (CLIP), Chinese University Prognostic Index (CUPI), Okuda, and Japanese Integrated System (JIS).

Common Mechanisms and Sites of Spread

CONTIGUOUS SPREAD

HCC may directly extend to involve the diaphragm and gallbladder. Extension into bile ducts is uncommon but may occur, potentially resulting in confusion with cholangiocarcinoma.

LIGAMENTS AND MESENTERIES

Spread of HCC via the perihepatic ligaments is rare.

LYMPHATIC SPREAD

Lymphatic spread may occur via the deep pathway to the hepatoduodenal ligament lymph nodes or terminal nodes of the IVC (juxtaphrenic). Spread may also occur via the superficial pathway to the anterior diaphragmatic nodes, inferior phrenic nodes, gastrohepatic ligament (left gastric) nodes, and falciform ligament (deep superior epigastric) nodes. The anterior periportal nodes within the hepatoduodenal ligament eventually drain to the celiac nodes, whereas the posterior periportal nodes drain to the retropancreatic nodes and the aortocaval nodes. Enlarged regional lymph nodes are common in patients with chronic liver disease. Therefore, size is an unreliable indicator of nodal metastases from HCC.

HEMATOGENOUS SPREAD

Liver, lung, lymph nodes, adrenal glands, ovaries, and bones (osteolytic, see Fig. 10-18) are potential metastatic sites. Venous extension is common into the portal vein (see Figs. 10-20 and Fig. 10-28). Hepatic vein extension is less common and can extend above the diaphragm.

PERITONEAL SPREAD

Peritoneal spread of HCC is uncommon but may occur.

Key Structures to Assess

The portal and hepatic veins should be assessed for evidence of tumor invasion. HCC is frequently multifocal; therefore, it is important to look for additional tumors. When tumor resection is contemplated, it may be helpful to determine the volume of liver to remain as a percentage of the total liver volume. A

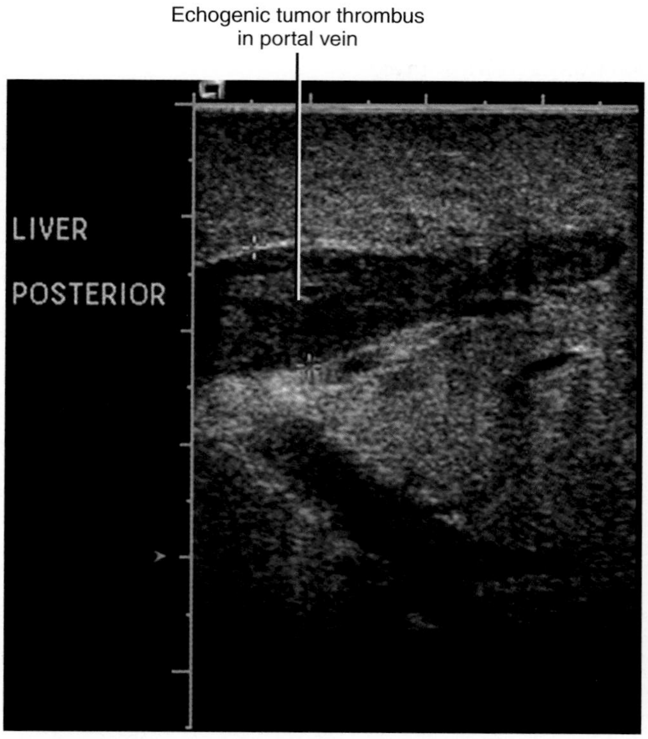

Echogenic tumor thrombus in portal vein

Figure 10-28 Intraoperative ultrasound of liver of a patient with hepatocellular carcinoma extending into portal vein.

residual volume of less than 25% to 30% may be insufficient to sustain the patient after resection. Invasion of the diaphragm, peritoneal metastases, or unfavorable vascular or biliary anatomy may preclude resection and should be reported when present. It is helpful to alert the surgeon to imaging findings of cirrhosis because the degree of liver failure present has a significant impact on whether a patient will tolerate surgery for HCC. Currently, the severity of liver failure is assessed according to the Child–Pugh classification, which is based on clinical and laboratory assessment.

Gallbladder Cancer

Tumor Markers
CA 19-9 is reasonably sensitive and specific for gallbladder cancer (approximately 79%). Carcinoembryonic antigen (CEA) (>4 ng/ml) is more specific but less sensitive.

Imaging Modalities
Gallbladder cancer may be incidentally discovered during right upper quadrant sonography. US can identify local disease, but further imaging evaluation is typically accomplished with CT or MRI. Nuclear scintigraphy and PET do not currently play a significant role.

Staging Highlights
The TNM system is in common use. Imaging is useful in detecting extension of tumor beyond the gallbladder. T3 disease perforates the serosa and/or directly invades an adjacent organ or structure (e.g., liver, stomach, colon, duodenum, pancreas, omentum, extrahepatic bile ducts). T4 disease involves the main portal vein or hepatic artery, or multiple extrahepatic organs and/or structures. Pericholecystic inflammation may lead to overstaging. Small vessels along the serosal surface of the gallbladder may mimic T3 disease.

Common Mechanisms and Sites of Spread
CONTIGUOUS SPREAD
Direct invasion is a common mode of spread to adjacent liver segments, most commonly segments IV and V (Fig. 10-29). Gallbladder cancer also can spread directly to the duodenum, stomach, transverse colon, and pancreas.

LIGAMENTS AND MESENTERIES
Gallbladder cancer occasionally spreads along the hepatoduodenal ligament, gastrohepatic ligament, or transverse mesocolon.

LYMPHATIC SPREAD
Lymph-node metastases are common and parallel the lymphatic drainage of the gallbladder. The lymphatic spread of gallbladder cancer is easy to remember, because it primarily involves the deep drainage pathway of the liver along the hepatoduodenal ligament. Therefore, metastases often are found in the hepatoduodenal

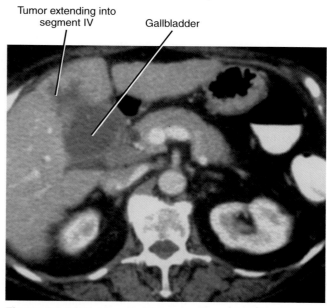

Figure 10-29 Enhanced axial computed tomographic scan of a patient with gallbladder carcinoma extending into segment IV of the left hemiliver.

ligament and portocaval nodes, and eventually in the celiac nodes and in the pancreaticoduodenal or aortocaval lymph nodes. As with many tumors, the rate of lymph-node metastases correlates with depth of invasion.

HEMATOGENOUS SPREAD
The most common sites of disease involvement are the liver (66%) and lungs (24%), although spread to other sites such as the bones (12%) can be seen. Hematogenous metastases are uncommon in the absence of advanced local disease. Venous blood drains from the gallbladder into segment IV of the liver. Therefore, metastatic spread to the liver preferentially involves segment IV.

PERITONEAL SPREAD
Peritoneal spread is not uncommon in gallbladder cancer.

Structures to Assess
The liver (particularly segments IV and V), stomach, colon, duodenum, pancreas, omentum, extrahepatic bile ducts, portal vein, hepatic artery, and peritoneum should be scrutinized for evidence of involvement with gallbladder cancer. The key lymph nodes to assess can be found in the hepatoduodenal ligament. Surgical resection is not a good option for patients with multiple liver metastases, peritoneal metastases, other distant metastases, extensive hepatoduodenal ligament involvement, or encasement or occlusion of major vessels such as the main portal vein or proper hepatic artery. Direct invasion of the colon, duodenum, or liver does not necessarily exclude the possibility of surgery.

Perihilar Cholangiocarcinoma

Tumor Markers

Serum CEA level (increased in 40%-60% of patients) and CA 19-9 (increased in >80% of patients in some reports) are often increased in patients with cholangiocarcinoma but are nonspecific, because they may be increased in a variety of nonmalignant hepatic and biliary diseases, as well as other tumors of the gastrointestinal tract. Serum levels of AFP are typically normal.

Imaging Modalities

US, CT, and MRI all play a role in the evaluation of cholangiocarcinoma. MRI has the capacity to provide a combined evaluation of the hepatic vasculature, hepatic parenchyma, bile ducts, and remainder of the abdomen (Fig. 10-30). Intraoperative US may facilitate resection. US, MRCP, CT cholangiography, or percutaneous transhepatic cholangiography may be beneficial in assessing extent of duct involvement. Endoscopic retrograde cholangiopancreatography (ERCP) is commonly used for diagnosis and biliary decompression, but we recommend that cross-sectional imaging be performed before stenting because decompression of the bile ducts and stent-induced inflammation may compromise staging. The role of PET has not been established for cholangiocarcinoma.

Staging Highlights

Two thirds of cholangiocarcinomas are perihilar in location. The Bismuth–Corlette classification of hilar tumors remains in common use (Fig. 10-31). Staging is also based on the TNM system. Subepithelial spread beyond gross tumor margins is common and difficult to detect with imaging. Therefore, understaging of cholangiocarcinoma is relatively common with imaging. Because surgical resection offers the best chance of cure, many surgeons will err on the side of resectability when imaging findings are inconclusive.

Common Mechanisms and Sites of Spread

CONTIGUOUS SPREAD

Perihilar tumors may spread by periductal infiltration or intraductal growth. Direct invasion of hepatic parenchyma is also relatively common (Fig. 10-32).

LIGAMENTS AND MESENTERIES

Cholangiocarcinoma often spreads along the hepatoduodenal ligament.

LYMPHATIC SPREAD

Perihilar cholangiocarcinoma spreads to the hepatoduodenal ligament and portocaval nodes, common hepatic nodes, and celiac nodes, as well as to the superior and posterior pancreaticoduodenal and paraaortic lymph nodes. Lymph-node metastases can occur to the region of the gastrohepatic ligament in setting of left-sided intrahepatic tumors. Enlarged nonmalignant lymph nodes are often present after stenting or in patients with sclerosing cholangitis and may mimic nodal metastases.

HEMATOGENOUS SPREAD

With the exception of the liver, hematogenous spread to distant sites is uncommon at time of presentation. The most frequent sites of distant recurrence after resection are the lungs and bones. Cholangiocarcinoma tends to encase the portal vein and may occasionally invade it (Fig. 10-33).

PERITONEAL SPREAD

Peritoneal spread is difficult to detect but may appear as enhancing peritoneal or omental thickening or nodularity on CT and MRI.

Structures to Assess

The proximal extent of ductal involvement by tumor is the most important factor determining resectability. Hepatic parenchymal invasion, involvement of the portal veins and hepatic arteries, and peritoneal metastases are also important features. One should report the presence of hepatic lobar atrophy, which implies vascular or biliary involvement of the affected lobe. Any combination of involvement of the right- and left-sided hepatic parenchyma or right- and left-sided vessels or secondary bile ducts may complicate surgical resection. For example, a patient with a tumor that involves the right portal vein and left secondary biliary confluence would be considered a poor surgical candidate at many institutions. Involvement of main portal vein, invasion of adjacent structures (e.g., diaphragm), distant metastases, peritoneal disease, or unfavorable variant vascular anatomy also may complicate or preclude surgery. Recent years have seen a trend in treatment toward aggressive surgical resection for cholangiocarcinoma because other treatment options are of limited efficacy. Therefore, criteria for unresectability are constantly being revised and vary among institutions.

Pancreatic Cancer (Ductal Adenocarcinoma)

Tumor Markers

CA 19-9 is the most widely used tumor marker for pancreatic cancer, although levels of this marker are often normal in patients with potentially curable tumors and may be increased in patients with other pancreatic or biliary diseases. CEA may be increased as well but is also nonspecific. CA-125 also may be increased in the setting of pancreatic cancer.

Imaging Modalities

In the United States, contrast-enhanced CT is the primary noninvasive imaging modality used for the diagnosis and staging of pancreatic cancer. MRI may be useful when CT is contraindicated or inconclusive. US is insufficiently sensitive for staging pancreatic cancer, and ERCP does not provide information regarding extraductal disease. Endoscopic US may be useful for obtaining tissue or when other imaging studies are unrevealing or equivocal. PET cannot accurately assess extent of primary local disease (e.g., vascular involvement) but may be useful for detecting distant metastases or locally recurrent disease.

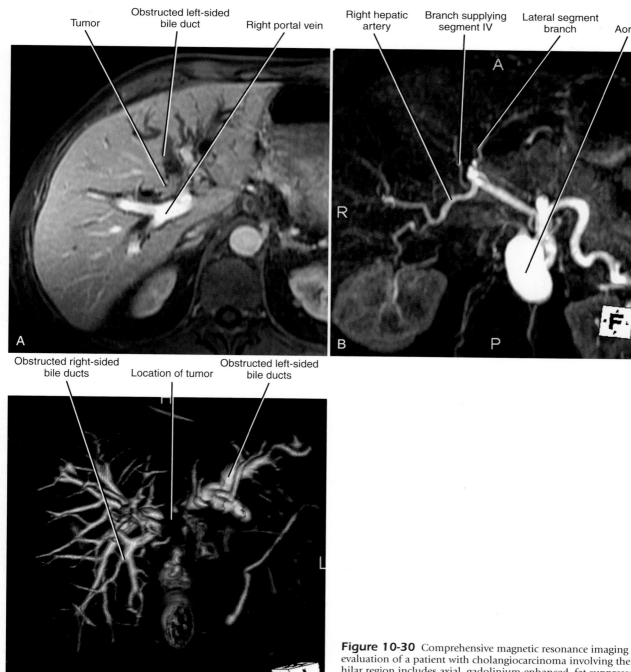

Figure 10-30 Comprehensive magnetic resonance imaging evaluation of a patient with cholangiocarcinoma involving the hilar region includes axial, gadolinium-enhanced, fat-suppressed, T1-weighted image (A); maximum intensity projection reconstruction of arterial phase acquisition (B); and volume-rendered magnetic resonance cholangiopancreatography image (C).

PET may have difficulty distinguishing inflammation (i.e., pancreatitis) from tumor.

Staging Highlights

The TNM staging system is widely used for pancreatic cancer. T3 and T4 tumors extend beyond the pancreas. T3 lesions do not involve the celiac axis or superior mesenteric artery (SMA) but may involve venous structures and may be resectable. T4 tumors involve the celiac axis or SMA and are not usually resected.

Common Mechanisms and Sites of Spread
CONTIGUOUS SPREAD

Duodenal and common bile duct involvement is common but does not preclude resection. Tumors arising in the pancreatic head often spread along the pancreaticoduodenal arteries and grow to involve the celiac axis and SMA. Direct renal or ureteral invasion is uncommon but may occur in advanced cases.

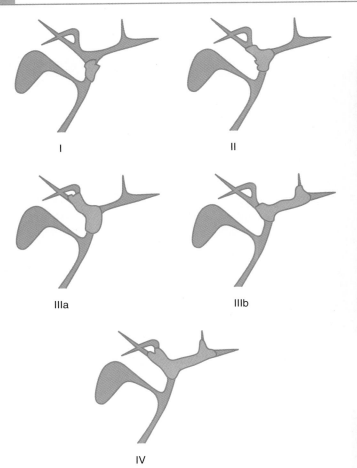

Figure 10-31 Bismuth–Corlette Classification System for Perihilar Cholangiocarcinoma.

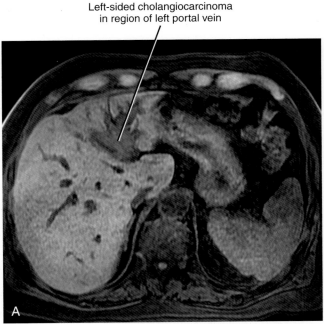

Left-sided cholangiocarcinoma in region of left portal vein

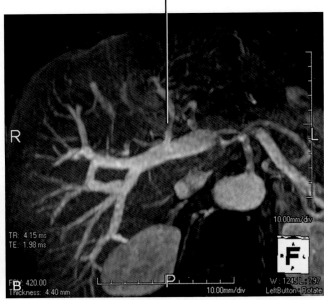

Focal narrowing of left portal vein caused by encasement by tumor shown in (**A**)

Figure 10-33 Cholangiocarcinoma encasing the left portal vein demonstrated on unenhanced, axial, T1-weighted, fat-suppressed, magnetic resonance imaging (**A**) and maximum intensity projection reconstruction of gadolinium-enhanced portal phase images (**B**).

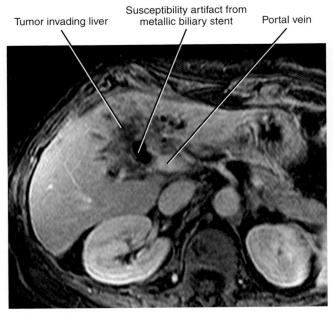

Tumor invading liver   Susceptibility artifact from metallic biliary stent   Portal vein

Figure 10-32 Axial gadolinium-enhanced magnetic resonance image of a patient with advanced perihilar cholangiocarcinoma invading hepatic parenchyma.

LIGAMENTS AND MESENTERIES

Pancreatic cancer may spread in the subperitoneal space via the transverse mesocolon, small-bowel mesentery, hepatoduodenal ligament, and gastrosplenic ligament. Tumors arising in the pancreatic tail tend to extend along the splenorenal ligament.

LYMPHATIC SPREAD

The pattern of lymphatic spread depends on the tumor location (Fig. 10-34). Tumors of the superior pancreatic head will spread anteriorly along the superior pancreaticoduodenal artery to the subpyloric nodes or posteriorly along the bile duct to the hepatoduodenal ligament nodes. Tumors of the inferior pancreatic head and uncinate process will spread along the inferior pancreaticoduodenal vessels to the SMA and eventually the paraaortic nodes. Tumors of the pancreatic tail spread to the pancreaticosplenic nodes and along the splenic artery to the celiac nodes.

HEMATOGENOUS SPREAD

Common sites of distant spread include liver and lungs. Uncommon sites include adrenal glands, bone, skin, and the central nervous system.

PERITONEAL SPREAD

Peritoneal metastases are not unusual but may be difficult to detect with imaging. The presence of ascites should arouse suspicion of peritoneal involvement.

Structures to Assess

The SMA and celiac axis must be closely scrutinized for evidence of encasement, because this will render the patient unresectable at most institutions (Fig. 10-35). Loss of the normal fat planes that surround the celiac axis and SMA origins implies tumor involvement. Tumor that is contiguous with greater than 50% (180 degrees) of an artery's circumference is unlikely to be resectable. Venous invasion does not necessarily render a patient unresectable because such patients can potentially undergo venous resection and reconstruction. Partial encasement of the superior mesenteric vein may result in a teardrop shape of the vein. An intact fat plane or normal pancreatic parenchyma separating tumor from the vein suggests lack of involvement.

Dilatation of the gastrocolic trunk and associated mesenteric venous collaterals may imply downstream portal vein involvement by tumor. Likewise, dilatation of the superior pancreaticoduodenal veins (a somewhat subjective determination) implies involvement of the larger, more central veins. The inferior pancreaticoduodenal veins are typically difficult to see in normal patients, so clear visualization of these veins implies more central venous involvement.

Multiplanar reformations created from thin-section, contrast-enhanced, multislice CT images may be useful for demonstrating vascular involvement by pancreatic cancer. Unfortunately, CT has traditionally been better at predicting unresectability than resectability. Limitations of preoperative imaging include the inability to reliably distinguish between pancreatic inflammation and tumor, and the relatively low sensitivity for small peritoneal metastases. Sensitivity and specificity for lymph-node metastases is likewise disappointing for cross-sectional imaging techniques.

Circumferential encasement or occlusion of the portal or superior mesenteric vein, extension of tumor along the hepatoduodenal ligament, tumor extension beyond the capsule into the retroperitoneum, or tumor encasement or invasion of the celiac artery or SMA may prevent tumor resection. Some surgeons are willing to perform a venous reconstruction in the setting of venous involvement. The finding of enlarged peripancreatic lymph nodes does not necessarily prevent resection, although it may be associated with a poorer prognosis. Duodenal and common bile duct involvement is common but does not alone represent inoperable disease. Distant metastases or peritoneal implants preclude curative resection, although patients may still undergo palliative surgery to bypass duodenal obstruction.

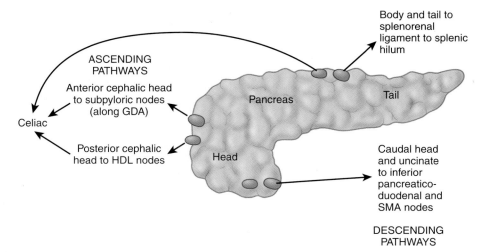

Figure 10-34 The lymphatic drainage pathways of the pancreas. *GDA,* Gastroduodenal artery; *HDL,* hepatoduodenal ligament; *SMA,* superior mesenteric artery.

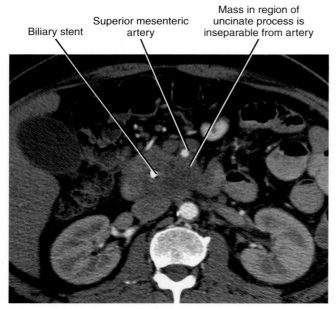

Figure 10-35 Enhanced axial computed tomographic scan of a patient with pancreatic cancer involving the superior mesenteric artery.

Gastric Cancer (Adenocarcinoma)

Tumor Markers

CEA level is increased in roughly a third of patients with primary gastric cancer. If CEA level is increased before surgery and returns to normal after surgery, CEA level can be monitored after surgery to aid in detection of tumor recurrence. The role of other tumor markers such as CA 19-9, AFP, CA-125, and β-HCG has been studied.

Imaging Modalities

Barium examination may be useful for detection of gastric cancer but is not useful for staging. CT is commonly performed before surgery for gastric cancer. More accurate staging of gastric cancer can be facilitated with gastric distension using either water or effervescent granules and an antiperistaltic agent. Multidetector CT with multiplanar reformations and virtual endoscopy improves primary tumor staging over standard axial images. This allows one to view the tumor in the most optimal plane to determine serosal extension or involvement of adjacent organs. MRI may yield results similar to CT for gastric cancer staging in experienced hands. Opposed-phase gradient-echo and dynamic gadolinium-enhanced MR images are helpful for detecting T3 and T4 disease. Endoscopic US is a relatively reliable method for the preoperative determination of T stage (depth of invasion) in gastric cancer and may offer improved (local) nodal staging over CT, but this technique may not be available at every institution (Fig. 10-36). PET may be helpful in detecting extraabdominal lymph-node metastases or clarifying postoperative findings seen on other imaging examinations. Intense uptake of FDG by the primary tumor may mask the presence of immediately adjacent lymph-node metastases. Mucinous carcinomas, signet

ring carcinomas, and poorly differentiated adenocarcinomas show lower FDG uptake than other types of gastric cancer.

Staging Highlights

Multiple staging systems have been used over the years for gastric adenocarcinoma, although the dominant current staging system is the AJCC TNM system. As with many other alimentary tract tumors, T stage is defined in terms of depth of invasion. Endoscopic US may provide the best imaging evaluation of T stage. CT and MRI can potentially detect tumor penetration of the serosa (T3) or invasion of adjacent structures (T4), but these modalities cannot distinguish reliably between T1 (tumor invades lamina propria or submucosa) and T2 (tumor invades muscularis propria or subserosa) disease. Lymph-node staging is now dependent on the number of lymph nodes positive for metastatic disease based on sampling a minimum of 15 regional nodes. The Japanese classification and staging system is also used for staging of gastric cancers. The Japanese system also stages the primary tumor based on depth of invasion, but N staging is more complex and detailed.

Common Mechanisms and Sites of Spread

CONTIGUOUS SPREAD

Gastric cancer commonly spreads directly to the esophagus or duodenum and can spread across fascial planes to the pancreas, liver, diaphragm, or adrenal gland.

LIGAMENTS AND MESENTERIES

Local subperitoneal spread is often via peritoneal reflections along the gastrocolic (to the colon), gastrosplenic (to the spleen), gastrophrenic (to the

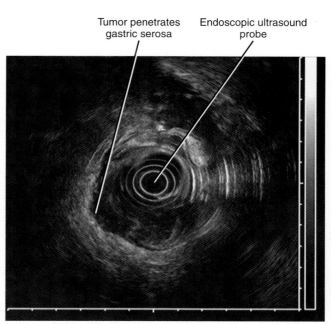

Figure 10-36 Endoscopic ultrasound image of stage T3 gastric adenocarcinoma. (Courtesy Jason Conway, M.D., Wake Forest University.)

diaphragm), or gastrohepatic (to the left hepatic lobe) ligaments (Fig. 10-37).

LYMPHATIC SPREAD

Lymph-node metastases are common with gastric adenocarcinoma. The location of nodal disease depends on the location of the primary tumor. The gastric lymphatic drainage consists of two systems: The intrinsic system includes the intramural networks, whereas the extrinsic system follows the arteries within the perigastric ligaments. The gastric nodes consist of three groups: (1) the left and right gastric nodes reside within the gastrohepatic ligament and drain the gastroesophageal junction and gastric body and antrum along the lesser curvature; (2) the right and left gastroepiploic nodes reside within the gastrocolic ligament and drain the greater curvature of the stomach; and (3) the subpyloric nodes lie close to the bifurcation of the gastroduodenal artery along the pyloric portion of the greater curvature and drain the pyloric portion of the stomach, the first part of the duodenum, the head of pancreas, and the right gastroepiploic nodes. All of these nodes, except the right gastroepiploic nodes, drain to the celiac lymph nodes (which are the principal nodes draining the stomach, duodenum, liver, gallbladder, dorsal portion of the pancreas, and spleen). Tumors that originate along the gastroesophageal junction and the lesser curvature of the stomach metastasize to the lymph nodes within the gastrohepatic ligament. Tumors arising from the lesser curvature of the antrum and pylorus drain along the hepatic artery to the celiac nodes. Tumors that originate along the greater curvature of the antrum spread to the nodes of the gastrocolic ligament and follow the right gastroepiploic vein to the gastrocolic trunk or the right gastroepiploic artery to the subpyloric nodes. They then drain to the preaortic nodes of the SMA or celiac artery. Figure 10-38 is a simplified diagram showing the lymphatic drainage of the stomach. In the staging of gastric cancer, certain distant lymph-node groups (e.g., supraclavicular nodes) are considered distant metastases.

HEMATOGENOUS SPREAD

Common sites of distant hematogenous metastases include the liver (because the stomach is drained by portal vein tributaries), lungs, adrenal glands, and bones.

PERITONEAL SPREAD

Gastric cancer is one of the tumors with propensity for intraperitoneal spread. One well-known result of this characteristic is the development of ovarian serosal metastases (Krukenberg tumor) (Fig. 10-39).

Structures to Assess

When imaging gastric cancer with CT or MRI, it is important to detect the presence of transserosal tumor. In the case of an intact serosa (T1 and T2 lesions), the gastric wall maintains a smooth outer border surrounded by clean perigastric fat. In T3 lesions, the serosal contour becomes indistinct or blurred, and soft-tissue stranding or nodularity may be seen in the perigastric fat (although these findings may be present in the setting of inflammation). Absence of a fat plane between the tumor and adjacent organs suggests, but is not definitive for, T4 disease. Peritoneal metastases are suggested by the presence of ascites, nodules or plaques along peritoneal surfaces, thickening or enhancement of the parietal peritoneum, or small-bowel wall thickening or distortion. Hematogenous or peritoneal metastases alter the therapeutic approach and should be looked for in every case.

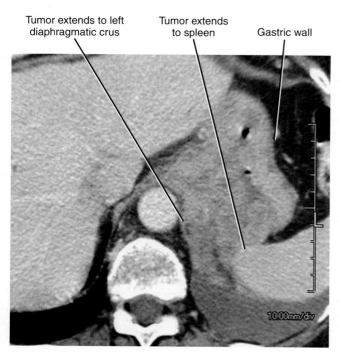

Figure 10-37 Enhanced axial computed tomographic scan of a patient with gastric cancer extending to the left hemidiaphragm and spleen.

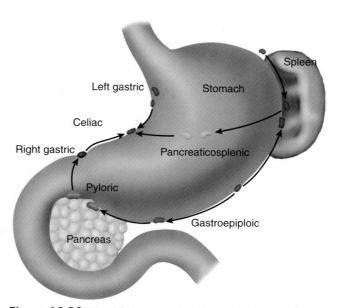

Figure 10-38 Simplified lymphatic drainage of the stomach.

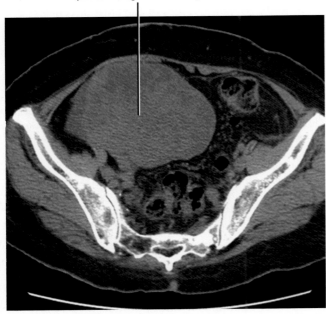

Heterogeneous mass replacing right ovary
(metastatic gastric cancer)

Figure 10-39 Unenhanced axial computed tomographic scan of a patient with metastatic gastric cancer involving the right ovary.

Colon Cancer (Adenocarcinoma)

Tumor Markers

CEA level is not sufficiently sensitive or specific to be a useful screening test for colon cancer. However, CEA level has utility for the detection of tumor recurrence after an attempt at curative resection. Return of increased CEA levels that had normalized after surgery may be a more sensitive indicator of recurrence than are imaging findings.

Imaging Modalities

Colonoscopy and barium enema can detect colon cancer but are not useful for staging. CT and MRI have only limited ability to accurately predict T stage and are primarily used to detect metastatic disease, particularly in the liver. CT and MRI can also detect lymphadenopathy but are nonspecific in this regard. PET and PET/CT are useful for the detection of distant metastases, although PET alone is limited in its ability to detect liver metastases smaller than 1 cm. As with gastric cancer, intense FDG uptake by the primary tumor may obscure immediately adjacent lymph-node metastases. PET and PET/CT may be useful in differentiating between postsurgical scarring and active recurrent tumor, although areas of inflammation may also demonstrate increased uptake of FDG. Technetium 99m (Tc-99m) CEA scan is an option in patients with increasing CEA level after surgery but without evidence of recurrent disease on imaging.

Staging Highlights

The Dukes classification system (and its various modifications) applied to colon cancer is still in use and was the dominant colorectal cancer staging system for many years. This system has the benefit of simplicity. Stage A disease is confined to the colonic wall and is equivalent to stage I disease of the TNM system of the AJCC. Stage B disease extends to or through the serosa and is comparable with TNM stage II disease. Stage C tumor is associated with lymph-node metastases (equivalent to TNM stage III disease), and Dukes stage D disease (not originally described by Dukes) involves distant metastases (equivalent to TNM stage IV disease). T staging of colon cancer under the TNM system depends on the depth of tumor invasion (Table 10-4; see Fig. 10-27). Lymph-node staging (N) based on the TNM system depends on the number of positive lymph nodes found at resection.

Common Mechanisms and Sites of Spread
CONTIGUOUS SPREAD

Colon cancer may spread directly to adjacent organs such as the kidneys, gallbladder, urinary bladder, uterus, duodenum and small bowel, spleen, and abdominal wall.

LIGAMENTS AND MESENTERIES

Spread from colon cancer may occur along the duodenocolic and gastrocolic ligaments to the duodenum and stomach, and via the transverse mesocolon to the pancreas. Tumors of the cecum and sigmoid colon can spread via the subperitoneal space to the broad ligament and subsequently to the female pelvic organs.

LYMPHATIC SPREAD

Lymphatic spread of colon cancer is initially to the epicolic and paracolic nodes (Fig. 10-40). The epicolic nodes lie on the colonic wall, antimesocolic beneath

Table 10-4   T Staging of Cancer of the Colon and Rectum Based on the American Joint Committee on Cancer TNM Staging System

Primary Tumor (T)	
TX	Primary tumor cannot be assessed
T0	No evidence of primary tumor
Tis	Carcinoma *in situ:* intraepithelial or invasion of lamina propria*
T1	Tumor invades submucosa
T2	Tumor invades muscularis propria
T3	Tumor invades through the muscularis propria into the subserosa, or into nonperitonealized pericolic or perirectal tissues
T4	Tumor directly invades other organs or structures, and/or perforates visceral peritoneum†, ‡

*Note: This includes cancer cells confined within the glandular basement membrane (intraepithelial) or lamina propria (intramucosal) with no extension through the muscularis mucosae into the submucosa.

†Note: Direct invasion in T4 includes invasion of other segments of the colorectum by way of the serosa; for example, invasion of the sigmoid colon by a carcinoma of the cecum.

‡Tumor that is adherent to other organs or structures, macroscopically, is classified T4. However, if no tumor is present in the adhesion, microscopically, the classification should be pT3. The V and L substaging should be used to identify the presence or absence of vascular or lymphatic invasion.

Adapted from Greene F, Page D, Fleming I et al, editors. *American Joint Committee on Cancer Staging Manual,* ed 6, New York, 2002, Springer-Verlag.

the peritoneal lining, whereas paracolic nodes lie along the marginal vessels on the mesocolic side. Lymphatic spread is then to the intermediate nodes in the mesocolon and from there to the principal nodes (preaortic nodes) at the mesenteric root of the SMA and inferior mesenteric artery (IMA) (Fig. 10-41). Key lymph nodes in the setting of cancer of the appendix, cecum, and ascending colon are the nodes in the ileocolic mesentery, along the ileocolic vessels, and the preaortic SMA nodes. Tumors of the transverse colon spread to nodes in the transverse mesocolon (along the middle colic vessels) and subsequently its root. Tumors of the proximal transverse colon and hepatic flexure spread to the nodes that follow the right or middle colic vessels and the region of the gastrocolic trunk. Tumors of the distal transverse colon and splenic flexure spread to the nodes that follow the left middle colic vessels. Tumors of the proximal descending colon can potentially spread to the lymph nodes within the left paraduodenal fossa (see Fig. 10-40). Tumors of the descending colon and sigmoid colon metastasize to the nodes along the vessels in the descending mesocolon and subsequently to the preaortic nodes at the origin of the IMA.

HEMATOGENOUS SPREAD

Hematogenous spread of tumor most often affects the liver. Colon cancer also frequently metastasizes to the lungs and occasionally to the bones, adrenal glands, and brain, among other sites.

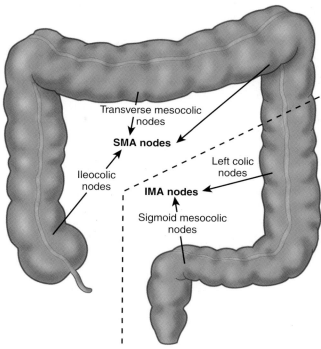

Figure 10-41 Most common lymphatic drainage patterns of the colon. IMA, Inferior mesenteric artery; *SMA,* superior mesenteric artery.

PERITONEAL SPREAD

Intraperitoneal spread of colon cancer is relatively common (see Fig. 10-26). As with gastric cancer, colon cancer may metastasize to the ovaries via the peritoneal cavity.

Structures to Assess

When reviewing imaging studies of patients with adenocarcinoma of the colon, one should try to assess whether tumor violates the serosa or invades adjacent structures. As with pancreatic cancer, distinguishing between tumor and inflammation or desmoplastic reaction may be difficult with imaging. Any extension via the relevant ligaments and mesenteries should be noted, and the draining lymph nodes should be examined for evidence of enlargement. Lymph-node metastases from right-sided colon cancers can obstruct the right ureter. Thus it is important to look for evidence of hydronephrosis. The most important role of cross-sectional imaging in known or suspected colon cancer, however, is the detection of distant hematogenous metastases. The portal circulation provides a direct venous conduit from the bowel to the liver, so liver metastases are particularly common in patients with colon cancer, and the liver should always be evaluated carefully. The presence of distant metastases may alter the goal of surgery (palliative vs. curative). However, the number and location of hepatic metastases should be carefully noted on imaging studies, as patients with liver metastases from colon cancer may still undergo curative resection of the primary tumor and liver disease. Also, patients who cannot undergo hepatic resection of metastases may be eligible for other treatments such as radiofrequency ablation.

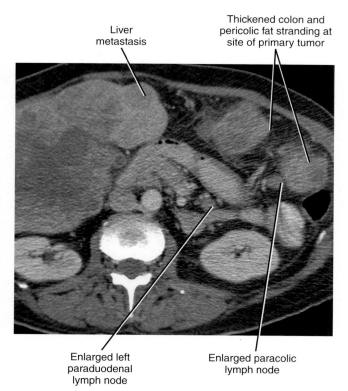

Figure 10-40 Enhanced axial computed tomographic image of a patient with adenocarcinoma of the colon with liver and lymph-node metastases.

Rectal Cancer

Tumor Markers

CEA values are in reference range in most patients with rectal cancer. CEA level is useful for monitoring patients with rectal cancer after treatment. Patients with recurrent rectal cancer often have increased levels of CEA even when presurgical levels were normal.

Imaging Modalities

Transrectal US is often performed for T staging rectal cancer and may be the most accurate modality available at most institutions, particularly for superficial tumors. Unfortunately, US cannot evaluate the mesorectal fascia or lymph nodes beyond the immediate vicinity of the probe. MRI performed with an endorectal coil provides high-resolution images that can improve the accuracy of MRI for determining depth of invasion, possibly to the level achievable with transrectal US. However, endorectal coil placement may be difficult in some patients with rectal cancer. High-field-strength scanners with state-of-the-art surface coils can also improve T staging, particularly when gadolinium chelates and rectal contrast are administered. MRI is also the best tool for assessment of the circumferential resection margin before total mesorectal excision (TME). CT is frequently used in follow-up after treatment for rectal cancer but is not generally used for T staging, except to detect extension beyond the serosa. PET/CT plays a similar role in rectal cancer as it does in colon cancer. PET and PET/CT are particularly helpful in differentiating presacral tumor recurrence from benign postoperative changes. No imaging modality is particularly good at reliably distinguishing between benign and malignant lymph nodes in the setting of rectal cancer.

Staging Highlights

Staging of rectal cancer under the AJCC TNM system is the same as for colon cancer. Dukes classification system described earlier for colon cancer was originally developed for rectal cancer staging.

Common Mechanisms and Sites of Spread

CONTIGUOUS SPREAD

Rectal cancer can spread directly to the seminal vesicles, prostate, uterus, bladder, sacrum, and vagina (see Fig. 10-2).

LYMPHATIC SPREAD

Conspicuous mesorectal lymph nodes are highly suspicious for tumor in the setting of rectal cancer. Cancer of the upper rectum spreads cephalad in lymphatic channels along the superior rectal vessels within the sigmoid mesocolon to the preaortic IMA lymph nodes (Fig. 10-42). The lower rectum and upper anal canal lymph drainage follows the middle rectal vessels to the internal iliac and obturator nodes. Nodal involvement continues cephalad to the common iliac nodes and paraaortic nodes. Lymph drainage from this region can also go to the ischiorectal fossa and follow the inferior rectal and internal iliac nodes. Lymphatic spread from the anus is to the superficial inguinal nodes, deep inguinal nodes, external iliac nodes, common iliac nodes, and eventually the paraaortic nodes.

HEMATOGENOUS SPREAD

The liver is the most frequent site of hematogenous spread, followed by the lungs (pulmonary metastases are more typical with distal rectal tumors). Other sites of spread, such as the bones and adrenal glands, can also be seen.

Structures to Assess

When interpreting imaging studies in patients with rectal cancer, it is helpful to be familiar with some of the surgical treatment options. A small minority of patients with superficial tumors (T1) not associated with lymph-node metastases may be treated with local excision, whereas involvement of the anal sphincter often necessitates abdominoperineal resection (although preoperative radiation and chemotherapy may allow a sphincter-sparing procedure to be performed). If the lower half of the rectum is involved, a TME has become the preferred surgical technique in recent years, resulting in fewer abdominoperineal resections. TME involves removing the rectum, mesorectum, and mesorectal fascia en bloc in combination with a low-stapled anastomosis.

Before TME, it is important to determine the tumor margin relative to the mesorectal fascia (Figs. 10-43 and 10-44). It has been shown that the distance from the tumor to the circumferential mesorectal resection plane (represented by the mesorectal fascia on imaging) is the best predictor of local tumor recurrence. In general, MRI is the most accurate method of determining involvement of the circumferential resection margin. Patients with tumor close to or involving the resection margin at TME may benefit from neoadjuvant therapy (i.e., radiation or chemotherapy) or more extensive surgery.

In all patients, an attempt should be made to assess the depth of tumor invasion, the longitudinal extent of tumor, the precise location of the tumor relative to the peritoneal reflection and anus, and the presence of abnormal lymph nodes. Involvement of the pyriformis and obturator internus muscles, sacrum, sciatic nerve, and pelvic organs should be noted.

Renal Cell Carcinoma

Tumor Markers

No currently widely available assays exist for tumor markers relevant to renal cell carcinoma.

Imaging Modalities

Intravenous pyelography and retrograde urography are insensitive for detection and rarely helpful for staging renal cell carcinoma. US can detect renal masses and differentiate between benign cysts and solid or complex lesions. US can also demonstrate thrombus within the renal vein or IVC in many

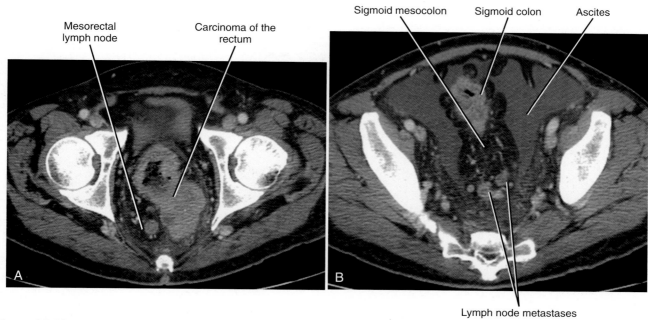

Figure 10-42 Axial enhanced computed tomographic image of pelvis in a patient with rectal cancer and mesorectal (**A**) and sigmoid mesocolon (**B**) lymph-node metastases.

patients. CT is the most frequently performed test for the evaluation of a patient with known or suspected renal cell carcinoma and is often the only test required before surgery. MRI is useful for patients who cannot undergo CT scanning and is the best means of evaluating for the extent of intracaval tumor thrombus. PET does not play a significant role in the diagnosis of primary renal tumors because many renal tumors are not FDG avid, although PET may eventually find a role in the detection of metastases and recurrent disease (Fig. 10-45).

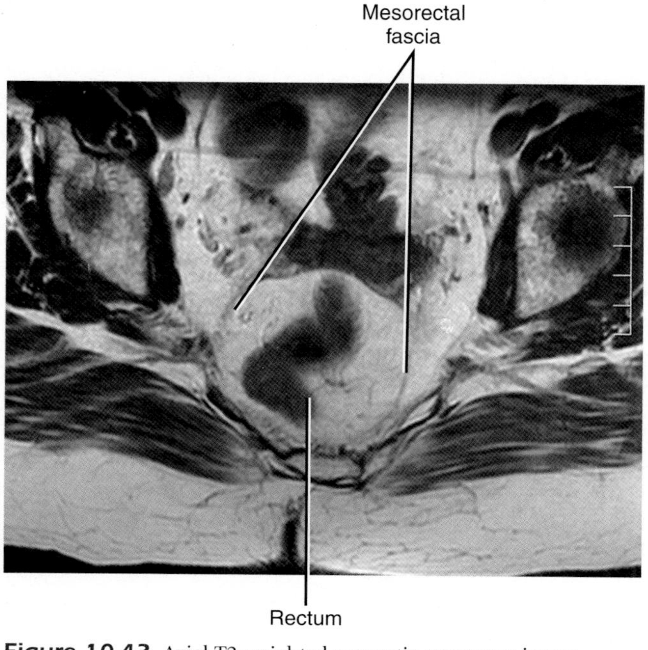

Renal vein or IVC extension is usually well-demonstrated on contrast-enhanced CT examinations and US imaging with color Doppler. However, when the tumor thrombus enhances to the same degree as the surrounding venous blood, venous extension may be missed. Disproportionate enlargement of the affected renal vein or IVC may be one sign of involvement in such a case, although the extent of tumor may be difficult to discern. The presence of enlarged capsular veins should also prompt scrutiny of the renal vein for evidence of invasion. MRI can image the renal vein using a variety of noncontrast- and contrast-enhanced techniques such as dark-blood, time-of-flight, phase-contrast, steady state free precession, and gadolinium-enhanced MRA (Fig. 10-46). This armamentarium ensures that the full extent of tumor thrombus is visualized, and that false-positive and -negative results because of imaging artifacts are minimized. Currently, neither MRI nor CT offers clear advantages over the other for lymph-node staging.

Staging Highlights

The Robson staging system remains in use for renal cell carcinoma (Table 10-5). The advantages of this system are that it is simple and widely known. The AJCC TNM staging system is also widely used (Table 10-6) and has many similarities to the Robson classification. Unlike the Robson system, T staging using the TNM system requires precise knowledge of the tumor size and extent of venous involvement.

Figure 10-43 Axial T2-weighted magnetic resonance image through the pelvis demonstrating normal mesorectal fascia.

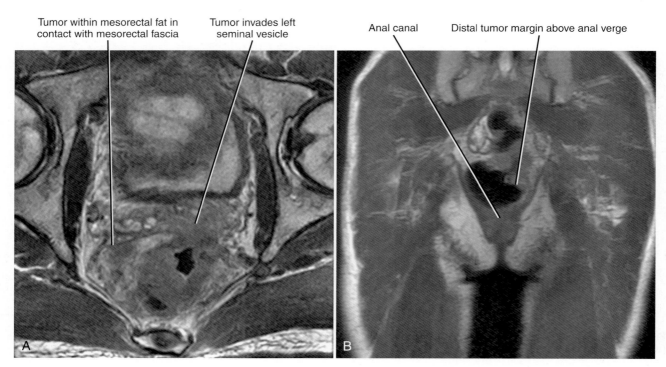

Figure 10-44 Axial (**A**) and coronal (**B**) T2-weighted magnetic resonance images of a patient with rectal cancer performed on 3-Tesla scanner.

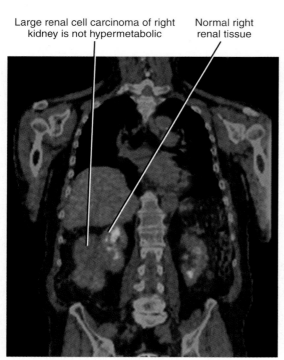

Figure 10-45 Fused coronal fluoro-2-deoxy-D-glucose positron emission tomography/computed tomographic image in a patient with nonhypermetabolic right renal cell carcinoma.

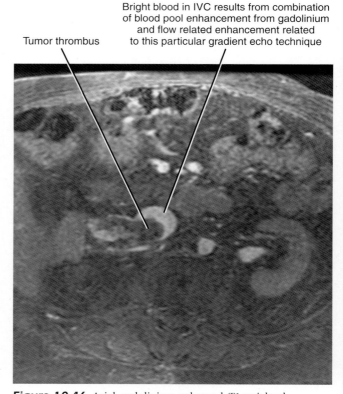

Figure 10-46 Axial, gadolinium-enhanced, T1-weighted, gradient-echo image in a patient with renal cell carcinoma extending into the inferior vena cava (IVC). Compare this with T2-weighted technique presented in Figure 10-21.

Table 10-5   Robson Classification of Renal Cell Carcinoma

Stage	Finding
I	Tumor within renal capsule
II	Tumor spread to perinephric fat
IIIa	Venous extension
IIIb	Regional lymph-node metastases
IIIc	Venous extension and regional lymph-node metastases
IVa	Direct invasion beyond renal fascia
IVb	Distant metastases

Table 10-6   T Staging of Cancer of the Kidney

Primary Tumor (T)	
TX	Primary tumor cannot be assessed
T0	No evidence of primary tumor
T1	Tumor 7 cm or less in greatest dimension, limited to the kidney
T1a	Tumor 4 cm or less in greatest dimension, limited to the kidney
T1b	Tumor more than 4 cm but not more than 7 cm in greatest dimension, limited to the kidney
T2	Tumor more than 7 cm in greatest dimension, limited to the kidney
T3	Tumor extends into major veins or invades adrenal gland or perinephric tissues but not beyond Gerota's fascia
T3a	Tumor directly invades adrenal gland or perirenal and/or renal sinus fat but not beyond Gerota's fascia
T3b	Tumor grossly extends into the renal vein or its segmental (muscle-containing) branches, or vena cava below the diaphragm
T3c	Tumor grossly extends into the vena cava above diaphragm or invades the wall of the vena cava
T4	Tumor invades beyond Gerota's fascia

Adapted from Greene F, Page D, Fleming I et al, editors. *American Joint Committee on Cancer Staging Manual*, ed 6, New York, 2002, Springer-Verlag.

Common Mechanisms and Sites of Spread
CONTIGUOUS SPREAD
Large tumors may spread directly to the adrenal glands or through the renal fascia to adjacent organs such as the liver, colon (most often on the left in region of descending colon), small bowel (most often descending duodenum on the right), psoas muscle, spleen, and pancreas. It is common for large right renal masses to indent the liver without actually invading.

LYMPHATIC SPREAD
Renal hilar and paraaortic lymph nodes are most frequently affected (Fig. 10-47), although lymphatic disease may spread to the cisterna chyli and ascend as far as the supraclavicular nodes.

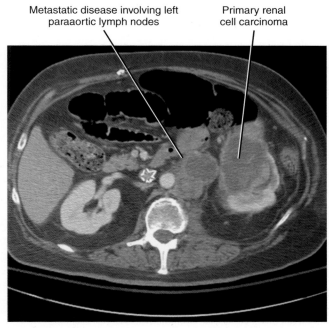

Metastatic disease involving left paraaortic lymph nodes

Primary renal cell carcinoma

Figure 10-47 Enhanced axial computed tomographic image of a patient with renal cell carcinoma metastatic to the left paraaortic lymph nodes.

HEMATOGENOUS SPREAD
Renal cell carcinoma may metastasize to the lungs and pleura, liver, bones, adrenal glands, pancreas, mediastinum, and brain (Figs. 10-48 and 10-49). Bone metastases are often lytic, and patients typically present with bone pain. Because of the lack of osteoblastic activity, bone metastases from renal cell carcinoma may go undetected on a Tc-99m bone scan. Venous extension into the renal vein lumen and IVC is relatively common, although invasion of the caval wall is rare. Intravenous tumor growth tends to follow the direction of blood flow.

Structures to Assess
Because of the many treatment options, surgical approaches (open vs. laparoscopic), and surgical techniques (partial vs. radical nephrectomy) available for the treatment of renal cell carcinoma, imaging results must provide a thorough description of the tumor extent and relevant anatomy. Tumor size, location, and number should be provided. The contralateral kidney should be examined for evidence of additional tumors. The renal capsule and renal fascia should be assessed for evidence of tumor involvement. Unfortunately, signs such as perinephric stranding and fat obliteration are unreliable indicators of Robson stage II disease, though the presence of a discrete soft-tissue mass in the perinephric space suggests extracapsular extension. Presence of a tumoral pseudocapsule on CT or MR images suggests lack of perirenal fat invasion. Involvement of adjacent organs with renal cell carcinoma may also be difficult to confirm on CT and MRI. A clear fat plane between the tumor and an adjacent structure such as the liver is often absent in the setting of invasion. However, large tumors often obliterate fat planes and distort adjacent organs by mass effect rather than invasion.

Enhancing left adrenal mass. Enhancement was progressive and persisted on delayed images (did not wash out)

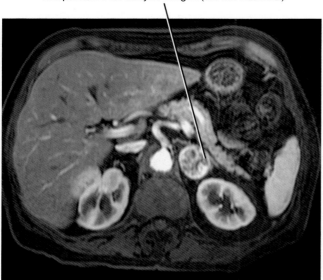

Figure 10-48 Axial, gadolinium-enhanced, T1-weighted, fat-suppressed, magnetic resonance image through the left adrenal gland in a patient with right-sided renal cell carcinoma (not shown) and contralateral adrenal gland metastasis. A biopsy of the mass was performed only after excluding pheochromocytoma.

Normal pancreatic body   Heterogenous enhancing mass in pancreatic body/tail

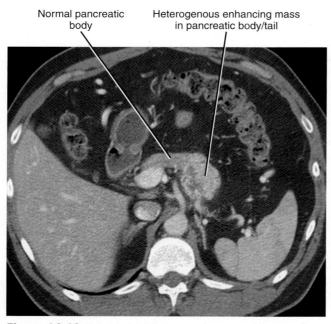

Figure 10-49 Enhanced axial computed tomographic scan of a patient with renal cell carcinoma (not shown) and metastasis to the pancreas.

The renal vein and IVC should be assessed for evidence of tumor involvement in every patient with renal cell carcinoma. Excretory phase images should be evaluated for evidence of calyceal or renal pelvis invasion. Relevant lymph-node drainage pathways should be searched. Unfortunately, enlarged lymph nodes in the setting of renal cell carcinoma are reactive at least

as often as they are neoplastic. The ipsilateral adrenal gland should be examined for evidence of direct extension, and both glands should be searched for evidence of hematogenous metastases. A normal ipsilateral adrenal gland demonstrated on CT potentially allows for adrenal-sparing surgery. However, an abnormal adrenal gland on CT has a relatively low positive predictive value because of the overall high incidence of benign adrenal lesions in the general population. Although adrenal metastases from clear cell carcinoma may potentially demonstrate low signal intensity on unenhanced CT or signal loss on opposed-phase MRI because of intracellular lipid, most lipid-rich adrenal masses in the setting of renal cell carcinoma are the result of adrenal hyperplasia or adenoma. When a well-defined focus of differing density or signal intensity is present in a lipid-containing adrenal mass, one should consider the possibility of a "collision tumor" (Fig. 10-50). A search for distant metastases should be conducted. Vascular and collecting system anomalies should be commented on. The relation between the tumor and the ipsilateral ureter is important to determine when percutaneous ablation techniques are a consideration. The contralateral kidney should be assessed for evidence of synchronous tumors, which are relatively common.

Tumor size and location dictate surgical approach. Small tumors may be candidates for nephron-sparing resection (partial nephrectomy), whereas larger lesions may necessitate radical nephrectomy. Patients with extracapsular disease or collecting system involvement will not benefit from nephron-sparing surgery. The presence of venous involvement will also alter the surgical approach. Intracaval tumor thrombus that extends above the hepatic venous confluence necessitates an intrathoracic approach and cardiopulmonary bypass. Caval wall invasion should be distinguished from tumor thrombus within the IVC, because the former will necessitate venous reconstruction. IVC invasion can best be detected by demonstrating tumor on both sides of the caval wall.

Bladder Cancer (Transitional Cell Carcinoma)

Tumor Markers
Currently, no serum tumor markers are in widespread use for the diagnosis of bladder cancer. A variety of urinary biomarkers are under investigation.

Imaging Modalities
Bladder cancer can be diagnosed with cystography, intravenous or retrograde pyelography, US, CT, and MRI, although only CT and MRI have the potential to offer accurate and complete staging information. Of these two latter modalities, MRI is the most useful for assessment of local invasion by bladder cancer. Cystoscopy offers the potential for tissue sampling but cannot assess the pelvic viscera, sidewalls, and lymph nodes. Urinary excretion of FDG limits the utility of PET for the evaluation of local disease.

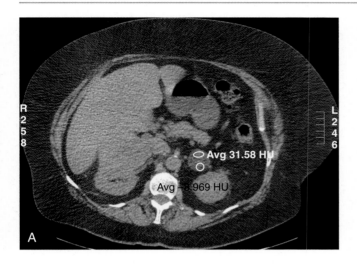

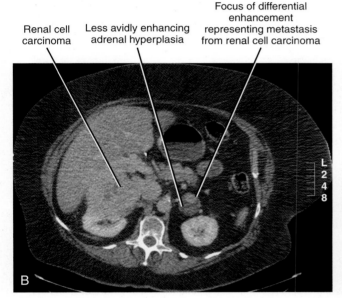

Renal cell carcinoma

Less avidly enhancing adrenal hyperplasia

Focus of differential enhancement representing metastasis from renal cell carcinoma

Figure 10-50 Axial unenhanced (**A**) and contrast-enhanced (**B**) computed tomographic images of a patient with renal cell carcinoma metastatic to the left adrenal mass consisting largely of adrenal hyperplasia. Imaging findings confirmed at adrenalectomy.

Staging Highlights

Bladder tumors are staged according to the AJCC TNM system. T staging is dependent on depth of tumor invasion and involvement of adjacent structures as shown in Table 10-7, which omits some of the T-stage subcategories. Nodal staging is based on the size and multiplicity of lymph nodes.

Common Mechanisms and Sites of Spread

CONTIGUOUS SPREAD

Bladder cancer can directly invade the prostate, seminal vesicles, uterus, vagina, rectum, and pelvic sidewall (Fig. 10-51). Bladder cancer may also spread along the urethra or urachus.

Table 10-7   T Staging of Cancer of the Urinary Bladder

Primary Tumor (T)	
TX	Primary tumor cannot be assessed
T0	No evidence of primary tumor
Ta	Noninvasive papillary carcinoma
Tis	Carcinoma *in situ;* "flat tumor"
T1	Tumor invades subepithelial connective tissue
T2	Tumor invades muscle
pT2a	Tumor invades superficial muscle (inner half)
PT2b	Tumor invades deep tissue (outer half)
T3	Tumor invades perivesical tissue
pT3a	microscopically
pT3b	macroscopically (extravesical mass)
T4	Tumor invades any of the following: prostate, uterus, vagina, pelvic wall, abdominal wall
T4a	Tumor invades prostate, uterus, vagina
T4b	Tumor invades pelvic wall, abdominal wall

Adapted from Greene F, Page D, Fleming I et al, editors. *American Joint Committee on Cancer Staging Manual,* ed 6, New York, 2002, Springer-Verlag.

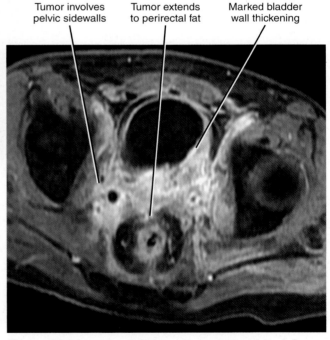

Tumor involves pelvic sidewalls

Tumor extends to perirectal fat

Marked bladder wall thickening

Figure 10-51 Axial, gadolinium-enhanced, T1-weighted, fat-suppressed, magnetic resonance imaging through the pelvis of a patient with locally advanced bladder cancer.

LYMPHATIC SPREAD

Lymphatic spread occurs first to the perivesical and presacral nodes, and then to the internal iliac, obturator, and external iliac nodes. From the pelvis, spread occurs to the paraaortic nodes. Ten-millimeter oval or 8-mm round lymph nodes are generally considered suspicious for metastatic disease.

HEMATOGENOUS SPREAD

Hematogenous metastases are primarily to the lung, liver, and bones, although other sites of involvement may occur (Fig. 10-52).

Structures to Assess

The bladder wall should be assessed carefully. Because bladder cancer typically enhances earlier than bladder wall, imaging-based T staging of bladder cancer is best accomplished with dynamic contrast-enhanced imaging. The important T-staging distinction is among T1 (superficial), T2 (muscle invasive), and T3 (extra vesical) tumors. Extravesical tumor extension may be suggested on CT and MRI when the outer bladder contour is irregular or when stranding or soft-tissue infiltration is present in the perivesical fat. Inflammation and granulation tissue after biopsy or transurethral resection of bladder cancer can mimic tumor and result in overstaging. The location of the tumor with respect to the ureters and urethra and the presence of ureteral obstruction should be noted. The prostate, seminal vesicles, pelvic sidewall, rectum, vagina, and uterus should be examined for evidence of direct invasion. Regional and paraaortic lymph nodes should be assessed for evidence of enlargement. Because synchronous upper tract tumors are not rare (2%) in the

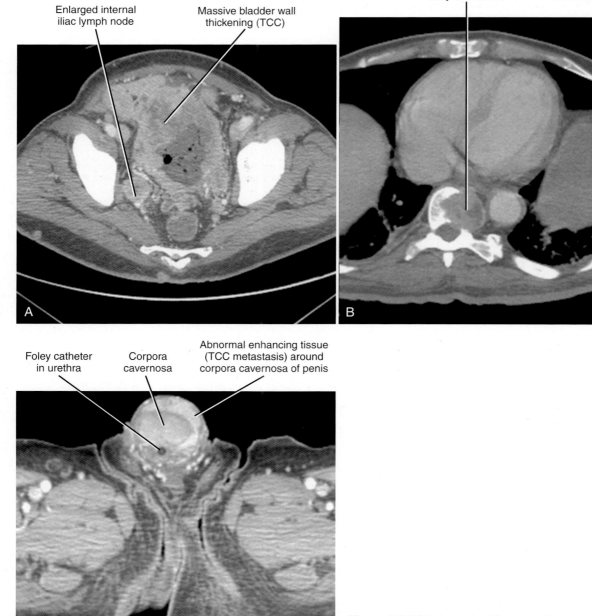

Figure 10-52 Enhanced axial computed tomographic images of a patient with transitional cell carcinoma (TCC) of the bladder (**A**), and metastatic disease to the spine (**B**) and penis (**C**).

setting of transitional carcinoma of the bladder, the upper urinary tracts should be assessed carefully. Depth of bladder wall invasion is predictive of tumor recurrence, the presence of metastases, and overall survival. Patients with deep muscle invasive tumors and lymph node metastases have a poor prognosis.

Endometrial Cancer

Tumor Markers

Serum CA-125 levels are increased in approximately 20% of patients with endometrial carcinoma and may indicate occult extrauterine disease.

Imaging Modalities

US is useful for the detection of endometrial cancer in patients with abnormal uterine bleeding and can be used to estimate the depth of myometrial invasion. However, CT and MRI are superior in demonstrating adenopathy and distant disease. CT can also be used to detect recurrence after hysterectomy. MRI using a combination of T2-weighted and dynamic gadolinium-enhanced images is the best imaging modality for local staging of endometrial cancer. MRI is helpful in determining the depth of myometrial invasion and presence of cervical invasion, in the detection of pelvic lymphadenopathy and peritoneal metastases, and in excluding myometrial invasion in patients with early-stage disease who wish to preserve fertility (Fig. 10-53). The role of PET in the setting of endometrial cancer remains to be established.

Staging Highlights

The International Federation of Gynecology and Obstetrics (FIGO) staging system remains in common use and is based on depth of myometrial invasion, involvement of the cervix, and extrauterine spread (Table 10-8). As shown in Table 10-8, the TNM staging of endometrial carcinoma has many similarities to the FIGO classification.

Common Mechanisms and Sites of Spread

CONTIGUOUS SPREAD

Endometrial cancer may spread directly to the cervix, vagina, colon, rectum, bladder, and adnexa.

LIGAMENTS AND MESENTERIES

Endometrial cancer can spread via the broad ligaments to the pelvic sidewall.

LYMPHATIC SPREAD

Endometrial cancer typically spreads to the pelvic lymph nodes and subsequently to the paraaortic nodes (Fig. 10-54). The presence of lymphadenopathy is correlated with the depth of myometrial invasion of the primary tumor. The risk for lymph-node metastases increases significantly with deep myometrial (>50% of myometrial thickness) or cervical invasion. Tumors of the upper fundus can spread via lymphatic channels paralleling the gonadal vessels to the paraaortic lymph nodes of the upper abdomen.

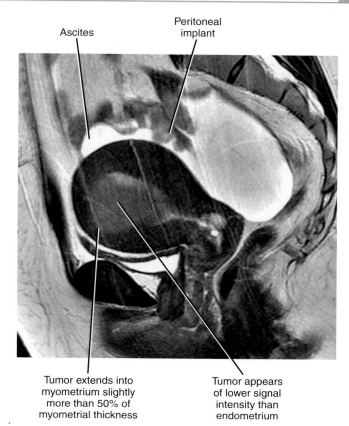

Ascites

Peritoneal implant

Tumor extends into myometrium slightly more than 50% of myometrial thickness

Tumor appears of lower signal intensity than endometrium

Figure 10-53 Sagittal T2-weighted magnetic resonance image through pelvis of a patient with endometrial cancer with deep myometrial invasion.

HEMATOGENOUS SPREAD

Distant metastatic sites include lungs, liver, bones, and brain, although it is rare for endometrial carcinoma to present with distant hematogenous metastatic disease.

PERITONEAL SPREAD

Endometrial cancer occasionally spreads to the peritoneum (see Fig. 10-23).

Structures to Assess

When CT or MR imaging is performed in the setting of endometrial carcinoma, attention should be directed toward the detection of deep myometrial invasion, extrauterine extension, enlarged lymph nodes, peritoneal implants or ascites, and distant metastases. CT is less accurate than MRI for determining depth of myometrial invasion and is typically not used for this purpose.

The primary role of MRI in the assessment of endometrial carcinoma is assessing the depth of myometrial invasion. An intact junctional zone on T2-weighted images with sharp delineation between the high-signal-intensity endometrium and the relatively low-signal-intensity junctional zone implies stage IA disease. Disruption of the junctional zone or evidence of poorly enhancing tumor extending into the normally avidly enhancing myometrium on dynamic contrast-enhanced T1-weighted images suggests myometrial

Table 10-8   T Staging of Cancer of the Corpus Uteri

Primary Tumor (T) (Surgical-Pathologic Findings)

TNM Categories	FIGO Stages	
TX		Primary tumor cannot be assessed
T0		No evidence of primary tumor
Tis	0	Carcinoma *in situ*
T1	I	Tumor confined to corpus uteri
T1a	IA	Tumor limited to endometrium
T1b	IB	Tumor invades less than one half of the myometrium
T1c	IC	Tumor invades one half or more of the myometrium
T2	II	Tumor invades cervix but does not extend beyond uterus
T2a	IIa	Tumor limited to the glandular epithelium of the endocervix. There is no evidence of connective tissue stromal invasion
T2b	IIB	Invasion of the stromal connective tissue of the cervix
T3	III	Local and/or regional spread as defined below
T3a	IIA	Tumor involves serosa and/or adnexa (direct extension or metastasis) and/or cancer cells in ascites or peritoneal washings
T3b	IIIB	Vaginal involvement (direct extension or metastasis)
T4	IVA	Tumor invades bladder mucosa and/or bowel mucosa (bullous edema is not sufficient to classify a tumor as T4)

Adapted from Greene F, Page D, Fleming I et al, editors. *American Joint Committee on Cancer Staging Manual*, ed 6, New York, 2002, Springer-Verlag.

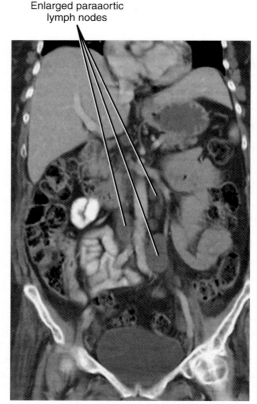

Enlarged paraaortic lymph nodes

Figure 10-54 Coronal reformatted image from enhanced computed tomographic scan in a patient with endometrial cancer metastatic to the paraaortic lymph nodes.

invasion (Fig. 10-55). Stage IIA disease may manifest as widening of the endocervical channel in continuity with the main tumor. When the normally hypointense cervical stroma is disrupted on T2-weighted images, stage IIB disease is suggested. Uterine contour changes contiguous with tumor (and not attributed to fibroids) suggest serosal involvement (FIGO stage III).

Cervical Cancer

Imaging Modalities

The initial diagnosis of cervical cancer is rarely made with imaging. MRI is the preferred imaging modality for local staging of cervical cancer. CT and MRI have demonstrated similar accuracy in the evaluation of pelvic lymph nodes in the setting of cervical cancer, and both modalities can demonstrate pelvic sidewall involvement or invasion of other organs such as the ureters or rectum. PET has been shown to improve detection of lymph-node metastases compared with CT and MRI,

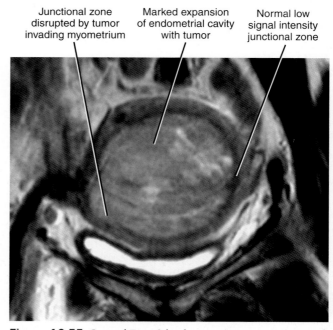

Junctional zone disrupted by tumor invading myometrium   Marked expansion of endometrial cavity with tumor   Normal low signal intensity junctional zone

Figure 10-55 Coronal T2-weighted magnetic resonance image of a patient with endometrial cancer. Imaging appearance correlated precisely with surgical and pathologic findings.

and may be useful for detection of tumor recurrence after treatment.

Staging Highlights

The FIGO classification for staging of cervical carcinoma is widely used (Table 10-9). The AJCC T staging parallels that of FIGO. The most important distinction to be made when staging cervical cancer with MRI is between stage IIA and IIB disease. This is because patients without parametrial involvement may be candidates for hysterectomy (with or without adjuvant therapy). Patients with more advanced disease are typically managed with radiation and chemotherapy.

Common Mechanisms and Sites of Spread

CONTIGUOUS SPREAD

Squamous cell carcinoma of the cervix frequently spreads directly to the uterine corpus and vagina, and surrounding pelvic organs and structures such as the bladder and rectum.

LIGAMENTS AND MESENTERIES

Cervical cancer often spreads within the cardinal ligaments to obstruct the ureters. Cervical cancer also spreads within the uterosacral ligaments.

LYMPHATIC SPREAD

As with many other tumors, the incidence of nodal involvement correlates with stage. Cervical cancer typically spreads to the paracervical, internal iliac, obturator, external iliac, sacral, common iliac, and eventually the paraaortic lymph nodes. As with other pelvic malignant tumors, the supraclavicular nodes may be involved in advanced disease. Tumor that involves the lower vaginal may metastasize to the inguinal nodes.

HEMATOGENOUS SPREAD

Hematogenous spread usually occurs late in the progression of disease. As with many other pelvic malignant tumors, cervical cancer can spread to the lungs, liver, and bones.

PERITONEAL SPREAD

Cervical cancer rarely involves the peritoneum.

Structures to Assess

When staging cervical cancer with MRI, it is important to evaluate the extent of tumor with respect to the vagina and to determine whether parametrial or pelvic sidewall involvement is present. Patients with stage IIB or higher disease (parametrial or pelvic sidewall involvement, paraaortic lymphadenopathy, or distant metastases) are generally spared hysterectomy. An intact, low-signal-intensity (on T2-weighted images) ring of cervical stroma has a negative predictive value (no parametrial involvement) of greater than 90%. Parametrial involvement (stage IIB disease) is suggested on MRI when there is evidence of disruption of the cervical fibrous stroma with evidence of tumor extending into the parametrial fat. Distal ureter obstruction on any imaging modality is strongly suggestive of pelvic

Table 10-9   T Staging of Cervical Carcinoma

TNM Categories	FIGO Stages	Primary Tumor (T)
TX		Primary tumor cannot be assessed
T0		No evidence of primary tumor
Tis	0	Carcinoma *in situ*
T1	I	Cervical carcinoma confined to uterus (extension to corpus should be disregarded)
*T1a	IA	Invasive carcinoma diagnosed only by microscopy. Stromal invasion with a maximum depth of 5.0 mm measured from the base of the epithelium and a horizontal spread of 7.0 mm or less. Vascular space involvement, venous or lymphatic, does not affect classification
T1a1	IA1	Measured stromal invasion 3.0 mm or less in depth and 7.0 mm in horizontal spread
T1a2	IA2	Measured stromal invasion more than 3.0 mm and not more than 5.0 mm with a horizontal spread 7.0 mm or less
T1b	IB	Clinically visible lesion confined to the cervix or microscopic lesion greater than T1a/IA2
T1b1	IB1	Clinically visible lesion 4.0 cm or less in greatest dimension
T1b2	IB2	Clinically visible lesion more than 4.0 cm in greatest dimension
T2	II	Cervical carcinoma invades beyond uterus but not to pelvic wall or to lower third of vagina
T2a	IIA	Tumor without parametrial invasion
T2b	IIB	Tumor with parametrial invasion
T3	III	Tumor extends to pelvic wall and/or involves lower third of vagina, and/or causes hydronephrosis or nonfunctioning kidney
T3a	IIIA	Tumor involves lower third of vagina, no extension to pelvic wall
T3b	IIIB	Tumor extends to pelvic wall and/or causes hydronephrosis or nonfunctioning kidney
T4	IVA	Tumor invades mucosa of bladder or rectum, and/or extends beyond true pelvis (bullous edema is not sufficient to classify a tumor as T4)

*All macroscopically visible lesions—even with superficial invasion—are T1b/IB
Adapted from Greene F, Page D, Fleming I et al, editors. *American Joint Committee on Cancer Staging Manual*, ed 6, New York, 2002, Springer-Verlag.

sidewall involvement (stage IIIB disease) (Fig. 10-56). The bladder and rectum are in close proximity to the cervix and should be assessed for evidence of direct invasion. Lymph nodes should be assessed for evidence of metastatic disease (currently, the best modality is probably PET). Lymph nodes greater than 8 to 10 mm in diameter are considered suspicious. The presence of

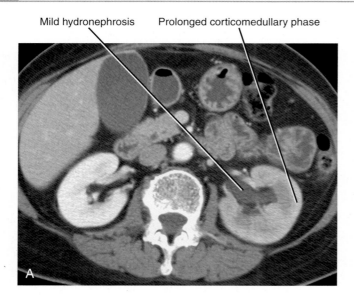

Mild hydronephrosis   Prolonged corticomedullary phase

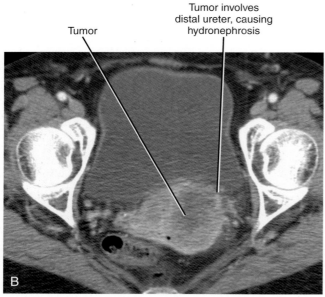

Tumor involves
distal ureter, causing
hydronephrosis

Tumor

Figure 10-56 Enhanced axial computed tomographic scan through the kidneys **(A)** and pelvis **(B)** of a patient with stage IIIB cervical carcinoma.

necrosis in lymph nodes on CT or MRI is highly suggestive of metastatic disease in the setting of squamous cell carcinoma. Always evaluate the supraclavicular lymph nodes when evaluating advanced disease.

Ovarian Cancer

Tumor Markers

CA-125 is the primary tumor marker increased in the setting of ovarian cancer. However, increased levels may also be present with pregnancy, endometriosis, menstruation, jaundice, pancreatitis, cirrhosis, pelvic inflammatory disease, and nongynecologic malignant tumors such as lung, appendiceal, and signet ring carcinomas. CA-125 is particularly unreliable in premenopausal women but has an 80% positive predictive value in postmenopausal women with adnexal mass. CA-125 is useful for monitoring response to treatment if increased before surgery. Certain germ cell tumors of the ovary may be associated with increased levels of β-HCG, AFP, or lactate dehydrogenase (LDH).

Imaging Modalities

Transvaginal US excels at detecting and characterizing ovarian masses, and is useful for triage of adnexal abnormalities to surgery, follow-up, or other therapy. CT is primarily used to detect metastases to the peritoneum and other organs, as well as to identify evidence of pelvic sidewall and ureteral involvement. MRI offers the highest specificity for characterizing adnexal masses, and is roughly equivalent to CT for detecting peritoneal and lymph-node metastases. PET may be a useful adjunct to other imaging modalities in the patient with suspected recurrent ovarian cancer.

Staging Highlights

The FIGO staging system is commonly used to classify ovarian cancer. This classification is presented in Table 10-10. The T staging of ovarian cancer according to the AJCC classification is similar to the FIGO system.

Common Mechanisms and Sites of Spread

CONTIGUOUS SPREAD

Direct extension of ovarian cancer occurs to the fallopian tube, uterus, and sigmoid colon.

LIGAMENTS AND MESENTERIES

Ovarian carcinoma can spread within the broad ligaments to the extraperitoneal pelvic spaces and eventually to the large-bowel (rectum, sigmoid colon, and cecum) or small-bowel mesentery.

LYMPHATIC SPREAD

Lymphatic spread of ovarian cancer often parallels the gonadal vessels to the paraaortic lymph nodes. Ovarian cancer may also spread via the uterine lymphatic drainage pathways to pelvic lymph nodes. Tumor that involves the pelvic sidewall also can metastasize to pelvic (internal iliac, obturator, external iliac) and retroperitoneal lymph nodes in the manner of most other pelvic tumors. Tumor spread may rarely follow the round ligaments to the inguinal lymph nodes.

HEMATOGENOUS SPREAD

Ovarian cancer preferentially spreads via the intraperitoneal and lymphatic pathways. Hematogenous metastases are not often present on imaging studies at the time of presentation. When hematogenous metastases are found, the liver is the most common site, followed by the lungs and pleura. Adrenal, splenic, bone, and brain metastases are less common. Ovarian sarcomas are more likely to utilize the hematogenous route than nonsarcomatous ovarian tumors.

PERITONEAL SPREAD

Peritoneal spread is common with ovarian cancer (particularly with epithelial tumors) and represents the most common mechanism of spread (Figs. 10-24 and 10-57).

Table 10-10   T Staging of Ovarian Carcinoma

		Primary Tumor (T)
TNM Categories	**FIGO Stages**	
TX		Primary tumor cannot be assessed
T0		No evidence of primary tumor
T1	I	Tumor limited to ovaries (one or both)
T1a	IA	Tumor limited to one ovary; capsule intact, no tumor on ovarian surface. No malignant cells in ascites or peritoneal washings*
T1b	IB	Tumor limited to both ovaries; capsules intact, no tumor on ovarian surface. No malignant cells in ascites or peritoneal washings*
T1c	IC	Tumor limited to one or both ovaries with any of the following: capsule ruptured, tumor on ovarian surface, malignant cells in ascites or peritoneal washings
T2	II	Tumor involves one or both ovaries with pelvic extension and/or implants
T2a	IIA	Extension to and/or implants on uterus and/or tube(s). No malignant cells in ascites or peritoneal washings
T2b	IIB	Extension to and/or implants on other pelvic tissues. No malignant cells in ascites or peritoneal washings
T2c	IIC	Pelvic extension and/or implants (T2a or T2b) with malignant cells in ascites or peritoneal washings
T3	III	Tumor involves one or both ovaries with microscopically confirmed peritoneal metastasis outside the pelvis
T3a	IIIA	Microscopic peritoneal metastasis beyond pelvis (no macroscopic tumor)
T3b	IIIB	Macroscopic peritoneal metastasis beyond pelvis 2 cm or less in greatest dimension
T3c	IIIC	Peritoneal metastasis beyond pelvis more than 2 cm in greatest dimension and/or regional lymph node metastasis

*Note: The presence of nonmalignant ascites is not classified. The presence of ascites does not affect staging unless malignant cells are present.
Note: Liver capsule metastasis T3/Stage III; liver parenchymal metastasis M1/Stage IV. Pleural effusion must have positive cytology for M1/Stage IV.
Adapted from Greene F, Page D, Fleming I et al, editors. *American Joint Committee on Cancer Staging Manual*, ed 6, New York, 2002, Springer-Verlag.

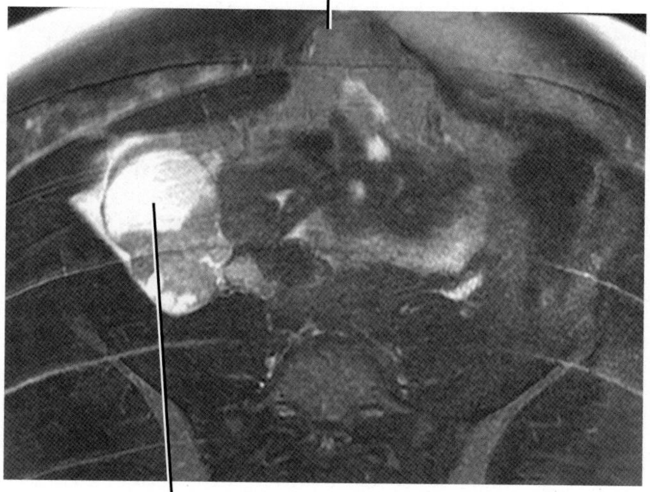

Structures to Assess
Imaging studies should be specifically evaluated for evidence of tumor involving the fallopian tube(s), uterus, and pelvic sidewall. The peritoneum should be examined closely, particularly in the regions of the cul-de-sac, adjacent to the sigmoid colon, right paracolic gutter, right subphrenic space, and omentum. The presence of ascites or pleural fluid should be noted. The rectum, sigmoid colon, cecum, and small-bowel mesentery should be examined for evidence of subperitoneal spread. Pelvic and retroperitoneal lymph nodes (especially at the level

Thick rind of peritoneal metastatic tumor

Thick-walled cystic ovarian mass (carcinoma) with surrounding fluid

Figure 10-57 Axial T2-weighted magnetic resonance imaging of the pelvis in a patient with ovarian carcinoma metastatic to the peritoneum.

of L2) and the liver should be assessed for evidence of metastases. The appendix, stomach, pancreas, and colon should be examined to ensure that these are not the original source of the ovarian tumor (tumor metastatic to ovary).

Prostate Cancer

Tumor Markers
Prostate-specific antigen (PSA) is a commonly performed screening test for prostate carcinoma and is useful to assess efficacy of treatment and to detect tumor recurrence. Prostate inflammation, injury, or benign prostatic hyperplasia (BPH) may also result in increased serum PSA levels. Prostate cancer generally results in a more rapid increase (velocity) in PSA level than BPH. A threshold serum PSA level of less than 4 ng/ml is typically used for prostate cancer screening, but up to a third of patients with prostate cancer have "normal" PSA levels.

Imaging Modalities
The two most useful modalities for prostate imaging are transrectal US and MRI, although no imaging modality currently available can be considered ideal. Transrectal US is used primarily to guide prostate biopsy and therapy rather than to stage prostate cancer. MRI has been promoted as a valuable staging modality by some centers with extensive clinical and research experience, although results in routine clinical practice are somewhat variable. MRI of the prostate at 1.5 Tesla is best performed with an endorectal coil and may be combined with dynamic contrast-enhanced imaging, spectroscopy,

and diffusion-weighted imaging. On dynamic contrast-enhanced MRI, prostate cancer may demonstrate early enhancement and early washout of gadolinium compared with the normal peripheral zone. However, this pattern is not always present. MR spectroscopy is based on detecting an altered ratio of choline (seen as a combined peak with creatine at 1.5 Tesla) to citrate (a metabolite of healthy prostate) but is tedious to perform and interpret, requires specialized equipment and software, and continues to undergo investigation and refinement. Most centers that perform MRI of the prostate rely primarily on T2-weighted imaging without fat suppression in multiple planes to detect and stage the tumor. CT is beneficial as a metastatic survey or for radiation oncology treatment planning. Tc-99m bone scintigraphy is useful to detect skeletal metastases, although it is not routinely performed in all patients (Fig. 10-58). The yield of bone scanning is greater in patients with increased PSA levels, stage T3 or T4 disease, high Gleason score, or bone pain. To date, PET has not played a significant role in the staging of prostate cancer.

Staging Highlights

Prostate cancer is commonly staged according to the AJCC TNM classification (Table 10-11). The goal of MRI of the prostate is usually to detect extracapsular tumor (T3 or T4 disease) that will preclude surgery (Fig. 10-59). Microscopic extracapsular tumor cannot be detected with current imaging techniques.

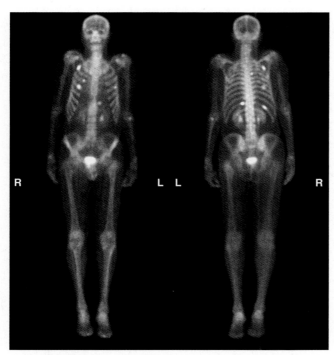

Figure 10-58 Whole-body technetium 99m bone scan demonstrating multiple rib metastases in a patient with prostate cancer.

Table 10-11   T Staging of Prostate Carcinoma

Primary Tumor (T)	
Clinical	
TX	Primary tumor cannot be assessed
T0	No evidence of primary tumor
T1	Clinically inapparent tumor neither palpable nor visible by imaging
T1a	Tumor incidental histologic finding in 5% or less of tissue resected
T1b	Tumor incidental histologic finding in more than 5% of tissue resected
T1c	Tumor identified by needle biopsy (eg, because of elevated PSA)
T2	Tumor confined within prostate*
T2a	Tumor involves one half of one lobe or less
T2b	Tumor involves more than one half of one lobe but not both lobes
T2c	Tumor involves both lobes
T3	Tumor extends through the prostate capsule**
T3a	Extracapsular extension (unilateral or bilateral)
T3b	Tumor invades seminal vesicle(s)
T4	Tumor is fixed or invades adjacent structures other than seminal vesicles: bladder neck, external sphincter, rectum, levator muscles, and/or pelvic wall
Pathologic (pT)	
pT2†	Organ confined
pT2a	Unilateral, involving one half of one lobe or less
pT2b	Unilateral, involving more than one half of one lobe but not both lobes
pT2c	Bilateral disease
pT3	Extraprostatic extension
pT3a	Extraprostatic extension††
pT3b	Seminal vesicle invasion
pT4	Invasion of bladder, rectum

*Note: Tumor found in one or both lobes by needle biopsy, but not palpable or reliably visible by imaging, is classified as T1c.
**Note: Invasion into the prostatic apex or into (but not beyond) the prostatic capsule is classified not as T3 but as T2.
†Note: There is no pathologic T1 classification.
††Note: Positive surgical margin should be indicated by an R1 descriptor (residual microscopic disease).
Adapted from Greene F, Page D, Fleming I et al, editors. *American Joint Committee on Cancer Staging Manual,* ed 6, New York, 2002, Springer-Verlag.

Gleason score is based on the histologic differentiation of the tumor, and correlates with tumor aggressiveness and stage. Gleason score cannot be determined with imaging, although attempts have been made to correlate tumor enhancement after intravenous gadolinium administration with tumor aggressiveness.

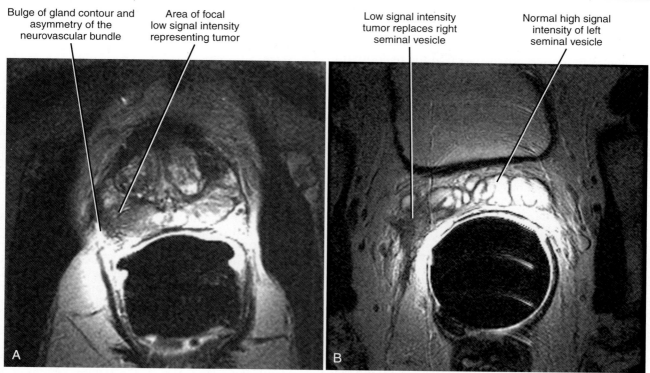

Bulge of gland contour and asymmetry of the neurovascular bundle

Area of focal low signal intensity representing tumor

Low signal intensity tumor replaces right seminal vesicle

Normal high signal intensity of left seminal vesicle

Figure 10-59 Axial T2-weighted endorectal magnetic resonance images through the prostate (**A**) and seminal vesicles (**B**) in a patient with T3b prostate cancer.

Common Mechanisms and Sites of Spread

CONTIGUOUS SPREAD

Prostate cancer spreads via direct invasion to the bladder, seminal vesicles, and rectum. Prostate cancer usually spreads first to the seminal vesicles and then to the anterior wall of the rectum near the rectosigmoid junction. On occasion, prostate cancer extends directly through Denonvillier's fascia.

LYMPHATIC SPREAD

Lymphatic spread via the pelvic lymph channels is extremely common. External iliac, internal iliac, and obturator nodes are frequently involved. Metastases to the internal iliac chains tend to be small (often <5 mm). Similar to other pelvic tumors, lymphatic spread of prostate cancer ascends from the pelvis to the paraaortic lymph nodes, to the cisterna chyli, and subsequently to the paraspinal or supraclavicular nodes, or both. Interest exists in the use of ultrasmall paramagnetic iron oxide particles to detect metastases in normal-size lymph nodes using MRI. However, such agents are not currently approved for use in the United States.

HEMATOGENOUS SPREAD

The most common site for hematogenous spread of prostate cancer is to bone (with most being osteoblastic), although it may spread to the lungs, breast, liver, adrenal glands, central nervous system, and elsewhere. The propensity of prostate cancer to preferentially involve the spine is believed related to the spread of tumor cells via the vertebral venous (Batson's) plexus.

Structures to Assess

The most important structures to assess on MR images of the prostate are the peripheral zone of the gland, prostate capsule, neurovascular bundles, seminal vesicles, bladder, rectum, pelvic lymph nodes, and bones. The peripheral zone of the prostate is normally high signal intensity on T2-weighted images. Areas of low signal intensity imply tumor, although focal fibrosis or hemorrhage (hemorrhage is bright on T1-weighted images) may also cause this finding. The prostate capsule manifests as a thin line of low signal intensity surrounding the gland on T2-weighted images. MRI findings that suggest extracapsular extension are listed in Box 10-4.

Convincing evidence of extracapsular tumor extension will often preclude surgery. Erectile dysfunction may occur because of injury to the neurovascular bundles (cavernous nerve) during prostatectomy. A similar outcome may result from irradiation of tumor in the apex of the gland (because of its close proximity to the penile root).

BOX 10-4   Findings Suggestive of Extracapsular Extension of Prostate Cancer on Magnetic Resonance Imaging

Focal irregular capsular bulge
Asymmetry of the neurovascular bundles
Obliteration of the rectoprostatic angle
Tumor within the periprostatic fat
Low T1- and T2-weighted signal intensity within the seminal vesicle(s) (T3b)

Testicular Cancer

Tumor Markers

AFP and β-HCG levels are increased in the majority of men with nonseminomatous germ cell tumors. AFP levels are most often increased in patients with embryonal carcinoma or yolk sac tumors. AFP level is not increased in pure seminoma or pure choriocarcinoma, whereas a minority of patients with seminoma will have an increased β-HCG level. Markedly increased levels of β-HCG are usually associated with choriocarcinoma. LDH level is increased in many patients with pure seminoma and nonseminomatous tumors. LDH may be the only increased tumor marker in patients with pure seminoma.

Imaging Modalities

US excels at detecting testicular carcinoma but plays little role in staging. CT and MRI are useful for identifying distant metastatic disease. PET may be useful in select patients but has not been part of the standard imaging evaluation for testicular cancer to date.

Staging Highlights

Imaging does not play a significant role in preoperative local staging of testicular cancer. The AJCC tumor (T) stage for testicular cancer is based on pathologic findings after orchiectomy. CT or MRI may be useful for identifying evidence of lymphnode or hematogenous metastases. Lymph-node (N) staging is based on lymph-node size and multiplicity. Nonregional lymph node metastases are considered distant metastases (M1a). A special category (S) exists for testicular cancer that takes into account the levels of the serum tumor markers LDH, β-HCG, and AFP.

Common Mechanisms and Sites of Spread

LYMPHATIC SPREAD

Testicular tumors tend to metastasize via the lymph channels, which parallel the testicular vessels, draining into the paraaortic lymph nodes at the level of the renal hila (Fig. 10-12). The tumor subsequently involves the paraaortic/paracaval, supraclavicular, and mediastinal nodes. Metastases from the right testis tend to involve the paracaval group. Metastases from the left testis tend to be left paraaortic, although there is frequent crossover from left to right and vice versa. Most lymph-node metastases occur ventral to the lumbar vessels. Inguinal and pelvic lymph nodes may become involved if testicular cancer extends beyond the tunica albuginea to invade the scrotum.

HEMATOGENOUS SPREAD

Lungs, liver, and brain are common sites of metastatic involvement. Hematogenous spread typically occurs after lymphatic dissemination, the exception being choriocarcinoma, which has a propensity for hematogenous spread.

Structures to Assess

Retroperitoneal lymph nodes (particularly at the level of the renal hila), liver, and lungs should be examined closely.

Lymphoma

Lymphoma represents a unique malignant disease that warrants separate consideration from other tumors arising from the abdomen and pelvis. No serologic tumor markers are useful for diagnosing lymphoma.

Imaging

Imaging is critical in determining the extent of disease. This is probably best accomplished with PET/CT (Fig. 10-60). PET has a higher sensitivity and specificity than CT alone. PET and PET/CT are rapidly replacing gallium imaging for lymphoma evaluation. Imaging is useful for initial staging before treatment and for detecting recurrence. The use of PET to monitor response to therapy is being investigated.

Staging

Lymphoid neoplasms are not staged using the TNM system. Instead, the Ann Arbor staging system is in widespread use, as follows*:

- Stage I: Involvement of a single lymph node region (I); or localized involvement of a single extralymphatic organ or site in the absence of any lymph node involvement (IE).
- Stage II: Involvement of two or more lymph node regions on the same side of the diaphragm (II); or localized involvement of a single extralymphatic organ or site in association with regional lymph node involvement with or without involvement of other lymph node regions on the same side of the diaphragm (IIE).
- Stage III: Involvement of lymph node regions on both sides of the diaphragm (III), which also may be accompanied by extralymphatic extension in association with adjacent lymph node involvement (IIIE) or by involvement of the spleen (IIIS) or both (IIIE,S).
- Stage IV: Diffuse or disseminated involvement of one or more extralymphatic organs, with or without associated lymph node involvement; or isolated extralymphatic organ involvement in the absence of adjacent regional lymph node involvement, but in conjunction with disease in distant site(s). Any involvement of the liver or bone marrow, or nodular involvement of the lung(s).

Because of the propensity of non-Hodgkin's lymphomas (NHLs) for hematogenous spread, therapy for NHL tends to be systemic. Therefore, staging is not as critical for NHL as it is for Hodgkin's lymphoma (HL).

---

*Adapted from Greene F, Page D, Fleming I et al, editors. *American Joint Committee on Cancer Staging Manual*, ed 6, New York, 2002, Springer-Verlag.

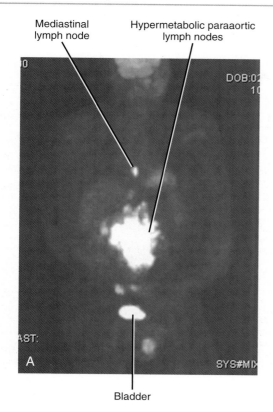

Mediastinal lymph node

Hypermetabolic paraaortic lymph nodes

Bladder

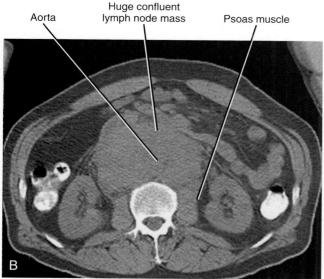

Aorta

Huge confluent lymph node mass

Psoas muscle

Figure 10-60 Maximum intensity projection image from a positron emission tomography scan (**A**) and axial unenhanced computed tomography (**B**) of a patient with newly diagnosed non-Hodgkin's lymphoma and extensive paraaortic lymphadenopathy.

Hodgkin's versus Non-Hodgkin's Lymphoma

Lymphoma is commonly divided into HL and NHL types. Each of these types of lymphoma is divided further into subtypes. Further classifying lymphoma is important for determining prognosis and therapy. However, the radiologist does not necessarily need to

Table 10-12   Typical Features of Hodgkin's versus Non-Hodgkin's Lymphoma

Features	Hodgkin's Lymphoma	Non-Hodgkin's Lymphoma
Typical spread	Contiguous	Noncontiguous
Nodes commonly involved	Cervical, mediastinal, hilar	Mesenteric and retrocrural
Retroperitoneal and mesenteric nodes	Uncommon	Common

know many details of these subtypes beyond the fact that they exist. Some notable differences exist between HL and NHL. These are summarized in Table 10-12.

HL spreads via the lymphatics from one nodal group to contiguous nodal groups and typically presents with supradiaphragmatic disease (>80%). Within the abdomen, some of the more common sites of involvement with HL are the paraaortic lymph nodes, the spleen, and the liver. Liver involvement almost always is associated with splenic and nodal disease. A normal-size spleen does not exclude involvement with HL, and splenomegaly is present in a third of patients without splenic involvement. Pulmonary involvement is more common in HL than in NHL.

NHL spreads hematogenously to involve noncontiguous sites. Extranodal disease is often present at the time of diagnosis of NHL. NHL often appears as bulky retroperitoneal and mesenteric lymphadenopathy on abdominal CT scans (Fig. 10-61). NHL may involve virtually any organ including the bowel, pancreas, kidneys, bone marrow, pelvic organs, and skin (Figs. 10-3 and 10-62).

Massive mesenteric lymph nodes surrounding the vessels of the small bowel mesentery

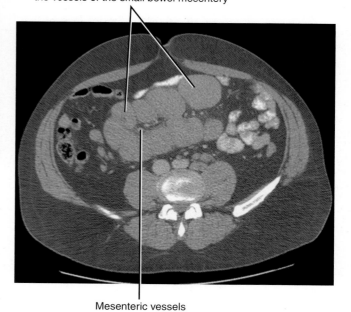

Mesenteric vessels

Figure 10-61 Axial computed tomographic scan through the lower abdomen in a patient with non-Hodgkin's lymphoma and adenopathy of the small-bowel mesentery.

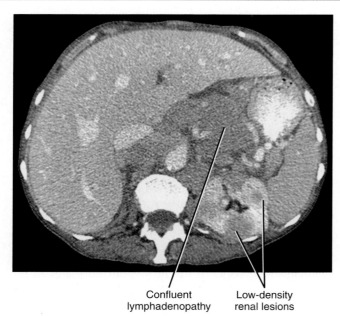

Confluent
lymphadenopathy

Low-density
renal lesions

Figure 10-62 Enhanced axial computed tomographic scan through the upper abdomen of a patient with non-Hodgkin's lymphoma of multiple organs and lymph-node groups.

Suggested Readings

Akin O, Hricak H: Imaging of prostate cancer, *Radiol Clin North Am* 45:207-222, 2007.

Akin O, Mironov S, Pandit-Taskar N et al: Imaging of uterine cancer, *Radiol Clin North Am* 45:167-182, 2007.

Barwick TD, Rockall AG, Barton DP et al: Imaging of endometrial adenocarcinoma, *Clin Radiol* 61:545-555, 2006.

Borbath I, Van Beers BE, Lonneux M et al: Preoperative assessment of pancreatic tumors using magnetic resonance imaging, endoscopic ultrasonography, positron emission tomography and laparoscopy, *Pancreatology* 5:553-561, 2005.

Chen J, Cheong J-H, Yun MJ et al: Improvement in preoperative staging of gastric adenocarcinoma with positron emission tomography, *Cancer* 103:2383-2390, 2005.

Engels JT, Balfe DM, Lee JKT: Biliary carcinoma: CT evaluation of extrahepatic spread, *Radiology* 172:35-40, 1989.

Gambhir SS, Czernin J, Schwimmer J et al: A tabulated summary of the FDG PET literature, *J Nucl Med* 42:15S-20S, 2001.

Greene F, Page D, Fleming I et al, editors: *American Joint Committee on Cancer staging manual*, ed 6, New York, 2002, Springer-Verlag.

Grubnic S, Vinnicombe SJ, Norman AR et al: MR evaluation of normal retroperitoneal and pelvic lymph nodes, *Clin Radiol* 57:193-200, 2002.

Harisinghani MG, Saini S, Weissleder R et al: MR lymphangiography using ultrasmall superparamagnetic iron oxide in patients with primary abdominal and pelvic malignancies: radiologic-pathologic correlation, *AJR Am J Roentgenol* 172:1347-1351, 1999.

Heidenreich A, Ravery V: Preoperative imaging in renal cell cancer, *World J Urol* 22:307-315, 2004.

Hong SS, Kim TK, Sung K-B et al: Extrahepatic spread of hepatocellular carcinoma: a pictorial review, *Eur Radiol* 13:874-882, 2003.

Katyal S, Oliver JH 3rd, Peterson MS et al: Extrahepatic metastases of hepatocellular carcinoma, *Radiology* 21:698-703, 2000.

Katz MH, Savides TJ, Moossa AR et al: An evidence-based approach to the diagnosis and staging of pancreatic cancer, *Pancreatology* 5:576-590, 2005.

Koh DM, Hughes M, Husband JE: Cross-sectional imaging of nodal metastases in the abdomen and pelvis, *Abdom Imaging* 31:632-643, 2006.

Kostaglu l, Agress H, Goldsmith SJ: Clinical role of FDG PET in evaluation of cancer patients, *Radiographics* 23:315-340, 2003.

Kumar R, Maillard I, Schuster SJ et al: Utility of fluorodeoxyglucose-PET imaging in the management of patients with Hodgkin's and non-Hodgkin's lymphomas, *Radiol Clin North Am* 42:1083-1100, 2004.

Kumaran V, Gulati MS, Paul SB et al: The role of dual-phase helical CT in assessing respectability of carcinoma of the gallbladder, *Eur Radiol* 12: 1993-1999, 2002.

Lane J, Buck JL, Zeman RK: Primary carcinoma of the gallbladder: a pictorial essay, *Radiographics* 9:209-228, 1989.

Lim JS, Yun MJ, Kim M-J et al: CT and PET in stomach cancer: preoperative staging and monitoring of response to therapy, *Radiographics* 26:143-156, 2006.

Lin EC, Lear J, Quaife RA: Metastatic peritoneal seeding patterns demonstrated by FDG positron emission tomographic imaging, *Clin Nucl Med* 26:249-250, 2001.

Meyers MA: Distribution of intra-abdominal malignant seeding: dependency on dynamics of flow of ascetic fluid, *AJR Am J Roentgenol* 119:198-206, 1973.

Meyers MA: *Dynamic radiology of the abdomen*, ed 5, New York, 2000, Springer-Verlag.

Mironov S, Akin O, Pandit-Taskar N et al: Ovarian cancer, *Radiol Clin North Am* 45:149-166, 2007.

Misra S, Chaturvedi A, Misra NC et al: Carcinoma of the gallbladder, *Lancet Oncol* 4:167-176, 2003.

Niederhuber JF: Colon and rectum cancer. Patterns of spread and implications for workup, *Cancer* 15:4187-4192, 1993.

Nishi M, Omori Y, Miwa K: *Japanese Research Society for Gastric Cancer (JRSGC): Japanese classification of gastric carcinoma*, Tokyo, Japan, 1995, Kanehara.

Oliphant M, Berne AS, Meyers MA: The subperitoneal space of the abdomen and pelvis: planes of continuity, *AJR Am J Roentgenol* 167: 1433-1439, 1996.

Rademaker J: Hodgkin's and non-Hodgkin's lymphomas, *Radiol Clin North Am* 45:69-83, 2007.

Ray B, Hajdu SI, Whitmore WF: Distribution of retroperitoneal lymph node metastases in testicular germinal tumors, *Cancer* 33:340-348, 1974.

Rohren EM, Turkington TG, Coleman RE: Clinical applications of PET in oncology, *Radiology* 231:305-332, 2004.

Setty BN, Holalkere NS, Sahani DV et al: State-of-the-art cross-sectional imaging in bladder cancer, *Curr Probl Diagn Radiol* 36:83-96, 2007.

Sironi S, Buda A, Picchio M et al: Lymph node metastasis in patients with clinical early-stage cervical cancer: detection with integrated FDG PET/CT, *Radiology* 238:272-279, 2006.

Turlakow A, Yeung HW, Salmon AS et al: Peritoneal carcinomatosis: role of (18)F-FDG PET, *J Nucl Med* 44:1407-1412, 2003.

Vinnicombe SJ, Norman AR, Nicolson V et al: Normal pelvic lymph nodes: evaluation with CT after bipedal lymphangiography, *Radiology* 194:349-355, 1995.

Woodward PJ, Hosseinzadeh K, Saenger JS: From the archives of the AFIP: radiologic staging of ovarian carcinoma with pathologic correlation, *Radiographics* 24:225-246, 2004.

Yang WT, Lam WW, Yu MY et al: Comparison of dynamic helical CT and dynamic MR imaging in the evaluation of pelvic lymph nodes in cervical cancer, *AJR Am J Roentgenol* 175:759-766, 2000.

Yoshimitsu K, Honda H, Shinozaki K et al: Helical CT of the local spread of carcinoma of the gallbladder: evaluation according to the TNM system in patients who underwent surgical resection, *AJR Am J Roentgenol* 179: 423-428, 2002.

Zhang J, Gerst S, Lefkowitz RA et al: Imaging of bladder cancer, *Radiol Clin North Am* 45:183-205, 2007.

Zhang J, Lefkowitz RA, Bach A: Imaging of kidney cancer, *Radiol Clin North Am* 45:119-147, 2007.

CHAPTER 11

Common Inherited and Metabolic Disorders

Andrew Deibler and John R. Leyendecker

Metabolic and inherited disorders are routinely encountered in pediatric radiology, where they often dominate the disease spectrum, and thus are more easily brought to mind when formulating differential diagnoses. In adult radiological practice, by contrast, most disease processes are acquired and a few general disease categories predominate, namely, neoplastic, traumatic, infectious, and inflammatory diseases. With few exceptions, no isolated finding on an abdominal imaging examination is pathognomonic for an inherited or metabolic disorder. However, an atypical distribution or multiplicity of a common lesion, or the coexistence of particular imaging findings should invite consideration of this disease category. As our knowledge of inherited diseases increases, it is likely that the list of inherited disorders and syndromes will continue to grow.

The goal of this chapter is to provide a practical, organ-system–based approach to commonly encountered inherited and metabolic diseases (Tables 11-1 and 11-2). Because of the vast number of potential hereditary syndromes, the focus has been kept on describing some of the more commonly encountered or discussed syndromes with typical abdominal imaging manifestations in adults. A detailed description of the germline mutations and other specific genetic features for each of the inherited conditions is beyond the scope of this chapter, but the Suggested Readings at the end of this chapter list several excellent references for further information. To avoid redundancy, we do not discuss the imaging appearance of the specific abnormalities that comprise each entity in any detail. Instead, the imaging appearances of the various cysts, tumors, and other abnormalities that may comprise a particular syndrome are discussed in detail in the organ-specific chapters in Section III of this textbook.

■ HEPATOBILIARY ABNORMALITIES

Diffuse Liver Disease

The liver is a complex organ involved in endocrine, exocrine, synthetic, and excretory function. Therefore, the liver is often a final common pathway for disease expression in inherited and metabolic disorders. Potential imaging features of metabolic disease that affects the liver diffusely include hepatomegaly, steatosis, and fibrosis. The presence of these findings in a young patient

without known risk factors, such as alcoholism, may signal an underlying inherited or metabolic disorder.

Steatosis

The excess deposition of fat within hepatocytes can result from a large number of acquired factors and inherited metabolic derangements. Hepatic steatosis manifests on imaging studies as increased liver echogenicity (ultrasound) or decreased liver density (computed tomography [CT]). With MRI, the steatotic liver appears as higher than normal signal intensity on non–fat-suppressed T1-weighted images. On in- and opposed-phase gradient-echo images (chemical shift imaging), the steatotic liver loses signal on opposed-phase images relative to in-phase images. Some better known metabolic and inherited causes of hepatic steatosis are listed in Box 11-1.

Iron Deposition

As with fat deposition, iron can be deposited in the liver as a result of a large number of acquired and hereditary disorders. Excess hepatic iron deposition manifests as increased attenuation on CT images, although the findings may be subtle. Magnetic resonance imaging (MRI) is more sensitive for the detection of excess iron in the liver, manifesting as decreased signal intensity on T1- and T2-weighted magnetic resonance (MR) images. The signal intensity loss on MR images worsens with increasing echo time.

Most cases of hereditary (a.k.a. primary) hemochromatosis involve a mutation in the *HFE* gene that results in excess intestinal absorption of dietary iron. The excess iron is deposited directly within a variety of organs, typically excluding the spleen. Hereditary hemochromatosis

---

BOX 11-1   Select Metabolic and Inherited Causes of Hepatic Steatosis and Steatohepatitis

Abetalipoproteinemia
Cystic fibrosis (Fig. 11-1)
Diabetes mellitus
Endogenous corticosteroid excess
Glycogen storage disease
Hyperlipidemia
Obesity
Wilson disease

Table 11-1   Alphabetical List of Select Inherited and Metabolic Disorders with Imaging Manifestations in the Adult

Disorder	Abdominal Region	Extraabdominal Regions
Autosomal dominant polycystic kidney disease (ADPKD)	Innumerable renal cysts Enlarged kidneys Nephrolithiasis (up to 20%) Hepatic cysts (50% or more) Hepatomegaly Cysts of other organs (e.g., pancreas, seminal vesicle) Diverticulosis Hernias	Intracranial aneurysms (up to 15%) Valvular heart disease Aortic coarctation Arachnoid cysts
Autosomal recessive polycystic kidney disease (ARPKD)	Congenital hepatic fibrosis Varices Splenomegaly Caroli disease and choledochal cyst Bile duct hamartomas Renal cysts	
Caroli disease	Saccular intrahepatic biliary ductal dilatation Intrahepatic biliary calculi Hepatic fibrosis (Caroli syndrome) Renal tubular ectasia ADPKD (rare association)	
Congenital hepatic fibrosis	Periportal fibrosis Varices Splenomegaly Caroli disease and choledochal cyst Bile duct hamartomas ARPKD	
Cowden disease	Hamartomatous polyps Malignant pelvic tumors	Hemangiomas Neuromas Breast cancer Thyroid abnormalities Glycogenic acanthosis
Cystic fibrosis (CF)	Hepatic fibrosis Hepatic steatosis Biliary ductal strictures, dilatation, calculi Microgallbladder Pancreatic enlargement, atrophy, fatty replacement Pancreatic cysts Pancreatitis Thickened appendix and appendicitis Peptic ulcer disease Meconium ileus equivalent Intussusception Gastrointestinal malignancies Nephrolithiasis Testicular abnormalities	Bronchiectasis Pulmonary infections
Diabetes mellitus	Hepatic steatosis Emphysematous urinary tract infections Diabetic nephropathy Renal papillary necrosis	Arthropathy Osteomyelitis Ischemic heart disease Vascular disease
Familial adenomatous polyposis syndrome (FAP)	Innumerable adenomatous colon polyps Colon cancer Gastric fundic gland retention polyps Gastric adenomas Duodenal and small-bowel adenomatous polyps (tend to cluster around major papilla) Periampullary cancer Extraintestinal malignancies	

Table 11-1   Alphabetical List of Select Inherited and Metabolic Disorders with Imaging Manifestations in the Adult—cont'd

Disorder	Abdominal Region	Extraabdominal Regions
Gardner syndrome	Same as FAP Desmoid tumors Retroperitoneal fibrosis	Mandibular osteomas Dental abnormalities
Gaucher disease (β-glucocerebrosidase deficiency) type I	Hepatosplenomegaly Hepatic fibrosis (uncommon) Hepatocellular carcinoma Lymphoproliferative disease Extramedullary hematopoiesis Splenic infarcts Splenic nodules	Osteonecrosis Long-bone deformities Osteopenia
Glycogen storage disease type I	Hepatomegaly Hepatic adenomas Hepatocellular carcinoma Renal enlargement	Osteoporosis
Glycogen storage disease type III	Hepatosplenomegaly Cirrhosis Hepatic adenomas Hepatocellular carcinoma	Cardiomegaly
Hereditary hemochromatosis	Iron deposition predominantly in liver and pancreas Cirrhosis Hepatocellular carcinoma	Myocardial iron deposition Congestive heart failure
Hereditary hemorrhagic telangiectasia (HHT)	Liver vascular malformations Enlarged hepatic artery Vascular malformations of other abdominal organs	Pulmonary arteriovenous malformations Central nervous system (CNS) vascular malformations
Lynch syndrome (hereditary nonpolyposis colorectal cancer syndrome [HNPCC])	Colorectal cancer Gastric cancer Small-bowel cancer Hepatobiliary cancer Endometrial cancer Urinary tract cancer Ovarian cancer	CNS tumors
Multiple endocrine neoplasia (MEN) type 1	Enteropancreatic neuroendocrine tumors (gastrinomas most common, often malignant and metastatic) Zollinger–Ellison syndrome Nephrolithiasis (secondary to parathyroid tumors) Adrenal cortical adenoma (up to 40%) Stomach and duodenal carcinoid tumor	Primary hyperparathyroidism Anterior pituitary adenoma (30%) Thymic and bronchial carcinoid tumor (3%) Thyroid adenoma Multiple lipomas
MEN type 2	Pheochromocytoma (50% of MEN 2, usually adrenal, 50% bilateral) Mucosal and intestinal ganglioneuromatosis (MEN 2B)	Medullary thyroid carcinoma Primary hyperparathyroidism (MEN 2A)
Neurofibromatosis type 1 (NF-1)	Pheochromocytoma and paragangliomas Neurofibromas and plexiform neurofibromas Malignant peripheral nerve sheath tumor Ganglioneuromas Gastrointestinal carcinoid tumors Gastrointestinal stromal tumor	Optic glioma Bone dysplasia Cutaneous and subcutaneous neurofibromas Plexiform neurofibromas Malignant peripheral nerve sheath tumor Spinal deformities

Continued

Table 11-1   Alphabetical List of Select Inherited and Metabolic Disorders with Imaging Manifestations in the Adult—cont'd

Disorder	Abdominal Region	Extraabdominal Regions
Peutz–Jeghers syndrome	Hamartomatous polyps (most common in small bowel but may occur in stomach and colon) Intussusception Bowel obstruction Sex cord tumors with annular tubules (SCTAT; benign ovarian neoplasm) Adenoma malignum (aggressive adenocarcinoma of cervix) Sertoli cell tumor of testes Intestinal and extraintestinal malignant tumors (e.g., small intestine, stomach, pancreas, colon, ovary)	Extraabdominal malignant tumors (e.g., lung, breast, esophagus)
Sickle cell disease*	Small, calcified spleen (autoinfarction) Splenomegaly (sequestration or extramedullary hematopoiesis) Cholelithiasis Cirrhosis Hemosiderosis Renal enlargement or infarction Renal papillary necrosis Renal medullary carcinoma (sickle trait)	Acute chest syndrome Interstitial lung disease Cranial vasculopathy Marrow expansion Extramedullary hematopoiesis Bone infarction Osteomyelitis
Tuberous sclerosis complex	Multiple angiomyolipomas (up to 80% of adults) Renal cysts (20%) Lymphangiomas Splenic cysts Colorectal hamartomatous polyps	Cortical tubers (brain) Subependymal nodules Giant cell astrocytomas Cardiac rhabdomyomas Pulmonary lymphangioleiomyomatosis Nonrenal hamartomas Bone cysts
Turcot syndrome	Colorectal adenomatous polyposis Colorectal cancer	Malignant CNS tumors
von Hippel–Lindau disease	Renal cell carcinoma (up to 70%, often multicentric) Renal cysts (50%-70%) Pancreatic cysts Microcystic (serous) cystadenoma Pheochromocytoma (7%-20%, often bilateral) Enteropancreatic neuroendocrine tumors Epididymal cysts Epididymal papillary cystadenoma Broad ligament papillary cystadenoma	Retinal and CNS hemangioblastomas

Lists do not represent diagnostic criteria; they represent findings that may be present on imaging studies and findings for which patients are at increased risk. Not all findings listed will be present in all patients.
*Manifestations depend on homozygous or heterozygous state.

involves the liver and pancreas on imaging studies (best appreciated with MRI) (Fig. 11-2). Patients with hereditary hemochromatosis are at significant risk for cirrhosis and hepatocellular carcinoma (HCC).

Most nonhereditary cases of iron deposition within the liver involve the reticuloendothelial system (RES) rather than the hepatocytes. This form of hemosiderin deposition is particularly common in anemia of chronic disease or in patients who receive multiple blood transfusions. Patients with end-stage renal disease often demonstrate hemosiderin deposition within the liver, spleen, and bone marrow. Patients with thalassemia who have not received multiple blood transfusions may demonstrate increased iron deposition in the hepatocytes because of increased intestinal absorption of iron, mimicking hereditary hemochromatosis. Patients with transfusion-dependent thalassemia will have excess iron deposited in the RES, as well as the hepatocytes. The presence of iron deposition within the renal cortex in addition to the liver and spleen (best demonstrated as low signal intensity on T2- or T2*-weighted MR images) should prompt consideration of a hemolytic disorder rather than hereditary hemochromatosis or hemosiderosis resulting from multiple blood transfusions (Fig. 11-3).

Pearl: Iron deposition in the liver and pancreas that spares the spleen suggests hereditary (primary) hemochromatosis. Iron deposition that involves the liver and spleen that spares the pancreas suggests other form of hemosiderosis (e.g., multiple blood transfusions). Iron deposition that involves the renal cortex suggests hemolysis (e.g., paroxysmal nocturnal hemoglobinuria [PNH], sickle cell disease, mechanical heart valve).

Table 11-2   Abdominal Imaging Combinations That Suggest Inherited Disorder

Combination of Findings Present	Disorders to Consider
Multiple renal cysts Large kidneys Liver cysts	Autosomal dominant polycystic kidney disease
Multiple renal cysts Renal cell carcinoma(s) Pancreatic cyst(s)/mass(es) Normal-size kidneys Adrenal mass(es) or paraganglioma(s)	von Hippel–Lindau disease
Multiple fat-containing renal lesions Renal cysts Perinephric hematoma Fat-containing liver lesion(s) Lung cysts	Tuberous sclerosis complex
Renal cysts Normal-size kidneys Stigmata of portal hypertension Biliary sacculations/cysts	Congenital hepatic fibrosis
Colorectal polyps Mesenteric or abdominal wall mass	Gardner syndrome
Diminutive or calcified spleen Cholelithiasis/cholecystitis Hemosiderosis Renal papillary necrosis Interstitial lung disease Bone infarcts	Sickle cell disease
Small or absent gallbladder Hepatic steatosis Pancreatitis/pancreatic atrophy (fat replaced) Fecalization of small-bowel contents	Cystic fibrosis
Hepatosplenomegaly Cirrhosis Extramedullary hematopoiesis	Gaucher disease
Pancreatic mass(es) Adrenal mass(es) (not adenoma)	Multiple endocrine neoplasia von Hippel–Lindau disease
Multiple cutaneous and subcutaneous nodules Mesenteric mass(es) Adrenal mass(es) (not adenoma) Spinal deformities Multiple intramural bowel masses	Neurofibromatosis type 1
Vascular malformations of the liver and gastrointestinal tract Enlarged hepatic artery	Hereditary hemorrhagic telangiectasia

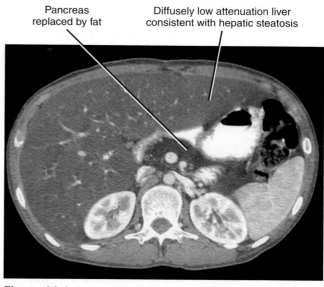

Figure 11-1 Enhanced axial computed tomographic scan of a patient with cystic fibrosis demonstrating severe hepatic steatosis and replacement of pancreatic parenchyma with fat.

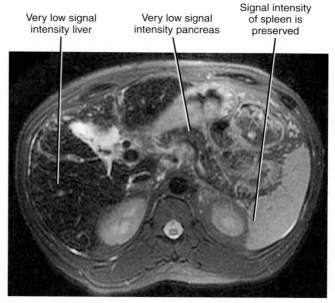

Figure 11-2 Axial T2-weighted magnetic resonance image through liver and pancreas of a patient with primary hemochromatosis.

intervening fibrosis. Potential inherited and metabolic causes of cirrhosis are listed in Box 11-2. Cirrhosis can also result from either hereditary hemochromatosis or hepatic steatosis complicated by steatohepatitis.

Cirrhosis

Cirrhosis represents a nonspecific response of the liver to any of a large number of hepatotoxins, functional derangements, or metabolic abnormalities consisting of hepatocellular injury, nodular regeneration, and

Fibropolycystic Liver Disease

Maldevelopment of the ductal plate of the liver may cause a spectrum of conditions collectively termed *fibropolycystic liver disease*. One or more of these conditions can coexist in an individual patient and can be associated with concomitant renal cystic disease.

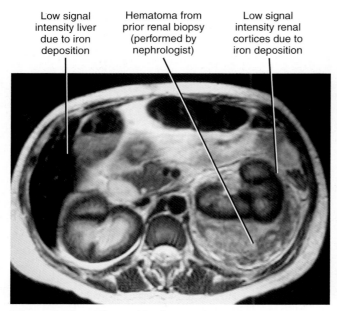

Figure 11-3 Axial T2-weighted magnetic resonance imaging through the kidneys of a patient with paroxysmal nocturnal hemoglobinuria.

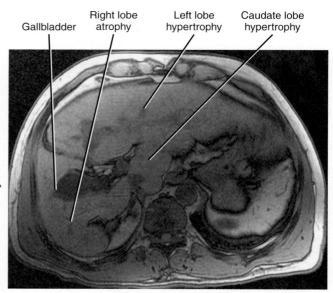

Figure 11-4 Axial unenhanced T1-weighted magnetic resonance image through the liver of a young man with Gaucher disease–associated cirrhosis.

BOX 11-2   Select Nonacquired Causes of Cirrhosis

α1 antitrypsin deficiency
Amino acid disorders (e.g., tyrosinemia)
Bile acid disorders
Carbohydrate disorders (e.g., fructose intolerance, galactosemia, glycogen storage disease)
Congenital hepatic fibrosis
Cystic fibrosis
Gaucher disease (Fig. 11-4)
Hemochromatosis (Fig. 11-5)
Hypercoagulable disorders (e.g., factor V Leiden, PNH)
Lipid disorders (e.g., abetalipoproteinemia)
Porphyrias
Urea cycle abnormalities
Wilson disease

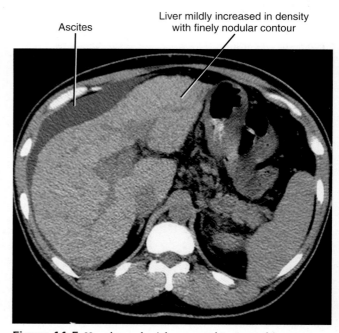

Figure 11-5 Unenhanced axial computed tomographic scan through the liver of a patient with primary hemochromatosis-associated cirrhosis.

Congenital Hepatic Fibrosis

Congenital hepatic fibrosis is closely associated with autosomal recessive polycystic kidney disease. In such cases, the severity of hepatic involvement observes an inverse relation with the degree of the renal involvement. Congenital hepatic fibrosis results in periportal fibrosis progressing to portal hypertension, splenomegaly, and formation of varices. Congenital hepatic fibrosis can lead to typical morphologic changes of cirrhosis such as right lobe atrophy and left lateral segment and caudate lobe hypertrophy. However, enlargement, rather than atrophy, of the medial segment has been described as a distinguishing feature of congenital hepatic fibrosis versus viral or alcoholic cirrhosis. Congenital hepatic fibrosis can coexist with Caroli disease.

Polycystic Liver Disease

Polycystic liver disease can occur as an extrarenal manifestation of autosomal dominant polycystic kidney disease (ADPKD) or as a genetically distinct entity without renal cysts. Biliary cysts occur in approximately 25% to 50% of patients with ADPKD and are usually randomly distributed throughout the hepatic parenchyma (Fig. 11-6). The cysts of ADPKD have similar imaging characteristics to sporadic hepatic cysts, when not complicated by hemorrhage or

Liver nearly replaced
by cysts of variable size

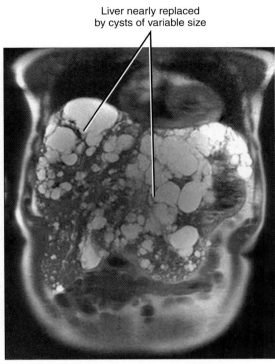

Figure 11-6 Coronal T2-weighted magnetic resonance image through the liver in a patient with polycystic liver disease.

Peribiliary cysts   Large complicated cyst

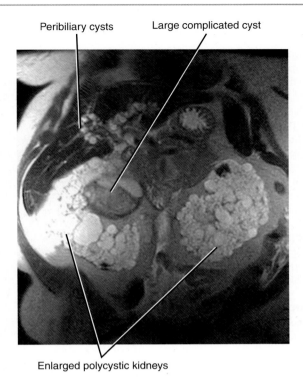

Enlarged polycystic kidneys

Figure 11-7 Coronal T2-weighted magnetic resonance image through the abdomen of a patient with autosomal dominant polycystic liver disease and peribiliary cysts.

infection. As with biliary hamartomas (to which these cysts are thought to be related), the cysts in ADPKD do not communicate with the biliary tree. Like their renal counterparts, these hepatic cysts can be complicated by infection, rupture, or rapid enlargement caused by intracystic hemorrhage, all of which may result in symptoms of acute abdominal pain. Cysts in polycystic liver disease can also compress and obstruct hepatic veins and inferior vena cava, portal veins, or bile ducts. Occasionally, a periportal distribution of liver cysts is seen with ADPKD (Fig. 11-7).

Caroli Disease
Caroli disease manifests as saccular intrahepatic biliary dilatation, leading to biliary stasis, stones, and cholangitis. Caroli disease can be distinguished from polycystic liver disease, because the "cysts" in Caroli disease communicate with the bile ducts. The dilated bile ducts in Caroli disease engulf the portal triads, resulting in what is known as the "central dot" sign on cross-sectional imaging studies. Caroli disease can coexist with congenital hepatic fibrosis, and there have been rare reports of Caroli disease associated with ADPKD. These associations likely relate to the role of the ductal plate in producing each of these abnormalities.

Pearl: The central dot sign helps distinguish Caroli disease from other cystic processes within the liver.

Biliary Hamartomas
Biliary hamartomas, also known as von Meyenburg complex, are small hepatic lesions composed of biliary epithelial-lined ductlike structures and fibrous stroma.

Biliary hamartomas are typically less than 15 mm in size, multiple, and mimic tiny cysts on CT and MR studies (Fig. 11-8). Because these lesions also result from maldevelopment of the ductal plate, it is not surprising that these lesions can be seen in association with the hereditary ductal plate abnormalities discussed earlier.

Innumerable tiny high signal intensity
foci scattered throughout liver

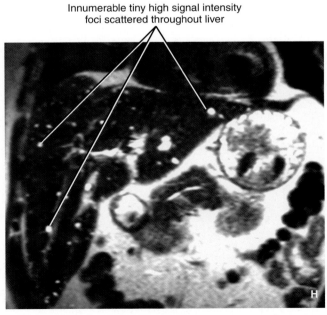

Figure 11-8 Coronal T2-weighted magnetic resonance image through the liver of a patient with multiple bile duct hamartomas.

Hepatic Neoplasms

Hepatic Adenoma

Hepatic adenoma is a benign liver tumor that most radiologists associate with young women who take oral contraceptives or men who take anabolic steroids. However, hepatic adenomas can also be found in up to half of patients with glycogen storage disorder type I and a quarter of patients with glycogen storage disease type III (Fig. 11-9). Hepatic adenomas in patients with glycogen storage disease tend to be multiple and carry a small risk for degeneration into HCC. Although rare, the incidence of malignant transformation is difficult to precisely determine from the literature.

Hepatic Angiomyolipoma

Hepatic angiomyolipomas (AMLs) occur with increased frequency in patients with tuberous sclerosis complex (TSC).

Hepatocellular Carcinoma

Most cases of HCC occur in patients with acquired liver disease (e.g., related to viral hepatitis or alcohol-induced cirrhosis). However, any of the earlier-described causes of cirrhosis, such as glycogen storage disease, hemochromatosis, or Wilson disease, can lead to the development of HCC (Fig. 11-10). HCC can rarely result from malignant transformation of a hepatic adenoma. Metabolic disorders such as galactosemia and tyrosinemia are causes of HCC in young patients.

Vascular Malformations

Hereditary Hemorrhagic Telangiectasia

Hereditary hemorrhagic telangiectasia (HHT) is the most common cause of diffuse vascular malformations of the liver. Patients rarely present with symptoms

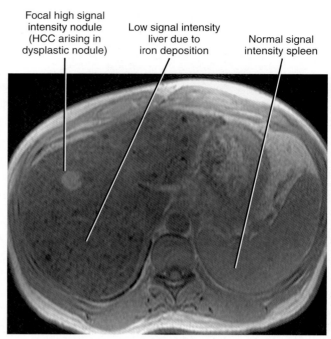

Focal high signal intensity nodule (HCC arising in dysplastic nodule)

Low signal intensity liver due to iron deposition

Normal signal intensity spleen

Figure 11-10 Axial T1-weighted magnetic resonance image through the liver of a patient with primary hemochromatosis-induced cirrhosis and hepatocellular carcinoma.

related to liver involvement. Instead, liver vascular malformations are usually discovered incidentally in patients with complications related to involvement of other organ systems such as the lungs or gastrointestinal tract. Intrahepatic shunting may occur between the hepatic artery and portal or hepatic veins, or between the portal vein and hepatic vein. The hepatic artery often becomes much enlarged in patients with HHT (Fig. 11-11). Malformations vary in size from microscopic shunts to large confluent vascular masses. The reported prevalence of hepatic vascular malformations

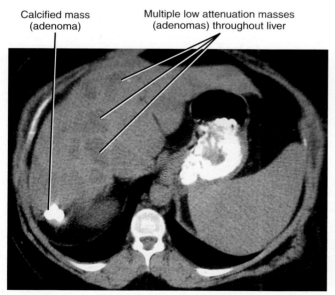

Calcified mass (adenoma)

Multiple low attenuation masses (adenomas) throughout liver

Figure 11-9 Unenhanced axial computed tomographic scan through the liver of a patient with type I glycogen storage disease and hepatic adenomatosis.

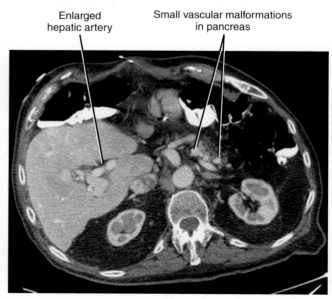

Enlarged hepatic artery

Small vascular malformations in pancreas

Figure 11-11 Axial enhanced computed tomographic image of a patient with hereditary hemorrhagic telangiectasia.

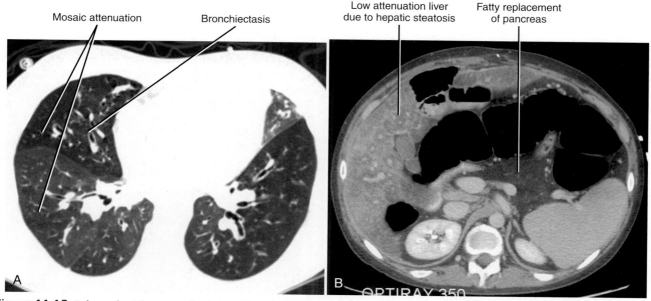

Mosaic attenuation   Bronchiectasis

Low attenuation liver due to hepatic steatosis   Fatty replacement of pancreas

Figure 11-12 Enhanced axial computed tomographic scan through the lungs **(A)** and upper abdomen **(B)** of a young adult patient with cystic fibrosis demonstrating bronchiectasis and mosaic attenuation at the lung bases **(A)**, and hepatic steatosis and fatty replacement of the pancreas **(B)**.

in patients with HHT also varies considerably, but the reported prevalence appears to be increasing as imaging technology improves. Although uncommon, complications of hepatic vascular malformations include heart failure, portal hypertension, encephalopathy, abdominal pain, and biliary abnormalities (likely caused by biliary ischemia). Intrahepatic shunting of blood can lead to development of nodular regenerative hyperplasia that may be confused with cirrhosis.

Pearl: Patients with hepatic involvement of HHT will often have a markedly enlarged hepatic artery.

◼ PANCREATIC ABNORMALITIES

Diffuse Pancreatic Abnormalities

Fatty Replacement
Patients with cystic fibrosis typically demonstrate diffuse fatty replacement of the pancreas such that normal pancreatic parenchyma is difficult to visualize on imaging studies (Fig. 11-12). Shwachman–Diamond syndrome is an inherited disorder of children characterized by pancreatic exocrine insufficiency and bone marrow failure that can be confused with cystic fibrosis. As with cystic fibrosis, fatty replacement of the pancreas is characteristic.

Diffuse Cystic Disease
Patients with von Hippel–Lindau disease (vHL) may have multiple epithelial cysts of variable size distributed throughout the pancreatic parenchyma (Fig. 11-13). In severe cases, the entire parenchyma appears replaced by cysts on imaging studies. Patients with cystic fibrosis may develop diffuse replacement of the pancreas by small cysts (pancreatic cystosis).

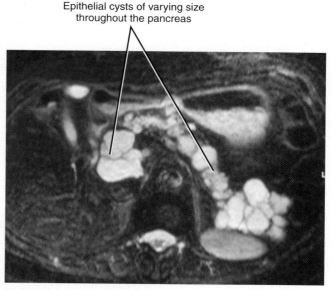

Epithelial cysts of varying size throughout the pancreas

Figure 11-13 Axial, fat-suppressed, T2-weighted image through the pancreas of a patient with von Hippel–Lindau disease.

Pancreatitis
Hereditary pancreatitis is an uncommon cause of acute pancreatitis characterized by recurrent bouts of acute pancreatitis in childhood and frequent progression to chronic pancreatitis. Hereditary pancreatitis is associated with a 40% cumulative lifetime risk for pancreatic cancer. Acute and chronic pancreatitis have also been reported in patients with other inborn errors of metabolism such as disorders of lipid metabolism, homocystinuria, and acute intermittent porphyria.

Iron Deposition

Iron deposition in the pancreas is typical of but not specific for hereditary hemochromatosis (see Fig. 11-2). Iron deposition in the pancreas is best demonstrated on T2*-weighted MRI. Evidence of iron deposition in RES organs such as the spleen and bone marrow suggests a cause other than hereditary hemochromatosis.

Focal Pancreatic Abnormalities

Pancreatic Cysts

True epithelial pancreatic cysts are relatively rare lesions compared with pancreatic pseudocysts and cystic mucinous neoplasms. The presence of pancreatic epithelial cysts may serve as a clue to the underlying cause of multiple renal cysts. vHL and ADPKD are syndromes associated with true pancreatic cysts and renal cysts (Fig. 11-14). Although pancreatic cysts in the setting of vHL tend to occur relatively commonly

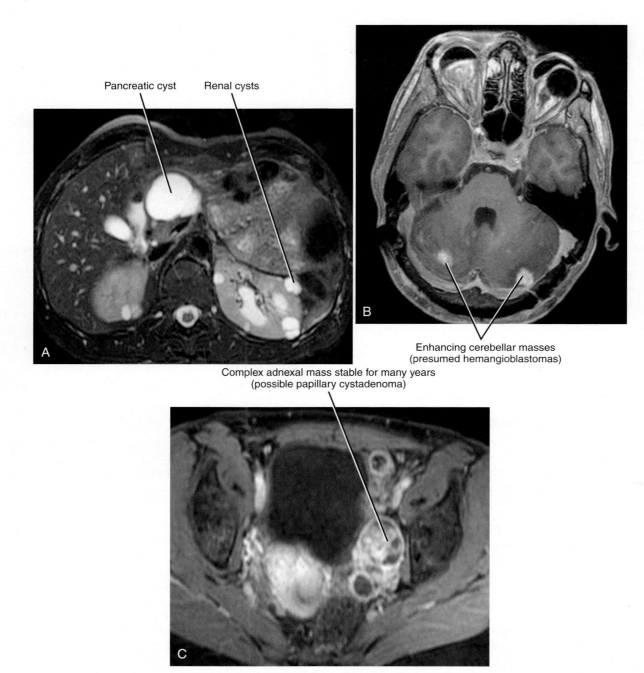

Figure 11-14 Axial T2-weighted magnetic resonance (MR) image through the abdomen **(A)**, enhanced axial T1-weighted MR image through the brain **(B)**, and enhanced axial, T1-weighted, fat-suppressed MR image through the pelvis **(C)** of a patient with von Hippel–Lindau disease.

and are numerous, most patients with ADPKD do not have pancreatic cysts evident on imaging studies.

Serous Cystadenoma
Serous cystadenoma of the pancreas most often occurs sporadically in older women but can be associated with vHL.

Neuroendocrine Tumors
Pancreatic and duodenal neuroendocrine tumors occur sporadically or in association with syndromes such as multiple endocrine neoplasia type 1 (MEN 1) and vHL. At CT and MRI, enteropancreatic neuroendocrine neoplasms associated with a hereditary syndrome tend to be smaller than nonsyndromic tumors at presentation and are often multiple. Neuroendocrine tumors in MEN 1 tend to be functional, with gastrinomas accounting for 60% of tumors. Insulinomas are the second most common tumor type in MEN 1 and can coexist with gastrinomas. Neuroendocrine tumors are present in approximately 12% of patients with vHL and are usually nonfunctioning, with the majority of small (<2-3 cm) tumors being benign. Therefore, small incidental neuroendocrine tumors are often followed with imaging rather than resected initially in patients with vHL (Fig. 11-15). Neuroendocrine tumors of the pancreas may rarely occur in the setting of neurofibromatosis type 1 (NF-1) and TSC.

▪ GASTROINTESTINAL ABNORMALITIES

Gastrointestinal Tumors

Malignant Neoplasms
A small percentage of gastrointestinal malignant neoplasms occur in association with a known inherited disorder. Hereditary nonpolyposis colorectal cancer (HNPCC, also known as Lynch syndrome) is an autosomal dominant disorder predisposing patients to colon cancer, as well as a variety of gynecologic, abdominal, and urologic cancers. Factors that suggest HNPCC include multiple synchronous or metachronous colon cancers, diagnosis of colon cancer before age 50 years, and concurrent tumors in other locations such as the endometrium, ovary, or bladder.

Gastrointestinal polyposis syndromes account for less than 1% of new colon cancer diagnoses. Syndromes with an increased risk for colon cancer include familial adenomatous polyposis syndrome (FAP) and its variants, and to a lesser extent, juvenile polyposis and Peutz–Jeghers syndrome (Fig. 11-16). Gastrointestinal stromal tumors (GISTs) are associated with NF-1 and Carney triad (GIST, pulmonary chondromas (Fig. 11-17), pheochromocytoma).

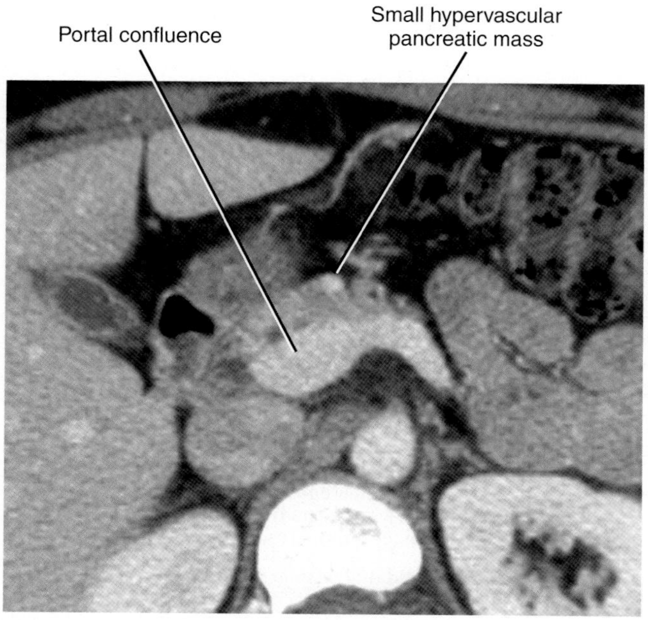

Portal confluence

Small hypervascular pancreatic mass

Figure 11-15 Screening axial-enhanced computed tomography through the pancreas of a patient with von Hippel–Lindau disease demonstrating small hypervascular mass in pancreas subsequently confirmed with magnetic resonance imaging. A decision was made to observe this lesion with imaging.

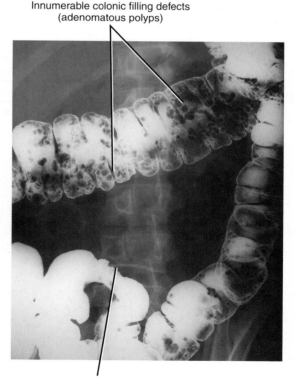

Innumerable colonic filling defects (adenomatous polyps)

Fixed narrowing (carcinoma) of sigmoid colon

Figure 11-16 Double-contrast barium enema of patient with Gardner variant of familial adenomatous polyposis showing diffuse colonic adenomatous polyposis and carcinoma of sigmoid colon. (Courtesy Dr. David Ott.)

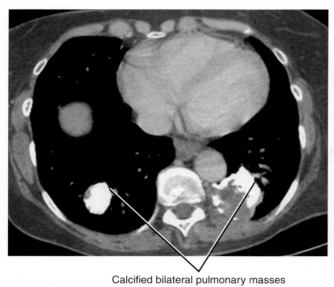

Calcified bilateral pulmonary masses

Figure 11-17 Enhanced axial computed tomographic scan of a patient with pulmonary chondromas related to Carney triad. The patient previously had resection of gastrointestinal stromal tumor and pheochromocytoma.

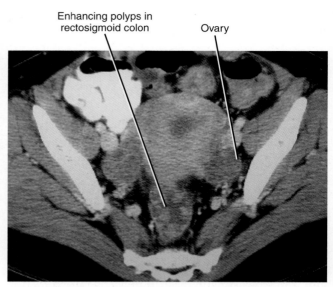

Enhancing polyps in rectosigmoid colon   Ovary

Figure 11-18 Enhanced axial computed tomographic scan through the pelvis of a woman with familial adenomatous polyposis syndrome demonstrating numerous enhancing polyps in rectosigmoid colon.

Polyps

A number of inherited disorders are associated with gastrointestinal polyps (Table 11-3). Patients with FAP experience development of innumerable colonic polyps, and almost all individuals with this disorder experience development of colon cancer by age 40 years if proctocolectomy is not performed (Fig. 11-18). FAP is usually inherited as an autosomal dominant trait (*adenomatous polyposis coli [APC]* gene mutation) but can occur because of a sporadic mutation. Gardner and Turcot syndromes are subclassifications of FAP with additional associations (see Fig. 11-16). Patients with FAP are also at risk for development of duodenal and ampullary carcinomas, a major cause of morbidity in

Table 11-3   Inherited Gastrointestinal Polyposis Syndromes

Syndrome	Primary Type of Polyps	Other Manifestations
Familial adenomatous polyposis (FAP)	Adenomatous (colon, stomach, duodenum, small bowel)	Colon cancer Periampullary carcinoma
Gardner variant of FAP	Adenomatous	Desmoid tumors Retroperitoneal fibrosis Mandibular osteomas Dental abnormalities Extraintestinal cancers
Turcot variant of FAP	Adenomatous	Malignant central nervous system tumors
Attenuated adenomatous polyposis coli	Adenomatous	
Familial juvenile polyposis	Hamartomatous (primarily stomach, colon)	Colon cancer Gastric cancer Small-bowel cancer Pancreatic cancer Intussusception
Peutz–Jeghers syndrome	Hematomatous (most prevalent in small bowel but also occur in stomach and colon)	Hyperpigmented macules Extraintestinal hamartomas Intestinal and extraintestinal malignant tumors (e.g., pancreatic cancer)
Cowden disease	Hamartomatous (proximal gastrointestinal tract through rectum)	Skin and oral lesions common Hemangiomas Neuromas Breast cancer Thyroid abnormalities Glycogenic acanthosis Malignant pelvic tumors

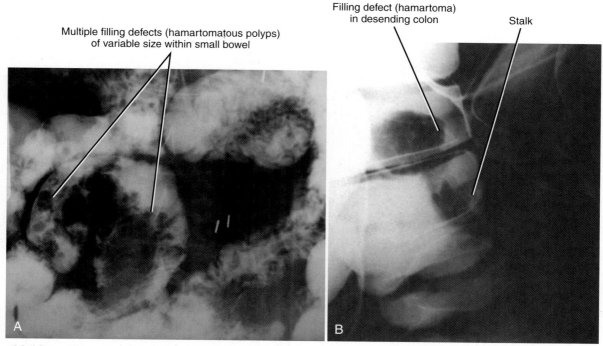

Multiple filling defects (hamartomatous polyps) of variable size within small bowel

Filling defect (hamartoma) in desending colon

Stalk

Figure 11-19 Small bowel barium examination (**A**) and barium enema (**B**) of a patient with Peutz–Jeghers syndrome demonstrating multiple bowel hamartomas. (Courtesy Dr. David Ott)

patients who have had prior colectomy. Attenuated familial APC syndrome is a variant of FAP that refers to patients who have fewer than 100 colorectal polyps at presentation and delayed onset of colorectal cancer.

The hamartomatous polyposis syndromes are considerably less common than the adenomatous syndromes and include familial juvenile polyposis syndrome, Peutz–Jeghers syndrome, Cowden syndrome, and Bannayan–Ruvalcaba–Riley syndrome (Fig. 11-19). Cowden disease and Bannayan–Ruvalcaba–Riley syndrome may result from mutation of the same (*PTEN*) gene and are considered by some to represent a single entity (PTEN hamartoma syndrome). Tuberous sclerosis is not considered a hamartomatous polyposis syndrome but may be associated with rectal hamartomatous polyps.

Other Gastrointestinal Abnormalities

Zollinger–Ellison Syndrome

Zollinger–Ellison (ZE) syndrome is defined as hypergastrinemia caused by the presence of a gastrin-secreting tumor, usually located in the pancreas or duodenum. Characterized by the presence of multiple peptic ulcers in the stomach and proximal small bowel, ZE syndrome may occur sporadically or in association with an inherited disorder. MEN 1 is the most common of these disorders to cause ZE syndrome, responsible for 20% of cases, although ZE syndrome has also been reported to occur in NF-1. Gastric and proximal small-bowel fold thickening and ulceration may be detected at upper gastrointestinal series or CT, and contrast-enhanced CT

may be able to demonstrate a hypervascular mass in the pancreas or duodenum.

C1 Esterase Inhibitor Deficiency

C1 esterase inhibitor deficiency, or hereditary angioedema, is an inherited cause of recurrent attacks of abdominal pain and nonpitting edema of the skin. The upper respiratory and gastrointestinal tracts may be affected, and abdominal pain, nausea, and vomiting predominate in a quarter of patients. Diffuse or segmental fold thickening of the stomach, small bowel, or both caused by submucosal edema may be seen on CT and barium examinations during an acute attack. Symptoms and imaging findings often resolve spontaneously several days after an attack. Laryngeal edema occurs in a significant number of patients and may be fatal. Angioedema with similar clinical and radiographic manifestations to C1 esterase inhibitor deficiency may occur in patients taking angiotensin-converting enzyme inhibitors.

Cystic Fibrosis

Gastrointestinal abnormalities, such as gastroesophageal reflux disease, peptic ulcer disease, and distal intestinal obstruction syndrome (meconium ileus equivalent), are a major feature of cystic fibrosis. Distal intestinal obstruction syndrome is caused by inspissated enteric contents in the setting of pancreatic exocrine dysfunction (Fig. 11-20). Appendiceal thickening, appendicitis, and intussusception are also features of the disease that may be seen in adults. An increased incidence of inflammatory bowel disease and gastrointestinal malignancy has been reported in adult patients with cystic fibrosis.

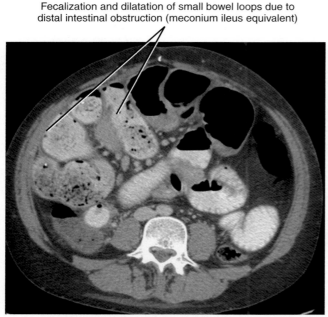

Fecalization and dilatation of small bowel loops due to distal intestinal obstruction (meconium ileus equivalent)

Figure 11-20 Enhanced axial computed tomographic scan through the lower abdomen of a young adult patient with cystic fibrosis with abdominal pain demonstrating distal intestinal obstruction.

Patients with cystic fibrosis may also have biliary ductal strictures, dilatation, and calculi, and microgallbladder (Fig. 11-21).

Neurofibromatosis

Multiple neurofibromas may originate in the intestinal wall and result in long-segment nodular mural thickening. Plexiform neurofibromas may involve the bowel and mesentery, and GISTs occasionally occur in patients with NF-1 (Fig. 11-22).

■ GENITOURINARY DISORDERS

Renal Cystic Disease

A comprehensive list of syndromes associated with multiple renal cysts is extremely long, although many of the entities included on such a list are unlikely to be encountered by a typical radiologist outside of a pediatric practice. This section discusses some of the more common renal cystic diseases likely to be encountered in adults. These diseases are compared in a summary table (Table 11-4).

Autosomal Dominant Polycystic Kidney Disease

ADPKD is rarely mistaken for other forms of polycystic kidney disease, typically showing a striking pattern of bilateral renal enlargement with replacement of normal renal parenchyma by innumerable cysts of varying complexity. The coexistence of polycystic liver disease is

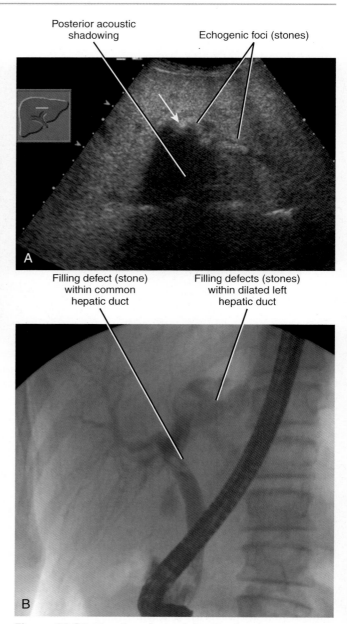

Figure 11-21 Hepatic sonogram **(A)** and endoscopic retrograde cholangiopancreatogram **(B)** of a patient with cystic fibrosis shows multiple stones within the left hepatic duct **(A)** and common hepatic duct **(B)**. (Courtesy Dr. Hisham Tchelepi.)

another hallmark of the syndrome (Fig. 11-23). Pancreatic cysts, cardiac valve abnormalities, cerebral aneurysms, abdominal hernias, and intestinal diverticulosis are additional potential abnormalities in ADPKD. Despite several anecdotal associations, the risk for development of renal cell carcinoma (RCC) is generally not considered to be increased in patients with ADPKD. Classic-appearing ADPKD is sometimes seen in patients with tuberous sclerosis. Ultrasound is usually used to screen patients genetically at risk for ADPKD. When at least two unilateral or bilateral cysts in an individual younger than 30 years, two cysts in each kidney in an

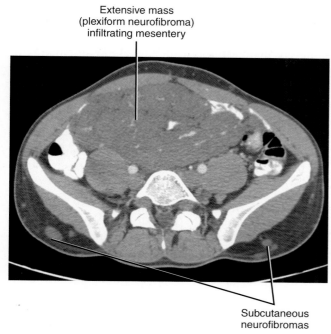

Extensive mass
(plexiform neurofibroma)
infiltrating mesentery

Subcutaneous
neurofibromas

Figure 11-22 Enhanced axial computed tomographic scan of a patient with neurofibromatosis type 1 and large mesenteric plexiform neurofibroma.

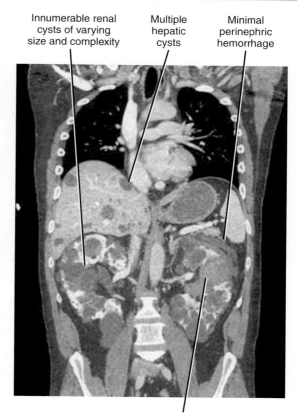

Innumerable renal
cysts of varying
size and complexity

Multiple
hepatic
cysts

Minimal
perinephric
hemorrhage

Hemorrhage in
collecting system
due to ruptured cyst

Figure 11-23 Coronal reformation of enhanced computed tomographic scan of a patient with autosomal dominant polycystic kidney disease who presented with acute left flank pain.

Table 11-4   Differentiation of Common Renal Cystic Diseases on Abdominal Imaging Studies

Disease	Features
Autosomal dominant polycystic kidney disease (ADPKD)	Innumerable bilateral renal cysts Symptomatic renal cysts (hemorrhage, infection, mass effect, rupture, stone formation) Renal enlargement Renal dysfunction Hepatic cysts (25%-50%) Pancreatic cysts (less than 10%) Splenic cysts (infrequent)
von Hippel–Lindau (vHL) disease	Fewer renal cysts than typical ADPKD Renal cell carcinoma (RCC) common Pancreatic cysts frequent Hepatic cysts rare Pancreatic neuroendocrine tumors Pancreatic serous cystadenomas Pheochromocytomas Central nervous system hemangioblastomas
Tuberous sclerosis complex	Fewer renal cysts than ADPKD Multiple, bilateral angiomyolipomas Lymphangiomas Perinephric hemorrhage
Autosomal recessive polycystic kidney disease/congestive heart failure	Periportal hepatic fibrosis Bile duct abnormalities Fewer macroscopic renal cysts Renal calcifications
Acquired cystic disease of dialysis	Small or normal-size kidneys End-stage renal disease on dialysis Increased risk for RCC (more than ADPKD but less than vHL disease)

individual 30 to 59 years of age, or four cysts in each kidney are present in an individual 60 years or older with a positive family history, a presumptive diagnosis of ADPKD is made. These criteria cannot be applied to CT or MRI because their increased sensitivity for the detection of cysts would likely result in a large number of false-positive examinations. Unilateral (or segmental) renal cystic disease is pathologically similar to ADPKD but differs in that it involves only one kidney and is not inherited.

von Hippel–Lindau Disease

vHL is an autosomal-dominant disorder related to a mutation in a tumor-suppressor gene. More than half of patients with vHL experience development of multiple, bilateral renal cysts that tend to increase with age. Up to 66% of cysts in patients with vHL harbor variously layered epithelium with papillary tufts. This histologic feature confers a significant risk for development of early, multiple, and bilateral RCCs. Therefore, presymptomatic screening of patients with vHL with CT or MRI is generally performed on a yearly basis to detect early RCC. Within the abdomen, additional manifestations of vHL include pheochromocytomas,

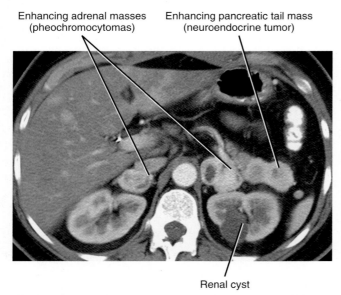

Figure 11-24 Enhanced axial computed tomographic scan of a patient with von Hippel–Landau disease demonstrates bilateral adrenal pheochromocytomas, a pancreatic neuroendocrine tumor, and renal cysts. The patient also had bilateral renal cell carcinomas found at surgery (not shown).

pancreatic cysts, neuroendocrine tumors, and pancreatic serous cystadenomas (see Figs. 11-14, 11-15, and 11-24). Serous cystadenoma of the epididymis can occur in male individuals and papillary serous cystadenoma of the broad ligament can occur in female individuals with vHL.

Tuberous Sclerosis Complex

TSC is a neurocutaneous disorder composed of seizures, intracranial abnormalities, and multiple hamartomatous neoplasms, of which renal AML is a hallmark (Fig. 11-25). Up to 80% of patients with TSC have renal manifestations. Fourteen to 32% of patients show multiple renal cysts, which are usually fewer in number than found in vHL or ADPKD. The cysts in TSC are rarely symptomatic. A tendency for the cysts in TSC to enlarge over time has been demonstrated. The coexistence of multiple renal cysts and AMLs is highly suggestive of TSC. Renal cystic involvement may rarely mimic ADPKD.

Other Cystic Disease of the Kidney

Juvenile nephronophthisis (JNPHP) and *medullary cystic renal disease* are rare entities that are characterized by the presence of small cysts located at the corticomedullary junction and renal medulla. These diseases typically lead to end-stage renal disease. Medullary cystic renal disease usually presents later than JNPHP and, unlike JNPHP, is not associated with extrarenal malformations. The kidneys and cysts of medullary cystic renal disease tend to be small.

Glomerulocystic kidney disease is characterized by tiny cortical cysts (smaller than 1 cm), may occur in patients with a family history of ADPKD, and may be associated with ductal plate abnormalities of the liver.

The strange designation of *pluricystic kidney of the multiple malformation syndromes* is conferred on the kidney when multiple renal cysts occur in association with

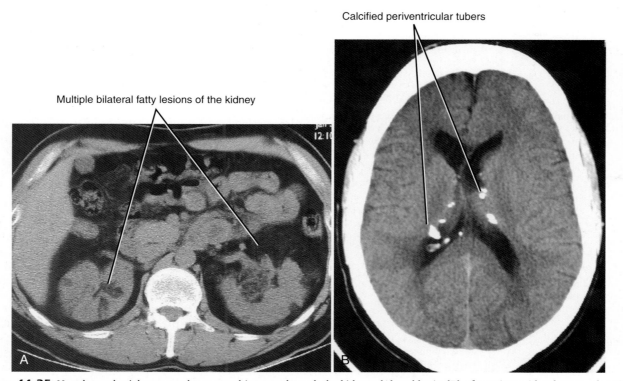

Figure 11-25 Unenhanced axial computed tomographic scans through the kidneys (**A**) and brain (**B**) of a patient with tuberous sclerosis complex and multiple renal angiomyolipomas.

various rare inheritable and noninheritable extrarenal syndromes such as Meckel–Gruber syndrome and its variants, a variety of trisomies, and other syndromes unlikely to be encountered outside of a pediatric practice.

Acquired Cystic Disease of Dialysis: Differentiation from Inherited Cystic Disease

Patients with end-stage renal disease on long-term dialysis (hemodialysis or peritoneal dialysis) can experience development of multiple renal cysts that may be confused with inherited renal cystic disease. Acquired cystic disease can be differentiated from ADPKD leading to chronic renal insufficiency, because the former entity is typically (but not always) associated with small or normal-size kidneys, whereas the kidneys in the latter entity are usually markedly enlarged (Fig. 11-26). In addition, the individual cysts in acquired cystic disease of dialysis do not usually enlarge to the extent typical of ADPKD. Approximately 7% of patients with acquired cystic disease of dialysis experience development of RCC. Acquired cystic disease can be distinguished from renal cysts associated with vHL and TSC because the latter entities are associated with characteristic renal and extrarenal tumors as described earlier.

Solid Renal Neoplasms

Renal Cell Carcinoma

RCC is by far the most common solid neoplasm of the kidney and is being diagnosed with increasing frequency in asymptomatic patients. RCC may arise de novo from solid adenomatous rests or may develop secondarily from the epithelial lining of a cyst. This latter mechanism is observed in vHL, in which multiple simple renal cysts may harbor papillary elements with preneoplastic potential from an early age. RCC is a major cause of morbidity and mortality in patients with vHL (Fig. 11-27).

Other hereditary conditions have been described with increased risk for RCC. TSC imparts a slightly increased risk for RCC, occurring in approximately 2% to 4% of patients. Hereditary papillary renal carcinoma is an autosomal dominant syndrome that places individuals at increased risk for development of bilateral, multifocal papillary RCCs. Birt–Hogg–Dubé syndrome is an autosomal dominant disorder predisposing patients to skin hamartomas, lung cysts, and RCC (features also present in some patients with TSC). Hereditary leiomyomatosis and renal cell cancer is a hereditary cancer syndrome in which unilateral solid RCC and concurrent uterine or skin leiomyomas occur. Renal medullary carcinoma, an aggressive malignant neoplasm with an extremely poor prognosis, has been described in young patients with sickle-cell trait.

Angiomyolipoma

AML is a relatively uncommon hamartomatous lesion composed of fat, muscle, and vascular tissue that may arise sporadically or in association with TSC. Approximately 34% to 80% of patients with TSC experience development of AMLs (see Fig. 11-25). Other manifestations of TSC include facial angiofibromas, ungual fibromas, shagreen patches, retinal

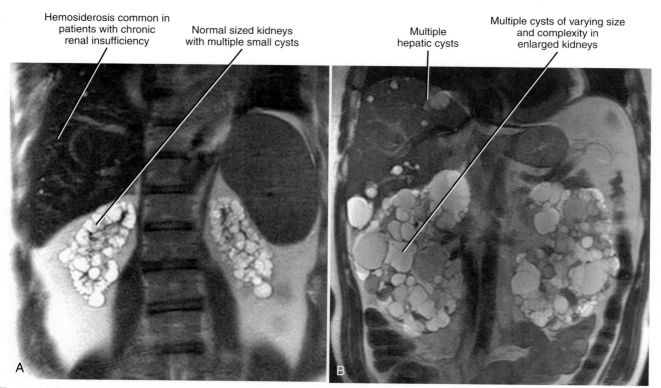

Hemosiderosis common in patients with chronic renal insufficiency

Normal sized kidneys with multiple small cysts

Multiple hepatic cysts

Multiple cysts of varying size and complexity in enlarged kidneys

Figure 11-26 Coronal T2-weighted magnetic resonance images in two different patients to compare acquired cystic disease of dialysis (**A**) with autosomal dominant polycystic kidney disease (**B**).

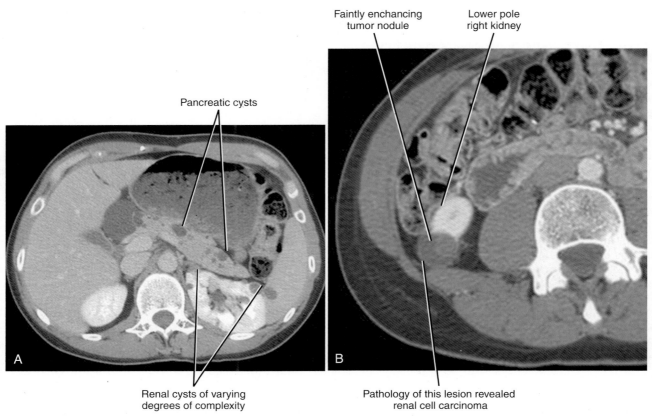

Figure 11-27 Axial enhanced computed tomographic scans through the pancreas (**A**) and kidneys (**B**) of a patient with von Hippel–Lindau disease and renal cell carcinoma (**B**).

hamartomas and astrocytomas, cortical tubers, subependymal nodules and astrocytomas, cardiac rhabdomyomas, and lymphangiomyomatosis. Minor features of TSC include enamel pits, hamartomatous rectal polyps, bone cysts, nonrenal hamartomas, renal cysts, and RCC. Pleuroparenchymal involvement occurs almost exclusively in female individuals with tuberous sclerosis.

Oncocytoma
Oncocytomas are generally considered benign renal neoplasms that can occur in the setting of familial renal oncocytoma and Birt–Hogg–Dubé.

Urinary Calculi

A variety of metabolic disorders predispose individuals to the development of urinary calculi (Box 11-3). Innate metabolic derangements combine with environmental factors (e.g., diet) to promote the formation of urinary stones. Hypercalciuria, hyperoxaluria, hypocitraturia, and hyperuricosuria from a variety of causes can lead to the formation of calcium-containing stones. Many individuals who suffer from urinary calculi fall under the category of idiopathic hypercalciuria. More than likely, this category represents a diverse group of metabolic disorders of the gut, bones, and kidneys. Approximately half of patients with idiopathic hypercalciuria have a

family history of kidney stones. Cushing syndrome, primary hyperparathyroidism, and renal tubular acidosis represent some metabolic diseases associated with renal calculi. Uric acid stones may develop in patients with gout, obesity, and diabetes. Cystinuria is a genetic (autosomal recessive) abnormality that results in increased urinary excretion of cystine, ornithine, lysine, and arginine. However, because of the insolubility of cystine, these patients are predisposed to formation of cystine stones. Some evidence suggests that the incidence of renal calculi is increased in patients with cystic renal disease such as ADPKD.

Medullary nephrocalcinosis is a particular form of calculous disease that describes formation of calcifica-

---

BOX 11-3 Metabolic Abnormalities Associated with Urinary Calculi

Cushing syndrome
Cystinuria
Diabetes
Gout
Hyperparathyroidism
Hyperuricosuria
Idiopathic hypercalciuria
Obesity
Primary hyperoxaluria
Renal tubular acidosis

tions within the renal pyramids from a variety of causes, including medullary sponge kidney, distal renal tubular acidosis, and hypercalcemic states such as hyperparathyroidism. Medullary nephrocalcinosis manifests as increased echogenicity of the renal pyramids on sonograms and increased density of the pyramids on radiographs and unenhanced CT images (Fig. 11-28).

■ ADRENAL

Adrenal Masses

Pheochromocytoma/Paraganglioma

Pheochromocytomas are catecholamine-producing neoplasms that arise from the adrenal medulla. Paragangliomas (sometimes referred to as extraadrenal pheochromocytomas) are tumors arising from the neural crest cells of the paraganglia neuroendocrine system. The classically held belief that only 10% of pheochromocytomas are bilateral and 10% are hereditary is tempered by recent data suggesting that up to 24% of sporadic cases are carriers for inherited endocrine syndromes such as MEN 2, vHL, and less often NF-1 (see Fig. 11-24). The definition of nonsyndromic pheochromocytoma continues to evolve as germline mutations not associated with well-established hereditary cancer syndromes are elucidated. An example of a more recent familial addition to this lineup is hereditary paraganglioma syndrome. Syndromic pheochromocytoma tends to be multifocal, bilateral, and benign, presenting at an earlier age than sporadic pheochromocytoma.

The risk for intraabdominal paraganglioma is estimated to be less than 1% in NF-1, 10% to 20% in vHL, 50% in MEN 2, and up to 80% in hereditary paraganglioma syndrome. The syndrome of pheochromocytoma, GIST, and pulmonary chondroma is referred to as Carney triad.

Adrenal Adenoma and Carcinoma

Hypersecreting adrenal adenoma can be associated with Cushing syndrome or Conn syndrome. In Cushing syndrome, excess cortisol secretion is associated with obesity, hypertension, and diabetes. Atrophy of the contralateral adrenal gland because of inhibition of pituitary adrenocorticotropic hormone (ACTH) secretion may occasionally be present. In Conn syndrome, an aldosterone-secreting adrenal adenoma leads to hypertension and, in some patients, hypokalemia. Conn syndrome may also result from adrenal hyperplasia in a third of patients. Adrenocortical carcinoma is associated with Beckwith–Wiedemann syndrome.

■ SPLEEN

Splenomegaly

The differential diagnosis for splenomegaly is quite long. Among the metabolic and inherited disorders that can be associated with splenomegaly are Gaucher disease, glycogen storage disease, various hemoglobinopathies, congenital hepatic fibrosis, cystic fibrosis, immunodeficiency diseases, and amyloidosis.

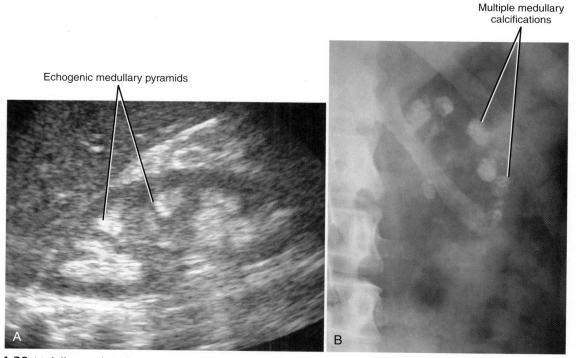

Figure 11-28 Medullary nephrocalcinosis in two different patients demonstrating the appearance on sonography (**A**) and radiography (**B**). (Courtesy Dr. Raymond Dyer.)

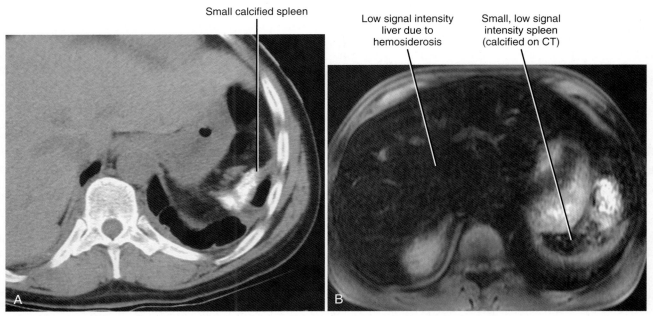

Figure 11-29 Unenhanced axial computed tomographic (CT) scan (**A**) and T1-weighted, fat-suppressed, magnetic resonance imaging (**B**) through the upper abdomen of a patient with sickle cell disease demonstrates small, calcified spleen and hemosiderosis.

Splenic Infarction

Splenic infarcts commonly occur in patients with sickle cell disease. The spleen often becomes shrunken and calcified over time (referred to as autosplenectomy) (Fig. 11-29).

Suggested Readings

Akhan O, Karaosmanoglu AD, Ergen B: Imaging findings in congenital hepatic fibrosis, *Eur J Radiol* 61:18-24, 2007.

Bisceglia, M, Galliani, CA, Senger C et al: Renal cystic diseases: a review, *Adv Anat Pathol* 13:26-56, 2006.

Brancatelli G, Federle MP, Vilgrain V et al: Fibropolycystic liver disease: CT and MR imaging findings, *Radiographics* 25:659-670, 2005.

Buetow PC, Miller DL, Parrino TV et al: Islet cell tumors of the pancreas: clinical, radiologic, and pathologic correlation in diagnosis and localization, *Radiographics* 17:453-472, 1997.

Bülow S, Berk T, Neale K: The history of familial adenomatous polyposis, *Fam Cancer* 5:213-220, 2006.

Casper KA, Donnelly LF, Chen B et al: Tuberous sclerosis complex: renal imaging findings, *Radiology* 225:451-456, 2002.

Choyke PL, Glen GM, Walther MM et al: von Hippel-Lindau disease: genetic, clinical, and imaging features, *Radiology* 194:629-642, 1995.

Choyke PL, Glen GM, Walther MM et al: Hereditary renal cancers, *Radiology* 226:33-46, 2003.

Chow E, Macrae F: A review of juvenile polyposis syndrome, *J Gastroenterol Hepatol* 20:1634-1640, 2005.

Cruz-Correa M, Giardiello FM: Familial adenomatous polyposis, *Gastrointest Endosc* 58:885-894, 2003.

Fields TM, Michel SJ, Butler CL et al: Abdominal manifestations of cystic fibrosis in older children and adults, *AJR Am J Roentgenol* 187:1199-1203, 2006.

Fricke BL, Donnelly LF, Casper KA et al: Frequency and imaging appearance of hepatic angiomyolipomas in pediatric and adult patients with tuberous sclerosis, *AJR Am J Roentgenol* 182:1027-1030, 2004.

Galiatsatos P, Foulkes WD: Familial adenomatous polyposis, *Am J Gastroenterol* 101:385-398, 2006.

Garcia-Tsao G: Liver involvement in hereditary hemorrhagic telangiectasia (HHT), *J Hepatol* 46:499-507, 2007.

Georgiades CS, Neyman EG, Barish MA et al: Amyloidosis: review and CT manifestations, *Radiographics* 24:405-416, 2004.

Grazioli L, Federle MP, Ichikawa T et al: Liver adenomatosis: clinical, histopathologic, and imaging findings in 15 patients, *Radiology* 216:395-402, 2000.

King LJ, Scurr ED, Murugan N et al: Hepatobiliary and pancreatic manifestations of cystic fibrosis: MR imaging appearances, *Radiographics* 20:767-777, 2000.

Lakhani VT, You YN, Wells SA: The multiple endocrine neoplasia syndromes, *Annu Rev Med* 58:253-265, 2007.

Levy AD, Patel N, Dow N et al: From the archives of the AFIP: abdominal neoplasms in patients with neurofibromatosis type 1: radiologic-pathologic correlation, *Radiographics* 25:455-480, 2005.

Lindor NM, Petersen GM, Hadley DW et al: Recommendations for the care of individuals with an inherited predisposition to Lynch syndrome: a systematic review, *JAMA* 296:1507-1517, 2006.

Lonser RR, Glenn GM, Walther M et al: von Hippel-Lindau disease, *Lancet* 361:2059-2067, 2003.

Madani G, Papadopoulou AM, Holloway B et al: The radiological manifestations of sickle cell disease, *Clin Radiol* 62:528-538, 2007.

Moe OW: Kidney stones: pathophysiology and medical management, *Lancet* 367:333-344, 2006.

Neumann HP, Berger DP, Sigmund G et al: Pheochromocytomas, multiple endocrine neoplasia type 2, and von Hippel-Lindau disease, *N Engl J Med* 329:1531-1538, 1993.

Rakowski SK, Winterkorn EB, Paul E et al: Renal manifestations of tuberous sclerosis complex: incidence, prognosis, and predictive factors, *Kidney Int* 70:1777-1782, 2006.

Ravine D, Gibson RN, Walder RG et al: Evaluation of ultrasonographic diagnostic criteria for autosomal dominant polycystic kidney disease 1, *Lancet* 343:824-827, 1994.

Rizk D, Chapman AB: Cystic and inherited kidney diseases, *Am J Kidney Dis* 42:1305-1317, 2003.

Robertson MB, Choe KA, Joseph PM: Review of the abdominal manifestations of cystic fibrosis in the adult patient, *Radiographics* 26:679-690, 2006.

Rosser T, Panigrahy A, McClintock W: The diverse clinical manifestations of tuberous sclerosis complex: a review, *Semin Pediatr Neurol* 13:27-36, 2006.

Scarsbrook AF, Thakker RV, Wass JA et al: Multiple endocrine neoplasia: spectrum of radiologic appearances and discussion of a multitechnique imaging approach, *Radiographics* 26:433-451, 2006.

Schreibman IR, Baker M, Amos C et al: The hamartomatous polyposis syndromes: a clinical and molecular review, *Am J Gastroenterol* 100:476-490, 2005.

Shapiro, SE, Cote, GC, Lee JF et al: The role of genetics in the surgical management of familial endocrinopathy syndromes, *J Am Coll Surg* 197:818-831, 2003.

Summerfield JA, Nagafuchi Y, Sherlock S et al: Hepatobiliary fibropolycystic diseases. A clinical and histological review of 51 patients, *J Hepatol* 2:141-156, 1986.

Taouli B, Ghouadni M, Correas JM et al: Spectrum of abdominal imaging findings in von Hippel-Lindau disease, *AJR Am J Roentgenol* 181:1049-1054, 2003.

Torreggiani WC, Keogh C, Al-Ismail et al: von Hippel-Lindau disease: a radiological essay, *Clin Radiol* 57:670-680, 2002.

Torres VE, Harris PC, Pirson Y: Autosomal dominant polycystic kidney disease, *Lancet* 369:1287-1301, 2007.

Watson P, Riley B: The tumor spectrum in Lynch syndrome, *Fam Cancer* 4:245-248, 2005.

Zbar B, Glenn G, Lubensky I et al: Hereditary papillary renal cell carcinoma: clinical studies in 10 families, *J Urol* 153:907-912, 1995.

Zeitoun D, Brancatelli G, Colombat M et al: Congenital hepatic fibrosis: CT findings in 18 adults, *Radiology* 231:109-116, 2004.

PROBLEM SOLVING: ANATOMIC REGIONS

CHAPTER 12

Liver

John R. Leyendecker

■ CLINICAL CONSIDERATIONS

Laboratory Tests Relevant to Hepatic Imaging

The liver is a biochemically complex organ, performing important metabolic and synthetic functions in the body. Therefore, it is not surprising that more basic laboratory tests are available to assess liver function than are available for any other organ in the abdomen and pelvis. In isolation, many of these tests are nonspecific. However, familiarity with these tests may add specificity to an imaging examination, direct the search for abnormalities, or aid the radiologist in recommending the appropriate next imaging examination to the referring physician. For these reasons, we provide a brief (alphabetical) summary of common laboratory tests relevant to liver imaging.

Albumin

Albumin is synthesized in the liver and is a measure of hepatic synthetic function. Low levels of serum albumin can be caused by impaired hepatic synthesis, urinary or enteric losses, or extravascular distribution (e.g., in ascites). Because the half-life of serum albumin is approximately 20 days, serum albumin levels are often normal in patients with acute liver abnormalities.

Alkaline Phosphatase

An increased level of the liver isoenzyme alkaline phosphatase (ALP) implies the presence of cholestasis but does not indicate the level of obstruction. Hepatobiliary origin of ALP can be suggested when γ-glutamyl transpeptidase (GGT) level is also increased. Disproportionately increased ALP levels can be seen with infiltrative malignancy.

α-Fetoprotein

The α-fetoprotein (AFP) level is commonly used to screen for or confirm the presence of hepatocellular carcinoma (HCC). The normal serum level of AFP is less than 10 ng/ml. For screening purposes, a level greater than 20 ng/ml may be considered abnormal, but this cutoff has a low positive predictive value because minor increases of AFP are common in patients with chronic liver disease. Increasing AFP levels over time should be considered suspicious, and a level exceeding 400 ng/ml is often considered diagnostic of HCC when correlated with typical imaging findings. Unfortunately, many HCCs, particularly small tumors, are not associated with an AFP level this high, and as many as 20% to 40% of patients with HCC have a normal serum AFP level. AFP levels can also be increased in patients with germ cell tumors and rarely with some gastrointestinal (GI) malignancies.

Aminotransferases (ALT, AST)

Alaninaminotransferase (ALT) and aspartate aminotransferase (AST) are sensitive indicators of hepatocellular injury (necrosis or inflammation). Levels of 500 to 1500 IU are common in acute viral or drug-induced hepatitis. Mild increase of ALT and AST concentrations can be seen with alcoholic hepatitis and biliary obstruction. Passage of a common bile duct stone can result in a transient severe increase in aminotransferase levels. An AST/ALT ratio greater than 1.5 to 2 may suggest alcoholic liver disease.

Antismooth Muscle Antibody

An increased antismooth muscle antibody level can be present in the setting of autoimmune hepatitis.

Bilirubin

The serum bilirubin level is often increased in cases of hepatocellular disease and biliary obstruction. Contrary to popular belief, the ratio of conjugated to unconjugated bilirubin may be an unreliable indicator of biliary obstruction. It can be more helpful to correlate bilirubin levels with other indicators of cholestasis, such as ALP or 5′ nucleotidase, when biliary obstruction is suspected.

γ-Glutamyl Transpeptidase

GGT level is a nonspecific indicator of liver disease but is often increased in alcohol induced liver injury. Serum GGT levels often parallel ALP levels.

Immunoglobulins

Diffuse increase of immunoglobulin (Ig) levels can be seen in patients with chronic liver disease of various causes. Specific increase of IgG can be present in patients with autoimmune hepatitis. IgM levels may be increased in the setting of primary biliary cirrhosis, and IgA may be disproportionately increased in alcoholic liver disease.

5′ Nucleotidase

The enzyme 5′ nucleotidase is found in bile canalicular membranes and is a specific marker of cholestasis. However, it is a less sensitive screening test for cholestasis than is ALP.

Prothrombin Time

A measurement of prothrombin time represents an assessment of fibrinogen (factor I), prothrombin (factor II), and clotting factors V, VII, and X. These factors are produced by the liver and have a relatively short half-life. Therefore, acute hepatocellular injury can result in an increased prothrombin time, and prothrombin time correlates with the severity of liver damage. Vitamin K deficiency and coumarin-like medications also affect prothrombin time. An increased prothrombin time in association with a normal serum albumin level (another indicator of hepatic synthetic function with a significantly longer half-life) implies acute, rather than chronic, hepatic dysfunction.

■ LIVER ANATOMY

Brief Review of Segmental Anatomy

Knowledge of segmental anatomy of the liver is critical because the hepatic segments represent discrete regions that can be surgically isolated and removed. Localization of an abnormality to the correct segment is a necessary part of surgical planning. Several systems are currently in use describing the anatomic segments of the liver (Table 12-1). The Couinaud–Bismuth system is currently the most often used nomenclature, although many surgeons are transitioning to the Brisbane terminology. According to the Brisbane 2000 Terminology of Liver Anatomy, the liver is divided into a right hemiliver (commonly referred to as the *right lobe*) and a left hemiliver (commonly referred to as the *left lobe*) by a vertical plane along the course of the middle hepatic vein that intersects the gallbladder fossa. The right hemiliver is divided into anterior and posterior sections (also known as *segments* under the terminology of Goldsmith and Woodburne) by a vertical plane along the right hepatic vein. The medial and lateral sections of the left hemiliver are divided by the fissure for the ligamentum teres, which contains the falciform ligament. The caudate lobe (segment I) protrudes from the right hemiliver between the portal vein and inferior vena cava (IVC).

The liver is further divided into segments by a transverse plane (scissura) along the right and left portal vein branches. Each segment has its own blood supply and biliary drainage. These segments are illustrated for multidetector computed tomography (CT) in Figure 12-1. For purposes of this textbook, we refer to the right and left lobes of the liver and use predominately the Couinaud–Bismuth terminology for segments, because this terminology is most familiar to radiologists. However, it is important to be familiar with systems of nomenclature in common use at one's own institution to facilitate accurate communication.

Clinically Relevant Vascular Anatomy of the Liver

Hepatic Veins

The right, middle, and left hepatic veins converge at the hepatic venous confluence and drain blood from the liver into the IVC just below the right atrium. The hepatic venous confluence has a variety of configurations, but most commonly, the middle and left hepatic veins share a common trunk before entering the IVC (Fig. 12-2). Segment I (caudate lobe) has a separate venous drainage directly to the IVC.

The middle hepatic vein is of particular importance to hepatic surgeons. In patients undergoing right hepatic resection or right hemiliver donation, the surgeon typically bisects the liver approximately 1 cm to the right of the middle hepatic vein. When such surgery is contemplated, this line serves as a landmark for determining the relative volumes of the right and left lobes. When living liver donation is being considered, it is important to note large tributaries of the middle hepatic vein that drain the right lobe (e.g., segments V and VIII), because these will be transected in the case of right hemiliver transplantation and may require reimplantation in the recipient.

Many individuals have accessory hepatic veins that drain the inferior right hepatic lobe directly into the IVC. In some patients, more than one inferior accessory vein is present. These have a similar relevance to hepatic transplant surgery as large tributaries of the middle hepatic vein. In general, tributaries and accessory hepatic veins in

Table 12-1   Nomenclature in Common Use for Describing Liver Anatomy

Brisbane	Couinaud–Bismuth	Goldsmith and Woodburne
Right Hemiliver	Right Lobe	Right Lobe
Anterior Section		*Anterior Segment*
Segment VIII (upper)	Segment VIII (upper*)	
Segment V (lower)	Segment V (lower*)	
Posterior Section		*Posterior Segment*
Segment VII (upper)	Segment VII (upper)	
Segment VI (lower)	Segment VI (lower)	
Left Hemiliver	Left Lobe	Left Lobe
Medial Section		*Medial Segment*
Segment IVa (upper)	Segment IVa (upper)	
Segment IVb (lower)	Segment IVb (lower)	
Lateral Section		*Lateral Segment*
Segment II (upper)	Segment II (upper)	
Segment III (lower)	Segment III (lower)	
Caudate	Segment I	Segment I

*Upper refers to above the transverse scissura described by the right and left portal veins; lower refers to below the transverse scissura described by the right and left portal veins.

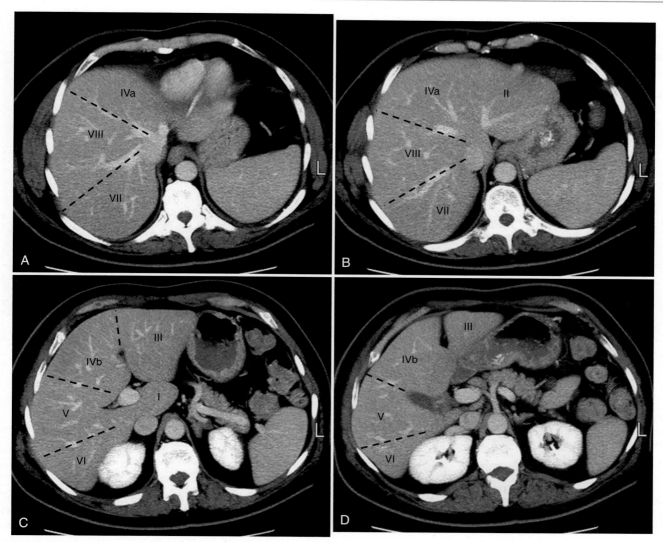

Figure 12-1 Segmental anatomy of the liver (Couinaud–Bismuth terminology). **A, B,** Taken above the transverse scissura of the portal vein. **C, D,** Taken below the transverse scissura of the portal vein.

the range of 5 to 10 mm in diameter that cross a transection plane are considered significant. Inferior accessory hepatic veins can also serve as a collateral pathway to circumvent intrahepatic vena cava obstruction (Fig. 12-3).

Portal Veins

The portal vein forms from the confluence of the splenic and superior mesenteric veins, and normally contributes a substantial portion of the hepatic blood flow (at least 75%). The main portal vein travels within the hepatoduodenal ligament as it enters the liver hilum. The portal vein typically bifurcates into right and left branches, each of which subsequently branches into anterior and posterior branches (right portal vein) or medial and lateral branches (left portal vein) (Fig. 12-4). These major branches further bifurcate to supply their respective hepatic segments. The portal vein branch to the caudate lobe can originate from either the left or the right portal vein.

The branching pattern of the portal vein may have important implications for the liver surgeon. It is important to recognize portal vein branching variants in

patients scheduled for liver resection or donor hemihepatectomy to prevent inadvertent interruption of the portal blood supply to the remaining liver. A variety of portal vein branching variations have been described. Portal trifurcation refers to simultaneous branching of the main portal vein into right posterior segment, right anterior segment, and left portal vein branches (Fig. 12-5). Additional variants are possible involving the lack of a common trunk for the right posterior and anterior segment branches, including origin of the right posterior segment branch from the main portal vein and origin of the right anterior segment branch from the left portal vein (Figs. 12-6 and 12-7). Other, less frequent anomalous portal branching patterns are possible. Some studies have demonstrated a somewhat weak concordance between anomalous portal vein branching and variant bile duct anatomy. However, bile duct anomalies can be present in the absence of variant portal venous branching, and the presence of a normal/classic portal vein branching pattern does not preclude anomalous biliary anatomy. Anomalous branching of the portal

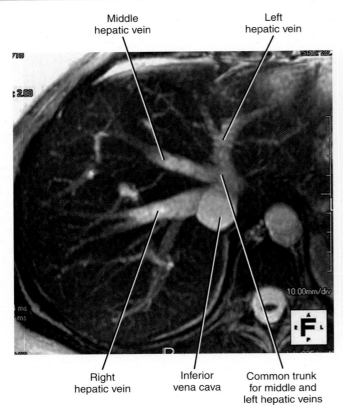

Figure 12-2 Typical hepatic venous anatomy shown on axial maximum intensity projection magnetic resonance image (balanced steady state free precession sequence).

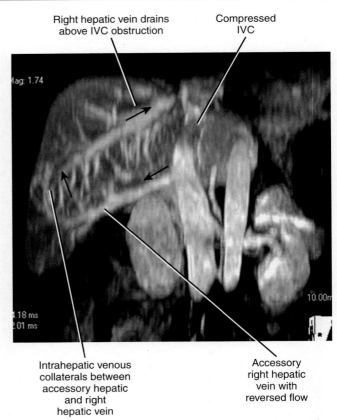

Figure 12-3 Coronal maximum intensity projection image from contrast-enhanced magnetic resonance imaging in a patient with a large mass (focal nodular hyperplasia) obstructing inferior vena cava (IVC). *Arrows* show direction of blood flow.

vein has also been associated with malposition of the gallbladder. Additional congenital variants of the portal vein include prepancreatic portal vein (often associated with situs inversus), double portal vein, and agenesis of the main portal vein or one of its major branches.

Hepatic Artery

The hepatic artery travels in the hepatoduodenal ligament anterior to the portal vein and supplies the liver with oxygen-rich arterial blood and approximately 25% of the total hepatic blood flow. The common hepatic artery typically originates from the celiac axis together with the splenic and left gastric arteries. After giving off the gastroduodenal artery, the proper hepatic artery bifurcates into the right and left hepatic arteries, which further branch to supply the hepatic segments. The caudate lobe can receive its blood supply from branches of either the right or left hepatic artery.

Correctly mapping out the hepatic arterial anatomy is important before liver and biliary surgery, hepatic chemoembolization, or placement of a chemoinfusion pump. Hepatic artery variants are extremely common. The term *replaced* is used when the entire right hepatic artery, entire left hepatic artery, or entire common hepatic artery arises from an atypical location. The terms *accessory* or *partially replaced* are used when only part of the arterial blood supply to the right or left lobe arises from an atypical location.

Fortunately, most replaced or accessory arteries can be identified by looking in only two locations. The replaced or accessory left hepatic artery arising from the left gastric artery can be found traveling in the fissure for the ligamentum venosum (Fig. 12-8). The replaced or accessory right hepatic artery can usually be identified in the portocaval space (Fig. 12-9). The most common hepatic artery variants are the left hepatic artery (or a portion thereof) arising from the left gastric artery and the right hepatic artery (or a portion thereof) originating from the superior mesenteric artery. Other variants include origin of the hepatic artery directly from the aorta; origin of one of the hepatic arteries before the origin of the gastroduodenal artery; trifurcation of the hepatic artery into left, right, and gastroduodenal arteries; and origin of the left hepatic artery from the celiac axis.

The artery supplying segment IV of the liver is often overlooked but is important to identify in patients who may be undergoing hemihepatectomy (including living hemiliver donors) (Fig. 12-10). In particular, it is important to note whether the segment IV artery arises from the left or right hepatic artery. When arising from the right hepatic artery, additional steps are needed to preserve the segment IV artery during right hepatectomy. A segment IV artery arising from the right hepatic artery has occasionally been referred to as a middle hepatic artery. The posterior part of segment IV can also receive blood supply from caudate artery branches.

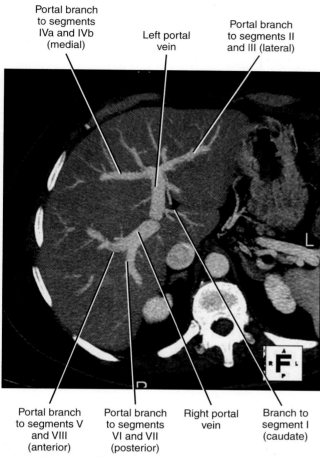

Portal branch to segments IVa and IVb (medial)

Left portal vein

Portal branch to segments II and III (lateral)

Portal branch to segments V and VIII (anterior)

Portal branch to segments VI and VII (posterior)

Right portal vein

Branch to segment I (caudate)

Figure 12-4 Axial maximum intensity projection image from an enhanced computed tomographic scan shows standard portal vein branching pattern.

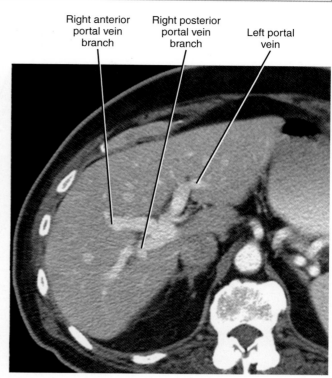

Right anterior portal vein branch

Right posterior portal vein branch

Left portal vein

Figure 12-5 Contrast-enhanced axial computed tomographic scan of a patient with portal trifurcation.

Nonportal Venous Supply to the Liver

Every practicing radiologist is familiar with the dual blood supply to the liver via the hepatic artery and portal vein. However, relatively little attention has been paid in Western radiology training to venous structures other than the main portal vein that drain from extrahepatic sites into the liver. Although these vessels contribute relatively little in the way of critical blood supply to the liver, they are a common source of vexing imaging findings that can generate unnecessary additional tests or invasive procedures.

Four major groups of veins drain into the liver aside from the main portal vein: paraumbilical, cholecystic, gastric, and parabiliary. Most radiologists associate the paraumbilical veins (also referred to as the superior and inferior veins of Sappey) with portal hypertension; in which case, they serve to divert portal blood flow to the systemic circulation. However, the paraumbilical veins normally drain toward the liver and into the hepatic parenchyma along the falciform ligament. These veins may be responsible for fatty infiltration or perfusion-related pseudolesions in this location (Fig. 12-11). Paraumbilical veins communicate with the epigastric veins

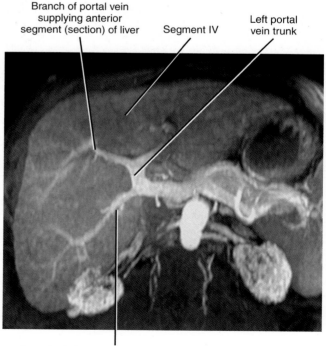

Branch of portal vein supplying anterior segment (section) of liver

Segment IV

Left portal vein trunk

Branch of portal vein supplying posterior segment (section) of liver

Figure 12-6 Oblique axial maximum intensity projection reconstruction of a gadolinium-enhanced magnetic resonance scan of a patient with variant portal venous anatomy.

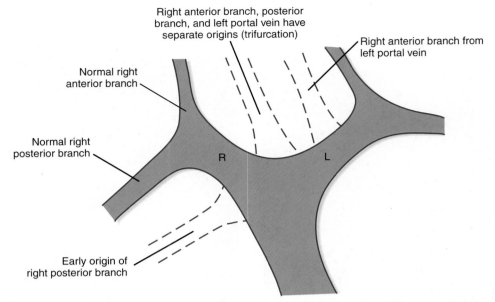

Figure 12-7 Common portal vein branching patterns. Variants are denoted by *dashed lines;* normal anatomy by *solid lines.*

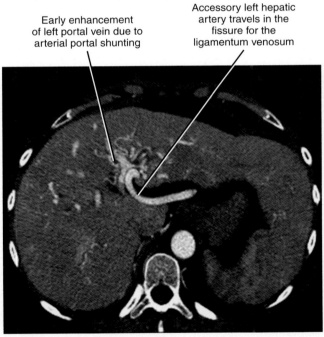

Figure 12-8 Enhanced axial computed tomographic image through the liver of a patient with hereditary hemorrhagic telangiectasia demonstrating the typical location of an accessory or replaced left hepatic artery arising from the left gastric artery. The artery is enlarged because of intrahepatic arteriovenous shunting.

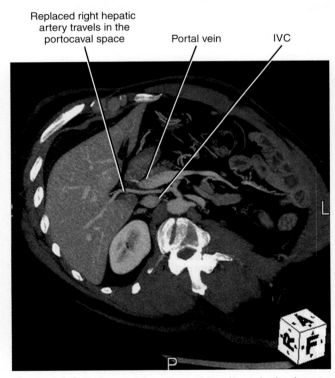

Figure 12-9 Oblique axial maximum intensity projection image of a replaced right hepatic artery arising from the superior mesenteric artery (SMA). *IVC,* Inferior vena cava.

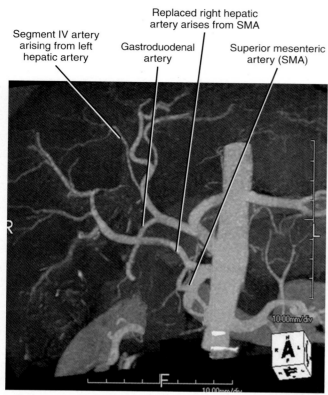

Segment IV artery arising from left hepatic artery

Replaced right hepatic artery arises from SMA

Gastroduodenal artery

Superior mesenteric artery (SMA)

Figure 12-10 Oblique coronal maximum intensity projection image from a computed tomographic angiogram demonstrating the segment IV artery and a replaced right hepatic artery arising from the superior mesenteric artery (SMA).

and can serve as a collateral pathway in the setting of superior vena cava or IVC obstruction. This helps explain the occasional finding of focal enhancement in the region of the falciform ligament on early-phase CT or magnetic resonance imaging (MRI) in patients with caval obstruction (Fig. 12-12). Hepatic inflow via the cystic (or cholecystic) vein may result in a perfusion-related pseudolesion in the region of the gallbladder fossa during enhanced CT and MRI, or may manifest as areas of focal fatty sparing adjacent to the gallbladder fossa in the setting of hepatic steatosis (Fig. 12-13). Gastric veins that drain into the liver are another potential source of perfusion-related pseudolesions, focal fatty infiltration, or focal fatty sparing involving segments II, III, and IV (Fig. 12-14). The last major group of systemic inflow veins is the parabiliary veins, better known for their role in bypassing portal vein occlusion (cavernous transformation of the portal vein). These veins drain the region of the pancreatic head and duodenum, course along the common bile duct in the hepatoduodenal ligament, and enter the liver at the hilum. They are responsible for perfusion-related pseudolesions and focal fatty infiltration or sparing adjacent to the liver hilum in the caudate and left hepatic lobes (Fig. 12-15).

It is not entirely predictable when small veins entering the liver will result in an area of enhanced perfusion during the arterial phase, a perfusion defect during the portal phase, an area of focal fatty infiltration, or an area of fatty sparing. The incidence of hepatic pseudolesions

will likely increase as quicker CT scanners and rapid bolus injection of intravenous contrast result in better temporal discrimination of vascular phases. Knowledge of the presence and typical locations of inflow vessels may prevent an errant diagnosis of tumor when such imaging findings are encountered.

■ NORMAL IMAGING APPEARANCE OF THE LIVER

Ultrasound

With sonography, normal hepatic parenchyma is of moderate, homogeneous echogenicity. The liver is normally slightly more echogenic than normal renal cortex and less echogenic than pancreas. Increased periportal echogenicity helps distinguish portal veins from the hepatic veins. The intrahepatic bile ducts are of smaller caliber than the portal veins, lack flow with color Doppler imaging, and are normally relatively inconspicuous.

Computed Tomography

With CT, normal hepatic parenchyma is of homogeneous density, with attenuation values in the range of 45 to 65 HU. The normal liver is typically 5 to 10 HU denser than the normal spleen on an unenhanced CT image. The normal liver can vary considerably in shape between individuals. Typical liver volumes as determined by CT are approximately 1700 and 1400 ml for male and female individuals, respectively, although this also varies considerably between individuals. The degree of parenchymal enhancement after administration of intravenous contrast material varies with injection rate, injected volume, and the timing of image acquisition after contrast administration. Peak liver enhancement increases with contrast volume and concentration, and decreases with increasing body weight. Peak hepatic parenchymal enhancement lags behind that of the renal cortex and pancreas. Table 12-2 presents the timing of the various phases of a dynamic contrast-enhanced CT examination in a typical patient.

Magnetic Resonance Imaging

The appearance of the normal liver on an MRI examination depends on the pulse sequence applied. On T1-weighted images, the normal liver is of higher signal intensity than the normal spleen but of lower signal intensity than the normal pancreas. On T2-weighted images, the liver is of lower signal intensity than the spleen. The relative signal intensity of the normal liver should not vary significantly between in-phase and opposed-phase gradient-echo images in the absence of abnormal iron or fat deposition. On a T1-weighted sequence after intravenous gadolinium chelate administration, the liver increases in relative signal intensity. Notably, there is no standard MR unit of signal intensity comparable with the Hounsfield unit.

Segment IV perfusion anomaly
only visible during portal phase.
This area was initially normal
in appearance on every other
MR sequence, including in
and opposed phase imaging.

No signal abnormality on in phase
image in segment IV

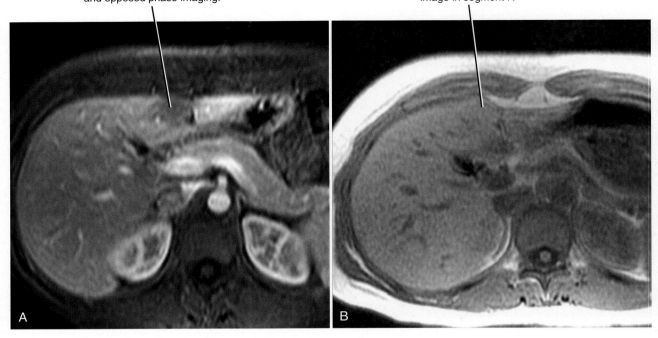

Area of signal loss on opposed phase image
represents new region of focal hepatic steatosis
2 years after perfusion abnormally was discovered.

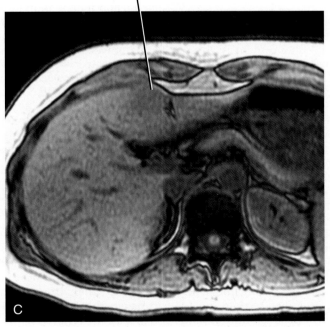

Figure 12-11 Axial portal-phase gadolinium-enhanced **(A)**, in-phase **(B)**, and opposed-phase **(C)** T1-weighted magnetic resonance (MR) images through the liver in a young woman with segment IV perfusion anomaly. **B, C,** Images were obtained 2 years after **(A)**.

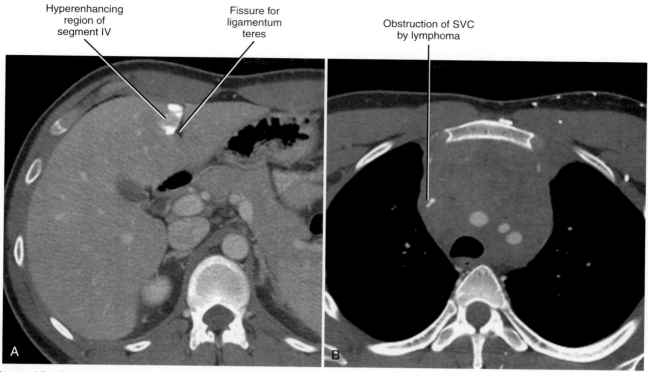

Figure 12-12 Axial contrast-enhanced computed tomographic scan through the abdomen (A) and chest (B) shows hyperenhancement in region of segment IV adjacent to falciform ligament in a patient with superior vena cava (SVC) obstruction by lymphoma.

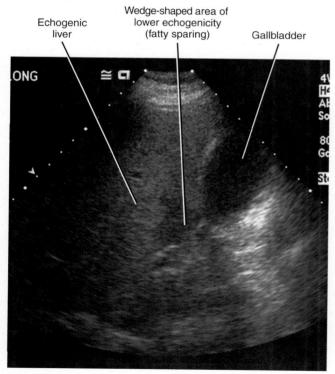

Figure 12-13 Sonogram through the liver and gallbladder of a patient with hepatic steatosis and focal sparing near the gallbladder (confirmed with magnetic resonance imaging, not shown).

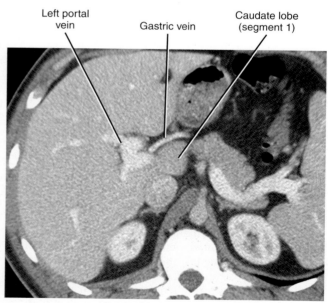

Figure 12-14 Enhanced axial computed tomographic scan showing a gastric vein entering the liver. This vein could be seen draining into segment IV on other images (not shown), although it was initially confused with an accessory left hepatic artery.

Focal perfusion anomaly   Small parabiliary vein entering liver   Left adrenal mass

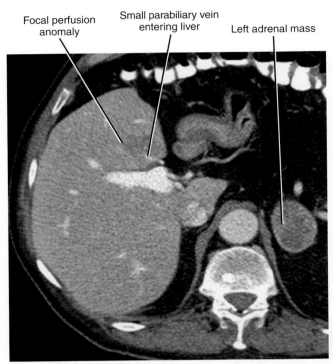

Figure 12-15 Axial portal-phase computed tomographic scan shows parabiliary vein entering the liver associated with small perfusion anomaly.

Table 12-2   Timing of Hepatic Enhancement Phases after Start of Contrast Bolus

Phase	Timing
Early arterial (for computed tomography angiographic studies)	20-25 seconds
Late arterial	30-40 seconds
Portal venous	60-90 seconds
Equilibrium	3-5 minutes

These estimates vary depending on type of scanner and injection protocol.

■ DIFFUSE ABNORMALITIES OF THE LIVER

Approach to Diffuse Liver Abnormalities

Diffuse hepatic abnormalities may manifest on imaging examinations as altered echogenicity (ultrasound [US]), attenuation (CT), signal intensity (MRI), enhancement, architecture, or size of the liver. When a diffuse process results in homogeneous alteration in the imaging appearance of the liver, it may become apparent only after direct comparison of the hepatic parenchyma to some internal (e.g., the vessels) or external (e.g., the spleen) reference.

When faced with a possible diffuse abnormality of the liver, it is often worthwhile to ask the following questions:

1. Is the echogenicity, attenuation, or signal intensity increased or decreased? Causes of diffusely altered appearance of the liver are listed in Table 12-3.

Table 12-3   Causes of Diffusely Altered Appearance of the Liver

Imaging Examination	Decreased	Increased
Echogenicity (US)	Hepatitis, tumor	Steatosis, fibrosis, tumor
Attenuation (CT)	Steatosis, hepatitis, tumor	Iron, glycogen, amiodarone (Fig. 12-16), iodine
T1W SI (in-phase MRI)	Iron,* edema	Steatosis, gadolinium, manganese
T1W SI (opposed-phase MRI)	Steatosis, iron*	Gadolinium, manganese
T2W SI (MRI)†	Iron	Edema, fibrosis, fat

*Signal loss because of iron will worsen as echo time increases.
†Echo train spin-echo sequence without fat suppression.
CT, Computed tomography; MRI, magnetic resonance imaging; SI, signal intensity; T1W, T1-weighted; T2W, T2-weighted; US, ultrasound.

Ascites   Dense liver (> 70 HU)

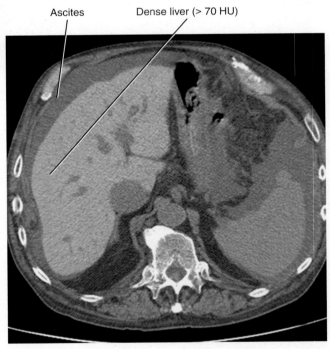

Figure 12-16 Unenhanced axial computed tomographic image through the abdomen of patient taking the drug amiodarone.

2. Are discrete small nodules visible? The most common cause of nodular liver is cirrhosis. The presence of discrete nodules in a noncirrhotic patient shifts the differential diagnosis toward granulomatous, infectious, or neoplastic causative agents (Fig. 12-17).

3. Are the vessels displaced, occluded, or enlarged? The presence of displaced or invaded vessels implies a space-occupying process such as neoplasm. Steatosis does not significantly alter the vascular architecture of the liver. Enlarged or thrombosed vessels can result in diffusely abnormal hepatic enhancement patterns. Table 12-4 lists some hemodynamic disturbances of the liver that result in diffusely abnormal enhancement.

Subtle diffuse nodularity of liver echotexture
prompted further evaluation with MRI

Innumerable high signal
intensity nodules
throughout entire liver

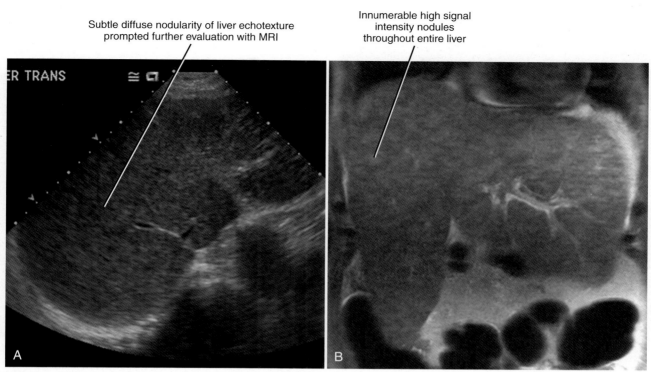

A   B

Figure 12-17 Transverse right upper quadrant ultrasound (**A**) and coronal T2-weighted magnetic resonance (**B**) images obtained in a patient with increased liver function tests and unsuspected diffuse hepatic metastases. *MRI,* Magnetic resonance imaging.

Table 12-4   Hemodynamic Disturbances of the Liver

Condition	Enhancement Pattern and Associated Findings
Hepatic congestion (Fig. 12-18)	Heterogeneous, mosaic-like pattern of enhancement associated with enlargement of the inferior vena cava (IVC) and hepatic veins. Reflux of contrast into the IVC and hepatic veins can be present, although this finding alone is not specific for cardiac dysfunction. Doppler ultrasound can demonstrate pulsatility of the portal vein (Fig. 12-19).
Budd–Chiari syndrome	Decreased early peripheral enhancement and increased enhancement of the central portions of the liver, particularly the caudate lobe. Nonenhancing hepatic vein or IVC thrombus may be present.
Main portal vein occlusion (Fig. 12-20)	Preferential early enhancement of the liver periphery with diminished central and caudate lobe enhancement. This pattern approximates the opposite of that seen with Budd–Chiari syndrome.
Right or left portal vein occlusion (Fig. 12-21)	Increased enhancement of liver on side of occlusion during arterial phase with straight border along middle hepatic vein. Steatosis involving one lobe of liver may develop over time (Fig. 12-22).
Hereditary hemorrhagic telangiectasia (Fig. 12-23)	Multiple intrahepatic vascular malformations and arteriovenous shunts can result in a bizarre, diffusely heterogeneous early enhancement pattern. Marked enlargement of the hepatic artery is often present.

Mosaic pattern of
hepatic enhancement

Distended IVC

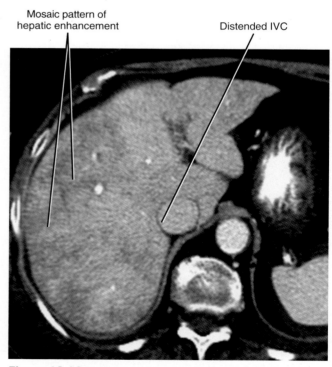

Figure 12-18 Enhanced axial computed tomographic image in a patient with congestive heart failure.

Pulsatile waveform

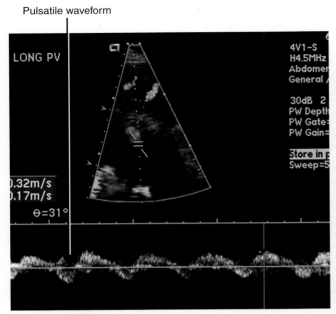

Figure 12-19 Doppler ultrasound of portal vein in a patient with congestive heart failure.

Straight line of demarcation along plane of middle hepatic vein

Relatively increased enhancement of left lobe

Acute thrombus in left portal vein

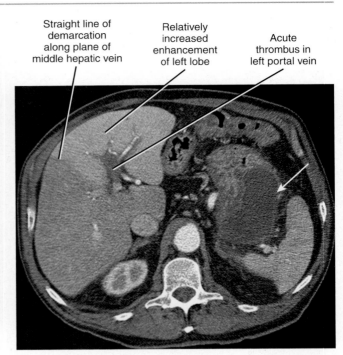

Figure 12-21 Early-phase enhanced axial computed tomographic scan through the abdomen of a patient with acute thrombosis of the left portal vein. Note pseudocyst along greater curvature of stomach *(arrow)* caused by pancreatitis.

Increased enhancement in liver periphery

Diminished central enhancement on arterial phase images

Low attenuation thrombus in right portal vein

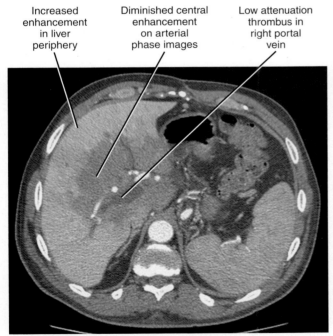

Figure 12-20 Early-phase enhanced axial computed tomographic scan of a patient with acute main and intrahepatic portal vein thrombosis demonstrating the typical early enhancement pattern. On portal-phase images (not shown), liver enhancement was homogeneous.

Straight line demarcating border between left and right lobes

Left lobe has no fatty infiltration

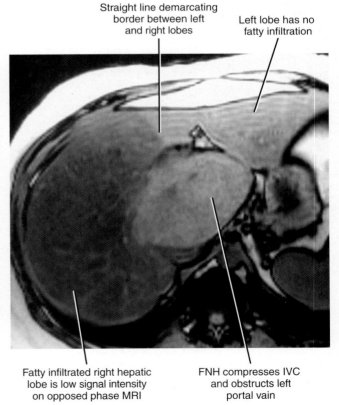

Fatty infiltrated right hepatic lobe is low signal intensity on opposed phase MRI

FNH compresses IVC and obstructs left portal vain

Figure 12-22 Axial opposed-phase gradient-echo magnetic resonance imaging (MRI) of the liver in a patient with a large focal nodular hyperplasia (FNH) obstructing the left portal vein. *IVC,* Inferior vena cava.

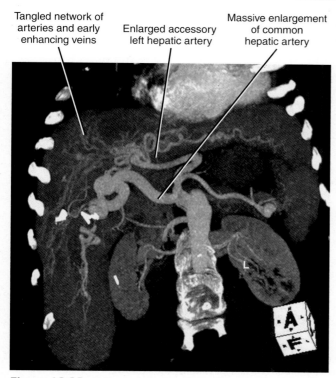

Tangled network of arteries and early enhancing veins

Enlarged accessory left hepatic artery

Massive enlargement of common hepatic artery

Figure 12-23 Oblique coronal maximum intensity projection image of the upper abdomen of a patient with hereditary hemorrhagic telangiectasia demonstrating bizarre tangle of intrahepatic arteries and veins, and massive enlargement of hepatic arteries. This is the same patient as in Figure 12-8.

Specific Deposition Disorders of the Liver

Steatosis

More commonly referred to as fatty liver, hepatic steatosis is often dismissed as a clinically insignificant radiologic finding. However, diffuse fatty infiltration of the liver can be associated with increased liver function tests, and if left unchecked, some types of steatosis can progress to steatohepatitis (manifesting as diffuse fatty infiltration, abnormal liver function tests, and hepatomegaly) and cirrhosis. For this reason, steatosis is a finding worthy of reporting. Hepatic steatosis results from a variety of hepatic insults in addition to dietary indiscretion (Box 12-1).

Sonography is the least specific cross-sectional imaging modality for the diagnosis of hepatic steatosis. The diagnosis may be suggested when the hepatic parenchyma demonstrates increased echogenicity associated with sound attenuation, resulting in poor depth of penetration and poor visualization of the hepatic veins, portal triads, and diaphragm (Fig. 12-24).

CT is more specific for the diagnosis of steatosis, which is suggested when the hepatic parenchyma is at least 10 HU lower in attenuation than the spleen on an unenhanced scan or 25 HU lower on a portal-phase contrast-enhanced CT scan. A liver attenuation of less than 40 HU on an unenhanced CT scan is also suggestive of steatosis. Steatosis can be subjectively diagnosed when hepatic vessels stand out as hyperdense against

BOX 12-1   Hepatic Steatosis: Associations and Causes in Adults

Obesity
Ethanol abuse
Diabetes
Hyperlipidemia
Corticosteroids and other medications (e.g., tetracycline, chemotherapy)
Viral hepatitis
Pregnancy
Malabsorption
Radiation treatment
Starvation
Parenteral hyperalimentation
Ischemia
Hereditary and metabolic disorders
Carbon tetrachlorides

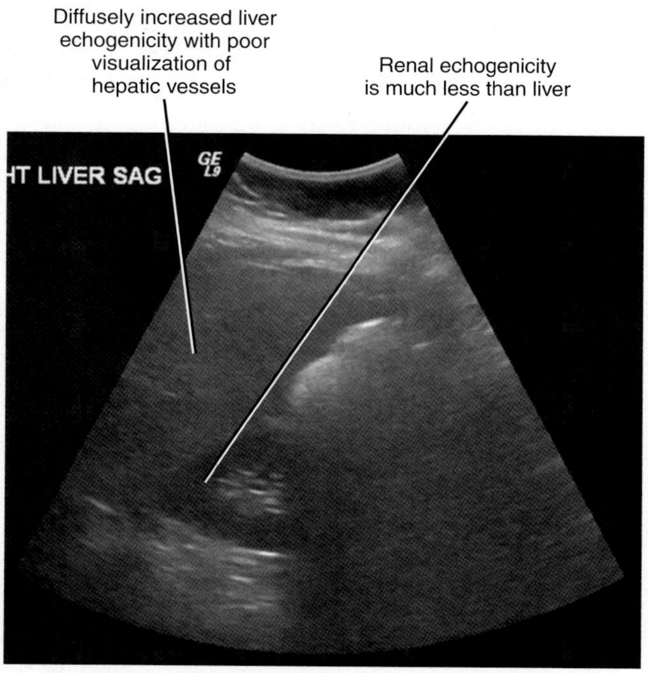

Diffusely increased liver echogenicity with poor visualization of hepatic vessels

Renal echogenicity is much less than liver

Figure 12-24 Longitudinal right upper quadrant sonogram through the liver and right kidney of a patient with hepatic steatosis.

the low-attenuation background of fatty liver parenchyma (Fig. 12-25). This degree of steatosis may create the appearance of an enhanced scan.

Chemical-shift MRI is highly specific for the diagnosis of hepatic steatosis. Areas of fatty infiltration will lose signal intensity on opposed-phase gradient-echo images relative to in-phase images (Fig. 12-26). Chemical-shift imaging is much more sensitive to the presence of steatosis than fat saturation or short tau inversion recovery MRI, because the latter techniques do not suppress the signal from water protons. MR spectroscopy has been used to further quantify the degree of fatty infiltration of the liver.

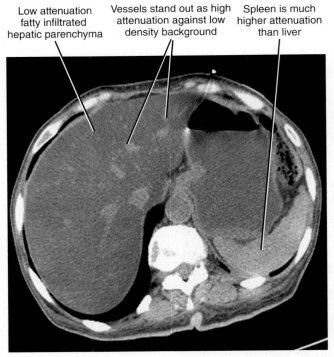

Low attenuation fatty infiltrated hepatic parenchyma

Vessels stand out as high attenuation against low density background

Spleen is much higher attenuation than liver

Figure 12-25 Unenhanced axial computed tomographic scan of a patient with hepatic steatosis.

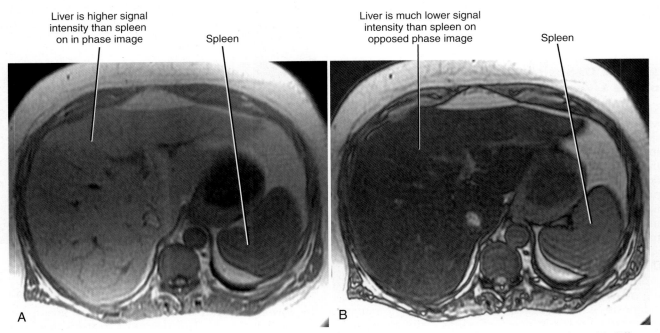

Liver is higher signal intensity than spleen on in phase image

Spleen

Liver is much lower signal intensity than spleen on opposed phase image

Spleen

A

B

Figure 12-26 Axial in-phase (**A**) and opposed-phase (**B**) gradient-echo magnetic resonance images of the liver in a patient with diffuse hepatic steatosis.

Steatosis may manifest in a variety of patterns and distributions (Box 12-2) (Fig. 12-27). Regardless of the pattern or imaging modality used to image the patient with hepatic steatosis, areas of uncomplicated fatty infiltration should not cause mass effect or displace vessels. One additional feature of hepatic steatosis is its capacity to change or fluctuate significantly over a relatively short period (<1 month) given changes in patient

BOX 12-2   Patterns of Hepatic Steatosis

Diffuse
Diffuse with focal sparing
Focal
Multifocal
Geographic
Perivascular

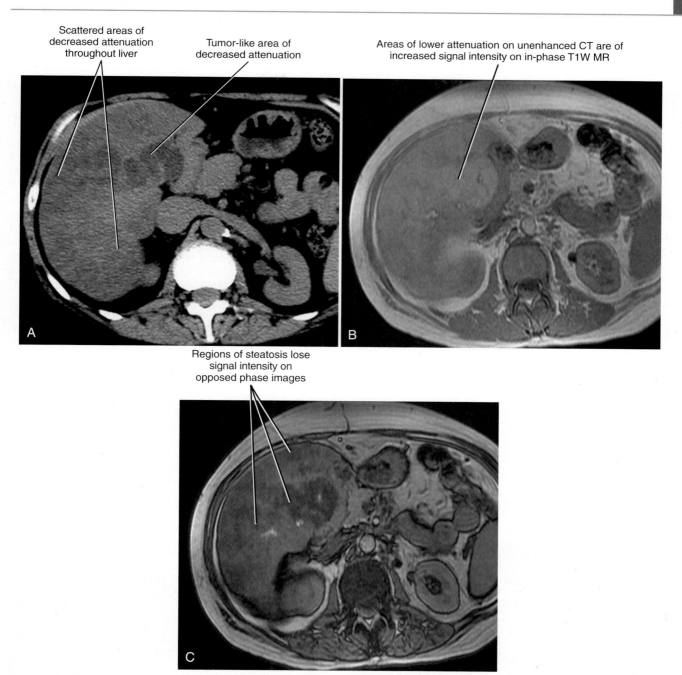

Figure 12-27 A, Unenhanced axial computed tomographic and in-phase (**B**) and opposed-phase (**C**) magnetic resonance (MR) images through the liver of a patient with heterogeneously distributed hepatic steatosis. MR imaging was performed to ensure findings on computed tomography (CT) represented fatty infiltration rather than tumor. *T1W*, T1-weighted.

behavior or exposure. Resolution can occur in response to correction of the underlying metabolic abnormality or removal of the responsible hepatic toxin, whereas progression can result from continued exposure.

Pearl: Areas of uncomplicated fatty infiltration should not cause mass effect or displace vessels.

Diffusely infiltrating lymphoma can mimic hepatic steatosis but can be distinguished with chemical-shift MRI. Acute hepatitis from causes other than steatosis may cause a relatively low-attenuation liver on CT, but such a liver may be decreased or normal in echogenicity with sonography and often will be associated with

periportal edema and gallbladder wall thickening. Table 12-5 summarizes imaging findings that suggest hepatic steatosis.

Iron Deposition

Iron may be deposited in the liver in two general ways. Deposition of iron directly into the hepatocytes occurs with primary or hereditary hemochromatosis, an autosomal recessive disorder resulting in abnormally increased intestinal absorption of iron. Hereditary hemochromatosis affects the liver, pancreas, heart, joints, endocrine glands, and skin. The spleen is typically

Table 12-5   Imaging Findings of Hepatic Steatosis

US	• Increased echogenicity • Obscuration of vessels, diaphragm, and posterior liver
CT	• Attenuation lower than spleen • Hepatic vessels appear denser than liver parenchyma
MRI	• Parenchyma loses signal intensity on out-of-phase images (MRI)*
All modalities	• No mass effect • No displacement of vessels • Rapid fluctuation over time

*Iron deposition may also cause signal loss on opposed-phase images if the out-of-phase echo time is longer than the in-phase echo time (common with 3.0-Tesla magnetic resonance scanners).
CT, Computed tomography; MRI, magnetic resonance imaging; US, ultrasound.

unaffected by hereditary hemochromatosis. The presence of excess iron causes organ damage, resulting in cirrhosis, diabetes, heart failure, and arthralgias. These patients are also at increased risk for HCC (Fig. 12-28).

Pearl: The spleen is typically unaffected by hereditary hemochromatosis.

Iron may also be taken up by the reticuloendothelial system (RES). RES iron deposition is commonly seen in patients with hemolytic anemia or those who require multiple blood transfusions. Iron deposition related to anemia or blood transfusions typically affects the spleen and bone marrow in addition to the liver. Once the RES system becomes saturated with iron, iron can be deposited in the parenchymal cells of various organs as with primary hemochromatosis. Therefore, although the presence of iron within organs such as the pancreas is a helpful differentiating feature between hereditary hemochromatosis and other iron deposition disorders, it is not an entirely specific finding. Increased hepatic iron can also be present in patients with paroxysmal nocturnal hemoglobinuria (PNH) or hemolytic anemia (e.g., sickle cell disease, prosthetic heart valve). With these disorders, excessive iron may be detected within the renal cortex in addition to the RES of the spleen and liver. Patients with PNH are prone to vascular thrombosis; therefore, if PNH is suspected, one should be sure to look for evidence of hepatic vein or portal vein thrombosis.

Iron deposition within the liver is not easily detected with ultrasonography, although the secondary effects (cirrhosis, HCC) may be evident. Unenhanced CT of patients with increased hepatic iron may demonstrate a dense liver (>70 HU) (Fig. 12-29). However, increased liver attenuation on unenhanced CT is not specific for the presence of iron, because patients receiving amiodarone therapy, patients exposed to a prior intravenous iodine dose, and some patients with glycogen storage disease may also have increased attenuation of their liver on CT (see Fig. 12-16).

MRI is more specific for iron deposition, demonstrating signal loss on all pulse sequences because of the ferromagnetic properties of iron (Figs. 12-30 and 12-31). $T2^*$-weighted images (gradient-echo images obtained with a relatively long TE) are highly sensitive to the presence of iron and may be used to quantify the amount of iron present. We frequently consult the in-phase and opposed-phase gradient-echo images routinely obtained as part of our liver protocol to confirm the presence of

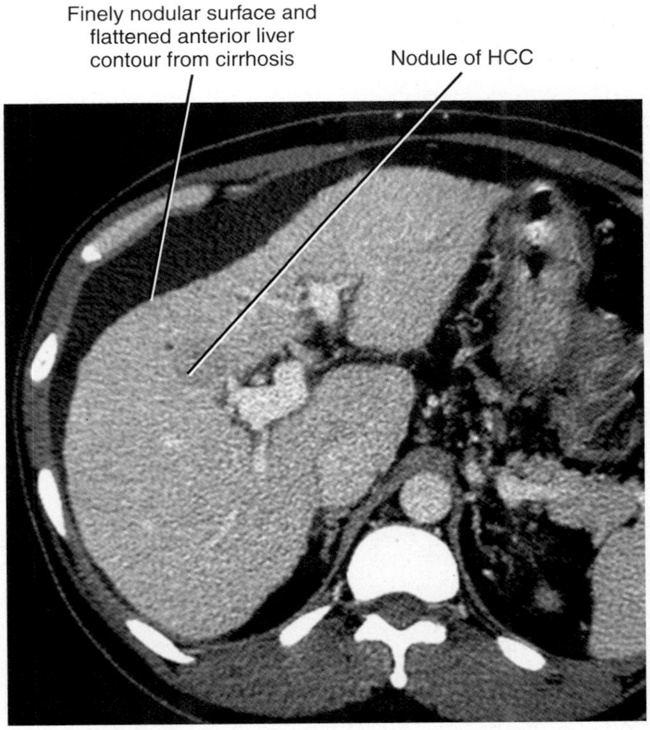

Finely nodular surface and flattened anterior liver contour from cirrhosis

Nodule of HCC

Figure 12-28 Axial portal-phase contrast-enhanced computed tomographic scan through the liver of a patient with cirrhosis and focus of hepatocellular carcinoma (HCC) secondary to primary hemochromatosis.

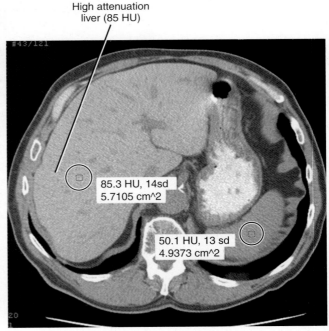

High attenuation liver (85 HU)

85.3 HU, 14sd
5.7105 cm^2

50.1 HU, 13 sd
4.9373 cm^2

Figure 12-29 Unenhanced axial computed tomographic image in a patient with primary hemochromatosis. This patient also eventually developed hepatocellular carcinoma.

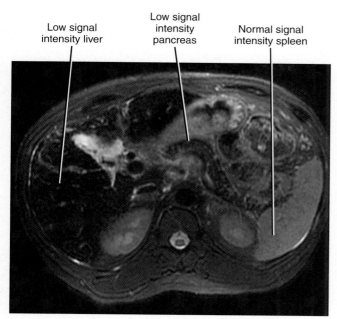

Figure 12-30 Axial T2-weighted magnetic resonance imaging through the upper abdomen of a patient with primary hemochromatosis.

iron, because the liver will appear to lose signal on the longer TE images in such cases.

MRI can also demonstrate excess iron within the pancreas and heart in patients with hereditary hemochromatosis (see Fig. 12-30). As with the liver, these organs will demonstrate a decrease in signal intensity on most imaging sequences, most noticeable on T2*-weighted images. Once the diagnosis of hereditary hemochromatosis has been established, it is important to assess the liver for evidence of organ damage (cirrhosis) and the presence of HCC (see Fig. 12-28). Nodules or masses within the liver that demonstrate increased signal intensity on T2-weighted images or nodular enhancement after

administration of intravenous gadolinium chelate should be viewed with suspicion. Table 12-6 summarizes the imaging findings of hepatic iron deposition disorders.

Uncommon Deposition Disorders

A variety of disorders may result in abnormal deposition of substances other than fat or iron within the liver. However, most deposition disorders have nonspecific manifestations on imaging studies. Patients with hepatolenticular degeneration (Wilson disease) have abnormal accumulation of copper within the liver, as well as the brain and cornea. Because of the high atomic number of copper, patients with this disorder may demonstrate a hyperdense liver with CT, although this is uncommon. With all modalities, none of the imaging findings of Wilson disease is specific. More commonly, patients with Wilson disease manifest nonspecific evidence of chronic liver disease such as steatosis and cirrhosis.

Patients with *amyloidosis* have deposition of protein-mucopolysaccharide complexes in various organs, including the liver. Hepatic amyloidosis may manifest as hepatomegaly or areas of low attenuation on CT. However, no specific findings exist that allow a definitive imaging diagnosis of amyloidosis.

Although glycogen deposited within the liver as a result of *glycogen storage disease* may appear hyperattenuating on

Table 12-6 Imaging Findings of Hepatic Iron Deposition

US	• Insensitive for detection of iron
CT	• Dense liver (>70 HU) on unenhanced CT
MRI	• Dark liver and pancreas on T2- and T2*-weighted images (hereditary hemochromatosis) • Dark liver and spleen on T2- and T2*-weighted images (transfusion related or hemolytic anemia) • Liver parenchyma loses signal intensity as echo time increases

CT, Computed tomography; *MRI,* magnetic resonance imaging; *US,* ultrasound.

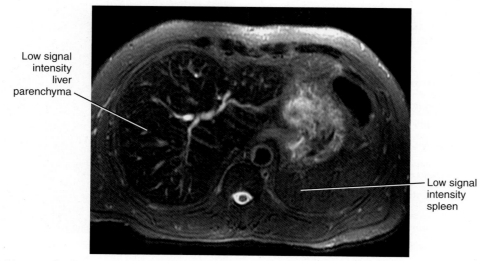

Figure 12-31 Axial T2-weighted magnetic resonance image of a patient with hemosiderosis associated with end-stage renal disease.

CT images, a low-density liver resulting from associated hepatic steatosis is more common. As with other storage diseases, hepatomegaly may be present. Patients with glycogen storage disease type I (von Gierke) or type III are at risk for development of hepatic adenomas.

Making Sense of Cirrhosis

Cirrhosis is characterized by fibrosis and nodular regeneration of the liver. These pathologic changes of cirrhosis are nonspecific, representing the end result of a variety of hepatic insults. Although alcohol is responsible for many cases of cirrhosis in the United States, the prevalence of viral hepatitis has been increasing. In addition to leading to impaired hepatic function, cirrhosis significantly increases a patient's risk for HCC. The typical practicing radiologist can expect to see many cases of cirrhosis and its complications during his/her career. Unfortunately, the combination of fibrosis, liver regeneration, architectural distortion, and altered hepatic hemodynamics makes the imaging assessment of the cirrhotic liver challenging.

Causes of Cirrhosis

Cirrhosis is a nonspecific diagnosis that is the end result of a variety of hepatic insults leading to hepatocellular injury. Most cases of cirrhosis apparent on imaging studies are due to alcohol abuse or viral hepatitis. Table 12-7 lists various categories of causes of cirrhosis.

Cirrhosis is usually preceded by hepatitis. This inflammatory process of the liver may be caused by toxic, metabolic, immune, infectious, or other types of insult. In the acute phase, hepatitis may be characterized clinically by some combination of fever, right upper quadrant pain, malaise, jaundice, elevated liver function tests, and hepatomegaly. Acute hepatitis uncommonly manifests sonographically as hepatomegaly with decreased echogenicity of the hepatic parenchyma and relatively increased echogenicity of the portal vein walls (sometimes referred to as the "starry-sky" appearance), although some studies show this is a nonspecific finding. Periportal edema manifests as periportal sonolucency. Thickening (edema) of the gallbladder wall may be noted. With CT, the periportal edema appears as fluid attenuation tracking along the portal vessels in the place of periportal fat

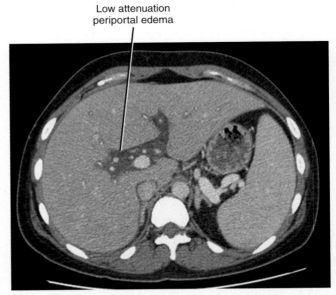

Low attenuation periportal edema

Figure 12-32 Axial enhanced computed tomographic scan through the upper abdomen of a patient with periportal edema caused by acute viral hepatitis.

(Fig. 12-32). Alcoholic and nonalcoholic steatohepatitis may be associated with low-attenuation hepatic parenchyma caused by fatty infiltration. Chronic active (viral) hepatitis is frequently associated with lymphadenopathy in the hepatoduodenal ligament (Fig. 12-33). With MRI, the periportal edema present in acute hepatitis manifests as high periportal signal intensity on T2-weighted images. The liver may also demonstrate mildly increased signal intensity on T2-weighted and decreased signal intensity on T1-weighted images, although these changes are likely to be subtle. Associated steatosis will be most evident with in- and opposed-phase MRI.

Table 12-7 Causes of Cirrhosis

General Category	Common Examples
Infection	Viral hepatitis
Drugs and toxins	Alcohol, methotrexate
Biliary abnormalities	Primary sclerosing cholangitis, primary biliary cirrhosis
Metabolic disorders	Hereditary hemochromatosis
Cardiovascular disorders	Congestive heart failure, Budd–Chiari syndrome
Steatohepatitis	Nonalcoholic steatohepatitis
Granulomatous disorders	Sarcoidosis

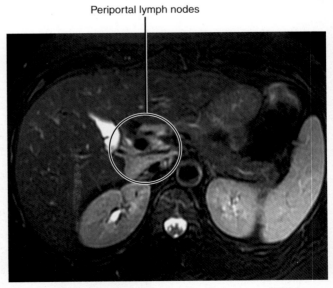

Periportal lymph nodes

Figure 12-33 Axial T2-weighted magnetic resonance (MR) image shows hepatoduodenal ligament lymph nodes in a patient with hepatitis C. High signal intensity is normal for lymph nodes on fat-suppressed T2-weighted MR images.

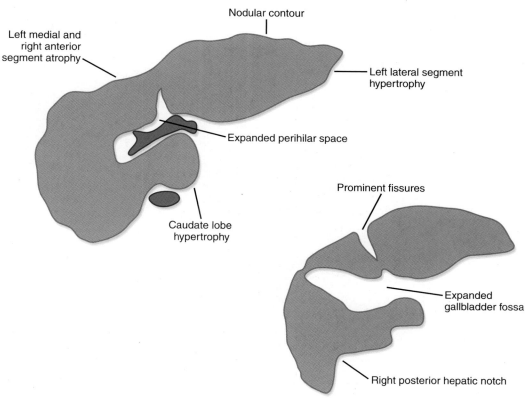

Figure 12-34 labels:
- Nodular contour
- Left medial and right anterior segment atrophy
- Left lateral segment hypertrophy
- Expanded perihilar space
- Caudate lobe hypertrophy
- Prominent fissures
- Expanded gallbladder fossa
- Right posterior hepatic notch

Figure 12-34 Typical morphologic changes of cirrhosis.

Gross Morphologic Findings and Patterns of Cirrhosis

Figure 12-34 illustrates some typical morphologic changes of cirrhosis that may be present on imaging studies. Not all findings will be present in all cases of cirrhosis, and early in its course, morphologic changes of cirrhosis may be undetectable with imaging. It is also important to emphasize that not all cirrhotic livers will be reduced in volume. Some cirrhotic livers will appear normal in size or enlarged (Fig. 12-35). A quantitative approach to diagnosing cirrhosis has been advocated by some. In our experience, however, calculation of such ratios as the caudate-right lobe ratio is rarely necessary to suggest the diagnosis of cirrhosis because other morphologic findings are usually sufficient. For readers who prefer objective criteria, we include an illustration of the modified caudate-right lobe ratio (Fig. 12-36). A modified caudate-right lobe ratio of at least 0.9 has been shown to have an accuracy rate of almost 75% for the diagnosis of cirrhosis when applied to MR images and should be expected to work equally well for CT. Examination of the left lateral segment (lateral section) of the liver with a high-frequency linear US transducer may identify subtle nodularity of the liver or rounding of the contour of the left lateral segment that may aid in suggesting a diagnosis of cirrhosis (Fig. 12-37).

A cirrhotic liver consists of regenerative nodules with intervening fibrosis, regardless of cause. As a result, significant overlap of imaging findings exists between the various causes of cirrhosis. Despite this overlap, certain imaging appearances are more commonly associated

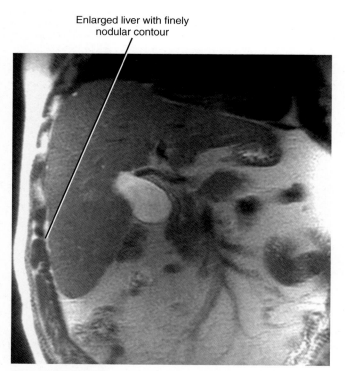

Enlarged liver with finely nodular contour

Figure 12-35 Coronal T2-weighted magnetic resonance imaging (MRI) in a patient with cirrhosis caused by alcohol abuse and hepatitis C.

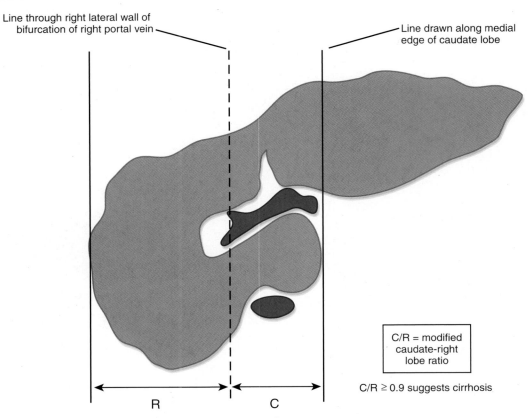

Figure 12-36 The modified caudate-right lobe ratio for diagnosing cirrhosis.

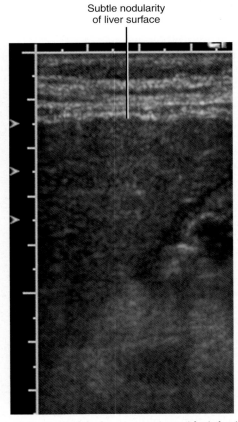

Figure 12-37 Sonogram of left lateral segment (section) of the liver in a patient with cirrhosis performed with a high-frequency linear transducer.

with a particular causative factor. For example, enlargement of the caudate lobe and a right posterior hepatic notch are more common with alcoholic cirrhosis than with viral-induced cirrhosis, although this combination of findings is not specific. Unfortunately, a specific imaging diagnosis is not possible in the majority of cases of cirrhosis, and multiple contributing causes may be present in any given patient (e.g., alcohol and viral hepatitis). Therefore, imaging findings should always be correlated with clinical data before rendering a specific diagnosis. Table 12-8 lists imaging findings that can suggest the cause of cirrhosis.

Extrahepatic Findings in Cirrhosis

When imaging findings suggest the diagnosis of cirrhosis, one should be sure to look for the host of extrahepatic findings that may be present. Stigmata of portal hypertension include *splenomegaly, ascites,* and *varices* (Fig. 12-40).

Table 12-8 Imaging Findings Suggestive of (But Not Specific for) Cause of Cirrhosis

Causative Factors	Imaging Findings
Primary sclerosing cholangitis (Fig. 12-38)	• Lobulated liver contour • Marked caudate lobe hypertrophy • Left lateral and right posterior segment atrophy • Rounded appearance of liver • Segmental intrahepatic bile duct dilatation • Intraductal biliary calculi
Primary biliary cirrhosis (Fig. 12-39)	• Generalized liver hypertrophy • Periportal halo on magnetic resonance images*
Hereditary hemochromatosis (see Figs. 12-28 and 12-30)	• Iron deposition in liver and pancreas but not spleen†
Schistosomiasis	• Periportal and subcapsular fibrosis (thick periportal bands) • Lobulation of the liver contour • Subcapsular and periportal calcifications
Congenital hepatic fibrosis (considered distinct from cirrhosis)	• Medial segment atrophy • Biliary sacculations • Renal tubular ectasia

*Low signal intensity surrounding the intrahepatic portal vein branches, most conspicuous on portal- and equilibrium-phase gadolinium-enhanced images.
†Liver iron deposition is not uncommon in cirrhosis of other causes; however, the pancreas is uninvolved in such cases.

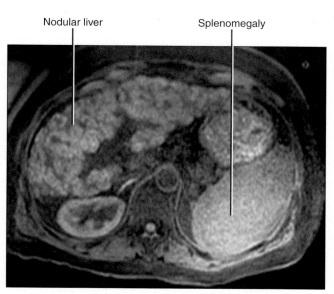

Figure 12-39 Axial, unenhanced, fat-suppressed, T1-weighted magnetic resonance image through the upper abdomen of a patient with primary biliary cirrhosis.

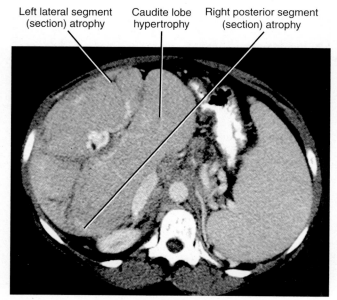

Figure 12-38 Axial enhanced computed tomographic scan of a patient with primary sclerosing cholangitis. Note the round shape of the liver.

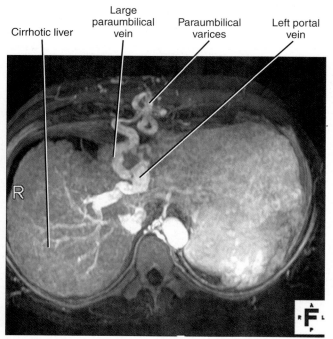

Figure 12-40 Axial maximum intensity projection image of portal-phase gadolinium-enhanced magnetic resonance imaging through the upper abdomen of a patient with cirrhosis and portal hypertension resulting in large paraumbilical varices.

Table 12-9 outlines some of the more common venous collateral pathways encountered in patients with portal hypertension. *Enlarged lymph nodes* are commonly seen in the hepatoduodenal ligament and elsewhere in the setting of cirrhosis. Siderotic deposits within the spleen *(Gamna–Gandy bodies)* may be noted on MRI (Fig. 12-41). These

Table 12-9 Common Collaterals of Portal Hypertension

Varices	Typical Supply*	Comments
Esophageal and para-esophageal	Left gastric (coronary) vein	Predominately (but not exclusively) drain* to azygous/hemiazygous system
Gastric	Left gastric vein and short gastric veins	Isolated gastric varices and enlarged gastroepiploic veins suggest splenic vein occlusion
Left renal vein shunts	Gastric (gastrorenal shunt) and splenic (splenorenal shunt) veins	Communication with the left renal vein is usually visible Enlargement of the left renal vein may be present
Paraumbilical	Left portal vein	Drain cephalad to the internal thoracic veins or caudally to the superior epigastric veins (and eventually inferior epigastric and external iliac veins)
Extraperitoneal	Mesenteric veins	Drain to gonadal, paravertebral, and other extraperitoneal veins

*In this table, *supply* and *drainage* refer to the abnormal (portal to systemic) pattern induced by portal hypertension.

lesions are most conspicuous on long TE gradient-echo images and appear as small, very-low-signal intensity foci scattered throughout the spleen. Patients with advanced cirrhosis may manifest *bowel wall thickening.* Edematous thickening of the ascending colon is particularly characteristic, although other segments of large or small bowel may be involved. Colon thickening related to cirrhosis and portal hypertension should not be confused with inflammatory or neoplastic processes. Thickening related to cirrhosis can be seen along the dependent wall of the colon or involving the haustrations. Air-distended nondependent portions of the colon often maintain a thin wall in the setting of portal hypertension (Fig. 12-42).

Imaging Mimics of Cirrhosis

One should be aware of entities that may simulate some of the morphologic features of cirrhosis. Patients with liver metastases who have been treated with chemotherapy may occasionally develop morphologic changes in the liver that simulate cirrhosis (Fig. 12-43). This has most frequently been described with *breast carcinoma,* although other tumors may behave similarly. Some chemotherapy agents can also directly cause hepatotoxicity. *Diffuse metastatic disease* replacing normal hepatic parenchyma can simulate cirrhosis by creating a nodular architecture that may be associated with stigmata of portal hypertension. The liver contour may appear irregular in patients with *pseudomyxoma peritonei,* and mucin may simulate simple ascites in such patients, potentially creating confusion with cirrhosis (Fig. 12-44). An appearance of cirrhotic liver morphology may also be created after *partial hepatectomy* or in the setting of congenital segmental atrophy, although there should be no nodularity or fibrosis of

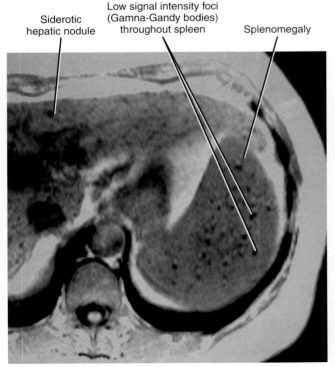

Figure 12-41 Axial T1-weighted image of the abdomen in a patient with cirrhosis and portal hypertension demonstrating Gamna–Gandy bodies in the spleen.

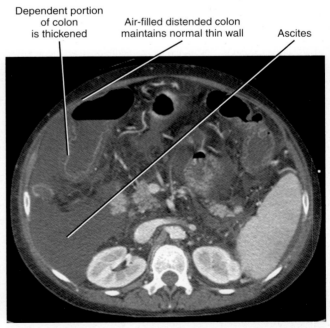

Figure 12-42 Axial enhanced computed tomography through the abdomen of a patient with cirrhosis and portal hypertension demonstrating edema of colon.

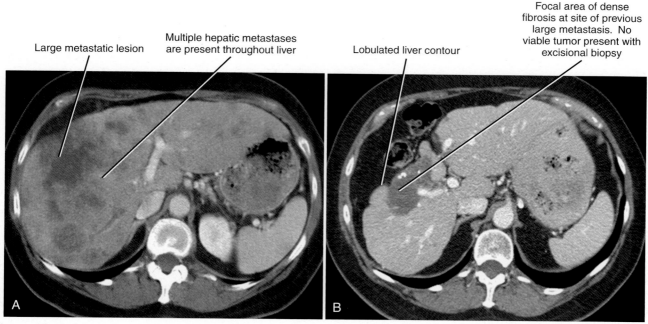

Large metastatic lesion

Multiple hepatic metastases are present throughout liver

Lobulated liver contour

Focal area of dense fibrosis at site of previous large metastasis. No viable tumor present with excisional biopsy

Figure 12-43 Axial enhanced computed tomographic images through the liver in a patient with breast cancer metastases before treatment (A) and several years after treatment (B). Note that the liver has developed a cirrhotic appearance after therapy (B).

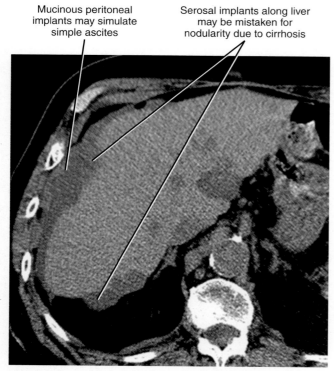

Mucinous peritoneal implants may simulate simple ascites

Serosal implants along liver may be mistaken for nodularity due to cirrhosis

Figure 12-44 Unenhanced axial computed tomographic scan through the upper abdomen of a patient with mucinous peritoneal metastatic disease.

such a liver in the absence of true cirrhosis. Areas of scarring and liver regeneration after fulminant hepatitis and *nodular regenerative hyperplasia* (regenerative nodules that occur in the absence of fibrosis) may likewise simulate cirrhosis. Granulomatous diseases such as

sarcoidosis can mimic cirrhosis early in their course (because of innumerable nodules throughout the liver) or progress to cirrhosis over time (Fig. 12-45).

Pitfall: Diffuse or treated metastatic disease that involves the liver can simulate cirrhosis.

Parenchymal Findings Associated with Cirrhosis

The cirrhotic hepatic architecture is typically heterogeneous and hyperechoic with grayscale US. Unenhanced CT and MRI may show heterogeneity because of areas of *fibrosis, fatty infiltration,* or *iron deposition* (Fig. 12-46). Contrast-enhanced CT and MRI often reveal heterogeneous enhancement because of hemodynamic alterations, as well as differential enhancement of cirrhotic nodules and fibrosis.

Regenerative nodules are present in all cirrhotic livers but are not always obvious with imaging. MRI is better than US or CT for demonstrating regenerative nodules throughout the liver (Fig. 12-47). With CT, most benign regenerative nodules are isoattenuating. Hyperattenuating nodules may reflect the presence of iron or glycogen. Most regenerative nodules are nearly isointense to hepatic parenchyma on T1- and T2-weighted MR images. Regenerative nodules can occasionally contain lipid or hemosiderin, both of which are detectable with chemical-shift (in-phase and opposed-phase) imaging. Lipid containing regenerative nodules will be of increased signal intensity on T1-weighted images and lose signal on opposed-phase images (Fig. 12-48). The presence of lipid within a cirrhotic nodule does not ensure benignity because nodules of HCC may contain lipid. Siderotic nodules demonstrate decreased signal intensity on T1- and T2-weighted images, and are of particularly low signal

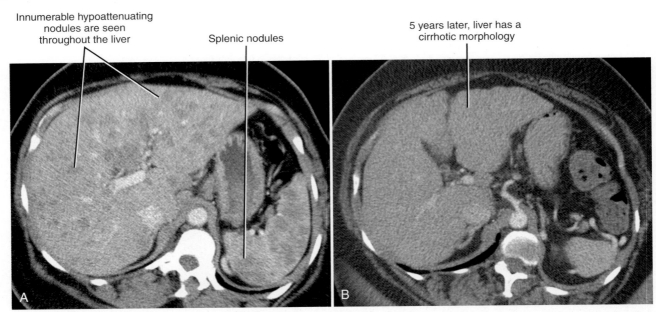

Innumerable hypoattenuating nodules are seen throughout the liver

Splenic nodules

5 years later, liver has a cirrhotic morphology

Figure 12-45 Enhanced axial computed tomographic images through the upper abdomen of a patient with sarcoidosis performed at time of diagnosis (**A**) and 5 years later (**B**).

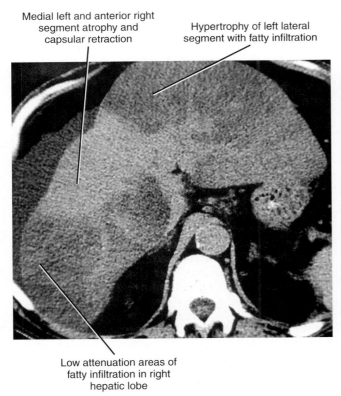

Medial left and anterior right segment atrophy and capsular retraction

Hypertrophy of left lateral segment with fatty infiltration

Low attenuation areas of fatty infiltration in right hepatic lobe

Figure 12-46 Axial unenhanced computed tomographic image through the liver in a patient with cirrhosis and hepatic steatosis.

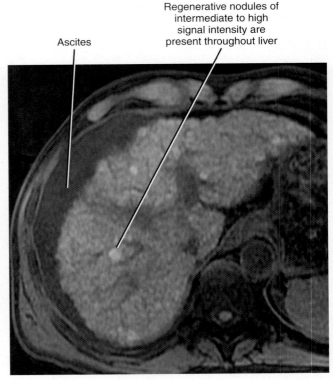

Ascites

Regenerative nodules of intermediate to high signal intensity are present throughout liver

Figure 12-47 Axial, T1-weighted, unenhanced, fat-suppressed magnetic resonance image in a patient with cirrhosis.

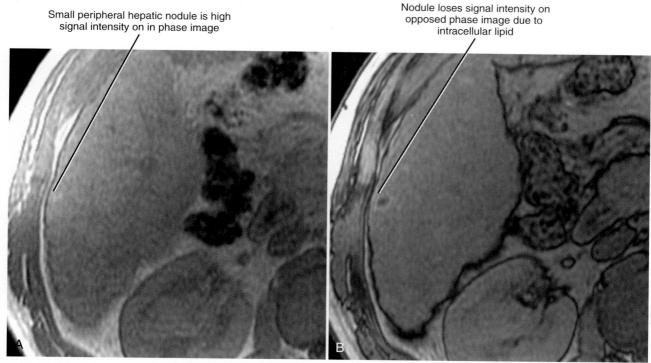

Small peripheral hepatic nodule is high
signal intensity on in phase image

Nodule loses signal intensity on
opposed phase image due to
intracellular lipid

Figure 12-48 Axial in-phase (**A**) and opposed-phase (**B**) gradient-echo magnetic resonance images of a patient with cirrhosis and a steatotic nodule.

intensity on T2*-weighted (long TE gradient-echo) images (Fig. 12-49).

The fibrosis that surrounds the regenerative nodules in a cirrhotic liver typically appears as hypoattenuating to isoattenuating on CT. The fibrous septa are better appreciated on MRI, which shows them to be hypointense on unenhanced T1-weighted images and hyperintense relative to the nodules on T2-weighted images (particularly when edema or inflammation is present) (Fig. 12-50). After administration of extracellular intravenous contrast agents, hepatic fibrosis will usually enhance gradually and

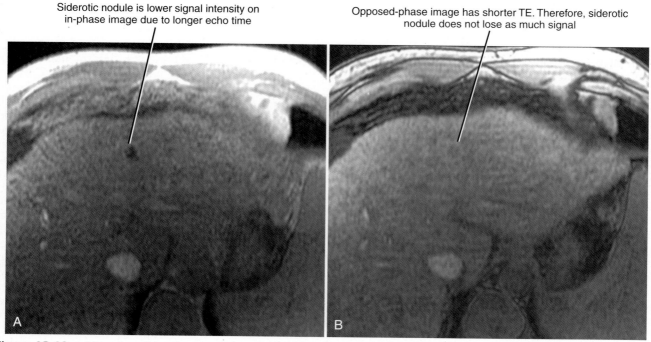

Siderotic nodule is lower signal intensity on
in-phase image due to longer echo time

Opposed-phase image has shorter TE. Therefore, siderotic
nodule does not lose as much signal

Figure 12-49 Axial in-phase (**A**) and opposed-phase (**B**) gradient-echo magnetic resonance images of a patient with cirrhosis and a siderotic nodule.

Fibrosis appears as low
signal intensity bands on
T1-weighted image

Fibrosis appears as high
signal intensity bands on
T2-weighted image

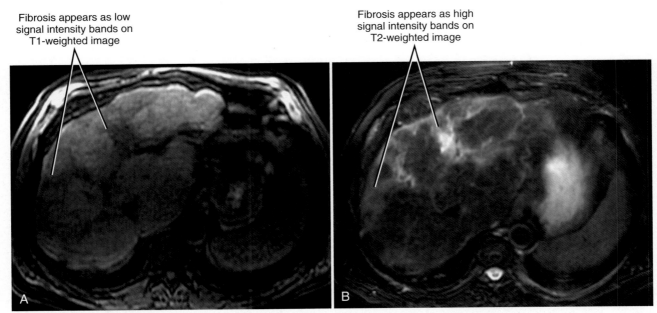

Figure 12-50 Axial fat-suppressed T1- (**A**) and T2-weighted (**B**) magnetic resonance images of a cirrhotic liver.

progressively, although early enhancement has been observed in rare cases.

Approximately 15% of patients with advanced cirrhosis experience development of *confluent hepatic fibrosis*. With US, confluent fibrosis is typically heterogeneous and hyperechoic in appearance. On CT images, confluent fibrosis appears hypoattenuating on unenhanced images and mildly hyperattenuating on contrast-enhanced equilibrium-phase images. With MRI, confluent fibrosis appears hypointense compared with hepatic parenchyma on T1-weighted images and mildly hyperintense on T2-weighted images. As with CT, areas of confluent fibrosis often demonstrate gradual enhancement after administration of extracellular gadolinium chelates with increased signal intensity relative to liver parenchyma on equilibrium-phase images. Areas of confluent fibrosis tend to be wedge shaped, extending out from the hepatic hilum toward the liver capsule. The left medial segment (IV) and right anterior segments (V, VIII) are most commonly involved. Capsular retraction is often present. Confluent fibrosis can be difficult to distinguish from sclerosing or infiltrative HCC, although the latter entity tends to demonstrate earlier enhancement with washout in the portal phase.

Cirrhotic Nodules: When to be Concerned

It is generally agreed that HCC in the setting of cirrhosis develops as a result of a progression from benign regenerative nodule to dysplastic nodule to malignant tumor with various degrees of differentiation. Much investigation has focused on differentiating benign from premalignant or malignant nodules, but it is becoming increasingly apparent that considerable overlap in imaging appearances exists. It has also become clear that the sensitivity of available imaging modalities for detection of small HCCs is limited. However, because of the high prevalence of hepatitis and cirrhosis-associated HCC

worldwide, imaging continues to play an important role in the detection and characterization of cirrhotic nodules. Until recently, invasive techniques such as CT arterial portography or intraarterial injection of iodized oil were routinely used to preoperatively detect small HCCs. However, with the advent of multidetector CT scanners and improved MRI sequences, these techniques are rarely performed for diagnosis in the United States.

In general, cirrhotic nodules that are isoechoic with sonography, isoattenuating on CT, and isointense or hypointense on T1- and T2-weighted MR images are considered benign provided they do not demonstrate increased flow with color Doppler imaging or enhancement after intravenous administration of extracellular contrast agents.

Dysplastic nodules represent an intermediate step in the progression from regenerative nodule to HCC. However, imaging findings associated with dysplastic nodules tend to be nonspecific and highly variable. With CT, the majority of dysplastic nodules go undetected despite use of dynamic, multiphase, contrast-enhanced techniques. We tend not to make a definitive diagnosis of dysplastic nodule on US or CT, although we will occasionally suggest the diagnosis based on MRI when we see the classic findings of high signal intensity on T1-weighted images, low signal intensity on T2-weighted images, and enhancement similar to hepatic parenchyma after gadolinium administration (Fig. 12-51). In reality, many nodules that demonstrate high signal intensity on T1-weighted images are not dysplastic, although some dysplastic nodules are isointense or hypointense to surrounding liver on T1-weighted images. Therefore, when a nodule demonstrates imaging characteristics that distinguish it from the background of regenerative nodules without displaying typical features of HCC, it may be more appropriate to refer to such a nodule as "atypical" and worthy of close follow-up.

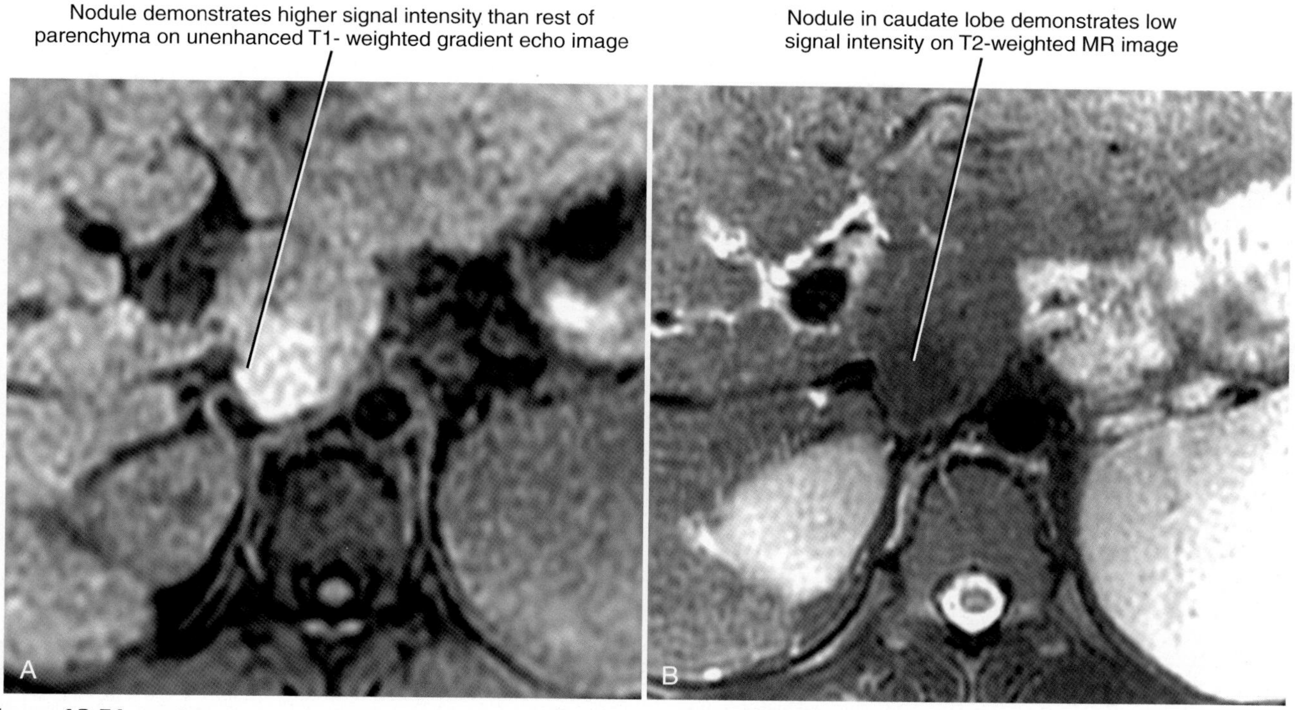

Nodule demonstrates higher signal intensity than rest of parenchyma on unenhanced T1- weighted gradient echo image

Nodule in caudate lobe demonstrates low signal intensity on T2-weighted MR image

Figure 12-51 Axial T1- (**A**) and T2-weighted (**B**) images of the liver in a patient with cirrhosis. The atypical nodule in the caudate lobe showed no abnormal enhancement after contrast administration and remained stable on subsequent follow-up imaging studies. *MR,* Magnetic resonance.

When arterial phase enhancement is present within a dysplastic nodule, confident distinction from HCC is not possible based on imaging appearance.

An uncomplicated HCC is often hypoechoic relative to surrounding liver with sonography (Fig. 12-52). HCC may also appear hyperechoic, particularly in the setting of fatty metamorphosis of the tumor (Figs. 12-53). In such a case, HCC can be confused with hemangioma. Therefore, a confident sonographic diagnosis of hemangioma is difficult to make in the setting of cirrhosis. Doppler sonography of HCC may reveal hypervascularity with high velocity signals. Larger HCCs tend to be

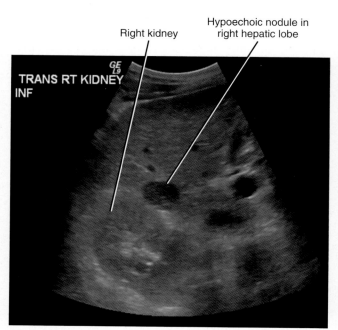

Right kidney

Hypoechoic nodule in right hepatic lobe

Figure 12-52 Transverse ultrasound image at the level of the right kidney in a patient with hepatitis C demonstrates a hypoechoic nodule in the liver. Subsequent biopsy confirmed hepatocellular carcinoma.

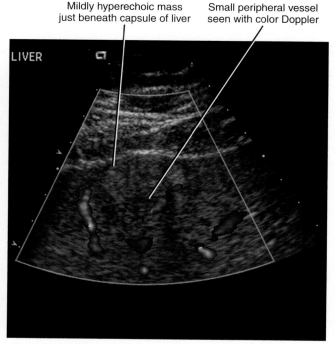

Mildly hyperechoic mass just beneath capsule of liver

Small peripheral vessel seen with color Doppler

Figure 12-53 Ultrasound of the liver in a patient with cirrhosis and hepatocellular carcinoma just beneath the liver capsule. Note that this lesion is mildly hyperechoic relative to the liver.

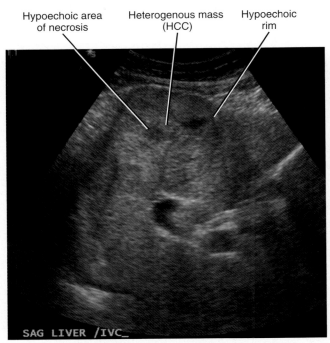

Hypoechoic area of necrosis — Heterogenous mass (HCC) — Hypoechoic rim

Figure 12-54 Transverse sonogram through the liver of a patient with cirrhosis demonstrates large heterogeneous mass (hepatocellular carcinoma [HCC]) within the left lobe (left hemiliver). This patient was treated with chemoembolization.

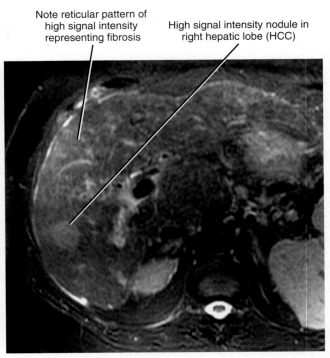

Note reticular pattern of high signal intensity representing fibrosis — High signal intensity nodule in right hepatic lobe (HCC)

Figure 12-55 Axial T2-weighted magnetic resonance imaging of the liver in a patient with cirrhosis and hepatocellular carcinoma (HCC). This lesion was successfully treated with radiofrequency ablation.

heterogeneous on US images (Fig. 12-54). With unenhanced CT, HCC can appear to be of similar, increased, or decreased attenuation compared with surrounding hepatic parenchyma. HCC can also be of similar, increased, or decreased signal intensity compared with surrounding liver on T1- and T2-weighted MR images. However, increased signal intensity of a nodule on T2-weighted images in a patient with cirrhosis is particularly worrisome for HCC (Fig. 12-55). Another concerning feature of a cirrhotic nodule is the "nodule within nodule" sign (Fig. 12-56). This refers to the presence of a nodular focus of HCC within a dysplastic nodule. This sign may manifest as either a hyperintense focus within a hypointense nodule on T2-weighted images, a hyperintense focus within a hypointense siderotic nodule on T2*-weighted images, or as a focus of arterial phase enhancement within an otherwise hypoenhancing or isoenhancing nodule. Additional features associated with malignant nodules are listed in Table 12-10, and include washout of contrast on portal-phase images, rim enhancement, and evidence of growth on successive examinations.

■ FOCAL ABNORMALITIES OF THE LIVER

Approach to Focal Liver Abnormalities

When confronted with a focal liver abnormality, it is helpful to have an organized, systematic approach to analyzing the lesion. Although it may be potentially entertaining to impress your colleagues with

across-the-room, shoot-from-the-hip diagnoses, it is not the least bit entertaining to see a patient undergo an unnecessary hepatectomy for a benign lesion because the radiologist did not perform a sufficient analysis of the lesion before surgery. Therefore, it may be beneficial to ask the following questions about a potential liver lesion:

1. *Is it real, a normal variant, or an artifact?* Focal fat, fatty sparing, vascular phenomena, normal anatomic structures, and a host of technical artifacts may all simulate hepatic neoplasms (Fig. 12-57).
2. *Is it truly arising from the liver?* Implants on the peritoneal surface of the liver or large tumors arising from adjacent organs may mimic hepatic parenchymal lesions (Fig. 12-58). Distinguishing these entities is important because, for example, a patient with a parenchymal metastasis from colon cancer may benefit from hepatic resection. A peritoneal implant from colon cancer along the liver surface requires an alternative approach to treatment.
3. *Is it likely benign or malignant?* Do not forget to consider the possibility of an atypical appearance of a benign lesion. In some patients, imaging follow-up may be a better option than biopsy.
4. *What is the lesion composed of?* Look for fluid, solid tissue, fat, calcium, and hemorrhage.
5. *What is the shape of the lesion and what type of margins does it have?* Perfusion anomalies and abnormalities of focal fat deposition often have straight rather than rounded borders.
6. *How does the lesion enhance?* Be certain to correlate lesion enhancement with the phase of imaging (i.e., arterial, portal, equilibrium, delayed).

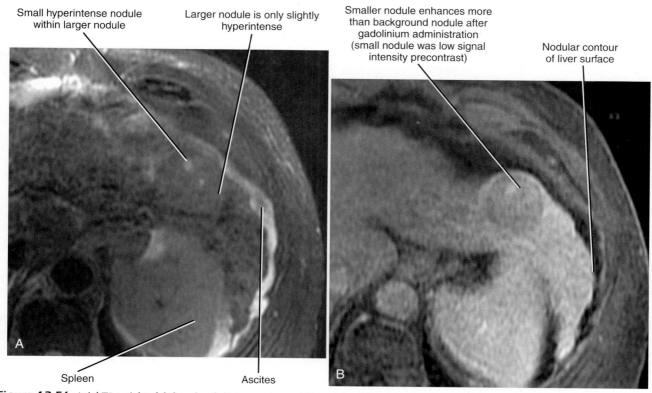

Small hyperintense nodule within larger nodule

Larger nodule is only slightly hyperintense

Smaller nodule enhances more than background nodule after gadolinium administration (small nodule was low signal intensity precontrast)

Nodular contour of liver surface

Spleen

Ascites

Figure 12-56 Axial T2-weighted (**A**) and gadolinium-enhanced T1-weighted (**B**) magnetic resonance images of a "nodule within nodule" in a patient with cirrhosis.

Table 12-10   Concerning Features of a Nodule in the Setting of Cirrhosis

US	Hypoechoic rim Increased vascularity with color Doppler imaging Growth over several months
CT	Arterial-phase enhancement Portal-phase washout Rim enhancement Nodule-within-nodule appearance Growth over several months
MRI	Arterial-phase enhancement Portal-phase washout Rim enhancement Nodule-within-nodule appearance High signal intensity on T2-weighted images Growth over several months

CT, Computed tomography; MRI, magnetic resonance imaging; US, ultrasound.

7. *Is the lesion(s) single or multiple?* Avoid satisfaction of search. Always look for more lesions.
8. *Is there evidence of biliary, vascular, or extrahepatic involvement?* These findings will add specificity and may affect subsequent management.
9. *Does the proposed diagnosis fit the clinical picture and patient risk factors?* An HCC is more likely than cholangiocarcinoma in a patient with chronic viral hepatitis and cirrhosis, even if the lesion appearance is atypical for HCC. Of course, it is also appropriate to keep in mind the possibility of something unusual or bizarre.

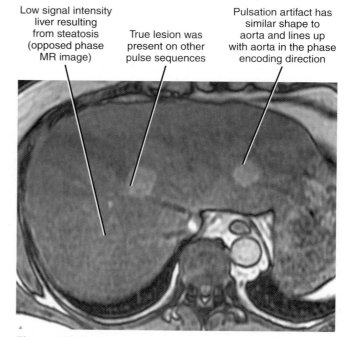

Low signal intensity liver resulting from steatosis (opposed phase MR image)

True lesion was present on other pulse sequences

Pulsation artifact has similar shape to aorta and lines up with aorta in the phase encoding direction

Figure 12-57 Axial, opposed-phase, T1-weighted, gradient-echo image in a patient with hepatic steatosis with one true hepatic mass and one artifact related to vascular pulsation. *MR,* Magnetic resonance.

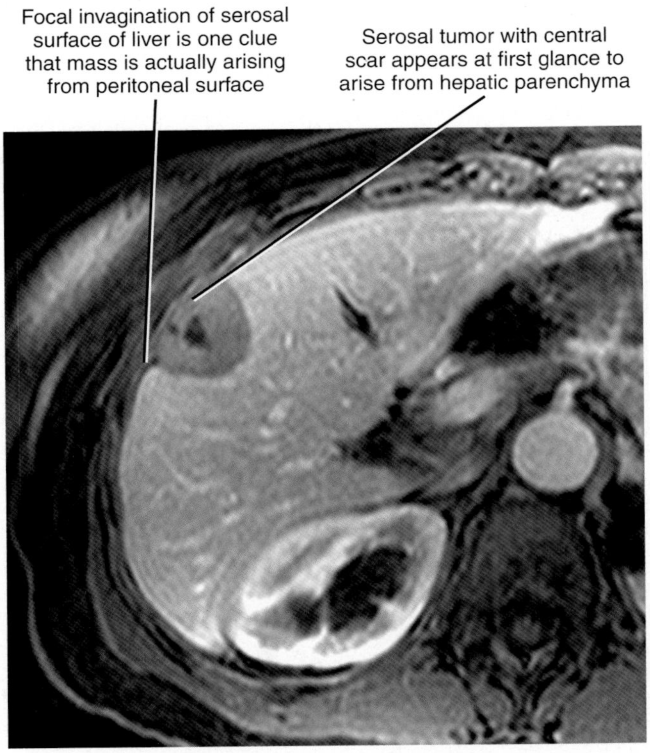

Focal invagination of serosal surface of liver is one clue that mass is actually arising from peritoneal surface

Serosal tumor with central scar appears at first glance to arise from hepatic parenchyma

Figure 12-58 Axial, gadolinium-enhanced, T1-weighted, magnetic resonance image of a patient with multiple gastrointestinal stromal tumor metastases involving the peritoneum. This one mimics a parenchymal hepatic lesion.

10. *Is there a better test to evaluate the lesion?* It is unnecessary and reckless to render a definitive diagnosis in every case.

By adhering to a systematic approach, one can minimize potentially dangerous misinterpretations and maximize diagnostic accuracy. The following sections examine some of the above questions in more detail.

Is the Lesion Real? Pseudolesions of the Liver

This chapter uses the term *pseudolesion* to describe a focal imaging finding of little or no clinical significance (if recognized) that does not result from a neoplastic, inflammatory, or infectious process. Pseudolesions may be the result of focal fat and fatty sparing, normal variations in hepatic perfusion, and technical imaging artifacts. Box 12-3 lists some general imaging characteristics of pseudolesions of the liver.

Focal Fatty Infiltration and Sparing

Hepatic steatosis does not always involve the entire liver. Focal areas of steatosis may appear geographic, wedge shaped, round, perivascular, or segmental. Fatty infiltration that involves a particular vascular distribution may be a sign of altered hepatic perfusion. We always emphasize that fatty infiltration involving a vascular territory should always prompt a search for a vascular abnormality (see Fig. 12-22). Systemic venous inflow to the liver (see earlier discussion in Liver Anatomy section) may result in focal areas of fatty infiltration or focal fatty sparing in the portion of liver supplied by systemic veins.

BOX 12-3   Typical Imaging Features of Hepatic Pseudolesions

No mass effect
Normal vessels course through the lesion without deviating
Subcapsular location without distortion of liver contour
Typical location (e.g., segment IV, near falciform ligament)
Wedge shape
No evidence of neovascularity
Normal uptake of liver-specific contrast agents (MRI, nuclear medicine)
Not visible with other modalities (e.g., targeted ultrasound)
No increased metabolic activity (PET)

Therefore, fatty infiltration is often seen in segment IV along the falciform ligament or hepatic hilum. In some cases, the responsible vessels may be seen entering the liver on a high-quality imaging examination. Focal fatty infiltration typically appears as an area of increased echogenicity with sonography and decreased attenuation on noncontrast-enhanced computed tomography (NCCT). Focal fatty infiltration is often triangular in shape and capsular based (Fig. 12-59). The lesion must not distort the liver contour, displace vessels, or demonstrate other evidence of mass effect to be characterized as focal fatty infiltration. Intravenous contrast agents should be taken up normally by such areas, although transiently diminished enhancement during the portal phase is seen occasionally.

Triangular subcapsular area of low attenuation in segment IV

Portal vein bifurcation

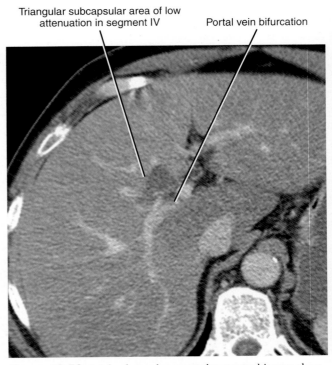

Figure 12-59 Axial enhanced computed tomographic scan showing focal fatty infiltration in segment IV of the liver.

Round or irregular areas of focal fatty infiltration well within the liver parenchyma are encountered occasionally. In such cases, it may be necessary to pursue further characterization with MRI. MRI can confirm the presence of focal fat through the use of chemical-shift (in- and opposed-phase) imaging. Perivascular fatty infiltration is an uncommon variant that can be seen around hepatic veins, portal veins, or both. The distribution of focal fatty infiltration may fluctuate over time or disappear completely on follow-up studies.

Pearl: Fatty infiltration involving a vascular territory should always prompt a search for a vascular abnormality.

Focal fatty sparing manifests as an island(s) of normal liver surrounded by diffuse hepatic steatosis. Fatty sparing is most often seen in the subcapsular region along the gallbladder fossa and the posteromedial aspect of segment IV (Fig. 12-60). As with focal fatty infiltration, regions of fatty sparing should not demonstrate evidence of mass effect, abnormal vascularity, or abnormal enhancement with contrast agents. The typical locations of focal fatty infiltration and sparing are shown in Figure 12-61.

Transient Hepatic Attenuation and Transient Hepatic Intensity Differences

The terms *transient hepatic attenuation difference* (THAD) and *transient hepatic intensity difference* (THID) may mean different things to different people, but most commonly, they refer to a transient variation (usually increase) in attenuation (CT) or signal intensity (MRI) relative to the normal liver during the early phase of a multiphase, dynamic, contrast-enhanced examination. This phenomenon is referred to as transient when significant differential enhancement does not persist into the portal venous and equilibrium phases. THADs and THIDs are usually caused by some derangement of blood flow to the affected part of the liver. This often results from diminished or disrupted portal flow or arterioportal shunting. THADs and THIDs often occur in the absence of tumor, although a variety of tumors, benign and malignant, may be associated with these phenomena. It is important to distinguish benign THADs and THIDS from those associated with malignant

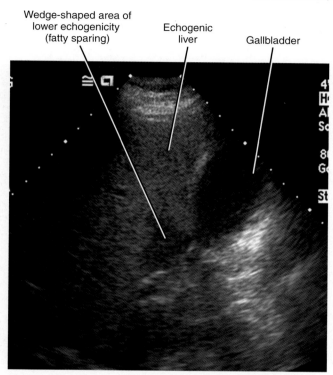

Figure 12-60 Sonogram through the liver and gallbladder of a patient with hepatic steatosis and focal sparing near the gallbladder (confirmed with magnetic resonance imaging, not shown).

hepatic lesions. The differentiation between a hemangioma associated with a THAD or a THID and an HCC is usually straightforward. Hemangiomas are typically much brighter on T2-weighted images than most HCCs. A background of cirrhosis favors a diagnosis of HCC. Furthermore, hemangiomas tend to retain intravenous contrast to the same degree as the hepatic vessels on later phases of contrast-enhanced imaging, whereas HCCs typically washout and become the same or lower attenuation or signal intensity than background liver (Fig. 12-62).

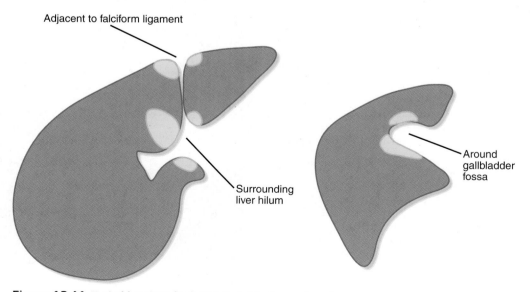

Figure 12-61 Typical locations for focal fatty infiltration and sparing.

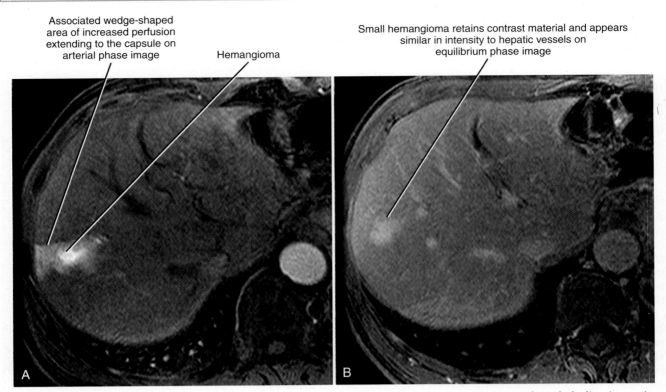

Associated wedge-shaped area of increased perfusion extending to the capsule on arterial phase image

Hemangioma

Small hemangioma retains contrast material and appears similar in intensity to hepatic vessels on equilibrium phase image

Figure 12-62 Axial arterial- **(A)** and equilibrium-phase **(B)** gadolinium-enhanced magnetic resonance images through the liver in a patient with a small hemangioma associated with a transient hepatic intensity difference. Lesion was bright on T2-weighted images (not shown).

THADs and THIDs that are not associated with any mass can appear wedge shaped, extend to the capsule, or conform to a vascular distribution. Whenever a THAD or THID is detected in the distribution of a vessel, such as a hepatic or portal vein branch, or bile duct, one should examine the images for evidence of vascular or biliary obstruction (Fig. 12-63). In many cases, an underlying cause for the THAD or THID is not evident on the imaging study. When not associated with a tumor, normal vessels may be seen traversing a THID or THAD without evidence of mass effect. MRI is the most definitive noninvasive imaging means of excluding a mass in the setting of THAD or THID. When no tumor is present, the affected area should exhibit normal hepatic signal intensity on T1- and T2-weighted images. The affected liver should also normally accumulate superparamagnetic iron oxide particles and gadolinium-based liver-specific contrast agents during the hepatobiliary phase in the absence of a mass. One should keep in mind that some tumors are visible only on arterial-phase CT or MR images. Therefore, it may be reasonable to follow an area of suspected THID or THAD when an underlying cause is not discernible.

Perfusion Defects

Perfusion defects during the portal phase of a contrast-enhanced CT or MRI are thought to result from mixing of unenhanced blood from nonportal venous inflow with enhanced portal blood flow. The most common location for a perfusion defect during the portal phase is in segment IV adjacent to the falciform ligament (just as with focal fatty infiltration) (see Fig. 12-11, *A*). As with many other pseudolesions,

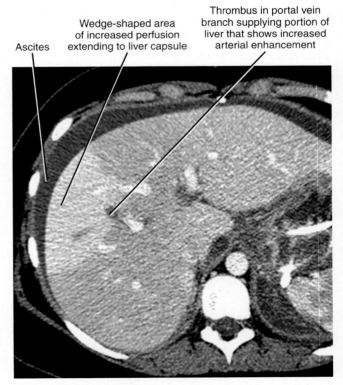

Ascites

Wedge-shaped area of increased perfusion extending to liver capsule

Thrombus in portal vein branch supplying portion of liver that shows increased arterial enhancement

Figure 12-63 Axial early-phase contrast-enhanced computed tomographic image shows increased enhancement peripheral to segmental portal vein thrombosis.

a benign perfusion defect should not demonstrate mass effect or capsular distortion. The affected area should enhance similar to the rest of the liver on other phases of enhancement and should demonstrate normal hepatic signal intensity on T1- and T2-weighted MR images.

, *Pitfall: Focal fatty infiltration, fatty sparing, THADs, THIDs, and perfusion abnormalities can simulate neoplastic lesions.*

Technical Artifacts

A variety of technical artifacts may result in pseudolesions of the liver. Modality-specific imaging artifacts and pitfalls are discussed in more detail in Section I of this textbook.

Is the Lesion Benign or Malignant?

Worrisome Features of Focal Hepatic Lesions

Sometimes a definitive diagnosis for a focal lesion cannot be rendered based only on the imaging appearance. In such cases, it may be sufficient for purposes of clinical management to characterize the lesion as likely benign or likely malignant. A lesion that is considered likely benign can often be managed with imaging follow-up rather than tissue sampling or excision. A lesion that demonstrates worrisome features on imaging may require biopsy or further imaging evaluation. Figure 12-64 illustrates some imaging features associated with increased likelihood of malignancy.

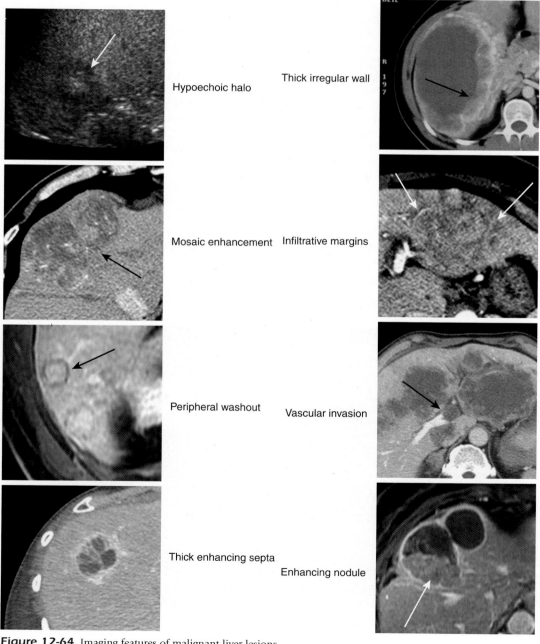

Hypoechoic halo

Thick irregular wall

Mosaic enhancement   Infiltrative margins

Peripheral washout   Vascular invasion

Thick enhancing septa

Enhancing nodule

Figure 12-64 Imaging features of malignant liver lesions.

When attempting to characterize a focal hepatic mass, one should always assess the status of the hepatic vessels and bile ducts. This is important for identifying variant anatomy before intervention, as well for detection of vascular or biliary obstruction or invasion. Tumor invasion of the hepatic or portal veins results in increased echogenicity of the veins on US, increased attenuation of the veins on NCCT, and abnormal signal intensity of the veins on MRI. Doppler US may demonstrate arterial signal within tumor thrombus, and tumor thrombus will enhance on CT or MRI after administration of intravenous contrast agents. The portal vein is more commonly invaded by tumor than the hepatic veins, and HCC is the most common tumor to invade the portal and hepatic veins. Cholangiocarcinoma more commonly encases portal vein branches, although portal invasion is occasionally seen with advanced tumors.

Bile duct obstruction can result from a wide variety of hepatic tumors, including primary liver neoplasms, as well as metastatic disease to the liver or porta hepatis lymph nodes. Intraductal extension of tumor is considerably less common and is most likely to occur with cholangiocarcinoma. Other tumors that can rarely invade into the bile ducts include HCC and metastases.

One additional feature of a lesion that warrants consideration is growth rate. Lesion stability over many years favors a benign diagnosis. Stability over a matter of months is not sufficient evidence of benignity because some malignant tumors grow slowly. To exclude diagnosis of a slow-growing neoplasm, one should compare the current examination not only with the most recent prior study but also with the oldest available examination. Many times, slow-growing tumors have gone unrecognized despite frequent imaging because the growth was not noticeable between consecutive imaging studies. Rapid growth favors infection or a complicating factor such as hemorrhage of a preexisting lesion. However, we have occasionally been surprised by the rapidity with which some malignant tumors, particularly metastases, grow (Fig. 12-65).

Malignant Mimics of Benign Lesions

Not all malignant lesions appear worrisome at first glance. A well-defined hyperechoic lesion discovered with US is likely to be a hemangioma in the absence of hepatitis, cirrhosis, or known malignant tumor elsewhere. One must be diligent to exclude these risk factors when a hyperechoic mass is detected because lesions such as HCC and some metastases may be hyperechoic (Fig. 12-66). Although the presence of a hypoechoic rim is highly suggestive of a malignant lesion, not all malignant lesions have this sonographic feature. If any doubt exists about a hyperechoic liver lesion, one should recommend additional imaging.

An area of increased echogenicity (US) or decreased attenuation (CT) adjacent to the falciform ligament usually represents focal fatty infiltration. However, cancers occasionally metastasize to this location in the absence of obvious lesions elsewhere. We have noticed this most often with breast cancer (Fig. 12-67).

Neuroendocrine metastases are known for mimicking hemangiomas on T2-weighted MRI because of their long T2 relaxation times (Fig. 12-68). Intravenous gadolinium chelate administration will often resolve the issue, although some neuroendocrine metastases may mimic the peripheral enhancement or delayed contrast retention typical of a hemangioma. Again, a history of primary extrahepatic tumor is helpful in

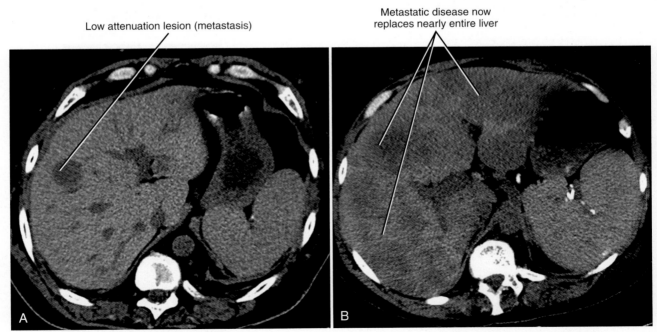

Low attenuation lesion (metastasis)

Metastatic disease now replaces nearly entire liver

Figure 12-65 Unenhanced axial computed tomographic images through the liver initially **(A)** and approximately 8 weeks later **(B)** demonstrating rapid growth of poorly differentiated metastatic bladder cancer.

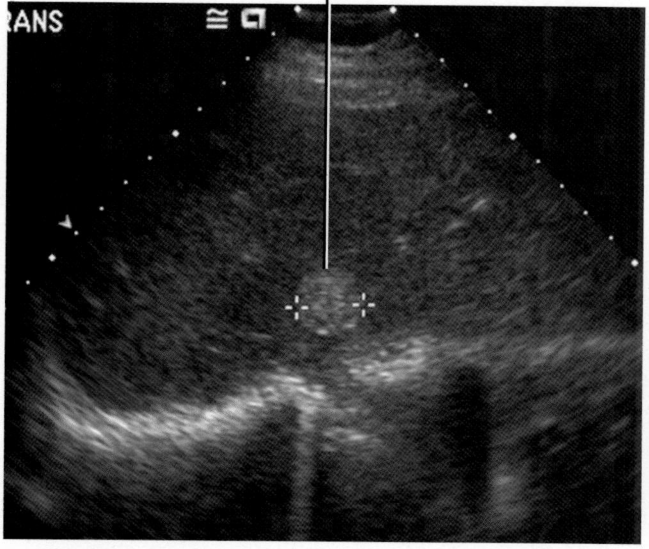

Uniformly echogenic round solitary lesion in liver

Figure 12-66 Transverse sonogram of the liver in a patient with right upper quadrant pain demonstrates an echogenic mass in the right hepatic lobe. This was thought to represent a hemangioma by expert sonologists on two separate occasions. The patient was diagnosed with adenocarcinoma of the colon with metastases to the liver shortly after this scan. The lesion shown here was partially calcified on unenhanced computed tomography (not shown).

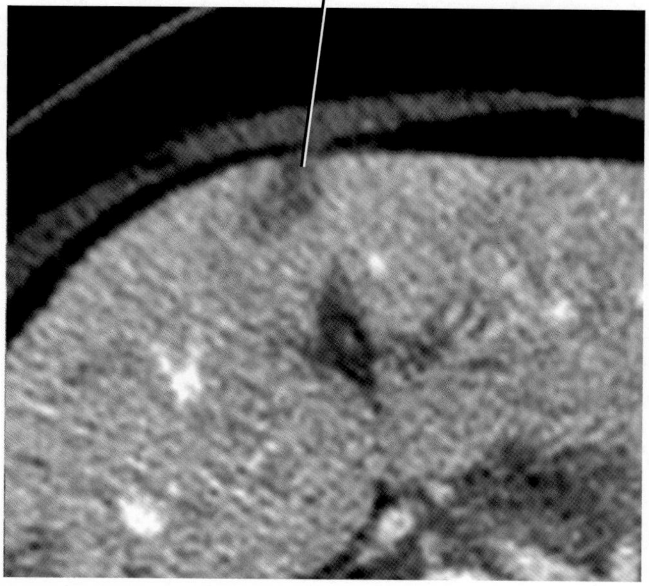

Low attenuation lesion in segment IV
(breast cancer metastasis)

Figure 12-67 Axial enhanced computed tomography through the liver of a patient with metastatic breast cancer involving segment IV.

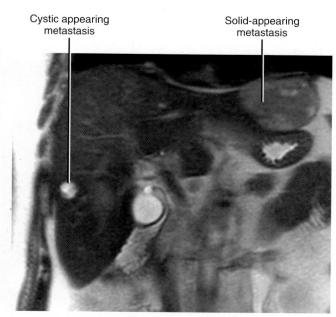

Cystic appearing metastasis   Solid-appearing metastasis

Figure 12-68 Coronal T2-weighted magnetic resonance image through the liver of a patient with metastatic neuroendocrine tumor metastases, some of which appear cystic.

scar should distinguish necrotic malignant tumors from FNH. Tumors that experience substantial necrosis may retain an irregular peripheral rim of viable tissue. Enhancement of this peripheral tissue after administration of an extracellular contrast agent can appear similar to the peripheral enhancement of a hemangioma or abscess (Fig. 12-70). However, it should become clear on dynamic imaging that the lesion fails to progressively enhance in the manner of a hemangioma. In addition, necrotic malignant tumors rarely demonstrate the discontinuous nodular enhancement typical of a hemangioma. Metastases that have responded favorably to systemic chemotherapy can become entirely cystic in appearance, although some tumor types (e.g., sarcomas) can appear cystic before any treatment (Fig. 12-71). Gastrointestinal stromal tumors (GISTs) that respond favorably to treatment with imatinib are particularly known for imitating simple cysts.

Fibrolamellar HCC is generally considered a rare mimic of FNH, because both entities can have central scars (see Fig. 12-69). Unlike the central scar of FNH, the central scar of fibrolamellar HCC is typically not bright on T2-weighted MR images, frequently calcifies, and does not typically demonstrate significant enhancement unless much delayed images are obtained.

Pitfall: Treated or necrotic tumors can simulate benign liver lesions such as cysts and hemangiomas.

Pitfall: Some metastases and HCCs can simulate FNH.

Benign Mimics of Malignant Lesions
Most hemangiomas have a typical imaging appearance that leads to the correct diagnosis without need for histologic confirmation. Large hemangiomas, however, often have an atypical appearance resulting from a central nonenhancing region of hyalinization, hemorrhage,

alerting one to this potential pitfall. Tumors that respond to chemotherapy may become partially or entirely necrotic. Central necrosis can resemble the scar of focal nodular hyperplasia (FNH) on noncontrast CT and MRI (Fig. 12-69). The enhancement pattern of the viable tumor and lack of enhancement of the central

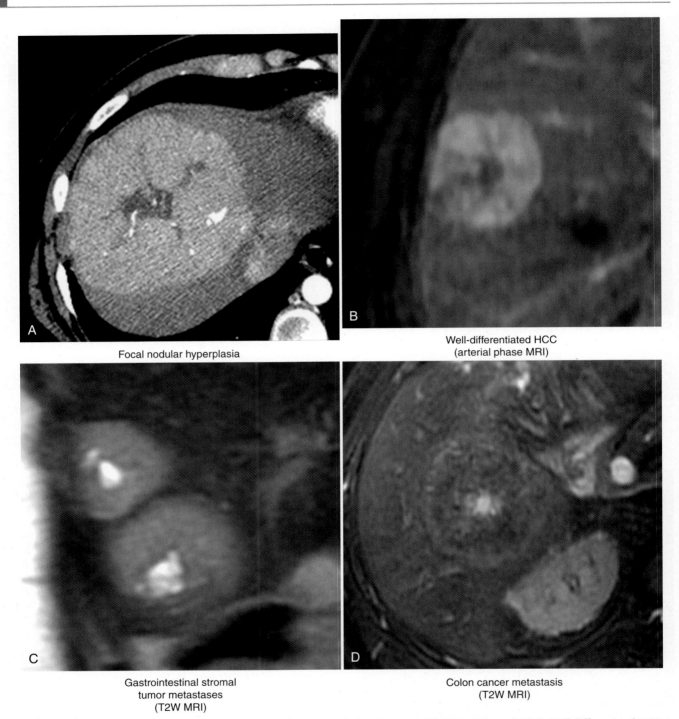

Focal nodular hyperplasia

Well-differentiated HCC
(arterial phase MRI)

Gastrointestinal stromal
tumor metastases
(T2W MRI)

Colon cancer metastasis
(T2W MRI)

Figure 12-69 Malignant mimics of focal nodular hyperplasia. **A,** Typical appearance of FNH on enhanced CT. **B,** Well-differentiated HCC on arterial phase MRI. **C,** Metastases from gastrointestinal stromal tumor on T2W MRI. **D,** Colon cancer metastasis on T2W MRI. *CT,* Computed tomography; *HCC,* hepatocellular carcinoma; *MRI,* magnetic resonance imaging; *T2W,* T2-weighted.

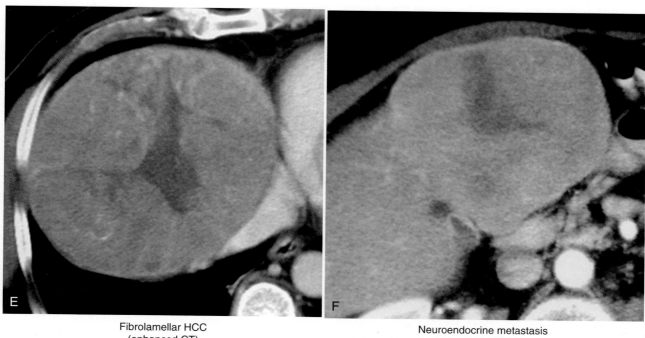

Fibrolamellar HCC
(enhanced CT)

Neuroendocrine metastasis
(enhanced CT)

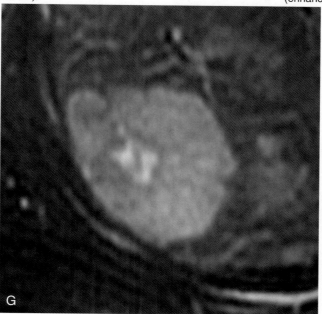

Neuroendocrine metastasis
(T2W MRI)

Figure 12-69, cont'd E, Fibrolamellar subtype of HCC on enhanced CT. F, Metastasis from neuroendocrine tumor on enhanced CT. G, Metastasis from neuroendocrine tumor on T2W MRI.

Peripheral enhancement looks similar to hemangioma enhancement. However, this enhancement did not progress centrally on subsequent images

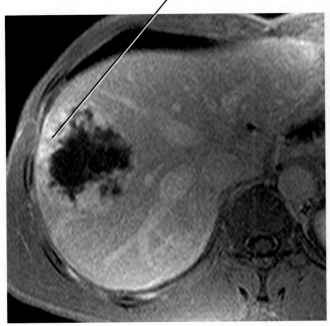

Figure 12-70 Axial gadolinium-enhanced magnetic resonance image of the liver in a patient with metastatic gastrointestinal stromal tumor (GIST) that could be confused with hemangioma.

Note simple cystic appearance of lesion (metastatic sarcoma)

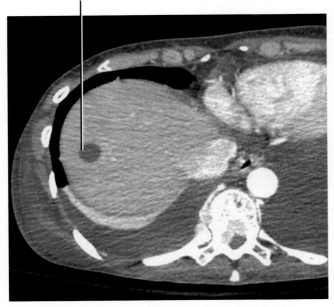

Figure 12-71 Enhanced axial computed tomographic image through the liver dome of a patient with soft-tissue sarcoma metastasis to the liver simulating a simple cyst.

thrombosis, or cystic degeneration (Fig. 12-72). This central "scar" does not typically enhance even on equilibrium-phase images, and it appears brighter than the periphery on T2-weighted MR images. Careful attention to the pattern of contrast enhancement of the lesion periphery will

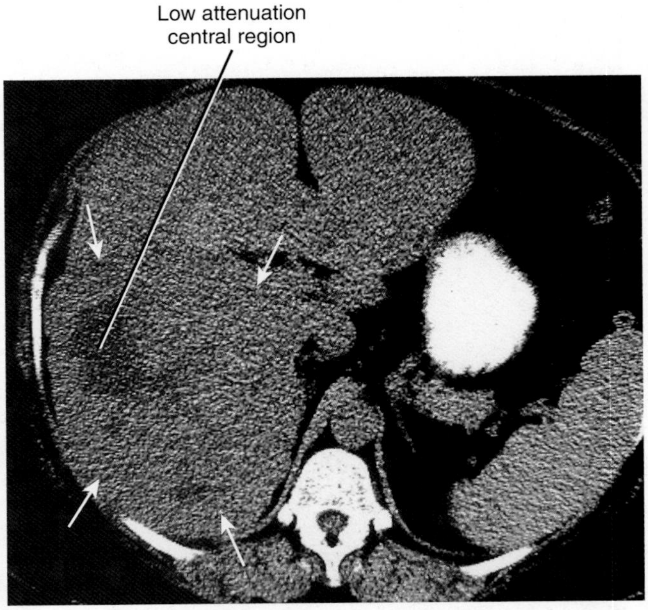

Low attenuation central region

Figure 12-72 Unenhanced axial computed tomographic image of a patient with giant hemangioma (*arrows*) demonstrating central area of low attenuation that did not enhance following contrast administration.

often reveal the typical interrupted, nodular, progressive enhancement pattern with delayed retention of contrast material characteristic of hemangioma. Atypical hemangioma can be distinguished from cholangiocarcinoma because the early peripheral enhancement that may be seen with the latter entity is usually not nodular or interrupted. On T2-weighted MRI, the central scar in cholangiocarcinoma is often dark rather than bright.

Small "flash-fill" hemangiomas may occasionally be confused with metastases or HCC. Clinical history is important to determine whether the patient has a known primary tumor or chronic liver disease. Unlike most HCCs, small hemangiomas will retain contrast into the equilibrium phase after intravenous administration of an extracellular contrast agent. Sclerosed hemangiomas have undergone extensive fibrosis with near-complete obliteration of the vascular spaces. Such lesions can mimic more aggressive tumors of the liver and may require biopsy for definitive diagnosis (Fig. 12-73). On CT and MR images, sclerosed hemangiomas tend to demonstrate geographic margins, capsular retraction, and reduction in size and loss of enhancement in previously enhancing regions over time. Nodular or rim enhancement can also be present. A heterogeneously hyperechoic appearance has been described for sonography.

Lesions of FNH that lack a characteristic central scar may be indistinguishable from HCC or metastatic disease on standard imaging examinations. In such cases, demonstration of Kupffer cell activity within the lesion with ferumoxide-enhanced MRI or sulfur colloid nuclear scintigraphy may help establish the diagnosis of FNH. More recently, gadobenate dimeglumine–enhanced MRI or gadoxetate disodium–enhanced MRI with imaging during the hepatobiliary phase (1-3 hours after contrast administration for gadobenate and 20 minutes after contrast administration for gadoxetate) has shown promise for differentiating FNH from other liver neoplasms (Fig. 12-74).

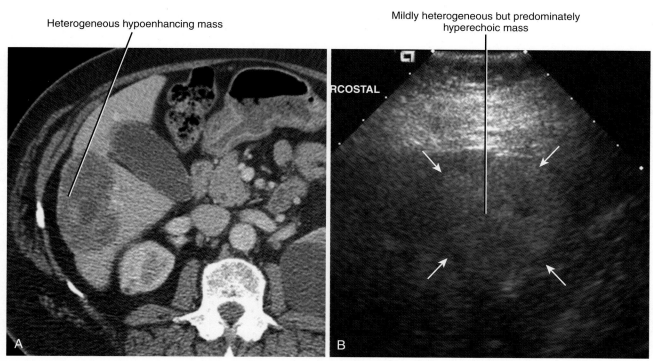

Figure 12-73 Enhanced axial computed tomographic scan (**A**) and sonogram (**B**) through the upper abdomen of a patient with a renal mass (renal cell carcinoma) and a sclerosed hemangioma initially thought to represent a metastasis. The lesion was densely fibrotic, and two biopsy sessions were necessary to exclude metastasis. Additional typical hemangiomas were present in the liver (not shown).

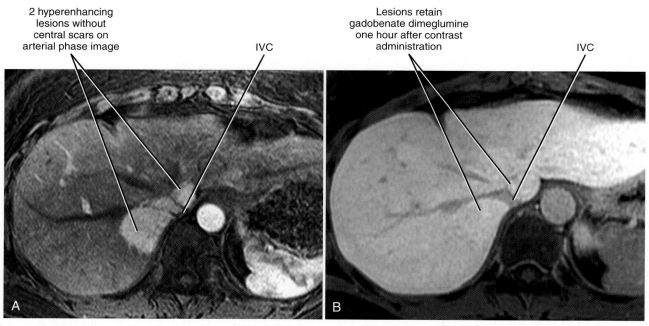

Figure 12-74 Axial arterial-phase magnetic resonance image (**A**) and hepatobiliary-phase image (**B**) performed with gadobenate dimeglumine through the liver of a young woman with ocular melanoma and hypervascular liver lesions discovered on computed tomographic scan (not shown). Lesions were diagnosed as probable focal nodular hyperplasia based on retention of gadobenate dimeglumine and followed with imaging. Lesions remained stable for over two subsequent years.

Hepatic adenoma is a histologically benign tumor of the liver. However, currently, no imaging test can reliably differentiate liver adenoma from malignant tumor.

Focal fatty infiltration or sparing may occasionally appear as one or more discrete hepatic nodules on imaging with US or CT, mimicking metastatic disease

(Fig. 12-75). Chemical-shift MRI is helpful in establishing the correct nature of the lesions.

Nodular regenerative hyperplasia in the setting of chronic Budd–Chiari syndrome may demonstrate increased signal intensity on T2-weighted images and early enhancement after iodinated contrast or gadolinium-based contrast

Hypodense lesion (focal fatty infiltration)
in segment IV near porta hepatis

Area in question is slightly hyperintense
relative to liver on in-phase T1WI

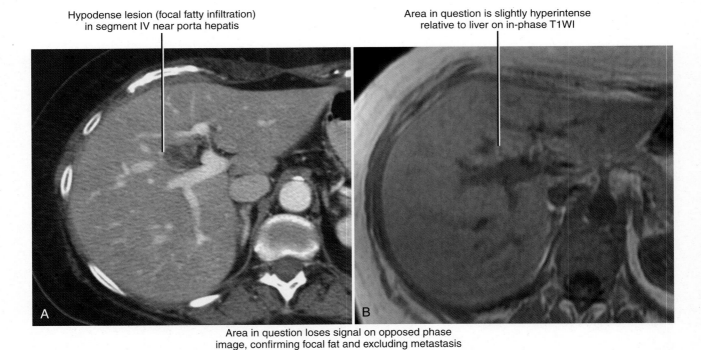

Area in question loses signal on opposed phase
image, confirming focal fat and excluding metastasis

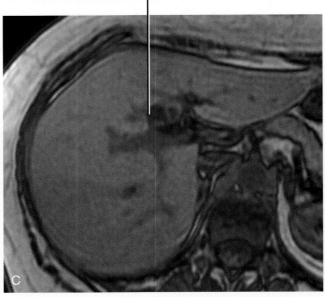

Figure 12-75 Axial enhanced computed tomography **(A)**, in-phase magnetic resonance imaging (MRI) **(B)**, and opposed-phase MRI **(C)** through the liver of a patient with lung cancer and a small liver mass. MRI was performed to help distinguish between focal fat and metastasis. *T1WI*, T1-weighted imaging.

administration, potentially resulting in confusion with HCC or metastatic disease (Fig. 12-76). Unlike the enhancement of HCC nodules, the nodular enhancement of regenerative hyperplasia typically persists into the portal phase. In addition, some nodules of Budd–Chiari syndrome may demonstrate a characteristic central scar.

Infarcted regenerative nodules may occasionally be found in patients with cirrhosis, often in association with shock from gastrointestinal hemorrhage. Infarcted regenerative nodules are typically isoattenuating to hypoattenuating on unenhanced CT and are heterogeneously enhancing or hypoenhancing after intravenous contrast administration. Such lesions can demonstrate increased

signal intensity on T2-weighted images, causing them to be confused with HCC in the setting of cirrhosis.

Echinococcus multilocularis (alveolaris) is a form of hydatid disease that has a more aggressive course. This lesion typically has an infiltrating appearance that may simulate a solid malignant neoplasm, although cystic features may be present. As with *Echinococcus granulosus*, calcifications may be present.

Pyogenic abscess, inflammatory pseudotumor, and eosinophilic necrosis are some additional benign entities that may be confused with malignant tumors of the liver. Eosinophilic necrosis is thought to be the result of eosinophil-induced tissue damage associated with

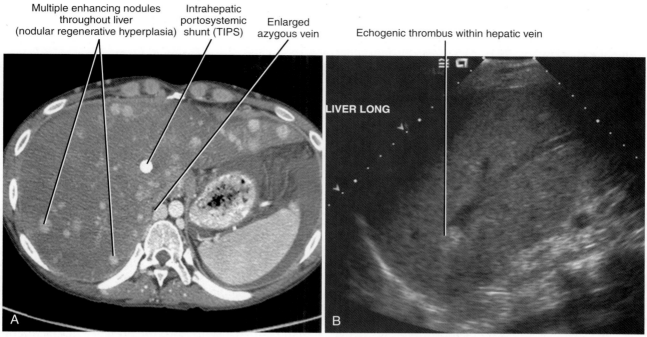

Multiple enhancing nodules throughout liver (nodular regenerative hyperplasia)   Intrahepatic portosystemic shunt (TIPS)   Enlarged azygous vein

Echogenic thrombus within hepatic vein

LIVER LONG

Figure 12-76 Enhanced axial computed tomographic image (**A**) and longitudinal sonogram (**B**) through the liver of a patient with inferior vena cava (IVC) and hepatic vein thrombosis (Budd–Chiari syndrome) and nodular regenerative hyperplasia. Note lack of visible IVC in **A**.

eosinophilia-related conditions such as parasitic disease, allergic conditions, and some neoplasms. Lesions of eosinophilic necrosis have been reported as more likely than metastases to be undetectable on arterial-phase CT images. In addition, nonspherical shape, indistinct margins, and homogeneous appearance on portal-phase images favors eosinophilic necrosis over metastatic disease.

What Is the Lesion Composed of?

Calcification

Calcification may be easily detected with CT, appearing as areas of high attenuation. One must be careful because substances other than calcium may cause regions of high attenuation within the liver. In particular, a liver tumor that has been treated with intraarterial chemoembolization using iodized oil may mimic a densely calcified mass (Fig. 12-77). With US, calcification appears as areas of increased echogenicity that may be associated with posterior acoustic shadowing when sufficiently large, although this constellation of findings may be mimicked by gas within a lesion (e.g., abscess) (see Fig. 12-66). MRI is relatively insensitive for detection of calcification. However, the presence of calcification can sometimes be inferred on MR images when areas of signal void are present within a lesion on all sequences. Areas of calcification will not enhance after gadolinium chelate administration.

Small, scattered, densely calcified foci within the liver are most commonly the result of granulomatous disease and can generally be dismissed if no other associated parenchymal abnormality is present. When multiple

Overall increase in liver attenuation resulting from nonselective embolization

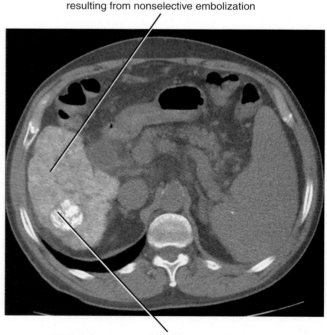

Well-defined mass with high attenuation material (oil-based contrast medium) that might be confused with calcification

Figure 12-77 Unenhanced axial computed tomographic scan through the liver of a patient with cirrhosis and hepatocellular carcinoma recently treated with chemoembolization using an oil-based contrast medium.

masses containing variable amounts of calcification are present within the liver, metastatic disease from adeno-carcinoma (most often colon cancer) is the most likely consideration (Fig. 12-78). Metastases from other tumors, such as teratoma, can also demonstrate calcification. Fibrolamellar HCC should be considered for a large solitary lesion with coarse central calcification. Fewer than 10% of hemangiomas demonstrate calcifications (Fig. 12-79). Box 12-4 lists noncystic liver lesions that may contain calcification.

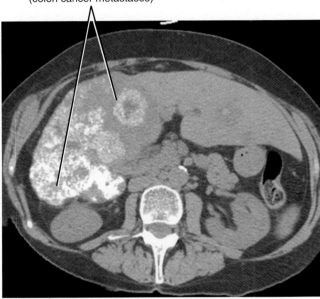

Multiple calcified liver masses (colon cancer metastases)

Figure 12-78 Unenhanced axial computed tomographic image through the liver of a patient with metastatic adenocarcinoma of the colon.

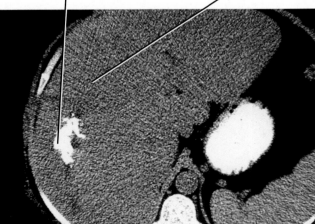

Central area of very high attenuation (calcification)

Borders of giant hemangioma are difficult to see in absence of intravenous contrast. Mass replaces much of right hemiliver

Figure 12-79 Unenhanced axial computed tomographic image through the liver of a patient with a giant hemangioma containing central calcification.

BOX 12-4   Noncystic Liver Lesions That Can Contain Calcification

Chronic/remote infection or hematoma
Fibrolamellar HCC (central scar)
Healed granulomas (small, punctuate)
Hepatocellular carcinoma
Metastases (e.g., mucinous tumors, malignant teratoma, others)
Adenoma
Hemangioma

Fat

Intralesional fat serves as an excellent discriminator of solid hepatic mass lesions. With US, the presence of macroscopic fat typically increases the echogenicity of a lesion. Unfortunately, sonography cannot be used to prove that fat is present within a lesion given the range of processes that increase echogenicity in the absence of fat. Macroscopic quantities of fat are readily detected with CT and characterized by the presence of low-attenuation regions within a mass measuring less than −20 HU. With MRI, the presence of macroscopic fat within a lesion can be confirmed by imaging with and without fat suppression.

When fat and water are present together in similar amounts within the cytoplasm of tumor cells (something that has been occasionally referred to as microscopic fat), the attenuation of the mass may be relatively low (e.g., less than 20 HU) but greater than fat density on unenhanced CT. The use of magnetic resonance chemical-shift imaging techniques (in- and opposed-phase gradient-echo imaging) greatly facilitates the detection of intracytoplasmic lipid or small clusters of adipocytes within tumors. When a tumor contains sufficient intracellular lipid or adipocytes mixed with other tissue elements, it will lose signal intensity on opposed-phase images compared with in-phase images.

Box 12-5 lists some hepatic lesions that can contain fat or intracellular lipid. It is important to note that fat or lipid is not always present in the lesions listed in Box 12-5. Hepatic adenoma, FNH, and HCC, in particular, often lack imaging evidence of intralesional macroscopic or microscopic fat. In some cases (e.g., FNH), lipid is only rarely present in sufficient quantities to be detected with imaging.

BOX 12-5   Fat- and Lipid-Containing Lesions of the Liver

Focal fatty infiltration
Hepatocellular adenoma
Focal nodular hyperplasia
Hepatocellular carcinoma
Steatotic regenerative nodule
Angiomyolipoma
Metastases from fat-containing primary tumors
Lipoma or pseudolipoma (Fig. 12-80)
Teratoma
Myelolipoma
Extramedullary hematopoiesis

Fat-attenuation lesion along the liver capsule
with central dot of higher density

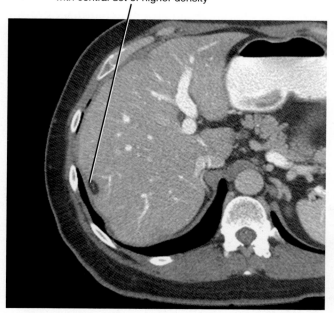

Figure 12-80 Enhanced axial computed tomographic image of the liver in a patient with an incidentally discovered fatty lesion with a typical appearance of pseudolipoma of Glisson's capsule.

Focal fatty infiltration is by far the most common fatty lesion of the liver and is discussed in more detail in the section on hepatic pseudotumors. The presence of microscopic fat within FNH is atypical and relatively rare but should not dissuade one from the diagnosis if other typical features are present. Hepatocellular adenomas can contain hepatocytes rich in lipid. This manifests as low attenuation on CT and signal loss on opposed-phase MRI (Fig. 12-81). Unlike other benign lesions of the liver characterized by intracytoplasmic lipid, hepatocellular adenomas have a propensity for hemorrhage. Unfortunately,

there are currently no imaging characteristics of hepatic adenoma that allow definitive differentiation from HCC, although it is more common to encounter a lipid-containing HCC than a benign adenoma, particularly in the setting of cirrhosis (Fig. 12-82). Evidence of vascular invasion or a significantly increased serum AFP level also strongly favors the diagnosis of HCC and may preclude the need for biopsy in some situations. Hepatic lesions other than HCC that contain macroscopic fat are extremely rare. In the case of angiomyolipoma associated with tuberous sclerosis, metastatic teratoma, and

Small foci of low attenuation corresponded to areas of signal loss on opposed-phase MRI (not shown)

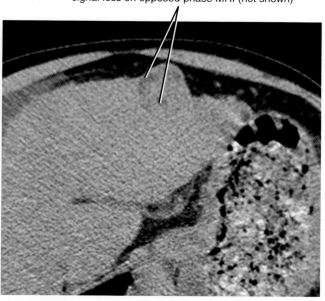

Figure 12-82 Unenhanced axial computed tomographic scan through the liver of a patient with cirrhosis and hepatocellular carcinoma demonstrating foci of lipid-containing tumor. *MRI,* Magnetic resonance imaging.

Multiple liver masses (adenomas) are slightly higher in signal intensity than normal liver

Masses (adenomas) lose signal intensity on opposed phase images

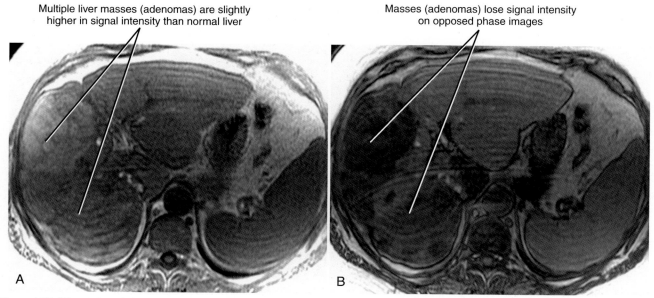

A   B

Figure 12-81 Axial in- **(A)** and opposed-phase **(B)** gradient-echo magnetic resonance images through the liver of a patient with hepatic adenomatosis.

extramedullary hematopoiesis, clinical history may be of assistance in at least suggesting the correct diagnosis. Fat-containing metastases are rare but can occur with fat-containing primary neoplasms (Fig. 12-83).

Hemorrhage

Virtually any focal hepatic lesion may undergo hemorrhage. However, some lesions are more prone to hemorrhage than others, making the presence of hemorrhage a potentially useful discriminator. The imaging appearance of hemorrhage depends on its chronicity. Acute

hemorrhage often appears as a nonspecific area of increased echogenicity with sonography and increased attenuation with CT. As an area of hemorrhage evolves over time, it becomes less echogenic and lower in attenuation. Hemorrhage often appears as an area of increased signal intensity on T1-weighted MR images. Repeated episodes of hemorrhage may impart a complex, heterogeneous appearance to a lesion with any imaging modality. The solid liver lesions most likely to demonstrate evidence of hemorrhage include hepatic adenoma, HCC, and metastases. Despite the vascular

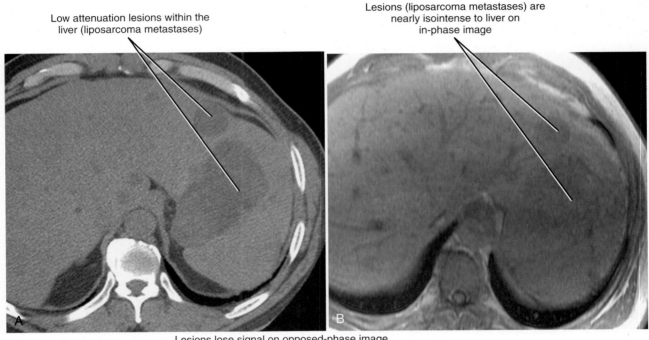

Low attenuation lesions within the liver (liposarcoma metastases)

Lesions (liposarcoma metastases) are nearly isointense to liver on in-phase image

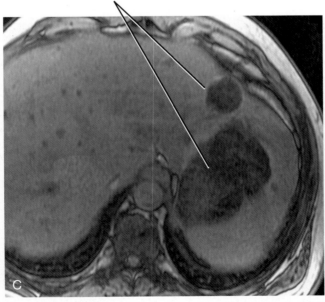

Lesions lose signal on opposed-phase image, indicating the presence of lipid or fat. Without appropriate history, these lesions could be confused with hepatocellular adenomas

Figure 12-83 Unenhanced axial computed tomographic image (**A**) and in- (**B**) and opposed-phase (**C**) magnetic resonance images through the upper abdomen of a patient with metastatic liposarcoma demonstrating fat-containing metastases.

nature of hemangiomas, hemorrhage is uncommonly encountered. When it occurs, however, it can be catastrophic.

Fluid (Cystic Masses)

Fluid is usually anechoic to hypoechoic with sonography, and the echogenicity varies with the complexity of the fluid. On CT images, fluid is usually low attenuation unless complicated by hemorrhage or contrast extravasation. With MRI, simple fluid is of low signal intensity on T1-weighted images and high signal intensity on T2-weighted images, although a wide range of signal intensities are possible with both types of sequences depending on the composition of the fluid. Typically, fluid does not enhance after intravenous contrast administration. Fluid-containing lesions in the liver can be divided into simple cystic lesions and complex cystic lesions.

SIMPLE CYSTIC LESIONS

A simple cyst appears to contain simple fluid with all cross-sectional imaging modalities; lacks wall thickening, irregularity, or nodularity; has minimal or no septation; and does not demonstrate evidence of enhancement. Simple cysts have well-defined margins with clear delineation between the lesion and surrounding parenchyma.

With US, a simple cyst is anechoic, demonstrates a well-defined wall, and has enhanced through-transmission (Fig. 12-84). Mild lobulation is usually not cause for concern in hepatic cysts. Simple cysts do not demonstrate evidence of altered perfusion of the surrounding hepatic parenchyma or internal flow with color Doppler imaging.

With CT, simple cysts are of fluid attenuation (−10 to 20 HU), are sharply marginated, and do not enhance with intravenous contrast agents.

On MRI, a simple cyst demonstrates relatively low signal intensity on a T1-weighted image, high signal intensity on a T2-weighted image, and no enhancement after gadolinium administration (Fig. 12-85). On heavily T2-weighted images, simple cysts maintain high signal intensity, whereas the background liver becomes dark.

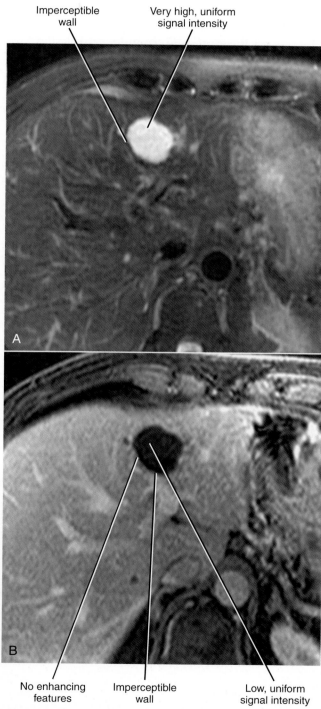

Imperceptible wall

Very high, uniform signal intensity

No enhancing features

Imperceptible wall

Low, uniform signal intensity

Figure 12-85 Axial T2-weighted (**A**) and gadolinium-enhanced (**B**) magnetic resonance images of simple hepatic cyst. Despite a definitive imaging diagnosis before surgery, this cyst was removed during surgery for a malignant tumor elsewhere.

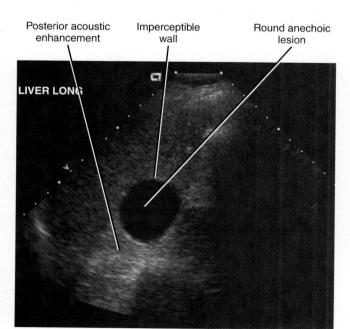

Posterior acoustic enhancement

Imperceptible wall

Round anechoic lesion

LIVER LONG

Figure 12-84 Grayscale ultrasound image of a simple hepatic cyst.

A definitive diagnosis of simple cyst on either CT or MRI requires administration of an intravenous contrast agent to exclude enhancement of the wall or internal components, because some neoplasms and infectious processes may mimic simple cysts on unenhanced images. In most cases, US is the least expensive and safest method of confirming the nature of a simple cyst. Other entities such as biliary hamartoma and biloma can mimic a simple hepatic cyst (Fig. 12-86).

COMPLEX CYSTIC LESIONS

When we use the expression "complex cystic lesion," we refer to a predominantly cystic mass exhibiting imaging features that preclude the diagnosis of simple cyst. Some of these complicating imaging features are listed in Box 12-6.

CT may occasionally fail to adequately demonstrate the internal architecture of a complex cystic lesion, although this is becoming less of a problem with the introduction of multidetector scanners. When a lesion is in a favorable location, US is an excellent method of demonstrating complicating features such as septa, mural nodules, internal debris, and internal vascularity. MRI is an excellent alternative to evaluate a complex cystic lesion when US is not possible or is inconclusive.

Hepatic metastases can appear as complex cystic masses with imaging (Fig. 12-87). In particular, sarcomas, GISTs, ovarian cystadenocarcinomas, pancreatic mucinous cystadenocarcinomas, colon adenocarcinomas, neuroendocrine tumors, melanomas, and squamous cell carcinomas are among the tumors that may

---

BOX 12-6   Imaging Characteristics of Complex Cystic Lesions

Internal echoes detected by sonography
Higher than fluid attenuation on CT images
Areas of high signal intensity on T1-weighted MR images
Areas of low or intermediate signal intensity on T2-weighted MR images
Wall thickening, irregularity, or nodularity
Enhancing components
Thick or multiple septa
Fluid–fluid levels
Intralesional air or calcification

---

produce cystic or necrotic metastases. Metastases that have responded to treatment with systemic chemotherapy or chemoembolization may also appear cystic. The presence of multiple lesions, irregularly thickened enhancing walls, or known primary extrahepatic tumor helps distinguish cystic metastases from other complex cystic lesions. Distinction from hepatic abscess may be difficult in some cases based on the imaging appearance alone. Therefore, if the nature of a complex cystic lesion is in doubt because of an ambiguous imaging appearance and clinical presentation, percutaneous aspiration should be performed and the material analyzed for the presence of tumor or infection before an attempt at drain placement.

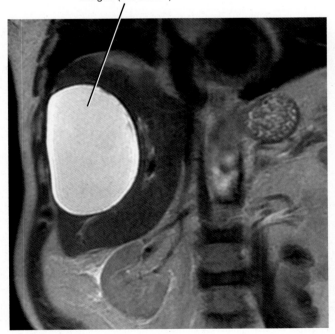

Homogeneous high SI lesion with no perceptible wall or enhancement on contrast-enhanced images (not shown)

Figure 12-86 Coronal T2-weighted magnetic resonance image at the level of the liver demonstrating a large biloma that developed after resection of a hepatocellular carcinoma. *SI*, Signal intensity.

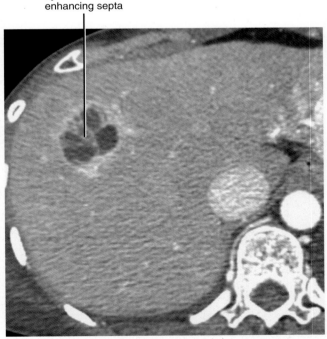

Cystic lesion with enhancing septa

Figure 12-87 Enhanced axial computed tomographic image through the liver of a patient with metastatic sarcoma.

Table 12-11 lists and compares a variety of complex cystic lesions of the liver.

Shape and Margins

Analysis of the shape and margins of a lesion may provide some indication as to the cause or aggressiveness of the lesion. Neoplastic processes are rarely triangular and do not typically have straight borders. Rather, the presence of a straight border implies a vascular phenomenon such as THAD, infarct, or fatty infiltration or sparing (although these changes could be a secondary manifestation of a neoplasm). Although lobulated lesion margins are typical of cavernous hemangioma, FNH, and fibrolamellar HCC, some HCCs, metastases, and peripheral cholangiocarcinomas may also demonstrate lobulated margins, making the presence of lobulation a relatively weak discriminator. Poorly defined margins imply an infiltrating process and virtually exclude the diagnoses of cyst, hemangioma, FNH, and uncomplicated hepatic adenoma. Although infiltrating margins may be present in malignant tumors such as HCC, cholangiocarcinoma, and some metastases, poorly defined margins are not exclusive to neoplastic processes. Some infectious processes such as *Echinococcus multilocularis* infection or inflammatory processes such as inflammatory pseudotumor may mimic infiltrating malignant neoplasms.

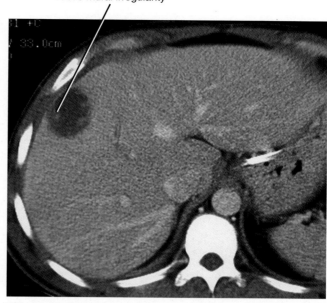

Figure 12-88 Enhanced axial computed tomographic image through the liver of a patient with an amoebic hepatic abscess.

Table 12-11   Comparison of Complex Cystic Lesions of the Liver

Lesion	Possible Clinical Settings	Possible Imaging Findings
Abscess (Figs. 12-88 to 12-90)	• Immunosuppression • Fever, chills, leukocytosis • Colitis, diverticulitis, appendicitis, cholangitis, recent surgery	• "Bull's-eye" appearance • Continuous enhancing wall of uniform thickness • Cluster sign • Gas • Perilesional edema • Mobile internal debris (US)
Aneurysm or pseudo-aneurysm	• Prior intervention or trauma	• Round shape • Flow with Doppler US • Central arterial-phase enhancement • Mural thrombus
Biliary cyst-adenoma (Fig. 12-91)	• Incidental finding in middle-aged woman	• Thin enhancing wall and septa • Enhancing nodules (cystadenocarcinoma)
Hematoma	• Prior intervention or trauma • Acute onset of pain	• Fluid–fluid level • High attenuation (CT) • High SI on T1W MRI
Hydatid disease (Fig. 12-92)	• Travel in endemic area	• Floating lily sign (US) • Peripherally arranged daughter cysts
Necrotic neoplasm (Fig. 12-93)	• Known primary cancer elsewhere • Positive tumor markers	• Multiple lesions (metastases) • Thick, irregular enhancing wall

CT, Computed tomography; *MRI,* magnetic resonance imaging; *SI,* signal intensity; *T1W,* T1-weighted; *US,* ultrasound.

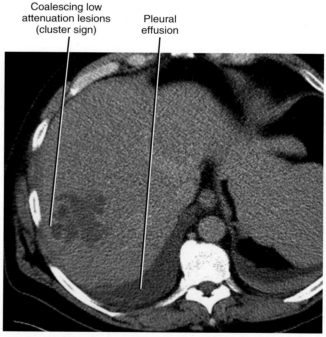

Figure 12-89 Axial computed tomographic image through the liver of a patient with a pyogenic liver abscess.

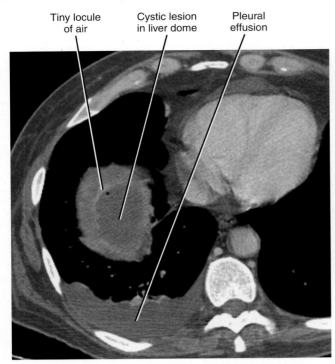

Tiny locule of air — Cystic lesion in liver dome — Pleural effusion

Figure 12-90 Enhanced axial computed tomographic image through the liver dome of a patient with a large pyogenic abscess. Tiny solitary locule of air within the fluid collection suggested the correct diagnosis (abscess was treated with percutaneous catheter drainage).

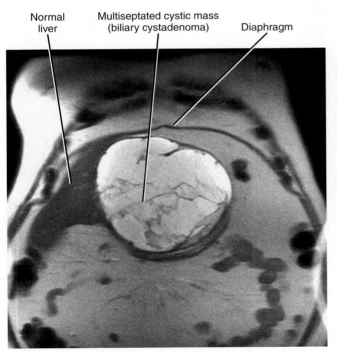

Normal liver — Multiseptated cystic mass (biliary cystadenoma) — Diaphragm

Figure 12-91 Coronal T2-weighted magnetic resonance image through the anterior left hepatic lobe of a woman with a biliary cystadenoma. No malignant features were found at surgery.

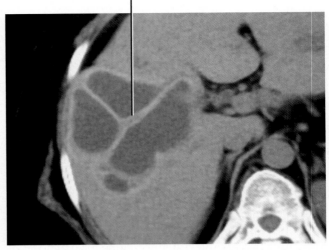

Multiseptated cystic mass with appearance of individual (daughter) cysts within larger cyst

Figure 12-92 Unenhanced axial computed tomographic image through the liver of a patient with hydatid (echinococcal) cyst.

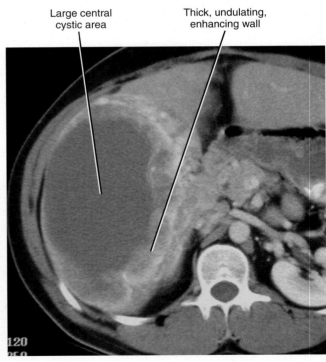

Large central cystic area — Thick, undulating, enhancing wall

Figure 12-93 Enhanced axial computed tomographic image through the liver of a patient with metastatic gastrointestinal stromal tumor (GIST).

The liver contour adjacent to a lesion may provide some additional specificity. When a solid subcapsular lesion distorts the liver contour outward, a neoplastic process should be considered. Retraction of the liver capsule is another feature that may be associated with particular processes and tumors (Box 12-7).

BOX 12-7   Focal Lesions That May Cause Retraction of the Liver Capsule

Cholangiocarcinoma (Fig. 12-94)
Metastasis (adenocarcinoma)
HCC (includes fibrolamellar variant)
Hemangioma (associated with thrombosis/fibrosis)
Epithelioid hemangioendothelioma
Hepatic infarction (nonacute)
Liver laceration (nonacute)
Treated liver tumor (systemic therapy, embolization, or ablative therapy) (Fig. 12-95)
Recurrent pyogenic cholangitis

Liver metastasis

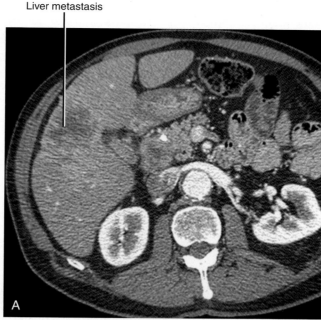

Note capsular retraction adjacent to treated metastasis

Capsular retraction | Low attenuation area of fatty infiltration (free of tumor at surgery) | Site of tumor | Low attenuation area of fatty infiltration (free of tumor at surgery)

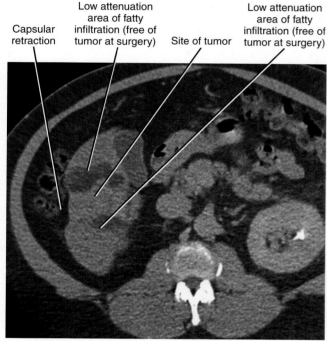

Figure 12-94 Unenhanced axial computed tomographic image through the lower liver of a patient with peripheral cholangiocarcinoma. Note fatty infiltration adjacent to tumor, likely the result of altered hemodynamics surrounding the tumor.

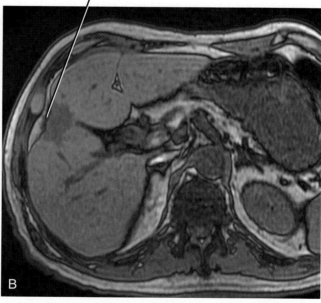

Figure 12-95 Enhanced axial computed tomographic image (**A**) performed before chemotherapy and T1-weighted magnetic resonance image (**B**) performed after chemotherapy for metastatic carcinoma involving the liver.

How Does the Lesion Enhance?

Enhancement Patterns

In this section, the term *enhancement* refers to the enhancement characteristics of a hepatic lesion as determined by multiphase dynamic imaging after rapid intravenous bolus administration of contrast material. In all cases, we are referring to the behavior of extracellular contrast agents such as the widely used iodinated CT agents or extracellular gadolinium chelates. Although sonographic contrast agents are not distributed in the extracellular space in the manner of most CT and MR contrast agents, some of the enhancement patterns described in this section can be applied to tumors examined with contrast-enhanced sonography. For all practical purposes, extracellular gadolinium chelates

behave in a similar manner to iodinated CT contrast media on multiphase contrast-enhanced scans. MR images are heavily represented in this section, however, because gadolinium-enhanced MRI better demonstrates tissue enhancement than contrast-enhanced CT.

Pearl: For all practical purposes, extracellular gadolinium chelates behave in a similar manner to iodinated CT contrast media on multiphase contrast-enhanced scans.

Nonenhancing Masses

Nonenhancing lesions are those that do not exhibit any detectable enhancement on any phase of imaging. Most nonenhancing masses are cystic in nature and include simple cysts, hemorrhagic cysts, bilomas, and hematomas. Nonenhancement of an area of solid tissue implies infarction. Hepatic infarction typically requires interruption of both the portal and arterial blood supply to a portion of the liver. Hepatic infarcts are often subcapsular in location and wedge shaped or irregularly shaped rather than round or oval (Fig. 12-96). Hepatic neoplasms or regenerative nodules may occasionally undergo spontaneous or treatment-related infarction. Radiofrequency ablation sites often appear as nonenhancing focal lesions that demonstrate mildly increased attenuation on unenhanced CT images, decreased signal intensity on T2-weighted MR images, and increased signal intensity on T1-weighted MR images (Fig. 12-97).

Hypoenhancing/Hypovascular Masses

Hypovascular or hypoenhancing lesions demonstrate enhancement to a lesser degree than that of liver parenchyma on arterial- and portal-phase images (Box 12-8). Lymphoma and metastatic disease are typical examples of hypoenhancing tumors. Many cancers can produce hypovascular metastases, including adenocarcinomas of the GI tract, lung cancer, prostate cancer, and transitional cell carcinoma. Hemangiomas are usually not included in the category of hypoenhancing masses. However, some hemangiomas enhance in a delayed manner and may appear hypoenhancing if sufficiently delayed imaging is not performed. Occasionally, primary hepatic neoplasms such as HCC can be hypoenhancing on all phases of a multiphase contrast-enhanced CT or MRI. In such cases, definitive imaging characterization can be difficult or impossible.

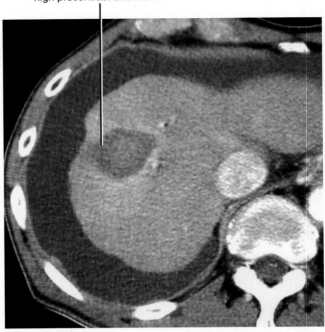

Nonenhancing lesion with relatively high precontrast attenuation

Figure 12-97 Enhanced axial computed tomographic scan through the liver of a patient who had previously undergone radiofrequency ablation of a hepatocellular carcinoma of the liver dome.

BOX 12-8 Typical Hypoenhancing Masses
Metastasis
Lymphoma
Slow-filling hemangioma
Regenerative nodule
Eosinophilic necrosis

Pitfall: Some hemangiomas enhance in a delayed manner and may appear hypoenhancing if sufficiently delayed imaging is not performed.

Lesions with Early Enhancement

Early enhancement describes lesions that enhance significantly more than liver parenchyma on arterial-phase images because of substantial arterial blood supply. Some hypervascular lesions appear to washout relative to liver parenchyma on portal-phase and later images to become hypoenhancing or nearly isoenhancing. HCC is a classic example of this type of enhancement pattern, although hepatic adenoma may also demonstrate this enhancement pattern (Fig. 12-98). In both cases, larger lesions typically enhance heterogeneously (referred to as mosaic enhancement). FNH typically exhibits brisk arterial-phase enhancement (more than hepatic adenoma) but usually appears isoenhancing to slightly hyperenhancing on portal-phase images. FNH also typically retains hepatobiliary gadolinium-based contrast agents such as gadobenate dimeglumine and gadoxetate disodium on delayed hepatobiliary phase images (Fig. 12-99). Some cases of FNH demonstrate radiating septa on early-phase images. Flash-fill hemangiomas

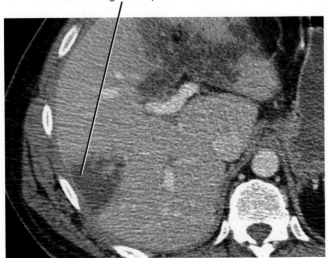

Wedge-shaped area of nonenhancing liver along liver capsule

Figure 12-96 Enhanced axial computed tomographic image through the liver of a patient who had undergone pancreatic resection with subsequent development of liver infarcts.

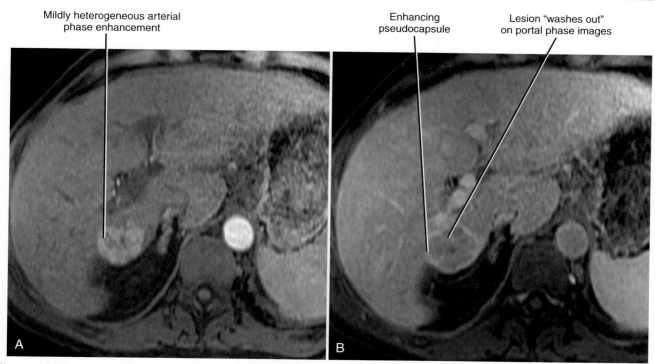

Mildly heterogeneous arterial phase enhancement

Enhancing pseudocapsule

Lesion "washes out" on portal phase images

Figure 12-98 Axial arterial- (**A**) and portal venous–phase (**B**) gadolinium-enhanced magnetic resonance images of a patient with hepatocellular carcinoma demonstrating typical enhancement pattern.

demonstrate arterial-phase enhancement that persists on subsequent phases (paralleling enhancement of the hepatic vessels) and are bright on T2-weighted images (Fig. 12-100). A variety of metastatic lesions can demonstrate early enhancement, including some metastases from breast carcinoma, renal cell carcinoma, thyroid carcinoma, neuroendocrine tumor, pheochromocytoma, and melanoma (Fig. 12-101). Nodular regenerative hyperplasia occurs commonly in the setting of Budd–Chiari syndrome. These nodules typically

enhance avidly in the arterial phase with enhancement often persisting into the portal phase (see Fig. 12-76). A central scar resembling that of FNH is sometimes present. Lesions that show early enhancement after contrast administration are summarized in Box 12-9.

Progressively Enhancing Lesions
Progressively enhancing lesions enhance increasingly from arterial to delayed phases. Box 12-10 lists lesions that tend to enhance progressively. Such lesions may

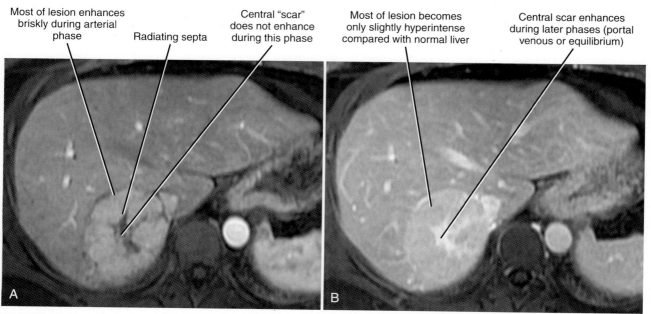

Most of lesion enhances briskly during arterial phase

Radiating septa

Central "scar" does not enhance during this phase

Most of lesion becomes only slightly hyperintense compared with normal liver

Central scar enhances during later phases (portal venous or equilibrium)

Figure 12-99 Typical enhancement pattern of focal nodular hyperplasia. Axial arterial- (**A**), equilibrium- (**B**),

Continued

Bile ducts enhance
during this phase

Lesion retains contrast material and
appears isointense to mildly hyperintense
compared with normal liver

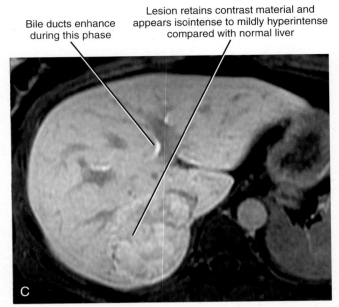

Figure 12-99, cont'd and hepatobiliary-phase (**C**) gadobenate dimeglumine-enhanced T1-weighted magnetic resonance image in a young woman with a typical lesion of focal nodular hyperplasia.

demonstrate centripetal enhancement (from the periphery toward the center) or noncentripetal enhancement. An example of the former type of progressive enhancement would be the typical cavernous hemangioma. The most specific enhancement pattern for hemangioma is that of peripheral, nodular, discontinuous enhancement that progresses centrally, persists on equilibrium-phase images, and parallels enhancement of hepatic vessels (Fig. 12-102). A lesion need not enhance completely to be called a hemangioma with confidence, provided these typical enhancement features are present.

Peripheral cholangiocarcinoma may demonstrate early peripheral enhancement with subsequent delayed enhancement of the central portion of the lesion. Peripheral cholangiocarcinoma can be easily distinguished from hemangioma, however, because the peripheral enhancement of cholangiocarcinoma is typically neither nodular nor discontinuous (Fig. 12-103). In addition, peripheral cholangiocarcinomas can demonstrate peripheral washout on equilibrium phase images and are usually not nearly as bright on T2-weighted magnetic resonance images as hemangiomas.

Small arterially enhancing lesion (hemangioma)

Liver lesion (hemangioma)
has same signal intensity
as other vascular structures

Hepatic vein   Portal vein

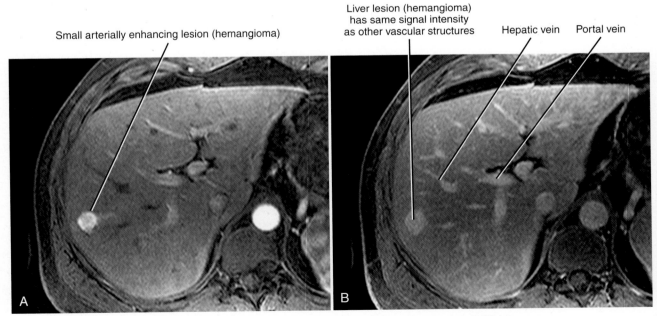

Figure 12-100 Axial arterial- (**A**) and portal-phase (**B**) gadolinium-enhanced magnetic resonance (MR) images

Lesion (hemangioma) has very high signal
intensity on T2-weighted images

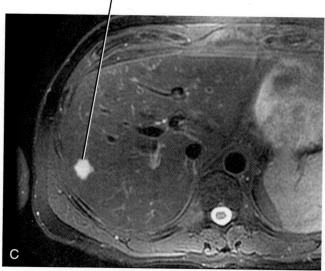

Figure 12-100, cont'd and T2-weighted MR image **(C)** through the liver of a patient with a typical small hemangioma.

Small arterially enhancing lesion
(neuroendocrine metastasis)

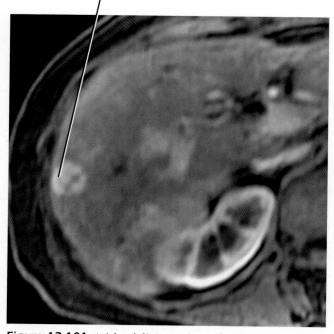

Figure 12-101 Axial gadolinium-enhanced magnetic resonance image of a liver metastasis from a neuroendocrine tumor.

Confluent fibrosis often enhances in a progressive manner. This enhancement pattern helps distinguish fibrosis from HCC in the setting of cirrhosis. Some metastatic tumors can demonstrate progressive enhancement on CT and MR images, including breast carcinoma and GISTs.

Pearl: *A lesion need not enhance completely to be called a hemangioma with confidence, provided other typical enhancement features are present.*

BOX 12-9   Lesions with Early Enhancement

Hepatocellular carcinoma
Hepatic adenoma
Flash-fill hemangioma
Focal nodular hyperplasia
Nodular regenerative hyperplasia
Hypervascular metastasis
Angiosarcoma
Arterioportal shunts, THAD/THID

BOX 12-10   Progressively Enhancing Liver Lesions

Hemangioma
Cholangiocarcinoma
Metastasis
Peliosis hepatis
Fibrosis

Peripherally Enhancing Lesions

Although we have included peripherally enhancing lesions as a separate category, many of the lesions discussed here also demonstrate evidence of early or progressive enhancement. These lesions are listed in Box 12-11. As mentioned earlier, cavernous hemangiomas classically demonstrate early peripheral enhancement that is discontinuous, nodular, and centripetal (Fig. 12-104). Peripheral cholangiocarcinoma and some metastatic lesions demonstrate early peripheral enhancement with peripheral washout on delayed images. Centrally necrotic tumors typically demonstrate a thick, irregular wall of enhancing viable tissue without

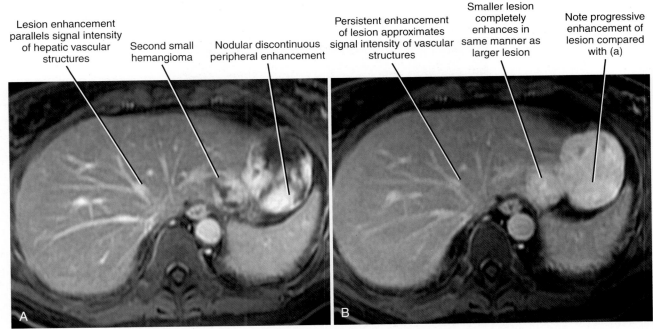

Figure 12-102 Axial portal- **(A)** and equilibrium-phase **(B)** gadolinium-enhanced magnetic resonance imaging of the liver shows typical enhancement pattern of cavernous hemangioma.

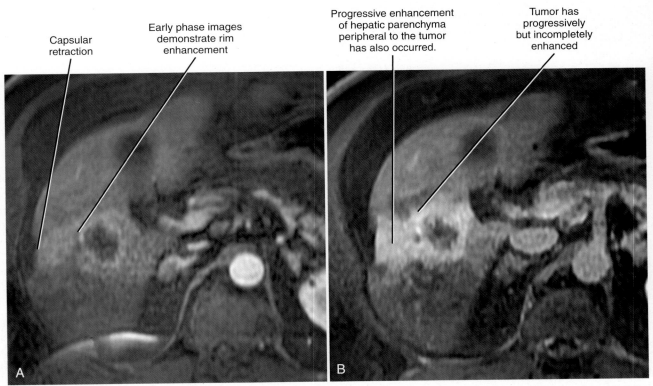

Figure 12-103 Axial arterial- **(A)** and equilibrium-phase **(B)** magnetic resonance images through the liver of a patient with peripheral cholangiocarcinoma (same patient as in Fig. 12-94).

BOX 12-11   Peripherally Enhancing Liver Lesions

Abscess
Cholangiocarcinoma
Hemangioma
Metastasis
Necrotic tumor
Thermal ablation site (first few months)
Peliosis hepatis

Lesion in caudal right lobe of liver
demonstrates target-like enhancement

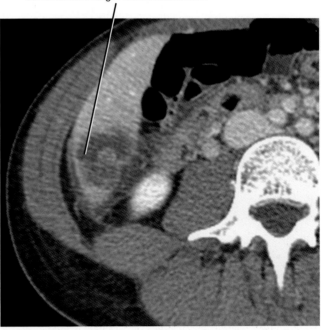

Figure 12-105 Portal-phase magnetic resonance image through the liver of a middle-aged woman with epithelioid hemangioendothelioma demonstrating target-like enhancement of the lesion.

Nodular discontinuous
peripheral enhancement

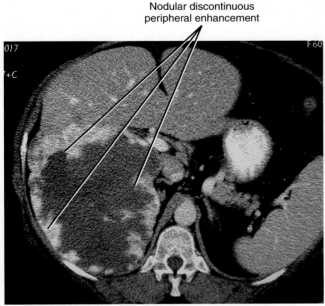

Figure 12-104 Enhanced axial computed tomographic image through the upper abdomen of a patient with a giant hemangioma with typical early enhancement pattern (same patient as in Fig. 12-72).

evidence of progressive or delayed central enhancement. Necrotic tumor can often be distinguished from abscess, because the peripheral enhancement in the latter tends to be thinner and more regular. Symptoms and clinical history are also useful in distinguishing these entities. Rate of growth can be an unreliable indicator of infection, because some aggressive metastases can demonstrate significant growth in a matter of weeks, and we have seen some abscesses persist for months because of inadequate treatment. A thermal ablation site may demonstrate peripheral rimlike enhancement caused by hyperemia lasting several months.

Other Features on Contrast-Enhanced Images

Other features that may be demonstrated with extracellular contrast agents include differential central enhancement (often referred to as a central "scar"), an enhancing capsule or pseudocapsule on later phases of enhancement, and target-like enhancement. Target-like enhancement has been described as a feature of epithelioid hemangioendothelioma (Fig. 12-105). An enhancing

pseudocapsule is most closely associated with HCC, although hepatic adenoma may also demonstrate this feature (see Fig. 12-98). Lesions that demonstrate peripheral washout with central enhancement on equilibrium-phase images should be assumed malignant until proved otherwise (Fig. 12-106).

Pearl: Lesions that demonstrate peripheral washout with central enhancement on equilibrium-phase images should be assumed malignant until proved otherwise.

Differential central enhancement occurs when the center of a lesion enhances in a clearly different manner from the peripheral portions of the lesion. This may be the result of hemorrhage, necrosis, fibrosis, or vascular supply. When differential central enhancement is present, the center of the lesion usually has different echogenicity, attenuation, or signal intensity from the periphery on noncontrast-enhanced US, CT, or MR images, respectively. The imaging appearance of the central "scar" of a lesion should always be interpreted in the context of the imaging appearance of that entire lesion. Table 12-12 lists lesions that may have a central "scar," and many of these lesions are illustrated in Figure 12-69. When the central "scar" is due to hemorrhage or necrosis (adenoma, HCC, metastasis), it will not enhance after intravenous contrast administration. Fibrous scars (cholangiocarcinoma, fibrolamellar carcinoma) may eventually enhance given enough time (usually greater than 10 minutes). The fibrovascular "scar" of FNH enhances after the arterial phase but within a few minutes of contrast administration.

Liver lesion (metastatic adenocarcinoma) demonstrates peripheral washout on equilibrium phase image

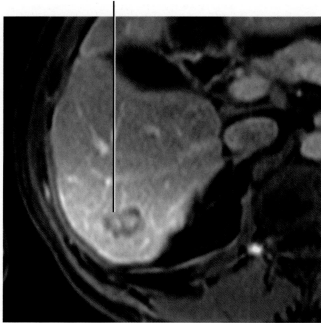

Figure 12-106 Axial equilibrium-phase gadolinium-enhanced magnetic resonance image through the right hepatic lobe of a patient with metastatic adenocarcinoma (colon primary).

Lesion is nearly isointense to liver with exception of central region

High SI central scar on T2W image

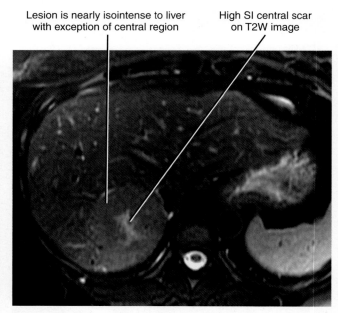

Figure 12-107 Axial T2-weighted (T2W) magnetic resonance image through the liver of a patient with focal nodular hyperplasia (FNH) demonstrating typical appearance of the central scar. *SI,* Signal intensity.

Table 12-12   Liver Lesions with a Central "Scar"

Lesion	T2W SI* of "Scar"	Enhancement† of "Scar"	Other Features of "Scar"
FNH (Fig. 12-107)	Bright	Mildly delayed enhancement (usually enhances after late arterial phase but within first few minutes)	
Atypical hemangioma	Bright	None	
HCC	Usually bright	None	
Metastasis	Usually bright	None	
Hepatic adenoma	Variable	None	
Cholangio-carcinoma	Often dark	Delayed enhancement (>5 minutes)	
Fibrolamellar HCC	Dark	Very delayed enhancement (>10 minutes, if at all)	Calcification common

*Typical signal intensity (SI) of central "scar" on T2-weighted (T2W) images.
†Enhancement pattern after intravenous administration of extracellular iodine- or gadolinium-based agents on computed tomography and magnetic resonance imaging.
HCC, Hepatocellular carcinoma.

Solitary or Multiple? Causes of Innumerable Liver Lesions

Innumerable Cystic-Appearing Lesions

Table 12-13 lists the causes of multiple cystic-appearing lesions of the liver. The size, distribution, and appearance of the cysts in addition to extrahepatic findings usually allow the various causes to be distinguished.

Innumerable Noncystic Liver Lesions

Table 12-14 lists the causes of innumerable noncystic liver lesions. Microabscesses may be pyogenic or fungal. Widespread pyogenic hepatic abscesses may be a manifestation of septicemia or arise from biliary infection. Fungal abscesses are typically present in immunosuppressed patients and are usually the result of *Candida albicans* infection. Other causative agents include *Cryptococcus* infection, histoplasmosis, mucormycosis, and aspergillosis. Candidal abscesses usually present as multiple small (approximately ≤1 cm), round lesions distributed throughout the liver. Splenic and renal involvement may also be present. With sonography, candidal microabscesses may appear uniformly hypoechoic, uniformly hyperechoic (often after therapy), or have a hyperechoic center with surrounding hypoechoic rim ("bull's-eye" appearance). A fourth US appearance described as "wheel-within-a-wheel" results from a central hypoechoic necrotic area surrounded by an echogenic zone of inflammatory cells and an outer hypoechoic fibrotic rim. With CT, candidal microabscesses tend to be low in attenuation on precontrast and postcontrast images. Some lesions may have a central area of higher

Table 12-13   Innumerable Cystic-Appearing Liver Lesions

Diagnosis	Distinguishing Features
Autosomal dominant polycystic kidney/liver disease (ADPKD) (Fig. 12-108)	• Variable cyst size from very small to very large • Variable appearance on ultrasound, computed tomography, or magnetic resonance imaging because of variable cyst composition and complexity • Calcification may be present • Renal cystic disease often present
Biliary hamartomas (von Meyenburg complex) (Fig. 12-109)	• Cysts are small (<1.5 cm) • Uniform in appearance • Uniformly distributed • No communication with biliary tree • Hyperechoic with ultrasound
Peribiliary cysts	• Distributed along bile ducts • Chronic liver disease or ADPKD
Choledochal cysts (Caroli disease)	• Communicate with biliary tree • Central "dot" sign*
Cystic metastases	• Primary neoplasm elsewhere • Rim enhancement may be present
Abscesses (Fig. 12-110)	• Immunocompromised patient • Signs/symptoms of infection may be present • Rim enhancement may be present • Spleen may be involved

*Central "dot" sign refers to the presence of portal triad structures (the central dots) enveloped by bile duct on axial computed tomographic and magnetic resonance images.

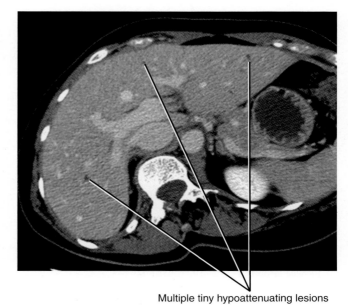

Multiple tiny hypoattenuating lesions

Figure 12-109 Enhanced axial computed tomographic image through the liver of a patient with bile duct hamartomas. Diagnosis was suggested before surgery but confirmed during surgery for unrelated reasons.

Innumerable cysts of variable size throughout the liver

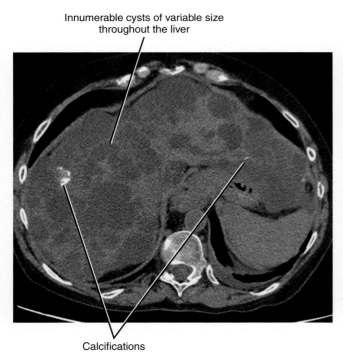

Calcifications

Figure 12-108 Unenhanced axial computed tomographic image through the liver of a patient with autosomal dominant polycystic kidney disease and extensive cystic disease of the liver.

Multiple hypoattenuating lesions of variable size with some clustering

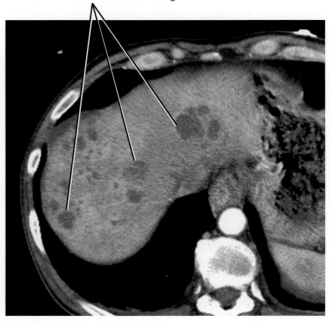

Figure 12-110 Enhanced axial computed tomographic image through the liver of a patient with multiple pyogenic hepatic abscesses.

Table 12-14 Innumerable Noncystic Liver Lesions

Diagnosis	Distinguishing Features
Metastases	• Primary neoplasm elsewhere • Early rim enhancement and late peripheral "washout" may be present
Hepatocellular carcinoma (Fig. 12-111)	• Evidence of cirrhosis • Arterial-phase enhancement • Portal-phase "washout" • Venous invasion
Regenerative nodules of cirrhosis	• Evidence of cirrhosis or portal hypertension • Enhancement similar to normal liver
Nodular regenerative hyperplasia (see Fig. 12-76)	• Evidence of Budd–Chiari syndrome
Infection Fungal Mycobacterial *Bartonella henselae* Brucellosis	• Immunocompromised state • Spleen often involved • Low-density lymph nodes (mycobacteria) • Hyperenhancing nodes (Bartonella)
Sarcoidosis (see Fig. 12-45)	• Spleen often involved • Pulmonary manifestations • Lymphadenopathy
Nodular fatty infiltration	• Signal loss on opposed-phase gradient-echo magnetic resonance images (chemical-shift imaging)
Lymphoma/leukemia	• Lymphadenopathy

Multiple lesions replacing
entire right lobe of liver

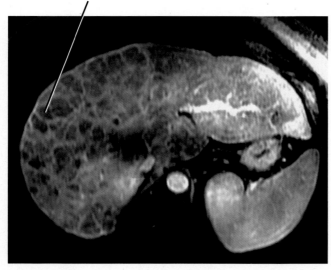

Figure 12-111 Axial portal-phase gadolinium-enhanced magnetic resonance image through the liver of a patient with multifocal hepatocellular carcinoma.

attenuation. As with other abscesses, candidal microabscesses appear as high-signal-intensity lesions on T2-weighted images. In the subacute phase, a dark ring may surround the lesions on all MR sequences. Rim enhancement is not a prominent feature of candidal microabscesses but may be present in some cases. Lesions may change appearance or resolve completely after therapy.

Mycobacterial infections of the liver rarely manifest on imaging studies. When present, imaging findings are nonspecific and include lesions of variable echogenicity with US or hypoattenuating lesions with CT. Healed tuberculosis may manifest as small, diffuse hepatic calcifications.

Bacillary angiomatosis is a rare manifestation of *Bartonella henselae* infection that may be present in patients with acquired immunodeficiency syndrome (AIDS). Imaging features of this entity are nonspecific and may mimic a variety of other opportunistic infections that afflict patients with AIDS. *Bartonella henselae* also causes cat-scratch disease in immunocompetent individuals. Clinical history and the presence of painful lymphadenopathy are helpful in establishing the diagnosis. Hepatic involvement in the immunocompetent individual usually heals spontaneously.

Sarcoidosis involving the liver frequently manifests as nonspecific hepatomegaly and is frequently associated with typical pulmonary findings, lymphadenopathy, and splenomegaly. However, sarcoidosis may occasionally manifest as a diffuse multinodular pattern in the liver, spleen, or both. The nodules (granulomas) are typically small (usually < 2 cm), hypoechoic on US, low density on NCCT, and low signal intensity on T1- and T2-weighted MR images. The nodules may become isodense to surrounding liver on contrast-enhanced CT.

Secondary lymphoma of the liver is usually of the non-Hodgkin's type. Lymphoma typically appears as hypoechoic areas on US images when focal but may be undetectable when diffuse. On noncontrast CT, mass-like lymphoma is lower in attenuation than normal liver, whereas diffuse infiltration may go undetected, even after intravenous contrast administration. Lymphoma enhances variably but typically enhances relatively homogeneously and only mildly, although a thin enhancing rim may be present. Lymphoma is generally hypointense on T1-weighted MR images and hyperintense to normal liver on T2-weighted images. As with CT, enhancement of lymphoma after gadolinium chelate administration is variable but usually mild and homogeneous. Because of the relatively nonspecific imaging appearance of lymphoma, obtaining an appropriate history of lymphoma or immunosuppression is extremely helpful. A new mass in a solid organ of an immunocompromised patient is often lymphoma.

Summary of Focal Hepatic Lesions

Many of the features discussed in the preceding section are summarized in Table 12-15. Only the more typical appearances of lesions are discussed; most of the lesions listed can have atypical appearances that overlap with other entities.

Table 12-15   A Quick Guide to Typical Features of Select Focal Hepatic Lesions (in Alphabetical Order)

Diagnosis	Key Points
Abscess, amebic (see Fig. 12-88)	**Clinical** • Caused by entamoeba histolytica • Found in developing tropical areas of the world • Cause of right upper quadrant pain and diarrhea • Majority found in the right hepatic lobe • Associated right pneumonitis, atelectasis, pleural effusion, or elevation of the right hemidiaphragm • Serology is positive in up to 90% of individuals **Imaging** *General* • Well-defined, round or oval, unilocular or multilocular • Look for evidence of colitis *US* • Hypoechoic with homogeneously distributed low-level echoes and distal acoustic enhancement; this latter feature helps distinguish abscess from a solid lesion. *CT* • Abscess cavity is usually hypoattenuating with a well-defined, continuous wall; some mural irregularity may be present. *MRI* • Abscess cavity is lower SI than hepatic parenchyma on T1WIs and hyperintense on T2WIs. *Contrast Enhancement** • Enhancement of the wall
Abscess, pyogenic (Figs. 12-89, 12-90, and 12-110)	**Clinical** • Caused by ascending biliary infection, infection associated with biliary obstruction, portal venous spread of infection from the intestinal tract, septicemia, infection from adjacent organ such as gallbladder or colon, or introduction of infection by penetrating trauma or surgery. • Causes right upper quadrant pain and tenderness, fever, and leukocytosis **Imaging** *General* • Abscesses of biliary origin are frequently multiple and scattered; abscesses of portal origin are often solitary. *US* • Variable echogenicity on ultrasound; early abscesses are often hyperechoic, whereas mature abscesses may demonstrate decreased echogenicity. • No flow within abscess cavity with color Doppler sonography. • Air manifests as areas of increased echogenicity. • Swirling of abscess contents sometimes visible in real time. *CT* • Generally hypoattenuating; a low-attenuation region surrounding the wall may be present ("double target" sign), representing periabscess edema and inflammation. • Multiple small abscesses coalescing into a larger collection ("cluster" sign). *MRI* • Cavity usually low SI on T1WIs and high SI on T2WIs. • Perilesional edema may be present as a rim of high SI parenchyma surrounding the abscess wall on T2WIs. • Air manifests as areas of signal void on MR that become more conspicuous on longer TE gradient-echo (T2*-weighted) sequences. • Debris–fluid levels of varying signal intensity may be present. *Contrast Enhancement** • Continuous, uniform, enhancing wall after intravenous contrast administration
Adenoma (hepatic adenoma, hepatocellular adenoma) (see Fig. 12-81)	**Clinical** • Much more common in women • Associated with oral contraceptive or anabolic steroid use or glycogen storage disease (Ia) • Frequently hemorrhage • Malignant transformation rare **Imaging** *General* • Intralesional hemorrhage or steatosis common • Pseudocapsule common *US* • Variable echogenicity • Echogenic foci related to fat or calcification *CT* • Variable attenuation depending on presence of fat, hemorrhage, or calcifications *MRI* • High SI areas on T1WI caused by hemorrhage or fat • Focal or diffuse signal loss on OOP images caused by intracellular lipid • Heterogeneous but generally increased SI on T2WI *Contrast Enhancement** • Early mosaic enhancement • Persistent enhancement of pseudocapsule • Less uptake of RES agents (e.g., SPIO) than focal nodular hyperplasia • Usually hypointense to liver on hepatobiliary phase images after gadobenate dimeglumine or gadoxetate disodium administration

Continued

Table 12-15 A Quick Guide to Typical Features of Select Focal Hepatic Lesions (in Alphabetical Order)—cont'd

Diagnosis	Key Points
Angiosarcoma (hemangio-sarcoma)	**Clinical** • Very rare • Associated with prior Thorotrast, polyvinyl chloride, or arsenic exposure, primary hemochromatosis or neurofibromatosis • Can occur in setting of cirrhosis • Can rupture or hemorrhage • Poor prognosis: high rate of recurrence and metastasis **Imaging** *General* • Often multifocal *US* • Variable/mixed echogenicity *CT* • Hypoattenuating on unenhanced CT *MRI* • Predominantly lower SI than liver on T1WI • Predominantly higher SI than liver on T2WI • Areas of hemorrhage bright on T1WI *Contrast Enhancement** • Enhancement may be heterogeneous or nodular • Enhancement is progressive and persistent • May demonstrate ring enhancement • May mimic hemangioma
Biliary cystadenoma or cystadenocarcinoma (see Fig. 12-91)	**Clinical** • Uncommon premalignant tumor (cystadenoma) of biliary origin that typically arises from the intrahepatic bile ducts. • Usually seen in middle-aged women. • Cause of right upper quadrant pain, jaundice, and a palpable mass. • Tumors with ovarian stroma are typically found in women and have a more indolent course and better prognosis. • Tumors without ovarian stroma are more common in male individuals and tend to be more aggressive. • Cyst fluid may be bilious, mucinous, serous, hemorrhagic, or a combination of these components. **Imaging** *General* • Typical lesion is multiseptated with relatively large cystic spaces; a microcystic variant exists; rarely unilocular. • Mural nodularity favors, but is not specific for, carcinoma. • Tend to be solitary and have a moderate preference for the right hepatic lobe. • Imaging cannot reliably differentiate biliary cystadenoma from cystadenocarcinoma. *US* • Multiseptated mass containing anechoic fluid, although some locules may demonstrate internal echoes. • Septal calcifications can appear as hyperechoic foci. *CT* • Locules range from fluid attenuation to high density (because of hemorrhage). • Fine mural or septal calcifications may be visible. *MR* • Fluid is variable SI on T1- and T2-weighted images depending on its composition. *Contrast Enhancement** • The tumor capsule, septa, and mural nodules enhance after intravenous contrast administration. • The fluid-filled spaces do not enhance, even on delayed images with hepatobiliary contrast agents, because these lesions do not communicate with the biliary tree.
Cholangiocarcinoma (peripheral) (see Figs. 12-94 and 12-103)	**Clinical** • Risk factors: primary sclerosing cholangitis, choledochal cyst, biliary lithiasis, congenital hepatic fibrosis, and *Clonorchis sinensis* **Imaging** *General* • Satellite nodules common • Can grow into or along bile ducts • Can be associated with capsular retraction • Dilated bile ducts variably present • Calcifications uncommon but can be present *US* • Variable echogenicity: more often hyperechoic than hypoechoic *CT* • Well-defined • Lobular margins *MRI* • Hypointense to liver on T1WI • Mildly hyperintense to liver on T2WI • Central portion of tumor often hypointense on T2WI because of fibrosis *Contrast Enhancement** • Early rim enhancement common • Progressive and persistent enhancement on subsequent phases of enhancement • Peripheral washout on delayed images

Table 12-15   A Quick Guide to Typical Features of Select Focal Hepatic Lesions (in Alphabetical Order)—cont'd

Diagnosis	Key Points
Cyst, simple (see Figs. 12-84 and, 12-85)	**Clinical** • Extremely common • Usually asymptomatic, incidentally discovered • More common in women • Peribiliary cysts seen in chronic liver disease or autosomal dominant polycystic kidney disease **Imaging** *General* • Multiple cysts common • Sharply demarcated thin wall with all modalities • May occasionally have thin septation *US* • Anechoic • Posterior acoustic enhancement *CT* • Uniform low attenuation (usually less than 10 HU) *MRI* • Low SI on T1WI • Very high SI on T2WI *Contrast Enhancement** • No enhancement
Epithelioid hemangioen-dothelioma (see Fig. 12-105)	**Clinical** • Rare • Most common in middle-aged women • Variable prognosis **Imaging** *General* • Lesions often peripheral, extending to capsule • Often multifocal • Lesions become confluent as they enlarge • Occasionally have calcifications • Can metastasize *US* • Typically hypoechoic • Peripheral hypoechoic rim may be present *CT* • Decreased attenuation on unenhanced CT *MRI* • Lower SI than liver on T1WI • Higher SI than liver on T2WI *Contrast Enhancement** • Target pattern of enhancement: nonenhancing center, enhancing inner rim, poorly enhancing outer rim
Fibrolamellar hepatocellular carcinoma (see Fig. 12-69)	**Clinical** • More common in young adults • AFP level usually normal • Cirrhosis usually absent • No gender predilection • Better prognosis than conventional hepatocellular carcinoma **Imaging** *General* • Usually large, lobulated mass • Central scar common *US* • Variable echogenicity • Echogenic central scar *CT* • Well-defined mass with radiating septa • Central scar may be hypodense or calcified *MRI* • Hypointense to liver on T1WI • Hyperintense to liver on T2WI • Central scar is hypointense to liver and lesion on T1WI and T2WI • Hypointense radiating septa *Contrast Enhancement** • Heterogeneous enhancement • Scar does not enhance or enhances very late (usually later than most standard protocols image)

Continued

Table 12-15 A Quick Guide to Typical Features of Select Focal Hepatic Lesions (in Alphabetical Order)—cont'd

Diagnosis	Key Points
Focal nodular hyperplasia (see Figs. 12-69, 12-74, 12-99, 12-107, and 12-112)	**Clinical** • Common incidental, asymptomatic lesion • More common in women **Imaging** *US* • Nearly isoechoic to liver • Hypoechoic central scar (may occasionally be hyperechoic) *CT* • Nearly isodense on unenhanced CT images • Low-attenuation central scar *MRI* • Nearly isointense to liver on T1WI and T2WI • High SI central scar on T2WI (low SI on T1WI) • Rarely can demonstrate signal loss on OOP images *Contrast Enhancement** • Brisk arterial-phase enhancement • Radiating septa on early-phase contrast-enhanced enhanced images • Nearly isodense/isointense on subsequent phases • Enhancement of central scar on equilibrium-phase images • Tumor isointense or hyperintense to liver on hepatobiliary phase images (1-3 hours) after gadobenate dimeglumine or gadoxetate disodium administration • Significant uptake of SPIO *NM* • Uptake of technetium-99m (Tc-99m) sulfur colloid common (60% have at least equal uptake to liver) • Retention of iminodiacetic acid common
Hemangioma (cavernous hemangioma) (see Figs. 12-62, 12-72, 12-79, 12-100, 12-102, and 12-104)	Clinical • Common • Usually incidental, asymptomatic • Rupture, hemorrhage are rare • Can grow slowly • Occasionally associated with focal nodular hyperplasia Imaging General • Solitary or multiple • Calcification rare • Larger lesions have lobular border • Larger lesions may have central scar US • Well-defined, homogeneously hyperechoic when small • Posterior acoustic enhancement often present • Sometimes have less echogenic center and uniform echogenic border (atypical appearance) CT • Well-defined, hypoattenuating on unenhanced CT MRI • Hypointense on T1WI • Hyperintense on T2WI • When present, central scar very hyperintense Contrast Enhancement* • Small lesions often enhance homogeneously and early • Small lesions often associated with wedge-shaped THID or THAD • Enhancement intensity similar to that of vessels • Enhancement persists into equilibrium phase • Classic pattern: peripheral, nodular, discontinuous enhancement that progresses centrally • Central scar, when present, does not enhance NM • Tc-99m red blood cell scan demonstrates focal defect on early dynamic imaging and persistent activity on delayed images

Table 12-15   A Quick Guide to Typical Features of Select Focal Hepatic Lesions (in Alphabetical Order)—cont'd

Diagnosis	Key Points
Hepatocellular carcinoma (hepatoma) (see Figs. 12-28, 12-52, 12-53, 12-54, 12-55, 12-69, 12-82, 12-98, and 12-111)	**Clinical** • Common risk factors: cirrhosis, viral hepatitis, hemochromatosis • AFP level often, but not always, elevated • M > F **Imaging** *General* • May be focal, multifocal, or diffusely infiltrating • Nodule-within-nodule appearance suggests hepatocellular carcinoma arising within a cirrhotic/dysplastic nodule • Intralesional steatosis or foci of fat may be present • Venous invasion by tumor common (portal vein > hepatic vein) *US* • Variable echogenicity (most small lesions are hypoechoic) • Hypoechoic halo may be present • Large lesions tend to be of heterogeneous echogenicity • Hypervascularity and high-velocity flow with Doppler *CT* • Small lesions often not visible in cirrhotic liver on unenhanced CT • Low-attenuation regions because of fat or necrosis *MRI* • Isointense or hypointense on T1WI • Isointense or hyperintense on T2WI *Contrast Enhancement** • Early mosaic enhancement • Washout on portal phase • Enhancing capsule on equilibrium phase • Arterioportal shunting • Less uptake of SPIO than surrounding liver
Hydatid disease (*Echinococcus granulosus*) (see Fig. 12-92)	**Clinical** • Classic form of hepatic hydatid cyst. • Caused by the cestode *E. granulosus,* found mostly in Mediterranean countries, Africa, South America, India, Australia, and New Zealand • Affected patients may demonstrate eosinophilia, and serologic tests can help establish the diagnosis but may be negative in a significant number of patients. • Cysts can rupture or become secondarily infected **Imaging** *General* • Larvae enter the liver via the portal vein and form slow-growing cysts surrounded by a fibrous capsule that can calcify • Peripherally arranged daughter cysts form, resulting in multiple cysts in the majority of cases • Lesions may grow to occupy a significant portion of the affected lobe • Air within cyst suggests secondary infection *US* • Well-defined anechoic cyst with enhanced through-transmission • Floating or dependent debris (hydatid sand) may be present • Double echogenic lines separated by a hypoechoic layer or a floating membrane may be noted ("water lily" sign) • Calcifications may be visible as echogenic foci, or the wall may be densely echogenic because of calcification *CT* • Low-attenuation unilocular or multilocular cystic mass • Daughter cysts are arranged peripherally and may appear as lower attenuation • Rim calcification or more extensive calcification may be present *MRI* • Uncomplicated cyst appears as high signal intensity on T2-weighted images with a low-signal- intensity rim (pericyst) around the cyst • Hypointense floating membranes may be present *Contrast Enhancement** • Mild enhancement of the cyst wall

Continued

Table 12-15 A Quick Guide to Typical Features of Select Focal Hepatic Lesions (in Alphabetical Order)—cont'd

Diagnosis	Key Points
Metastasis (see Figs. 12-17, 12-43, 12-65 to 12-71, 12-83, 12-87, 12-93, 12-95, 12-101, and 12-106)	**Clinical** • Most common malignant liver tumor • Liver is common site of metastatic disease • Blood supply tends to be from hepatic artery • Most common primary tumor sites include colon, stomach, pancreas, breast, lung, melanoma, and gallbladder **Imaging** *General* • Highly variable appearance • Cystic metastases: cystadenocarcinoma of ovary and pancreas, mucinous adenocarcinoma of colon, sarcomas, squamous cell carcinoma, treated metastases *US* • Hypoechoic halo on US (also seen with other tumors such as hepatocellular carcinoma) • Hyperechoic metastases: gastrointestinal primaries, neuroendocrine tumors, choriocarcinoma, renal cell carcinoma • Hypoechoic metastases: breast cancer, lung cancer, lymphoma, esophageal, gastric, and pancreatic cancer *CT* • Usually isodense or hypodense to liver on unenhanced CT • Calcified metastases: colon cancer, osteogenic sarcoma, chondrosarcoma, malignant teratoma, neuroblastoma, treated metastases *MRI* • Usually hypointense to liver on T1WI • Hemorrhagic metastases, metastatic melanoma, and fat-containing metastases (liposarcoma or malignant teratoma) may be hyperintense to liver on T1WI • Usually hyperintense to liver on T2WI • Neuroendocrine or cystic metastases can be bright on T2WI (mimic of hemangioma on T2WI) *Contrast Enhancement** • Typical hypervascular liver metastases: neuroendocrine tumors, renal cell carcinoma, thyroid cancer, melanoma, breast cancer, pheochromocytoma • Typical hypovascular liver metastases: colon cancer, lung cancer, prostate cancer, stomach cancer, transitional cell carcinoma, pancreatic cancer, lymphoma • Rim enhancement common • The combination of central enhancement and peripheral washout on delayed contrast-enhanced images is suggestive of metastases but can be seen with cholangiocarcinoma *NM* • Multiple hypermetabolic foci with 18-fluoro-2-deoxy-D-glucose positron emission tomography

*Unless otherwise stated, contrast enhancement implies enhancement after intravenous injection of extracellular iodinated media for computed tomography (CT) or extracellular gadolinium-based media for magnetic resonance imaging (MRI).
AFP, α-Fetoprotein; *NM*, nuclear medicine; *OOP*, out-of-phase; *RES*, reticuloendothelial system; *SI*, signal intensity; *SPIO*, superparamagnetic iron oxide; *T1WI*, T1-weighted image; *T2WI*, T2-weighted image; *THAD*, transient hepatic attenuation difference; *THID*, transient hepatic intensity difference; *US*, ultrasound.

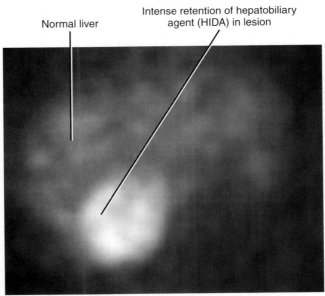

Normal liver

Intense retention of hepatobiliary agent (HIDA) in lesion

Figure 12-112 Hepatobiliary iminodiacetic acid (HIDA) scan obtained 51 minutes after radionuclide administration in a patient with focal nodular hyperplasia (same patient as in Fig. 12-107).

Suggested Readings

Alobaidi M, Shirkhoda A: Benign focal liver lesions: discrimination from malignant mimickers, *Curr Probl Diagn Radiol* 33:239-253, 2004.

Alobaidi M, Shirkhoda A: Malignant cystic and necrotic liver lesions: a pattern approach to discrimination, *Curr Probl Diagn Radiol* 33:254-268, 2004.

Awaya H, Mitchell DG, Kamishima T et al: Cirrhosis: modified caudate-right lobe ratio, *Radiology* 224:769-774, 2002.

Baron RL, Peterson MS: From the RSNA refresher courses: screening the cirrhotic liver for hepatocellular carcinoma with CT and MR imaging: opportunities and pitfalls, *Radiographics* 21(spec no):S117-S132, 2001.

Basaran C, Karcaaltincaba M, Akata D et al: Fat-containing lesions of the liver: cross-sectional imaging findings with emphasis on MRI, *AJR Am J Roentgenol* 184:1103-1110, 2005.

Bismuth H: Surgical anatomy and anatomical surgery of the liver, *World J Surg* 6:3-9, 1982.

Brancatelli G, Federle M, Ambrosini R et al: Cirrhosis: CT and MR imaging evaluation, *Eur J Radiol* 61:57-69, 2007.

Brancatelli G, Federle MP, Vilgrain V et al: Fibropolycystic liver disease: CT and MR imaging findings, *Radiographics* 25:659-670, 2005.

Chen JS, Yeh BM, Wang ZJ et al: Concordance of second-order portal venous and biliary tract anatomies on MDCT angiography and MDCT cholangiography, *AJR Am J Roentgenol* 184:70-74, 2005.

Danet IM, Semelka RC, Braga L: MR imaging of diffuse liver disease, *Radiol Clin North Am* 41:67-87, 2003.

Danet IM, Semelka RC, Leonardou P et al: Spectrum of MRI appearances of untreated metastases of the liver, *AJR Am J Roentgenol* 181:809-817, 2003.

Dodd GD 3rd, Baron RL, Oliver JH 3rd et al: End-stage primary sclerosing cholangitis: CT findings of hepatic morphology in 36 patients, *Radiology* 211:357-362, 1999.

Dodd GD 3rd, Baron RL, Oliver JH 3rd et al: Spectrum of imaging findings of the liver in end-stage cirrhosis: part I, gross morphology and diffuse abnormalities, *AJR Am J Roentgenol* 173:1031-1036, 1999.

Dodd GD 3rd, Baron RL, Oliver JH 3rd et al: Spectrum of imaging findings of the liver in end-stage cirrhosis: part II, focal abnormalities, *AJR Am J Roentgenol* 173:1185-1192, 1999.

Doyle DJ, Khalili K, Guindi M et al: Imaging features of sclerosed hemangioma, *AJR Am J Roentgenol* 189:67-72, 2007.

Elsayes KM, Narra VR, Yin Y et al: Focal hepatic lesions: diagnostic value of enhancement pattern approach with contrast-enhanced 3D gradient echo MR imaging, *Radiographics* 25:1299-1320, 2005.

Erbay N, Raptopoulos V, Pomfret EA et al: Living donor liver transplantation in adults: vascular variants important in surgical planning for donors and recipients, *AJR Am J Roentgenol* 181:109-114, 2003.

Gallego C, Velasco M, Marcuello P et al: Congenital and acquired anomalies of the portal venous system, *Radiographics* 22:141-159, 2002.

Geraghty EM, Boone JM, McGahan JP et al: Normal organ volume assessment from abdominal CT, *Abdom Imaging* 29:482-490, 2004.

Gupta AA, Kim DC, Krinsky GA et al: CT and MRI of cirrhosis and its mimics, *AJR Am J Roentgenol* 183:1595-1601, 2004.

Hamer OW, Aguirre DA, Casola G et al: Fatty liver: imaging patterns and pitfalls, *Radiographics* 26:1637-1653, 2006.

Hashimoto M, Heianna J, Tate E et al: Small veins entering the liver, *Eur Radiol* 12:2000-2005, 2002.

Hur J, Park M-S, Yu J-S et al: Focal eosinophilic necrosis versus metastasis in the liver: the usefulness of two-phase dynamic CT, *AJR Am J Roentgenol* 184:1085-1090, 2005.

Itai Y, Hachiya J, Makita K et al: Transient hepatic attenuation differences on dynamic computed tomography, *J Comput Assist Tomogr* 11:461-465, 1987.

Itai Y, Matsui O: Nonportal splanchnic venous supply to the liver: abnormal findings on CT, US and MRI, *Eur Radiol* 9:237-243, 1999.

Itai Y, Saida Y: Pitfalls in liver imaging, *Eur Radiol* 12:1162-1174, 2002.

Jeong YY, Yim NY, Kang HK: Hepatocellular carcinoma in the cirrhotic liver with helical CT and MRI: imaging spectrum and pitfalls of cirrhosis-related nodules, *AJR Am J Roentgenol* 185:1024-1032, 2005.

Kanematsu M, Kondo H, Goshima S et al: Imaging liver metastases: review and update, *Eur J Radiol* 58:217-228, 2006.

Karcaaltincaba M, Akhan O: Imaging of hepatic steatosis and fatty sparing, *Eur J Radiol* 61:33-43, 2007.

Kim HJ, Kim AY, Kim TK et al: Transient hepatic attenuation differences in focal hepatic lesions: dynamic CT features, *AJR Am J Roentgenol* 184:83-90, 2005.

Kim M-J, Mitchell DG, Ito K: Portosystemic collaterals of the upper abdomen: review of anatomy and demonstration on MR imaging, *Abdom Imaging* 25:462-470, 2000.

Koseoglu K, Ozsunar Y, Taskin F et al: Pseudolesions of the left liver lobe during helical CT examinations: prevalence and comparison between unenhanced and biphasic CT findings, *Eur J Radiol* 54:388-392, 2005.

Leifer DM, Middleton WD, Teefey SA et al: Follow-up of patients at low risk for hepatic malignancy with a characteristic hemangioma at US, *Radiology* 214:167-172, 2000.

Li D, Hann LE: A practical approach to analyzing focal lesions in the liver, *Ultrasound Q* 21:187-200, 2005.

Mortele KJ, Ros PR: Imaging of diffuse liver disease, *Semin Liver Dis* 21:195-212, 2001.

Mortele KJ, Ros, PR: Cystic focal liver lesions in the adult: differential CT and MR imaging features, *Radiographics* 21:895-910, 2001.

Prasad SR, Wang H, Rosas H et al: Fat-containing lesions of the liver: radiologic-pathologic correlation, *Radiographics* 25:321-331, 2005.

Reinhold C, Hammers L, Taylor CR et al: Characterization of focal hepatic lesions with duplex sonography: findings in 198 patients, *AJR Am J Roentgenol* 164:1131-1135, 1995.

Strasberg S: The Brisbane 2000 terminology of liver anatomy and resections, *J Hepatobiliary Pancreat Surg* 12:351-355, 2005.

Tchelepi H, Ralls PW: Ultrasound of focal liver masses, *Ultrasound Q* 20:155-169, 2004.

Tchelepi H, Ralls PW, Radin R et al: Sonography of diffuse liver disease, *J Ultrasound Med* 21:1023-1032, 2002.

Valls C, Iannaccone R, Alba E et al: Fat in the liver: diagnosis and characterization, *Eur Radiol* 16:2292-2308, 2006.

Wenzel JS, Donohoe A, Ford KL III et al: Primary biliary cirrhosis: MR imaging findings and description of MR imaging periportal halo sign, *AJR Am J Roentgenol* 176:885-889, 2001.

Yang DM, Kim HS, Cho SW et al: Various causes of hepatic capsular retraction: CT and MR findings, *Br J Radiol* 75:994-1002, 2002.

Yoshimitsu K, Honda, H, Kuroiwa T et al: Unusual hemodynamics and pseudolesions of the noncirrhotic liver at CT, *Radiographics* 21:S81-S96, 2001.

Young ST, Paulson EK, Washington K et al: CT of the liver in patients with metastatic breast carcinoma treated by chemotherapy: findings simulating cirrhosis, *AJR Am J Roentgenol* 163:1385-1388, 1994.

CHAPTER 13

Gallbladder and Bile Ducts

John R. Leyendecker and Hisham Tchelepi

■ CLINICAL CONSIDERATIONS

Disorders of the biliary tree and gallbladder commonly require imaging evaluation for diagnosis and management, although imaging findings are often nonspecific when patients present with suspected biliary disease. For example, gallbladder wall thickening may be entirely incidental and benign (adenomyomatosis), life-threatening (gallbladder cancer), or unrelated to primary gallbladder disease (congestive heart failure). When interpreting nonspecific imaging findings, it is helpful to interpret them within the appropriate clinical context. For this reason, we briefly discuss clinical presentations of common diseases of the gallbladder and biliary tract.

Acute Cholecystitis

Acute cholecystitis usually begins with colicky pain that localizes to the right upper quadrant, occasionally radiating to the right scapula. Nausea and vomiting are often present, and pain can be exacerbated by deep inspiration. The gallbladder can be palpable and tender, and involuntary guarding eventually develops. A positive Murphy sign is said to be present when severe pain and guarding occur with palpation of the right upper quadrant during deep inspiration. Once gangrenous cholecystitis develops, the Murphy sign may be absent. High fever, rebound tenderness, and ileus are associated with gangrene or perforation. Leukocytosis in the range of 10,000 to 15,000 cells/mm³ is usually present with acute cholecystitis, and serum transaminase and alkaline phosphatase levels are often slightly increased. Sonography is the preferred imaging modality for the initial evaluation of patients with suspected acute cholecystitis.

When there is marked hyperbilirubinemia, one should suspect common bile duct stones, although a mild increase of serum bilirubin level (e.g., 4 mg/dl) can occur in the absence of choledocholithiasis. Increased serum amylase and lipase levels usually indicate associated pancreatitis.

Choledocholithiasis

The patient with common bile duct stones classically presents with jaundice and abdominal pain, although symptoms may be transient and intermittent. The presence of fever and chills suggests cholangitis or coexistent acute cholecystitis. The serum bilirubin level tends to be increased more with choledocholithiasis than with acute cholecystitis but usually does not exceed 15 mg/dl. A normal bilirubin level does not exclude the diagnosis of choledocholithiasis. Increased levels of alkaline phosphatase, 5'-nucleotidase, and leucine aminopeptidase are typical of choledocholithiasis, although increased levels of these substances may occur with bile duct obstruction from any cause. Transaminases are usually mildly increased (two to three times normal) but may occasionally be high, particularly in the setting of acute cholangitis.

Cholangitis

Acute Cholangitis

Acute cholangitis is generally diagnosed clinically and requires urgent medical therapy. Left untreated, acute cholangitis can progress to hepatic abscess formation and septicemia. Most cases result from ascending infection from bowel or bacterial seeding via the portal venous system. Gram-negative enteric bacteria are the typical offending organisms. Risk factors for the development of acute cholangitis include choledocholithiasis, biliary-enteric anastomosis, biliary stricture or obstruction, and recent biliary procedure (e.g., endoscopic retrograde cholangiopancreatogram [ERCP]). The Charcot triad of fever, jaundice, and right upper quadrant pain represents the classic presentation, although one or more feature may be absent in any given patient. Patients with acute cholangitis typically experience less pain than patients with acute cholecystitis. Laboratory studies often reveal leukocytosis, increased serum alkaline phosphatase level, and hyperbilirubinemia (so-called cholestatic pattern). A mild transaminitis may develop. Up to a third of blood cultures will be positive in the setting of acute cholangitis.

Recurrent Pyogenic Cholangitis

Recurrent pyogenic cholangitis (RPC) is characterized by recurrent bouts of cholangitis associated with intrahepatic stones and biliary strictures. This disorder is predominantly found in Asia (and was previously called *oriental cholangiohepatitis*), although Asian immigrants elsewhere in the world can present with RPC. Symptoms include right upper quadrant pain, fever, and mild jaundice. Leukocytosis and a cholestatic pattern of liver function tests are often present. If left unchecked, cirrhosis or liver failure may ensue. Additional complications of RPC include choledochoduodenal fistula, stone-related pancreatitis, and cholangiocarcinoma.

Acquired Immune Deficiency Syndrome Cholangitis (Human Immunodeficiency Virus Cholangiopathy)

This biliary disorder affects human immunodeficiency virus (HIV)–positive patients and is most often associated with secondary *Cryptosporidium* or cytomegalovirus infection. Patients can present with severe right upper quadrant pain. Alkaline phosphatase level will often be increased in the presence of a normal serum bilirubin concentration. CD4 cell count is usually less than 100 cells per microliter and often less than 50 cells per microliter in patients with acquired immune deficiency syndrome (AIDS) cholangitis.

Primary Sclerosing Cholangitis

Primary sclerosing cholangitis (PSC) occurs most commonly in patients with inflammatory bowel disease. Average age at diagnosis is 40 years, and the disease is more prevalent in men. Ulcerative colitis is more closely associated with PSC than other forms of inflammatory bowel disease. However, fewer than 10% of patients with ulcerative colitis will experience development of PSC. Symptoms can include fatigue, pruritus, and jaundice, although patients are often asymptomatic early in course of the disease. The serum alkaline phosphatase level is typically increased, and increase of serum bilirubin is variably present. Unlike primary biliary cirrhosis (PBC), the mitochondrial antibody test is negative in PSC. Up to 15% of patients (or approximately 1% per year) eventually experience development of cholangiocarcinoma. The progression of PSC is highly variable, with some patients remaining asymptomatic for many years and others progressing rapidly to cirrhosis and portal hypertension. Carcinoembryonic antigen (CEA) or CA 19-9 levels, or both, may be increased in the setting of cholangiocarcinoma.

Cholangiocarcinoma

Patients with cholangiocarcinoma often have painless jaundice. Serum bilirubin levels are frequently greater than 10 mg/dl, and alkaline phosphatase is usually markedly increased. CEA or CA 19-9 levels may also be increased at presentation but are not specific for cholangiocarcinoma. Making a definitive diagnosis of cholangiocarcinoma is often frustrating and challenging. Bile cytology, bile duct brushings, transluminal biopsy, and even percutaneous fine-needle aspiration all have relatively low sensitivity for cholangiocarcinoma, rendering a negative result unreliable.

■ ANATOMY OF THE BILIARY SYSTEM

Standard Biliary Anatomy

The right-sided intrahepatic bile ducts draining their respective hepatic segments converge to form the right anterior segment duct (draining segments V and VIII) and right posterior segment duct (draining segments VI and VII). These ducts join to form the relatively short right hepatic duct. The right hepatic duct joins the left hepatic duct formed from the segmental ducts draining the left lobe of the liver (segments II, III, and IV) to form the common hepatic duct. This biliary confluence is typically extrahepatic and anterior to the portal vein bifurcation. The caudate lobe (segment I) duct can drain into either the right or left system. The common hepatic duct joins with the cystic duct to form the common bile duct. The common bile duct travels in the hepatoduodenal ligament and drains into the duodenum at the ampulla (of Vater). The pancreatic duct can join the bile duct before the duodenal wall (long common channel) or within the duodenal wall. The pancreatic and common bile ducts can also drain into the duodenum through separate ostia.

Variant Biliary Anatomy

Variations in biliary anatomy are common; less than two thirds of individuals exhibit standard bile duct anatomy (one of the authors has a right posterior segment duct draining into his left hepatic duct). The most common biliary anatomic variants involve aberrant confluence of the right posterior segment duct (Figs. 13-1 to 13-3). Variations in bile duct anatomy do not necessarily parallel variations in portal venous anatomy. Variations of the cystic duct include a long parallel course with low insertion into the common duct, insertion into the left side of the common duct, and drainage into a right hepatic duct. Rarely, an accessory hepatic duct may enter the gallbladder. Agenesis, duplication, and ectopic location of the gallbladder may also rarely occur.

Pearl: The most common biliary anatomic variants involve aberrant confluence of the right posterior segment duct.

Gallbladder Anatomy

The gallbladder is divided into a fundus, body, infundibulum, and neck. The cystic duct joins with the common hepatic duct to drain the gallbladder. The site of union of the cystic duct with the common hepatic duct is variable, but usually the cystic duct joins with the common hepatic duct at an acute angle on the right side.

Several anatomic structures are in close proximity to the gallbladder. The gallbladder neck is intimately associated with the lateral proximal duodenum, and the gallbladder fundus resides near the hepatic flexure of the colon. The body and fundus of the gallbladder are

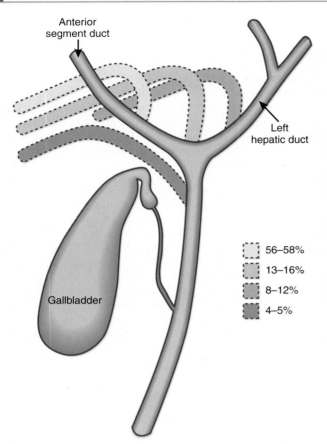

Anterior segment duct

Left hepatic duct

Gallbladder

56–58%
13–16%
8–12%
4–5%

Figure 13-1 Common variations of the biliary confluence that involve the right posterior segment duct.

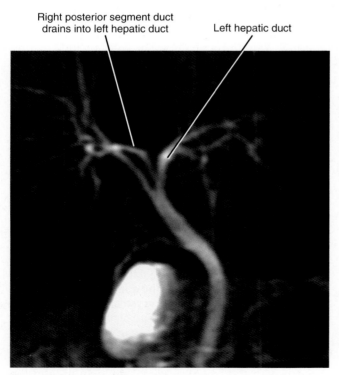

Right posterior segment duct drains into left hepatic duct

Left hepatic duct

Figure 13-2 Thick-slab coronal magnetic resonance cholangiopancreatography demonstrating anomalous confluence of the right posterior segment duct.

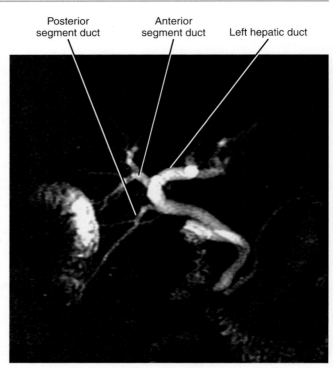

Posterior segment duct

Anterior segment duct

Left hepatic duct

Figure 13-3 Coronal thick-slab magnetic resonance cholangiopancreatography demonstrating low insertion of right posterior segment duct.

also immediately adjacent to segments IVb and V of the liver. Veins drain directly into adjacent liver from the body and fundus of the gallbladder.

■ NORMAL IMAGING APPEARANCE OF THE BILIARY SYSTEM

The normal intrahepatic bile ducts course along with the portal veins and appear as thin structures that may be visible on either side of the accompanying vein on imaging studies. The right and left hepatic ducts are usually less than 3 mm in diameter. With improvements in imaging techniques, intrahepatic ducts are routinely visible with a variety of imaging modalities. The common bile duct usually measures less than 6 mm in diameter, although larger ducts are occasionally visible in patients without bile duct obstruction. There is significant variability in the literature regarding the location from which extrahepatic bile-duct measurements are taken. With ultrasound (US), the bile duct is typically measured at the level of the right hepatic artery, although the maximum duct diameter may be a more useful measurement. Advanced age has been associated in some studies with increased common duct diameter, although most elderly patients have a common bile duct diameter less than 6 mm. Likewise, several studies have linked prior cholecystectomy with increased bile duct diameter, although several other studies have failed to confirm a clinically relevant effect of cholecystectomy on common bile duct diameter. When the common bile duct is dilated from choledocholithiasis, the bile duct will return to normal in three fourths of patients after choledochostomy.

For better or worse, many radiologists have adopted 6 mm as the common bile duct diameter threshold beyond which further evaluation is indicated, particularly when clinical evidence for pancreaticobiliary disease exists. Many radiologists will also accept a common bile duct diameter of 8 or even 10 mm in an elderly patient in the absence of other radiological or clinical evidence for pancreaticobiliary disease. Be aware that the effect of age and prior cholecystectomy on bile duct diameter is a subject of controversy

With US, intrahepatic bile ducts appear as thin, anechoic tubes, although usually only the first- (right and left hepatic ducts) and second-order bile ducts are readily visible with US. The ducts usually appear on the ventral side of the portal vein with US, although color Doppler or spectral analysis may be necessary to distinguish between blood vessels and bile ducts. Harmonic imaging may improve conspicuity of the bile duct and its contents.

With computed tomography (CT), the intrahepatic ducts are thin structures with nearly imperceptible walls that parallel the portal veins. The bile within the ducts normally measures fluid attenuation and appears homogeneous. On magnetic resonance (MR) images, the normal bile ducts parallel simple fluid on all pulse sequences. The signal intensity of the gallbladder contents varies on T1-weighted images but usually appears relatively bright on T2-weighted images.

The normal gallbladder wall measures less than 3 mm in thickness. A small fundal gallbladder division (Phrygian cap) may be present as an incidental finding.

■ GALLSTONES AND SLUDGE

Gallstones

Gallstones are common, particularly in the Western hemisphere. They can be associated with biliary colic, acute or chronic cholecystitis, bile duct obstruction, cholecystenteric fistula formation, and gallbladder carcinoma.

Abdominal radiographs show gallstones as rounded densities in the right upper quadrant. However, radiographs may miss up to 85% of gallstones. Occasionally, gas within gallstones is visible on radiographs. Signs of rare complications of cholelithiasis such as pneumobilia, gallstone ileus, or emphysematous cholecystitis can occasionally be detected with abdominal radiographs.

Transabdominal US is highly sensitive for the diagnosis of uncomplicated cholelithiasis. Larger (>5 mm) stones appear as echogenic foci with strong posterior acoustic shadowing (Fig. 13-4). The color comet tail artifact ("twinkle artifact") can be helpful for confirming the presence of a stone, and the intensity of this artifact is related to the surface characteristics of the stone. Isolated stones smaller than 5 mm may not demonstrate acoustic shadowing but can be differentiated from polyps by their mobility. In general, when echogenic foci are detected with sonography, one should image in several different patient positions to confirm mobility of the abnormality (Fig. 13-5). Large stones or collections

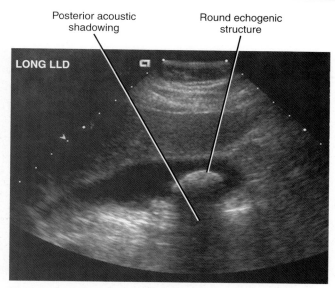

Posterior acoustic shadowing   Round echogenic structure

Figure 13-4 Sonogram of the gallbladder demonstrating typical appearance of a gallstone.

of smaller stones may completely fill the gallbladder, making the gallbladder difficult to identify. The WES (wall-echo-shadow) complex has been described as a means of differentiating gallstones filling the gallbladder from other abnormalities such as emphysematous cholecystitis or porcelain gallbladder, or structures such as the colon (Fig. 13-6). Before invoking the WES complex, one must ensure that the wall is seen as a distinct entity. When air or calcium is present in the gallbladder wall, a normal wall is not visualized. Instead, only an echogenic line and posterior shadow are seen. Stones impacted within the neck or cystic duct of the gallbladder may not be outlined by anechoic bile and can be missed. Therefore, it is always important to examine the neck region and cystic duct to detect evidence of posterior acoustic shadowing and color comet tail artifact. Cystic duct stones, in particular, are a relatively frequent cause of false-negative US results for cholelithiasis.

Pitfall: Stones impacted within the neck or cystic duct of the gallbladder may not be outlined by anechoic bile and can be missed. Therefore, it is always important to examine the neck region and cystic duct to detect evidence of posterior acoustic shadowing and color comet tail artifact.

CT is considerably less sensitive than US but more sensitive than radiographs for detection of gallstones. CT is primarily used in patients with abdominal pain when acute cholecystitis is not the prime consideration and should not be relied on to exclude the presence of gallstones. On CT, gallstones range from hypodense (pure cholesterol stones) to hyperdense and may occasionally contain gas. It is not unusual for even large stones to be missed on technically excellent CT images (Fig. 13-7).

Pitfall: It is not unusual for even large gallstones to be missed on technically excellent CT images.

Although MRI is rarely performed as the primary means of diagnosing cholelithiasis, MRI is highly sensitive for the detection of gallstones, particularly when

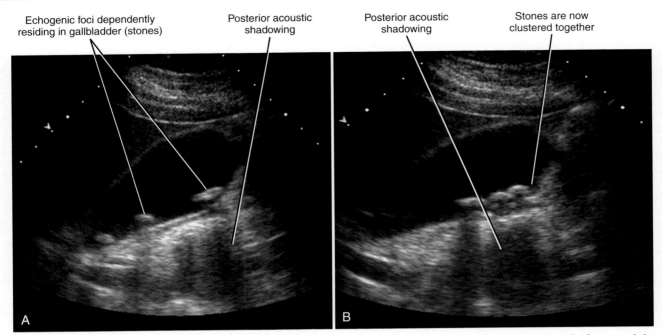

Echogenic foci dependently residing in gallbladder (stones)

Posterior acoustic shadowing

Posterior acoustic shadowing

Stones are now clustered together

A

B

Figure 13-5 Sonographic images performed immediately after changing patient position to left lateral decubitus (**A**) and a few seconds later (**B**) demonstrate mobility of stones within the gallbladder.

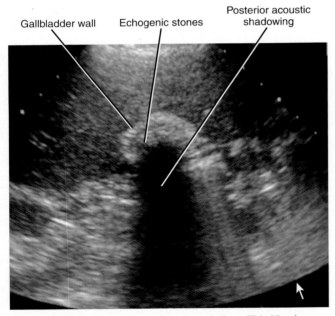

Gallbladder wall   Echogenic stones   Posterior acoustic shadowing

Figure 13-6 Transverse sonogram through the gallbladder demonstrates the wall-echo-shadow complex in a patient with a contracted, stone-filled gallbladder.

motion-insensitive T2-weighted images are performed. Gallstones are typically very low signal intensity on T2-weighted images and variable (very dark to very bright) signal intensity on T1-weighted images.

Occasionally, dropped gallstones will be encountered on imaging examinations after cholecystectomy (usually laparoscopic cholecystectomy). These most often accumulate in the subhepatic space but may be found as far away as the pelvis (Fig. 13-8). The most frequent complication of dropped gallstones is abscess formation. Abscesses related to dropped gallstones can present months to years after cholecystectomy.

Other Substances That Fill the Gallbladder

Biliary Sludge

Sludge consists of precipitated material within the bile that cannot be resolved into individual particles on imaging studies. With sonography, sludge appears as dependent, low-level echoes within the gallbladder lumen (Fig. 13-9). Sludge is usually amorphous, lacks internal vascularity, does not shadow, and slowly changes shape and position with patient movement. When sludge fills the entire gallbladder lumen, it produces echogenicity similar to liver. This observation led the expression "hepatization of the gallbladder." Occasionally, sludge can take on a rounded, masslike appearance mimicking a gallbladder polyp or cancer (tumefactive sludge). Tumefactive sludge will change appearance between serial US examinations. About half of patients with gallbladder sludge will experience spontaneous resolution, whereas at most 15% of patients will progress to cholelithiasis.

Milk of Calcium

Milk of calcium bile is occasionally detected with abdominal radiography or CT. Milk of calcium bile appears as dependently layering high-attenuation (>150 HU) material within the gallbladder. Milk of calcium bile can cause signal loss in the dependent part of the gallbladder on T2-weighted MRI scans. With US, milk of calcium bile appears echogenic and can exhibit posterior acoustic shadowing.

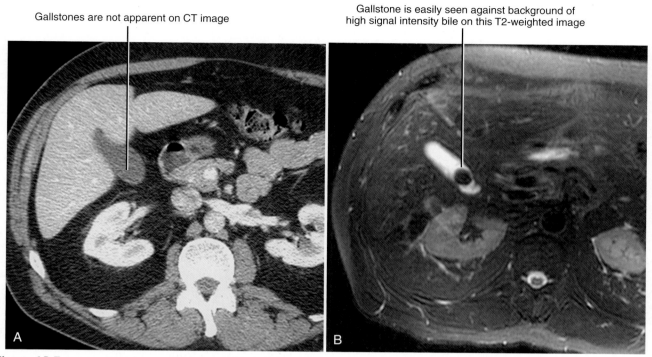

Gallstones are not apparent on CT image

Gallstone is easily seen against background of high signal intensity bile on this T2-weighted image

A

B

Figure 13-7 Enhanced axial computed tomographic (CT) **(A)** and T2-weighted magnetic resonance **(B)** images through the upper abdomen of a patient with cholelithiasis. The single large stone within the gallbladder was not appreciated on the CT examination.

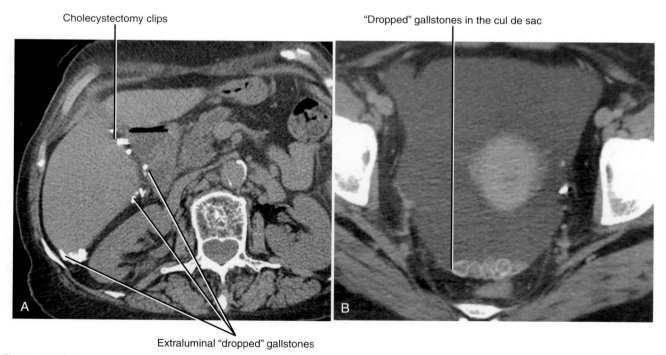

Cholecystectomy clips

"Dropped" gallstones in the cul de sac

A

B

Extraluminal "dropped" gallstones

Figure 13-8 Unenhanced computed tomographic images of the upper abdomen **(A)** and pelvis **(B)** in two separate patients found to have retained peritoneal gallstones after laparoscopic cholecystectomy.

Vicarious Excretion

Vicarious excretion of iodinated intravenous contrast material will also appear as high-density material within the gallbladder with radiography and CT. A history of recent intravenous contrast administration is helpful in differentiating this phenomenon from other causes of dense bile. Imaging with MRI during the hepatobiliary phase after administration of gadobenate dimeglumine or gadoxetate disodium will often reveal accumulation of these contrast media in the gallbladder.

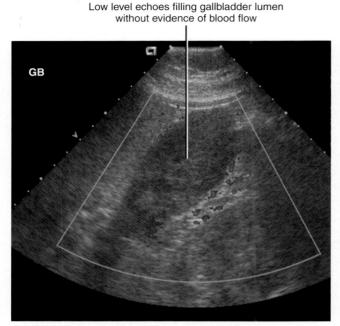

Low level echoes filling gallbladder lumen
without evidence of blood flow

Figure 13-9 Ultrasound image through the gallbladder of a patient with gallbladder sludge.

Hemorrhage

Blood within the gallbladder typically has a density greater than 30 HU but does not appear as dense as typical cases of milk of calcium or vicarious excretion of iodinated contrast material (Fig. 13-10). Hemorrhage appears as echogenic material within the gallbladder lumen with US.

■ THICK-WALLED GALLBLADDER

Diffuse thickening of the gallbladder wall is one of the most common abnormalities seen on an US examination of the right upper quadrant. This is due to the myriad of processes that result in gallbladder wall thickening. Many of the causes of gallbladder wall thickening are listed in Table 13-1.

■ CHOLECYSTITIS

Cholecystitis refers to inflammation of the gallbladder. A number of variants of cholecystitis warrant discussion.

Chronic Cholecystitis

Chronic cholecystitis results from chronic irritation or repeated episodes of acute inflammation leading to mural fibrosis. Chronic cholecystitis can be asymptomatic, is usually associated with gallstones, and is commonly found in cholecystectomy specimens after surgery for symptomatic cholelithiasis. When sufficiently severe, it can manifest on imaging studies as gallbladder wall thickening in the presence of gallstones. Features present with acute cholecystitis, such as pericholecystic fluid, gallbladder distention, Murphy sign, and hyperemia are absent in chronic cholecystitis, although acute and chronic cholecystitis may coexist.

Cholescintigraphy is often normal in the setting of chronic cholecystitis, although delayed (>1 hour) filling of the gallbladder is seen in some patients. Patients with symptomatic chronic cholecystitis may demonstrate a low gallbladder ejection fraction.

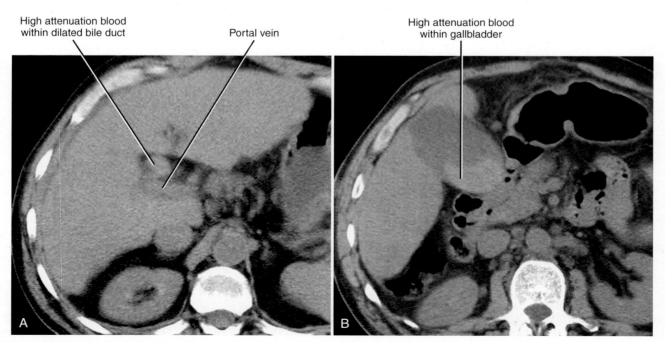

High attenuation blood
within dilated bile duct   Portal vein

High attenuation blood
within gallbladder

Figure 13-10 Unenhanced computed tomographic images of the liver after radiofrequency of hepatocellular carcinoma near the liver dome show high-attenuation blood within the common hepatic duct (**A**) and gallbladder (**B**).

Table 13-1   Causes of Gallbladder Wall Thickening

Cause	Diagnostic Clues (Variably Present)
Adenomyomatosis (Fig. 13-11)	• Comet tail artifacts on ultrasound (US) • Cystic spaces within wall on US, computed tomography (CT), or magnetic resonance imaging (MRI)
Adjacent inflammation	• Inflammation of the hepatic flexure of the colon, duodenum, right kidney, or pancreas
Carcinoma (Fig. 13-12)	• Irregular thickening of gallbladder wall • Intraluminal mass • Mass extending into liver • Porcelain gallbladder
Cholangiopathy/cholangitis (e.g., acquired immune deficiency syndrome cholangiopathy, sclerosing cholangitis)	• Associated abnormalities of the bile ducts
Cholecystitis (Fig. 13-13)	• Gallstone impacted in gallbladder neck or cystic duct • Sonographic Murphy sign • Hyperemia of gallbladder wall with Doppler US • Striation of gallbladder wall with US • Hyperemia of adjacent liver with CT or MRI • Stranding in pericholecystic fat on CT or MRI • Pericholecystic fluid • Intramural gas
Cirrhosis	• Cirrhotic morphology of liver • Splenomegaly • Varices • Ascites • Biphasic flow or reversal of flow in portal vein with color Doppler
Congestive heart failure (Fig. 13-14)	• Cardiomegaly • Pleural effusions • Distention of the inferior vena cava and hepatic veins • Exaggerated hepatic venous waveforms with Doppler imaging • Pulsatility of the portal vein waveform with Doppler imaging • Heterogeneous enhancement pattern of liver with delayed enhancement of hepatic veins on contrast-enhanced CT and MRI
Gallbladder torsion (Fig. 13-15)	• Marked gallbladder distention • Abnormal gallbladder position • Twisting of cystic duct and artery • Right angle bend in bile duct at cystic duct insertion
Hepatitis (Fig. 13-16)	• Hepatomegaly • Periportal edema with CT or MRI • Small anechoic gallbladder lumen • Hepatoduodenal ligament lymphadenopathy
Hypoalbuminemia	• Ascites and generalized edema
Nondistention	• Recent meal • Collapsed gallbladder
Varices (Fig. 13-17)	• Serpiginous vessels around the gallbladder wall

Acute Cholecystitis

Acute inflammation of the gallbladder usually results from gallbladder obstruction secondary to impaction of a gallstone in the gallbladder neck or cystic duct. Eventually, gallbladder distention, ischemia, superinfection, or necrosis develops. Most cases of acute cholecystitis can be accurately diagnosed by US in the appropriate clinical setting (i.e., fever, right upper quadrant pain, and leukocytosis). False-positive results occur in the setting of gallbladder wall thickening in the absence of acute inflammation (see Table 13-1). For this reason, careful attention to the clinical setting is important. The sonographic findings of acute cholecystitis are listed in Table 13-2.

CT and MRI are usually not performed specifically to exclude acute cholecystitis. Occasionally, however, CT and MRI establish a diagnosis of acute cholecystitis when performed for other reasons. These modalities demonstrate many of the signs listed in Table 13-2 with the addition of stranding in the pericholecystic fat (see Fig. 13-13, *B*). Hyperemia manifests as intense enhancement of the gallbladder wall after administration of intravenous contrast agents (Fig. 13-18). Increased enhancement of adjacent liver can be present in severe cases (Fig. 13-19).

Occasionally, the diagnosis of acute cholecystitis remains in doubt despite multiple cross-sectional imaging studies. In such a situation, nuclear scintigraphy

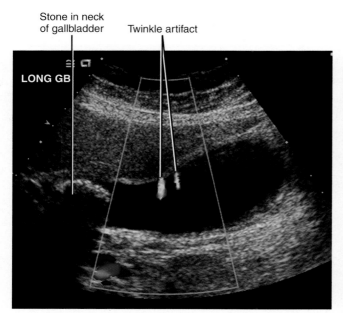

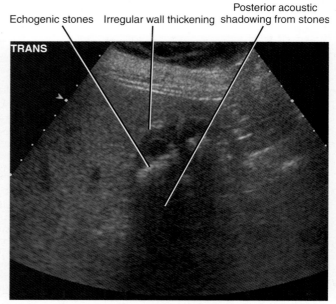

Figure 13-11 Longitudinal sonogram through the gallbladder (GB) of a patient with cholelithiasis and adenomyomatosis of the gallbladder.

Figure 13-12 Ultrasound image through the gallbladder of a patient with gallbladder cancer. Findings were initially thought to represent cholecystitis, but carcinoma was found at surgery.

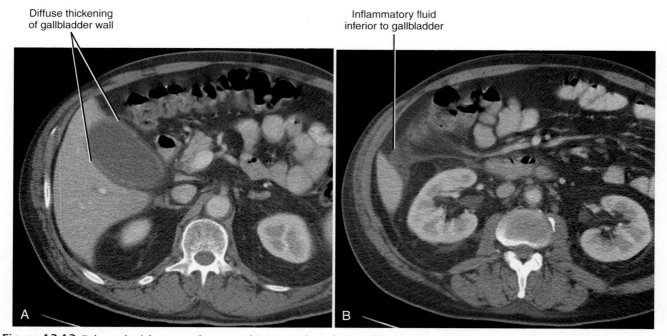

Figure 13-13 Enhanced axial computed tomographic images through the gallbladder (**A**) and inferior to the gallbladder (**B**) in a patient with acute cholecystitis.

with Tc-99m iminodiacetic acid derivatives remains a valuable tool. The important scintigraphic finding of acute cholecystitis is nonvisualization of the gallbladder despite sufficient delay (3-4 hours) or morphine augmentation with visualization of the bile ducts and duodenum. False-positive results can occur in the setting of chronic cholecystitis or noncontracting gallbladder.

Acalculous Cholecystitis

Acute cholecystitis can develop in the absence of stones, particularly in critically ill or elderly patients. With sonography, acalculous cholecystitis manifests as gallbladder wall thickening and distention, often in association with intraluminal sludge or pericholecystic fluid. The diagnosis of acute acalculous cholecystitis is important

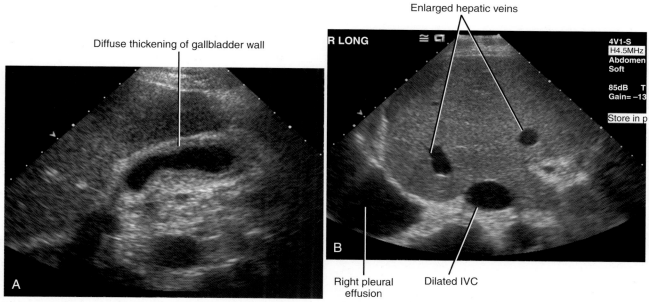

Figure 13-14 Ultrasound image through the gallbladder **(A)** and liver **(B)** of a patient with congestive heart failure. *IVC,* Inferior vena cava.

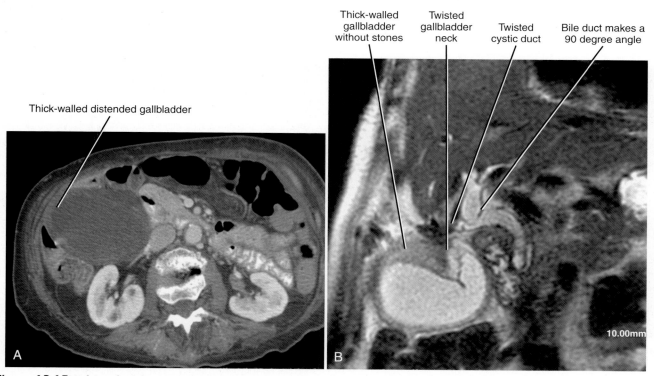

Figure 13-15 Enhanced axial computed tomographic image **(A)** and coronal T2-weighted magnetic resonance (MR) image **(B)** through the gallbladder of an elderly woman with acute onset of right upper quadrant pain. The diagnosis of gallbladder torsion was made with MR imaging and confirmed at surgery.

to make because timely intervention can be lifesaving. Unfortunately, acalculous cholecystitis can be difficult to distinguish from other causes of gallbladder wall thickening on imaging studies. Gallbladder scintigraphy can be extremely helpful in establishing the diagnosis of acalculous cholecystitis, although sensitivity may be slightly less than for calculous cholecystitis. When the diagnosis remains uncertain despite exhaustive imaging evaluation, gallbladder aspiration is a reasonable next step.

Diffuse gallbladder wall thickening

Gallbladder lumen is not dilated

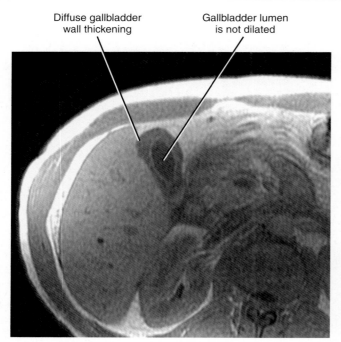

Figure 13-16 Axial T1-weighted magnetic resonance image through the gallbladder of an asymptomatic patient with acute hepatitis C.

Serpiginous vessels surrounding gallbladder

Anechoic gallbladder lumen

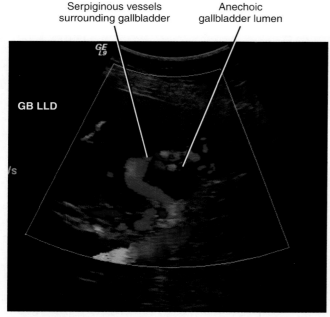

Figure 13-17 Color Doppler sonogram through the gallbladder of a patient with chronic portal vein thrombosis and gallbladder varices.

Gangrenous Cholecystitis

Severe acute inflammation of the gallbladder can progress to necrosis if left untreated. This represents a serious condition that eventually leads to gallbladder perforation, peritonitis, or abscess formation. The gangrenous gallbladder is also at increased risk for rupture during cholecystostomy. With imaging, the gangrenous gallbladder demonstrates the imaging findings listed in Box 13-1

Table 13-2 Sonographic Signs of Acute Cholecystitis

Primary signs	• Cholelithiasis • Stone impacted in gallbladder neck • Sonographic Murphy sign*
Secondary signs	• Gallbladder wall thickening (>3 mm) • Pericholecystic fluid • Sludge
Tertiary signs	• Leukocytosis • Fever

* The sonographic Murphy sign refers to reproducible tenderness induced by pressure applied with the ultrasound transducer that is maximal directly over the imaged gallbladder.

Enhancement and thickening of the gallbladder wall

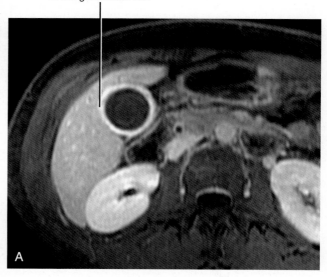

A

Large low signal intensity gallstone impacted in gallbladder neck

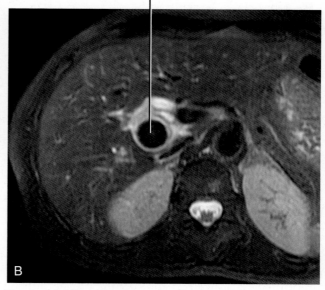

B

Figure 13-18 Axial gadolinium-enhanced (**A**) and T2-weighted (**B**) magnetic resonance images through the gallbladder of a patient with acute cholecystitis. A large stone can be seen impacted in the gallbladder neck on the T2-weighted image (**B**).

Increased enhancement of liver around gallbladder   Secondary inflammation of adjacent duodenum

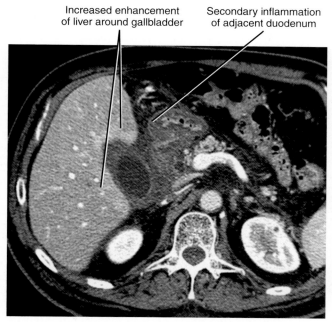

Figure 13-19 Enhanced axial computed tomographic image through the liver and gallbladder of a patient with acute cholecystitis demonstrating hyperenhancement of the adjacent liver.

BOX 13-1   Imaging Findings That Suggest Gangrenous Cholecystitis

Sonolucencies or striations in gallbladder wall with US
Intramural fluid collections on CT or MRI
Sloughed membranes in the gallbladder lumen
Pericholecystic abscess
Disruption of the gallbladder wall
Lack of gallbladder wall enhancement on CT or MRI
Hepatic hyperenhancement adjacent to gallbladder on CT or MRI
Rim sign on Tc-99m iminodiacetic acid derivative scan*

* Rim sign refers to increased hepatic uptake of radionuclide adjacent to the gallbladder fossa.

---

and shown in Figure 13-20. Some of these imaging findings can be present in cases of acute uncomplicated cholecystitis as well. Notably, the Murphy sign may be absent in patients with severe complicated cholecystitis.

Pitfall: The Murphy sign may be absent in patients with gangrenous cholecystitis.

Emphysematous Cholecystitis

Emphysematous cholecystitis represents a severe form of cholecystitis that occurs with or without coexistent cholelithiasis. The perforation rate is relatively high with this condition, and patients should be managed with urgent cholecystectomy. Individuals with diabetes are particularly prone to this disease. The diagnosis is made when gas is identified within the wall of the gallbladder in a patient with suspected cholecystitis. Gas can be present

Striated thickened gallbladder wall   Gallstones

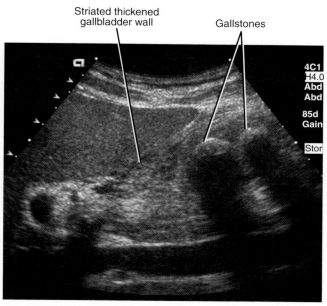

Figure 13-20 Longitudinal sonogram of a patient with cholelithiasis and acute gangrenous cholecystitis.

within the gallbladder lumen in such cases, although intraluminal gas can also be introduced via other means such as ERCP. When severe, the abnormal gas collections can be visible in the right upper quadrant on abdominal radiographs. Intramural gas is readily identified on CT images as areas of very low attenuation within the gallbladder wall (Fig. 13-21). MRI is relatively insensitive to

Gas outlining gallbladder wall   Gallbladder lumen

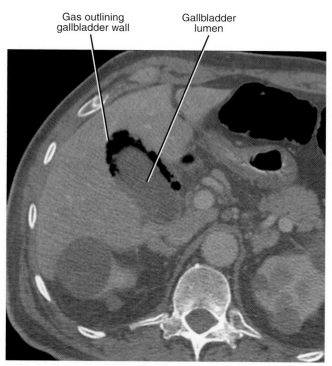

Figure 13-21 Enhanced axial computed tomographic image through the upper abdomen displayed with wide window settings demonstrates gas in the gallbladder wall of a patient with acute emphysematous cholecystitis.

the detection of small amounts of gas, although a sufficient amount of gas manifests on MR images as areas of susceptibility artifact. With US, intramural gas appears as echogenic foci with posterior acoustic shadowing or reverberation artifact (Fig. 13-22). Gas within the gallbladder wall can be differentiated from a contracted gallbladder filled with stones because the normal gallbladder wall is not evident in the former process. When gas is extensive, the gallbladder may be difficult to see or may be mistaken for bowel. Emphysematous cholecystitis must be kept in mind when the gallbladder cannot be visualized in the setting of suspected acute cholecystitis. Identifying echogenic gas bubbles with the bile ducts with US or an abscess in the adjacent hepatic parenchyma can be helpful in establishing a diagnosis of emphysematous cholecystitis. Emphysematous cholecystitis cannot be differentiated from uncomplicated acute cholecystitis with nuclear scintigraphy alone. Advanced adenomyomatosis can demonstrate shadowing on US examinations, resulting in confusion with emphysematous cholecystitis.

Pearl: With US, gas within the gallbladder wall can be differentiated from a contracted gallbladder filled with stones because the normal gallbladder wall is not evident with emphysematous cholecystitis.

Hemorrhagic Cholecystitis

Severe cholecystitis can induce bleeding within the gallbladder wall and lumen. Hemorrhage may result in echogenic material filling the gallbladder lumen on US or moderately high-attenuation material filling the lumen on CT (see Fig. 13-10). Intraluminal hemorrhage can be difficult to distinguish from sludge balls with US.

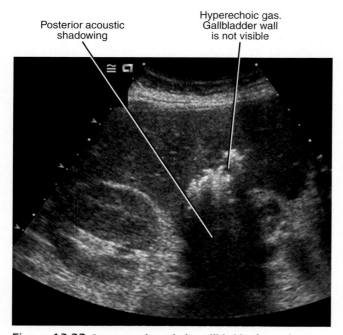

Posterior acoustic shadowing

Hyperechoic gas. Gallbladder wall is not visible

Figure 13-22 Sonogram through the gallbladder fossa of a patient with emphysematous cholecystitis.

Xanthogranulomatous Cholecystitis

Xanthogranulomatous cholecystitis (XGC) is a rare chronic inflammatory process that involves the gallbladder characterized by intramural collections of lipid-laden macrophages. XGC is associated with cholelithiasis and can coexist with gallbladder carcinoma in a small minority of cases. The imaging features of XGC include wall thickening and the presence of xanthogranulomatous foci within the wall that manifest as areas of decreased echogenicity with US, low attenuation with CT, and high signal intensity with T2-weighted MRI. As with acute cholecystitis, early enhancement of the adjacent liver parenchyma may occur with XGC. Because XGC can extend into the liver and have associated enlarged hepatoduodenal lymph nodes, it can closely mimic gallbladder carcinoma. Although the distinction between XGC and gallbladder carcinoma on imaging examinations can be difficult, some imaging findings can suggest XGC. In particular, a well-defined internal gallbladder border with continuous luminal surface enhancement and the presence of intramural hypoechoic (US), low-attenuation (CT), or high-signal-intensity (T2-weighted MRI) areas should prompt consideration of this entity.

■ GALLBLADDER MASSES

Gallbladder masses unrelated to stones or sludge are occasionally encountered during sonography of the right upper quadrant. It is important to be able to distinguish between clinically insignificant masses and those masses that require surgical intervention. In particular, one must pay close attention to asymmetric wall thickening or polypoid masses that have a wide base because these findings are suggestive of gallbladder carcinoma. Not all malignant masses of the gallbladder demonstrate increased vascularity with color Doppler imaging, and a small percentage of gallbladder carcinomas will be missed by US because of the confounding presence of multiple stones (see Fig. 13-12).

Adherent Stones

Small stones occasionally fail to demonstrate posterior acoustic shadowing and can resist movement with changes in patient position. At times, shadowing can be elicited by using a higher frequency transducer and setting the focal zone to the depth of the stone. Twinkle artifact is helpful in suggesting the presence of an adherent stone, although cholesterol polyps in the nondependent portion of the gallbladder can produce the same artifact.

Tumefactive Sludge (Sludge Balls)

Gallbladder sludge may mimic the appearance of a fixed polypoid lesion of the gallbladder with US. Clues to the true nature of the abnormality include lack of intrinsic vascularity, mobility, and change in shape over time. Lack of vascularity must be interpreted with caution because hypovascular tumors can demonstrate this feature. In some cases, sludge can be slow to move with changes in patient position. Short-term follow-up imaging (e.g., several days or weeks later) usually demonstrates a significant change in appearance of tumefactive sludge, whereas a polypoid mass will remain unaltered.

Polyps

Unlike most gallstones, polyps usually do not shadow (unless calcified) and remain fixed to the gallbladder wall (Fig. 13-23). Cholesterol polyps are the most common polypoid gallbladder mass encountered on US images. They are benign, frequently multiple, and less than 1 cm in diameter. Inflammatory polyps are less common, frequently multiple, and occur in the setting of chronic cholecystitis. Adenomatous polyps are neoplastic lesions with malignant potential. Larger gallbladder polyps (>10 mm) may demonstrate intrinsic vascularity with color Doppler imaging. Enhancement can be detected with contrast-enhanced CT or MRI (Fig. 13-24).

The size of a polyp is the critical factor in deciding further management. Polyps less than 5 mm in diameter usually require no further evaluation or management. The management of polyps between 5 and 10 mm is more controversial, although a more aggressive approach than sonographic follow-up is seldom recommended. Polyps larger than 1 cm have a significant chance of harboring malignant tumor, and cholecystectomy is generally recommended. Sessile lesions and lesions that demonstrate growth on imaging are cause for concern.

No polyps are detected within the gallbladder on unenhanced images

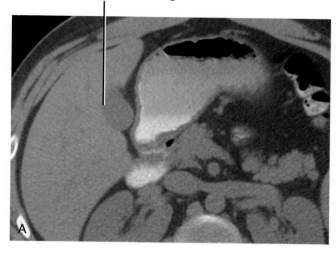

Multiple enhancing polyps become evident after contrast administration

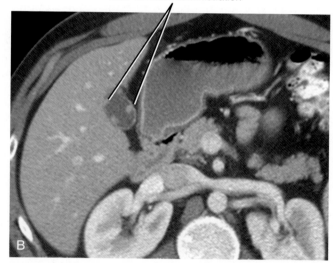

Figure 13-24 Unenhanced (**A**) and enhanced (**B**) axial computed tomographic images through the gallbladder of a patient with multiple gallbladder polyps.

Fixed, nondependent lesion of intermediate echogenicity

No posterior shadowing

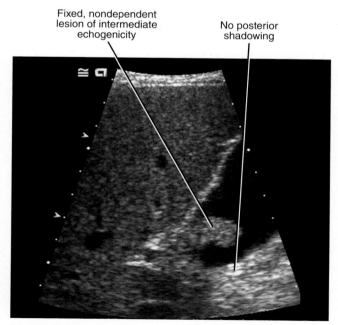

Figure 13-23 Longitudinal sonogram through the gallbladder neck of a patient with a gallbladder polyp.

Adenomyomatosis

Adenomyomatosis is characterized by enlarged Rokitansky–Aschoff sinuses and thickening of the muscularis layer of the gallbladder. As a result, adenomyomatosis (which should not be confused with adenomyosis, a condition that affects the uterus) manifests as gallbladder wall thickening with intramural cystic spaces. Adenomyomatosis most commonly affects the fundus but can also involve the gallbladder diffusely. When the body of the gallbladder is affected, it may become stenotic, resulting in an "hourglass" appearance. This can lead to focal cholelithiasis or cholecystitis involving only the fundus of the gallbladder. Focal adenomyomatosis manifesting as a mass is sometimes referred to as an adenomyoma. The presence of cystic spaces and mural-based comet tail artifacts on US images help to establish the diagnosis (see Fig. 13-11).

Carcinoma

Most gallbladder carcinomas are adenocarcinomas. As mentioned earlier, gallbladder carcinoma can appear as diffuse thickening of the gallbladder wall. Gallbladder carcinoma can also present as a focal mass that extends in a polypoid manner into the gallbladder lumen. Gallbladder carcinoma frequently invades segments IV and V of the adjacent liver. Carcinoma that causes diffuse gallbladder wall thickening associated with invasion of the liver can be confused with acute cholecystitis with abscess formation and vice versa (Fig. 13-25). The presence of large or necrotic lymph nodes in the porta hepatis favors a diagnosis of cancer (Fig. 13-26). A malignant mass can obliterate the gallbladder lumen, making the gallbladder difficult to locate. Malignant polypoid masses within the gallbladder are usually larger than 1 cm in diameter and can demonstrate internal vascularity with color Doppler imaging or enhancement after administration of intravenous contrast material (CT and MRI). The staging and patterns of spread of gallbladder carcinoma are discussed in Chapter 10.

> *Pitfall: Carcinoma that causes diffuse gallbladder wall thickening associated with invasion of the liver can be confused with acute cholecystitis with abscess formation.*

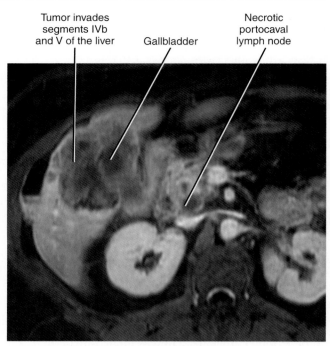

Figure 13-26 Axial gadolinium-enhanced magnetic resonance image through the gallbladder of a patient with advanced gallbladder carcinoma invading segments IVb and V of the liver. A necrotic portocaval lymph node is present.

Metastasis

The gallbladder can become secondarily involved with tumor by direct invasion from adjacent organs such as the liver or colon and hematogenous spread (most commonly with melanoma). Sessile masses, in particular, are concerning for metastases. Appropriate history is obviously helpful in establishing the diagnosis of metastatic disease to the gallbladder.

◼ DILATED BILE DUCTS

Approach to Dilated Bile Ducts

Dilated bile ducts are commonly encountered on cross-sectional imaging studies performed for evaluation of suspected biliary obstruction, as well as for reasons unrelated to the biliary system. One needs to systematically answer several questions in the interpretation of such images.

1. *Are the ducts really dilated?* Determining whether bile ducts are dilated is often a subjective matter. Box 13-2 lists a few tips for helping in this assessment on sonograms. Remember, no measurement is infallible, and it should be put in the proper clinical context and correlated with other imaging findings. Also, a normal diameter duct does not exclude disease. Wall thickening, nodularity, or filling defects of the bile duct are abnormal findings regardless of the duct diameter. Because of the improved spatial resolution of imaging studies, bile ducts previously seen only when abnormal are now

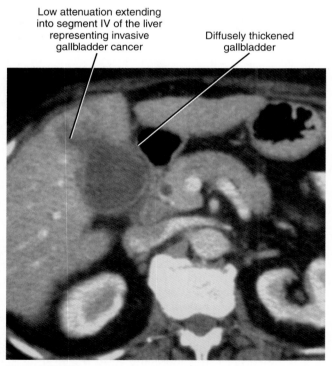

Figure 13-25 Enhanced axial computed tomographic image through the gallbladder of a patient with gallbladder cancer invading the liver. The images were initially thought to represent acute cholecystitis with early hepatic abscess formation.

routinely visualized. The correlation between bile duct diameter and age or history of cholecystectomy is controversial. Color Doppler imaging can be useful in distinguishing between dilated bile ducts and normal vascular structures with sonography (Fig. 13-27).

2. *Are the ducts obstructed?* Once the bile ducts have been determined to be dilated, the next step in analysis is to determine whether the ducts are obstructed. The clinical scenario is helpful in making this determination. Jaundice and a cholestatic pattern of laboratory abnormalities favor obstruction. Patients with opioid addiction often have a dilated common bile duct in the absence of a lesion because of sphincter of Oddi spasm. Imaging findings that support the diagnosis of obstruction include evidence of an obstructing mass or stone, abnormal hepatic perfusion on contrast-enhanced CT or MRI, or abrupt change(s) in bile duct caliber. Lack of pneumobilia in a patient with a biliary stent or surgical biliary-enteric anastomosis raises the possibility of obstruction. Occasionally, it is necessary to perform additional tests to determine whether dilated bile ducts are truly obstructed (Table 13-3). The tests listed must be interpreted with caution, however. Delayed biliary-to-bowel transit on a hepatobiliary nuclear medicine scan may be related to opiates, chronic cholecystitis, or a hypertonic sphincter of Oddi. Incomplete filling of the intrahepatic bile ducts on ERCP may be the result of patient positioning (e.g., the left ducts are often not filled completely when the patient is supine). Filling defects may be related to pneumobilia rather than stones, and not all strictures are functionally obstructive. Finally, poor excretion of hepatobiliary agents may be related to poor hepatic function (e.g., cirrhosis) rather than obstruction.

3. *What level is the obstruction?* Determining the level of biliary obstruction is a step often accomplished in concert with establishing the presence of obstruction. In most cases, the level of obstruction involving the common bile duct is identified by an abrupt change

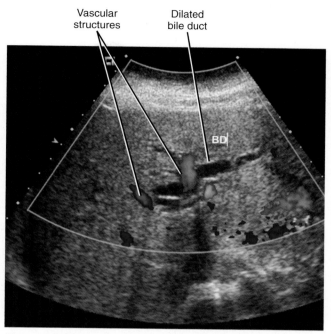

Vascular structures   Dilated bile duct

Figure 13-27 Right upper quadrant sonogram performed with color Doppler imaging demonstrating dilated intrahepatic bile ducts.

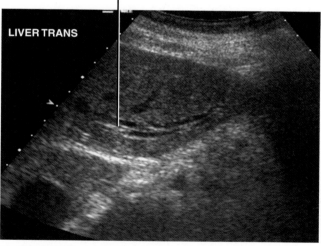

Dilated bile duct paralleling portal vein. Note similar size of these two structures

LIVER TRANS

Figure 13-28 Ultrasound images through the left hepatic lobe of a patient with obstructing choledocholithiasis.

BOX 13-2   Dilated Bile Ducts: Some Suggested Sonographic Criteria

Visualization of peripheral (third order and above) ducts
Parallel channel sign on grayscale images (Fig. 13-28)
Right and left hepatic ducts greater than 2 mm in diameter (Fig. 13-29)
Intrahepatic ducts greater than 40% of the adjacent portal vein diameter
Common bile duct diameter
- ≤5 mm normal
- 6-9 mm equivocal (correlate with laboratory and clinical data)
- ≥10 mm abnormal (additional evaluation indicated)

---

in caliber of the bile duct on imaging studies. With US, the ability to visualize the precise level of obstruction often depends on the location of the obstruction, patient body habitus, distribution of bowel gas, and the technical prowess of the sonographer or sonologist. CT and MRI are highly accurate and roughly equivalent at determining the level of obstruction. The level of obstruction can be determined by percutaneous or endoscopic cholangiography, although high-grade obstruction may prevent a complete evaluation of the biliary tree, because only those structures that fill with contrast medium will be visualized.

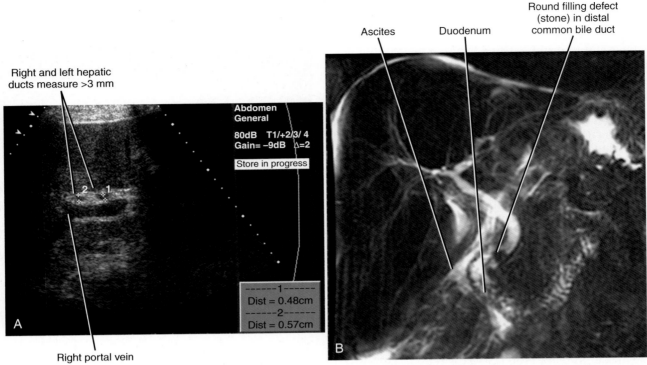

Figure 13-29 Ultrasound image (**A**) just proximal to the biliary confluence demonstrates mild dilatation of the right and left hepatic ducts. The distal common bile duct could not be visualized. Magnetic resonance cholangiopancreatography performed to evaluate this finding (**B**) confirmed choledocholithiasis. The stones were successfully managed endoscopically.

Table 13-3   Potential Methods of Confirming Bile Duct Obstruction

Test	Findings That Suggest Obstruction
Technetium 99m iminodiacetic acid derivative scan	• Good hepatic extraction without biliary excretion • Delayed biliary-to-bowel transit (partial) • Poor bile duct clearance of radiotracer
Transhepatic cholangiography	• No passage of contrast material into duodenum • Presence of stricture or filling defect
Endoscopic retrograde cholangiography	• Incomplete filling of bile ducts • Presence of stricture or filling defect

4. *What is causing the obstruction?* Obstructions are usually caused by one of four major causes: stones (choledocholithiasis), benign strictures, malignant strictures, and extrinsic compression. Remember that the majority of common bile duct stones are found in the distal (intrapancreatic) duct. A stone within the mid or proximal portion of the bile duct is unlikely to be a cause of obstruction. Therefore, a search for a more distal obstructive lesion (stone or tumor) should be sought in such cases.

Choledocholithiasis

Choledocholithiasis is the most common cause of bile-duct obstruction. The literature reports a wide range of sensitivities and specificities of the various imaging modalities for the detection of choledocholithiasis. The wide range of reported numbers can be explained, in part, by the wide range of expertise and techniques utilized by the reporting institutions. When determining which modality to use to evaluate a patient with suspected choledocholithiasis, one should not rely exclusively on numbers reported in the literature because factors such as the condition of the patient, relative risk of the procedure, local expertise, and available equipment warrant equal consideration.

Detection of common bile duct stones with US depends on the availability of a suitable sonographic window and the persistence and skill level of the sonographer or sonologist. With US, the diagnosis of common bile duct stones requires a sincere effort to visualize the entire duct to the level of the ampulla. This may require adjustments in patient position (including left lateral decubitus and upright), the use of compression to collapse or displace bowel, and considerable patience. As would be expected, intraductal stones appear as echogenic foci with posterior acoustic shadowing along the course of the bile duct (Fig. 13-30). Small stones are often outlined by anechoic bile, whereas larger or impacted stones can occupy the entire duct lumen. Very small stones sometimes do not produce shadowing.

With CT, stone detection depends on stone attenuation. On unenhanced scans, attention to technique may also improve sensitivity. Thin (<5 mm) reconstructed images obtained during a single breath hold without oral contrast will reveal radiodense stones as foci that appear higher density than the surrounding bile (Fig. 13-31). Impacted stones that are not outlined by bile may appear

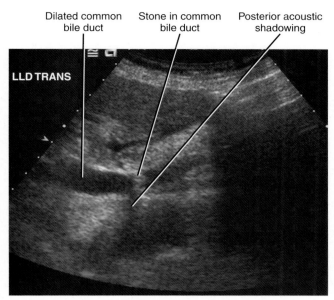

Dilated common bile duct Stone in common bile duct Posterior acoustic shadowing

LLD TRANS

Figure 13-30 Ultrasound images through the left hepatic lobe (A) and common bile duct (B) of a patient with choledocholithiasis.

as high-density foci associated with proximal bile duct dilatation. Many stones are not densely calcified; therefore, a casual glance at the duct may not be sufficient to exclude stones. Unfortunately, many stones are identified only retrospectively on CT after being identified on alternate imaging studies. The role of oral and intravenous biliary contrast agents administered with CT for the diagnosis of cholelithiasis has not been established.

MRCP has been a major advance for the noninvasive diagnosis of choledocholithiasis. Most centers use a combination of thin-section and thick-slab heavily T2-weighted imaging in multiple planes to detect bile duct stones. Most intraductal calculi appear as round or faceted low-signal-intensity foci surrounded by high-signal-intensity bile on T2-weighted images (Fig. 13-32). Small stones (<5 mm) and those impacted at the ampulla may be difficult to detect with MRI. Occasionally, intraductal stones will be bright on T1-weighted images; thus, these images should also be obtained and examined.

Endoscopic US is a sensitive method for detecting extrahepatic bile duct stones. Verma and colleagues' review examined five randomized, prospective, blinded trials comparing MRCP with endoscopic US for the detection of choledocholithiasis and found no statistically significant difference between the two techniques in terms of sensitivity, specificity, positive and negative prediction values, and likelihood ratios. Other studies have suggested that endoscopic US is more sensitive than MRCP for detection of stones measuring less than 5 mm.

Not all choledocholithiasis occurs in the extrahepatic ducts. Any process that results in intrahepatic biliary obstruction and stasis may result in the formation of intrahepatic bile duct stones. Some diseases associated with intrahepatic choledocholithiasis include PSC, Caroli disease, RPC/hepatitis, sickle cell disease, and cystic fibrosis.

Not all real or apparent intraductal abnormalities are related to calculi. Box 13-3 lists some entities that may be confused with choledocholithiasis.

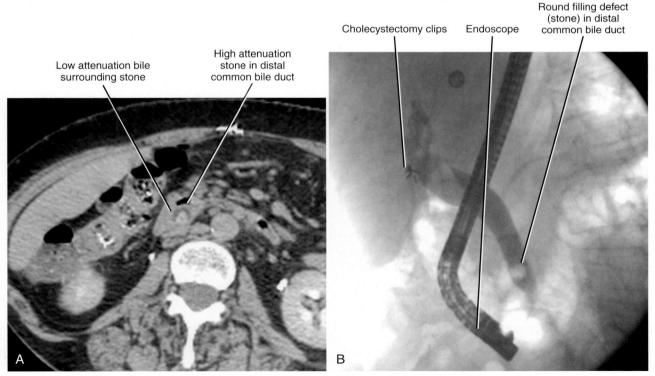

Low attenuation bile surrounding stone High attenuation stone in distal common bile duct

Cholecystectomy clips Endoscope Round filling defect (stone) in distal common bile duct

A B

Figure 13-31 Axial computed tomographic (A) and endoscopic retrograde cholangiopancreatogram (B) images of a patient with retained common bile duct stone after cholecystectomy.

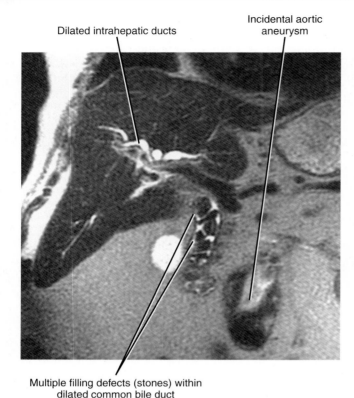

Dilated intrahepatic ducts

Incidental aortic aneurysm

Multiple filling defects (stones) within dilated common bile duct

Figure 13-32 Coronal thin-slice T2-weighted magnetic resonance image through the common bile of a patient with extensive choledocholithiasis.

BOX 13-3   Causes of False-Positive Diagnosis of Choledocholithiasis

Pneumobilia
Hemobilia
Surgical clips (associated with ring-down artifact)
Calcified right hepatic artery
Crossing vessel (usually right hepatic artery or varices)
Neoplasm

Benign Strictures

Nonneoplastic narrowing of the bile duct can be caused by intrinsic abnormalities (e.g., inflammatory stricture or fibrosis) or extrinsic abnormalities (e.g., compression by an adjacent structure or process) of the duct. The most important distinction to be made with imaging when ductal narrowing is identified is between benign stricture and malignant neoplastic stricture (Table 13-4). Box 13-4 lists some potential causes of nonneoplastic bile-duct stricture.

Neoplastic Strictures

Neoplastic strictures may be caused by primary neoplasm of the bile duct (e.g., cholangiocarcinoma), malignant tumor of the ampulla, hematogenous metastasis to the bile duct (e.g., from breast, colon, or melanoma

Table 13-4   Features of Benign and Malignant Biliary Strictures

Feature	Benign	Malignant
Transition	Gradually tapering (Fig. 13-33)	Abrupt (Fig. 13-34)
Contour	Smooth	Irregular
Wall	Thin (<5 mm), uniform	Thick (>5 mm), nonuniform
Length	Shorter	Longer
Enhancement	Isoenhancing or hypoenhancing	Portal phase hyperenhancement

BOX 13-4   Causes of Nonneoplastic Bile-Duct Stricture

Cholecystitis (Mirizzi syndrome)
Choledocholithiasis
Congenital abnormality
Infectious cholangitis (pyogenic cholangitis, parasites, HIV cholangiopathy)
Ischemia (often in patients with liver transplant with hepatic artery thrombosis)
Pancreatitis
After instrumentation or prior surgery
Primary sclerosing cholangitis

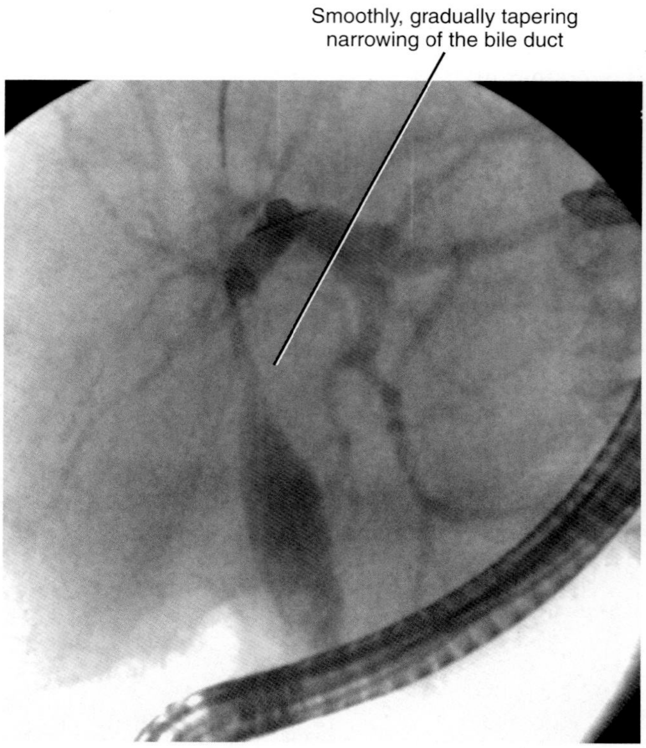

Smoothly, gradually tapering narrowing of the bile duct

Figure 13-33 Endoscopic retrograde cholangiopancreatogram image of a benign (inflammatory) biliary stricture.

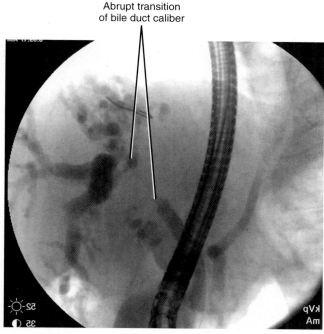

Abrupt transition
of bile duct caliber

Figure 13-34 Endoscopic retrograde cholangiopancreatogram image of malignant stricture caused by cholangiocarcinoma.

primaries), or extrinsic tumor invading the bile duct (e.g., pancreatic or duodenal carcinoma). Occasionally, adjacent lymph nodes enlarged by metastatic disease will obstruct the bile duct. Neoplastic processes that involve the intrapancreatic bile duct or ampullary region are often associated with pancreatic duct dilatation (double duct sign), although choledocholithiasis is known to cause this appearance as well on occasion. Some tumor markers (e.g., CEA, CA 19-9, CA-125) may be helpful in suggesting the presence of malignant tumor, although none is entirely specific.

Managing the Patient with Biliary Obstruction: What Is the Next Step?

Once a patient has been sufficiently evaluated with imaging to determine that biliary obstruction is present, the next step in evaluation depends on the suspected cause of obstruction. If a diagnosis of choledocholithiasis has been established, ERCP with attempted stone extraction is usually appropriate. If a malignant tumor is suspected, attempts at biliary decompression can be combined with tissue sampling. When surgical resection of a malignant biliary tumor is contemplated, it is helpful to complete all imaging staging examinations before biliary decompression, because the extent of tumor may be more difficult to assess after decompression of the bile ducts and creation of an inflammatory response related to the decompression procedure or stent. Distal biliary obstruction is usually managed endoscopically, whereas hilar obstruction occasionally requires percutaneous decompression. The diagnostic yield of bile cytology is relatively low,

so attempts at bile duct brushing or biopsy are usually made at the time of biliary stenting. If endoscopic or transductal attempts at tissue sampling are insufficient to establish a diagnosis, percutaneous biopsy is often the next step. Metallic self-expanding stents are often placed in patients with malignant biliary obstruction when they are not candidates for surgical resection. Nonmetallic removable stents or external biliary drains can be used to temporarily relieve obstruction in patients with benign disease or in whom further surgical management is anticipated.

> **Pearl:** When surgical resection of a malignant biliary tumor is contemplated, it is helpful to complete all imaging staging examinations before biliary decompression, because the extent of tumor may be more difficult to assess after decompression of the bile ducts and creation of an inflammatory response related to the decompression procedure or stent.

Choledochal Cysts

Cystic dilatation of a portion of the biliary tree is known as a choledochal cyst. No universally accepted caliber exists beyond which a bile duct becomes a choledochal cyst. Most physicians classify choledochal cysts according to the Todani classification system (Fig. 13-35). Fusiform dilation of the extrahepatic bile duct (type I) is the most common type of choledochal cyst (Fig. 13-36). Type II cysts are bile duct diverticula and are rare. Type III cysts, also known as *choledochoceles*, involve the intraduodenal portion of the bile duct. A choledochocele may be identified on cross-sectional imaging studies as a fluid-filled structure protruding into the duodenum near the ampulla. Type IV cysts are multiple (type IVa cysts involve intrahepatic and extrahepatic ducts, whereas type IVb cysts involve extrahepatic ducts). One proposed mechanism of biliary cyst formation invokes an anomalous junction of the common bile and pancreatic ducts, resulting in a long common channel (>1.5 cm) that facilitates reflux of pancreatic enzymes into the biliary tree. The anomalous pancreaticobiliary junction can be demonstrated with ERCP, CT, or MRCP.

Type V cysts are commonly referred to as Caroli disease and are thought to possibly result from a ductal plate abnormality that affects the large intrahepatic ducts. Fusiform dilatation of the extrahepatic bile duct can be present (Fig. 13-37). Caroli syndrome refers to the association of intrahepatic duct dilatation (Caroli disease) and periportal fibrosis, which can result in cirrhosis and portal hypertension. Caroli disease is associated with intraductal stone formation and cholangitis.

Choledochal cysts are usually diagnosed in childhood, although some cases do not present until later in life. Complications include bile duct obstruction associated with pain and jaundice, choledocholithiasis, cholangitis, pancreatitis, cyst rupture, and development of carcinoma. US is particularly useful for identifying cholangiocarcinoma arising within a preexisting choledochal cyst.

Saccular dilatation of intrahepatic bile ducts may simulate cystic disease of the liver. In particular, intrahepatic choledochal cysts may appear as multiple hepatic cysts

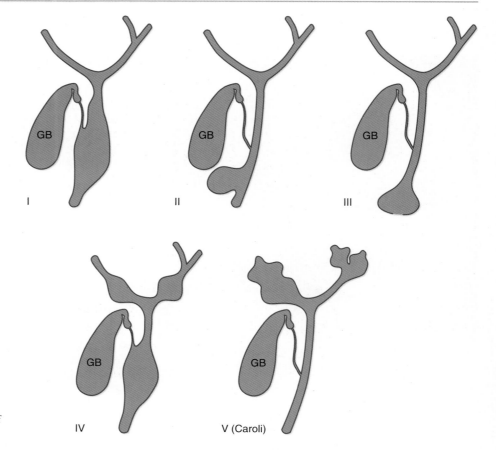

Figure 13-35 Todani classification of choledochal cysts. *GB,* Gallbladder.

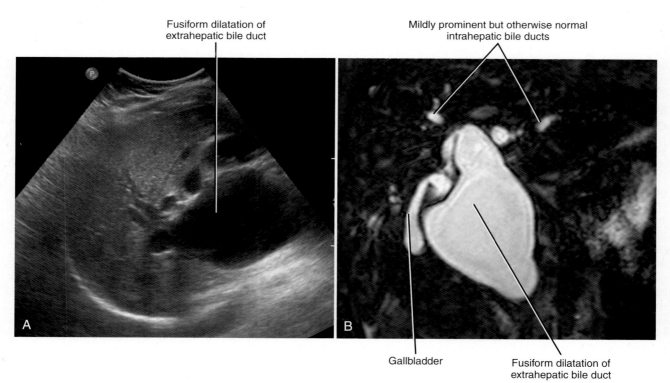

Figure 13-36 Ultrasound image (**A**) and coronal single-shot T2-weighted magnetic resonance image (**B**) show a type I choledochal cyst.

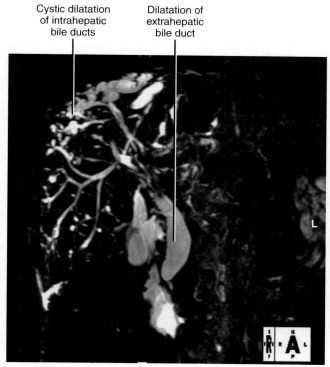

Cystic dilatation of intrahepatic bile ducts

Dilatation of extrahepatic bile duct

Figure 13-37 Coronal partial volume maximum intensity projection image from, a respiratory-triggered thin-slice magnetic resonance cholangiopancreatography of a patient with Caroli disease and fusiform dilatation of the extrahepatic bile duct.

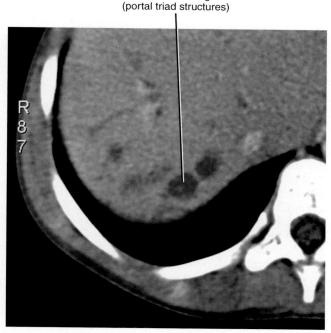

"Central dot" sign (portal triad structures)

Figure 13-38 Enhanced axial computed tomographic image through the liver of a patient with intrahepatic choledochal cysts.

with any of the cross-sectional modalities. Key features of Caroli disease that distinguish it from polycystic liver disease include communication of the cystic abnormalities with the biliary tree and the "central dot sign." This latter sign refers to the presence of portal triad structures (the central dot) surrounded by ectatic bile duct and may be visualized with sonography, CT, or MRI (Fig. 13-38). Although the central dot sign is not entirely specific, having been described in other entities such as peribiliary cysts, we have found it helpful in our own practice.

■ CHOLANGITIS AND CHOLANGIOPATHIES

Acute Infectious Cholangitis

Acute infectious, or ascending, cholangitis results from bacterial infection of the bile, usually in the presence of biliary stasis. Imaging often reveals dilated bile ducts, a finding that alone lacks specificity. Ductal irregularities can be visible with various cholangiographic techniques (ERCP, CT cholangiography, MRCP), and circumferential bile duct wall thickening may be present on US, CT, and MRI examinations. Administration of intravenous contrast agents can show mural enhancement on CT or MR images. The presence of purulent material within the bile ducts causes internal echoes to be visible with US, raises the attenuation of the bile on CT, or manifests as a decrease in signal intensity of the bile on T2-weighted images with MRI. Nodular, patchy, wedge-shaped, or geographic areas of hepatic parenchymal enhancement

can be visible on arterial-phase CT or MR images. Wedge-shaped areas of increased signal intensity representing edema in the distribution of affected ducts can be present on T2-weighted MR images.

Acute cholangitis can progress to multiple small hepatic abscesses, and communication between the abscesses and the biliary tree can sometimes be demonstrated at imaging. Pneumobilia caused by gas-forming organisms is a rare feature of acute infectious cholangitis, and pneumobilia is more likely to be of enteric origin (e.g., from a biliary-enteric anastomosis or fistula). Imaging findings associated with acute infectious cholangitis often resolve after appropriate treatment.

Primary Sclerosing Cholangitis

PSC is an immune-mediated chronic and progressive inflammatory disease of the bile ducts of unknown cause that can be complicated by cholestasis, cirrhosis, and cholangiocarcinoma. The majority of patients with PSC have inflammatory bowel disease (usually ulcerative colitis), although only a minority (fewer than 10%) of patients with inflammatory bowel disease experience development of PSC. PSC can also be associated with other systemic sclerosing disorders such as retroperitoneal fibrosis. PSC is more common in men than in women.

Imaging of the bile ducts in patients with PSC shows irregular circumferential bile duct thickening, focal biliary strictures, and dilatations that involve the intrahepatic or extrahepatic ducts. In most cases, PSC involves both intrahepatic and extrahepatic ducts, although the gall-bladder is abnormal in fewer than 20% of patients (unlike HIV cholangiopathy in which gallbladder thickening is common). Some patients with PSC experience development of intrahepatic choledocholithiasis. ERCP, percutaneous transhepatic cholangiography, and MRCP show mural irregularity of the bile ducts early in the disease course with eventual progression to multifocal short strictures, creating the classic beaded appearance of the ducts (Fig. 13-39). Marked ductal dilatation is not a feature of PSC because of periductal fibrosis and inflammation. Although ERCP has superior spatial resolution to MRCP, the intrahepatic ducts beyond areas of severe stricture may not be visible with the former technique. Duct wall thickening and enhancement are visible on enhanced CT and MR images of some patients (Fig. 13-40). When present, morphologic changes of the liver visible with imaging include lobulation of the liver contour, posterior and lateral segment atrophy, and marked caudate lobe hypertrophy. This combination of findings gives the liver a rounded appearance that is suggestive of PSC (see Fig. 12-38).

> *Pearl:* The combination of lobulation of the liver contour, posterior and lateral segment atrophy, and marked caudate lobe hypertrophy gives the liver a rounded appearance that is suggestive of PSC.

Patients with PSC are at increased risk for the development of cholangiocarcinoma. Although reported numbers vary, the lifetime prevalence rate of cholangiocarcinoma for patients with PSC is likely about 15%. The development of a mass, the presence of disproportionately dilated ducts in one part of the liver, development of a dominant stricture, or an increase

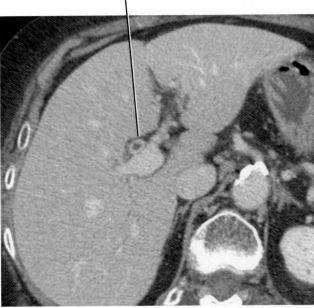

Uniform circumferential thickening of the right hepatic duct

Figure 13-40 Enhanced axial computed tomographic image through the liver of a patient with primary sclerosing cholangitis demonstrating thickening of the right hepatic duct.

in ductal dilatation or stricture length on successive examinations raises the possibility of cholangiocarcinoma. Unfortunately, the detection of cholangiocarcinoma at a potentially curable stage remains an elusive goal of imaging. Although often increased in patients who have experienced development of cholangiocarcinoma in the setting of PSC, serum CA 19-9 levels are of limited benefit for screening. Many tumors are at an advanced stage when detected despite attempts at clinical, biochemical, and imaging surveillance. Although liver transplantation remains an option for patients with PSC, the disease can recur in the donor liver after liver transplantation. Box 13-5 lists a variety of disorders that can mimic PSC on imaging studies.

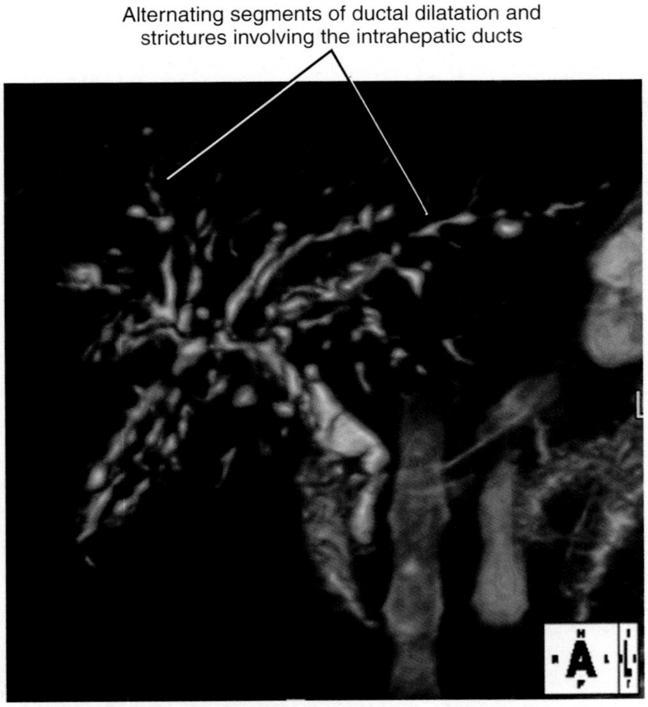

Acquired Immune Deficiency Syndrome/Human Immunodeficiency Syndrome Cholangiopathy

The inflammatory cholangitis AIDS/HIV cholangiopathy is most often associated with opportunistic infection in the clinical setting of advanced HIV infection.

Alternating segments of ductal dilatation and strictures involving the intrahepatic ducts

Figure 13-39 Volume-rendered image from a respiratory-triggered T2-weighted magnetic resonance cholangiopancreatography demonstrates typical changes of primary sclerosing cholangitis.

BOX 13-5   Mimics of Primary Sclerosing Cholangitis

Infectious cholangitis/cholangiopathy (including HIV)
Sclerosing cholangiocarcinoma
Biliary ischemia
Intraarterial chemotherapy infusion
Autoimmune pancreatitis
Langerhans cell histiocytosis

US is useful in cases of suspected AIDS cholangiopathy because normal US results make the diagnosis unlikely. Abnormal imaging findings are similar to those of PSC, and include intrahepatic and extrahepatic bile duct wall thickening, focal strictures and dilatations, common bile duct dilatation caused by papillary stenosis, and diffuse gallbladder wall thickening.

Recurrent Pyogenic Cholangitis (Formerly Known as Oriental Cholangiohepatitis)

RPC is typically characterized by recurrent episodes of acute pyogenic cholangitis, segmental intrahepatic biliary stricture and dilatation, and intrahepatic choledocholithiasis (calcium bilirubinate stones) (Fig. 13-41). Common bile duct thickening may be present, although common bile duct stricture is not typical. Segmental hepatic atrophy, biliary cirrhosis, and cholangiocarcinoma can eventually develop. RPC has been associated with parasitic disease of the liver (e.g., *Clonorchis sinensis*), although the precise cause of RPC is still a matter of speculation.

Autoimmune Pancreatitis

Patients with autoimmune pancreatitis can develop a sclerosing inflammatory process of the bile ducts related to infiltration by IgG4-positive plasma cells. Bile-duct abnormalities associated with autoimmune pancreatitis consist of wall thickening, strictures, and dilatation, and can mimic PSC. Gallbladder involvement can occur with autoimmune pancreatitis. Unlike PSC, the biliary abnormalities associated with autoimmune pancreatitis are reversible after steroid therapy.

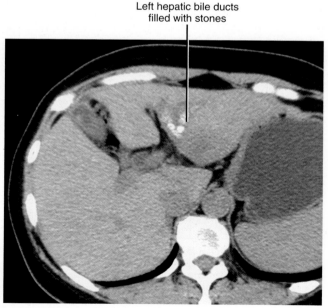

Left hepatic bile ducts filled with stones

Figure 13-41 Unenhanced axial computed tomographic image through the liver of a patient with recurrent pyogenic cholangitis involving the left hepatic lobe.

Primary Biliary Cirrhosis

PBC is a chronic, progressive, cholestatic inflammatory disorder of the bile ducts that presents as cirrhosis. Visualized bile ducts appear normal on US, CT, and MRI in the setting of PBC. Therefore, PBC does not resemble other forms of cholangitis on imaging studies, and diagnosis is based on the clinical presentation and liver biopsy.

■ TUMORS AND TUMOR-LIKE CONDITIONS OF THE EXTRAHEPATIC BILE DUCT

Tumors and tumor-like conditions that affect the extrahepatic bile duct usually present as either a polypoid mass or a mass that causes stenosis.

Lesions That Present as a Polypoid Mass

Bile duct adenomas, papillomatosis, neurofibromas, inflammatory polyps, heterotopic tissue, cholangiocarcinomas, and some metastases can present as a polypoid mass or masses within the extrahepatic bile duct. Bile-duct adenomas are usually of tubular histology and have similar features to intestinal adenomas. Biliary papillomatosis refers to the presence of multiple papillary adenomas within the biliary system. Intrahepatic and extrahepatic bile-duct dilatation is often present on imaging studies of patients with papillomatosis with obstructive jaundice. Polypoid lesions within the dilated bile ducts may be visible on US, CT, and MRI. Imaging findings related to secondary cholangitis may also be present.

Lesions That Present as a Stenosing Mass

Granular cell tumor, carcinoid tumor, heterotopic tissue, cholangiocarcinoma, and some metastases can present as a stenosing mass that involves the extrahepatic bile duct. Granular cell tumors of the extrahepatic bile duct often cause painless jaundice and mimic cholangiocarcinoma. Bile-duct strictures caused by granular cell tumors tend to be short and abrupt, and the mucosa remains smooth and intact.

■ CHOLANGIOCARCINOMA AND ITS MIMICS

Cholangiocarcinoma is a malignant tumor of biliary epithelium that is refractory to medical management and is associated with poor prognosis. Histologically, most cholangiocarcinomas are sclerosing adenocarcinomas, and predisposing factors include PSC, choledochal cyst, and RPC. These tumors can arise from the peripheral intrahepatic ducts (peripheral cholangiocarcinoma), the perihilar/biliary confluence region (Klatskin tumor), or common hepatic or common bile ducts (Fig. 13-42). Cholangiocarcinomas have a propensity toward periductal infiltration, although masslike hepatic parenchymal invasion and intraductal spread also occur.

Most cholangiocarcinomas originate at or near the biliary confluence, and patients present with painless jaundice and proximal bile duct dilatation caused by bile-duct obstruction. A mass may be visible at the level of obstruction, although a mass is not always detectable with US, CT, or MRI (Fig. 13-43). Dilation of the right and left intrahepatic ducts that cannot be seen to join at the expected region of the confluence is a typical appearance on US, CT, and MRI. This finding is particularly useful for locating the tumor when a distinct mass cannot be identified. Lobar atrophy implies involvement of the vessels or bile duct of the affected lobe.

When a mass is visible, it tends to be hypodense on noncontrast CT, hypointense on precontrast T1-weighted MR images, and isointense or mildly hyperintense on T2-weighted MR images. Larger masses may demonstrate central hypointensity on T2-weighted images related to dense fibrous tissue. After administration of intravenous contrast material, cholangiocarcinomas often demonstrate peripheral enhancement during the arterial phase with central enhancement on more delayed images.

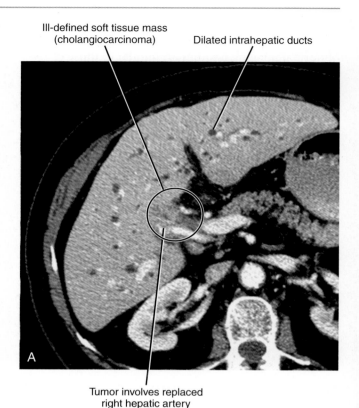

Ill-defined soft tissue mass (cholangiocarcinoma)

Dilated intrahepatic ducts

Tumor involves replaced right hepatic artery

A

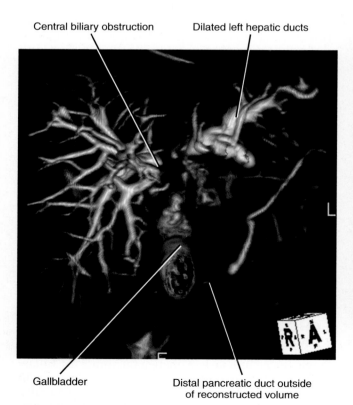

Central biliary obstruction

Dilated left hepatic ducts

Gallbladder

Distal pancreatic duct outside of reconstructed volume

Figure 13-42 Volumetric rendering of a respiratory-triggered T2-weighted magnetic resonance cholangiopancreatography in a patient with a hilar cholangiocarcinoma.

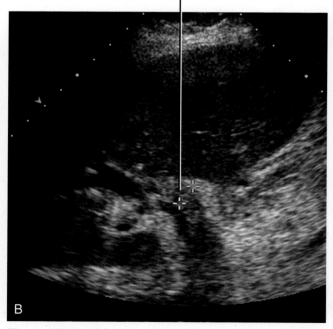

Mildly echogenic mass in porta hepatis in expected location of bile duct

B

Figure 13-43 Enhanced axial computed tomographic (**A**) and ultrasound (**B**) images through the porta hepatis of a patient with cholangiocarcinoma demonstrate a soft-tissue mass causing biliary obstruction.

Occasionally, cholangiocarcinoma manifests on cross-sectional imaging examinations as bile duct wall thickening. Thickening of the bile duct wall exceeding 5 mm is concerning for cholangiocarcinoma.

Because cholangiocarcinomas are often subtle tumors that exhibit periductal and perineural infiltration, imaging often understages these tumors. A carefully performed US or MRI examination in a cooperative patient can accurately assess vascular invasion and bile duct involvement in most patients with cholangiocarcinoma, although MRI is likely more sensitive for detection of liver metastases and peritoneal involvement (Fig. 13-44). Cholangiocarcinoma can invade vascular structures such as the portal vein, although vascular encasement is more typical than invasion. When cholangiocarcinoma invades the portal vein, confusion

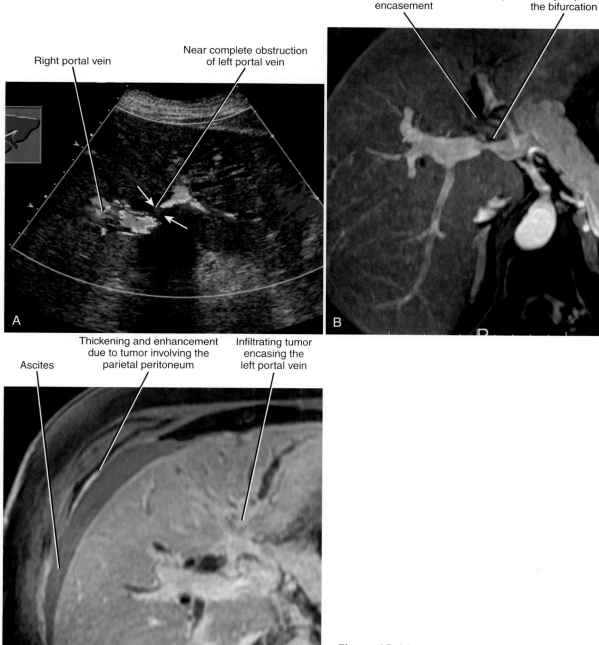

Figure 13-44 Ultrasound image through the liver hilum (**A**), axial partial volume maximum intensity projection magnetic resonance (MR) image (**B**), and delayed enhanced axial MR image (**C**) of a patient with hilar cholangiocarcinoma encasing the portal veins and involving the peritoneum.

with hepatocellular carcinoma (HCC) may occur. More information about the spread and staging of cholangiocarcinoma may be found in Chapter 10.

Because of the desmoplastic nature of many cholangiocarcinomas, progressive enhancement after intravenous contrast administration is considered to be a typical feature. For this reason, many radiologists obtain delayed images through the liver and bile ducts approximately 10 to 20 minutes after extracellular CT or MRI contrast administration. Although delayed imaging can be helpful in characterizing a lesion suspected to represent cholangiocarcinoma, delayed imaging does not always improve the sensitivity of a contrast-enhanced imaging examination. Tumors that are initially hypodense or hypointense compared with liver parenchyma can enhance to the point of isodensity or isointensity on delayed CT and MR images, respectively. Also, enhancement of the periportal tissues is common on delayed gadolinium-enhanced MR images, a phenomenon that may obscure enhancing tumor.

The utility of fluoro-2-deoxy-D-glucose positron emission tomography for the detection and staging of cholangiocarcinoma has not been clearly established, although evidence exists to suggest that positron emission tomography may be helpful for the detection of lymph-node involvement and distant metastases.

Several entities have been known to mimic cholangiocarcinoma. A rare malignant neoplasm exists that combines histologic and imaging features of HCC and cholangiocarcinoma. Gallbladder carcinoma or metastatic adenocarcinoma of the gastrointestinal origin can demonstrate a contrast enhancement pattern similar to that displayed by cholangiocarcinoma, and can invade and/or obstruct the bile ducts on rare occasions. Benign fibrosis has been known to mimic cholangiocarcinoma, although this is a difficult diagnosis to confirm before surgery. Box 13-6 lists additional potential mimics of intrahepatic and extrahepatic cholangiocarcinoma.

BOX 13-6   Mimics of Cholangiocarcinoma

Metastatic adenocarcinoma of gastrointestinal origin
(e.g., stomach, colon)
Gallbladder carcinoma
Hepatocellular carcinoma
Neuroendocrine tumor
Inflammatory stricture
Sclerosing cholangitis
Granular cell tumor
Biliary adenoma
Biliary papilloma
Heterotopic tissue (e.g., pancreatic)
Granulomatous diseases

Suggested Readings

Bowie JD: What is the upper limit of normal for the common bile duct on ultrasound: how much do you want it to be? *Am J Gastroenterol* 95:897-900, 2000.

Choi SH, Han JK, Lee JM et al: Differentiating malignant from benign common bile duct stricture with multiphase helical CT, *Radiology* 236:178-183, 2005.

Chun KA, Ha HK, Yu ES et al: Xanthogranulomatous cholecystitis: CT features with emphasis on differentiation from gallbladder carcinoma, *Radiology* 203:93-97, 1997.

Corvera CU, Blumgart LH, Darvishian F et al: Clinical and pathologic features of proximal biliary strictures masquerading as hilar cholangiocarcinoma, *J Am Coll Surg* 201:862-869, 2005.

Feng B, Song Q: Does the common bile duct dilate after cholecystectomy? Sonographic evaluation in 234 patients, *AJR Am J Roentgenol* 165:859-861, 1995.

Gore RM, Yaghmai V, Newmark GM et al: Imaging benign and malignant disease of the gallbladder, *Radiol Clin North Am* 40:1307-1323, 2002.

Horrow MM, Horrow JC, Niakosari A et al: Is age associated with size of adult extrahepatic bile duct: sonographic study, *Radiology* 221:411-414, 2001.

Kaim A, Steinke K, Frank M et al: Diameter of the common bile duct in the elderly patient: measurement by ultrasound, *Eur Radiol* 8:1413-1415, 1998.

Kim JH, Kim MJ, Chung JJ et al: Differential diagnosis of periampullary carcinomas at MR imaging, *Radiographics* 22:1335-1352, 2002.

Lamah M, Karanjia ND, Dickson GH: Anatomical variations of the extrahepatic biliary tree: review of the world literature, *Clin Anat* 14:167-172, 2001.

Lazaridis KN, Gores GJ: Primary sclerosing cholangitis and cholangiocarcinoma, *Semin Liver Dis* 26:42-51, 2006.

Lee WJ, Lim HK, Jang KM et al: Radiologic spectrum of cholangiocarcinoma: emphasis on unusual manifestations and differential diagnosis, *Radiographics* 21:S97-S116, 2001.

Levy AD, Murakata LA, Rohrmann CA Jr: Gallbladder carcinoma: radiologic-pathologic correlation, *Radiographics* 21:295-314, 2001.

Levy AD, Murakata LA, Abbott RM et al: Benign tumors and tumorlike lesions of the gallbladder and extrahepatic bile ducts: radiologic-pathologic correlation, *Radiographics* 22:387-413, 2002.

Levy AD, Rohrmann CA Jr, Murakata LA et al: Caroli's disease: radiologic spectrum with pathologic correlation, *AJR Am J Roentgenol* 179:1053-1057, 2002.

Moon JH, Cho YD, Cha SW et al: The detection of bile duct stones in suspected biliary pancreatitis: comparison of MRCP, ERCP, and intraductal US, *Am J Gastroenterol* 100:1051-1057, 2005.

Parra JA, Acinas O, Bueno J et al: Xanthogranulomatous cholecystitis: clinical, sonographic, and CT findings in 26 patients, *AJR Am J Roentgenol* 174: 979-983, 2000.

Perret RS, Sloop GD, Borne JA: Common bile duct measurements in an elderly population, *J Ultrasound Med* 19:727-730, 2000.

Pickuth D, Spielmann RP: Detection of choledocholithiasis: comparison of unenhanced spiral CT, US, and ERCP, *Hepatogastroenterology* 47:1514-1517, 2000.

Puente SG, Bannura GC: Radiological anatomy of the biliary tract: variations and congenital abnormalities, *World J Surg* 7:271-276, 1983.

Puri SK, Gupta P, Panigrahi P et al: Ultrasonographic evaluation of common duct diameter in pre and post cholecystectomy patients, *Trop Gastroenterol* 22:23-24, 2001.

Reinhardt MJ, Strunk H, Gerhardt T et al: Detection of Klatskin's tumor in extrahepatic bile duct strictures using delayed 18F-FDG PET/CT: preliminary results for 22 patient studies, *J Nucl Med* 46:1158-1163, 2005.

Russell E, Yrizzary JM, Montalvo BM et al: Left hepatic duct anatomy: implications, *Radiology* 174:353-356, 1990.

Shea JA, Berlin JA, Escarce JJ et al: Revised estimates of diagnostic test sensitivity and specificity in suspected biliary tract disease, *Arch Intern Med* 154:2573-2581, 1994.

Shuto R, Kiyosue H, Komatsu E et al: CT and MR imaging findings of xanthogranulomatous cholecystitis: correlation with pathologic findings, *Eur Radiol* 14:440-446, 2004.

Soto JA, Alvarez O, Munera F et al: Diagnosing bile duct stones: comparison of unenhanced helical CT, oral contrast-enhanced CT cholangiography and MR cholangiography, *AJR Am J Roentgenol* 175:1127-1134, 2000.

Sperti C, Pasquali C, Fiore V et al: Clinical usefulness of 18-fluorodeoxyglucose positron emission tomography in the management of patients with nonpancreatic periampullary neoplasms, *Am J Surg* 191:743-748, 2006.

Todani T, Watanabe Y, Narusue M et al: Congenital bile duct cysts, classification, operative procedures, and review of thirty-seven cases including cancer arising from choledochal cyst, *Am J Surg* 134:263-269, 1977.

Trowbridge RL, Rutkowski NK, Shojania KG: Does this patient have acute cholecystitis? *JAMA* 289:80-86, 2003.

Verma D, Kapadia A, Eisen GM et al: EUS vs MRCP for detection of choledocholithiasis, *Gastrointest Endosc* 64:248-254, 2006.

Vilgrain V, Palazzo L: Choledocholithiasis: role of US and endoscopic ultrasound, *Abdom Imaging* 26:7-14, 2001.

CHAPTER **14**

Pancreas

John R. Leyendecker and Michael Oliphant

■ CLINICAL CONSIDERATIONS

Pancreatic Physiology

The pancreas serves exocrine and endocrine functions critical to normal digestion and metabolism. The exocrine components of the pancreas are arranged in clusters of acinar cells that produce and secrete an electrolyte-enhanced alkaline solution rich in digestive enzymes into the duodenum via the pancreatic duct. A variety of neural and hormonal regulators of pancreatic secretion exist, with cholecystokinin and secretin being the ones most familiar to radiologists. Because pancreatic secretion is minimized during fasting, fasting plays an important role in the management of pancreatic pseudocysts communicating with the pancreatic duct. Fasting is also recommended before secretin-augmented magnetic resonance cholangiopancreatography (MRCP), a method of assessing pancreatic exocrine function in patients with suspected chronic pancreatitis.

The endocrine components of the pancreas are arranged into pancreatic islets that are scattered throughout the pancreas with a concentration toward the tail. Islet cells produce hormones critical to carbohydrate metabolism. Normal pancreatic islets cannot be resolved with current imaging modalities, and their importance in imaging extends from the occasional development of islet cell neoplasms.

Acute Pancreatitis

Acute pancreatitis refers to acute onset of pancreatic inflammation instigated by one or more of a variety of innate or acquired mechanical, chemical, or metabolic factors. Gallstones expelled into the common bile duct incite the majority of cases of acute pancreatitis. Other causes of acute pancreatitis include alcohol abuse, drug reactions, pancreatic and ampullary neoplasms, hypertriglyceridemia, hypercalcemia (caused by hyperparathyroidism), hypothermia, congenital anomalies, trauma, and parasites. Rarely, pancreatitis results from bites or stings of a variety of venomous organisms (our personal favorite is the Gila monster). Despite the proliferation of sophisticated imaging technologies in the last century, establishing the diagnosis of pancreatitis remains a clinical pursuit. Serum amylase and lipase levels are routinely checked when patients have abdominal pain and a compelling (and sometimes not so compelling) history and physical examination. Mild increases of amylase level occur with causes of abdominal pain other than pancreatitis, although a threefold increase of amylase level is specific for pancreatitis. Amylase levels are typically greater in gallstone pancreatitis than in alcohol-related pancreatitis, and only minimal increase is noted in many patients with hyperlipidemic pancreatitis. Normal amylase levels can be found in a small minority of patients with acute pancreatitis.

Serum lipase levels increase within 8 hours of onset of acute pancreatitis. Lipase levels may be significantly increased despite only mild increase of amylase levels in a patient with pancreatitis. Lipase levels also tend to remain increased longer than amylase levels. Although lipase levels can be increased out of proportion to amylase levels in patients with alcoholic pancreatitis, this finding is not as specific as once thought. Mild lipase level increase can occur with other causes of abdominal pain such as cholelithiasis and choledocholithiasis, ruptured aortic aneurysm, and small-bowel obstruction. A serum lipase level greater than three times normal makes a nonpancreatic cause of increased levels unlikely.

Other laboratory findings that can be associated with severe pancreatitis include hypocalcemia, hyperglycemia, hypoalbuminemia, hyperlipidemia, coagulopathy, and leukocytosis.

A variety of systemic complications of severe acute pancreatitis can occur, including diabetes, shock/hypovolemia, adult respiratory distress syndrome, disseminated intravascular coagulation, fat necrosis, and polyarthritis.

Chronic Pancreatitis

Patients with chronic pancreatitis often suffer from chronic, sometimes severe, epigastric or diffuse abdominal pain that can radiate to the back. Patients who do not suffer from continuous or intermittent abdominal pain can present clinically with symptoms of pancreatic insufficiency, including steatorrhea, weight loss, or diabetes.

Pancreatic Cancer

The peak incidence of ductal adenocarcinoma of the pancreas is in the seventh and eighth decades of life, although patients with hereditary pancreatitis are prone to earlier development of pancreatic cancer. Smokers and patients with chronic pancreatitis also appear to be at increased risk for development of pancreatic cancer. Patients often have nonspecific symptoms such as abdominal pain, weight loss, anorexia, or depression. Jaundice results from malignant obstruction of the distal bile duct and can be associated with pruritus, light-colored stools, and a palpable but nontender gallbladder. Diabetes can eventually ensue but is rarely a presenting symptom. Migratory thrombophlebitis and polyarthralgias are rare manifestations. Carcinoembryonic antigen (CEA) or CA 19-9 levels can be increased in patients with ductal adenocarcinoma of the pancreas but are nonspecific. CA 19-9 levels are less helpful in the setting of biliary obstruction and are often normal in patients with small tumors.

Neuroendocrine Tumor (Islet Cell Tumor)

A variety of functioning and nonfunctioning endocrine tumors arise in the pancreas. Many pancreatic neuroendocrine tumors occur sporadically, although neuroendocrine tumors of the pancreas also constitute one component of multiple endocrine neoplasia syndrome type 1 (MEN-1). In the setting of MEN-1, neuroendocrine tumors have a tendency to be multiple.

Symptomatic nonfunctioning neuroendocrine tumors tend to be large at presentation, because patients have symptoms of mass effect rather than clinical sequelae of excess hormone secretion. The various functional neuroendocrine tumors of the pancreas are listed in Table 14-1 with their associated clinical manifestations.

Table 14-1   Pancreatic Neuroendocrine Tumors

Tumor	Hormone	Manifestations
Insulinoma	Insulin	Related to hypoglycemia or neuroglycopenia*
Glucagonoma	Glucagon	Necrolytic migratory erythema,† glucose intolerance
Gastrinoma	Gastrin	Peptic ulcer disease (Zollinger–Ellison syndrome)
VIPoma	Vasoactive intestinal polypeptide	Watery diarrhea, hypokalemia (WDHA syndrome)
Somatostatinoma	Somatostatin	Mild diabetes, diarrhea, steatorrhea
GRFoma	Growth hormone–releasing factor	Acromegaly
PPoma	Pancreatic polypeptide	No known typical clinical manifestations

*Headache, light-headedness, confusion, abnormal behavior, seizures.
†Dermatitis that begins in groin and spreads to thighs, buttocks, and extremities.

■ ANATOMY AND NORMAL IMAGING APPEARANCE

The Normal Pancreas

Grossly, the pancreas is a lobulated extraperitoneal organ that resides in the anterior pararenal space. As such, it is surrounded by areolar tissue and lacks a distinct capsule. The pancreas is divided into the head and uncinate process, the neck, the body, and tail (Fig. 14-1). The divisions between these portions represent arbitrary boundaries that aid in communicating the location of abnormalities. These divisions do not separate anatomically or functionally distinct units.

The superior mesenteric vein (SMV) serves as a useful anatomic landmark. The pancreatic head is generally

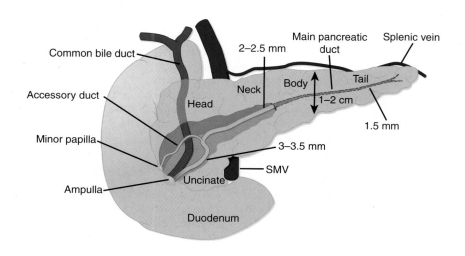

Figure 14-1 Typical pancreas. *SMV*, Superior mesenteric vein.

considered the portion of pancreas to the right of the SMV and resides within the c-loop of the duodenum. The uncinate process is the continuation of the head posterior to the SMV and normally has a triangular shape. The posteromedial border of the uncinate process should be concave or flat rather than rounded. The portion of pancreas immediately ventral to the SMV is considered the neck, whereas the body and tail continue to the left. No clear external landmark divides body and tail of the pancreas; therefore, most radiologists roughly divide the pancreas to the left of the SMV in half, designating the more midline portion the body. The pancreatic tail lies within the splenorenal ligament, which provides a conduit for tumor and inflammation between the pancreatic tail and the spleen. The exocrine pancreas generally diminishes with age, often becoming replaced by fat.

Lobulations of the lateral contour of the pancreatic head are commonly visualized on cross-sectional imaging studies of the pancreas. These protrusions of the pancreatic head are similar in echogenicity, attenuation, signal intensity, and enhancement characteristics to normal pancreas and should not be mistaken for pancreatic neoplasm.

The normal pancreatic echotexture is homogeneous and isoechoic to mildly hyperechoic compared with the normal liver on ultrasound (US) images (Fig. 14-2). Increased echogenicity of the pancreas occurs with fatty infiltration. The normal pancreatic parenchyma measures 40 to 50 HU on unenhanced computed tomographic (CT) images. The pancreas is higher in signal intensity than liver, spleen, or skeletal muscle on T1-weighted magnetic resonance (MR) images. The innately high signal intensity of the pancreas on fat-suppressed T1-weighted images makes such images valuable for detecting tumors (Fig. 14-3). The normal pancreas is only slightly higher in signal intensity than muscle on T2-weighted images. With

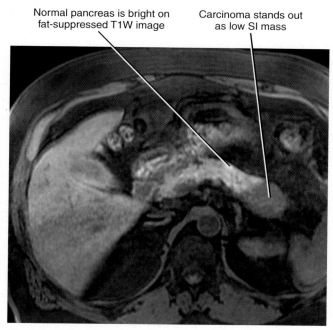

Normal pancreas is bright on fat-suppressed T1W image

Carcinoma stands out as low SI mass

Figure 14-3 Unenhanced, fat-suppressed, T1-weighted (T1W), axial magnetic resonance image through the tail of the pancreas in a patient with pancreatic cancer. *SI,* Signal intensity.

CT or magnetic resonance imaging (MRI), maximum pancreatic parenchymal enhancement occurs at 35 to 45 seconds after intravenous contrast administration or approximately 15 seconds after the contrast bolus arrives in the abdominal aorta.

Pancreatic Relationships

The pancreas is predominantly an extraperitoneal organ that resides in the anterior pararenal space immediately posterior to the lesser sac. The pancreas is separated from the stomach anteriorly by the lesser sac of the peritoneal cavity. The pancreatic tail courses in the splenorenal ligament along with the splenic vessels, rendering this portion of the pancreas intraperitoneal. The two layers of the transverse mesocolon (reflections of the posterior parietal peritoneum) split near the anterior surface of the pancreas providing a route for spread of tumor and inflammation between the pancreas and the transverse colon. The root of the small-bowel mesentery lies just inferior to the pancreas. These relationships provide anatomic continuity among the pancreas, transverse colon, and small bowel. The duodenum is intimately associated with the pancreas and frequently involved by tumor and inflammation arising within the pancreas. The intraperitoneal portion of the duodenum is connected to the pancreas by the dorsal mesoduodenum. The extraperitoneal portion is in the anterior pararenal space adjacent to the pancreas. The second portion of the duodenum courses along the right lateral pancreatic head. The third and fourth portions of the duodenum run dorsal to the pancreatic head, body, and tail.

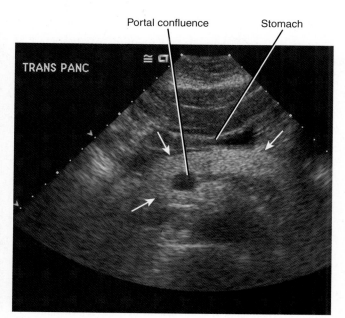

Portal confluence   Stomach

TRANS PANC

Figure 14-2 Transverse sonogram of the normal pancreas *(arrows)* in a patient without clinical evidence of pancreatic disease.

Pancreatic Duct Anatomy

The main pancreatic duct forms when the dorsal pancreatic duct and ventral pancreatic duct join during embryologic fusion of the dorsal and ventral pancreas. The main duct (duct of Wirsung) runs the length of the pancreas and receives small branch duct tributaries at right angles along its entire length. Until recently, the normal branch ducts were rarely visible on cross-sectional imaging studies. Although this is changing with higher resolution CT scanning and MRI, numerous conspicuous branch ducts should be considered an abnormal finding on cross-sectional imaging studies. The main pancreatic duct gradually tapers from pancreatic head toward the tail without abrupt changes in caliber. The course of the main pancreatic duct varies in the region of the pancreatic neck and head. Some of the more common variants in duct course include a gradual caudal bend toward the ampulla, a "hockey-stick" configuration, a sigmoid or S-shaped course, and a looped appearance. These meanderings of the pancreatic duct are rarely important provided the duct maintains a smoothly tapering and nondilated appearance. The main pancreatic duct normally enters the duodenum with the common bile duct via the major papilla. In many individuals, the dorsal pancreatic duct persists as a smaller caliber accessory duct that extends from the main pancreatic duct near the neck of the pancreas to enter the duodenum at the minor papilla approximately 2 cm proximal to the major papilla (see Fig. 14-1). With state-of-the-art equipment, the normal accessory pancreatic duct can be routinely identified on multidetector CT and high-resolution MRI examinations (this duct is also referred to as the duct of Santorini). Usually, the accessory duct appears as a small rudimentary structure with CT and MRI, although it can be dominant in a small percentage of individuals. On secretin-stimulated MRCP examinations, the pancreatic ducts begin to enlarge approximately 1 minute after secretin administration and reach maximum diameter after approximately 20 minutes.

Vascular Anatomy of the Pancreas and Peripancreatic Vessels

The blood supply to the pancreas comes from branches of the celiac artery and superior mesenteric artery (SMA). The head of the pancreas is richly supplied by three arteries forming an intricate vascular arcade. The gastroduodenal artery (GDA) is a branch of the common hepatic artery that arises from the celiac artery. The GDA gives off the posterior and anterior superior pancreaticoduodenal arteries. These arteries anastomose with the posterior and anterior inferior pancreaticoduodenal arteries, which are branches of the inferior pancreaticoduodenal artery branch of the SMA. The inferior pancreaticoduodenal vessels supply the uncinate process and caudad portion of the head of the pancreas. The third vessel is the dorsal pancreatic artery, a branch of the splenic artery. These intricate vascular arcades that surround the pancreas play a critical role in providing collateral blood supply in the event of celiac axis or proximal SMA obstruction. The body and tail of the pancreas are supplied by the dorsal pancreatic artery, a branch of the splenic artery, and multiple other branches of the splenic artery.

The veins draining the head of the pancreas initially course with the arteries but eventually deviate from these paths. The posterior superior pancreaticoduodenal vein drains to the main portal vein, and the anterior superior pancreaticoduodenal vein drains to the gastrocolic trunk, which drains into the SMV ventrally at the level of the midpancreatic head. The gastrocolic trunk is formed by the junction of the right gastroepiploic vein and the right or middle colic vein. The inferior pancreaticoduodenal vein drains into the proximal jejunal vein that drains into the SMV dorsally at the level of the uncinate process. The pancreaticoduodenal venous arcades serve as a potential portoportal collateral pathway in the event of portal vein obstruction. Enlargement of the pancreaticoduodenal veins in the setting of pancreatic carcinoma is a secondary sign of portal vein compromise by tumor (Fig. 14-4).

The venous drainage of the body and tail of the pancreas is to the splenic vein. The splenic vein then joins with the SMV to form the portal vein.

The pancreatic blood supply and drainage are identifiable on vascular-phase, thin-slice, axial CT images. The SMA and SMV normally lie to the left of the pancreatic head. A fat plane surrounds the artery, whereas a fat

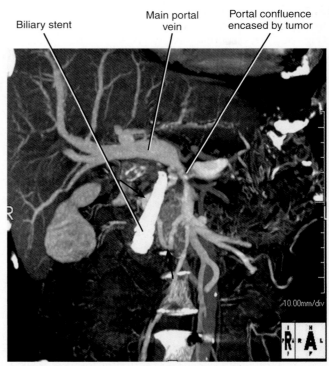

Biliary stent   Main portal vein   Portal confluence encased by tumor

Figure 14-4 Coronal reformation of a portal-phase enhanced computed tomographic scan through the upper abdomen of a patient with pancreatic cancer. Portal vein obstruction is bypassed by posterior pancreaticoduodenal veins *(arrows)*.

plane is only occasionally visible between the right lateral margin of the SMV and the pancreatic head. The GDA is easily identified on imaging studies coursing along the right anterolateral border of the pancreatic head. The anterior superior pancreaticoduodenal artery continues caudally from the GDA along the anterolateral pancreatic head. The anterior superior pancreaticoduodenal vein usually drains into the gastrocolic trunk or right gastroepiploic vein and tends to be horizontally oriented on axial CT and MR images. The gastrocolic trunk is easily and consistently found on cross-sectional imaging studies just anterior to the midpancreatic head (Fig. 14-5). The posterior superior pancreaticoduodenal artery (first branch of the GDA) and vein are seen in the

region of the distal bile duct between the pancreatic head and the proximal duodenum. The vein can often be seen in cross section on axial images and drains into the suprapancreatic portion of the portal vein within 2 cm of the portal confluence. The inferior pancreaticoduodenal vessels may be visible at the level of the uncinate process, although their small size makes them difficult to identify definitively.

Pearl: Enlargement of the pancreaticoduodenal veins in the setting of pancreatic carcinoma is a secondary sign of portal vein compromise by tumor..

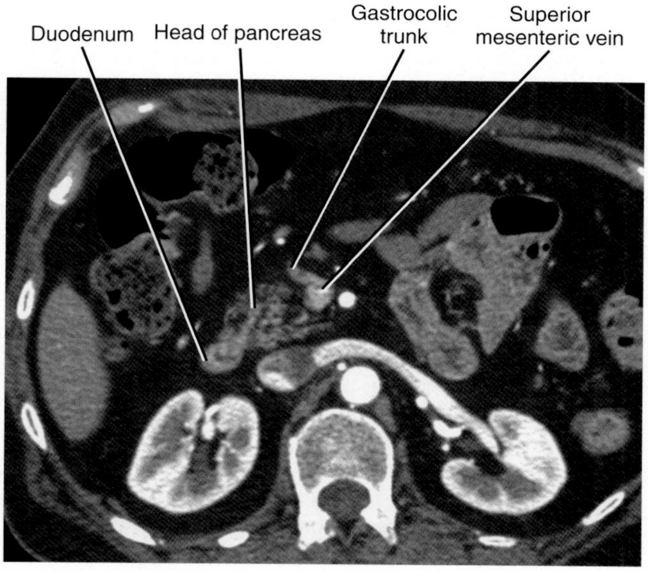

Developmental Anomalies of the Pancreas

The organogenesis of the pancreas occurs in concert with the formation of the liver and duodenum, and involves two separate components, dorsal and ventral, each with its own ductal system. During development, the ventral pancreas rotates posterior to the duodenum to join with the dorsal pancreas, forming a single organ. The two ductal systems also join to create the main pancreatic duct. Not surprising, given the complexity of this process, pancreatic variant anatomy is relatively common (Fig. 14-6).

Agenesis of the dorsal anlage (dorsal agenesis) occurs when only the pancreatic head and uncinate process develop, and the accessory duct (Santorini) is absent (Fig. 14-7). Dorsal agenesis may be incomplete, resulting in the presence of a variable portion of the dorsal pancreas and accessory duct. Dorsal agenesis can be associated with polysplenia.

Ectopic pancreatic tissue can be present within organs of entodermal origin (organs arising from the primitive gut). The gastric antrum and proximal duodenum are most commonly affected. In such cases, the ectopic tissue can consist of acinar cells, islet cells, and a small duct. Ectopic pancreas can also occur in other organs

Duodenum   Head of pancreas   Gastrocolic trunk   Superior mesenteric vein

Figure 14-5 Enhanced axial computed tomographic image through the abdomen demonstrates the gastrocolic trunk.

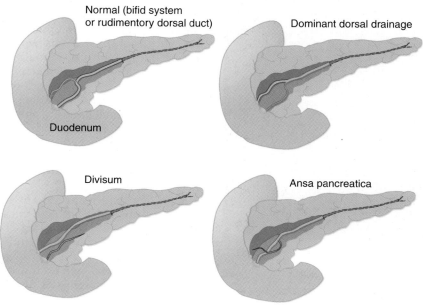

Figure 14-6 Variant pancreatic ductal anatomy.

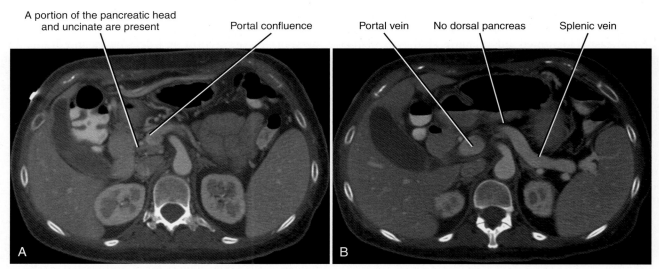

Figure 14-7 Enhanced axial computed tomographic images through the upper abdomen in a patient with dorsal agenesis of the pancreas show presence of the ventral pancreas (**A**) and complete absence of the dorsal pancreas (**B**).

such as the remainder of the small bowel, colon, appendix, Meckel's diverticulum, gallbladder, liver, and spleen. Rarely, ectopic pancreas occurs above the diaphragm. Abnormalities that affect the pancreas, such as neoplasia and inflammation, can also affect heterotopic pancreatic tissue.

Pancreas divisum is a relatively common anomaly (almost 10% of individuals) characterized by completely separate dorsal and ventral ductal systems draining the pancreas (Fig. 14-8). In divisum, the

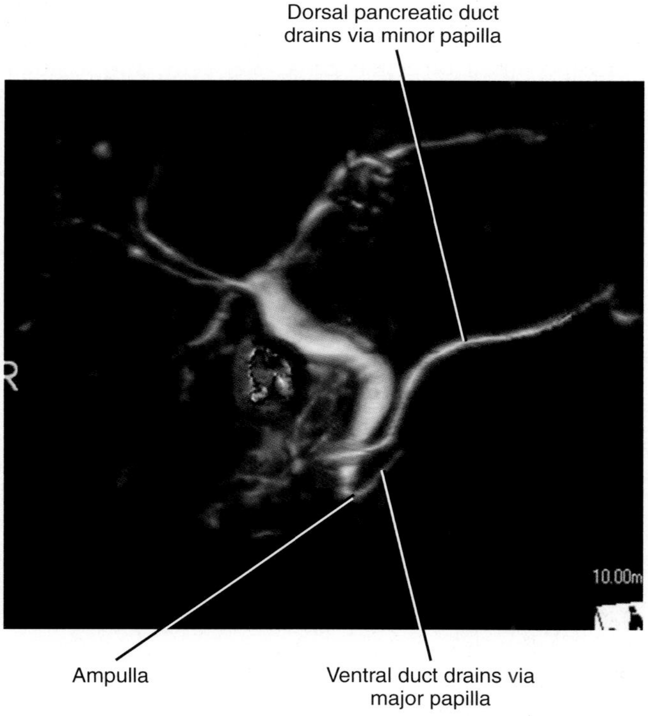

Figure 14-8 Volume-rendered magnetic resonance cholangiopancreatographic image demonstrating pancreas divisum in an asymptomatic patient.

dorsal duct drains the body and tail of the pancreas via the minor papilla, whereas the ventral pancreatic duct drains the caudad portion of the head and uncinate process via the major papilla. This variant has been implicated in the development of pancreatitis, although many cases of pancreas divisum are discovered incidentally on high-resolution CT or MR images. Occasionally, the dorsal and ventral moieties are separated by a fat plane, but frequently the pancreas is normal in size and shape.

Ansa pancreatica occurs when the normal communication between the accessory pancreatic duct and ventral (main) duct is replaced by a looping branch duct that courses from the region of the minor papilla to drain into the main pancreatic duct (see Fig. 14-6).

Annular pancreas is much less common than divisum. In the case of annular pancreas, the duodenum is completely encircled by pancreatic tissue. Pancreatic ducts can either encircle or drain directly into the duodenum. This anomaly manifests on upper gastrointestinal series in neonates as obstructive narrowing of the second portion of the duodenum. Occasionally, annular pancreas presents in adulthood as an incidental finding on CT or MRI (Fig. 14-9). The pancreatic tissue surrounding the descending duodenum maintains identical echogenicity, attenuation, signal intensity, and enhancement characteristics to the remainder of the pancreas. When the duodenum is not adequately distended with oral contrast material or fluid, the combination of collapsed duodenum and annular pancreas may simulate a neoplasm of the pancreatic head.

One final pancreatic variant rarely described in the literature involves complete encasement of the portal vein by pancreatic tissue (Fig. 14-10). In such cases, pancreatic parenchyma surrounds the portal vein on all sides, potentially simulating a mass lesion or encasement of the portal vein by tumor. The main pancreatic duct can course anterior or posterior to the portal vein in such cases. Surgical resection of the pancreas can be potentially complicated by this variant.

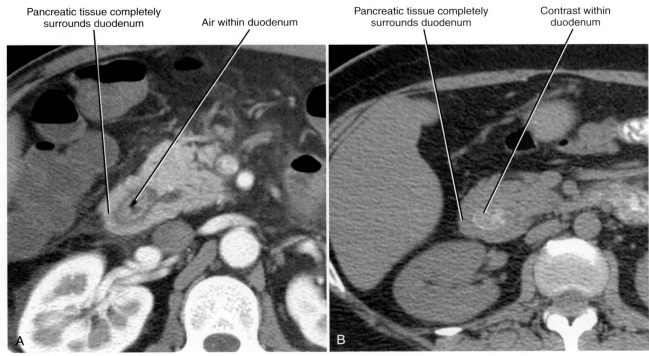

Pancreatic tissue completely surrounds duodenum | Air within duodenum

Pancreatic tissue completely surrounds duodenum | Contrast within duodenum

Figure 14-9 Annular pancreas. **A,** Contrast-enhanced computed tomography performed to evaluate the liver in a patient with cirrhosis shows an asymptomatic annular pancreas. **B,** A similar abnormality is seen on a noncontrast examination in a different patient.

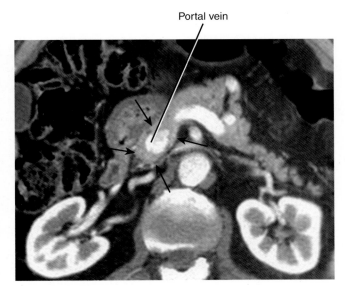

Portal vein

Figure 14-10 Enhanced axial computed tomographic image through the pancreas of a patient with complete encasement of the portal vein by normal pancreatic tissue *(arrows)*.

■ PANCREATITIS

Acute Pancreatitis

Acute pancreatitis ranges in severity from mild inflammation beyond the limits of detection of most standard imaging examinations to extensive pancreatic necrosis. Although most patients are diagnosed before imaging, acute pancreatitis is being increasingly diagnosed on imaging studies used to evaluate nonspecific abdominal complaints (often in the place of thorough clinical and laboratory assessment). In cases of pancreatitis established clinically, imaging serves to establish the potential cause, predict the disease course, and detect complications of pancreatitis.

Imaging Findings of Acute Pancreatitis
RADIOGRAPHY
Conventional radiographs are not able to directly image pancreatic inflammation and rarely yield a specific diagnosis of pancreatitis. However, radiographs are often abnormal in the setting of acute pancreatitis (Fig. 14-11). The most common radiographic abnormalities include a focal or generalized ileus, pleural effusion (often left sided), and basal atelectasis. The "colon cutoff sign" originally referred to gaseous distention of the right colon with abrupt termination of the gas column to the left of the hepatic flexure. This sign has been generalized to include areas of narrowing anywhere in the colon related to mesocolic involvement with pancreatitis. Dilatation of the descending duodenum ("sentinel-loop") can be a sign of pancreatic inflammation and is more suggestive of acute pancreatitis when accompanied by colonic involvement.

BARIUM
Barium examinations can demonstrate findings of acute pancreatitis or pathology mimicking acute pancreatitis such as peptic ulcer disease.

Upper gastrointestinal series can demonstrate widening of the duodenal c-loop because of an enlarged pancreatic head and thickening and spiculation of the duodenal mucosal folds, especially along the medial wall caused by mucosal edema.

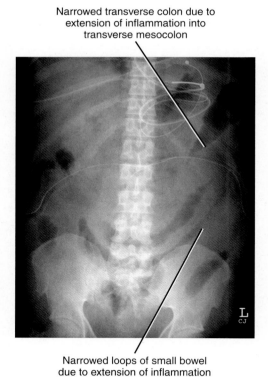

Narrowed transverse colon due to
extension of inflammation into
transverse mesocolon

Narrowed loops of small bowel
due to extension of inflammation
into small intestine mesentery

Figure 14-11 Abdominal radiograph of a patient with severe acute pancreatitis.

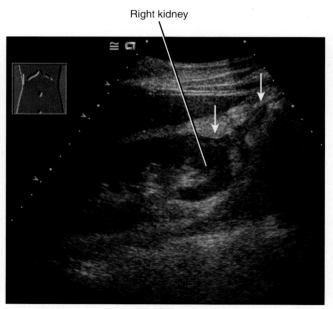

Right kidney

Figure 14-12 Longitudinal sonogram of the right kidney demonstrates inflammation *(arrows)* inferior to the right kidney secondary to acute pancreatitis.

Pancreatic inflammation can extend within the small-intestine mesentery, causing thickening of the small-bowel mucosal folds. These findings can extend to the cecum via the ileocolic mesentery.

Barium enema can demonstrate a dilated right and transverse colon, spasm (particularly common in the region of the splenic flexure), thickened spiculated fold pattern in the transverse colon, or effacement of the inferior haustra of the transverse colon.

ULTRASOUND

Diffuse acute pancreatitis manifests on US as decreased or heterogeneous echogenicity of the pancreas, which can appear enlarged. In the setting of pancreatitis, US has its greatest utility in the diagnosis of gallstones, choledocholithiasis, and biliary obstruction. Hypoechoic inflammation, acute fluid collections, and pseudocysts are easily revealed provided a suitable sonographic window exists (Fig. 14-12). Lesser sac collections are relatively easy to see anterior to the pancreas. Fluid accumulating in the superior recess of the lesser sac can be seen around the caudate lobe. Standard grayscale US is relatively insensitive for the diagnosis of pancreatic necrosis in the setting of acute pancreatitis. Table 14-2 lists some sonographic signs of acute pancreatitis.

COMPUTED TOMOGRAPHY

The initial diagnosis of acute pancreatitis is based on clinical and laboratory findings. However, pancreatitis occasionally presents with a confusing clinical

Table 14-2   Sonographic Abnormalities in Acute Pancreatitis

Finding	Prevalence Rate
Peripancreatic inflammation	60%
Heterogeneous parenchyma	56%
Decreased gland echogenicity	44%
Indistinct ventral margin	33%
Glandular enlargement	27%
Focal parenchymal echo change	23%
Peripancreatic fluid collection	21%
Focal mass (usually hypoechoic)	17%
Perivascular inflammation	10%
Pancreatic duct dilatation	4%
Venous thrombosis	4%

Adapted from Finstad TA, Tchelepi H, Ralls PW: Sonography of acute pancreatitis: prevalence of findings and pictorial essay, *Ultrasound Q* 21:95-104, 2005, by permission.

picture. In such cases, CT findings can suggest the correct diagnosis. Furthermore, enhanced CT is of benefit in the initial evaluation of pancreatitis to assess its severity and to identify complications. Intravenous contrast media improve detection of pancreatic necrosis or complications such as pseudoaneurysm formation or venous thrombosis. Occasionally, CT will establish a cause for pancreatitis such as choledocholithiasis or aberrant pancreatic ductal anatomy (Fig. 14-13).

The CT findings of uncomplicated acute pancreatitis include focal or diffuse pancreatic enlargement with infiltration or stranding in the peripancreatic fat (Fig. 14-14). Peripancreatic fluid collections commonly occur and either resolve over time or organize to form pseudocysts. After administration of intravenous contrast material, the inflamed pancreas can enhance heterogeneously. Confluent areas of nonenhancing tissue suggest pancreatic necrosis.

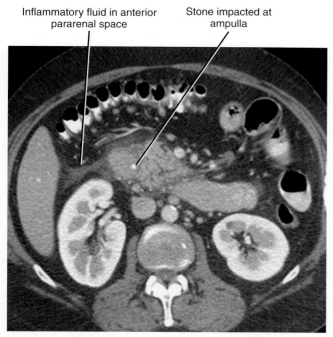

Inflammatory fluid in anterior pararenal space

Stone impacted at ampulla

Figure 14-13 Enhanced axial computed tomographic image through the abdomen of a patient with gallstone pancreatitis and a small calcified stone impacted at the ampulla.

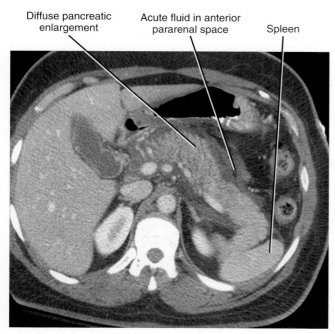

Diffuse pancreatic enlargement

Acute fluid in anterior pararenal space

Spleen

Figure 14-14 Enhanced axial computed tomographic image through the upper abdomen of a patient with acute pancreatitis.

MAGNETIC RESONANCE IMAGING

MRI is rarely essential to the acute management of patients with pancreatitis. MRI is considerably less sensitive than CT for detection of calcifications and gas bubbles, but it excels at demonstrating the biliary and pancreatic ductal systems and pancreatitis-related fluid collections. MRI is also more sensitive than other modalities for the detection of pancreatic hemorrhage. In patients with contraindications to iodinated contrast media, gadolinium-enhanced MRI may be helpful in detecting pancreatic necrosis and vascular complications. MRCP aids in detecting stones within the gallbladder, common bile duct, and pancreatic duct. MRCP can also be helpful for defining ductal anatomy in suspected cases of pancreas divisum or annular pancreas. Secretin-augmented MRCP has been suggested as a means of evaluating the pancreatic duct for stricture, disruption, or continuity with pseudocysts. Secretin should be administered in a closely monitored setting to patients with acute pancreatitis because of the potential to exacerbate pancreatic inflammation.

Pancreatic edema results in a higher-than-normal signal intensity pancreas on T2-weighted images and lower-than-normal signal intensity pancreas on T1-weighted images. When sufficiently severe, acute pancreatitis causes diminished enhancement of the pancreas with gadolinium-based contrast administration. Absent enhancement suggests pancreatic necrosis. Uncomplicated acute peripancreatic fluid collections appear as irregularly shaped areas of low signal intensity on T1-weighted images and of very high signal intensity on T2-weighted images. Areas of hemorrhage appear relatively bright on T1-weighted images. Fluid collections complicated by hemorrhage or infection have variable signal intensity on T1- and T2-weighted MR images.

Intraabdominal Spread of Acute Pancreatitis

In cases of severe pancreatitis, inflammatory fluid extends from the centrally located pancreas throughout the extraperitoneum of the abdomen, pelvis, and even mediastinum. Inflammation often initially extends bilaterally within the anterior pararenal space and dissects between the leaves of the posterior renal fascia. Because the anterior pararenal space is in continuity with the ligaments and mesenteries of the abdomen (according to the unifying concept of the subperitoneal space), pancreatitis can spread within the upper abdomen via the gastrosplenic ligament, gastrocolic ligament, and greater omentum. In this manner, inflammation spreads from the pancreas to organs such as the liver, stomach, and spleen. Spread within the gastrohepatic ligament can also extend through the esophageal hiatus into the mediastinum.

Pathways for spread of pancreatitis in the lower abdomen are within the transverse mesocolon to the transverse colon, and within the small intestine mesentery to the small bowel and right lower quadrant. Pancreatic inflammation can also extend caudally via the infrarenal space (confluence of the pararenal spaces beneath the kidneys) or the small-intestine mesentery into the pelvis. Extension along the left lateral pelvis can continue into the sigmoid mesocolon to the sigmoid colon. Inflammation can also extend from the pelvic sidewalls via the broad ligaments to the uterus and ovaries or posteriorly to the presacral space and mesorectum.

Complications of Acute Pancreatitis

Imaging plays an important role in the detection and management of complications related to pancreatitis. *Pancreatic pseudocysts* are collections of inflammatory fluid contained within a fibrous capsule (Fig. 14-15). Pseudocysts result from the maturation of acute peripancreatic fluid collections that fail to resolve over the course of several weeks. Many pseudocysts maintain a communication with the pancreatic duct, and this communication may be evident on thin-section CT or MRCP images. Pseudocysts that become symptomatic because of mass effect or infection are usually managed by percutaneous or endoscopic drainage. Pancreatic pseudocysts can exert mass effect on the posterior gastric wall visible with radiography or fluoroscopy (Fig. 14-16). The distinction between pseudocysts and other cystic pancreatic masses is discussed later in this chapter.

Pancreatic necrosis is present when one or more demarcated foci of pancreatic parenchyma fail to enhance on dynamic contrast-enhanced CT or MRI (≤30 HU at peak enhancement with CT) and occurs in up to a third of cases of acute pancreatitis (Fig. 14-17). Pancreatic necrosis increases mortality and may require necrosectomy when extensive. Focal acute fluid collections, fatty infiltration, or glandular atrophy should not be misinterpreted as pancreatic necrosis. Pancreatic necrosis can become infected, usually several weeks after onset of acute pancreatitis. Gas within an area of nonenhancing parenchyma suggests the diagnosis, although gas also results from fistulous communication with the bowel or prior intervention. Unlike pancreatic pseudocyst or

abscess, sterile or infected pancreatic necrosis is difficult to manage via catheter drainage because of the presence of copious solid debris.

Pancreatic necrosis can involve the central portion of the pancreas, potentially resulting in interruption of the pancreatic duct because of necrosis of the duct epithelium (Fig. 14-18). In such cases, a variable amount of

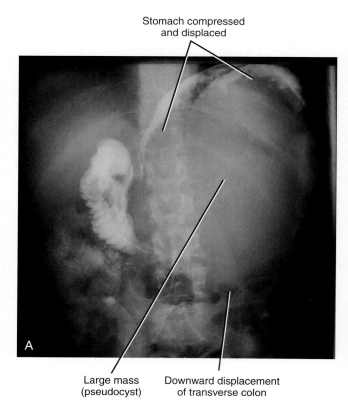

Stomach compressed and displaced

Large mass (pseudocyst)   Downward displacement of transverse colon

Pancreatic tail   Stomach   Large pseudocyst

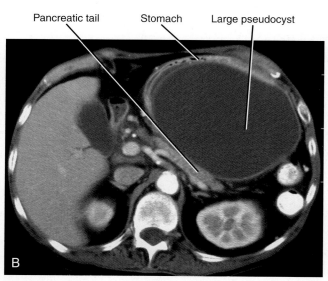

Figure 14-16 Frontal radiograph from upper gastrointestinal series (**A**) and enhanced axial computed tomographic image (**B**) through the abdomen of a patient with a previous episode of acute pancreatitis and a large pancreatic pseudocyst that displaces the stomach upward and the transverse colon downward. This localizes the mass to the left supramesocolic compartment.

Necrotic debris   High signal intensity collection in region of pancreatic tail

Figure 14-15 Axial T2-weighted magnetic resonance image through the level of the pancreatic tail in a patient with a large pancreatic pseudocyst.

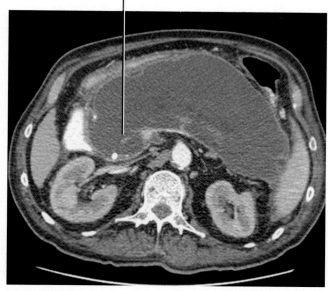

Almost no enhancing pancreatic parenchyma remains

Figure 14-17 Enhanced axial computed tomographic image through the upper abdomen of a patient with extensive pancreatic necrosis and a large pancreatiform fluid collection replacing nearly the entire pancreas within the anterior pararenal space.

the setting of disconnected pancreatic duct, although this finding is nonspecific, because disruption of a pancreatic branch duct can also cause an intrapancreatic fluid collection. Although a branch duct disruption can often be treated with placement of a pancreatic stent, main duct disconnection often requires surgery.

Pearl: Necrosis of the central portion of the pancreas can result in interruption of the pancreatic duct, isolation of the remaining viable pancreatic tissue in the tail, and leakage of pancreatic secretions into the peripancreatic spaces.

Pancreatic abscess is a well-defined collection of pus in or near the pancreas that demonstrates variable amounts of gas, a thick enhancing wall, and no central enhancement after administration of intravenous contrast material. Percutaneous aspiration may be necessary to confirm infection or identify an organism. Pancreatic abscess is more amenable to percutaneous drainage than infected pancreatic necrosis.

Hemorrhage associated with acute pancreatitis may occur within the pancreas, within the peripancreatic fat, or within a pancreatic pseudocyst. Hemorrhage within a pseudocyst results in internal echoes with US and increased attenuation of pseudocysts on CT images. Hemorrhage typically causes areas of increased signal intensity on T1-weighted MR images.

Venous thrombosis is relatively common in the setting of pancreatitis and most often involves the splenic vein because of its close relation with the pancreas. Splenic vein thrombosis should be suspected when the vein fails to enhance on CT or MR images after intravenous contrast administration, or when the vein fails to demonstrate flow with Doppler interrogation. Enlarged gastroepiploic veins often signify collateral flow in the setting of splenic vein thrombosis. Other veins to evaluate for evidence of thrombosis in the setting of pancreatitis include the superior mesenteric and portal veins (Fig. 14-19).

the pancreatic tissue proximal to the area of necrosis becomes isolated from the main ductal system. This potentially allows leakage of pancreatic secretions into the peripancreatic spaces. The imaging findings of a disconnected pancreatic duct include necrosis of at least 2 cm of pancreas, viable pancreatic tissue proximal to the disruption, and extravasation of contrast material injected at pancreatography. On CT and MR images, a large intrapancreatic fluid collection is often present in

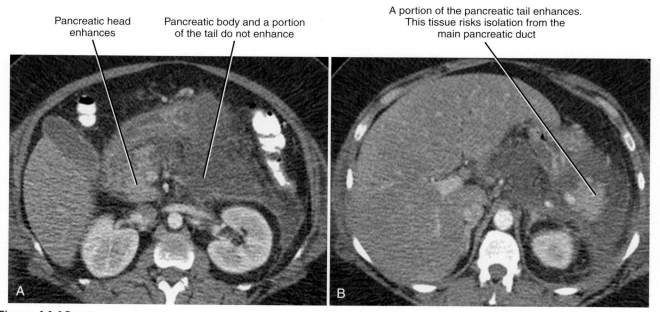

Pancreatic head enhances

Pancreatic body and a portion of the tail do not enhance

A portion of the pancreatic tail enhances. This tissue risks isolation from the main pancreatic duct

Figure 14-18 Enhanced axial computed tomographic images through the head **(A)** and tail **(B)** of the pancreas in a patient with necrosis involving the central pancreas.

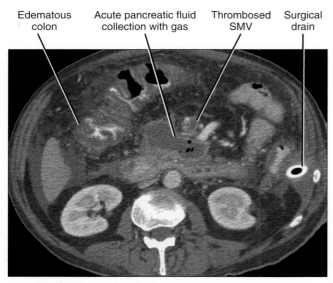

Edematous colon Acute pancreatic fluid collection with gas Thrombosed SMV Surgical drain

Figure 14-19 Enhanced axial computed tomographic image through the abdomen of a patient with severe necrotizing pancreatitis and superior mesenteric vein (SMV) thrombosis.

Pseudoaneurysm formation results from weakening of an arterial wall by pancreatic enzymes. Pseudoaneurysms are typically round and demonstrate arterial-phase enhancement on CT and MRI (Fig. 14-20). Depending on the timing of the scan, some pseudoaneurysms may not completely fill until the second contrast-enhanced phase of a dynamic study; therefore, all vascular phases should be routinely consulted. Pseudoaneurysms will demonstrate evidence of flow on color Doppler images. Whenever a round, potentially fluid-filled structure is

Pseudoaneurysm is partially filled with thrombus Pseudoaneurysm lumen demonstrating arterial phase enhancement Large pancreatic pseudocyst

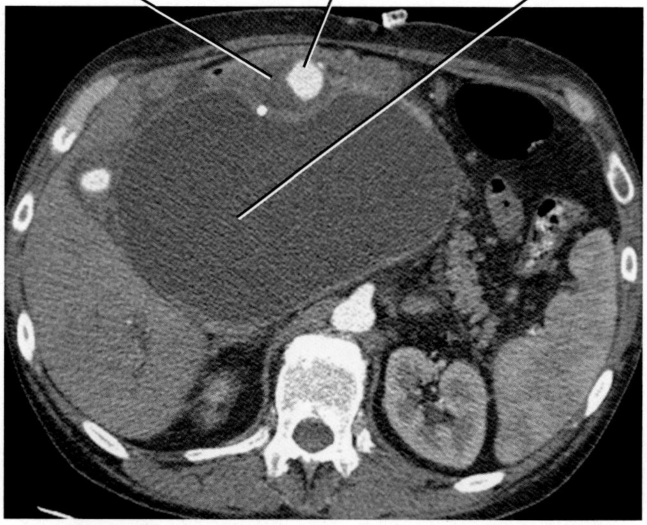

Figure 14-20 Enhanced axial computed tomographic image through the upper abdomen of a patient with a pseudoaneurysm of the gastroduodenal artery and a large pancreatic pseudocyst. This patient was managed successfully with coil embolization of the pseudoaneurysm and percutaneous drainage of the pseudocyst.

identified in the region of the pancreas in a patient with acute pancreatitis, one must always consider the possibility of pseudoaneurysm before attempting aspiration or drainage. Table 14-3 lists some additional potential complications resulting from pancreatitis.

Pitfall: Whenever a round, potentially fluid-filled structure is identified in the region of the pancreas in a patient with acute pancreatitis, one must always consider the possibility of pseudoaneurysm before attempting aspiration or drainage.

Computed Tomographic Severity Indices for Acute Pancreatitis

Several attempts have been made to use CT to prognosticate patient outcomes in the setting of acute pancreatitis. In our experience, a specific score regarding the severity of pancreatitis is rarely issued during routine scan review. Furthermore, the degree to which initial disease severity documented by imaging correlates with final patient outcome is debated. Nonetheless, we believe radiologists should be familiar with CT imaging findings that potentially portend an unfavorable prognosis in the setting of acute pancreatitis. CT classification schemes have been devised that rely on the detection of inflammatory changes in the pancreas and peripancreatic tissues, the degree of pancreatic necrosis, the location and number of inflammatory fluid collections, and the extension of inflammation into the retroperitoneal interfascial planes (Table 14-4). In general, a larger number and greater extent of inflammatory fluid collections and more extensive pancreatic necrosis are associated with a greater likelihood of a complicated or poor outcome. Investigators have shown that MRI criteria paralleling those used for CT can also be used to assess the severity and clinical course of acute pancreatitis. Advantages of MRI for assessing patients with acute pancreatitis include superior sensitivity for biliary stones and pancreatic hemorrhage compared with CT, although imaging acutely ill patients with MRI can be logistically more difficult.

Table 14-3 Potential Complications of Pancreatitis Visible on Imaging Studies

Pancreatic and peripancreatic	• Acute fluid • Pseudocyst • Necrosis • Infected necrosis • Abscess
Biliary	• Obstruction • Cholecystitis
Gastrointestinal	• Ileus • Obstruction • Hemorrhage • Fistulae
Vascular	• Venous thrombosis • Pseudoaneurysm • Hemorrhage
Extraabdominal	• Pleural effusions • Atelectasis • Bone infarction • Fat necrosis • Pulmonary opacities

Table 14-4   Select Computed Tomographic–Based Scoring Systems for Acute Pancreatitis

System	Finding and Assigned Points or Grade
CT severity index (Balthazar et al., *Radiology* 1990;174:331-336)	Pancreatic inflammation • Normal pancreas = 0 • Pancreatic enlargement = 1 • Inflammation involving pancreas and peripancreatic fat = 2 • Single fluid collection or phlegmon = 3 • Two or more fluid collections or retroperitoneal gas = 4 Degree of pancreatic necrosis • No necrosis = 0 • Necrosis < 30% = 2 • Necrosis = 30-50% = 4 • Necrosis > 50% = 6
Modified CT severity index (Mortele et al., *AJR Am J Roentgenol* 2004;183:1261-1265)	Pancreatic inflammation • Normal pancreas = 0 • Intrinsic pancreatic abnormalities with or without inflammatory changes in peripancreatic fat = 2 • Pancreatic or peripancreatic fluid collection or peripancreatic fat necrosis = 4 Pancreatic necrosis • None = 0 • Necrosis ≤ 30% = 2 • Necrosis > 30% = 4 Extrapancreatic complications (one or more of pleural effusion, ascites, vascular complications, parenchymal complications, or gastrointestinal tract involvement) = 2
EPIC (extrapancreatic inflammation on CT) (De Waele et al., *Pancreas* 2007;34:185-190)	Pleural effusion • None = 0 • Unilateral = 1 • Bilateral = 2 Ascites (perisplenic, perihepatic, interloop, or pelvic) • None = 0 • 1 location = 1 • >1 location = 2 Retroperitoneal inflammation • None = 0 • Unilateral = 1 • Bilateral = 2 Mesenteric inflammation • Absent = 0 • Present = 1
Retroperitoneal extension of inflammatory fluid (Ishikawa et al., *Eur J Radiol* 2006;60:445-452)	• Fluid confined to the anterior pararenal space or spreads into the retromesenteric plane adjacent to the anterior pararenal space = grade I • Fluid spreads farther into the lateroconal plane or retrorenal plane via the retromesenteric plane = grade II • Fluid spreads further caudally into the combined interfascial plane = grade III • Fluid escapes from the interfascial plane into the subfascial plane via the narrow connecting passageway = grade IV • Fluid intrudes directly into the posterior pararenal space across the lateroconal plane, retrorenal plane, or subfascial plane = grade V

CT, Computed tomography.

Pearl: A larger number and greater extent of inflammatory fluid collections and more extensive pancreatic necrosis are associated with a greater likelihood of a complicated or poor outcome in the setting of acute pancreatitis.

Chronic Pancreatitis

Chronic pancreatic inflammation leads to irreversible fibrosis, parenchymal atrophy, and loss of exocrine (and often endocrine) function, a condition referred to as chronic pancreatitis. The parenchymal and ductal changes of chronic pancreatitis can be visualized with a variety of imaging examinations, most notably endoscopic retrograde cholangiopancreatogram (ERCP), endoscopic ultrasound (EUS), MRI, and CT. For many years, ERCP has been considered the gold standard for the diagnosis of chronic pancreatitis, although newer techniques such as MRCP and EUS are becoming more commonplace. Compared with CT, MRCP can better demonstrate ectatic pancreatic ducts, although even copious pancreatic calcifications can be difficult to visualize with MRI. Transabdominal US, CT, and MRI are relatively insensitive for the detection of early or mild chronic pancreatitis. Box 14-1 lists the typical imaging findings of chronic pancreatitis.

The dilated pancreatic duct of chronic pancreatitis can mimic dilatation seen with other entities such as ductal adenocarcinoma or main duct type of intraductal papillary mucinous neoplasm (IPMN). With chronic pancreatitis, the pancreatic duct has an irregular caliber likened to a "chain of lakes" caused by alternating strictures and dilatations (Fig. 14-21). MRI with MRCP is

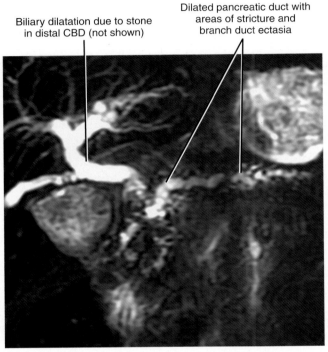

Biliary dilatation due to stone in distal CBD (not shown)

Dilated pancreatic duct with areas of stricture and branch duct ectasia

Figure 14-21 Coronal magnetic resonance cholangiopancreatography image of a patient with chronic pancreatitis. *CBD,* Common bile duct.

superior to CT and US for demonstrating ductal morphologic changes of chronic pancreatitis along the entire extent of the pancreas. When the pancreatic duct dilatation is due to malignant obstruction or excess mucin production without chronic pancreatitis, the duct tends to be less irregular in caliber. Even so, differentiation between chronic pancreatitis and pancreatic cancer on the basis of a single imaging study can sometimes be difficult.

Pitfall: Pancreatic duct obstruction caused by malignant tumor or dilatation caused by mucinous neoplasm can mimic the appearance of chronic pancreatitis on cross-sectional imaging examinations.

The intraductal calcifications of chronic pancreatitis result from proteinaceous debris that plugs the ducts and calcifies. Such calcifications are frequently multifocal within the main duct and branch ducts. When calcifications are sufficiently dense and numerous, the diagnosis of chronic pancreatitis can be suggested based on abdominal radiography. Calcifications appear as focal areas of increased echogenicity with or without shadowing with sonography. CT is superior to other cross-sectional

imaging modalities for the detection of pancreatic calcifications (Fig. 14-22). Although even extensive calcification of the pancreas can be missed on MR images, intraductal stones can occasionally be visualized as low-signal-intensity foci within the pancreatic duct on T2-weighted images. Calcification can occur in a variety of pancreatic neoplasms (microcystic [serous] adenoma, islet cell tumor, mucinous cystic neoplasm, and rarely, ductal adenocarcinoma), but neoplastic calcification usually has a particular appearance (e.g., stellate or curvilinear) that allows distinction from intraductal stones. Occasionally, a calcified splenic artery will mimic the calcifications of chronic pancreatitis on plain radiography and CT images.

Fibrosis results in nonspecific areas of increased echogenicity on transabdominal US images. EUS is a more sensitive imaging technique for the detection of parenchymal changes associated with chronic pancreatitis. The presence of pancreatic fibrosis reduces the signal intensity of the pancreas on T1-weighted MR images and decreases early pancreatic parenchymal enhancement after intravenous contrast administration on both CT and MR images. Peak enhancement of the pancreatic parenchyma is typically delayed in patients with chronic pancreatitis. CT and MRI are essentially equivalent for demonstrating pancreatic parenchymal atrophy. Although parenchymal atrophy is considered a typical imaging finding of chronic pancreatitis, focal pancreatic enlargement also occurs and can be confused with pancreatic cancer.

Pseudocysts also occur in the setting of chronic pancreatitis and are characterized by simple fluid characteristics of their contents and a uniform wall thickness on imaging studies (when not complicated by infection or hemorrhage). MRCP images may be useful in

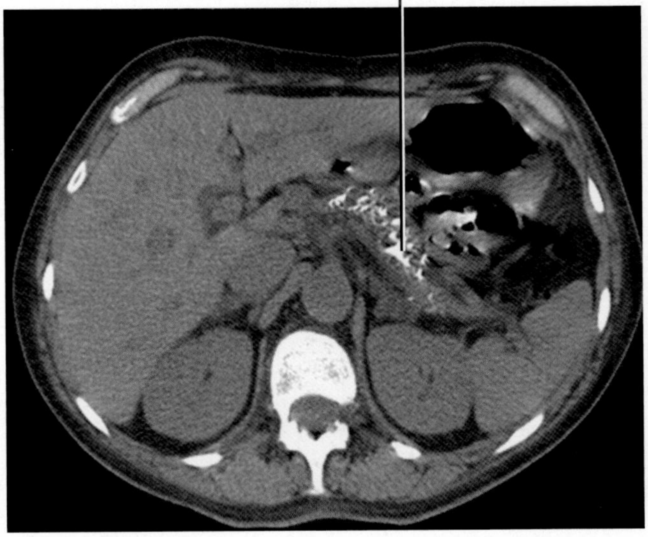

Multiple foci of pancreatic intraductal calcification

Figure 14-22 Unenhanced axial computed tomographic image through the pancreatic body and tail of a patient with chronic pancreatitis and numerous pancreatic intraductal calcifications.

documenting communication of a pseudocyst with the pancreatic duct. Internal enhancing septa and thickened irregular walls favor cystic neoplasm over pseudocyst.

Pearl: Internal enhancing septa, nodules, or thickened irregular walls favor cystic neoplasm over pancreatic pseudocyst.

Intravenously administered secretin increases the production of pancreatic juice, which is ultimately excreted into the duodenum and is a valuable adjunct in the evaluation of patients with chronic pancreatitis. Secretin administration during MRCP can be used to enhance visualization of the pancreatic duct, to detect variant ductal anatomy, and to assess pancreatic exocrine function (Fig. 14-23). Qualitative or semiquantitative (based on the degree to which signal intensity increases within a region of interest within the duodenum) analysis of duodenal filling can be used to diagnose diminished exocrine function. Alternatively, the apparent diffusion coefficient (ADC value) of the pancreas can be calculated over time after the administration of intravenous secretin. In the normal pancreas, the ADC value increases, reaching a peak at approximately 2 minutes. Patients with chronic pancreatitis have a lower baseline pancreatic ADC value, and the ADC value does not increase significantly after secretin stimulation in chronic pancreatitis. A delayed ADC peak can be seen in patients who abuse alcohol. Pancreatic exocrine insufficiency blunts the expected increase in signal intensity within the pancreas on T2-weighted images that is normally seen in response to the administration of secretin.

Groove Pancreatitis

The term *groove pancreatitis* refers to an uncommon form of chronic focal pancreatitis resulting in scarring and fibrosis in the dorsal mesoduodenum, which connects the head of the pancreas, duodenum, and common bile duct (Fig. 14-24). Involvement of the parenchyma of the superior pancreatic head can occur, although inflammation is often restricted to the space between the duodenum and pancreatic head. Groove pancreatitis appears as a hypoechoic mass with US, and as a hypoattenuating, poorly enhancing mass between the pancreatic head and duodenum with CT. With MRI, the mass demonstrates low signal intensity on T1-weighted images and at most mild hyperintensity on T2-weighted images. The fibrous nature of the mass causes delayed enhancement after gadolinium administration that is similar to the pattern seen with pancreatic carcinoma.

Duodenal stenosis, duodenal wall thickening, and Brunner gland hyperplasia are common findings with groove pancreatitis. Cystic lesions can be present within the duodenal wall (Fig. 14-25). Biliary stricture can occur and is characterized by smooth tapering of the common bile duct. Groove pancreatitis often mimics pancreatic carcinoma, although pancreatic cancer is more likely to cause obstructive jaundice and abrupt or irregular narrowing of the common bile duct. In suspected cases of groove pancreatitis, EUS-guided biopsy can be helpful in differentiating between inflammation and cancer.

Pitfall: Groove pancreatitis can mimic carcinoma of the pancreatic head, although groove pancreatitis is less likely to present with obstructive jaundice.

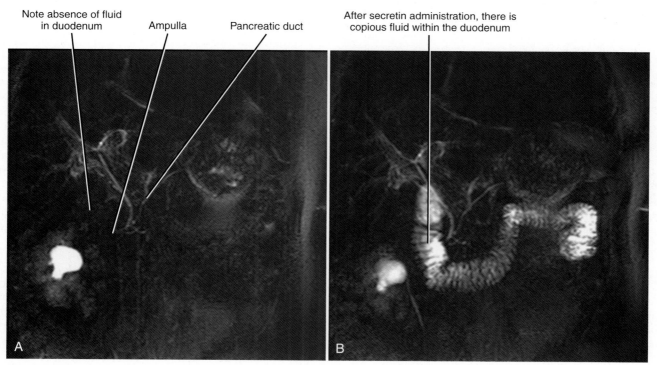

Note absence of fluid in duodenum   Ampulla   Pancreatic duct

After secretin administration, there is copious fluid within the duodenum

A

B

Figure 14-23 Coronal magnetic resonance cholangiopancreatography image before (**A**) and several minutes after (**B**) administration of intravenous secretin in a patient with normal pancreatic exocrine function.

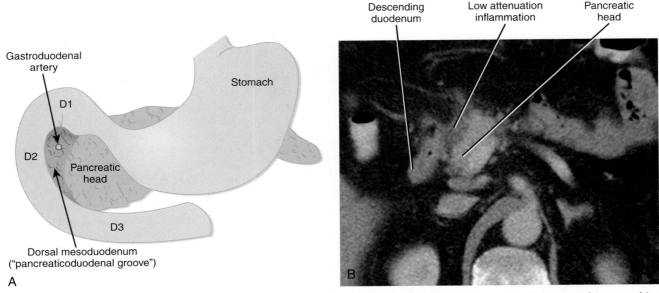

Figure 14-24 "Groove pancreatitis." **A,** Anatomy of the dorsal mesoduodenum, the site of groove pancreatitis. **B,** Computed tomographic image showing inflammation between the duodenum and pancreatic head.

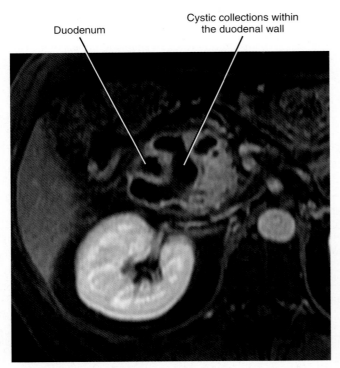

Figure 14-25 Enhanced T1-weighted fat-suppressed magnetic resonance image through the pancreatic head of a patient with cystic changes of the duodenal wall related to chronic pancreatic inflammation.

Autoimmune Pancreatitis

Autoimmune pancreatitis is an uncommon entity that, until recently, received relatively little attention from radiologists. Also known as lymphocytoplasmacytic sclerosing pancreatitis, this entity differs from alcohol-induced chronic pancreatitis in that the morphologic and functional abnormalities are reversible if the diagnosis is suggested and the patient appropriately treated with steroids. Autoimmune pancreatitis can be associated with other autoimmune abnormalities such as Sjögren syndrome. Serum γ-globulin level may be increased, but increased IgG levels are not entirely specific. The degree of increase of serum amylase and lipase levels is typically modest despite the imaging appearance of pancreatic inflammation. Because of the potential for dramatic clinical improvement after appropriate diagnosis and treatment, it is critical that radiologists consider this diagnosis in patients referred for pancreatic imaging.

Diffuse pancreatic enlargement, rather than parenchymal atrophy, is typical of autoimmune pancreatitis. Parenchymal and intraductal calcifications are usually absent, and the pancreatic duct tends to be diffusely and irregularly narrowed rather than dilated. Changes within the pancreatic duct are best demonstrated with ERCP and can be difficult to appreciate with CT, MRI, or transabdominal sonography. With CT, a low-attenuation rim surrounding the enlarged pancreas is typical but not always present, and pancreatic enhancement tends to be delayed. Inflammatory changes within the peripancreatic fat tend to be minimal, and pseudocysts are absent. With MRI, the pancreas may have lower-than-normal signal intensity on T1-weighted images, and a low-signal-intensity capsule-like rim may be visible on T1- and T2-weighted images. Focal, rather than diffuse, pancreatic enlargement can occasionally result from autoimmune pancreatitis, and differentiation from a neoplastic mass is difficult in such cases.

Obstructive jaundice is common in patients with autoimmune pancreatitis. The intrapancreatic portion of the common bile duct is usually narrowed, and bile duct abnormalities simulating sclerosing cholangitis may be visible on MRCP images in some patients. As with the pancreatic parenchymal abnormalities, the biliary abnormalities of autoimmune pancreatitis resolve after steroid therapy. Takahashi and colleagues report a variety of renal lesions in patients with autoimmune pancreatitis, including cortical nodules and wedge-shaped lesions that also resolved with steroid therapy.

Pearl: Autoimmune pancreatitis should be considered in patients with diffuse pancreatic enlargement without significant surrounding inflammatory fluid or pancreatic ductal dilatation. Biliary and renal abnormalities may also be present and typically respond to steroid therapy.

Pancreatitis and Cancer

Patients with chronic pancreatitis are at increased risk for development of pancreatic cancer. However, not all focal masses occurring in the presence of chronic pancreatitis represent malignant tumor. Differentiating between inflammatory masses of chronic pancreatitis and pancreatic cancer remains a challenge, because both conditions may present with similar symptoms, both entities can cause pancreatic parenchymal atrophy and duct dilatation, and both entities spread locally along similar pathways. Box 14-2 lists some imaging findings that favor the presence of pancreatic cancer over pancreatitis. Of course, there are exceptions to these rules, and tissue diagnosis remains the standard for differentiating between inflammation and cancer. Pancreatic carcinoma (because of its desmoplastic nature) and inflammatory mass of pancreatitis (because of the presence of fibrosis) can exhibit an identical enhancement pattern of progressive delayed enhancement after intravenous contrast administration. The attenuation value of a chronic inflammatory mass can also be identical to that of pancreatic cancer. Therefore, none of the features listed in Box 14-2 is entirely specific for pancreatic cancer.

Pitfall: Always remember that pancreatitis can mimic, coexist with, or be caused by neoplasm.

BOX 14-2   Imaging Findings That Should Prompt Consideration of Pancreatic Carcinoma

Soft-tissue mass in background of an atrophic gland
Segmental rather than diffuse atrophy of the pancreas
Dilatation of both the common bile duct and pancreatic duct (double duct sign)
Pancreatic duct dilated to a point of abrupt termination (duct cutoff)
No main pancreatic duct visualized within the mass
Main pancreatic duct-width/gland-width ratio > 0.5
Vascular invasion or encasement
Development of a new mass
Growth of a mass
Mass displaces calcifications or progressively obliterates the pancreatic duct over time
Metastases

■ DILATED PANCREATIC DUCT

Pancreatic ductal dilatation is a common finding on imaging studies. When confronted with pancreatic duct dilatation, one must determine whether the duct is truly dilated, whether the duct is obstructed or filled with mucin (in the case of IPMN), and whether the dilatation is due to benign or malignant disease. The normal pancreatic duct usually measures less than 3 mm in diameter and is continuous from the tail to the ampulla without abrupt alterations in caliber. Table 14-5 lists the major entities to be considered when encountering pancreatic ductal dilatation.

Table 14-5   Dilated Pancreatic Duct

Cause of Duct Dilatation	Imaging Features That May Be Present
Chronic pancreatitis (see Fig. 14-21)	• Alternating dilations and strictures (chain of lakes) • Strictures short and symmetrical • Ectatic branch ducts • Ratio of duct width to total gland width < 0.5 • Intraductal calcifications • Fistulas, pseudocysts
Intraductal papillary mucinous neoplasm (IPMN) (Figs. 14-26 and 14-27)	• Duct dilated to level of ampulla • Bulging ampulla • Ectatic branch ducts • Enhancing soft-tissue nodules (concerning for malignant IPMN)
Ductal adenocarcinoma (Fig. 14-28)	• Abrupt cutoff of duct • Dilated bile duct • Vascular encasement • Ill-defined mass with gradual progressive enhancement • Smoothly dilated duct • Strictures longer, more irregular • Ratio of duct width to total gland width > 0.5
Inflammatory stricture (Fig. 14-29)	• No visible mass • Short segment of narrowing
Ampullary stone	• Filling defect at ampulla (endoscopic retrograde cholangiopancreatography, magnetic resonance cholangiopancreatography) • Echogenic focus (with/without shadowing) at ampulla (ultrasound or endoscopic ultrasound)
Ampullary or periampullary tumor (Fig. 14-30)	• Mass in region of ampulla • Pancreatic duct dilated to ampulla

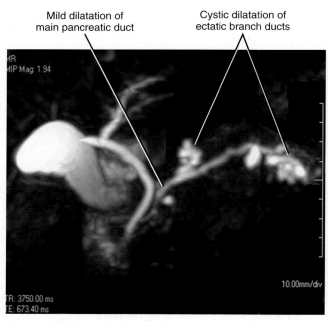

Figure 14-26 Coronal maximum intensity projection image of the pancreatic duct of a patient with intraductal pappilary mucinous neoplasm (IPMN).

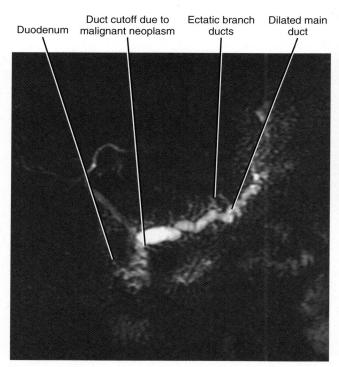

Figure 14-27 Coronal thick-slab magnetic resonance cholangio-pancreatographic image through the pancreas of a patient with long-standing pancreatic duct dilatation. Because of increasing duct dilatation and increasing soft-tissue mass on computed tomography and magnetic resonance imaging, patient underwent surgery and malignant intraductal papillary mucinous neoplasm was removed.

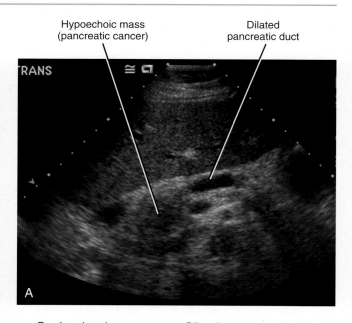

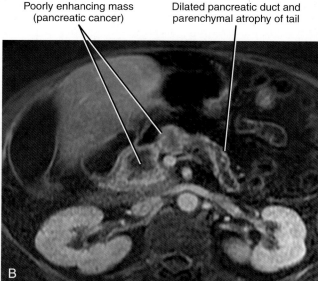

Figure 14-28 Transverse sonogram (A) and enhanced magnetic resonance imaging (B) through the upper abdomen of a woman with ductal adenocarcinoma of the pancreas.

■ PRACTICAL APPROACH TO CYSTIC LESIONS OF THE PANCREAS

The topic of cystic pancreatic masses instills in many individuals a sense of frustration or fear. This relatively simple subject would not warrant such emotions were it not for the ever-evolving and lengthening lexicon used to categorize these lesions. One might mistake the proliferation of terms used to refer to cystic pancreatic masses for a proliferation of distinct pathologic entities. In reality, there are relatively few lesions with which one must be familiar. Table 14-6 lists some neoplasms of the pancreas that can appear cystic, together with their various aliases, primarily for entertainment purposes. We have tried to list these lesions by their most fashionable name at the time of this writing, but be aware that things may have changed by the

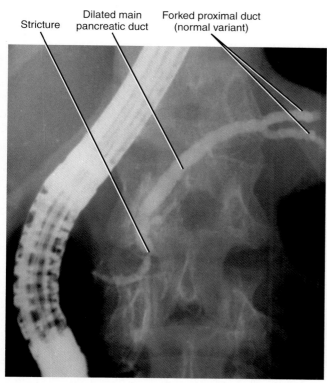

Stricture | Dilated main pancreatic duct | Forked proximal duct (normal variant)

Figure 14-29 Pancreatogram from an endoscopic retrograde chol-angiopancreatogram in a young woman with pancreatic duct stricture. Changes of acute and chronic pancreatitis were found at surgery.

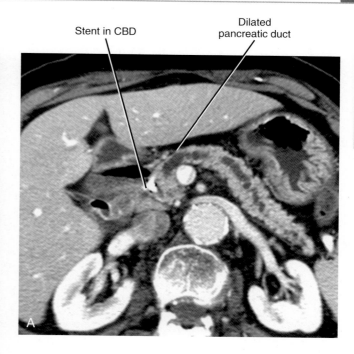

Stent in CBD | Dilated pancreatic duct

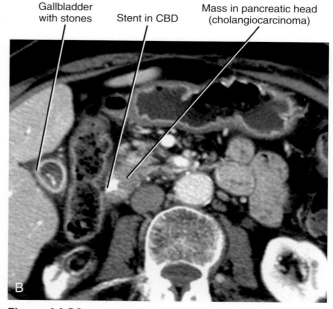

Gallbladder with stones | Stent in CBD | Mass in pancreatic head (cholangiocarcinoma)

Figure 14-30 Enhanced axial computed tomographic images through the body and tail (**A**) and head (**B**) of the pancreas of a patient with cholangiocarcinoma of the distal bile duct. *CBD,* Common bile duct.

time you read this. It is also quite likely that the list of names provided is incomplete.

Four Pancreatic Cystic Lesions You Must Know About

The following discussion addresses some common cystic lesions of pancreatic origin in more detail. Knowledge of these four entities will cover most cystic pancreatic lesions encountered in daily practice.

Microcystic Adenoma (Serous Cystadenoma)

Microcystic adenomas are benign neoplasms with no malignant potential that have a predilection to occur in middle-aged or older women. An association with von Hippel–Lindau disease has been reported, but most cases are sporadic. Microcystic adenomas are asymptomatic when small, and resection is indicated only for the relief of symptoms related to mass effect. The classic CT appearance of this lesion consists of a somewhat lobulated mass in the head of the pancreas composed of multiple small (<2 cm) cysts and a central calcified stellate scar (Fig. 14-31). The individual cysts of some lesions may be too small to clearly resolve with CT, and the cyst walls can enhance, occasionally giving the lesion the appearance of a solid enhancing mass after intravenous contrast administration. In such cases, EUS or MRI often show the true cystic nature of the lesion. When small individual cysts are resolved with imaging, microcystic adenoma classically resembles a honeycomb.

With transabdominal US, microcystic adenomas can appear as a multicystic mass, a mixed solid and cystic mass, or a solid-appearing echogenic mass depending on the size and number of cysts. Posterior acoustic enhancement is often visible because of the cystic nature of the mass. When present, the central scar appears echogenic on sonograms. Flow may be detected within the cyst walls with Doppler imaging. With MRI, these tumors are very high signal intensity on T2-weighted

Table 14-6   Pancreatic Cystic Neoplasms and Their Aliases

Tumor	Also Known As...
Microcystic adenoma*	• Microcystic cystadenoma • Serous cystadenoma • Serous cystic neoplasm/tumor • Serous microcystic adenoma • Glycogen-rich adenoma • Glycogen-rich cystadenoma
Mucinous cystic neoplasm†	• Macrocystic adenoma • Macrocystic cystadenoma • Mucinous macrocystic adenoma • Mucinous cystadenoma • Mucinous macrocystic neoplasm • Mucin hypersecreting carcinoma
Intraductal papillary mucinous neoplasm†	• Intraductal papillary mucinous tumor • Intraductal papillary neoplasm • Mucinous ductal ectasia • Mucin hypersecreting tumor • Mucin villous adenomatosis • Ductectatic tumor • Ductectatic mucinous tumor • Ductectatic cystadenoma
Solid pseudopapillary tumor‡	• Solid and papillary epithelial neoplasm • Solid and cystic papillary neoplasm • Solid cystic papillary epithelial neoplasm • Solid-cystic papillary tumor • Papillary cystic neoplasm (tumor) • Papillary solid-cystic neoplasm • Papillary cystic (and) solid tumor

*To further the confusion, this category also includes a subcategory of lesions with fewer and larger cysts known as macrocystic serous cystadenoma or serous oligocystic adenoma. A solid variant has also been described.
†Includes premalignant and malignant varieties.
‡Has variable cystic component because of hemorrhage, cystic degeneration, and necrosis, hence the variable appearance of "solid" and "cystic" in its name.

images regardless of cyst size. The cysts only occasionally hemorrhage and, therefore, are usually of relatively low signal intensity on T1-weighted images. The individual cyst walls or septa are best seen on gadolinium-enhanced T1-weighted images. The central scar can demonstrate delayed enhancement after intravenous contrast administration when not densely calcified.

Although the presence of a central scar and location within the pancreatic head are classic findings of microcystic adenoma, a central stellate scar is frequently absent, and lesions are not uncommonly found in the body and tail of the pancreas. Bile duct and pancreatic duct dilatation are not usually present (but can be present in some cases because of mass effect), and these tumors do not encase or invade vessels. Microcystic adenomas do not communicate with the pancreatic duct, although this feature may be difficult to confirm for lesions that are in close proximity to the duct.

A macrocystic variant of microcystic adenoma has been described, creating potential confusion with mucinous cystic neoplasm on imaging studies. Because this variant often consists of fewer individual cysts than the typical microcystic adenoma, and to avoid confusion with mucinous cystic neoplasms (also known as macrocystic adenoma), the term *oligocystic* is often used to describe this variant. CT findings typical of oligocystic serous cystadenoma that may be helpful in distinguishing this entity from pancreatic pseudocyst or mucinous cystic neoplasm include location in the pancreatic head, lobulated contour, and lack of wall enhancement (Fig. 14-32). A rare variant of microcystic adenoma that has been described is the solid serous adenoma. We predict that it is only a matter of time

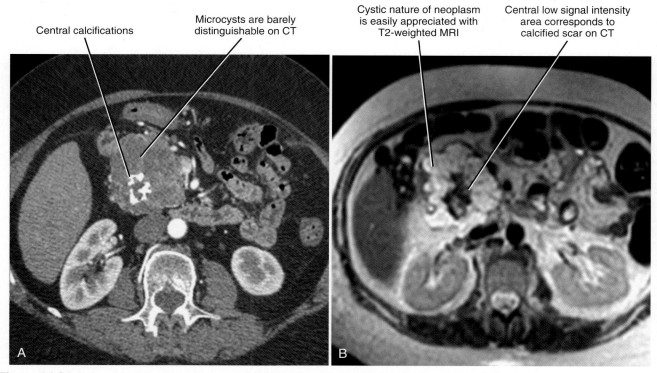

Figure 14-31 Enhanced axial computed tomographic (CT) **(A)** and T2-weighted magnetic resonance **(B)** images through the pancreatic head of an elderly woman with serous cystadenoma. *MRI,* Magnetic resonance imaging.

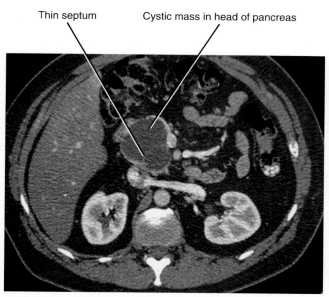

Thin septum   Cystic mass in head of pancreas

Figure 14-32 Enhanced axial computed tomographic image through the pancreatic head of a patient with oligocystic serous cystadenoma.

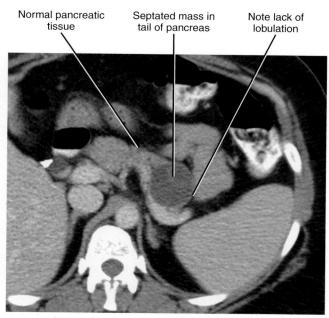

Normal pancreatic tissue   Septated mass in tail of pancreas   Note lack of lobulation

Figure 14-33 Enhanced axial computed tomographic image through the pancreatic tail of a patient with a mucinous cystic neoplasm of the pancreas.

before someone describes the solid and macrocystic microcystic adenoma.

Given that many microcystic adenomas do not demonstrate completely specific imaging characteristics, EUS may be extremely beneficial in establishing the diagnosis when glycogen-rich epithelial cells are obtained via aspiration.

Pearl: The diagnosis of microcystic (serous) adenoma should be considered when a lobulated mass consisting of multiple tiny cysts and a central scar is present in the pancreatic head of an older woman.

Mucinous Cystic Neoplasm

Mucinous cystic neoplasms (Fig. 14-33) are significantly more common in women than in men, have malignant potential (if not malignant at diagnosis), and as the name implies, are composed of mucin-filled cysts. These lesions can contain ovarian-type stroma. Unlike microcystic adenoma and IPMN, mucinous cystic neoplasms have a predilection for the pancreatic body and tail. These lesions may be unilocular or multilocular, and the individual cysts often exceed 2 cm in diameter. The outer wall of a mucinous cystic neoplasm tends to be thicker and less lobulated (smoother) than that of microcystic adenoma, and curvilinear calcifications may be visible in the wall or septa on CT images. Unlike IPMN, these lesions do not normally communicate with the pancreatic duct, although they can occasionally compress and obstruct the pancreatic duct.

Transabdominal US demonstrates the cystic nature of mucinous cystic neoplasms, although the cysts can contain echogenic debris or mural nodules. With MRI, most mucinous cystic neoplasms are bright on T2-weighted images with lower-signal-intensity septa or papillary projections. On T1-weighted images, signal intensity of the individual cysts varies based on the

amount of hemorrhage or protein present. The septa and papillary projections enhance on CT and MRI after intravenous contrast administration. The presence of enhancing nodules and thick septa suggests malignancy, and the presence of adjacent organ invasion or metastases confirms the malignant nature of a mucinous cystic neoplasm. EUS with cyst aspiration aids in establishing the diagnosis when aspirated cyst fluid contains high-viscosity mucin and increased levels of CA 19-9, CEA, or CA 72-4.

Pearl: The diagnosis of mucinous cystic neoplasm should be suggested when a smoothly marginated septated cystic mass not in communication with the pancreatic duct is present in the body or tail of the pancreas of a middle-aged woman.

Intraductal Papillary Mucinous Neoplasm

IPMN stands for *intraductal papillary mucinous neoplasm*. We like this term because it tells something about the tumor: that it is a neoplasm of cells that exhibit an intraductal papillary growth pattern and secrete mucin into the duct. It should not be surprising that one of the diagnostic clues to the diagnosis of IPMN is communication with the pancreatic duct, a feature lacking with mucinous cystic neoplasm and microcystic adenoma. Because an excess of mucin is secreted into the pancreatic duct, another clue to this diagnosis is a bulging papilla filled with mucin. Although this sign is often absent in cases of IPMN, when present, it is helpful in distinguishing IPMN from other causes of pancreatic duct dilatation. IPMN can be broadly categorized into several types: main duct, branch duct (or side branch), or mixed. Main duct involvement is associated with a greater incidence of malignancy, particularly when the duct diameter exceeds 1 cm or when intraductal nodules are present (see Fig. 14-27). Glandular atrophy is often present with main duct IPMN, potentially resulting in confusion with chronic pancreatitis.

Branch duct IPMN is most common in, but not exclusive to, older men. Lesions are commonly located in the pancreatic head or uncinate process and are often incidentally discovered (Fig. 14-34). The appearance of branch duct IPMN has been appropriately likened to a cluster of grapes. Individual cystic components may range from a few millimeters to several centimeters in diameter. Because of the ductal nature of the tumor, the cystic areas can have a tubular appearance. The mucin that gives IPMN its cystic appearance appears indistinguishable from simple fluid with US, CT, and MRI. Calcifications and hemorrhage are not common imaging features of IPMN. When attempting to establish the diagnosis of IPMN, emphasis should be on demonstrating communication of the cystic mass with the pancreatic duct. The major differential diagnostic consideration for a cystic mass communicating with the pancreatic duct is pancreatic pseudocyst.

Transabdominal US of branch duct IPMN demonstrates a multicystic mass but rarely allows definitive characterization. CT and MRI with MRCP may be helpful in demonstrating communication between the cystic mass and the pancreatic duct. Attempts to establish communication with the duct are facilitated through the use of thin-section multiplanar reconstructions (CT) or multiplanar acquisitions (MRI).

IPMN can be benign or malignant. Features that have been associated with malignant IPMN include enhancing mural nodules, a dilated (>10 mm) main pancreatic duct, and lesions larger than 3 cm. Overt features of malignancy include vascular encasement, invasion of adjacent structures or organs, and metastases. Smaller lesions without these features are sometimes followed with serial imaging, particularly when surgical resection is ill-advised because of age or comorbidities.

Pearl: One should consider the diagnosis of IPMN when a cystic lesion is discovered in the uncinate process of an elderly man, particularly when the lesion communicates with the pancreatic duct.

Pancreatic Pseudocyst

Pancreatitis-related pseudocyst (see Figs. 14-15 and 14-16) is the most common cystic lesion of the pancreas. As a result, these nonneoplastic lesions are the major differential consideration when encountering a cystic-appearing pancreatic mass. Although the presence or history of pancreatitis can be helpful in suggesting the diagnosis of pancreatic pseudocyst, one must always keep in mind that pancreatitis can coexist with or result from neoplastic pancreatic lesions. Therefore, peripancreatic inflammation supports but does not prove the diagnosis of pancreatic pseudocyst.

Pancreatic pseudocysts are usually unilocular, occasionally multilocular, and often multiple. With US, internal echoes or layering debris are often visible, and septa are less commonly observed. Color Doppler interrogation reveals no evidence of internal blood flow and is an important technique for excluding pseudoaneurysm. Uncomplicated pseudocysts measure fluid density on CT images, although hemorrhagic pseudocysts are common and appear higher than water density. The

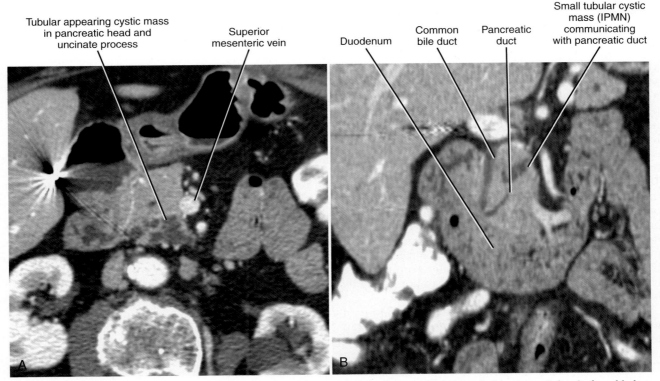

Figure 14-34 Enhanced axial computed tomographic image **(A)** and coronal reformation **(B)** through the pancreatic head of an elderly man with branch duct intraductal papillary mucinous neoplasm (IPMN).

fibrous capsule of a pseudocyst typically enhances after intravenous contrast administration but does not exhibit enhancing excrescences. Gas within a pseudocyst may result from infection, enteric communication, or recent intervention (Fig. 14-35). The diagnosis of infection in the absence of gas may be difficult to establish with imaging alone. Therefore, when an infected pseudocyst is suspected, fluid aspiration or drainage is appropriate.

Pitfall: Gas within a pancreatic pseudocyst does not always signify infection. Gas can result from an enteric communication or an intervention such as aspiration or ERCP.

With MRI, uncomplicated pseudocysts are low signal intensity on T1-weighted images and very high signal intensity on T2-weighted images. As with CT, there should be no enhancing nodules or enhancing septa within a pseudocyst. Hemorrhagic or proteinaceous pseudocysts demonstrate increased signal intensity on T1-weighted images and variable signal intensity on T2-weighted images. Occasionally, a layered appearance may be evident because of dependent settling of blood products or debris.

Pseudocysts can mimic any of the cystic neoplasms discussed to this point in this chapter. For example, main pancreatic duct dilatation can be present with either IPMN or pancreatic pseudocyst occurring in the setting of chronic pancreatitis. The latter entity is often associated with pancreatic calcifications, and pancreatic duct strictures are typically associated with chronic pancreatitis but not with IPMN. When present, a bulging

papilla indicates IPMN rather than chronic pancreatitis. Communication with the pancreatic duct occurs with either pseudocyst or IPMN, but when visible on CT or MR images, communication is helpful in excluding mucinous cystic neoplasm or microcystic adenoma. The presence of enhancing septa or nodules favors a cystic neoplasm over pseudocyst.

Pearl: A cystic pancreatic mass that communicates with the pancreatic duct is most likely to be a pancreatic pseudocyst or branch duct IPMN.

Cystic lesions of the pancreas are summarized in Table 14-7 and Box 14-3.

■ SOLID PANCREATIC MASSES

Most solid pancreatic masses encountered in a typical clinical radiology practice are either ductal adenocarcinomas or neuroendocrine tumors. Both ductal adenocarcinomas and neuroendocrine tumors have typical appearances that allow accurate preoperative characterization in the majority of cases. Because inflammatory processes and a variety of rare primary and secondary pancreatic neoplasms can mimic these entities, tissue sampling via percutaneous, endoscopic, or surgical techniques is still performed in most cases before treatment.

Although the majority of cystic pancreatic lesions are benign, the presence of a solid pancreatic mass is an ominous finding. Box 14-4 lists imaging findings that suggest the presence of a solid pancreatic neoplasm. Most of the imaging findings listed here can also be associated with acute or chronic inflammation in the absence of neoplasm.

Ductal Adenocarcinoma

Ductal adenocarcinoma of the pancreas arises from duct epithelium of the exocrine pancreas and is the most common solid neoplasm of the pancreas. These cancers tend to be dense fibrous tumors that occur most often in the head of the pancreas in patients older than 60 years. Patients usually present with some combination of pain, weight loss, and in the case of pancreatic head tumors, jaundice. Unfortunately, patients often present with locally advanced disease, and this carcinoma has a poor prognosis despite aggressive surgical options.

Sonography is rarely used as the sole preoperative imaging modality in patients with known pancreatic cancer, but one must be aware of the sonographic findings that can lead to discovery of an unsuspected tumor. With sonography, pancreatic cancer usually appears as an ill-defined, predominantly hypoechoic mass, although the relative appearance and conspicuity of a pancreatic carcinoma depends, in part, on the echogenicity of the surrounding unaffected pancreas. Doppler imaging rarely demonstrates significantly increased vascularity of the lesion. As with other cross-sectional imaging modalities, abrupt termination of a dilated pancreatic duct is a concerning finding that

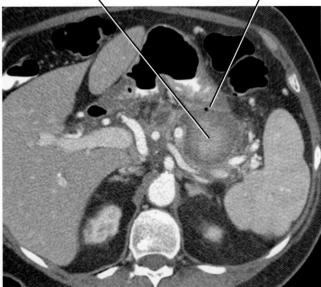

High density material within the pseudocyst represents contrast material injected at ERCP

Gas within pseudocyst introduced at time of ERCP

Figure 14-35 Enhanced axial computed tomographic image through the pancreas of a patient with a pancreatic pseudocyst who had recently undergone endoscopic retrograde cholangiopancreatography (ERCP). A communication between the pancreatic duct and pseudocyst resulted in gas and contrast material accumulation within the pseudocyst.

Table 14-7   Quick Guide to Cystic Neoplasms of the Pancreas and Their Mimics

Cystic Mass	Helpful Clinical Information	Helpful Imaging Features
Microcystic adenoma (also known as serous cystadenoma) (see Fig. 14-31)	Most often occurs in middle-aged or elderly women	• Lobulated contour • Thin capsule • Stellate scar (with/without calcification) • Honeycomb appearance • Subtle, thin septa • Cysts < 1.5 cm • More than six cysts • No mural nodules • Most common in pancreatic head
Mucinous cystic neoplasm (also known as macrocystic or mucinous cystadenoma) (see Fig. 14-33)	Most often occur in middle-aged women	• Cysts > 1.5 cm • Fewer than six cysts • Smooth outer contour • Enhancing septa • Mural nodules (suggests malignancy) • Curvilinear cyst wall calcification • No communication with pancreatic duct • Most common in pancreatic body or tail
Intraductal papillary mucinous neoplasm (see Fig. 14-34)	Most often occur in elderly men	• Communication with pancreatic duct • Grapelike cluster of small cysts • Dilated pancreatic duct • Bulging ampulla • Mural nodules (suggests malignancy)
Epithelial cyst (Fig. 14-36)	von Hippel–Lindau disease, autosomal dominant polycystic kidney disease	• Thin wall • Unilocular • No enhancement or internal flow • No communication with pancreatic duct
Solid pseudopapillary tumor	Most often occur in young Asian or African-American female individuals	• Solid and cystic mass • Intratumoral hemorrhage
Pseudocyst (see Figs. 14-15 and 14-16)	Acute or chronic pancreatitis	• Communication with duct • Evidence of pancreatitis • Rapid growth or resolution • No enhancing septa or excrescences
Duodenal diverticulum (Fig. 14-37)		• Communication with duodenum • Appearance changes over short intervals (minutes) • Often contains air

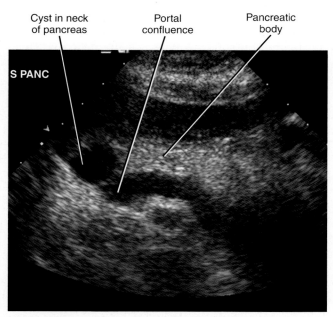

Cyst in neck of pancreas   Portal confluence   Pancreatic body

S PANC

Figure 14-36 Transverse sonogram through the pancreas of a patient with autosomal dominant polycystic kidney disease demonstrates an epithelial cyst.

should prompt a search for other signs of pancreatic tumor (see Fig. 14-28). Bile duct dilatation with abrupt termination of the common bile duct in the pancreatic head region without evidence of a stone is likewise suggestive of neoplasm. Gallbladder distention and sludge may be present, and the sonographic Murphy sign is usually negative in this setting.

Once a pancreatic cancer is suspected with US, one should look for signs that may complicate or preclude surgical resection. These include celiac axis or SMA encasement and venous invasion. Venous involvement may be suspected in the setting of enlarged venous collaterals, a dilated gastrocolic trunk, or failure to identify the splenic vein or SMV.

EUS is more sensitive than cross-sectional imaging modalities such as CT and MRI for small tumors in the pancreatic head region and has the advantage of facilitating biopsy. EUS is not typically relied on as a standalone staging modality, although it generally performs well for the detection of vascular invasion and abnormal regional lymph nodes. Intraoperative US may be a useful adjunct to laparotomy to detect the presence of unsuspected liver metastases before an attempt at a Whipple procedure.

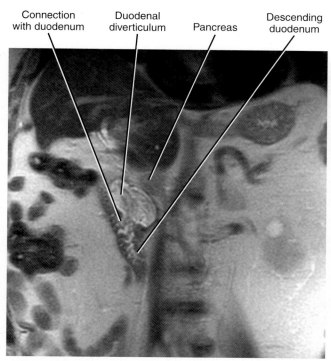

Connection with duodenum | Duodenal diverticulum | Pancreas | Descending duodenum

Figure 14-37 Coronal T2-weighted magnetic resonance image through the pancreatic head region demonstrates a duodenal diverticulum.

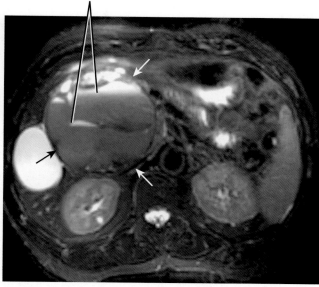

Fluid-fluid levels due to presence of blood products within cystic spaces

Figure 14-38 Axial T2-weighted magnetic resonance imaging through the pancreatic head of a patient with a cystic islet cell tumor *(arrows)*. Extensive cystic changes and hemorrhage were found at pathologic examination.

CT has become the primary imaging modality for the evaluation of patients with known or suspected pancreatic cancer. The key to detecting and staging pancreatic cancer with CT is meticulous attention to technique. Institutions and investigators do not necessarily agree on the best way to perform pancreatic CT for the detection and staging of pancreatic cancer. However, certain components should be present, even if the exact imaging parameters are disputed. Thin-section imaging allows detection of small lesions and creation of multiplanar or curved reformations. Intravenous contrast should be administered as a rapid intravenous bolus. Postcontrast-enhanced images should be obtained in such a way that maximizes tumor and vessel conspicuity.

This latter requirement typically involves imaging multiple times after contrast administration. Some individuals prefer an arterial-phase image, a pancreatic parenchymal–phase image (usually about 35-45 seconds

after contrast administration), and a portal-venous–phase image. Of these three phases, the arterial phase may be the least important, because arterial enhancement is probably still sufficient for staging purposes during the pancreatic parenchymal phase. However, an arterial phase image does permit the creation of impressive CT angiogram images. Many centers administer oral water before imaging in an effort to distend the duodenum with negative contrast, although this is variably successful.

BOX 14-3   Additional Rare Causes of Cystic Pancreatic Mass*

Ductal adenocarcinoma
Islet cell tumor (Fig. 14-38)
Lymphangioma
Metastasis
Echinococcus
Acinar cell carcinoma
Mature cystic teratoma
Inflammatory pseudotumor
Giant cell tumor

*Many of these lesions typically present as solid tumors.

BOX 14-4   Imaging Findings of Solid Pancreatic Neoplasm

Focal contour abnormality or pancreatic enlargement
Rounding of uncinate process
Loss of pancreatic lobulation
Parenchymal atrophy (body or tail)
Focal area of sparing in fat-replaced pancreas (Fig. 14-39)
Focal area of decreased echogenicity on US
(see Fig. 14-28)
Focal low-attenuation area on CT
Focal low-signal-intensity area on T1-weighted MRI
(see Fig. 14-3)
Focal high-signal-intensity area on T2-weighted MRI
Loss of fat plane around superior mesenteric artery
(Fig. 14-40)
Peripancreatic lymph-node enlargement
Pancreatic and/or biliary duct dilatation (double duct sign when both dilated) (Fig. 14-41)
Abrupt termination of a dilated pancreatic duct
(duct cutoff sign) (Fig. 14-42)
Focal area of differential enhancement on CT or MRI

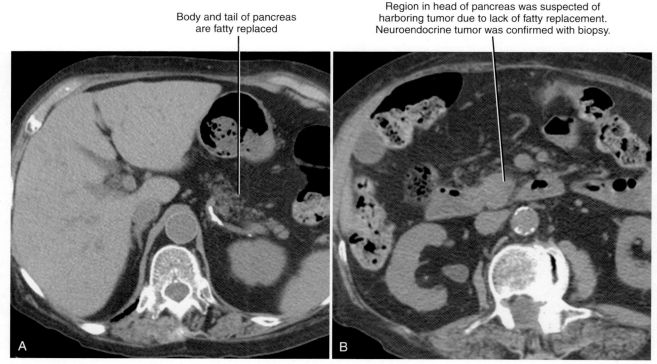

Body and tail of pancreas are fatty replaced

Region in head of pancreas was suspected of harboring tumor due to lack of fatty replacement. Neuroendocrine tumor was confirmed with biopsy.

Figure 14-39 Unenhanced axial computed tomographic images through the tail (**A**) and head (**B**) of the pancreas of a patient with a neuroendocrine tumor occurring in a background of fatty pancreas.

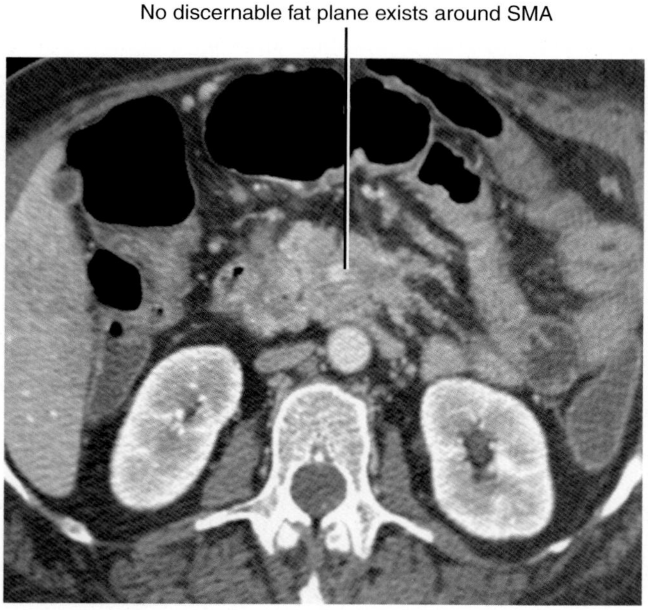

No discernable fat plane exists around SMA

Figure 14-40 Enhanced axial computed tomographic image through the upper abdomen of a patient with pancreatic cancer encasing the superior mesenteric artery (SMA).

Ductal adenocarcinoma tends to be isoattenuating compared with normal pancreas on unenhanced CT images, although necrotic or mucinous tumors may appear hypodense. Most pancreatic carcinomas will remain hypoattenuating relative to the pancreas during the arterial and parenchymal phases of imaging. Pancreatic carcinomas tend to be hypovascular, fibrous tumors that slowly and progressively enhance after intravenous contrast administration on CT and MR examinations (Fig. 14-43). This feature helps to distinguish adenocarcinomas from neuroendocrine tumors, which tend to be hyperenhancing on early-phase images.

MRI is capable of similar rates of pancreatic tumor detection and similar tumor staging accuracy compared with CT. However, MRI is seldom performed once an adequate-quality CT scan has been obtained in a patient with pancreatic cancer. MRI of the pancreas should include a combination of T1- and T2-weighted images in addition to T1-weighted, fat-suppressed, dynamic, gadolinium-enhanced images.

Because the normal pancreas is relatively bright on a fat-suppressed T1-weighted image, pancreatic carcinoma will appear as an area of lower signal intensity with this type of sequence (see Fig. 14-3). MRCP images clearly demonstrate dilatation of the pancreatic and common bile ducts when present. Abrupt termination of the pancreatic duct before the level of the ampulla, particularly when associated with common bile duct dilatation, is suggestive of pancreatic cancer (see Figs. 14-41 and 14-42).

PET is relatively sensitive for detection of pancreatic cancer (possibly exceeding 90%). However, PET lacks specificity, because pancreatic inflammation (i.e., acute or chronic pancreatitis) can also demonstrate increased activity.

Additional information on staging of pancreatic cancer is available in Chapter 10. Box 14-5 lists some imaging features that may complicate or preclude surgical

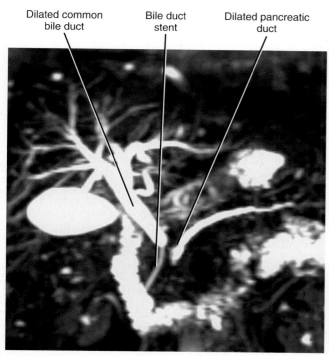

Dilated common bile duct   Bile duct stent   Dilated pancreatic duct

Figure 14-41 Coronal maximum intensity projection image from a respiratory-triggered magnetic resonance cholangiopancreatogram of a patient with ductal adenocarcinoma of the pancreas demonstrating the "double duct" sign.

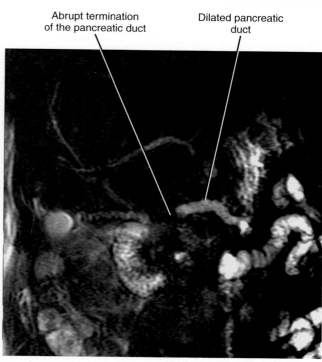

Abrupt termination of the pancreatic duct   Dilated pancreatic duct

Figure 14-42 Coronal thick-slab magnetic resonance cholangiopancreatographic image demonstrates the pancreatic duct "cutoff" sign in a patient with ductal adenocarcinoma of the pancreas.

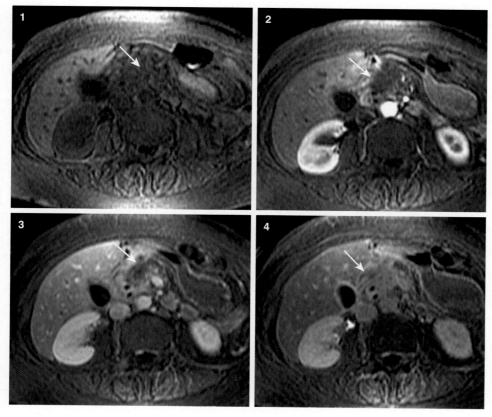

1 - precontrast
2 - arterial phase
3 - portal phase
4 - equilibrium phase

Figure 14-43 Four images from a multiphase, gadolinium-enhanced, magnetic resonance examination of the pancreas of a patient with ductal adenocarcinoma *(arrows)* demonstrating the slow, progressive enhancement pattern typical of pancreatic cancer. *1,* Precontrast; *2,* arterial phase; *3,* portal phase; *4,* equilibrium phase.

- Tumor contiguous with more than 50% (180 degrees) of the circumference of a major artery (celiac axis, common/proper hepatic artery, superior mesenteric artery) (Figs. 14-40 and 14-44)
- Distorted shape, thrombosis, or obliteration of a major vein (portal vein, SMV or portal confluence)†
- Distant metastases
- Peritoneal implants

*Determinants of resectability vary by institution and individual. Therefore, one should always consult with one's referring surgeons regarding what constitutes an unresectable tumor. Furthermore, tumors initially deemed unresectable may undergo neoadjuvant chemotherapy/radiation therapy to improve the chances for resection.
†Some surgeons will operate in the setting of venous involvement, opting to perform a vein graft if necessary.

resection. Involvement of the duodenum, splenic vein, or GDA is common but not considered a contraindication to surgical resection. Peripancreatic lymph-node metastases are associated with a relatively poor prognosis, but the suspicion of regional nodal metastases does not necessarily preclude surgery. Traditionally, CT and MRI have been better at predicting unresectability than resectability. That is, CT and MRI cannot completely eliminate the possibility that a patient with unresectable disease will undergo unnecessary surgery. However, when CT and MRI predict a patient is unresectable, the patient usually does, indeed, have incurable disease.

Ductal adenocarcinoma can have an atypical appearance on imaging studies because of the excess production of mucin, the presence of necrosis, or pancreatic duct obstruction (Fig. 14-45). Any of these processes may cause ductal adenocarcinoma to be confused with a different type of cystic neoplasm. A diffuse form of ductal adenocarcinoma has been described but is rarely encountered. Diffuse adenocarcinoma can be confused with pancreatic lymphoma or other diffuse process such as autoimmune pancreatitis. Pancreatic cancer may also be mimicked by pancreatitis. In fact, one of the greatest challenges in pancreatic imaging is the differentiation between pancreatic inflammatory mass and pancreatic neoplasm (Fig. 14-46). A further confounder is that pancreatic cancer may incite or coexist with pancreatitis. Both processes are associated with fibrosis that results in similar imaging appearances.

Neuroendocrine (Islet Cell) Tumors

Neuroendocrine tumors of the pancreas arise from amine precursor uptake and decarboxylation system cells. These tumors can produce a variety of substances that result in clinical manifestations. Alternatively, neuroendocrine tumors of the pancreas can be non-functioning (between 15% and 40%). Of the functioning pancreatic neuroendocrine tumors, insulinomas are most common, followed by gastrinomas. The majority of insulinomas are small, solid, and solitary at presentation, whereas gastrinomas have a propensity to be multiple at presentation. Approximately

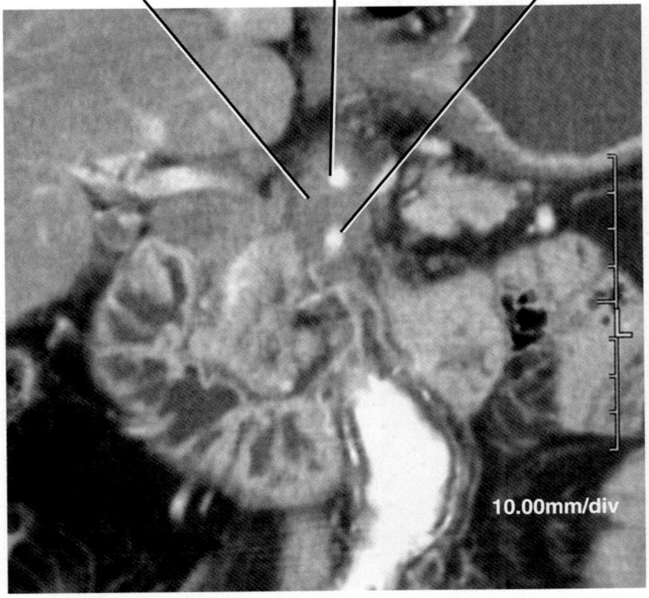

Tumor completely encases celiac artery and SMA   Celiac artery   Superior mesenteric artery

10.00mm/div

Figure 14-44 Coronal reformation of enhanced abdominal computed tomographic scan of a patient with unresectable pancreatic cancer. *SMA,* Superior mesenteric artery.

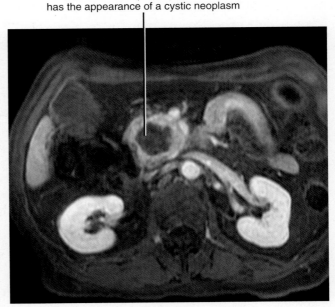

Necrotic mass (adenocarcinoma) has the appearance of a cystic neoplasm

Figure 14-45 Gadolinium-enhanced, T1-weighted, fat-suppressed, axial magnetic resonance image obtained during the equilibrium phase through the pancreatic head of a patient with necrotic ductal adenocarcinoma.

Inflammatory mass involving head of the pancreas simulates a neoplasm

Normal head of pancreas

Enhancing mass (gastrinoma) in pancreatic tail

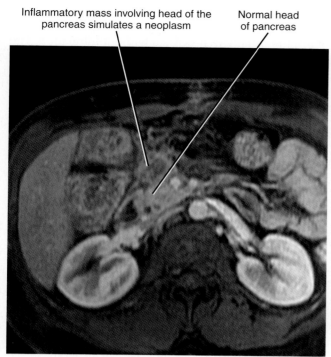

Figure 14-46 Gadolinium-enhanced, T1-weighted, fat-suppressed image through the pancreatic head of a patient with an inflammatory mass secondary to pancreatitis. This mass resolved over the subsequent year.

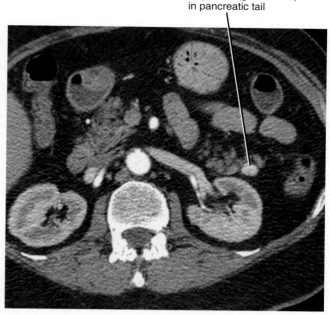

Figure 14-47 Arterial-phase enhanced axial computed tomographic image through the pancreatic tail of a patient with a gastrinoma. Two additional gastrinomas and a liver metastasis were confirmed at surgery.

10% of insulinomas, somewhat less than half of gastrinomas, and at least 80% of nonfunctioning neuroendocrine tumors are malignant at the time of diagnosis. The majority of functioning neuroendocrine tumors of the pancreas other than insulinomas and gastrinomas are malignant and relatively advanced at the time of presentation because of nonspecific clinical manifestations. Malignant islet cell tumors tend to spread to regional lymph nodes, metastasize hematogenously to the liver and bones, and can invade venous structures. Nonfunctioning tumors are more likely to calcify, or appear cystic or necrotic. Calcifications are more common in malignant than benign neuroendocrine tumors and more common than in ductal adenocarcinoma. Approximately 15% of islet cell tumors are found outside the confines of the pancreas.

Transabdominal US is relatively insensitive for the detection of islet cell tumors. When visible, intrapancreatic neuroendocrine tumors usually appear as hypoechoic masses with relatively well-defined borders.

Since the advent of multiphase contrast-enhanced CT, the majority (roughly 70-80%) of islet cell tumors have become detectable. Small lesions are usually not visible without the use of intravenous contrast material. Most tumors are hypervascular and most conspicuous during the early phases of enhancement (Fig. 14-47). The metastatic deposits of neuroendocrine tumors are also often hypervascular. Cystic, necrotic, and calcified regions may be identified in larger tumors (not typical of insulinomas).

The MRI findings of islet cell tumors include decreased signal intensity on T1-weighted images, hyperintensity on T2-weighted images (best demonstrated with fat-suppression techniques), and arterial-phase enhancement after gadolinium administration (Fig. 14-48). As with CT, enhancement can be homogeneous or ringlike. Neuroendocrine tumors can occasionally be hyperintense on delayed postcontrast T1-weighted images.

The preoperative localization of a functioning neuroendocrine tumor can be a challenge. Most insulinomas and roughly half of gastrinomas are pancreatic in location. The gastrinoma triangle defines a common territory for extrapancreatic gastrinomas to present and is bordered by the cystic duct–common hepatic duct confluence, second and third portions of the duodenum, and the neck of the pancreas, although gastrinomas can be found in other locations such as the stomach wall. Approximately a quarter of gastrinomas are associated with MEN-1 syndrome and often are found in the duodenal wall in such cases. When CT fails to demonstrate a tumor in the setting of suspected hyperfunctioning neuroendocrine tumor, MRI or EUS can be helpful. EUS appears to be highly sensitive for the detection of islet cell tumors and can be combined with biopsy in the same setting. A negative EUS study of the pancreas in combination with negative CT or MRI results strongly favors an extrapancreatic tumor. In some cases, however, laparotomy and intraoperative US are necessary to localize the tumor(s) (Fig. 14-49).

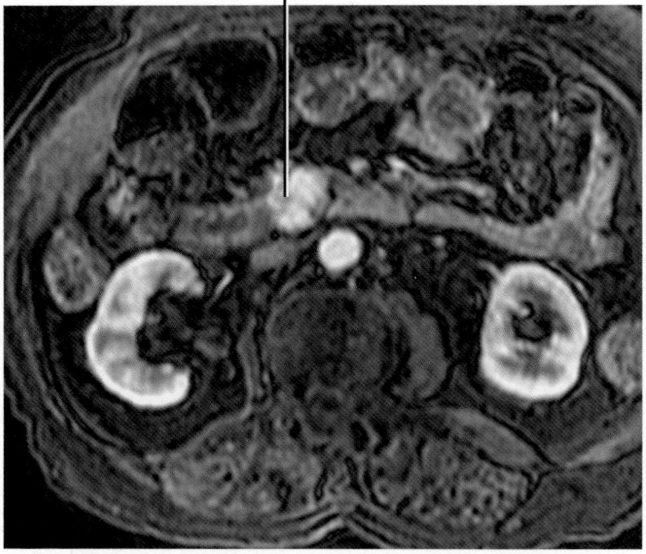

Hypervascular mass
(neuroendocrine tumor)

Figure 14-48 Gadolinium-enhanced arterial-phase magnetic resonance image through the caudal pancreatic head demonstrates a small hypervascular mass subsequently shown to represent a neuroendocrine tumor by endoscopic ultrasound (EUS)–guided biopsy.

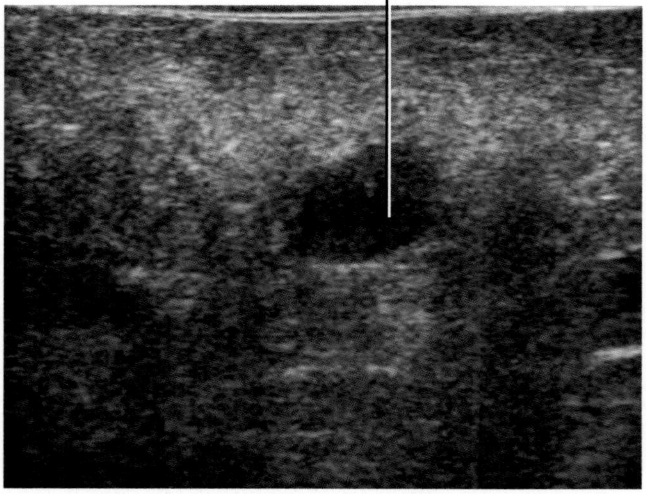

Hypoechoic mass
(neuroendocrine tumor)
in pancreatic body

Figure 14-49 Intraoperative sonogram of the pancreas demonstrates an 8-mm neuroendocrine tumor not visible on patient's preoperative computed tomographic scan.

Other Rare Pancreatic Tumors

Solid Pseudopapillary Tumor

Solid pseudopapillary tumor (SPT) is a rare, slow-growing, low-grade malignant tumor that has a favorable prognosis after surgical resection. These tumors primarily affect young women (mean age, 20-30 years) with a predilection for women of African-American or Asian descent. These tumors often have areas of necrosis and hemorrhage, and may display fluid–debris levels on CT and MR images. The absence of hemorrhage does not exclude this diagnosis, however. Lesions of SPT are usually well-defined without lobulation. The degree of necrosis or cystic change is variable, with tumors ranging from predominantly solid to nearly completely cystic. There may be some predilection for the tail of the pancreas, although these lesions can potentially be found throughout the pancreas. A well-defined hemorrhagic pancreatic mass in a young woman should suggest this diagnosis.

Acinar Cell Carcinoma

Acinar cell carcinoma of the pancreas is a rare (1% of exocrine tumors) pancreatic epithelial neoplasm with evidence of acinar differentiation. Patients are generally middle-aged and older. Although considered an aggressive tumor, prognosis of patients with acinar cell carcinoma is better than for ductal adenocarcinoma. Tumor cells can produce pancreatic enzymes such as lipase, resulting in systemic manifestations such as subcutaneous fat necrosis, bone infarction, or polyarthropathy. With CT and MRI, these tumors tend to be well-marginated and somewhat exophytic. Smaller tumors tend to be homogeneous, whereas larger tumors exhibit variable degrees of necrosis. Acinar cell carcinomas can invade adjacent organs but tend not to exhibit the poorly defined, infiltrating appearance of ductal adenocarcinoma.

Lymphoma

Pancreatic lymphoma usually results from secondary involvement and presents with lymphadenopathy of the mesentery and retroperitoneum. Primary lymphoma (non-Hodgkin's B-cell lymphoma) is extremely rare. Both mass-forming and infiltrative forms of primary pancreatic lymphoma have been reported. As with lymphoma involving other organs, lymphoma of the pancreas is relatively homogeneous in attenuation on CT images and enhances relatively poorly after intravenous contrast administration. Calcification and necrosis are not features of untreated pancreatic lymphoma. Clues that favor lymphoma over adenocarcinoma include absence of pancreatic duct dilatation and the presence of retroperitoneal lymphadenopathy outside of the nodal stations that drain the pancreas.

Metastatic Disease to the Pancreas

The presence of multiple pancreatic masses in a patient with a known primary malignant neoplasm elsewhere suggests the possibility of metastatic disease to the pancreas. Renal cell carcinoma, breast cancer, lung cancer, and melanoma are among the primary malignant neoplasms that metastasize to the pancreas. When solitary, metastatic disease to the pancreas can mimic other primary pancreatic neoplasms.

Other Tumors

Pancreatoblastomas are primarily childhood tumors that are extremely rare in adults. These tumors tend to be large and heterogeneous on imaging studies. *Giant cell tumors* of the pancreas can be divided into osteoclast-like and pleomorphic types, and often present as large necrotic or cystic masses. As with other organs, a variety of benign and malignant *mesenchymal tumors* can arise from the pancreas. *Carcinosarcomas* consist of a mixture of malignant epithelial and stromal elements. *Adenosquamous carcinoma* is a rare aggressive variant of ductal adenocarcinoma with a propensity to metastasize and a poor prognosis (Fig. 14-50).

Peripancreatic Mimics of Pancreatic Disease

When developing a differential diagnosis for a presumed pancreatic abnormality, it is important to consider peripancreatic mimics of primary pancreatic diseases. Some mimics to consider are listed in Box 14-6.

Hypoattenuating mass
(adenosquamous carcinoma)
in tail of pancreas

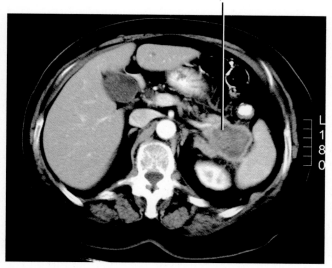

Figure 14-50 Enhanced axial computed tomographic image through the pancreatic tail of a patient with an adenosquamous carcinoma of the pancreas.

BOX 14-6   Peripancreatic Mimics of Pancreatic Disease

Aneurysm and pseudoaneurysm
Carcinoid tumor
Choledochal cyst
Desmoid tumor
Duodenal diverticulum
Duodenal duplication
Duodenitis
Gastric cancer
Intrapancreatic accessory spleen
Lymphadenopathy and lymphoma
Peptic ulcer disease
Pseudocyst
Renal infection
Retroperitoneal fibrosis
Retroperitoneal sarcoma
Varices

Suggested Readings

Adsay NV, Basturk O, Klimstra DS et al: Pancreatic pseudotumors: non-neoplastic solid lesions of the pancreas that clinically mimic pancreas cancer, *Semin Diagn Pathol* 21:260, 2004.

Balthazar EJ: Acute pancreatitis: assessment of severity with clinical and CT evaluation, *Radiology* 223:603-613, 2002.

Balthazar EJ: Pancreatitis associated with pancreatic carcinoma, *Pancreatology* 5:330-344, 2005.

Blasbalg R, Baroni RH, Costa DN et al: MRI features of groove pancreatitis, *AJR Am J Roentgenol* 189:73-80, 2007.

Boland GW, O'Malley ME, Saez M et al: Pancreatic-phase versus portal vein-phase helical CT of the pancreas: optimal temporal window for evaluation of pancreatic adenocarcinoma, *AJR Am J Roentgenol* 172:605-608, 1999.

Choi EK, Park SH, Kim DY et al: Unusual manifestations of primary pancreatic neoplasia: radiologic-pathologic correlation, *J Comput Assist Tomogr* 30:610-617, 2006.

Chung MJ, Choi BI, Han JK et al: Functioning islet cell tumor of the pancreas: localization with dynamic spiral CT, *Acta Radiol* 38:135-138, 1997.

Cohen-Scali F, Vilgrain V, Brancatelli G et al: Discrimination of unilocular macrocystic serous cystadenoma from pancreatic pseudocyst and mucinous cystadenoma with CT: initial observations, *Radiology* 228:727-733, 2003.

Crabo LG, Conley DM, Graney DO et al: Venous anatomy of the pancreatic head: normal CT appearance in cadavers and patients, *AJR Am J Roentgenol* 160:1039-1045, 1993.

Finstad TA, Tchelepi H, Ralls PW: Sonography of acute pancreatitis: prevalence of findings and pictorial essay, *Ultrasound Q* 21:95-104, 2005.

Fletcher JG, Wiersema MJ, Farrell MA et al: Pancreatic malignancy: value of arterial, pancreatic, and hepatic phase imaging with multi-detector row CT, *Radiology* 229:81-90, 2003.

Horton KM, Fishman EK: Multidetector CT angiography of pancreatic carcinoma: part 1, evaluation of arterial involvement, *AJR Am J Roentgenol* 178:827-831, 2002.

Horton KM, Fishman EK: Multidetector CT angiography of pancreatic carcinoma: part 2, evaluation of venous involvement, *AJR Am J Roentgenol* 178:833-836, 2002.

Horton KM, Hruban RH, Yeo C et al: Multi-detector row CT of pancreatic islet cell tumors, *Radiographics* 26:453-464, 2006.

Ibukuro K, Tsukiyama T, Mori K et al: Peripancreatic veins on thin-section (3mm) helical CT, *AJR Am J Roentgenol* 167:1003-1008, 1996.

Imbriaco M, Megibow AJ, Camera L et al: Dual-phase versus single-phase helical CT to detect and assess resectability of pancreatic carcinoma, *AJR Am J Roentgenol* 178:1473-1479, 2002.

Imbriaco M, Megibow AJ, Ragozzini A et al: Value of the single-phase technique in MDCT assessment of pancreatic tumors, *AJR Am J Roentgenol* 184:1111-1117, 2005.

Itoh S, Yamakawa K, Shimamoto K et al: CT findings in groove pancreatitis: correlation with histopathological findings, *J Comput Assist Tomogr* 18:911-915, 1994.

Karasawa E, Goldberg HI, Moss AA et al: CT pancreatogram in carcinoma of the pancreas and chronic pancreatitis, *Radiology* 148:489-493, 1983.

Kim JH et al: Differential diagnosis of periampullary carcinomas at MR imaging, *Radiographics* 22:1335-1352, 2002.

Kim T, Murakami T, Takamura M et al: Pancreatic mass due to chronic pancreatitis: correlation of CT and MR imaging features with pathologic findings, *AJR Am J Roentgenol* 177:367-371, 2001.

Kim YH, Saini S, Sahani D et al: Imaging diagnosis of cystic pancreatic lesions: pseudocyst versus nonpseudocyst, *Radiographics* 25:671-685, 2005.

Lawler LP, Horton KM, Fishman EK: Peripancreatic masses that simulate pancreatic disease: spectrum of disease and role of CT, *Radiographics* 23:1117-1131, 2003.

Leyendecker JR, Elsayes KM, Gratz BI et al: MR cholangiopancreatography: spectrum of pancreatic duct abnormalities, *AJR Am J Roentgenol* 179:1465-1471, 2002.

Leyendecker JR, Baginski SG: Complete pancreatic encasement of the portal vein (circumportal pancreas): imaging findings and implications of a rare pancreatic anomaly. *J Comput Assist Tomogr* 32:61-64, 2008.

Lu DS, Reber HA, Krasny RM et al: Local staging of pancreatic cancer: criteria for unresectability of major vessels as revealed by pancreatic-phase, thin-section helical CT, *AJR Am J Roentgenol* 168:1439, 1997.

Matos C, Metens T, Deviere J et al: Pancreatic duct: morphologic and functional evaluation with dynamic MR pancreatography after secretin stimulation, *Radiology* 203:435-441, 1997.

McNulty NJ, Francis IR, Platt JF et al: Multi-detector row helical CT of the pancreas: effect of contrast-enhanced multiphasic imaging on enhancement of the pancreas, peripancreatic vasculature, and pancreatic adenocarcinoma, *Radiology* 220:97-102, 2001.

Merkle EM, Bender G, Brambs HJ: Imaging findings in pancreatic lymphoma: differential aspects, *AJR Am J Roentgenol* 174:671-675, 2000.

Morana G, Guarise A: Cystic tumors of the pancreas, *Cancer Imaging* 6:60-71, 2006.

Mori H, Miyake H, Aikawa H et al: Dilated posterior superior pancreaticoduodenal vein: recognition with CT and clinical significance in patients with pancreaticobiliary carcinomas, *Radiology* 181:793-800, 1991.

Mortele KJ, Wiesner W, Intriere L et al: A modified CT severity index for evaluating acute pancreatitis: improved correlation with patient outcome, *AJR Am J Roentgenol* 183:1261-1265, 2004.

Procacci C, Carbognin G, Biasiutti C et al: Intraductal papillary mucinous tumors of the pancreas: spectrum of CT and MR findings with pathologic correlation, *Eur Radiol* 11:1939-1951, 2001.

Procacci C, Carbognin G, Accordini S et al: CT features of malignant mucinous cystic tumors of the pancreas, *Eur Radiol* 11:1626-1630, 2001.

Procacci C, Carbognin G, Accordini S et al: Nonfunctioning endocrine tumors of the pancreas: possibilities of spiral CT characterization, *Eur Radiol* 11:1175-1183, 2001.

Raptopoulos V, Steer ML, Sheiman RG et al: The use of helical CT and CT angiography to predict vascular involvement from pancreatic cancer: correlation with findings at surgery, *AJR Am J Roentgenol* 168:971-977, 1997.

Ross BA, Jeffrey RB Jr, Mindelzun RE: Normal variations in the lateral contour of the head of the pancreas mimicking neoplasm: evaluation with dual-phase helical CT, *AJR Am J Roentgenol* 166:799-801, 1996.

Sahani DV, Kalva SP, Farrell J et al: Autoimmune pancreatitis: imaging features, *Radiology* 233:345-352, 2004.

Sahani DV, Kadavigere R, Blake M et al: Intraductal papillary mucinous neoplasm of pancreas: multi-detector row CT with 2D curved reformations-correlation with MRCP, *Radiology* 238:560-569, 2006.

Sahani DV, Kadavigere R, Saokar et al: Cystic pancreatic lesions: a simple imaging-based classification system for guiding management, *Radiographics* 25:1471-1484, 2005.

Sandrasegaran K, Tann M, Jennings SG et al: Disconnection of the pancreatic duct: an important but overlooked complication of severe acute pancreatitis, *Radiographics* 27:1389-1400, 2007.

Shah S, Mortele KJ: Uncommon solid pancreatic neoplasms: ultrasound, computed tomography, and magnetic resonance imaging features, *Semin Ultrasound CT MR* 28:357-370, 2007.

Sidden CR, Mortele KJ: Cystic tumors of the pancreas: ultrasound, computed tomography, and magnetic resonance imaging features, *Semin Ultrasound CT MR* 28:339-356, 2007.

Sugiyama M, Haradome H, Atomi Y: Magnetic resonance imaging for diagnosing chronic pancreatitis, *J Gastroenterol* 42:108-112, 2007.

Takahashi N, Kawashima A, Fletcher JG, et al: Renal involvement in patients with autoimmune pancreatitis: CT and MR imaging findings. *Radiology* 242:791-801, 2007.

Tanaka M, Chari S, Adsay V et al: International consensus guidelines for management of intraductal papillary mucinous neoplasms and mucinous cystic neoplasm of the pancreas, *Pancreatology* 6:17-32, 2006.

Tatli S, Mortele KJ, Levy AD et al: CT and MRI features of pure acinar cell carcinoma of the pancreas in adults, *AJR Am J Roentgenol* 184:511-519, 2005.

To'o KJ, Raman SS, Yu NC et al: Pancreatic and peripancreatic diseases mimicking primary pancreatic neoplasia, *Radiographics* 25:949-965, 2005.

CHAPTER 15

Spleen

John R. Leyendecker

"I don't pay much attention to the spleen." This quote from an abdominal imager acquaintance of mine typifies the opinion of many radiologists regarding the spleen. The spleen lacks the complex metabolism of the liver, the strategic location of the pancreas, and the crucial role of the kidneys. Most radiologists do not perceive splenic anatomy as particularly intricate. Primary malignant neoplasms of the spleen are rare, whereas incidental nonspecific splenic lesions are relatively common. No wonder the spleen is so maligned (or at least ignored).

Despite the prevailing aversion among radiologists to all things splenic, the spleen is an important organ that deserves some consideration. The spleen is a lymphoid organ that serves to filter the blood and generate an immune response to provocative stimuli. Phagocytic cells within the spleen remove abnormal or damaged cells, foreign particles, and microorganisms from circulation. Individuals without a spleen are at risk for overwhelming infection. Variations in splenic morphology and location can be mistaken for true abnormalities, instigating unnecessary interventions.

■ ANATOMY

Splenic Size and Shape

The typical spleen measures less than 13 cm in length, up to 7 to 8 cm in width, and 4 cm in thickness. Normal splenic volume is usually less than 300 ml. The spleen generally has a smooth convex posterior, superior, and lateral surface. Splenic clefts are relatively common and may be confused with lacerations in the setting of trauma (Fig. 15-1). Unlike most lacerations, congenital clefts are sharply and smoothly marginated and not associated with perisplenic blood. Splenic bulges are common medially and may cause mass effect on the stomach or be mistaken for a splenic or renal mass.

> *Pitfall: Splenic clefts are relatively common and may be confused with lacerations in the setting of trauma. Unlike most lacerations, congenital clefts are sharply and smoothly marginated.*

Anatomic Relations and Peritoneal Reflections

The spleen usually resides within the left upper quadrant of the abdomen and is in close proximity to the diaphragm, left abdominal wall, greater curvature of the stomach, left kidney, tail of the pancreas, splenic flexure of the colon, and occasionally the lateral segment of the left hepatic lobe. The spleen forms within the dorsal mesogastrium and lies between the pancreas and stomach. It divides the dorsal mesogastrium into the splenorenal and gastrosplenic ligaments.

The splenorenal ligament connects the anterior left kidney to the splenic hilum and contains the splenic vessels and the tail of the pancreas. Pancreatic neoplasms and inflammation can spread from the pancreas directly to the spleen via this ligament. Between the spleen and greater curvature of the stomach, these same peritoneal folds form the gastrosplenic ligament, which contains the short gastric and left gastroepiploic vessels. This ligament facilitates spread of infection and tumor between the stomach and spleen. The spleen is also supported, in part, by the phrenicocolic ligament.

The spleen and its corresponding ligaments form the left lateral extent of the lesser sac. The spleen itself is invested in a fibroelastic capsule. This capsule is continuous with numerous trabeculae that extend into and compartmentalize the splenic parenchyma, and convey the trabecular vessels. As with the liver, a variably sized bare area is present that lacks a visceral peritoneal covering. The spleen may demonstrate considerable mobility on its mesentery. When the splenorenal ligament fails to fuse with the retroperitoneum, the spleen may be exceptionally mobile. This condition predisposes individuals to ectopic splenic location (i.e., "wandering" spleen) and torsion.

Vascular Anatomy of the Spleen

The blood supply to the spleen is via the splenic artery, which travels in the splenorenal ligament with the splenic vein. The splenic artery creates many smaller arteries in addition to the terminal splenic branches,

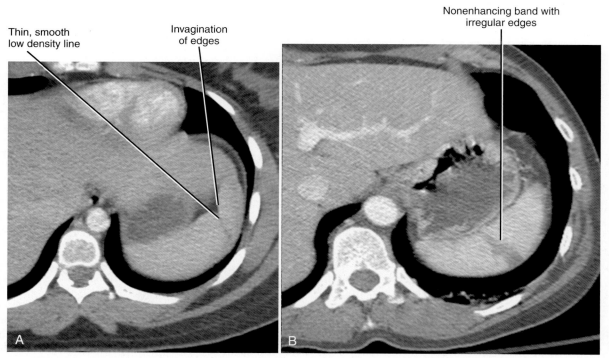

Figure 15-1 Thin, smooth low density line — Invagination of edges — Nonenhancing band with irregular edges

Figure 15-1 Enhanced axial computed tomographic scan of a patient with a splenic cleft (**A**) and a patient with a splenic laceration (**B**).

including several pancreatic branches, short gastric arteries (which travel in the gastrosplenic ligament), the left gastroepiploic artery, and occasionally a posterior gastric artery.

The splenic parenchyma consists of white pulp and red pulp. The white splenic pulp consists of lymphatic tissue surrounding the arterioles that exit the trabeculae. White pulp causes most lymphatic neoplasms of the spleen. The red pulp consists of splenic sinuses and the splenic chords, which contain blood cells supported by a reticular network. Nonhematolymphoid tumors tend to arise from cells of the red pulp. The interface between red and white pulp is referred to as the marginal zone. Blood flowing through the spleen may bypass the splenic cords and flow directly to the venous sinuses (closed circulation) or enter the splenic cords (open circulation). As part of the reticuloendothelial system, the spleen contains abundant numbers of phagocytic cells.

The splenic vein runs posterior to the body and tail of the pancreas, and represents a useful sonographic landmark for the position of the pancreas. In addition to draining the spleen, the splenic vein receives venous blood from short gastric veins, the left gastroepiploic vein, pancreatic veins, and usually the inferior mesenteric vein before joining the superior mesenteric vein at the portal confluence. The lymphatic drainage of the spleen is to the hilar and, ultimately, celiac lymph nodes.

Accessory Splenic Tissue

During development, several splenic islands coalesce within the dorsal mesogastrium. When some of these islands fail to join the bulk of the coalescing splenic tissue, accessory spleens or splenules result. Splenules are typically round, smooth, smaller than 2 cm, and functional. Despite being completely separate from the spleen, splenules share similar imaging characteristics with the normal spleen (Fig. 15-2). Occasionally, the branch of the splenic artery that supplies the splenule can be seen on imaging studies (Fig. 15-3). More than 95% of splenules are found in the splenorenal ligament (near or in the pancreatic tail), gastrosplenic ligament, splenic hilum, gastrocolic ligament, or greater omentum. However, accessory spleens have been localized as far away as the pelvis, and they are occasionally mistaken for adrenal, pancreatic, and peritoneal tumors (Fig. 15-4). Accessory spleens rarely reside lateral to the main spleen.

Pitfall: Splenules can mimic adrenal, pancreatic, and peritoneal tumors.

Pathologic processes that affect the spleen may also involve splenules (Fig. 15-5). Accessory spleens are important to identify before surgery in patients undergoing splenectomy for such disorders as idiopathic thrombocytopenic purpura. Failure to prospectively identify and remove accessory spleens in such a setting may result in return of hypersplenism. After splenectomy, residual accessory spleens often enlarge (Fig. 15-6). Accessory spleens may occasionally undergo torsion, infarction, or spontaneous rupture.

Splenosis is a condition that can result when splenic tissue gains entrance to the peritoneal cavity, usually caused by trauma, splenic rupture, or splenectomy (Fig. 15-7). Once within the peritoneal cavity, splenosis can migrate to any peritoneal recess similar to the peritoneal spread of tumor or infection. Splenosis does not receive blood supply from the splenic artery, resulting in

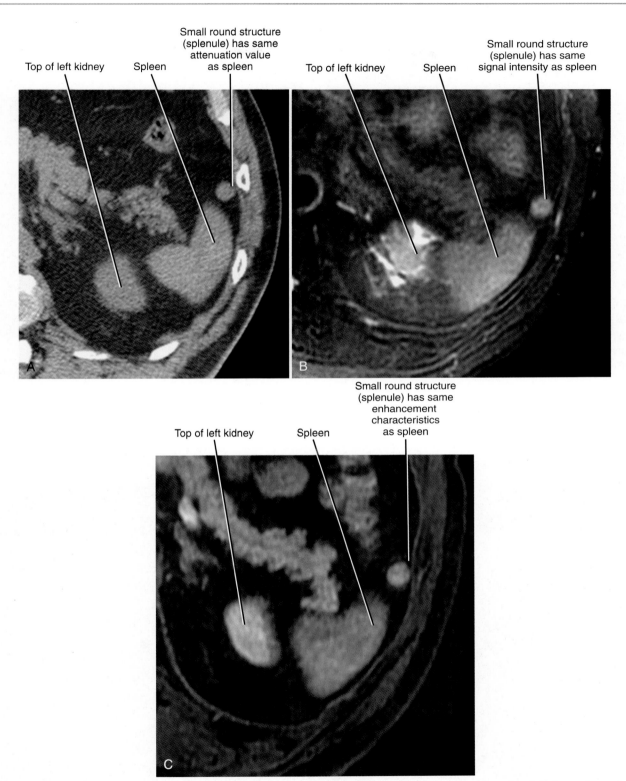

Figure 15-2 Unenhanced axial computed tomographic **(A)**, T2-weighted magnetic resonance (MR) **(B)**, and gadolinium-enhanced, fat-suppressed, T1-weighted MR image **(C)** of splenule.

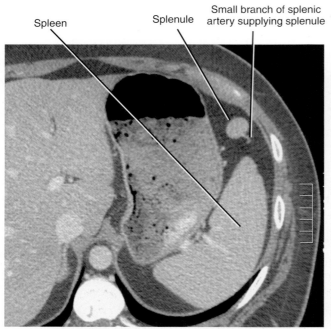

Spleen Splenule Small branch of splenic artery supplying splenule

Figure 15-3 Enhanced axial computed tomographic scan through the spleen shows arterial supply to a splenule. This vessel could be traced back to the splenic hilum on the complete data set.

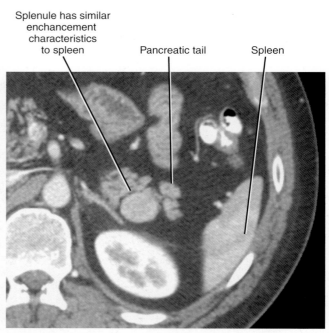

Splenule has similar enchancement characteristics to spleen Pancreatic tail Spleen

Figure 15-4 Enhanced axial computed tomographic scan through the upper abdomen shows a splenule in the region of the pancreatic tail. A splenule such as this can be mistaken for a pancreatic mass.

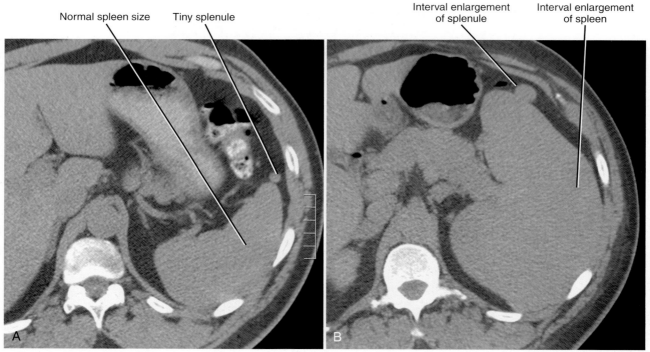

Normal spleen size Tiny splenule Interval enlargement of splenule Interval enlargement of spleen

Figure 15-5 Unenhanced axial computed tomographic scans through the spleen of a patient who was diagnosed with lymphoma between the time of the first scan **(A)** and the second scan **(B)**. Note increase in size of both the spleen and the splenule.

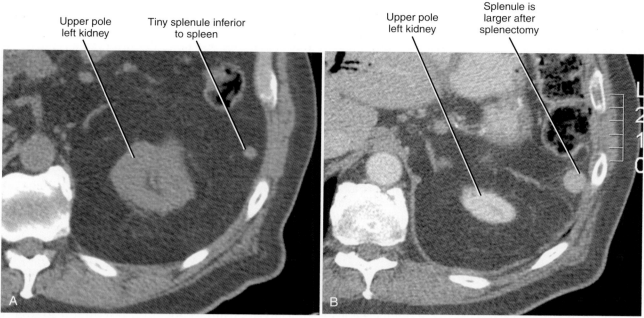

Figure 15-6 Axial computed tomographic scans through the upper abdomen of a patient before (**A**) and after (**B**) splenectomy. Note interval enlargement of splenule after splenectomy (**B**).

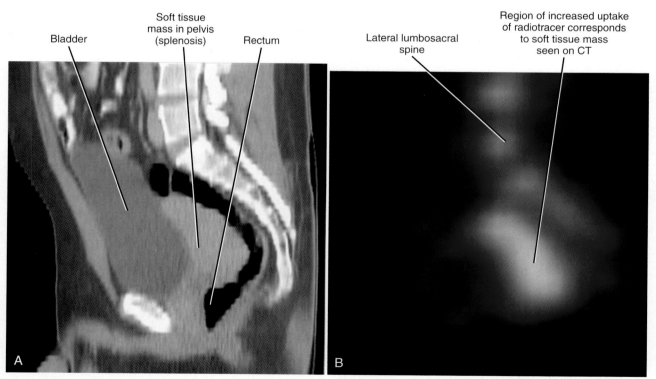

Figure 15-7 Sagittal reformation from unenhanced computed tomographic scan (**A**) and lateral single-photon emission computed tomographic (SPECT) image from technetium-99m–labeled, heat-damaged, red blood cell study (**B**) in a patient with splenosis in the pelvis.

different enhancement characteristics and poor function compared with the normal spleen and splenules. Splenosis may be confused with pathologic processes such as peritoneal metastatic disease or lymphadenopathy. Polysplenia, a congenital condition associated with a variety of other congenital abnormalities, can be distinguished from multiple accessory spleens by the absence of a normal dominant spleen in the former condition (Fig. 15-8).

Single-photon emission computed tomographic scanning after administration of technetium 99m (Tc-99m) sulfur colloid may demonstrate uptake of the radiopharmaceutical in an accessory spleen or splenosis. Similarly, uptake of superparamagnetic iron oxide by accessory spleens or splenosis may be demonstrated with MRI. Therefore, these tests may be beneficial when attempting to distinguish between ectopic splenic tissue and other causes of soft-tissue mass.

■ NORMAL IMAGING APPEARANCE OF THE SPLEEN

With sonography, the spleen is usually of homogeneous echogenicity. It is more echogenic than normal renal cortex and liver parenchyma. On unenhanced CT images, the spleen is normally slightly less dense (approximately 5-10 HU less) than the normal liver, ranging from 40 to 60 HU in attenuation. On unenhanced MRI, the spleen is lower in signal intensity than the normal liver on T1-weighted images and normally brighter than the liver than on T2-weighted images. The unenhanced T1 and T2 relaxation times of the spleen on MRI closely resemble those of many types of liver metastases.

During the arterial phase of dynamic multiphase, enhanced imaging with CT or MRI, the normal spleen enhances with a characteristic heterogeneous pattern that sometimes resembles the stripes of a zebra or tiger (Fig. 15-9). This heterogeneous enhancement pattern presumably results from differences in the rate of contrast (blood) flow through the different splenic compartments, with a portion of the blood percolating slowly through the splenic cords (open circulation of the spleen), and a percentage of splenic blood flow passing more rapidly through the splenic sinuses and into the venous sinuses that join to form the trabecular veins (closed circulation). Normal splenic enhancement usually becomes homogeneous after the first minute. The spleen avidly accumulates technetium sulfur colloid and heat-damaged red blood cells. Splenic uptake of superparamagnetic iron oxide particles results in significant signal loss on T2- and T2*-weighted MRI sequences.

Accessory spleens have the same imaging characteristics on ultrasound (US), CT, and MRI as the normal spleen (see Fig. 15-2). Enhancement of accessory spleens after intravenous contrast administration on CT and MR images may be similar in character and intensity to that of the normal spleen, a feature that helps distinguish accessory spleens from pancreatic, adrenal, or peritoneal neoplasms. However, when accessory spleens enhance to a lesser degree than the spleen, they may be more difficult to distinguish from other types of masses. They can be correctly identified with the same nuclear medicine techniques used to image normal spleen or with ferumoxides-enhanced MRI.

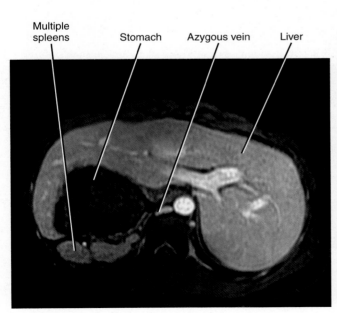

Figure 15-8 Axial, gadolinium-enhanced, T1-weighted, magnetic resonance imaging of a patient with polysplenia, abnormal situs, and azygous continuation of the inferior vena cava.

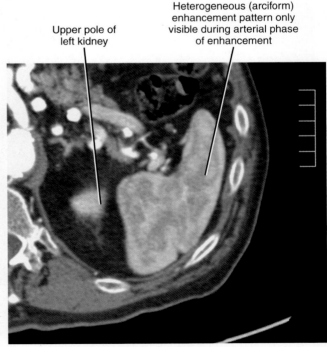

Figure 15-9 Axial arterial phase-enhanced computed tomographic scan through the upper abdomen of a patient with normal spleen shows normal heterogeneous early enhancement pattern.

Pearl: Splenules usually have the same imaging characteristics as the normal spleen and are supplied by branches of the splenic artery.

■ DIFFUSE SPLENIC ABNORMALITIES

Splenomegaly

The most frequently encountered abnormality of the spleen is splenomegaly. Normal splenic size and shape varies considerably between individuals, making a simple and accurate imaging definition of splenomegaly difficult to establish. A variety of measurement techniques have been proposed to define splenomegaly on imaging studies, although most radiologists rely on the readily determined splenic length for this purpose. Although a length of more than 13 cm is often regarded as evidence of splenomegaly in clinical practice, the range of lengths considered abnormal in the literature extends from 10 to 15 cm (Fig. 15-10). More complex multidimensional indices or volumes are rarely calculated in routine practice, and a subjective assessment of splenomegaly is often made. A rounded appearance or extension of the spleen below the right hepatic lobe or lower third of the left kidney is used by some as a rapidly obtained estimate of splenomegaly.

In most cases, splenomegaly is part of a systemic infectious, inflammatory, hematologic, or hemodynamic disease process. Therefore, one should be familiar with some of the general associations of splenomegaly (Table 15-1).

Table 15-1 Disorders Associated with Splenomegaly

Disorder	Associated Imaging Clues
Systemic infection	
Immune disorders	
Hematologic malignancy and myeloproliferative disorders (Fig. 15-11)	Bone marrow replacement, loss of normal arciform arterial enhancement pattern (lymphoma), lymphadenopathy
Anemias	Hemosiderosis of liver and spleen, iron deposition in renal cortex (hemolytic anemia), extramedullary hematopoiesis
Portal hypertension (Fig. 15-12)	Cirrhosis, portal venous obstruction, varices, Gamna-Gandy bodies,* ascites, hepatofugal portal flow
Congestive heart failure	Enlarged hepatic veins and inferior vena cava, cardiomegaly, pleural effusions, early mosaic liver enhancement
Amyloidosis	Loss of normal arciform arterial enhancement pattern
Sarcoidosis and other granulomatous diseases	Mediastinal and hilar adenopathy; multiple small nodules in spleen, liver, or both
Rheumatologic disorders (e.g., Felty syndrome)	Lymphadenopathy, arthritis
Storage diseases	
Splenic mass	
Acute splenic infarction	Lack of splenic parenchymal enhancement
Splenic hemorrhage	Other signs of trauma, extravascular blood products

*Small, siderotic nodules probably resulting from punctate hemorrhage.

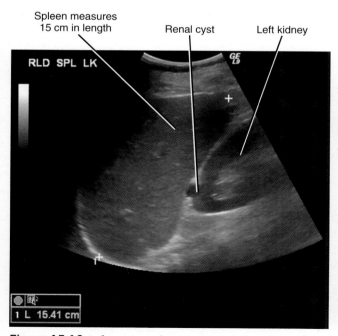

Figure 15-10 Left upper quadrant sonogram in a patient with splenomegaly.

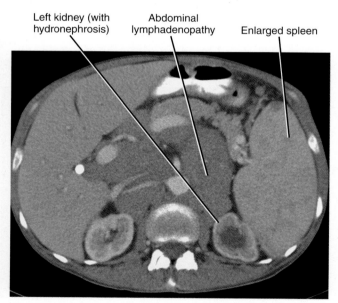

Figure 15-11 Enhanced axial computed tomographic scan of a patient with chronic lymphocytic leukemia.

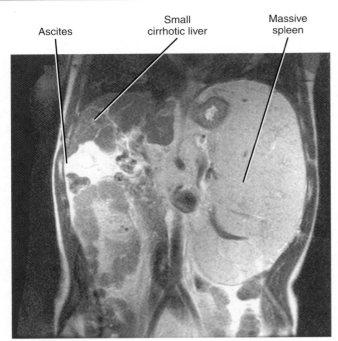

Ascites

Small cirrhotic liver

Massive spleen

Figure 15-12 Coronal T2-weighted magnetic resonance imaging of a patient with cirrhosis, portal hypertension, and splenomegaly.

Iron Deposition

One of the most common splenic abnormalities involves excess iron deposition within the reticuloendothelial system. This may be the result of excess red blood cell destruction and turnover as occurs with hemolytic anemias or may be caused by multiple blood transfusions. Excess splenic iron accumulation rarely occurs in the setting of hereditary (primary) hemochromatosis, making the spleen a potentially useful discriminator between hereditary and secondary forms

of hemochromatosis. Excess splenic iron accumulation associated with deposition of iron within the renal cortices may be seen with paroxysmal nocturnal hemoglobinuria or in some patients with prosthetic heart valves because of intravascular hemolysis. Sickle cell anemia may also be associated with splenic and renal cortical iron deposition, although the spleen is often small and may be calcified in this setting because of splenic infarction.

Splenic iron may increase the attenuation value of the spleen on CT, although CT is relatively insensitive for detection of splenic iron. MRI is considerably more sensitive, demonstrating a low-signal-intensity spleen on T2- and T2*-weighted images (Fig. 15-13). Splenic iron deposition should be suspected when the signal intensity of the spleen is equal to or lower than that of the liver on T2-weighted images. In- and opposed-phase gradient-echo images of the spleen will demonstrate relative signal loss of the spleen on the images with the longer echo time (usually the in-phase images at 1.5 Tesla) in the setting of excessive iron deposition (Fig. 15-14).

> *Pearl:* Splenic iron deposition should be suspected when the signal intensity of the spleen is equal to or lower than that of the liver on T2-weighted images. In- and opposed-phase gradient-echo images of the spleen will demonstrate relative signal loss of the spleen on the images with the longer echo time (usually the in-phase images) in the setting of excessive iron deposition.

■ FOCAL SPLENIC ABNORMALITIES

General Approach to Focal Splenic Lesions

Many focal splenic lesions have a nonspecific appearance on imaging. Often, the role of the radiologist who has just discovered a splenic abnormality is determining

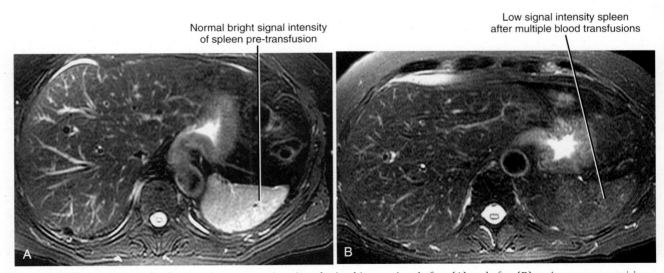

Normal bright signal intensity of spleen pre-transfusion

Low signal intensity spleen after multiple blood transfusions

Figure 15-13 Axial T2-weighted magnetic resonance imaging obtained in a patient before (**A**) and after (**B**) major surgery requiring multiple blood transfusions demonstrating transfusional hemosiderosis of the spleen.

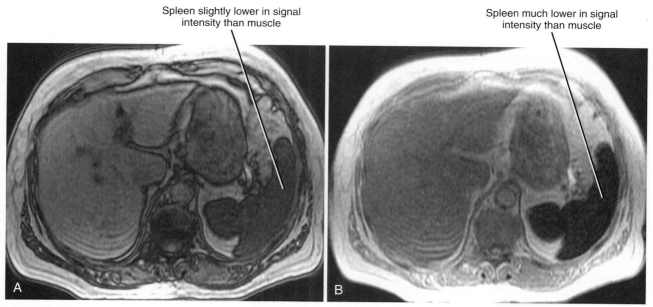

Spleen slightly lower in signal intensity than muscle

Spleen much lower in signal intensity than muscle

Figure 15-14 Axial opposed-phase (**A**) and in-phase (**B**) magnetic resonance images of a patient with splenic hemosiderosis. Note loss of signal intensity in the spleen on in-phase images because of the longer echo time (echo time [TE] = 2.1 milliseconds opposed phase; TE = 4.2 milliseconds in phase).

the next step in evaluation. If symptoms such as hypersplenism are present, splenectomy may be indicated regardless of the nature of the lesion, and an exhaustive imaging evaluation may not be necessary. In the case of an asymptomatic, simple-appearing, unilocular splenic cyst, the cause of the cyst (e.g., congenital, traumatic) may not be important, and management may consist of only observation. In patients with a splenic lesion and potentially life-limiting comorbidities, one must consider the risks and benefits of further evaluation against the likelihood that a definitive diagnosis will significantly alter patient management.

Perhaps the single most helpful tool when attempting to characterize a splenic abnormality is the clinical history. For example, multiple splenic lesions are reasonably likely to represent metastases in a patient with known metastatic melanoma, lymphoma in a patient with known lymphoma elsewhere, granulomas in a patient with sarcoidosis, and opportunistic infection in an immunocompromised patient. Pyogenic abscess should be a prime consideration in a patient with left upper quadrant pain, fever, leukocytosis, and a cystic-appearing splenic mass.

Pearl: Clinical history is often crucial to accurate characterization of a splenic abnormality.

Some splenic lesions have a sufficiently suggestive imaging appearance that close imaging follow-up may be a reasonable alternative to tissue diagnosis. We would include presumed splenic hemangioma, cyst/pseudocyst, or hamartoma in this category (Fig. 15-15). Occasionally, a suspected imaging diagnosis of hemangioma or hamartoma can be confirmed with a radionuclide imaging study such as Tc-99m–labeled red blood cell (hemangioma) or sulfur colloid (hamartoma) scintigraphy.

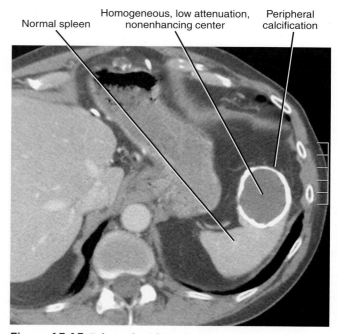

Normal spleen

Homogeneous, low attenuation, nonenhancing center

Peripheral calcification

Figure 15-15 Enhanced axial computed tomographic image through the upper abdomen of a patient with a peripherally calcified cyst (likely secondary) of the spleen. This lesion was unchanged over a 4-year period.

Predominantly Cystic-Appearing Lesions

In the category of predominantly cystic-appearing lesions, we consider lesions of the spleen that are predominantly or entirely cystic in appearance. We readily acknowledge that a wide variety of splenic masses may

---

BOX 15-1   Cystic-Appearing Masses of the Spleen

Primary (epithelial) cyst
Secondary cyst (caused by trauma, infection, inflammation)
Lymphangioma
Abscess
Necrotic tumor

---

have cystic components; however, in the interest of practicality, we include only some of the more common lesions likely to have a cystic appearance (Box 15-1).

Primary (epithelial) cysts of the spleen contain a cell lining and are considered congenital. These lesions often appear simple in nature, lacking nodules, septa, or enhancing components. *Secondary splenic cysts* result from trauma, infection, or inflammation (e.g., pancreatitis) and may be indistinguishable from primary cysts with imaging (see Fig. 15-15). *Hydatid cysts* can appear indistinguishable from other types of splenic cysts but are rare in nonendemic areas. The presence of daughter cysts distinguish hydatid cyst from other secondary splenic cysts. A thin rim of calcification may be present in primary or secondary splenic cysts and is not a useful discriminator (see Figs. 15-15 and 15-16). A patient's medical history may be the most useful means of discriminating among the various causes of a simple-appearing splenic cyst. Occasionally, a review of prior studies will reveal the process that led to cyst formation (e.g., pancreatitis, abscess, infarction, trauma).

Lymphangiomas consists of endothelial-lined channels, but unlike hemangiomas, lymphangiomas are not filled with blood. These lesions often involve the splenic capsule and can be multilocular or unilocular. Peripheral mural calcifications can be present. The fluid component appears simple on US, CT, and MRI, although the presence of hemorrhage or proteinaceous content can complicate the imaging appearance. Lymphangioma of the spleen can be associated with consumptive coagulopathy or extrasplenic lymphangiomas. Malignant degeneration is rare. The presence of solid elements within a presumed lymphangioma should raise concern for malignant degeneration.

Pyogenic abscess results from primary hematogenous or contiguous spread of infection, or secondary infection of a pre-existing abnormality. Splenic abscesses, in general, are more common in immunocompromised patients. Pyogenic abscess can be solitary or multiple and typically appear hypoechoic with US, low attenuation with CT, and high signal intensity on T2-weighted MR images. Grayscale US may demonstrate mobile or layering internal debris. The liquefied center lacks flow with color Doppler US and does not enhance with intravenous contrast material, although peripheral enhancement or enhancing septa may be present. The presence of gas within a cystic mass of the spleen is highly suggestive of pyogenic abscess but is an uncommon finding (Fig. 15-17). Imaging of the chest may show a left pleural effusion and left lower lobe atelectasis. Rupture of an abscess into the peritoneum can result in peritonitis.

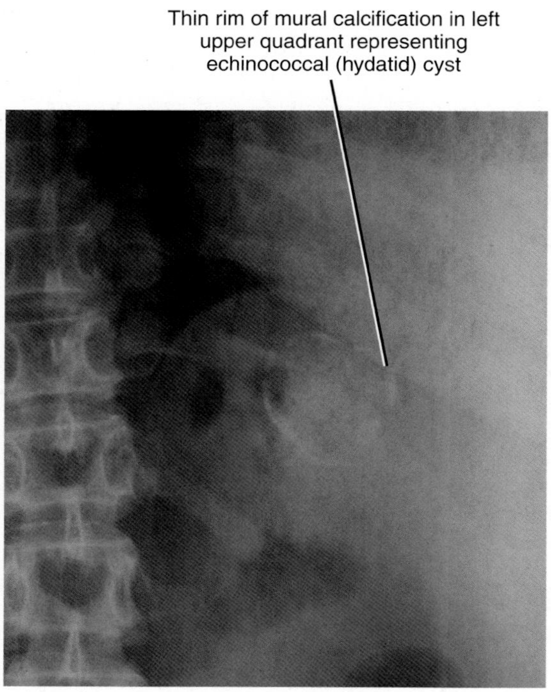

Thin rim of mural calcification in left
upper quadrant representing
echinococcal (hydatid) cyst

Figure 15-16 Frontal radiograph of a patient with hydatid cyst of the spleen demonstrating peripheral rimlike calcification.

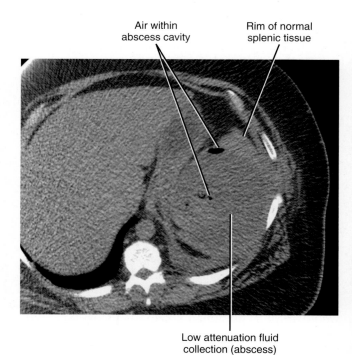

Air within abscess cavity

Rim of normal splenic tissue

Low attenuation fluid collection (abscess)

Figure 15-17 Unenhanced axial computed tomographic scan through the spleen of a patient with pyogenic splenic abscess. The patient was managed successfully with percutaneous catheter drainage.

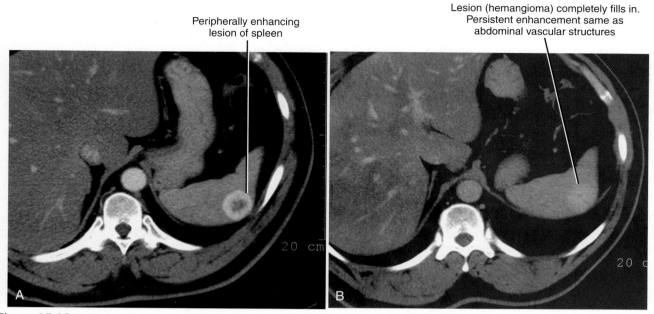

Peripherally enhancing
lesion of spleen

Lesion (hemangioma) completely fills in.
Persistent enhancement same as
abdominal vascular structures

Figure 15-18 Enhanced axial computed tomographic scan during portal (**A**) and equilibrium (**B**) phases through the spleen of a patient with isolated splenic hemangioma.

As in the liver, malignant lesions of the spleen can undergo necrosis and take on a partially cystic appearance. In most cases, necrotic malignant masses will have a complex appearance on imaging studies that differentiate them from benign splenic cysts.

Predominantly Solid-Appearing or Vascular Lesions

In the category of predominantly solid-appearing or vascular lesions, we consider lesions that are predominantly composed of solid or enhancing vascular tissue. *Hemangiomas* are the most common primary splenic neoplasm. Composed of endothelial-lined vascular spaces, hemangiomas are usually asymptomatic and are frequently discovered incidentally. Multiple lesions are commonly encountered. With US, most hemangiomas appear as an echogenic or complex mass with solid and cystic-appearing areas. Capillary hemangiomas may demonstrate increased flow with color Doppler US. With CT, these lesions are hypoattenuating relative to normal spleen and enhance after administration of intravenous contrast material. Although helpful in establishing the diagnosis when present, not all splenic hemangiomas demonstrate the centripetal, nodular enhancement pattern typical of many hepatic hemangiomas. Small lesions may enhance early and homogeneously, whereas some large hemangiomas may appear to replace the entire spleen. Splenic hemangiomas are similar in signal intensity to liver hemangiomas on MR images (Figs. 15-18 and 15-19). However, the signal intensity of splenic hemangiomas on T2-weighted MR images may not appear as bright as in the case of most liver hemangiomas because of the

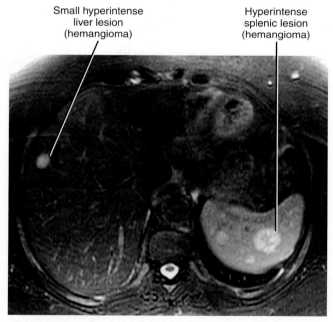

Small hyperintense
liver lesion
(hemangioma)

Hyperintense
splenic lesion
(hemangioma)

Figure 15-19 Axial, fat-suppressed, T2-weighted, magnetic resonance image through the liver and spleen of a patient with hepatic and splenic hemangiomas.

inherently bright normal splenic tissue. Splenic hemangiomas can develop areas of fibrosis, occasionally protrude beyond the margins of the splenic contour, and rarely calcify. Hemangiomas can also rupture with resultant peritoneal hemorrhage and can be associated with Kasabach–Merritt syndrome (anemia, thrombocytopenia, and coagulopathy) when large.

Pitfall: Not all splenic hemangiomas demonstrate the centripetal, nodular enhancement pattern typical of many hepatic hemangiomas.

Hamartomas, also known as nodular hyperplasia, represent an abnormal arrangement of normal splenic tissue elements and are usually asymptomatic. Hamartomas are typically well circumscribed and vary greatly in size. US usually shows a relatively homogeneous hyperechoic mass, although there may be hypoechoic or cystic areas present in some cases. Increased blood flow may be demonstrated with color Doppler imaging. These lesions can be difficult to detect on CT and MRI because they closely resemble splenic parenchyma in attenuation and signal intensity (Fig. 15-20). Coarse calcifications may rarely be present. On T2-weighted images, hamartomas are often mildly and heterogeneously hyperintense relative to the normal spleen. After intravenous administration of an extracellular contrast agent, hamartomas demonstrate mild-to-moderate heterogeneous enhancement that becomes isoenhancing to hyperenhancing relative to spleen on delayed images.

Splenic infarction may mimic a focal splenic mass, but differentiation of infarct from splenic tumor is relatively easy with imaging. Splenic infarcts tend to be wedge shaped with a broad base along the splenic capsule. The infarcted tissue does not enhance on contrast-enhanced CT and MRI examinations, although a characteristic thin rim of capsular enhancement is typically present (Fig. 15-21). US shows the infarcted region to be avascular and hypoechoic acutely, increasing in echogenicity over time as scarring develops.

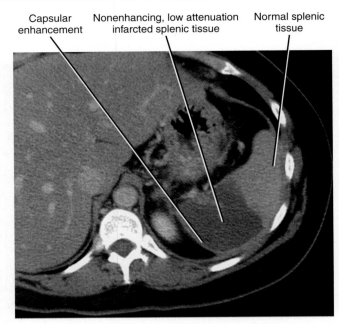

Capsular enhancement — Nonenhancing, low attenuation infarcted splenic tissue — Normal splenic tissue

Figure 15-21 Enhanced axial computed tomographic image through the upper abdomen in a patient with acute splenic infarction.

Extramedullary hematopoiesis may occasionally appear as a focal splenic mass (Fig. 15-22). Most cases occur in response to hemolytic anemia, bone marrow replacement, or myelodysplasia. Splenomegaly is common, and hemosiderosis (best demonstrated with MRI) may be present because of blood transfusions. Because of the nonspecific imaging appearance of extramedullary hematopoiesis, the presence of risk factors may be the most useful diagnostic clue. There may be a role for the use of Tc-99m sulfur colloid scintigraphy in making this diagnosis.

Lymphoma is the most common malignant tumor involving the spleen, but the spleen is usually secondarily rather than primarily involved. Primary lymphoma is rare and usually of the non-Hodgkin's type. A focal dominant mass is an uncommon manifestation of lymphoma (Fig. 15-23). When present, such masses are typically hypoechoic with US and of low attenuation on CT images. With MRI, lymphoma parallels the signal intensity of normal spleen somewhat, making it relatively inconspicuous on noncontrast-enhanced studies. After administration of extracellular contrast agents, focal lymphomatous masses tend to be poorly enhancing relative to normal spleen. However, early imaging is important because lymphoma may become isointense to spleen on delayed images. Lymphoma may be rendered more conspicuous on MR images after administration of superparamagnetic iron oxide particles because of suppression of the normal splenic signal intensity on T2- and T2*-weighted images.

Pitfall: Early imaging after administration of intravenous contrast is important for CT and MRI detection of splenic lymphoma because lymphoma may become isointense to spleen on delayed images.

Angiosarcoma is a rare, highly aggressive endothelial cell tumor with poor prognosis that usually affects older patients. Splenic involvement may be focal or diffuse, and metastatic disease involving liver, lungs, or bone is common at diagnosis. The spleen is usually enlarged.

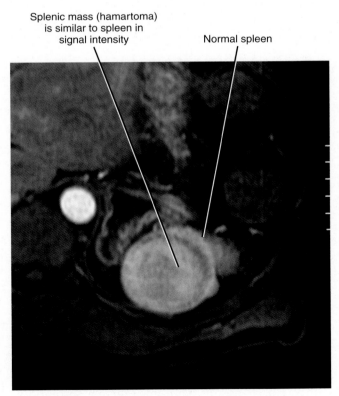

Splenic mass (hamartoma) is similar to spleen in signal intensity — Normal spleen

Figure 15-20 Gadolinium-enhanced, axial, fat-suppressed, T1-weighted image of the left upper quadrant of a patient with splenic hamartoma. The mass was difficult to see on unenhanced T1- and T2-weighted images (not shown).

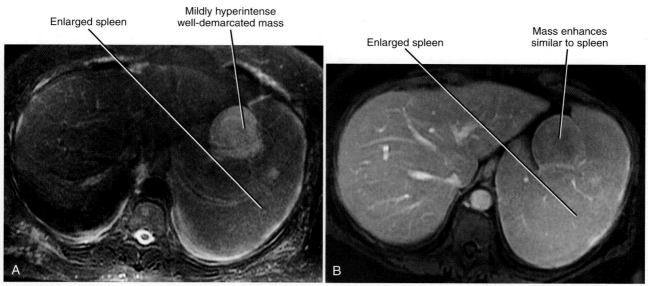

Figure 15-22 Axial, fat-suppressed, T2-weighted (**A**) and gadolinium-enhanced (**B**) magnetic resonance images through the spleen in a patient with idiopathic thrombocytopenic purpura and intrasplenic extramedullary hematopoiesis. The patient underwent splenectomy after this examination.

Angiosarcoma tends to be heterogeneous in appearance with all imaging modalities, in part because of areas of necrosis or hemorrhage. Calcifications can occasionally be present. Enhancement on CT and MR tends to be heterogeneous, and the areas of enhancing solid tissue may demonstrate increased flow with Doppler US. Spontaneous tumor rupture or hemorrhage can result in hemoperitoneum.

Splenic hematogenous metastases are uncommon in the absence of advanced metastatic disease elsewhere. Although melanoma is the tumor with the greatest predilection for splenic metastases, metastases from other tumors such as breast and lung cancer are more common because of the greater overall prevalence of those tumors. Metastases may have a highly variable appearance but most often appear as hypoechoic with US and low attenuation with CT (Fig. 15-24). Metastases often have nearly the same signal characteristics as normal spleen on unenhanced T1- and T2-weighted MR images. The use of dynamic imaging with gadolinium chelates or T2-weighted imaging after administration of superparamagnetic iron oxide particles may improve detection. Peritoneal implants on the serosal surface of the spleen may mimic parenchymal hematogenous metastases (Fig. 15-25).

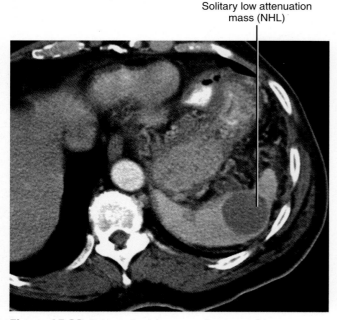

Figure 15-23 Enhanced axial computed tomographic scan through the spleen in a patient with a nonspecific solitary splenic mass. Biopsy showed non-Hodgkin's lymphoma (NHL).

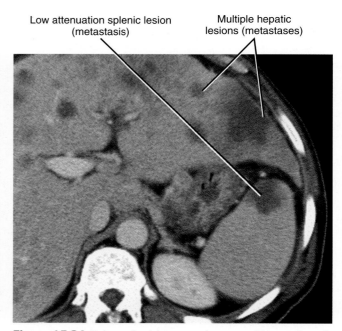

Figure 15-24 Enhanced axial computed tomographic scan through the spleen of a patient with gastric cancer metastases involving the liver and spleen.

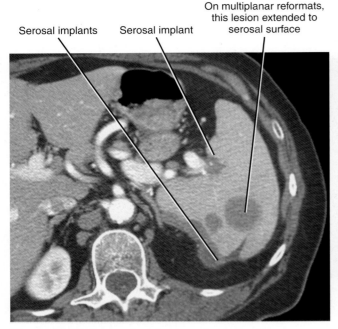

Serosal implants   Serosal implant   On multiplanar reformats, this lesion extended to serosal surface

Figure 15-25 Enhanced axial computed tomographic scan through the spleen of a patient with peritoneal cancer shows multiple splenic serosal implants. Despite the appearance of parenchymal lesions on this slice, all lesions could be shown to extend to the serosal surface on multiplanar reformations (not shown) and at surgery.

Pitfall: Metastases often have nearly the same signal characteristics as normal spleen on unenhanced T1- and T2-weighted MR images.

■ MULTIPLE SMALL SPLENIC LESIONS

A variety of abnormalities may result in multiple small splenic lesions. Some of these are listed in Box 15-2. You will no doubt note that most of these entities fit

---

BOX 15-2   Causes of Multiple Small Lesions throughout the Spleen

Bartonella henselae (cat scratch disease)
Brucellosis (Fig. 15-26)
Fungal abscesses (Fig. 15-27)
Gamna–Gandy bodies (Fig. 15-28)
Gaucher disease
Hemangioma (see Fig. 15-19)
Kaposi sarcoma
Leukemia
Littoral cell angioma
Lymphangioma
Lymphoma (Fig. 15-29)
Metastases
Mycobacteria infection
Peliosis
Pneumocystis carinii
Sarcoidosis (Fig. 15-30)

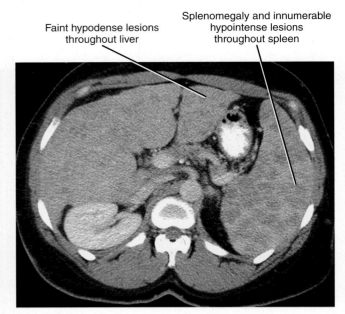

Faint hypodense lesions throughout liver   Splenomegaly and innumerable hypointense lesions throughout spleen

Figure 15-26 Enhanced axial computed tomographic scan through the upper abdomen of a patient with brucellosis.

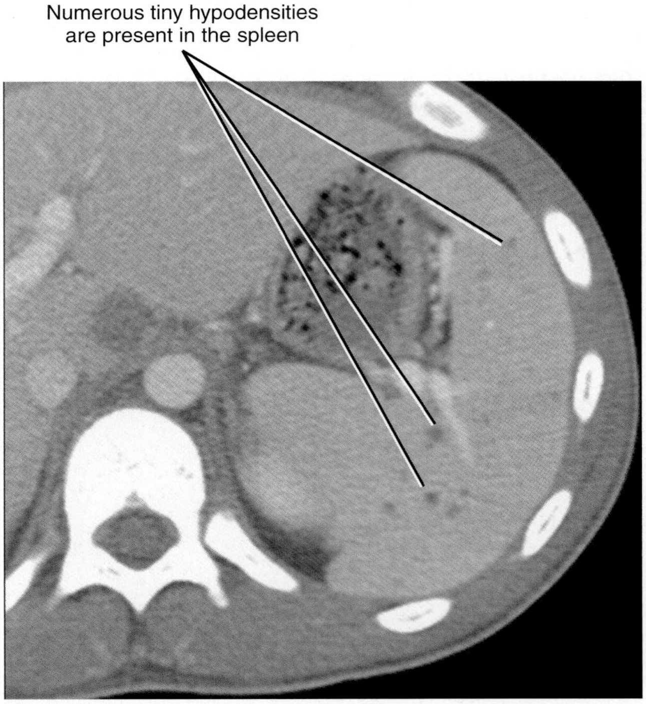

Numerous tiny hypodensities are present in the spleen

Figure 15-27 Enhanced axial computed tomographic image through the upper abdomen of an immunocompromised patient with multiple tiny fungal abscesses in the spleen. Lesions resolved after treatment.

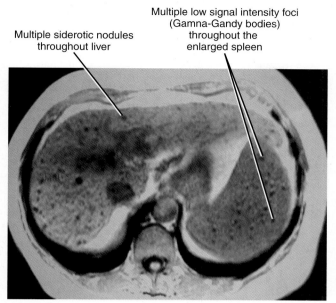

Multiple siderotic nodules throughout liver

Multiple low signal intensity foci (Gamna-Gandy bodies) throughout the enlarged spleen

Figure 15-28 Axial T1-weighted magnetic resonance image through the upper abdomen of a patient with cirrhosis, portal hypertension, multiple siderotic nodules throughout the liver, and Gamna–Gandy bodies in the spleen.

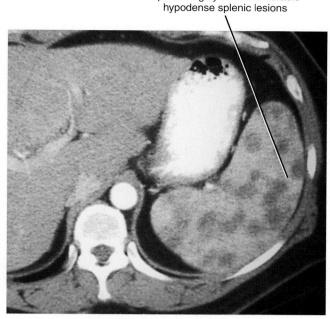

Splenomegaly and innumerable hypodense splenic lesions

Figure 15-30 Enhanced axial computed tomographic through the upper abdomen of a patient with sarcoidosis.

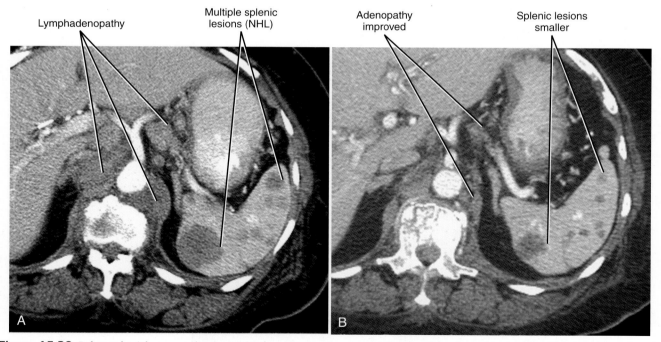

Lymphadenopathy

Multiple splenic lesions (NHL)

Adenopathy improved

Splenic lesions smaller

Figure 15-29 Enhanced axial computed tomographic scan through the upper abdomen of a patient with non-Hodgkin's lymphoma (NHL) involving the spleen before **(A)** and after **(B)** treatment.

BOX 15-3 General Processes That May Result in Multiple Small Splenic Lesions

Primary splenic neoplasm
Secondary splenic neoplasm
Infection
Granulomatous disease

Table 15-2 Clinical Scenarios Resulting in Multiple Small Splenic Lesions

Clinical Scenario	Causes to Consider
Acquired immune deficiency syndrome	Non-Hodgkin's lymphoma, Kaposi sarcoma (Fig. 15-31), mycobacterial infection, *Pneumocystis carinii*, peliosis, microabscesses
Cancer chemotherapy	Fungus, metastases
Organ transplant	Fungus, lymphoma, metastases
Disseminated cancer	Metastases
Anabolic steroid use	Peliosis
Chronic wasting state	Peliosis
Cirrhosis/portal hypertension	Gamna–Gandy bodies (see Fig. 15-28)

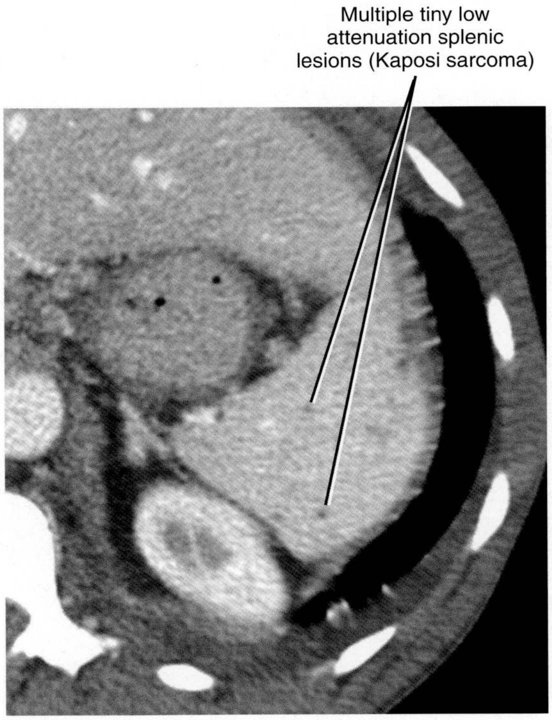

into one or more of the general categories listed in Box 15-3.

Many causes of small multifocal splenic lesions have a similar appearance regardless of imaging modality, making a definitive diagnosis based on imaging alone difficult or impossible. Therefore, differentiating the various causes of multiple small splenic lesions usually relies heavily on knowledge of the clinical scenario (Table 15-2).

The majority of small splenic lesions have a variable appearance with US, are hypoattenuating on contrast-enhanced CT, and are hypointense on gadolinium-enhanced, T1-weighted MR images, limiting the specificity of these techniques. However, a few relatively specific appearances may be encountered with imaging. For example, fungal abscesses can have a characteristic "target" appearance with US. Gamna–Gandy bodies are inconspicuous on CT and US images but appear dark on T2- and T2*-weighted MR images because of susceptibility effects. Occasionally, extrasplenic imaging findings are present that suggest the diagnosis. When multiple hepatic lesions are present in the setting of multiple splenic lesions, one should include fungal disease, metastases, lymphoma, and sarcoidosis in the differential diagnosis. Patients with sarcoidosis may have associated pulmonary findings and abdominal lymphadenopathy. Abdominal lymphadenopathy is also relatively common with non-Hodgkin's lymphoma and acquired immune deficiency syndrome (see Fig. 15-29).

Pearl: Fungal abscesses can have a characteristic "target" appearance on US images.

Multiple tiny low attenuation splenic lesions (Kaposi sarcoma)

Figure 15-31 Enhanced axial computed tomographic image through the spleen of a patient with acquired immune deficiency syndrome. Tiny splenic lesions were found to represent Kaposi sarcoma at autopsy.

■ RARE, VERY RARE, AND INCREDIBLY, MIND-BOGGLINGLY RARE THINGS THAT CAN OCCUR IN THE SPLEEN

Table 15-3 lists some rare conditions that can involve the spleen. In most of these cases, it is not possible to offer a definitive diagnosis based on imaging.

Table 15-3   Rare Splenic Conditions

Diagnosis	Relevant Information
Angiomyolipoma	Can contain adipose tissue, can be associated with renal angiomyolipoma
Castleman disease	Can have central calcification
Hemangioendothelioma	Can be solitary or multiple
Hemangiopericytoma	Can be solitary or multiple
Heterotopic pancreas	Can be source of mucinous pancreatic neoplasms
Inflammatory pseudotumor (inflammatory myofibroblastic tumor)	Can have central calcification, hypovascular
Leiomyosarcoma	Nonspecific appearance
Littoral cell angioma	Splenomegaly, multiple splenic lesions of similar size, hypersplenism
Malignant fibrous histiocytoma	Nonspecific appearance
Teratoma	See Figure 15-32
Peliosis	Associated with anabolic steroid use, hematologic disorders, and wasting diseases; can rupture

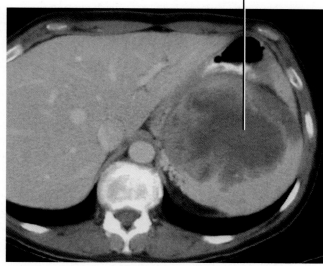

Large heterogeneous splenic mass

Figure 15-32 Enhanced axial computed tomographic image through the upper abdomen of a patient with splenic teratoma.

Suggested Readings

Abbott RM, Levy AD, Aguilera NS et al: Primary vascular neoplasms of the spleen: radiologic-pathologic correlation, *Radiographics* 24:1137-1163, 2004.

Bezerra AS, D'Ippolito G, Faintuch S et al: Determination of splenomegaly by CT: is there a place for a single measurement? *AJR Am J Roentgenol* 184:1510-1513, 2005.

De Schepper AM, Vanhoenacker F, Op de Beeck B et al: Vascular pathology of the spleen, part I, *Abdom Imaging* 30:96-104, 2005.

De Schepper AM, Vanhoenacker F, Op de Beeck B et al: Vascular pathology of the spleen, part II, *Abdom Imaging* 30:228-238, 2005.

Elsayes KM, Narra VR, Mukundan G et al: MR imaging of the spleen: spectrum of abnormalities, *Radiographics* 25:967-982, 2005.

Mainenti PP, Camera L, Nicotra S et al: Splenic hypoperfusion as a sign of systemic amyloidosis, *Abdom Imaging* 30:768-772, 2005.

Mortelé KJ, Mortelé B, Silverman SG: CT features of the accessory spleen, *AJR Am J Roentgenol* 183:1653-1657, 2004.

Paterson A, Frush DP, Donnelly LF et al: A pattern-oriented approach to splenic imaging in infants and children, *Radiographics* 19:1465-1485, 1999.

Ramani M, Reinhold C, Semelka RC et al: Splenic hemangiomas and hamartomas: MR imaging characteristics of 28 lesions, *Radiology* 202:166-172, 1997.

Robertson F, Leander P, Ekberg O: Radiology of the spleen, *Eur Radiol* 11:80-95, 2001.

Taura T, Takashima S, Shakudo M et al: Castleman's disease of the spleen: CT, MR imaging and angiographic findings, *Eur J Radiol* 36:11-15, 2000.

Urrutia M, Mergo PJ, Ros LH et al: Cystic masses of the spleen: radiologic-pathologic correlation, *Radiographics* 16:107-129, 1996.

CHAPTER 16

Gastrointestinal Tract

David J. DiSantis, Michael Oliphant, and John R. Leyendecker

It is unrealistic to think that we can thoroughly address every aspect of gastrointestinal (GI) anatomy and pathophysiology in a textbook of this scope and purpose. Consequently, we focus our discussion on diseases and quandaries likely to be encountered in a typical clinical practice. Our goal is to lead the reader from an imaging finding toward a specific diagnosis or manageable list of likely diagnoses. After a brief discussion of alimentary tract anatomy and imaging modalities, this chapter focuses on diagnostic possibilities for common imaging findings in each section of the alimentary tract, including wall thickening, luminal narrowing, dilatation, ulceration, and masses. This chapter does not always specify a modality when discussing the findings of specific abnormalities. This is to encourage thinking across all modalities, because most radiologists who interpret abdominal studies do not practice in a specific modality, and because many diseases of the alimentary tract manifest on more than one type of imaging study. Furthermore, advances in technology have allowed cross-sectional modalities such as computed tomography (CT) and magnetic resonance imaging (MRI) to create images remarkably similar to fluoroscopic studies (Fig. 16-1).

■ ANATOMY OF THE GASTROINTESTINAL TRACT

Alimentary Tube

Stomach

The stomach is divided into the cardia, fundus, body, and antrum, although no radiographically evident landmarks separate these regions. The stomach is joined to the duodenum via the muscular pyloric channel. The lumen contour of the stomach is characterized by rugal folds that are most conspicuous when the stomach is contracted and nearly completely obliterated when distended. On a double-contrast upper GI examination, a reticular surface pattern, the *areae gastricae,* can be visible. This pattern is variably present on fluoroscopic examinations and usually predominates in the gastric body or antrum. The mucosa of the stomach contains gastric glands and lymphoid tissue (mucosa-associated lymphoid tissue [MALT]). This lymphoid tissue can cause a distinct form of gastric lymphoma.

The *gastrohepatic ligament* (lesser omentum) extends from the lesser curvature of the stomach to the medial margin of the liver and can serve as a conduit for the spread of disease between the stomach and the liver. The gastrocolic ligament joins the greater curvature of the stomach and the transverse colon, whereas the gastrosplenic ligament joins the stomach and spleen. As with the other abdominal mesenteries, these ligaments facilitate the spread of inflammation and tumor between the contiguous organs.

Duodenum

The duodenum is divided into four parts. The first part, the *duodenal bulb,* lies in close proximity to the gallbladder. This close association explains how a cholecystoduodenal fistula can result from the erosion of a gallstone into the duodenum or perforation of a duodenal ulcer into the gallbladder. The duodenal bulb is the most mobile of the duodenal segments, because it is almost completely invested in peritoneum (the exception being its posterior surface near the gallbladder neck and inferior vena cava). The gastroduodenal artery courses posterior to the first portion of the duodenum, explaining the greater rate of GI hemorrhage associated with ulcers of the posterior duodenal wall.

The *second part of the duodenum* (referred to as the descending portion) borders the right lateral margin of the pancreatic head, and receives the common bile and pancreatic ducts at the major papilla. Therefore, abnormalities of the distal common bile duct, ampulla, or pancreatic head can involve the descending duodenum. The location of the major papilla is suggested on double-contrast barium examinations by the presence of several longitudinal or oblique folds. When there is a minor papilla as well, it is typically about 1 cm proximal and slightly anterior to the major papilla. The posterior surface of the descending duodenum is in continuity with the anterior pararenal space. The transverse colon passes anterior to the middle third of the descending duodenum. They are linked by the duodenocolic ligament, which serves as another bidirectional conduit for inflammation or tumor.

The *third portion of the duodenum* (the transverse portion) crosses midline from right to left, immediately ventral to the anterior wall of the aorta and dorsal to the origin of the superior mesenteric artery (SMA). This

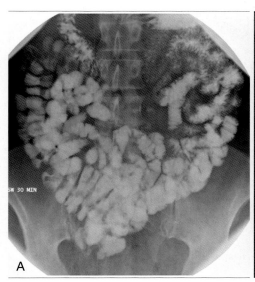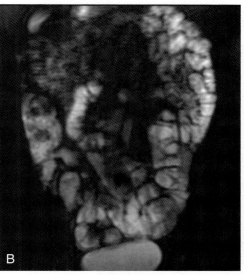

Figure 16-1 Images from a small-bowel series **(A)** and a magnetic resonance (MR) enterography examination **(B)** demonstrate similar appearances, although the spatial resolution of MR imaging lags behind fluoroscopy.

relation explains why aortoenteric fistulas typically involve the third portion of the duodenum. The transverse duodenum is also bordered superiorly by the pancreatic head and, like the second portion of the duodenum, occupies the anterior pararenal space. Contiguity with the pancreas permits frequent involvement of the duodenum with pancreatic cancers and pancreatitis.

The *fourth portion of the duodenum* becomes largely invested in peritoneum before joining the jejunum. A suspensory ligament (of Treitz) consisting of muscle fibers and fibrous tissue extends from the region of the celiac axis and left diaphragmatic crus to the duodenojejunal junction.

Mucus-secreting *Brunner glands* are found in the duodenum and most proximal jejunum but are largest and most numerous near the pylorus.

Jejunum and Ileum

The small bowel measures approximately 20 feet in length. The jejunum lies chiefly in the upper left portion of the abdomen, whereas the ileum occupies the lower right abdomen and enters the colon at the ileocecal valve. The jejunum is normally larger in diameter than the ileum, as seen by small-bowel series or enteroclysis. The small-bowel lumen measures up to 4 cm proximally and tapers to less than 3 cm distally. Although the duodenal-jejunal junction is demarcated by the suspensory ligament (of Treitz), the jejunal-ileal junction is not distinct, either histologically or radiologically. The proximal jejunum contains some Brunner glands but few Peyer patches. On imaging examinations, the *valvulae conniventes* are conspicuous in the proximal jejunum and nearly absent in the distal ileum. These folds may number up to seven per inch in the jejunum but only two to four per inch in the proximal ileum.

The distal ileum appears relatively featureless on barium examinations but can demonstrate tiny submucosal nodules that represent lymphoid follicles, particularly in young individuals or those with immune deficiency. These follicles measure 2 to 3 mm in diameter and

are often umbilicated. The arteries, veins, nerves, and lymphatics of the small bowel are conveyed within the fan-shaped small-bowel mesentery that normally extends obliquely from the region of the duodenal-jejunal junction to the right lower quadrant.

Colon and Rectum

The colon extends from the cecum to the rectum and consists of ascending, transverse, descending, and sigmoid segments. The *cecum* is a blind ending pouch extending caudal to the ileocecal valve, typically in the right lower quadrant. The cecum is variably covered in peritoneum and potentially mobile. The appendiceal lumen communicates with that of the cecum. The appendix is notoriously variable in length (up to 20 cm) and location, and can extend far cephalad into the right upper quadrant or caudally into the inguinal canal. It can cross the midline or curl behind the cecum (retrocecal appendix). The *ileocecal valve* consists of mucosal membrane and circular muscle fibers. It variably allows passage of contrast material on retrograde fluoroscopic studies and is often quite fatty on CT and MRI studies.

The ascending and descending colon and rectum are extraperitoneal, whereas the transverse and sigmoid colon are intraperitoneal, invested in, and suspended by the transverse and sigmoid mesocolons, respectively. The longitudinal muscle of the colon wall is arranged in three parallel bands (taeniae coli), and the contour of the colon is marked by haustrations. Fatty appendages *(appendices epiploicae)* attach to the serosal surface of the colon. These are normally inconspicuous unless outlined by ascites (Fig. 16-2). On double-contrast barium examination of the colon, one can sometimes see the fine innominate lines (underdistended colon), transverse folds (contracted colon), and lymph follicles that may have central umbilication (young patients) (Fig. 16-3). Lymph follicles can be associated with lymphoma, carcinoma, and inflammatory processes, and when conspicuous in older patients, should prompt a search for an associated abnormality.

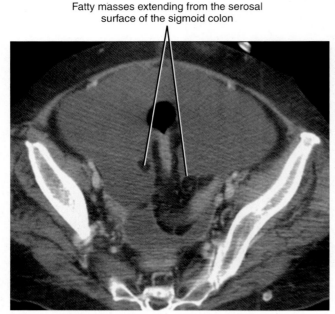

Fatty masses extending from the serosal surface of the sigmoid colon

Figure 16-2 Contrast-enhanced axial computed tomographic image through the pelvis of a patient with copious ascites demonstrating the normal epiploic appendages.

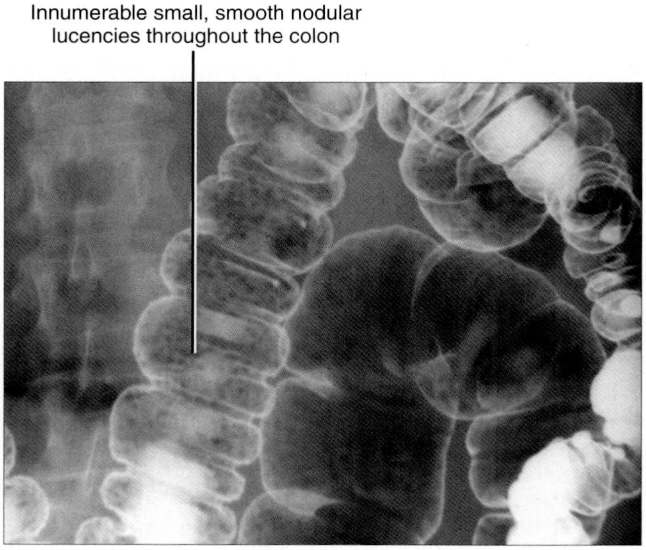

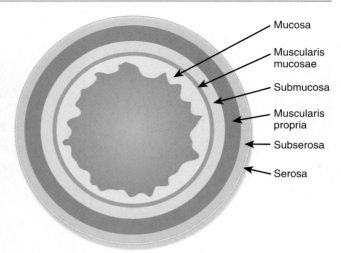

Figure 16-4 Schematic demonstrating layers of the bowel wall.

Mucosa
Muscularis mucosae
Submucosa
Muscularis propria
Subserosa
Serosa

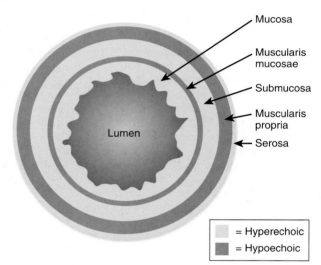

Mucosa
Muscularis mucosae
Submucosa
Muscularis propria
Serosa
Lumen

= Hyperechoic
= Hypoechoic

Figure 16-5 Ultrasound appearance of bowel wall under optimal conditions.

Innumerable small, smooth nodular lucencies throughout the colon

Figure 16-3 Appearance of lymph follicles on double-contrast barium enema.

Bowel Wall

The basic layers of the GI tract wall are illustrated in Figure 16-4. The mucosa is best depicted with double-contrast barium studies, although one can only infer information about the bowel wall with fluoroscopy. Using ultrasound (US) under ideal conditions, one can distinctly identify as many as five bowel wall layers (Fig. 16-5). In many circumstances, however, only a central echogenic area (mucosa and submucosa) surrounded by a hypoechoic rim (muscularis propria) can be distinguished.

CT and MRI are usually incapable of resolving the bowel wall to the same extent as US. With contrast-enhanced CT, the bowel wall displays stratification during the arterial phase with enhancing mucosa, hypoenhancing submucosa, and moderately enhancing muscularis propria all visible. Visualization of bowel wall layers depends on rate of injection and phase of imaging, and is better appreciated with intraluminal water rather than opaque oral contrast media. The presence of submucosal edema or hemorrhage contributes to a stratified appearance of the bowel.

The normal gastric wall is approximately 5 mm thick as measured between rugal folds in a distended state. The valvulae conniventes of the small bowel are normally less than 2 to 3 mm thick in distended loops, and the normal small bowel wall is only 1 to 2 mm thick when the lumen is sufficiently distended (diameter ≥ 2 cm). The normal colon wall thickness also measures only a few millimeters when adequately distended. Once considered an indicator of inflammatory bowel disease (Fig. 16-6), intramural fat can occur normally in the small intestine and colon of obese patients. This fatty layer becomes less conspicuous with luminal distention.

With any imaging modality, the normal bowel wall can appear thickened if the bowel lumen is not sufficiently distended. It is important to evaluate segments that are distended with gas, fluid, or enteric contrast material to decide whether apparent bowel wall thickening is real, keeping in mind that lumen narrowing can result from mural thickening. Coexisting findings such as adjacent edema, abnormal wall enhancement, or vascular engorgement on CT or MRI examinations can improve diagnostic confidence. Spurious wall thickening tends to be transient, and real-time imaging modalities such as fluoroscopy and US can determine whether an area of questionable wall thickening persists. With many CT and MRI protocols, multiphase or delayed acquisitions are performed, and comparing different phases can help confirm whether an area of bowel wall thickening is fixed or transient. Newer MRI protocols designed to assess the bowel often include rapid imaging sequences such as steady-state free precession that also allow the peristaltic activity of the bowel to be observed.

Bowel Rotation

Normal orientation of the intestinal tract occurs only after the embryologic gut completes a complex series of maneuvers. Failure of any one of these steps results in a variety of congenital abnormalities of the bowel. These developmental maneuvers include elongation of the gut and suspending mesentery, herniation of the gut into the base of the umbilical cord, rotation, and return of the developing gut to the abdominal cavity. It is important to recognize when the process of gut rotation and fixation has gone awry. Box 16-1

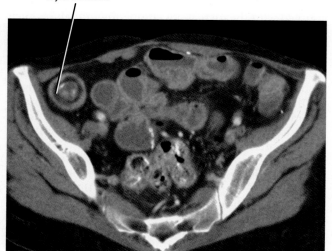

Figure 16-6 Axial image of the pelvis from a contrast-enhanced computed tomographic scan demonstrates submucosal fat in the distal ileum of a patient with Crohn's disease.

Fat attenuation submucosal layer in ileum

> **BOX 16-1   Clues to Rotational Abnormalities of the Bowel (Fig. 16-7)**
>
> Superior mesenteric vein positioned to the left of the SMA
> SMA initially courses to the right rather than left
> Small bowel located in the right abdomen, large bowel on the left (nonrotation)
> Malposition of the cecum too far medial or superior
> Duodenal-jejunal junction is inferiorly positioned or too far rightward
> "Corkscrew" orientation of duodenum and proximal small bowel
> "Whirling" of mesenteric vessels (suggests volvulus)
> Duodenum fails to cross midline between the aorta and SMA

lists imaging findings that suggest a gut rotational abnormality. The clinical significance of abnormal rotation and fixation of the bowel is the increased risk for intestinal volvulus, especially in neonates and infants.

■ IMAGING MODALITIES

Radiography (Plain Films)

Radiographs are still widely performed for the evaluation of abdominal complaints. Supine portable radiographs can confirm enteric tube placement, identify calcifications and foreign bodies, suggest a mass or organomegaly, and evaluate for obstruction. The combination of supine and upright radiographs is generally preferred to supine images alone for detection of extraluminal (i.e., intraperitoneal, intramural, or intravascular) gas and for assessment of the bowel gas pattern. Wall thickening can be inferred on abdominal radiography, although the bowel wall is not directly visible in the absence of peritoneal gas (Fig. 16-8). Bowel obstruction causes dilated gas-filled bowel loops proximal to the obstruction, with a lack of gas or bowel contents distal to the obstruction. Dilated fluid-filled bowel loops can escape radiographic detection, although obstruction can be suspected when bubbles of gas collect between mucosal folds ("string-of-pearls sign").

Pneumatosis intestinalis can be a subtle finding on radiographs, imparting a bubbly appearance to the bowel that is often mistaken for stool (Fig. 16-9). The presence of pneumatosis should prompt a search for portal venous gas, best seen overlying the periphery of the liver, often on the left of a supine patient. Often, radiographs will be inconclusive in the setting of abdominal pain, and further imaging evaluation will be necessary. Because abdomen radiographs can be the first imaging study for a patient with abdominal pain, timely and accurate interpretation can be critical to patient management and outcome.

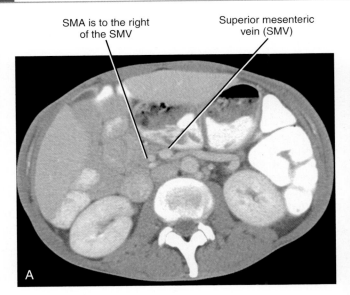

SMA is to the right of the SMV

Superior mesenteric vein (SMV)

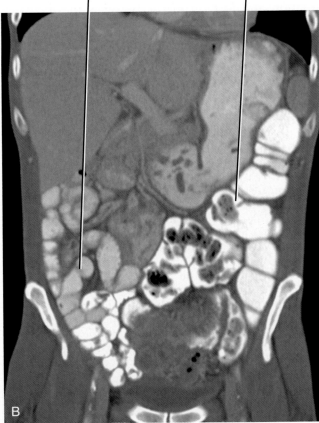

Small bowel is entirely positioned in the right abdomen

Colon is entirely positioned in the left abdomen

Figure 16-7 Nonrotation of the bowel on computed tomography (CT). **A,** Axial image of the midabdomen from a contrast-enhanced CT scan demonstrates a reversal of the normal relationship of the superior mesenteric artery (SMA) and superior mesenteric vein. **B,** Coronal reconstruction from the same examination demonstrates abnormal distribution of the large and small bowel.

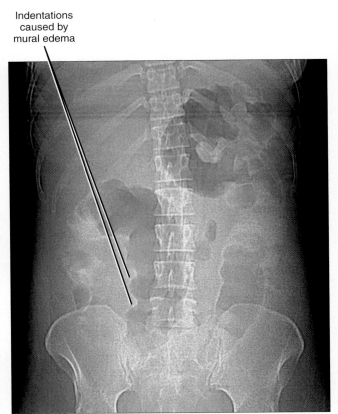

Indentations caused by mural edema

Figure 16-8 Supine abdominal radiograph of a patient with ulcerative colitis demonstrating thumbprinting of the colon.

Fluoroscopy

Clinical Utility

The use of fluoroscopy with various intraluminal contrast agents to diagnose abnormalities of the GI tract has decreased markedly in recent years. Together with a decline in usage has come a decline in expertise. The falling number of "barium gurus" will doubtless contribute to a further decline in barium studies. This trend, coupled with the increase of competing modalities such as multidetector CT and endoscopy, has led some radiologists to conclude that barium serves no purpose in today's modern radiology department. In some respects, this is a self-fulfilling prophecy, because individuals scantily trained to perform high-quality examinations are likely to provide little diagnostically useful information during fluoroscopy.

In reality, fluoroscopy plays a limited, but nonetheless important, role in GI problem solving (Box 16-2). As with other imaging modalities, such as US, the problem-solving yield of fluoroscopy can be improved by taking an interactive approach. The timely acquisition of spot films, attention to motility, appropriate patient positioning, and application of compression can markedly improve the diagnostic yield of fluoroscopic examinations. The appropriate usage of specialized techniques such as peroral pneumocolon and enteroclysis can further increase the diagnostic yield.

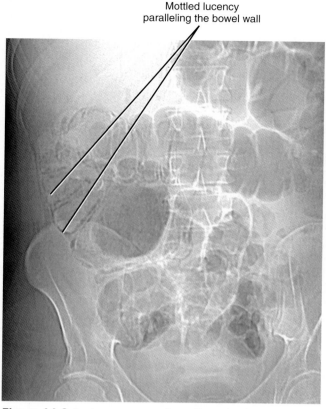

Mottled lucency
paralleling the bowel wall

Figure 16-9 Supine anteroposterior radiograph of the abdomen demonstrates appearance of pneumatosis involving the right colon.

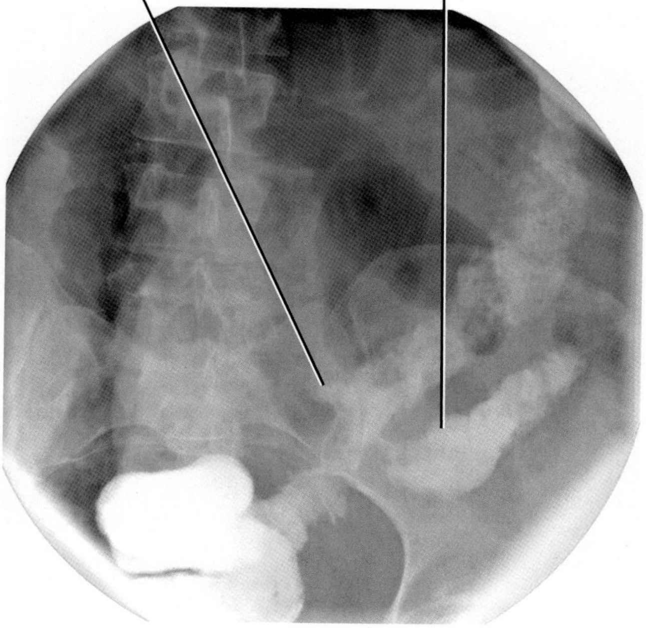

Site of
anastomosis

Extraluminal contrast material leaking
from anastomosis site

Figure 16-10 Single-contrast enema examination performed with a water-soluble agent in a patient with colocolonic anastomosis leak.

BOX 16-2   Indications for Which Fluoroscopy May Be the Preferred Technique

Enteric fistula
Enteric leak (Fig. 16-10)
Bowel obstruction versus pseudoobstruction
Assessment of anatomy and function of postoperative GI tract
Failed or incomplete endoscopy
When endoscopy cannot be performed

BOX 16-3   What to Look for during Fluoroscopy of the Gastrointestinal Tract

Abnormal bowel motility
Abnormal loop configuration or angulation
Separation or displacement of bowel loops
Malposition of bowel
Dilution or flocculation of contrast material
Ulceration
Narrowing
Dilatation
Loss of distensibility
Fold thickening
Fold irregularity or distortion
Diverticula
Filling defects
Extraluminal contrast material

There are some scenarios in which fluoroscopy can be potentially harmful. These include toxic megacolon and typhlitis. Water-soluble contrast is preferable to barium in cases of suspected bowel perforation, obstipation, chronic intestinal pseudoobstruction, fistula evaluation, and before abdominal surgery or endoscopy.

Fluoroscopic Findings
Box 16-3 and Table 16-1 list key findings visible with GI fluoroscopy. Of course, one must also remember to inspect regions and findings beyond the confines of the GI tract, such as abnormal gas collections, calcifications and other abnormal opacities, organ outlines, and skeletal abnormalities.

Ultrasound

In the United States, ultrasound is rarely used as a stand-alone technique for assessment of bowel. In most general radiology practices, it is more likely that a bowel abnormality will be discovered incidentally during an abdominal sonographic survey than as the

Table 16-1 **Fluoroscopic Findings and Their Significance**

Finding	Possible Significance
Thickened folds (single or double contrast)	Inflammation, infection, neoplastic infiltration, intramural hemorrhage, or submucosal edema
Radiating folds (single or double contrast)	Normal gastric cardia or pylorus, gastric or duodenal ulcer or ulcer scar
Linear density (double contrast)	Linear ulcer, edge of a protruding lesion, edge of an extrinsic lesion, extrinsic structure viewed through bowel, or coaptation artifact
Ring shadow (double contrast)	Gas-filled diverticulum, polyp surrounded by gas, gas-filled ulcer, gas bubble, or extrinsic structure viewed through bowel (e.g., pedicle)
Double ring shadow (double contrast) (Fig. 16-11)	Polyp on a stalk viewed end-on creates a double ring appearance; this has been referred to as the "Mexican hat sign"; do not confuse this with a barium droplet hanging from sessile polyp or barium pooled in an ulcer crater or diverticulum; in these latter cases, the center of the inner ring will be uniformly dense rather than lucent
Bowler hat (double contrast) (Fig. 16-12)	Sessile polyp (dome of hat points to lumen) or diverticulum (dome of hat points away from lumen)
Focal round density (double contrast)	Stalactite phenomenon (barium dripping from a protruding lesion of the nondependent surface), ulcer, diverticulum, barium precipitate, barium trapped in mucosal fold or pit, or extrinsic density (e.g., calcification)
Filling defect (single contrast) (Fig. 16-13)	Mucosal or submucosal mass, food, stool, foreign body, bubble, blood clot, redundant or nodular mucosa
Bull's-eye/target lesion (single or double contrast)	Hematogenous metastasis, ulcerated submucosal tumor, aphthous lesion, or ectopic pancreatic rest

Inner ring (stalk)   Outer ring (polyp)

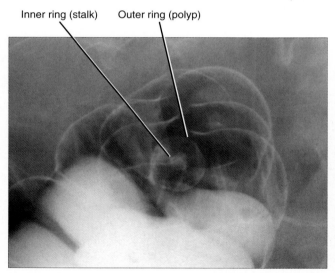

Figure 16-11 Image from a double-contrast barium enema demonstrates a pedunculated polyp creating a "double ring shadow."

Dome of "Bowler hat" points to lumen, signifying polyp rather than diverticulum

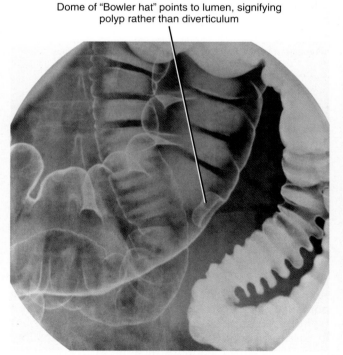

Figure 16-12 Image from a double-contrast barium enema demonstrates a sessile polyp of the transverse colon.

result of a directed search (Fig. 16-14). It is perhaps most important that one be able to distinguish between normal and abnormal bowel with US, because additional diagnostic tests will likely be necessary before a definitive diagnosis can be established.

Normal bowel is compressible by the US transducer, and peristalsis can be observed during real-time imaging. Water administered by mouth or per rectum aids in distinguishing bowel from other structures or conditions such as abscess. Normal bowel typically demonstrates some degree of stratification with US, and interruption of any of the bowel wall layers may be a sign of abnormality such as tumor. A thick hypoechoic ring (representing thickened bowel wall) surrounding a hyperechoic residual lumen, ulcerated mucosa, or both is referred to as the "pseudokidney sign." This appearance is reasonably predictive of bowel pathology.

When bowel wall thickening is present, one should attempt to distinguish between short-segment thickening

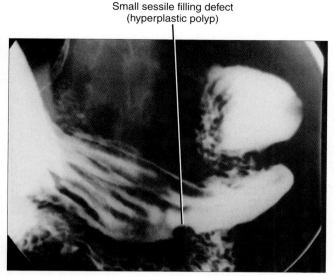

Small sessile filling defect
(hyperplastic polyp)

Figure 16-13 Spot film from a single-contrast barium examination of the stomach demonstrating a small hyperplastic antral polyp.

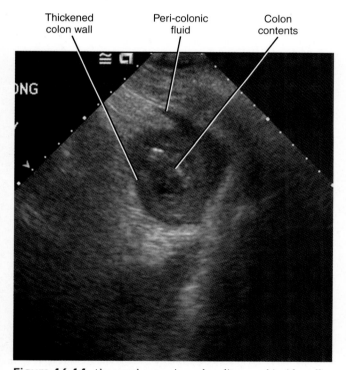

Thickened colon wall   Peri-colonic fluid   Colon contents

Figure 16-14 Abnormal-appearing colon discovered incidentally in a patient with pseudomembranous colitis undergoing ultrasound of the kidneys and bladder.

(more worrisome for a malignant process) and long-segment thickening (more likely with benign processes such as inflammation or infection). Bowel wall tumors are usually hypoechoic. Increased echogenicity in the fat adjacent to bowel may be a sign of inflammation. Gas trapped in ulcerated mucosa produces linear echogenic foci often associated with ring-down artifact. Pneumatosis produces echogenic foci in the bowel wall that can shadow. The normal bowel wall shows minimal signal with color Doppler. Completely absent flow with color

Doppler can be a sign of intestinal ischemia, whereas increased flow suggests inflammation or neoplasia.

Pearl: Short segments of bowel wall thickening are commonly associated with malignant processes, whereas long segments of thickening are more commonly associated with benign disease processes.

Pelvic bowel loops that are difficult to evaluate transabdominally may be better visualized with transvaginal US, although transvaginal US is rarely performed for this indication. Endorectal US is commonly performed for the staging of rectal carcinoma. Although endorectal US cannot assess distant disease, it is a relatively accurate method of determining T stage of rectal cancer. Loss or discontinuity of the normal layered appearance of the rectal wall implies tumor invasion. Endoscopic US is also useful for the diagnosis and staging of gastric tumors, and it has the advantage of facilitating biopsy of any abnormalities encountered.

Computed Tomography

With appropriate patient preparation, protocol design, and reconstruction techniques, CT is an excellent means of assessing the GI tract (Box 16-4). CT excels at the detection of inflammatory and neoplastic processes that affect the bowel, even when patient preparation and cooperation are less than optimal. CT has replaced other methods of detecting the presence, site, and cause of bowel obstruction. CT enterography (without small-bowel intubation) and enteroclysis (with small-bowel intubation) are used increasingly to evaluate small-bowel disorders, and CT colonography may soon become the preferred method of screening patients for colon polyps and cancer (Fig. 16-15). Currently, most nonpolypoid mucosal processes, small vascular malformations, motility disorders, and malabsorptive states cannot be reliably and routinely diagnosed with CT.

Magnetic Resonance Imaging

Indications for Magnetic Resonance Imaging of the Bowel

MRI of the bowel has a few significant advantages over CT that may increase utilization for evaluation of the GI tract. These include improved contrast conspicuity and lack of ionizing radiation. However, MRI examinations take significantly longer than the typical CT scan to perform and require greater patient cooperation. As scan

---

BOX 16-4   Gastrointestinal Disorders Readily Diagnosed with Computed Tomography

Inflammation
Obstruction
Ischemia
Neoplasia
Injury
Perforation

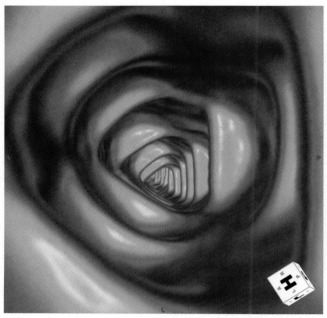

Figure 16-15 Endoluminal view from a computed tomography colonographic study. The colon lumen is distended with gas administered per rectum after a bowel prep.

Enhancing, thickened loop of ileum

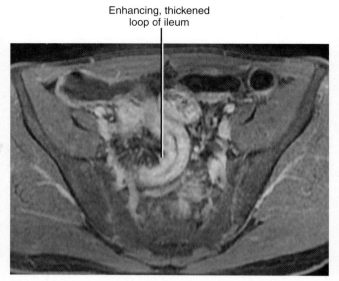

Figure 16-16 Axial fat-suppressed contrast-enhanced magnetic resonance image of a patient with inflamed distal ileum caused by Crohn disease.

times continue to shorten and expertise continues to grow, MRI will doubtless play a larger role in evaluating the GI tract in the near future.

Sequences useful for imaging bowel include single-shot echo train spin-echo sequences, balanced steady-state free precession sequences, and two- or three-dimensional gadolinium-enhanced fat-suppressed gradient-echo sequences. Administration of an anti-peristaltic agent immediately before contrast-enhanced imaging improves image quality. When performing gadolinium-enhanced imaging to evaluate the bowel wall, a negative contrast agent (dark on T1) that distends the bowel lumen is helpful. A variety of intraluminal contrast agents have been recommended for this purpose, including water, dilute barium, and polyethylene glycol. Additives such as mannitol, Psyllium husk, and locust bean gum have been used to improve bowel distention. Although expertly performed MRI of a cooperative patient is equivalent to CT for evaluation of many suspected GI abnormalities, there are a few indications for which MRI may be preferable to CT (Box 16-5).

Uterus   High signal intensity tumor fills the rectal lumen   Mesorectal fascia is intact

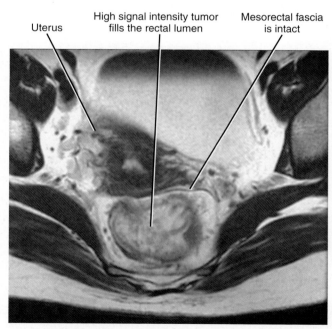

Figure 16-17 Axial T2-weighted magnetic resonance image through the pelvis of a patient with adenocarcinoma of the rectum.

BOX 16-5   Potential Indications for Magnetic Resonance Imaging of the Gastrointestinal Tract

Evaluation of disease activity and treatment response in Crohn disease (Fig. 16-16)
Evaluation of pelvic and perianal fistulae
Staging of rectal cancer (Fig. 16-17)
Suspected bowel abnormality during pregnancy (e.g., appendicitis, obstruction, neoplasm)

Nuclear Medicine

Nuclear scintigraphy has a limited but important role in evaluating the GI tract. Table 16-2 lists potential applications to consider.

Positron emission tomography (PET) utilizing F-18 fluorodeoxyglucose (^{18}F-FDG) is revolutionizing oncologic imaging. Because cancer cells often demonstrate higher metabolic activity than normal cells, the uptake of glucose by many cancer cell types is generally greater. ^{18}F-FDG is a glucose analog that is handled in much the same way by cells as glucose. Within the GI tract,

Table 16-2   Potential Indications for Nuclear Scintigraphy of the Gastrointestinal Tract

Radiopharmaceutical	Application
Tc-99m sulfur colloid	• Detection of active gastrointestinal hemorrhage • Evaluation of gastric emptying • Detection of gastroesophageal reflux
Tc-99m red blood cells	• Detection of active gastrointestinal hemorrhage
Tc-99m pertechnetate	• Diagnosis of bleeding Meckel's diverticulum • Detection of ectopic gastric mucosa in locations other than Meckel diverticulum
Tc-99m CEA-scan	• Detection of recurrent and metastatic colorectal cancer
In-111 pentreotide	• Detection of neuroendocrine tumors (e.g., carcinoid)

Tc-99m, Technetium 99m.

PET imaging with ^{18}F-FDG is used primarily to stage and assess response to therapy for esophageal and colorectal carcinoma. PET may also detect malignant tumors from non-GI sites that secondarily involve the bowel.

Capsule Endoscopy

Capsule endoscopy has supplanted small-bowel fluoroscopic studies in searching for mucosal lesions, particularly in patients with occult GI bleeding. It should not be used, however, if there is suspicion of bowel stricture or obstruction.

■ ABNORMALITIES OF THE STOMACH

Thickening

Deciding whether the gastric wall is too thick on an imaging study is a challenge, because the gastric wall varies in thickness between its nondistended and distended states. If the study is performed specifically to evaluate the stomach, every reasonable effort should be made to completely distend the lumen by using effervescent granules, water, or other oral contrast material. When only partial distention of the stomach can be achieved, changing the patient's position can redistribute the gastric contents to distend individual gastric segments. The gastric wall between rugal folds generally measures 5 mm or less. The gastric cardia looks thickened and masslike when not adequately distended, mimicking a carcinoma on CT. The distal antrum and pyloric channel are also common locations of spurious thickening on CT and MRI. Giving gas crystals and scanning the patient left-side-down can help to differentiate real from artifactual thickening. As a general rule, the prepyloric antral wall of the stomach should measure less than 5 mm. The antrum should be considered abnormal when this thickness exceeds 10 mm or if asymmetric thickness is present.

Normally the gastric wall is thinner in nondependent segments of the stomach that are well distended by gas. In addition, adherent debris that may add to the appearance of gastric wall thickening typically remains within the fluid-filled dependent portions. When wall thickening involves not only dependent, fluid-filled parts of the stomach but also nondependent, gas-filled portions on a CT or MRI scan, an underlying abnormality should be suspected (Fig. 16-18).

Pearl: When wall thickening involves not only dependent, fluid-filled parts of the stomach but also nondependent, gas-filled portions on a CT or MRI scan, an underlying abnormality should be suspected.

Thickening of the rugal folds has an extensive differential diagnosis (Table 16-3). Fortunately, many of the entities that cause rugal fold thickening are extremely rare, and many of the common causes will have other imaging findings that allow a specific diagnosis to be made.

Gastric adenocarcinoma can cause focal or diffuse gastric wall thickening, although the normal rugal fold pattern is typically not maintained at the site of tumor. Scirrhous carcinoma infiltrates the submucosa of the stomach, resulting in some combination of wall thickening, luminal narrowing, and reduced distensibility. Gastric lymphoma can have a variety of appearances including diffuse gastric wall thickening (see Fig. 16-18).

Luminal Narrowing

Gastric narrowing is often more apparent on barium examination of the stomach than on cross-sectional imaging studies, because most causes of gastric narrowing also result in reduced distensibility and hypomotility. The antrum is the most commonly narrowed gastric

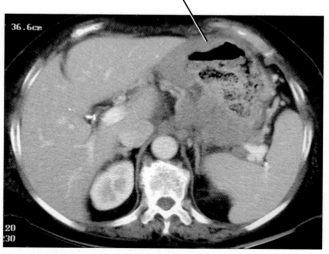

Wall thickening involves nondependent air-distended wall

Figure 16-18 Enhanced axial computed tomographic scan through the abdomen of a patient with B-cell lymphoma involving the stomach.

Table 16-3   Causes of Rugal Fold Thickening

Causes	Helpful Distinguishers
Common Causes	
Underdistention	• Collapsed lumen • Resolves with distention
Gastritis (most often *Helicobacter pylori*)	• Positive urea breath test • Predominates in body and antrum
Pancreatitis	• Pancreatic inflammation (CT/MR) • Peripancreatic fluid (CT/MR) • Increased serum amylase, lipase levels
Portal hypertension	• Cirrhosis (CT/MR) • Varices (CT/MR) • Splenomegaly
Varices	• Cirrhosis (CT/MR) • Splenic vein thrombosis (enhanced CT/MR) • Enhance like veins (enhanced CT/MR)
Lymphoma (Figs. 16-19 and 16-20)	• Adenopathy (CT/MR) • Distensible lumen
Rare Causes	
Zollinger–Ellison syndrome	• Postbulbar ulcers (UGI) • Gastric hypersecretion (UGI) • Gastrinoma (CT/MR)
Ménétrier disease	• Hypoproteinemia
Eosinophilic gastritis	• Small-bowel involvement • Peripheral eosinophilia
Amyloidosis	• Small-bowel involvement
Sarcoidosis	• Adenopathy (CT/MR) • Splenomegaly • Pulmonary manifestations

CT, Computed tomography; *MR,* magnetic resonance; *UGI,* upper gastrointestinal.

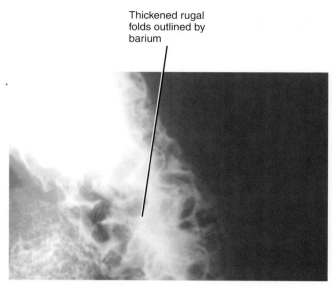

Thickened rugal folds outlined by barium

Figure 16-19 Spot film from a single-contrast barium examination of a patient with rugal fold thickening caused by gastric lymphoma.

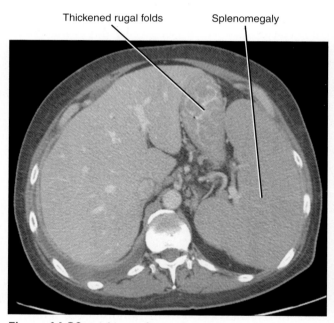

Thickened rugal folds   Splenomegaly

Figure 16-20 Axial image from a contrast-enhanced computed tomographic scan through the upper abdomen of a patient with lymphoma involving the stomach.

segment, and wall thickening often accompanies luminal narrowing. Clinical history plays an important role in distinguishing causes of gastric narrowing (e.g., history of caustic ingestion, radiation treatment, known primary neoplasm). Table 16-4 lists some causes of gastric narrowing.

Dilatation

Gastric dilatation is often associated with a history of nausea, vomiting, or both, although asymptomatic gastric distention is not uncommon. The causes of gastric dilatation can be divided into two major groups: (1) *functional obstruction* or atony from a wide variety of causes, such as prior vagotomy, medications, diabetes, uremia, ischemia, trauma, or scleroderma; and (2) *mechanical outlet obstruction* from abnormalities such as tumor, ulcer, inflammatory stricture, pancreatitis, bezoar, prolapsed polyp, or volvulus. A distended, gas-filled stomach can be seen in patients after resuscitation or instrumentation. When a dilated stomach is encountered on an imaging examination, one must always closely examine the gastric outlet, duodenum, and surrounding structures for possible causes.

Ulceration

With the widespread availability of endoscopy and development of effective methods of treating peptic ulcer disease, gastric ulcers are rarely encountered by radiologists. Many radiologists will have never diagnosed a gastric ulcer on an upper GI examination during their training.

Most gastric ulcers are found along the posterior wall of the antrum or body, or along the lesser curvature of the stomach. Anterior wall or greater curvature ulcers account for about 15% of gastric ulcers. Of course, this statistic is not particularly useful to the radiologist faced with one particular ulcer on a fluoroscopic study. It is

Table 16-4   Causes of Gastric Narrowing

Category	Disease Process
Neoplastic	• Carcinoma (scirrhous carcinoma) • Noncontiguous spread of tumor (e.g., colon cancer) • Hematogenous spread of tumor (e.g., lung cancer, breast cancer) • Lymphoma
Inflammatory	• Postpeptic scarring • Caustic ingestion • Radiation • Crohn disease • Eosinophilic gastritis • Sarcoidosis
Infectious	• Tuberculosis • Syphilis
Extrinsic compression	• Splenomegaly • Aortic aneurysm • Pancreatic pseudocyst
Other	• Amyloidosis

far more useful to know whether to recommend endoscopy for further evaluation when encountering a gastric ulcer. In general, endoscopy should be pursued if any ulcer is less than unequivocally benign in appearance (Table 16-5). Although the other signs are useful from a statistical standpoint, only the rarely seen *Hampton line* is believed to be an unequivocal sign of benignity.

Erosions are small, superficial linear or round ulcerations that often occur on the crests of gastric folds. Erosions are typically multiple and often demonstrate a radiolucent halo of edematous mucosa on double-contrast barium examinations. Box 16-6 lists some causes of gastric erosions. Note that many of the entities that cause erosions also can result in gastric wall thickening and narrowing when advanced.

Table 16-5   Features Suggestive of Benign versus Malignant Gastric Ulcers

Feature	Benign	Malignant
Location	Lesser curvature and distal stomach more common	Greater curvature and proximal stomach more common
Margins	Sharp, round	Irregular, elevated
Folds	Smooth, extend to edge of crater	Nodular, amputated, do not extend to crater edge
Mucosa	Area gastricae intact	Area gastricae distorted or obliterated
Profile	Projects beyond expected lumen contour	Projects within expected lumen contour
Signs	Hampton line*	Carman meniscus sign†
Clinical course	Heals with appropriate peptic ulcer therapy	Persists or progresses despite appropriate therapy for peptic ulcer disease

*Hampton line refers to a thin, straight lucent line across the neck of a contrast-filled ulcer representing intact mucosa.
†Carman meniscus sign is created when the heaped-up edges of a large shallow malignant ulcer are apposed during compression, trapping barium in a collection that is convex to the gastric lumen.

BOX 16-6   Causes of Gastric Erosions

Helicobacter pylori gastritis
Nonsteroidal antiinflammatory drugs
Granulomatous gastritis (e.g., Crohn disease, tuberculosis)
Caustic ingestion
Radiation
Acquired immune deficiency syndrome related (e.g., cytomegalovirus)

Masses

Pseudotumors

The stomach is a common site for a false-positive interpretation regarding a mass. Some common locations for gastric pseudotumors include the region of the gastric cardia, along the proximal lesser curvature, and in the distal antrum and pyloric region. Most often, the appearance of a mass is related to redundant, contracted, or nondistended gastric wall, and the issue can be satisfactorily resolved with further distention of the stomach. Ingested material or *bezoar* may also give the false impression of a gastric mass (Fig. 16-21). A pseudotumor can change dramatically in position, often does not have a consistent connection with the gastric wall, and may fail to demonstrate enhancement after intravenous contrast administration on CT and MR images. A true gastric neoplasm is a persistent finding on multiple phases, acquisitions, or examinations that has a consistent communication with the gastric wall and demonstrates enhancement. Movement alone is not a helpful sign because pedunculated gastric masses can change position. Unlike some bezoars, gastric neoplasms do not contain gas. A *pancreatic rest* can simulate an ulcerated submucosal mass. Ectopic pancreatic tissue usually occurs along the greater curvature of the distal gastric

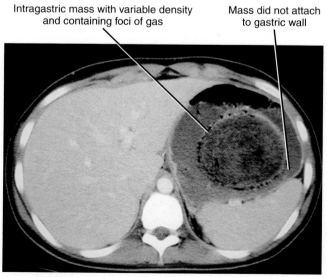

Intragastric mass with variable density and containing foci of gas

Mass did not attach to gastric wall

Figure 16-21 Axial image from a contrast-enhanced computed tomographic scan through the stomach of a patient with a large bezoar.

antrum or in the proximal duodenum. Pancreatic rests are usually small (1 cm or less), broad based, smooth, and have a central umbilication related to the primitive ductal system as seen on barium studies.

Pitfall: Pseudotumors of the stomach commonly occur in the region of the gastric cardia, along the proximal lesser curvature, and in the distal antrum and pyloric region.

Gastric Polyps

Gastric polyps are common mucosal masses of the stomach. Gastric polyps can be adenomatous, hyperplastic, or hamartomatous (Fig. 16-22). Most gastric polyps are hyperplastic, whereas in the duodenum, most polyps are adenomatous. Hyperplastic polyps are often small (<1 cm), smooth, sessile, and multiple. Adenomatous polyps are frequently solitary and more likely to be large (>2 cm) and pedunculated (Table 16-6).

Pearl: Most gastric polyps are hyperplastic, whereas most duodenal polyps are adenomatous.

Submucosal Mass

Submucosal masses typically have borders that are mildly obtuse with respect to the gastric wall, although some submucosal masses will appear pedunculated, potentially creating confusion with gastric polyps. Most benign submucosal masses are smooth with intact overlying gastric mucosa, although central ulceration or umbilication can occasionally create a bull's-eye appearance. Definitively characterizing a submucosal mass with imaging is difficult in most cases. Occasionally, some clues as to causative factors exist. Lipomas and lymphangiomas are compressible and can be seen to change shape. *Lipomas* are fat density, whereas lymphangiomas are cystic on CT images. A lesion that contains phleboliths represents a hemangioma. A solitary, smooth, round, submucosal soft-tissue mass or a large, exophytic, necrotic mass are statistically most likely to

Table 16-6   Adenomatous versus Hyperplastic Gastric Polyps

Feature	Adenomatous	Hyperplastic
Size	>1 cm	<1 cm
Shape	Lobulated	Smooth
Number	Solitary	Multiple
Base	Sessile or pedunculated	Sessile

represent *leiomyoma* or gastrointestinal stromal tumor *(GIST)* (Fig. 16-23). Box 16-7 lists some causes of submucosal mass.

Common Malignant Gastric Tumors

GASTROINTESTINAL STROMAL TUMOR

GISTs are histologically distinct from leiomyomas, although this distinction cannot be made with imaging. Likewise, the distinction between benign or malignant is difficult unless metastatic disease or frank invasion is present. Most GISTs are sporadic, but these tumors can be associated with *neurofibromatosis* (NF-1) and *Carney triad* (gastric GIST, pulmonary chondroma, extraadrenal paraganglioma). GISTs are usually solitary, often large, round tumors of the gastric wall. They can appear primarily exophytic (common), intramural, or endophytic (i.e., bulging into gastric lumen [least common]). GISTs are often necrotic, demonstrating mucosal ulceration or deep cavitation that can communicate with the gastric lumen. Up to 25% of lesions demonstrate calcifications on CT. GISTs usually are of intermediate signal intensity on T1-weighted MRI and intermediate to low signal intensity on T2-weighted MRI. Areas of central necrosis

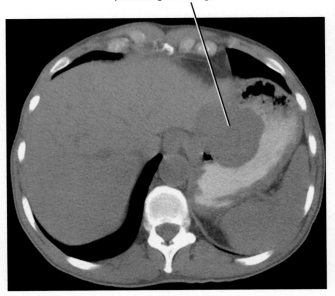

Large smooth, round, submucosal mass
protruding into the gastric lumen

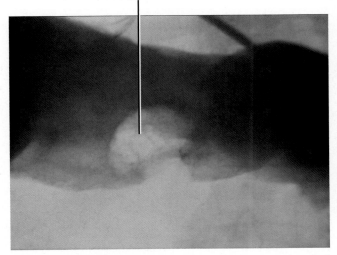

Filling defect on a short stalk
within the gastric antrum

Figure 16-22 Spot film from a single-contrast upper gastrointestinal examination demonstrates an antral polyp.

Figure 16-23 Axial image of the abdomen from computed tomography performed with positive oral contrast material but no intravenous contrast in a patient with a gastrointestinal stromal tumor of the stomach.

BOX 16-7 *Submucosal Gastric Masses*

Leiomyoma (leiomyosarcoma)
GIST
Lymphoma
Lipoma
Hemangioma
Neurogenic tumors (e.g., neurofibroma)
Metastasis
Varix

demonstrate increased signal intensity on T2-weighted images. Enhancement after intravenous contrast administration is variable on CT and MRI (necrotic areas do not enhance). GISTs tend to be ^{18}F-FDG avid. Therefore, PET is a useful modality for documenting early response to imatinib. Malignant tumors can spread to liver, peritoneum, and rarely, lymph nodes. Metastatic foci often resemble the primary tumor, although metastases treated with imatinib can mimic cysts.

> *Pearl: GISTs are often necrotic, demonstrating mucosal ulceration or deep cavitation that can communicate with the gastric lumen.*
> *Pitfall: Metastases treated with imatinib can mimic cysts.*

ADENOCARCINOMA

Most gastric cancers are adenocarcinomas. Adenocarcinomas can be polypoid, plaquelike, endophytic, exophytic, or infiltrative. Unlike stromal tumors, most adenocarcinomas present as endophytic masses or irregular focal wall thickening (Fig. 16-24). Ulceration is relatively common. Scirrhous carcinoma results in a thickened nondistensible stomach (*linitis plastica*

appearance). Gastric cancer can be associated with malignant ascites, peritoneal nodules, or regional lymphadenopathy.

LYMPHOMA

Lymphoma often presents with thicker and more diffuse circumferential involvement of the stomach than other tumors (see Fig. 16-18). Despite this, the stomach involved with lymphoma often remains distensible. As elsewhere in the body, lymphoma is a great mimicker of other diseases. When presenting as a large, solitary, ulcerated mass, lymphoma can be indistinguishable from a GIST. Hodgkin's lymphoma can be scirrhous or present as thickened rugal folds. MALT lymphoma is a low-grade B-cell lymphoma associated with *Helicobacter pylori* infection. MALT lymphoma can present as multiple round, confluent nodules. Lymphadenopathy in a distribution other than the gastric drainage is a clue that a gastric mass represents lymphoma, although lymphadenopathy is not a conspicuous feature of MALT lymphoma. Gastric outlet obstruction is uncommon with lymphoma.

> *Pearl: The stomach involved with lymphoma can remain distensible and rarely becomes obstructed.*

SECONDARY TUMORS

Malignant tumors can spread to the stomach via hematogenous spread, direct spread from contiguous organs, and peritoneal spread (Fig. 16-25). Breast cancer, lung cancer, and melanoma are among the more common malignant neoplasms to metastasize to the stomach. Hematogenous metastases can mimic primary gastric tumors such as adenocarcinoma or GIST, although the classic appearance is one of multiple centrally ulcerated submucosal masses (*bull's-eye lesions*). Breast cancer involving the stomach can cause a linitis plastica appearance. Pancreatic cancer and colon cancer can spread to

Irregular endophytic mass
in gastric antrum

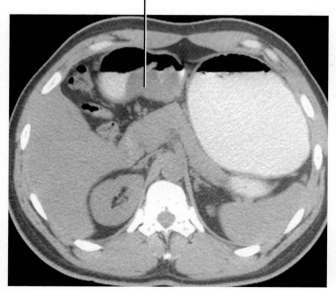

Figure 16-24 Axial image from a computed tomographic scan performed through the upper abdomen with positive oral contrast material in a patient with gastric adenocarcinoma.

Stomach

Exophytic, partially necrotic mass of gastric
fundus (melanoma metastasis)

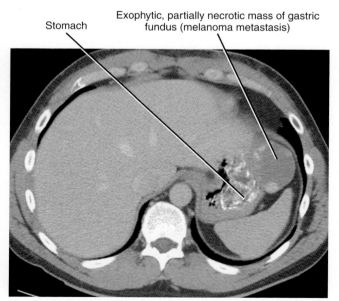

Figure 16-25 Axial image of the upper abdomen from contrast-enhanced computed tomographic scan of a patient with melanoma metastatic to the stomach.

the stomach directly, whereas other tumors can involve the stomach via the gastric mesenteries. Direct invasion of the stomach from a nongastric primary results in spiculation and/or tethering of the involved wall with distortion of the mucosal folds. CT reveals a soft-tissue mass obliterating the fat planes between the stomach and the organ of origin.

Cystic Masses of the Stomach

The most common cystic lesion to involve the stomach is *pseudocyst* of pancreatic origin. When changes of acute pancreatic inflammation are present, the diagnosis is usually straightforward. Pancreatic pseudocysts are of variable attenuation or signal intensity on CT and MRI, respectively. The contents of a pseudocyst should not enhance with intravenous contrast agents. Pseudocysts can occur adjacent to or within the gastric wall, and can communicate with the gastric lumen and pancreatic duct. On upper GI examination, pseudocysts can cause a smooth extrinsic impression on the gastric lumen, often along the posterior wall.

On CT, a *gastric duplication cyst* typically appears as a water-density mass along the greater curvature of the stomach that does not communicate with gastric lumen. Mural calcification can be present in some cases. MRI signal intensity varies with protein content. The contents of a gastric duplication cyst should not enhance, and no mural nodules should be present.

Occasionally, GISTs can undergo necrosis to the extent that they appear cystic, particularly with treatment. A juxtagastric abscess likewise can mimic a cystic gastric mass.

Other

Gastric Diverticula

Gastric diverticula arise most often from the posterior fundus of the stomach along the lesser curvature. Though usually asymptomatic, they can be confused with adrenal masses, gastric masses, gastric ulcers, or abscesses on CT and MR images (Fig. 16-26). Diverticula can be differentiated from these pathologic conditions because diverticula fill with gas or oral contrast material and demonstrate no enhancement centrally. Complications are rare and include bleeding and ulceration. Carcinoma rarely develops within a gastric diverticulum.

Gastric Volvulus

Clinical signs and symptoms of gastric volvulus include acute epigastric pain, retching producing minimal vomitus, and inability to pass a nasogastric tube. Among the complications of gastric volvulus are gastric outlet obstruction, ischemia, and perforation. Traumatic diaphragmatic hernia, paraesophageal hernia, and congenital diaphragmatic defects predispose to gastric volvulus. Abnormal rotation of the stomach can occur along its longitudinal axis (*organoaxial* rotation; Fig. 16-27), or it may twist about the gastrohepatic ligament (*mesenteroaxial* rotation; Fig. 16-28). Often

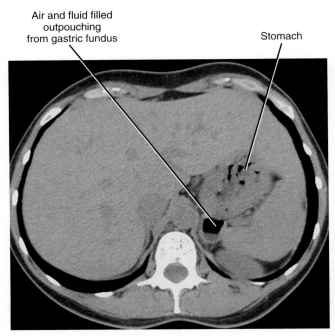

Air and fluid filled outpouching from gastric fundus

Stomach

Figure 16-26 Axial view of the upper abdomen from an unenhanced computed tomographic scan demonstrates air and fluid within a gastric diverticulum.

best demonstrated on fluoroscopic examination, diagnosis of gastric volvulus can be challenging on CT (Fig. 16-29). Box 16-8 lists imaging signs of gastric volvulus.

Acute gastric volvulus with vascular compromise is a surgical emergency. It is not uncommon, however, to find an elderly patient with an intrathoracic stomach that has varying degrees of rotation but minimal or no symptoms. Volvulus of an intrathoracic stomach can compromise cardiac function because of gastric distention.

Pneumatosis

Gas within the gastric wall can occur for a variety of reasons (Box 16-9). The appearance of pneumatosis can be simulated when air bubbles are dispersed within gastric contents and lodge between rugal folds. In such cases, close examination of the distended portions of the stomach wall will fail to reveal intramural gas. As with pneumatosis elsewhere, the presence of gas in the wall of the stomach should prompt a search for portal venous gas (Fig. 16-30).

■ ABNORMALITIES OF THE DUODENUM

Thickening

Duodenal fold thickening can be seen with duodenitis (and consequent Brunner gland hyperplasia), peptic ulcer disease (including Zollinger–Ellison syndrome), Crohn disease, and giardiasis. Patients with duodenal Crohn disease can have manifestations

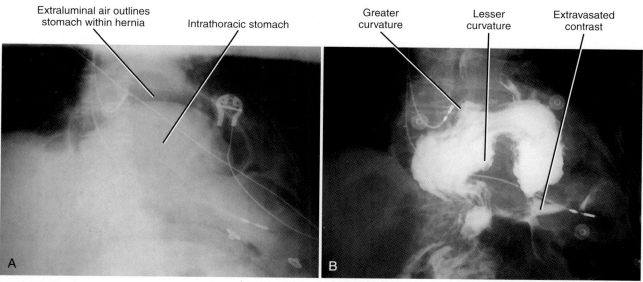

Figure 16-27 Intrathoracic gastric volvulus. **A,** Chest radiograph performed for chest pain demonstrates abnormal air within a large hiatal hernia. **B,** Image from an upper gastrointestinal examination demonstrates intrathoracic location of the stomach with inversion of the greater and lesser curvatures, indicating organoaxial volvulus of the stomach. Contrast is leaking from the stomach that has already perforated.

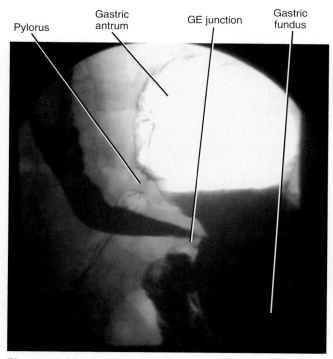

Figure 16-28 Spot image from an upper gastrointestinal examination demonstrates inversion of the gastroesophageal (GE) junction and the pylorus caused by twisting around the lesser omentum, indicating mesenteroaxial gastric volvulus.

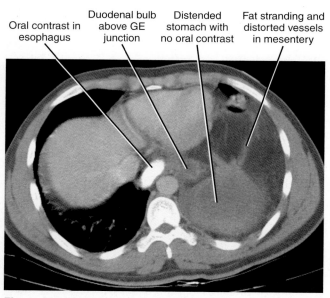

Figure 16-29 Axial image from computed tomography performed with oral and intravenous contrast demonstrates oral contrast in the esophagus that does not reach the stomach. The stomach is distended with wall thickening, elevating the left hemidiaphragm. Mesenteroaxial gastric volvulus was treated surgically. *GE,* Gastroesophageal.

BOX 16-8   *Imaging Signs of Gastric Volvulus*
Oral contrast does not enter or exit stomach
Nasogastric tube does not enter stomach
Antrum and pylorus are superior to the level of the fundus
Beaking of contrast column
Distended gas-filled viscus in chest
Double fluid level in chest
"Upside-down" stomach
Downward-pointing pylorus

in any portion of the GI tract. Fold thickening in giardiasis is typically restricted to the duodenum and proximal jejunum. Both giardiasis and Zollinger–Ellison syndrome can be associated with increased fluid production. Duodenal hematoma causes localized wall thickening and can occur in the setting of trauma or pancreatitis (Fig. 16-31). Hematoma causes

BOX 16-9   Causes of Gastric Wall Gas
Emphysematous gastritis (gas-producing organism)
Caustic ingestion
Trauma (including endoscopic)
Gastric infarction
Ulcer disease

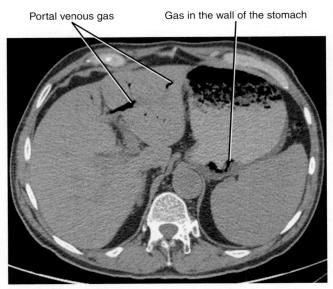

Portal venous gas   Gas in the wall of the stomach

Figure 16-30 Axial image of the upper abdomen from an unenhanced computed tomographic scan demonstrates gastric pneumatosis and portal venous gas. The cause of this finding was never definitively determined.

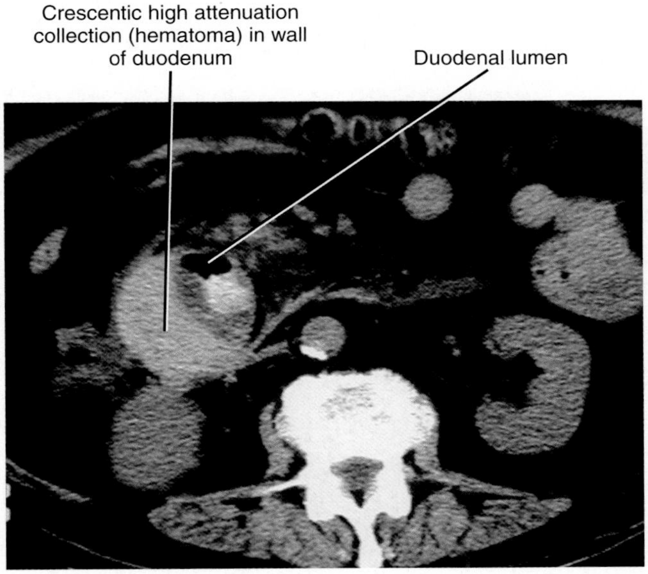

Crescentic high attenuation
collection (hematoma) in wall
of duodenum   Duodenal lumen

Figure 16-31 Axial image through the level of the descending duodenum from an unenhanced computed tomographic scan of a patient with acute pancreatitis demonstrates an intramural hematoma of the duodenum. The high-density material within the duodenal wall could be confused with intramural leakage of positive oral contrast material.

characteristic crescentic high attenuation within the submucosal region of the duodenal wall (ring sign). Pancreatitis can also result in intramural pseudocyst formation in the duodenum. Although duodenal thickening can be found in the setting of cirrhosis and portal hypertension, it rarely occurs in the absence of jejunal thickening. Annular pancreas can also mimic duodenal thickening (Fig. 16-32).

Luminal Narrowing

Narrowing of the duodenum most commonly results from inflammatory disease such as peptic ulcer disease, pancreatitis, or Crohn disease (Fig. 16-33). Neoplastic narrowing is most often due to duodenal carcinoma or pancreatic cancer (Fig. 16-34). Malignant tumors are more likely to cause an abrupt change in duodenal caliber, whereas a smoothly tapered narrowing is typical of a benign process. Annular pancreas is a relatively rare cause of duodenal narrowing in adults, as most cases manifest at an early age.

When duodenal narrowing is discovered on CT or MRI, one should always check for biliary or pancreatic duct dilatation. Focal dilatation of the duodenum can occur proximal to a site of extrinsic compression by a vascular structure (most often SMA or aortic aneurysm) or pseudocyst.

Dilatation

Any process that obstructs the duodenum can cause dilatation proximal to the obstruction (see Fig. 16-34). This includes pancreatic and duodenal carcinoma,

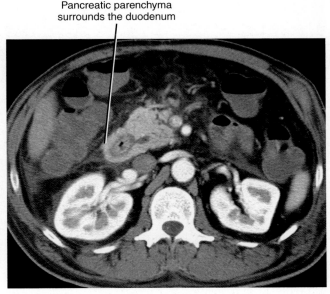

Pancreatic parenchyma
surrounds the duodenum

Figure 16-32 Axial image of the midabdomen from a contrast-enhanced computed tomographic scan of a patient with annular pancreas. This could be mistaken for duodenal thickening.

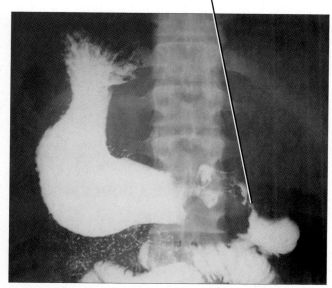

Narrowing of proximal duodenum associated with mucosal nodularity

Figure 16-33 Prone film from a single-contrast upper gastrointestinal series demonstrates severe narrowing of the proximal duodenum caused by Crohn disease.

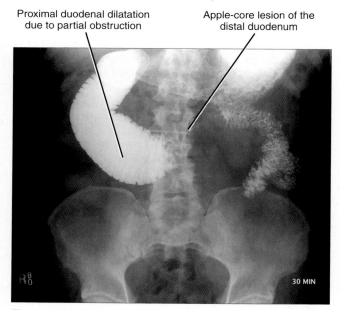

Proximal duodenal dilatation due to partial obstruction

Apple-core lesion of the distal duodenum

30 MIN

Figure 16-34 Supine image from an upper gastrointestinal series demonstrates high-grade duodenal obstruction from adenocarcinoma.

inflammatory stricture, and extrinsic compression. Compression of the third portion of the duodenum between the SMA and the aorta is a relatively common finding on imaging studies. *SMA syndrome* is present when this finding is accompanied by proximal dilatation of the duodenum and clinical symptoms of obstruction. SMA syndrome typically occurs in asthenic individuals who have experienced rapid weight loss. The obstruction may be relieved in the prone position. The duodenal compression in SMA syndrome is vertical and bandlike with intact mucosa. Features inconsistent with SMA syndrome include mucosal irregularity or ulceration, nodularity, shelflike margins, long-segment narrowing, and intraluminal filling defects.

Congenital *duodenal webs* are thin intraluminal membranes, usually in the descending duodenum, which can cause varying degrees of obstruction. Dilatation in the absence of obstruction can occur in patients with scleroderma, ileus, and motility disorders. In such cases, the dilatation is rarely restricted to the duodenum.

Ulceration

Like gastric ulcers, duodenal ulcers are associated with *H. pylori* infection. Unlike gastric ulcers, the overwhelming majority of duodenal ulcers are benign. Most peptic duodenal ulcers are found in the duodenal bulb along the anterior wall and measure less than 1 cm in diameter. Occasionally, duodenal ulcers can be so large as to replace the normal bulbar architecture and escape detection (giant duodenal ulcer). One clue to the presence of a giant duodenal ulcer is its persistent, rigid nature. Despite the extraordinary effort that many radiologists and radiology residents still exert in the quest for the portrait-quality air-contrast duodenal bulb image, duodenal ulcers are often best seen on single-contrast compression views.

At fluoroscopy, most duodenal ulcers appear as a small, persistent collection of barium. Radiating folds and deformity of the bulb can also suggest the presence of a duodenal ulcer. On CT or MRI, the only clue to the presence of an ulcer could be wall thickening or narrowing with inflammatory stranding of the surrounding fat. An actual ulcer crater is rarely seen on cross-sectional imaging. The presence of intraperitoneal (most common) or extraperitoneal gas associated with duodenal thickening or periduodenal fat stranding should suggest the presence of a perforated duodenal ulcer. Whether the extraluminal gas is primarily intraperitoneal or extraperitoneal depends on the site of perforation, with duodenal bulb perforation more likely to produce intraluminal gas and distal perforation more likely to produce extraperitoneal gas. One site of intraperitoneal gas that may be seen with perforated duodenal ulcer is the fissure for the ligamentum venosum.

Only approximately 5% of duodenal ulcers occur in a postbulbar location. The presence of a postbulbar ulcer does not establish the diagnosis of Zollinger–Ellison syndrome, although it should prompt further investigation.

Multiple aphthous ulcers can be an early manifestation of Crohn disease. Eventually, these can progress to deep fissuring ulcers. Unlike peptic aphthous ulcers, which have a predilection for the bulb, Crohn ulcers occur anywhere in duodenum. Most patients with duodenal Crohn disease have concomitant involvement of small bowel and colon.

Pearl: The majority of duodenal ulcers are histologically benign.

Mass

Pseudotumors and Masses of Extraduodenal Origin

The duodenum is a common site for pseudotumors and extraduodenal masses that mimic duodenal neoplasms. Prolapsed antral mucosa can form a mushroom-shaped mass at the base of the duodenal bulb that is transient in nature. Heterotopic gastric mucosa and pancreatic rests can also mimic duodenal neoplasm. Heterotopic gastric mucosa manifests as tiny, flat, polygonal filling defects in the bulb. Occasionally, a prominent major papilla will be mistaken for an ampullary neoplasm, although the former should not exceed 1.5 cm in diameter, and biliary or pancreatic duct dilatation should not be present in the absence of tumor.

Polyps

Although most gastric polyps tend to be hyperplastic, most duodenal polyps are adenomatous (hyperplastic polyps are rare in the duodenum). The duodenum is the second most common location of adenomatous polyps in *familial polyposis syndrome* after the colon. Villous adenomas often are found near the major papilla and have a characteristic reticular appearance (likened to pouring barium on a sponge). Duodenal lipomas can be depicted as smooth submucosal polypoid masses on fluoroscopic studies. They are usually soft and pliable, and are readily diagnosed with CT (fat attenuation) or MRI (fat signal intensity) (Fig. 16-35).

Cystic Lesions

Gut duplication cysts, pancreatic pseudocysts, cystic pancreatic neoplasms, and choledochoceles can cause smooth extrinsic impressions where they contact the duodenum. US, CT, and MRI depict these lesions well and characterize their relation to surrounding organs.

Malignant Tumors of the Duodenum

Adenocarcinoma is the most common malignant tumor of the duodenum and is more common than adenocarcinoma of the jejunum or ileum. Duodenal carcinomas affect older patients and usually occur at or beyond the ampulla. The first portion of the duodenum is rarely affected. Duodenal carcinomas can present as an irregular intraluminal mass, polypoid mass, plaquelike thickening, or apple-core lesion (see Fig. 16-34). Ulceration can occur, although a large cavitating mass of the duodenum is more likely to be lymphoma. Gastric outlet obstruction is common in cases of adenocarcinoma. Periampullary tumors can obstruct the pancreatic and bile ducts. With US, carcinoma appears hypoechoic,

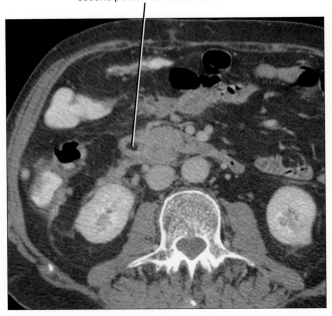

Fat density round lesion in second portion of duodenum

Figure 16-35 Axial image of the midabdomen from a contrast-enhanced computed tomographic scan of a patient with metastatic cancer and an incidental duodenal lipoma. The lipoma was visible on multiple studies over several years.

and water distention of the duodenal lumen helps visualize the tumor on all cross-sectional imaging studies. Intravenous contrast material also improves tumor conspicuity.

Other malignant tumors that involve the duodenum include gastric cancer, pancreatic cancer, ampullary cancer, distal bile duct cancer, metastatic disease, GIST, sarcoma, carcinoid, islet cell tumor (especially gastrinoma), and lymphoma. Duodenal lymphoma is usually associated with gastric involvement and rarely causes obstruction.

Nodular Duodenum

A variety of normal variants or pathologic conditions result in the appearance of a nodular duodenum on barium examinations (Table 16-7).

Other

Duodenal Diverticula

Duodenal diverticula are commonly seen on upper GI examinations and CT or MRI studies of the abdomen. They often arise from the medial aspect of the second or superior margin of the third portion of the duodenum and are frequently multiple. Lateral diverticula are uncommon but do occur. The major papilla may insert into a duodenal diverticulum, and periampullary diverticula can complicate endoscopic procedures. Gas, debris, blood clots, tablets, and other ingested materials can accumulate in duodenal diverticula. These diverticula can

Table 16-7   Nodular Appearance of the Duodenum at Fluoroscopy

Condition	Imaging Appearance or Diagnostic Clues
Brunner gland hyperplasia	• Single or multiple nodules
Lymphoid hyperplasia	• Small, uniform nodules
Celiac disease	• "Bubbly" appearance of the bulb • Dilated small bowel • Jejunization of ileum • Excess fluid
Multiple polyps	• Polyps elsewhere • Known polyposis syndrome
Heterotopic gastric mucosa	• Multiple small polygonal nodules • Clustering near base of duodenal bulb

mimic a cystic pancreatic mass, abscess, or pseudocyst on cross-sectional imaging studies (Fig. 16-36). Occasionally, they can be mistaken for duodenal perforation. Complications of duodenal diverticula include infarction or inflammation, perforation, bleeding, ulceration, and bacterial overgrowth leading to vitamin B_{12} deficiency (an uncommon occurrence). An intraluminal or "windsock" diverticulum appears as a thin, curved, radiolucent line outlining a featureless sac.

Pitfall: Duodenal diverticula can be mistaken for duodenal perforation or can mimic a cystic pancreatic mass, abscess, or pseudocyst on cross-sectional imaging studies.

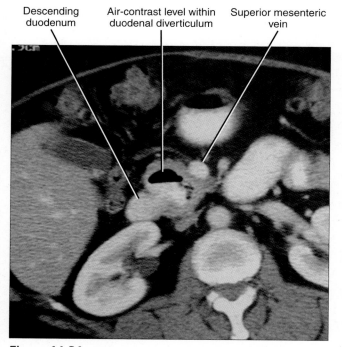

Descending duodenum   Air-contrast level within duodenal diverticulum   Superior mesenteric vein

Figure 16-36 Axial image of the region of the pancreatic head from a contrast-enhanced computed tomographic scan demonstrates oral contrast material and air within a duodenal diverticulum.

■ ABNORMALITIES OF THE JEJUNUM AND ILEUM

Thickening

Thickening of the small bowel is a relatively common finding on imaging studies. In many cases, the apparent thickening reflects suboptimal luminal distention. In general, if the small-bowel wall thickness is at least 3 mm despite optimal luminal distention, it is considered abnormal. The closely packed valvulae conniventes in the jejunum make this a frequent site of spurious thickening. The presence of perienteric fat stranding, vascular engorgement, regional adenopathy, or abnormal enhancement of the bowel wall improves the likelihood that true thickening is present. Unfortunately, the list of disease processes that can cause small-bowel wall or fold thickening is quite long.

Attempts have been made to classify small-bowel fold thickening seen with fluoroscopy into various patterns. Unfortunately, this approach has had its greatest utility in preparing radiology residents for the boards. Nevertheless, it is important to recognize when the small bowel is abnormal and to decide whether further evaluation is prudent. Furthermore, correlation between imaging examinations and clinical data will often allow one to offer a relatively short differential diagnosis.

On CT, the degree of wall thickening, a somewhat subjective determination, can help reduce the differential diagnosis. For example, thickening of the bowel wall to 10 mm or more is typically caused by neoplastic processes (e.g., lymphoma, adenocarcinoma), vasculitis, Crohn disease, or intramural hemorrhage.

Practical Approach to Small-Bowel Thickening

The traditional method of attempting to diagnose small-bowel disease through an analysis of mucosal fold patterns based on fluoroscopy is rarely sufficient and does not reflect real-life practice. It is far more realistic to attempt to render a diagnosis only after careful correlation of the fluoroscopic findings (if a small-bowel follow-through or enteroclysis was performed) with findings on other imaging studies (most commonly CT) and the patient's clinical data. Table 16-8 presents our recommended approach to small-bowel thickening. This approach is primarily applicable to CT, although many of the findings discussed have fluoroscopic or MRI correlates.

Pearl: Submucosal edema of the small-bowel wall with mucosal and serosal enhancement (target sign) or diffuse involvement suggests a benign cause for small-bowel wall thickening.

Luminal Narrowing

Small-bowel lumen narrowing in the absence of obstruction is usually the result of a previous or acute inflammatory process such as Crohn disease, vasculitis,

Table 16-8   Practical Approach to Small-Bowel Thickening

DISTRIBUTION

Proximal involvement (duodenum/jejunum): giardiasis, Whipple disease, cryptosporidiosis, celiac disease, adenocarcinoma

Distal involvement: Crohn disease, *Mycobacterium tuberculosis, Yersinia enterocolitica,* Campylobacter, Behçet syndrome, CMV, lymphoma, carcinoid tumor

Focal involvement: neoplasm (often malignant), intussusception, trauma, radiation, endometriosis, diverticulitis, granulomatous disease, perforated foreign body (e.g., fish bone)

Segmental involvement: Crohn disease, hemorrhage, lymphoma, radiation enteritis, infection, ischemia (embolic, venous thrombosis)

Diffuse involvement (Fig. 16-37): Hypoalbuminemia, nonocclusive mesenteric ischemia (low-flow states), vasculitis, angioedema, GVHD, infectious enteritis

Skip areas: Crohn disease

Stomach and small bowel: eosinophilic gastroenteritis, Crohn disease

Colon and small bowel: Crohn disease, MAC, CMV

WALL ANALYSIS

Submucosal edema ("target" sign, usually benign) (Fig. 16-38): angioedema (e.g., C1-esterase inhibitor deficiency, ACE inhibitors), hypoalbuminemia, right-sided heart failure, cirrhosis (jejunum and ascending colon most common), inflammatory bowel (Crohn disease), infectious enteritis, vasculitis (including radiation), ischemia

Homogeneous enhancement (Fig. 16-39): chronic inflammation caused by radiation, Crohn disease, lymphoma

High attenuation value (unenhanced CT): intramural hemorrhage

Poorly enhancing or nonenhancing (Fig. 16-40): ischemia with necrosis

Gas (pneumatosis): ischemia, mucosal disruption, idiopathic

MESENTERY

Vessels

- Vascular engorgement (comb sign) (Fig. 16-41): inflammation or infection

- Vascular occlusion (Fig. 16-42): mesenteric or portal vein thrombosis, mesenteric arterial thrombosis or embolism

- Vascular aneurysms/pseudoaneurysms: vasculitis, trauma

- Portal venous gas: ischemia, mucosal disruption

Fat

- Proliferation: Crohn disease ("creeping fat" resulting in separation of bowel loops)

- "Misty": inflammation, edema, infection, lymphoma, intestinal lymphangiectasia, lymphatic obstruction, idiopathic

- Enhancing mass: carcinoma, carcinoid, lymphoma, metastasis

Lymph Nodes

- Enlarged (Fig. 16-43): infection, inflammation, carcinoma, lymphoma

- Low attenuation value: Whipple disease, mycobacterial infection

- High attenuation value: Kaposi sarcoma

CORRELATION

Cirrhosis: bowel edema most commonly involving ascending colon and jejunum

CHF: bowel edema, ischemia

Trauma: shock bowel, submucosal hemorrhage, ischemia

Medications: ACE inhibitors (angioedema of bowel), vasopressors (nonocclusive mesenteric ischemia), anticoagulants (intramural hemorrhage)

Organ transplant patient (see Fig. 16-37): GVHD, opportunistic infection, lymphoma, posttransplant lymphoproliferative disorder (Fig. 16-44)

Immunosuppression/HIV: MAC, CMV, cryptosporidium parvum, lymphoma

Atherosclerotic disease: ischemia

Atrial fibrillation or endocarditis: emboli

Radiation therapy: radiation enteritis

ACE, Angiotensin-converting enzyme; *CHF,* congestive heart failure; *CMV,* cytomegalovirus; *GVHD,* graft-versus-host disease; *HIV,* human immunodeficiency virus; *MAC, Mycobacterium avium intracellulare* complex.

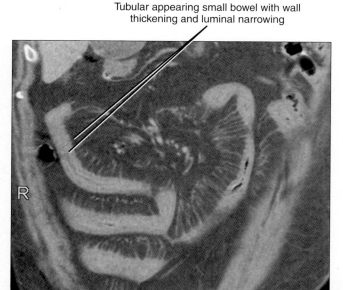

Tubular appearing small bowel with wall thickening and luminal narrowing

R

Figure 16-37 Coronal reformation of an enhanced computed tomographic (CT) scan through the abdomen of a patient who underwent bone marrow transplantation 4 months before this CT scan. This demonstrates the typical "tubular" appearance of graft-versus-host disease affecting the small bowel.

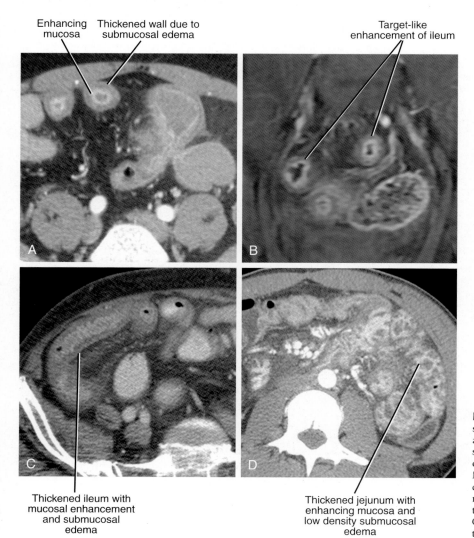

Enhancing mucosa   Thickened wall due to submucosal edema

Target-like enhancement of ileum

A

B

C

D

Thickened ileum with mucosal enhancement and submucosal edema

Thickened jejunum with enhancing mucosa and low density submucosal edema

Figure 16-38 Submucosal edema of the small bowel on computed tomography (CT) and magnetic resonance (MR) imaging. **A,** CT shows target-like enhancement in Crohn disease. **B,** Coronal fat-suppressed T1-weighted MR image of a different patient with Crohn disease also demonstrates target-like enhancement. **C,** Mucosal enhancement on CT of a patient with *Escherichia coli* ileitis. **D,** Enhanced CT in a young woman with angioedema of the small bowel.

Homogeneous wall
thickening

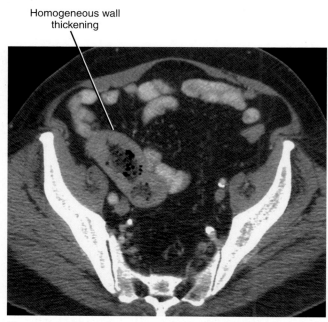

Figure 16-39 Axial image of the pelvis from a contrast-enhanced computed tomographic scan demonstrates homogeneous thickening of the wall of the distal ileum caused by lymphoma

Mesenteric vascular
engorgement ("comb" sign)

Wall thickening with
mucosal enhancement and
submucosal edema

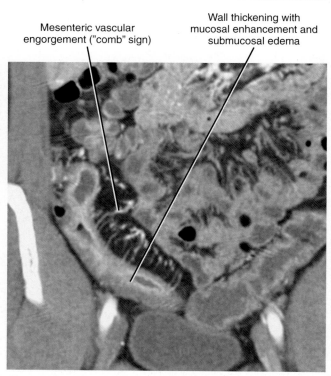

Figure 16-41 Coronal reformation of an enhanced computed tomographic scan through the abdomen and pelvis of a patient with Crohn disease demonstrating the "comb" sign.

Normal bowel wall enhances

Ischemic bowel wall
does not enhance

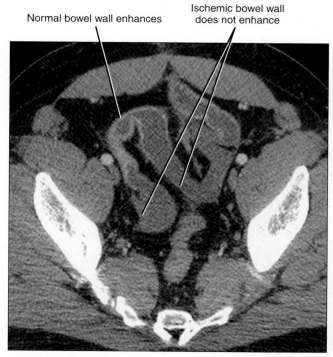

Figure 16-40 Axial image of the pelvis from a contrast-enhanced computed tomographic scan of a young male patient involved in a motor vehicle collision. Ischemic loops of ileum were found in the pelvis at surgery.

Distal small bowel
mural thickening

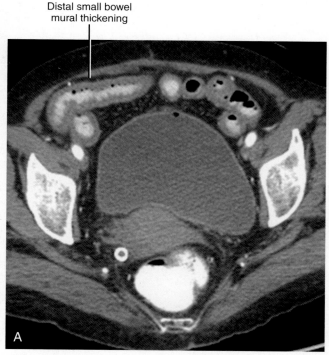

A

Figure 16-42 Acute mesenteric ischemia on computed tomography (CT). **A,** Axial image of the pelvis from contrast-enhanced computed tomographic scan.

(continued)

Abrupt occlusion of mid SMA due to embolus

Proximal SMA is patent

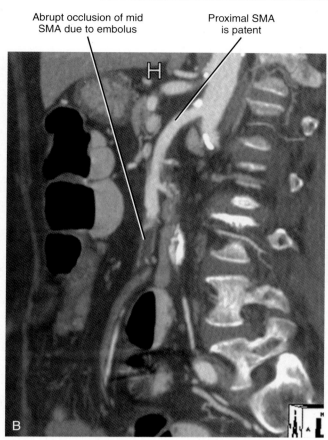

Figure 16-42, cont'd **B.** Sagittal reformation from the same scan of an elderly patient with cardiomyopathy and ischemic bowel secondary to superior mesenteric artery (SMA) embolus.

Homogeneous thickening of small bowel wall

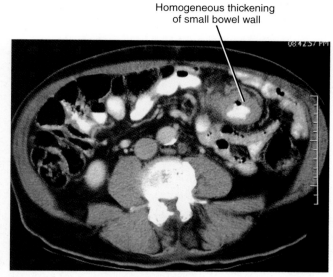

Figure 16-44 Axial image of the midabdomen from a contrast-enhanced computed tomographic scan of a patient who experienced development of posttransplant lymphoproliferative disorder involving the small bowel after kidney transplantation.

radiation treatment, or ischemia (Fig. 16-45). Acute pancreatitis usually affects the duodenum but can occasionally affect other segments of bowel. Serosal involvement with endometriosis or peritoneal metastases can cause focal small-bowel narrowing. Adhesions and hernias likewise can narrow the bowel lumen with or without obstruction. Primary carcinoma of the small bowel is rare but can present as an annular constricting lesion (Fig. 16-46). Associated wall thickening related to tumor infiltration will be present. Formation of

Homogeneous thickening of the ileum (lymphoma)

Lymphadenopathy

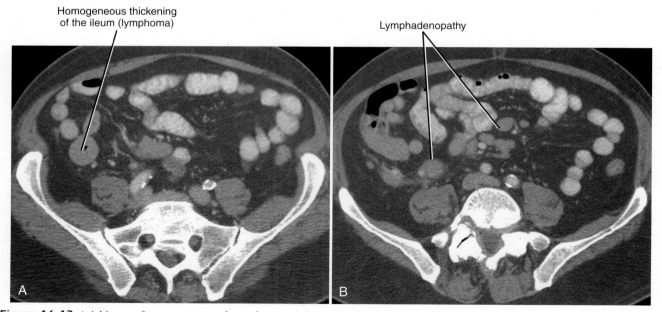

Figure 16-43 Axial images from a contrast-enhanced computed tomographic scan of a patient with small-bowel lymphoma. **A,** Image of the upper pelvis demonstrates homogeneous bowel wall thickening. **B,** A more inferior image demonstrates mesenteric adenopathy.

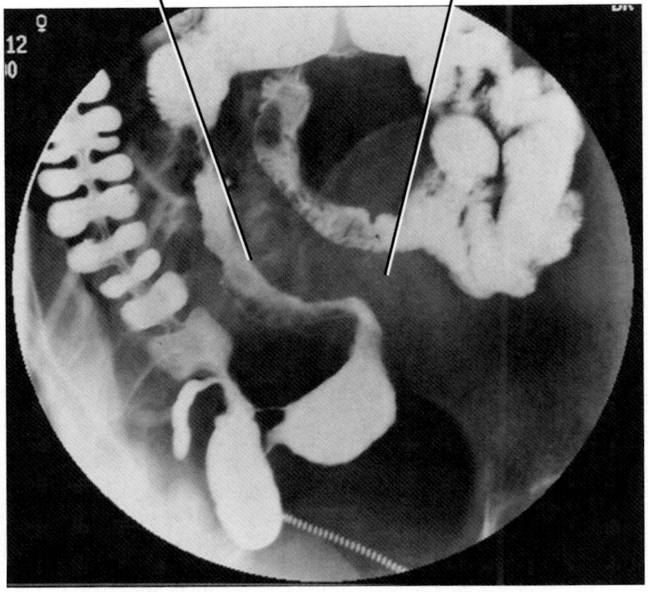

Long narrowed segment
of distal ileum

Separation of the bowel loops
in right lower quadrant

Figure 16-45 Spot film from a barium small-bowel series demonstrates stricture of the terminal ileum caused by Crohn disease.

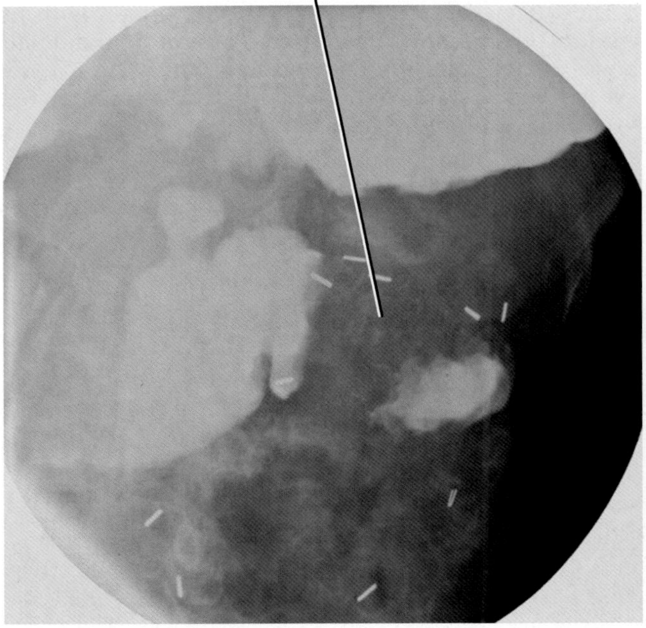

Annular constriction of the proximal
jejunum due to adenocarcinoma

Figure 16-46 Spot radiograph from an upper gastrointestinal series in a patient with adenocarcinoma of the proximal jejunum.

weblike stenoses of the small bowel is a rare complication of nonsteroidal antiinflammatory drugs and may be best demonstrated with enteroclysis. Carcinoid tumors involving the mesentery can narrow adjacent small bowel with a desmoplastic, tethering effect. Graft-versus-host disease can cause wall thickening and

luminal narrowing of the small bowel, resulting in a tubular appearance on CT and MRI (see Fig. 16-37).

Dilatation

Distinguishing Obstructive from Nonobstructive Causes of Bowel Dilatation

Dilated bowel is a frequent finding on imaging examinations. Distinguishing obstructed from nonobstructive bowel is a critical task for the radiologist that has a significant impact on patient management.

Clinical history can be essential to distinguish obstructed from nonobstructed bowel. Patients with recent trauma, surgery, or shock are at risk for ileus, as are patients with profound electrolyte derangements or who take medications, such as narcotics, known to affect bowel function. Vomiting, remote rather than recent history of surgery, or known intraabdominal malignancy are more suggestive of mechanical bowel obstruction.

Supine and upright radiographs are frequently the first imaging test ordered in the setting of suspected bowel obstruction. Plain film signs of small-bowel obstruction (SBO) include dilated small bowel in the absence of colonic dilatation, paucity of stool or gas in the colon and rectum, "string of pearls" sign (small gas bubbles in fluid-filled loops), and ladder-like arrangement of bowel loops containing gas-fluid levels (Fig. 16-47).

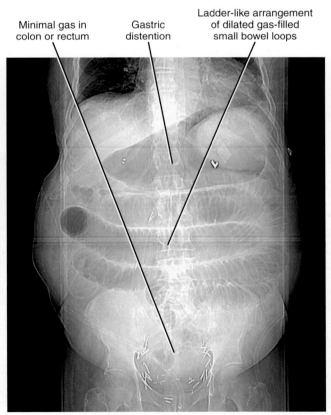

Minimal gas in
colon or rectum

Gastric
distention

Ladder-like arrangement
of dilated gas-filled
small bowel loops

Figure 16-47 Supine computed tomographic scout image of a patient with high-grade small-bowel obstruction caused by adhesions after appendectomy.

As a result of its ability to determine the location, cause, and complications of obstruction, CT has replaced fluoroscopy as the next test for patients with suspected SBO after abdominal radiographs. In many centers, CT has supplanted radiography for suspected SBO. Clear evidence of a transition point between dilated bowel and collapsed bowel remains the most reliable CT finding of obstruction. Occasionally, the transition point is associated with a hernia or mass, allowing a diagnosis of SBO to be characterized with relative certainty. The presence of orally administered contrast material in the colon excludes complete SBO. Be careful not to confuse rectally administered contrast material with that administered orally.

Pitfall: Do not confuse rectally administered contrast material with that administered orally when trying to evaluate bowel obstruction.

Fecalization of small-bowel contents is a relatively good indicator that a chronic partial SBO is present (Fig. 16-48). The site of obstruction is typically in the region of small-bowel feces. In classic chronic partial obstruction, the oral contrast column becomes progressively dilute until it is replaced by unopacified fluid and eventually small-bowel feces (Fig. 16-49). Occasionally, the appearance of small-bowel feces can be encountered in the region of the terminal ileum in patients without SBO.

Fluoroscopy now plays a limited role in the evaluation of patients with suspected SBO. Barium better reveals the site of obstruction, because water-soluble contrast dilutes as it travels through fluid-filled bowel. However, most surgeons do not want to perform bowel surgery on a patient who has large quantities of retained barium in the gut. Therefore, barium is rarely used when surgery is anticipated.

As with other modalities, the goal of fluoroscopy in the setting of suspected SBO is to identify a transition point. Timely transit of orally administered contrast material through the entire small bowel excludes significant obstruction. In patients with adynamic ileus, transit times of several hours are not unusual. As on CT, partial SBO can be difficult to identify on conventional small-bowel follow-through examinations. If a

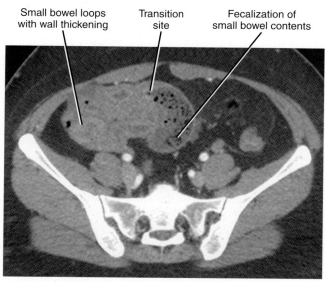

Small bowel loops with wall thickening   Transition site   Fecalization of small bowel contents

Figure 16-48 Axial image of the pelvis from a contrast-enhanced computed tomographic scan of a patient with chronic partial small-bowel obstruction caused by Crohn disease.

partial SBO is suspected but unconfirmed on small-bowel follow-through examination, enteroclysis may be helpful. Enteroclysis "stresses" the small bowel by distending the lumen, highlighting the site of partial obstruction.

Small-Bowel Obstruction

Once it has been determined that small-bowel dilatation results from obstruction, a systematic analysis should be performed. This analysis can be performed to varying degrees with any imaging modality but is best done with CT.

First, find the transition point. The task of finding the exact site of SBO is greatly facilitated through the use of picture archiving and communication systems and three-dimensional workstations. Before embarking on this task, it is helpful to identify the terminal ileum. If the terminal ileum is collapsed, then the

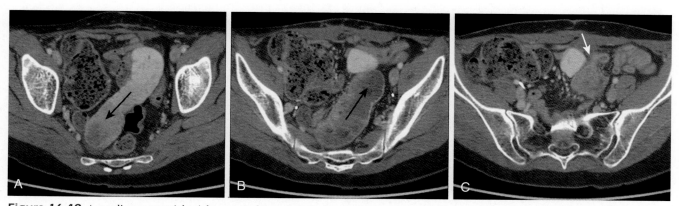

Figure 16-49 Ascending sequential axial computed tomographic images in a patient with high-grade small-bowel obstruction (SBO). Note that following the bowel in the direction from **(A)** more concentrated (higher attenuation) to **(B)** more dilute contrast material quickly leads to **(C)** the transition point (*short white arrow,* far right). *Long arrows* demonstrate antegrade direction within the bowel.

obstruction is located in the small bowel. The exact point of obstruction can be located by following the bowel to a site of caliber change. In the case of high-grade obstruction, this change is usually abrupt. For proximal obstruction, it may be most efficient to start at the ligament of Treitz, but if there are a large number of distended loops, it may be more efficient to evaluate the bowel retrograde, beginning at the terminal ileum. Window and level settings should make the bowel wall clearly visible to avoid jumping between adjacent loops.

Oral contrast material becomes progressively more dilute as it approaches the site of obstruction, and the most distal obstructed loops are often unopacified and fluid filled (see Fig. 16-49). Therefore, the transition site can often be rapidly localized by looking first where the oral contrast is most dilute or nonexistent. If the small-bowel feces sign is present, it will be near the level of obstruction. When the transition point cannot confidently be identified on axial images, multiplanar reconstructions can be beneficial.

Pearl: The site of transition in SBO often can be quickly localized by looking for distended bowel loops containing dilute or absent oral contrast material (if administered) or by looking for evidence of small-bowel feces (partial chronic obstruction).

Second, determine the degree and type of obstruction. Subsequent patient management depends, in part, on the severity of obstruction. A patient with a chronic partial obstruction may be managed conservatively, whereas most complete obstructions require surgery. The small-bowel feces sign on CT implies a chronic partial obstruction. The distinction between a complete obstruction and a high-grade partial obstruction can be difficult with any modality unless oral contrast material is seen to traverse the site of obstruction. In most cases, this distinction is irrelevant to patient management.

A high-grade obstruction may be difficult to detect on abdomen radiographs (particularly supine views) when the obstructed loops are fluid filled. However, high-grade obstruction can be inferred from an upright film when the "string of pearls" sign is present. A *closed loop obstruction* is a surgical emergency characterized on imaging by dilated loops of small bowel arranged in a C or U configuration. CT often depicts adjacent mesenteric stranding. The presence of a "beak" or "whirl" sign lends further support to the diagnosis of closed loop obstruction (Fig. 16-50). Intramural hemorrhage can increase the attenuation value of the bowel wall. With bowel ischemia, the involved segment will show decreased enhancement after intravenous contrast administration.

Pearl: A closed loop obstruction is characterized on imaging by dilated loops of small bowel arranged in a C or U configuration. CT often depicts adjacent mesenteric stranding. The presence of a "beak" or "whirl" sign lends further support to the diagnosis of closed loop obstruction. Be sure to check for signs of ischemia.

Third, determine the cause of obstruction. SBOs can be caused by intrinsic factors (e.g., strictures, tumors, intussusception) or extrinsic factors (e.g., hernias, adhesions). Table 16-9 lists some causes of SBO.

Fourth, look for complications. Patients with SBO may experience perforation that can manifest as free intraperitoneal gas, abscess formation, peritonitis (enhancing peritoneum), and free peritoneal fluid or bowel contents. Occasionally, oral contrast material will leak from the bowel, accumulating in the peritoneal recesses. If perforation is a chief concern, then any oral contrast administered for an imaging study should be water soluble. Bowel ischemia and necrosis cause lack of mural enhancement with intravenous contrast media, discontinuity of the bowel wall, or gas in the bowel wall or portal venous system. Prompt recognition of these complications can be key to avoiding an adverse patient outcome.

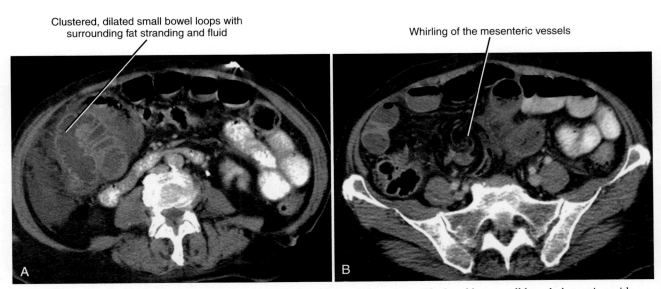

Clustered, dilated small bowel loops with surrounding fat stranding and fluid

Whirling of the mesenteric vessels

Figure 16-50 Axial computed tomographic images through the abdomen of a patient with closed loop small-bowel obstruction with volvulus. Clustered dilated small-bowel loops are seen in **A**, whereas "whirling" of the mesenteric vessels is seen in **B**.

Table 16-9   Causes of Small-Bowel Obstruction

Cause	Discriminators
Adhesions (Fig. 16-51)	• Previous surgery or abdominal inflammation • Acute angulation of bowel with abrupt transition
Abdominal wall hernia (Fig. 16-52)	• Dilated bowel entering and collapsed bowel exiting a wall defect
Internal hernia	• Clustering of dilated bowel loops in an unusual configuration or site • Crowding or twisting of mesenteric vessels • "Beaking" of bowel at transition point
Small-bowel volvulus (Fig. 16-53)	• Evidence of malrotated bowel • Closed loop obstruction • Twisting ("whirl") of mesenteric vessels
Stricture (Fig. 16-54)	• Gradual, smooth, fixed tapering of bowel without acute angulation • History of previous radiation, ischemia, or inflammation • "Small-bowel feces" sign
Tumor (Fig. 16-55)	• Enhancing mass near transition point
Intussusception (Fig. 16-56)	• Multilayered appearance of bowel with mesenteric fat interposed between layers
Inflammation	• Bowel wall thickening • Adjacent fat stranding • Increased enhancement with intravenous contrast • Increased flow with color Doppler
Extrinsic compression	• Displaced bowel loops • Extraintestinal mass visible near transition point
Foreign body	• Pneumobilia (gallstone ileus) • High-attenuation, nonanatomic structure near transition point

Nonobstructive Dilatation

Dilated small bowel does not necessarily indicate SBO (Fig. 16-57). Table 16-10 lists a differential diagnosis for nonobstructed, dilated small bowel.

Pitfall: Although diffuse dilatation of small bowel and colon is often found in patients with adynamic ileus, an obstructing distal colonic or rectal lesion can have a similar appearance on abdominal radiographs (Fig. 16-58).

Aneurysmal Dilatation of Bowel Caused by Necrotic Tumor

Neoplasms such as GIST, lymphoma, and certain hematogenous metastases involving the small bowel can cavitate, yielding focal aneurysmal dilatation of the bowel lumen (Fig. 16-59).

Mass

Intraluminal Mass or Filling Defect

Lesions that present as intraluminal masses or filling defects include bezoars, gallstones that have eroded into the bowel, and sometimes lipomas. Bezoars (masslike

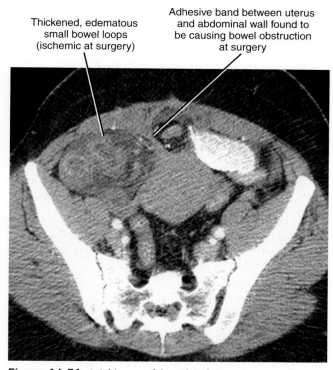

Thickened, edematous small bowel loops (ischemic at surgery)

Adhesive band between uterus and abdominal wall found to be causing bowel obstruction at surgery

Figure 16-51 Axial image of the pelvis from a contrast-enhanced computed tomographic scan of a woman with closed loop small-bowel obstruction caused by adhesive disease. The trapped small-bowel loops were severely ischemic at surgery.

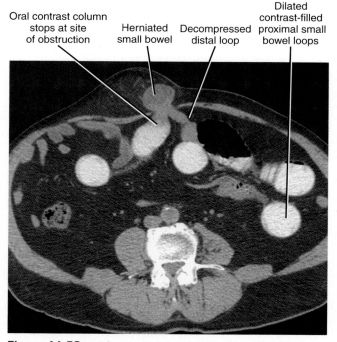

Oral contrast column stops at site of obstruction

Herniated small bowel

Decompressed distal loop

Dilated contrast-filled proximal small bowel loops

Figure 16-52 Axial computed tomographic image through the midabdomen of a patient with small-bowel obstruction caused by a small ventral hernia.

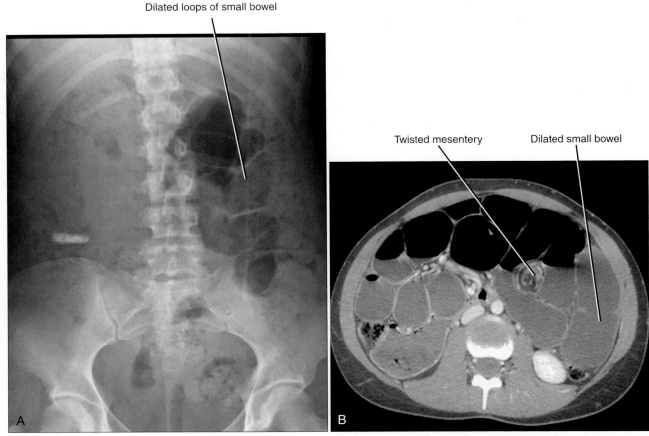

Dilated loops of small bowel

Twisted mesentery   Dilated small bowel

Figure 16-53 Abdominal radiograph (**A**) and axial enhanced computed tomographic image (**B**) of a patient who presented acutely with small-bowel volvulus showing dilated small-bowel loops and twisting of mesenteric vessels.

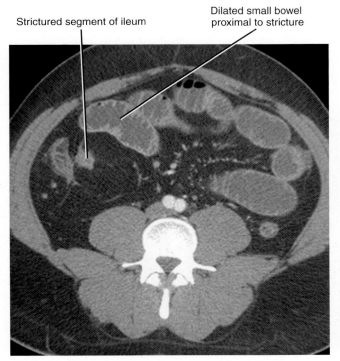

Strictured segment of ileum   Dilated small bowel proximal to stricture

Figure 16-54 Axial image of the abdomen from a contrast-enhanced computed tomographic scan of a patient with Crohn disease and chronic partial small-bowel obstruction caused by stricture.

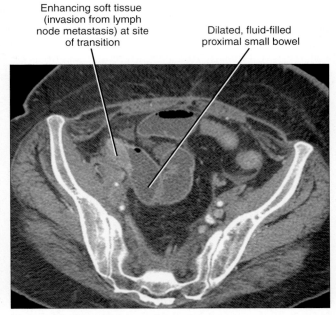

Enhancing soft tissue (invasion from lymph node metastasis) at site of transition   Dilated, fluid-filled proximal small bowel

Figure 16-55 Axial image of the pelvis from a contrast-enhanced computed tomographic scan of a patient with small-bowel obstruction caused by metastatic vulvar cancer.

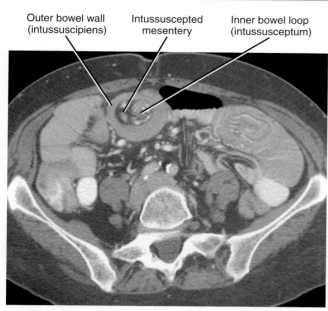

Outer bowel wall
(intussuscipiens)   Intussuscepted
mesentery   Inner bowel loop
(intussusceptum)

Figure 16-56 Axial image of the upper pelvis from a contrast-enhanced computed tomographic scan of a patient with small-bowel intussusception.

Table 16-10   Nonobstructive Causes of Small-Bowel Dilatation

Cause	Helpful discriminators
Adynamic ileus	• Colonic distention (beware of distal colonic obstruction) • Recent surgery, electrolyte imbalance, opiates
Ischemia	• Arterial or venous occlusion on CT or MRI • Poor perfusion of bowel wall on CT or MRI • Lack of flow with color Doppler
Celiac sprue	• Reversal of the normal jejunum-ileum fold pattern • Increased intestinal fluid (causes flocculation of barium) • "Bubbly" appearance of duodenal bulb • "Moulage sign" (amorphous cast of bowel on barium examination)
Scleroderma	• Crowding of folds despite lumen distention (hidebound) • Wide-mouthed sacculations along antimesenteric border • Patulous gastroesophageal junction with spontaneous reflux
Pseudoobstruction	• Lack of other cause for bowel dilatation

CT, Computed tomography; *MRI,* magnetic resonance imaging.

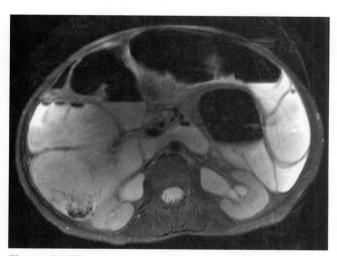

Figure 16-57 Axial T2-weighted magnetic resonance image through the abdomen shows massive diffuse bowel dilatation in a patient with chronic intestinal pseudoobstruction. This appearance was stable over many examinations over many years.

conglomerates of ingested material) are mobile, do not enhance, and lack an attachment to the bowel wall. Oral contrast material can fill the interstices of the mass, and bezoars can trap gas within. Occasionally, bezoars obstruct the small bowel or can form proximal to chronic partial SBO.

Gallstones that have eroded into the small-bowel lumen can lodge at the ileocecal valve. The triad of gas in the bile ducts, SBO, and an obstructive intraluminal gallstone is not nearly as common as some board examiners and teaching files may make you think.

Lipomas are submucosal lesions that can be pedunculated, accounting for their intraluminal appearance. Mobile, pliable, and composed of fat, they are easily distinguished from other tumors with CT and MRI.

Small-bowel polyps are uncommon and often associated with a polyposis syndrome (Fig. 16-60). Before advancing to an annular lesion, primary small-bowel carcinomas can appear as intraluminal filling defects on both barium studies and cross-sectional imaging.

Annular Masses

Masses that involve the bowel circumferentially include adenocarcinoma, metastatic disease, and lymphoma (Fig. 16-61). Moving from proximal to distal in the small bowel, adenocarcinoma decreases in incidence, whereas lymphoma increases.

Intramural/Submucosal Masses

The differential diagnosis for a submucosal mass in the small bowel parallels that for a submucosal mass in the stomach and includes GIST, leiomyoma, lipoma, hemangioma, schwannoma, and neuroendocrine tumors (Fig. 16-62). Many lesions that cause a bull's-eye appearance in the stomach can have a similar appearance in the small bowel. These include metastatic melanoma and lung carcinoma, lymphoma, and Kaposi sarcoma. The antimesenteric border of the bowel is most often involved by metastatic tumor. Carcinoid tumor is a submucosal lesion, although the primary tumor is often not seen with barium studies and CT. Instead, carcinoid often presents as a desmoplastic mesenteric mass resulting from lymphatic spread.

Markedly dilated gas-filled
small and large bowel

Irregular narrowing that completely
obstructs the rectum

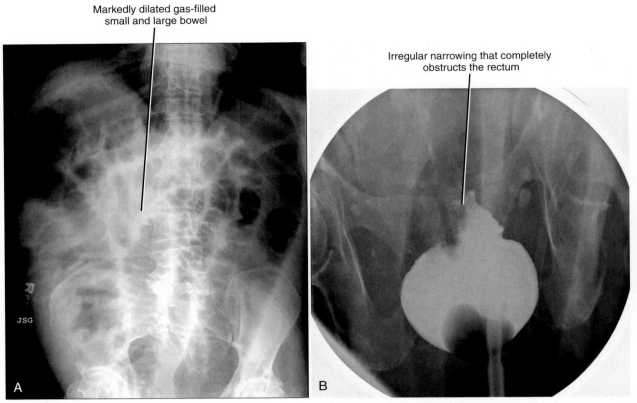

Figure 16-58 Supine abdominal radiograph **(A)** and barium enema examination **(B)** in a patient with obstructing rectal carcinoma. The abdominal radiographs were initially interpreted as ileus rather than obstruction.

Focal ("aneurysmal") dilatation of the bowel lumen due
to cavitary small bowel metastasis (melanoma)

Polyps in jejunum

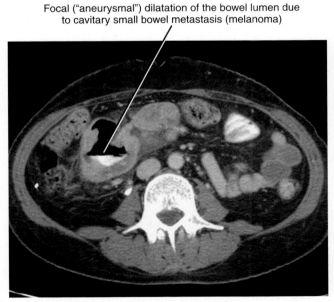

Figure 16-59 Axial image of the abdomen from a contrast-enhanced computed tomographic scan of a patient with metastatic melanoma involving the small bowel.

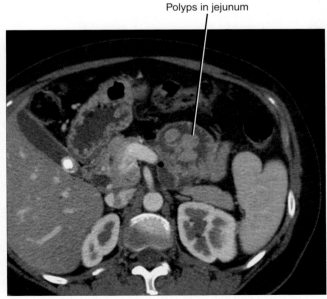

Figure 16-60 Axial image from a contrast-enhanced computed tomographic scan of a patient with Peutz–Jeghers syndrome demonstrates multiple hamartomatous polyps in the jejunum.

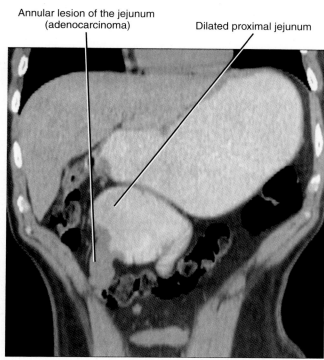

Annular lesion of the jejunum (adenocarcinoma)

Dilated proximal jejunum

Figure 16-61 Coronal reformation of a computed tomographic scan through the abdomen of a patient with adenocarcinoma of the jejunum.

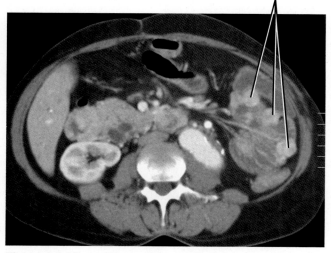

Multiple enhancing submucosal tumors (GIST)

Figure 16-62 Axial image of the abdomen from a contrast-enhanced computed tomographic scan of a patient with multiple gastrointestinal stromal tumors (GIST) involving the small bowel.

Serosal Masses

Masses involving the serosal lining of the small bowel most often result from peritoneal spread of tumor. Serosal metastases to the small bowel can tether bowel loops, with crowding of folds on the side of the implants. Other findings include increased space between bowel loops, angulation and kinking of the bowel, and narrowing of the lumen. Multiple implants are typical.

Breast cancer implants are more often scirrhous and desmoplastic than other metastases and can mimic carcinoid. Like desmoplastic neoplasms, implants of endometriosis can enhance on CT, are often multifocal, and cause adhesions and fibrosis.

Other

Pneumatosis

Small-bowel pneumatosis, with its varied causes (Box 16-10), can be innocuous or grave. Because bowel necrosis represents the most serious cause of pneumatosis, one should routinely evaluate the bowel for evidence of pneumatosis on imaging studies of any patient with unexplained abdominal pain, sepsis, intestinal bleeding, or suspected bowel ischemia or infarction.

Pneumatosis can create lucent curvilinear streaks or a mottled or bubbly appearance that parallels the location of bowel on plain films. Unfortunately, pneumatosis is easily mistaken for feces within the bowel lumen and is often overlooked on radiographs unless specifically sought. Finding associated portal venous gas helps confirm the presence of pneumatosis but provides no clue as to causative factors. Similarly, intraperitoneal gas in a patient who did not recently undergo surgery can mean either bowel perforation or benign pneumoperitoneum that can accompany intestinal pneumatosis. CT is more sensitive than plain films for the diagnosis of pneumatosis. When evaluating the bowel for pneumatosis on CT, view the images with bone or lung windows to better differentiate gas from fat, while clearly delineating the bowel wall. Intestinal contents can trap gas against the bowel wall and simulate pneumatosis. In such cases, the appearance of pneumatosis extends up the bowel wall only as far as the intestinal contents. Gas trapped between valvulae can also simulate pneumatosis. But when gas is present in both the dependent and nondependent walls of well-distended bowel, think pneumatosis. Although intramural bowel gas can be found incidentally in an asymptomatic patient and does not necessarily require urgent intervention, a search for an underlying cause is mandatory (Fig. 16-63).

When signs of bowel ischemia or necrosis are present (e.g., poor or absent wall perfusion, wall thickening, mesenteric stranding), one should immediately alert the referring physician and obtain a surgical consultation.

BOX 16-10   *Causes of Small-Bowel Pneumatosis*

Bowel obstruction
Bowel necrosis/infarction
Iatrogenic mucosal disruption (e.g., endoscopy, surgery)
Mucosal ulceration (e.g., inflammatory bowel disease)
Immunosuppressive agents (e.g., steroids)
Collagen vascular diseases (e.g., lupus, scleroderma)
Intrathoracic abnormality (e.g., chronic obstructive pulmonary disease, pneumothorax, barotrauma)

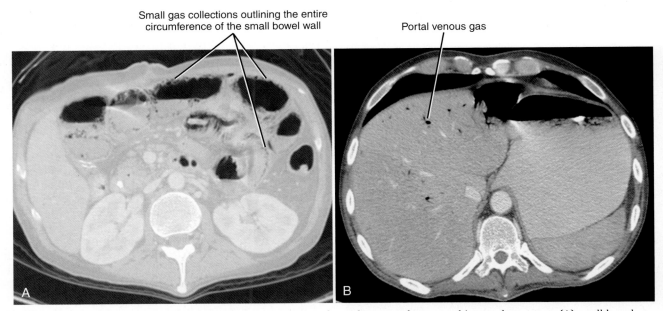

Small gas collections outlining the entire circumference of the small bowel wall

Portal venous gas

Figure 16-63 Two axial images of the abdomen from a contrast-enhanced computed tomographic scan demonstrate **(A)** small-bowel pneumatosis and **(B)** portal venous gas. An underlying cause for these findings was never found, and the patient recovered fully without intervention.

Knowing the clinical situation and patient risk factors is key to determining the significance of pneumatosis.

Pearl: When evaluating the bowel for pneumatosis on CT, view the images with bone or lung settings. Small foci of gas that involve the dependent wall of the small bowel, especially if visible in segments free of fluid and debris, are suspicious for pneumatosis.

Intussusception

Intussusception in adults is often a transient benign incidental finding, largely unappreciated before the widespread availability of CT (Fig. 16-64). Small bowel is the most common site of involvement in adults. More significant causes of intussusception in adults include benign or malignant tumors, diverticula, and polyps. The classic appearance of intussusception with fluoroscopy is that of a coiled spring caused by barium trapped between the intussusceptum and intussuscipiens. On axial CT images, intussusception has a *target appearance* because of mesenteric fat interposed between the intussusceptum and intussuscipiens (see Fig. 16-56). This multilayered appearance is also depicted with sonography, with the interposed fat appearing echogenic. When a segment of intussuscepted bowel is viewed with sonography, it can also resemble a kidney ("*pseudokidney*" sign). Proximal obstruction often accompanies clinically significant intussusception. If the length of the intussusception measures less than 3 to 5 cm and no proximal dilatation is present in an adult, it is unlikely to be of clinical significance.

Meckel's Diverticulum

This remnant of the vitelline (omphalomesenteric) duct is present in approximately 2% of individuals and typically arises from the antimesenteric border of the distal ileum within a few feet of the ileocecal valve. This true diverticulum is of variable length (usually 2-10 cm), is devoid of mucosal folds or valvulae, and can contain heterotopic gastric or intestinal mucosa, or pancreatic

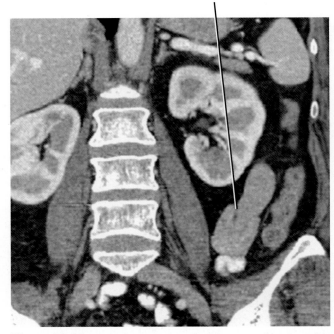

Short segment intussusception of small bowel without associated mass or obstruction

Figure 16-64 Coronal reformation of axial computed tomographic data obtained in a patient with incidental, transient intussusception.

tissue. Complications of Meckel's diverticulum include hemorrhage (usually in the presence of heterotopic gastric mucosa), inflammation (Meckel's diverticulitis), intestinal obstruction, and perforation (Fig. 16-65). Occasionally, these diverticula invert and become a lead point for intussusception. They can contain a calcified enterolith, and Meckel's diverticulitis can mimic appendicitis both clinically and on imaging studies.

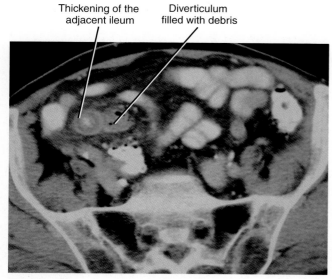

Figure 16-65 Axial image of the upper pelvis from contrast-enhanced computed tomographic scan of a patient with right lower quadrant pain. Meckel's diverticulitis was found at surgery.

The diagnosis of Meckel's diverticulum can be made with technetium 99m (Tc-99m) pertechnitate scintigraphy if sufficient heterotopic gastric mucosa is present. Administering pentagastrin can help by stimulating uptake of Tc-99m by gastric mucosa. Barium small-bowel studies are insensitive for the detection of Meckel's diverticulum, though enteroclysis can increase the chances of detection.

■ ABNORMALITIES OF THE COLON AND RECTUM

Thickening

Colonic mural thickening is a frequent imaging finding. Colonic thickening manifests on radiographs primarily as "thumbprinting," a term used to refer to thickened haustra outlined by gas within the colon lumen. Thickening of the colon wall is more clearly demonstrated by CT and MRI, although the colon lumen must be adequately distended to exclude spurious thickening. Normally, the colon wall is only a few millimeters thick as imaged in its moderately distended state.

The most common cause of colon wall thickening is the muscular hypertrophy associated with diverticulosis. This condition, also known as myochosis, primarily affects the sigmoid colon. Neoplastic thickening usually involves short segments of the colon. When neoplastic thickening is suspected, look for enlarged lymph nodes along the primary drainage pathways. Inflammatory thickening generally involves longer segments of the colon than neoplastic thickening, but scirrhous colon cancers and lymphoma can infiltrate longer segments, mimicking benign inflammatory processes.

Practical Approach to Colon Thickening

We use an analytic approach for colonic mural thickening that is similar to the one presented for the small bowel (Table 16-11).

Table 16-11 Practical Approach to Colon Thickening

PRIMARY DISTRIBUTION (Fig. 16-66)

Terminal ileum involved: Crohn disease, *Mycobacterium tuberculosis*, *Yersinia enterocolitica*, Campylobacter, histoplasmosis, Behçet syndrome, CMV, lymphoma

Ascending colon (Fig. 16-67): neutropenic colitis (typhlitis), amebiasis, portal hypertension, lymphoma

Transverse colon: subperitoneal (mesenteric) spread of gastric cancer (via gastrocolic ligament), or pancreatic tumor or inflammation (via transverse mesocolon)

Splenic flexure (Fig. 16-68): ischemia

Sigmoid colon (Fig. 16-69): diverticular disease, ischemia, radiation, endometriosis, "drop" metastases

Rectum (Fig. 16-70): radiation, infectious proctitis, stercoral colitis

Pancolonic (Fig. 16-71): ulcerative colitis, *Clostridium difficile* colitis

Short segment: malignant neoplasm, diverticulitis, trauma

Skip areas: Crohn disease

WALL ANALYSIS

Low-attenuation wall (Fig. 16-72) (submucosal edema or target sign): hypoalbuminemia, right-sided heart failure, cirrhosis, inflammatory and infectious colitides

Nonenhancing wall: ischemia, necrosis

Intensely enhancing mucosa: inflammation, ischemia

Dependent wall thickening: bowel wall edema

Pneumatosis (Fig. 16-73): idiopathic, ischemia, mucosal disruption.

MESENTERY

Vessels

- Vasa recta engorgement (comb sign): inflammation or infection

- Vascular occlusion: mesenteric or portal vein thrombosis, mesenteric arterial thrombosis or embolism, vasculitis

- Vascular aneurysms: vasculitis, atherosclerosis

- Portal venous gas: ischemia, mucosal disruption

- Varices: portal hypertension, venous thrombosis or occlusion

Fat

- Proliferation: Crohn disease

- Fat stranding: inflammation, edema, infection, lymphoma

Lymph Nodes

- Enlarged: infection, inflammation, carcinoma, metastases, lymphoma

- Low attenuation: mycobacterial infection

CLINICAL CORRELATION

Cirrhosis: associated with bowel edema most commonly involving ascending colon and jejunum

Congestive heart failure: associated with bowel edema, ischemia

Trauma: shock bowel, submucosal hemorrhage, ischemia

Medications

- Vasopressors: nonocclusive mesenteric ischemia

- Antibiotics: *C. difficile* colitis, hypersensitivity reactions

Continued

Table 16-11 Practical Approach to Colon Thickening—cont'd

Laboratory Values

- Eosinophilia: eosinophilic colitis, parasitic disease

- *C. difficile* toxin: *C. difficile* colitis

- Stool evaluation: parasites, amebiasis, bacterial colitides

- Serologic evaluation: amebiasis, salmonella

Immunosuppression/Human immunodeficiency virus: mycobacterium, cytomegalovirus

Cardiovascular disease: ischemia

Radiation therapy: radiation colitis

Organ transplantation: graft-versus-host disease, opportunistic infection, posttransplant lymphoproliferative disorder (distal small bowel/proximal colon)

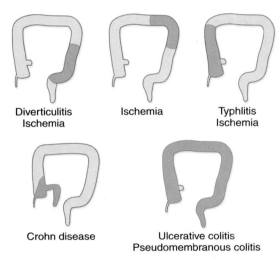

| Diverticulitis Ischemia | Ischemia | Typhlitis Ischemia |

| Crohn disease | Ulcerative colitis Pseudomembranous colitis |

Figure 16-66 Illustration demonstrating the typical or classic distributions of common colitides.

Seven Forms of Colitis to Know About

PSEUDOMEMBRANOUS COLITIS (CLOSTRIDIUM DIFFICILE COLITIS)

Pseudomembranous colitis is characterized by more wall thickening than found in most other forms of colitis (see Figs. 16-71*B* and 16-74). Colonic edema results from overgrowth of *Clostridium difficile*, usually secondary to antibiotic therapy (classically, but not exclusively, clindamycin). *C. difficile* produces an enterotoxin that causes mucosal damage.

Pseudomembranous colitis typically is pancolonic but sometimes involves only the right or left colon. Fibrinous plaques and fibropurulent debris coat the mucosa and can create a polypoid appearance. Thumbprinting is common. Enteric contrast material trapped between the thickened folds creates an accordion-like appearance on CT. Complications include toxic megacolon and perforation; thus, contrast enema should be avoided in severe cases. CT reveals intense mucosal enhancement with submucosal edema. Typically, relatively little pericolonic

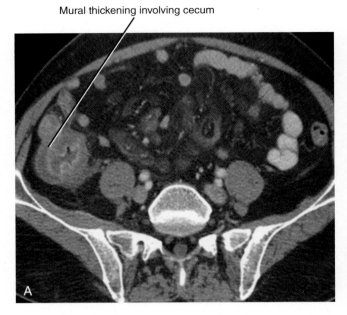

Mural thickening involving cecum

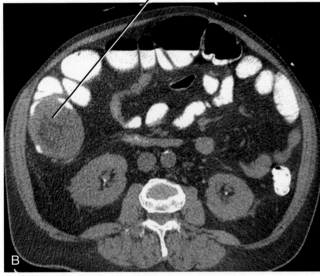

Marked thickening of the ascending colon due to lymphoma

Figure 16-67 Thickening of the ascending colon. **A,** Axial image from a contrast-enhanced computed tomographic (CT) scan of a patient with neutropenic colitis. **B,** Axial image from a CT performed with oral contrast material in a different patient with non–Hodgkin's lymphoma involving the ascending colon.

inflammation is present considering the degree of bowel wall thickening. Ascites is common, and pneumatosis and portal gas are occasionally seen. Note that CT can be normal, particularly with early pseudomembranous colitis.

Pearl: Pseudomembranous colitis typically appears as a pancolitis with a thick wall and relatively little pericolonic inflammation considering the degree of bowel wall thickening. An accordion-like appearance is classic but is not always present.

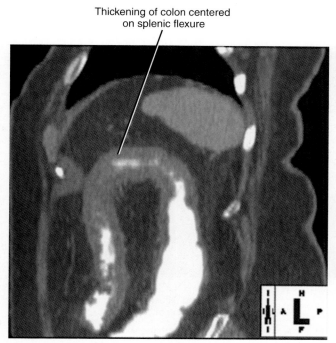

Thickening of colon centered
on splenic flexure

Figure 16-68 Oblique sagittal reconstruction of a computed tomographic scan of a patient with ischemic colitis involving the splenic flexure.

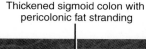

Thickened sigmoid colon with
pericolonic fat stranding

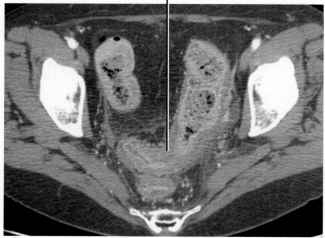

Figure 16-69 Axial image of the pelvis from a contrast-enhanced computed tomographic scan of a patient who received pelvic radiation therapy 8 weeks prior.

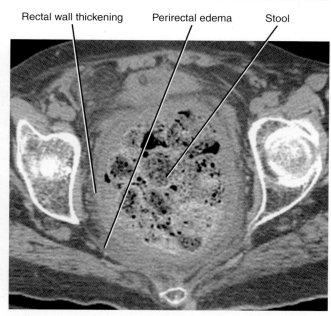

Rectal wall thickening   Perirectal edema   Stool

Figure 16-70 Axial image of the rectum from an unenhanced computed tomographic scan of a patient with stercoral colitis secondary to large fecal impaction.

CROHN DISEASE

About 20% of cases of Crohn disease are limited to the small bowel, 20% are limited to the colon, and 60% of cases involve both (Fig. 16-75). Skip lesions, separated by uninvolved segments, are the rule. The granulomatous inflammatory lesions cause ulceration, mural thickening, sinuses, fistulae, and strictures. Deep longitudinal and transverse ulcerations create the cobblestone pattern classically described for barium studies. CT and MR enterography depict areas of active inflammation, fistulae, strictures, and abscesses. The *target sign* (enhancing mucosa with submucosal edema) and the *comb sign* point to sites of active inflammation. Fibrofatty proliferation in the adjacent mesentery causes involved loops to stand out. One area of particular concern is the anal/perianal region, where fistulae and abscesses are common in patients with Crohn disease (Fig. 16-76). MRI excels at evaluating perianal fistulae in patients with Crohn disease.

ULCERATIVE COLITIS

Typically a pancolitis, ulcerative colitis (UC) is characterized by mucosal ulcerations that are shallower than those of Crohn disease. The rectum is virtually always involved, and the terminal ileum can be as well. Because the inflammation is not transmural, wall thickening is less marked than seen with Crohn disease (Fig. 16-77). Because colonoscopy is the prime diagnostic tool for suspected colitis, UC is rarely diagnosed with barium enema. When performed, air-contrast barium enema reveals a "granular" mucosal contour with tiny ulcerations pooling barium. Deeper ulcers excavate the submucosa (collar button or flask-shaped ulcers). Depending on chronicity, the colon can be shortened, straightened, and relatively ahaustral (see Figs. 16-71 and 16-78). When ulceration becomes confluent, islands of residual normal mucosa look masslike (*inflammatory pseudopolyps*) (Fig. 16-79). These should not be confused with the irregular heaps of regenerated mucosa (postinflammatory polyps) that can occur in the healing phase. Strictures occur in about 10% of patients and rarely cause obstruction. Colorectal carcinoma

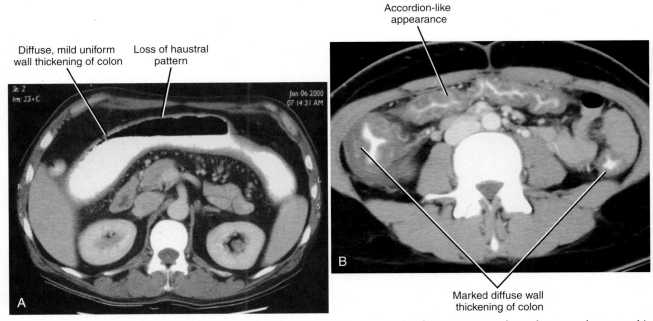

Figure 16-71 labels: Diffuse, mild uniform wall thickening of colon · Loss of haustral pattern · Accordion-like appearance · Marked diffuse wall thickening of colon

Figure 16-71 Thickening of the transverse colon. **A,** Axial image of the transverse colon from a contrast-enhanced computed tomographic (CT) scan of a patient with chronic ulcerative colitis. **B,** Axial CT image of the midabdomen from a contrast-enhanced CT scan of a patient with pseudomembranous colitis.

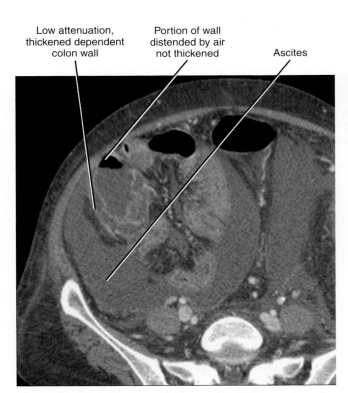

Figure 16-72 labels: Low attenuation, thickened dependent colon wall · Portion of wall distended by air not thickened · Ascites

Figure 16-72 Axial computed tomographic (CT) image through the pelvis from a contrast-enhanced CT scan of a patient with cirrhosis, portal hypertension, and bowel wall edema.

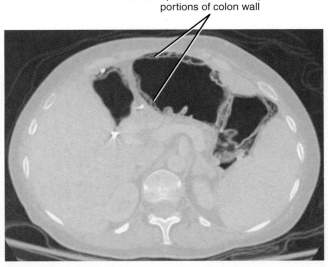

Figure 16-73 label: Gas in dependent and nondependent portions of colon wall

Figure 16-73 Axial computed tomographic image of the cecum viewed with lung window and level settings demonstrates pneumatosis of the colon. Serositis, adhesions, and perforation were present at surgery.

occurs with increased frequency in patients with inflammatory colitides, particularly UC (Fig. 16-80). Lesions often are plaquelike or scirrhous, and thus can be difficult to detect.

Toxic megacolon is a feared complication of UC (but can occur with other forms of colitis as well). Fulminant ulceration leads to colon wall thinning, marked distention, and sometimes disruption.

Marked colonic thickening with
"accordian-like" appearance

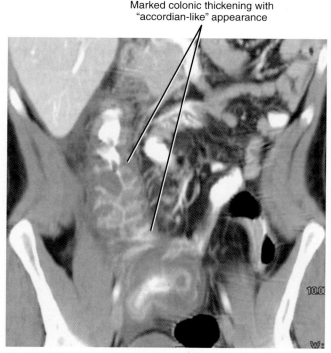

Figure 16-74 Coronal reformation of an enhanced computed tomographic scan of a patient with pseudomembranous colitis caused by *Clostridium difficile*.

Perirectal abscess

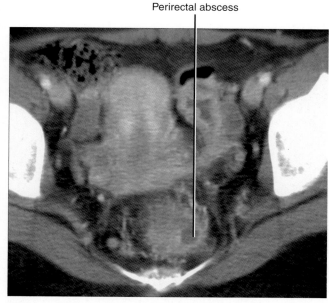

Figure 16-76 Axial image of the pelvis from a contrast-enhanced computed tomographic scan of a patient with Crohn disease and a perirectal abscess.

Excess pericolonic fat   Thickened, inflamed
ascending colon

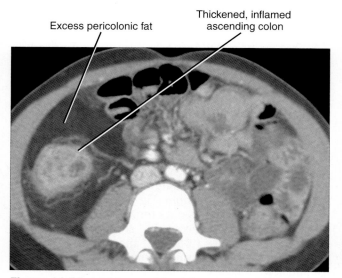

Figure 16-75 Axial image of the abdomen from a contrast-enhanced computed tomographic scan of a patient with active Crohn colitis.

Rectum involved   Mucosal enhancement
and mild wall thickening

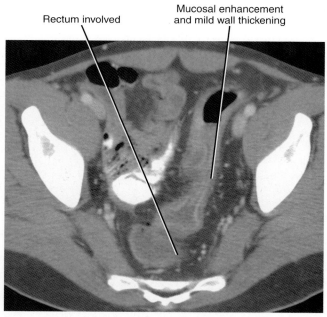

Figure 16-77 Axial image of the pelvis from a contrast-enhanced computed tomographic scan of a patient with newly diagnosed ulcerative colitis.

CT cannot depict the fine mucosal ulcerations of UC but does reveal mural thickening and lumen narrowing. The wall can have a stratified "target" appearance with a thickened hypoenhancing submucosa caused by edema (acute/subacute) or fat (chronic) (see Fig. 16-80). The rectal narrowing and proliferation of perirectal fat that widen the presacral space in patients with UC are readily apparent on CT images.

Pearl: The rectum is usually involved in patients with UC but usually spared in patients with ischemic colitis.

ISCHEMIC COLITIS

Ischemic colitis typically occurs in watershed areas such as the splenic flexure (between the SMA and inferior mesenteric artery [IMA] territories) and the rectosigmoid colon (between the IMA and internal iliac circulations)

Engorged mesenteric vessels | Ahaustral transverse colon | Mild mural thickening

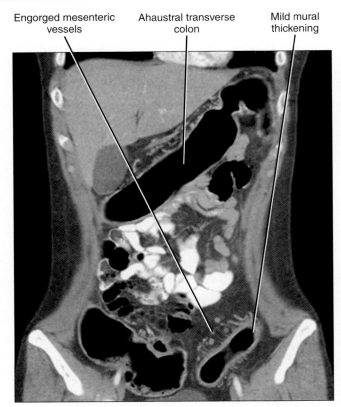

Figure 16-78 Coronal reformation from contrast-enhanced computed tomography of a patient with ulcerative colitis.

Mesorectal lymph node | Increased presacral fat | Stricturing adenocarcinoma of sigmoid colon | Submucosal fat

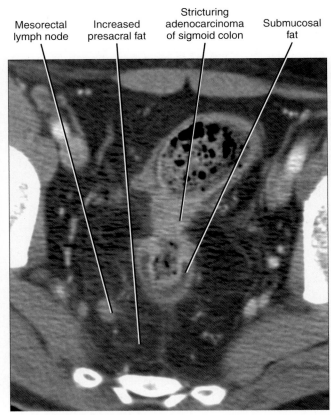

Figure 16-80 Axial image of the pelvis from a contrast-enhanced computed tomographic scan of a patient with ulcerative colitis and rectosigmoid carcinoma.

Multiple polypoid islands of spared mucosa

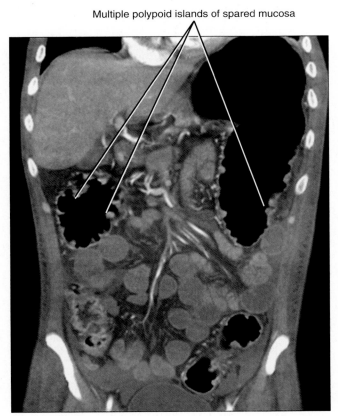

Figure 16-79 Coronal reformation of a contrast-enhanced computed tomographic scan of a patient with acute ulcerative colitis and inflammatory pseudopolyps.

(see Fig. 16-68). The length of involvement is variable, and the rectum is typically spared. Thumbprinting, pneumatosis, and portal venous gas can be evident on radiography in severe cases. Barium enemas demonstrate thumbprinting, transverse ridging, and sometimes ulceration. Particularly when ischemia is associated with obstruction, the mucosa can show slightly raised polygonal filling defects known as *colonic urticaria*. Ischemia leads to stricture in a minority of patients; interestingly, some strictures are reversible (Fig. 16-81).

CT most commonly depicts mural thickening in areas of ischemic colon. When seen in cross section, submucosal edema creates a "target" appearance with low-attenuation submucosa sandwiched between the mucosal and serosal layers.

Anything that compromises colonic blood flow is a potential cause of ischemic colitis. Congestive heart failure, thromboembolic disease, vasculitides, diabetes, radiation therapy, prior aortic graft, and bowel obstruction are frequent offenders. When fecal impaction leads to chronic lumen overdistension, pressure necrosis can cause localized ischemia (particularly in the rectum) known as stercoral colitis (see Fig. 16-70).

INFECTIOUS COLITIS
When patients have crampy abdominal pain and bloody diarrhea, colonoscopy, stool culture, histopathologic evaluation, and serology are now first-line diagnostic tools. If the abdomen physical examination is equivocal,

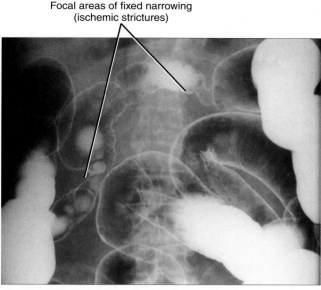

Figure 16-81 Double-contrast barium enema in a patient with ischemic colitis secondary to vasculitis.

Focal areas of fixed narrowing (ischemic strictures)

CT might be obtained. Barium enemas are no longer initial diagnostic studies in evaluating suspected colitides. With either CT or barium enema, the manifestations of infectious colitides are overlapping, variable, and nonspecific. That is not surprising, given the long list of bacteria, parasites, and viruses that can afflict the colon. CT most often reveals mural thickening/edema, with mucosal enhancement and pericolonic inflammatory change (Fig. 16-82). Barium enema demonstrates lumen narrowing, thickened haustra, "granular" mucosal pattern, and sometimes ulceration or fistulae. Table 16-12

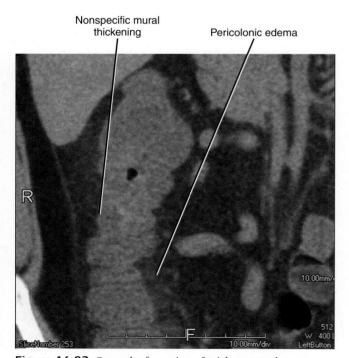

Nonspecific mural thickening

Pericolonic edema

Figure 16-82 Coronal reformation of axial computed tomographic data of a patient with *Campylobacter jejuni* colitis.

Table 16-12   Differentiating Select Infectious Colitides

Agent	Findings
Shigella	• Usually involves the left colon • Shallow or deep ulceration
Campylobacter	• Can involve both colon and small bowel • Left colon nearly always affected • Mimics both ulcerative colitis and Crohn colitis radiographically
Yersinia enterocolitica	• Typically right colon and terminal ileum • Enlarged lymphoid follicles and ulceration • Usually without stenosis
Salmonella	• Segmental or pancolitis • Distal ileum often involved • Superficial or deep ulcers
Escherichia coli	• Thumbprinting • Lumen narrowing and spasm • Mimics ischemic colitis
Tuberculosis	• Ileocolonic mural thickening • Changes often resemble those of Crohn disease • Low-attenuation lymph nodes
Actinomycosis	• Most often involves rectosigmoid and ileocecal regions • Inflammatory masses and fistulae • Closely simulates neoplasm
Gonorrhea, lymphogranuloma venereum, syphilis	• Ulcerative proctitis
Cytomegalovirus	• Seen commonly in patients with acquired immune deficiency syndrome • Typically affects distal ileum and right colon • Mural thickening and ulceration
Histoplasmosis	• Ileocecal ulceration and mural thickening • Occasional mesenteric adenopathy and hepatosplenomegaly
Amebiasis	• Right colon most severely involved • Terminal ileum spared • Deep mucosal ulcers and mural edema • Can mimic colon carcinoma

lists infectious agents that can cause colitis and their salient radiographic features.

NEUTROPENIC COLITIS
Known as typhlitis when limited to the cecum, neutropenic colitis is a common complication that affects patients undergoing chemotherapy or bone marrow transplantation. The cecum and right colon show thumbprinting and ulceration plus mural thickening (see Fig. 16-67A). Pneumatosis and pericolonic fluid and inflammation are common. Clinical setting is the key to distinguishing neutropenic colitis from similar-appearing colitides, such as pseudomembranous colitis.

DIVERTICULITIS
Colonic diverticula are actually acquired pseudodiverticula, containing no muscularis layer. The sigmoid colon is by far the predominate site of involvement. The

muscular hypertrophy and shortening that accompanies diverticulosis cause mural thickening on CT and an accordion or saw tooth pattern on barium studies. Stool can become inspissated in poorly emptying diverticula, with resultant inflammation, mucosal erosion, and localized perforation (diverticulitis).

CT is now the initial imaging evaluation for suspected diverticulitis. In addition to revealing diverticula in the involved area, CT demonstrates mural thickening, adjacent edema or fluid, and intramural or juxtacolonic abscesses (Fig. 16-83). Contrast enemas reveal lumen narrowing and spasm in the area of diverticulitis, with intramural or extrinsic mass effect if there is an abscess. Complications include fistulae (intramural, colovesical, colovaginal, coloenteric), abscess formation, peritonitis, bowel obstruction, and portal vein thrombophlebitis (sometimes with liver abscess). Look for portal venous gas, gas in the bladder lumen, and fluid, enteric contrast material, or gas outside the expected confines of the colon lumen.

Neoplastic Thickening of the Colon
Unfortunately, colonic mural thickening is a nonspecific finding seen in both malignant and benign disease. Some imaging clues, though, can help distinguish between malignant and benign causes with CT (Table 16-13). Of course, malignant and benign disease can coexist (e.g., colon edema/ischemia proximal to colon cancer or inflammation associated with perforated tumor) or overlap in imaging appearance. In such cases, the clinical setting is often the most useful clue.

The most common neoplastic causes of colonic thickening are adenocarcinoma and lymphoma. The classic appearance of adenocarcinoma is the "apple-core"

Table 16-13 Findings Helpful in Distinguishing Malignant from Benign Colonic Thickening with Computed Tomography

Malignant	Benign
Eccentric thickening	Concentric thickening
Isodense mural thickening	Stratified wall (submucosal edema)
Short-segment involvement	Longer segments involved
Abrupt caliber change, shouldering (Fig. 16-84)	Gradual tapering
Mesenteric adenopathy	Mesenteric fluid
Visible metastases	No metastases
No vascular engorement (Fig. 16-85)	Vascular engorgement (comb sign)

lesion (Fig. 16-86). Lymphoma has a highly variable appearance on imaging studies, including short- or long-segment mural thickening, solitary or multiple masses, or cavitary mass extending into the mesentery (see Fig. 16-67B). Lymphoma is typically associated with more adenopathy than adenocarcinoma, particularly outside the usual drainage pattern of the affected segment of colon.

Luminal Narrowing

Table 16-14 lists causes of luminal narrowing of the colon. Notably, many of the entities that cause mural thickening also cause luminal narrowing.

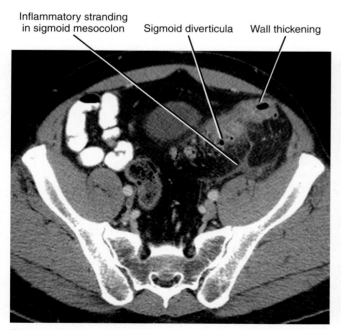

Inflammatory stranding in sigmoid mesocolon   Sigmoid diverticula   Wall thickening

Figure 16-83 Axial image of the pelvis from a contrast-enhanced computed tomographic scan of a patient with acute diverticulitis of the sigmoid colon.

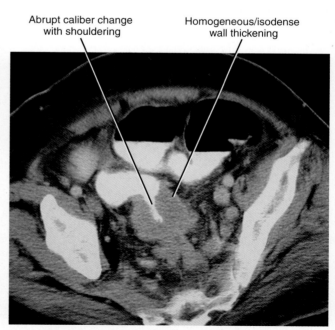

Abrupt caliber change with shouldering   Homogeneous/isodense wall thickening

Figure 16-84 Axial image of the pelvis from a contrast-enhanced computed tomographic scan of a patient with an obstructing carcinoma of the sigmoid colon.

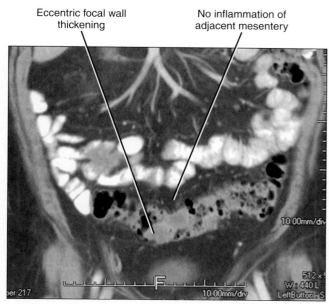

Eccentric focal wall thickening

No inflammation of adjacent mesentery

Figure 16-85 Coronal reformation of a contrast-enhanced computed tomographic scan in a patient with adenocarcinoma of the sigmoid colon arising in a segment of severe diverticulosis.

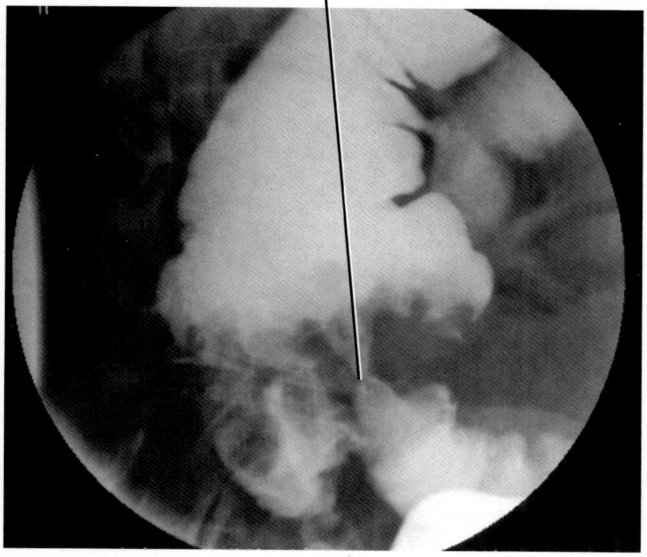

Severe constriction of the ileocecal region due to carcinoma

Figure 16-86 Single-contrast barium enema demonstrating the "apple-core" appearance of a carcinoma involving the cecum.

Colon Dilatation

Dilatation of the colon can be caused by obstructive and nonobstructive causative factors. Nonobstructive causes of colonic dilatation include ileus or pseudoobstruction, toxic megacolon, ischemia, and scleroderma. The imaging hallmark of scleroderma in the colon is wide-mouthed sacculations on the antimesenteric border of the transverse and descending colon. Patients with scleroderma can also experience development of benign

Table 16-14   Luminal Narrowing of the Colon

Causative Factor	Typical Findings
Radiation	• Circumferential wall thickening • Tapered luminal narrowing • Widened presacral space • History of radiation therapy
Ischemia (see Fig. 16-81)	• Watershed areas • Can be reversible
Carcinoma (see Fig. 16-84)	• Abrupt caliber change • Shouldering ("apple-core" appearance) • Irregular mucosal contour
Chronic ulcerative colitis	• Smoothly tapering • Sometimes reversible • Can be mimicked by a scirrhous neoplasm
Lymphogranuloma venereum	• Rectosigmoid region • Inguinal lymphadenopathy • Fistula formation
Endometriosis	• Serosal implants • Inferior surface of rectosigmoid region most common
Peritoneal metastases	• Most often involve sigmoid, transverse, and proximal ascending colon/cecum. • Serosal masses on computed tomography • Known gastrointestinal or gynecologic tumor
Tuberculosis	• Ileocecal region and right colon most common

pneumoperitoneum. Obstruction can be caused by tumor, stricture, adhesion, acute inflammation, or volvulus. Some important causes of colon dilatation are discussed in more detail in the following subsections.

Sigmoid Volvulus
In the United States, sigmoid volvulus afflicts the elderly, particularly the debilitated. Abdominal radiographs show the dilated, gas-filled sigmoid colon looping upward from the pelvis, often reaching high into the abdomen. The apposed walls of the sigmoid loop create a vertical stripe (the "coffee bean" sign) between the proximal and distal limbs. Contrast enema reveals a sharply tapering "bird beak" lumen contour, ending abruptly at the volvulus (Fig. 16-87). This tapering frequently is evident on CT as well. Whirling of mesenteric vasculature is an additional clue.

Cecal Volvulus
When the cecum twists around its long axis, it (along with adjacent ascending colon) shifts position into the mid or left abdomen. Plain films reveal the dilated, gas-filled cecum frequently in the left upper abdomen. Contrast enema reveals "bird beak"–like abrupt lumen tapering at the point of volvulus in the ascending colon. As with sigmoid volvulus, the "beaking" and whirled mesenteric vessels are depicted well on CT.

Cecal Bascule
Cecal bascule is a controversial entity, believed by some to be an anterior folding of the cecum and ascending colon without twisting. The dilated cecum

"Beaking" at site of obstruction
in distal sigmoid colon

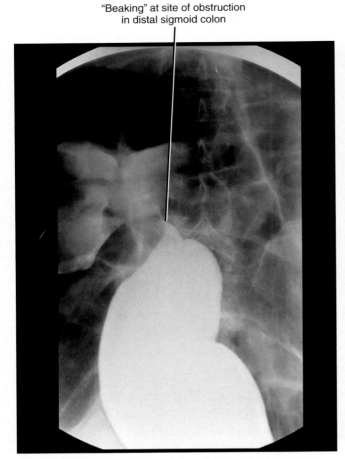

Figure 16-87 Spot image from a water-soluble contrast enema in a patient with sigmoid volvulus.

Marked dilatation of the transverse
colon with mucosal irregularity

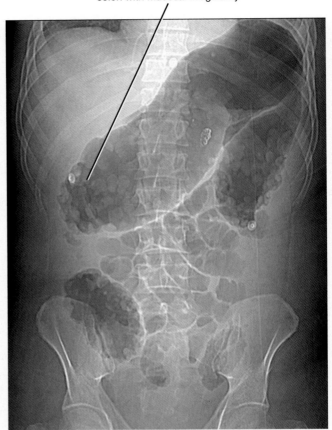

Figure 16-88 Abdominal radiograph showing marked dilatation of the transverse colon with mucosal irregularity (inflammatory pseudopolyps) in a patient with toxic megacolon associated with ulcerative colitis.

usually lies in the midabdomen. As with any cause of relatively prolonged cecal distension, a risk for perforation exists.

Toxic Megacolon

Toxic megacolon occurs most often with UC but can be seen with other colitides. A plain film of the abdomen is often diagnostic. Radiographic signs of toxic megacolon include a dilated ahaustral transverse colon (>6 cm in diameter) and a nodular colon lumen contour (islands of spared mucosa known as inflammatory pseudopolyps) (Fig. 16-88). Signs of intraperitoneal gas may be present, because up to half of patients will have colonic perforation. CT is excellent for detection of toxic megacolon, perforation, and pneumatosis.

If the radiographic findings are equivocal in a patient with suspected toxic megacolon, clinical clues can be helpful. Patients are typically acutely ill, and a history of colitis is often elicited. It is important not to perform a contrast enema on a patient with suspected toxic megacolon because of the thin, friable nature of the colonic tissues.

Pitfall: Do not perform contrast enema examinations on patients with suspected toxic megacolon, because perforation can result.

Masses

Polypoid Masses

Lesions that commonly present as polypoid masses in adults include hyperplastic, hamartomatous, and adenomatous polyps, inflammatory or postinflammatory pseudopolyps, and lipomas.

Hyperplastic polyps are usually small (<1 cm), lack malignant potential, and are frequently found in the distal colon and rectum. *Hamartomatous polyps* are nonneoplastic lesions that are associated with Peutz–Jeghers syndrome, Cowden disease, and Cronkhite–Canada syndrome.

Adenomatous polyps are neoplastic polyps that are classified as tubular, villous, tubulovillous, or flat. Villous adenomas have frondlike surfaces, creating a cauliflower-like appearance (similar to pouring barium on a sponge). Flat adenomas (carpet lesions) show a similar irregular surface appearance but are only slightly raised and, therefore, difficult to detect with imaging. Size matters for the likelihood of an adenomatous polyp to be malignant. The traditional teaching is that polyps smaller than 1 cm have a low likelihood of being malignant (about 1%). Polyps in the 1- to 2-cm range are associated with a likelihood of 10% to 20%. Polyps larger than 2 cm have about a 40% to 50% chance of being malignant.

Pearl: Polyps smaller than 1 cm have about 1% chance of being malignant. Polyps in the 1- to 2-cm range are associated with a likelihood of 10% to 20%. Polyps larger than 2 cm have about a 40% to 50% chance of being malignant.

Inflammatory pseudopolyps are actually islands of preserved mucosa surrounded by mucosal inflammation and ulceration. Inflammatory pseudopolyps are typically found in the colitides such as UC. Postinflammatory pseudopolyps (filiform polyps) result from tissue overgrowth during the healing phase of an ulcerating colitis. Such lesions are often linear, club shaped, or comma shaped.

Lipomas are really submucosal lesions, but they can become pedunculated and protrude into the colon lumen (Fig. 16-89). Lipomas are smoothly marginated and pliable (a feature demonstrated best with compression during fluoroscopy). CT easily demonstrates the fatty nature of lipomas (Fig. 16-90).

Colonic lymphoma is almost exclusively of the non–Hodgkin's variety and can present as a polypoid mass. Mantle cell lymphoma can present as multiple smooth nodules roughly 2 cm in diameter that carpet the colon lumen. Colitis cystica profunda is characterized by dilated mucous-filled glands that appear as rectal submucosal nodules.

Polypoid masses are easily distinguished from diverticula on cross-sectional imaging studies. On double-contrast barium studies, the distinction between a colon polyp and a diverticulum can be challenging, particularly once the patient leaves the department. Table 16-15 presents some helpful signs.

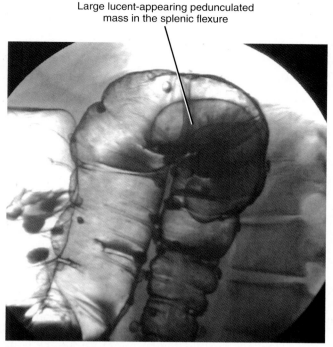

Large lucent-appearing pedunculated mass in the splenic flexure

Figure 16-89 Double-contrast barium enema spot film image of a patient with a large colonic lipoma. This mass readily changed shape and position during the examination. (Courtesy Dr. Shailendra Chopra)

Annular Masses

The most common annular lesion of the colon is adenocarcinoma. Adenocarcinoma often begins as a small polypoid mass (arising within a polyp), and progresses to become a large polypoid mass and, eventually, a circumferential apple-core lesion. CT and MRI clearly demonstrate the mural thickening associated with

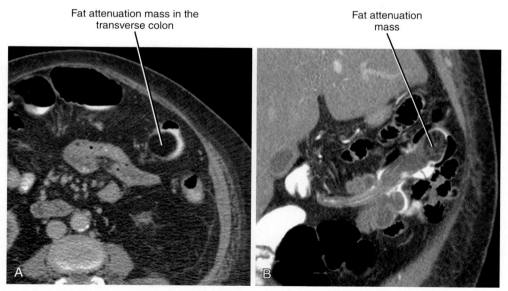

Fat attenuation mass in the transverse colon

Fat attenuation mass

Figure 16-90 Two colonic lipomas on computed tomography (CT). **A,** Axial image of the abdomen from a contrast-enhanced CT scan of a patient with a colonic lipoma. Despite its submucosal origin, the mass protrudes significantly into the colon lumen. **B,** Coronal oblique reformation of a contrast-enhanced CT scan of a different patient with an intussuscepting pedunculated lipoma of the transverse colon.

Table 16-15   Tips for Distinguishing Polyps from Diverticula on Double-Contrast Barium Enema

Polyp	Diverticulum
Displaces barium in the lumen	Fills with barium
Projects into lumen	Projects outside of lumen
"Bowler hat" points toward lumen (see Fig. 16-12)	Hat dome points away from lumen
Sharp inner margin and indistinct outer margin (sometimes difficult to determine)	Indistinct inner margin and sharp outer margin

carcinoma. Unlike inflammatory causes of colon wall thickening, adenocarcinoma typically lacks mural stratification on contrast-enhanced examinations. Adjacent lymphadenopathy and extraserosal extension are best demonstrated with CT or MRI. Synchronous lesions are common and should be specifically sought with imaging or endoscopy.

Lymphoma has a highly variable imaging appearance, including masslike, multinodular, and cavitary appearances. However, circumferential mural thickening with luminal narrowing is relatively common. Unlike adenocarcinoma, lymphoma can involve long segments of the colon but rarely obstructs the lumen. Circumferential colon thickening is a relatively uncommon manifestation of metastatic disease that can simulate primary adenocarcinoma.

Submucosal Masses

Submucosal colon masses can be caused by carcinoid tumor, lymphoma, GIST, hemangioma, lymphangioma, lipoma, and metastatic disease. Carcinoid tumors are usually small submucosal nodules in the rectum or large masses mimicking adenocarcinoma in the proximal colon. Rectal carcinoids can appear as submucosal masses 2 cm or larger and sometimes develop an ulcerated luminal surface. More advanced lesions can be annular with a sizeable extraluminal component. GISTs also have a predilection to occur in the rectum rather than in the more proximal colon.

Metastatic disease to the colon can result from hematogenous spread, direct extension, or peritoneal seeding. The most common hematogenous sources include lung, breast, and skin (melanoma). Hematogenous metastases can appear as ulcerated submucosal masses or create circumferential mural thickening and luminal narrowing. Direct extension of tumor to the colon has numerous origins, given the presence of colon in all four quadrants of the abdomen and pelvis. Peritoneal seeding of the colonic serosa can occur from many tumors but is most often of gynecologic or GI origin. Following the flow of peritoneal fluid, common sites of deposition include the pelvis, right lower quadrant, superior border of the sigmoid colon, and right paracolic gutter. A spiculated luminal contour, abnormal angulation, and luminal narrowing of the colon can all signify metastatic disease.

■ BRIEF GUIDE TO ABDOMINAL HERNIAS

Inguinal Hernia (Indirect Common, Direct Less Common)

Indirect

Most inguinal hernias are indirect, reflecting congenital patency of the processus vaginalis. The hernia sac extends through the inguinal ring, paralleling the spermatic cord and sometimes reaching the scrotum (Fig. 16-91). A convenient clue is that indirect hernias lie lateral to the inferior epigastric artery. They can contain small bowel and colon, and occasionally pelvic viscera such as the bladder or appendix.

Direct

Direct hernias are less common, protruding through a focus of weakness in the transversalis fascia, medial to inferior epigastric artery. They are shorter than indirect hernias, rarely causing incarceration of their contents. Occasionally, direct and indirect hernias coexist, flanking the inferior epigastric vessels as so-called saddlebag hernias.

Pearl: Indirect inguinal hernias occur lateral to the inferior epigastric arteries, whereas direct inguinal hernias protrude medial to these vessels.

Spigelian Hernia (Common)

Spigelian hernias protrude through the linea semilunaris along the lateral margin of the rectus muscle. The hernia sac pokes through the posterior layer of transversalis fascia, lying between the oblique muscle layers. Spigelian hernias usually contain omental fat and can include both small bowel and colon. Most occur at a level roughly halfway between the umbilicus and the pubic symphysis.

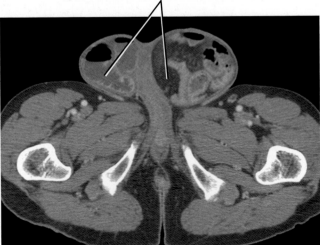

Small bowel and mesentary fill both inguinal canals and extend into the scrotum

Figure 16-91 Axial image of the perineum from a contrast-enhanced computed tomographic scan of a patient with bilateral inguinal hernias containing small bowel.

Umbilical Hernia (Common)

Umbilical hernias are common and usually contain omentum and sometimes small bowel or colon. Barium studies can demonstrate bowel within the hernia sac; cross-sectional imaging depicts the wall defect plus its contents.

Ventral Hernia (Common)

Ventral hernias are common and occur through a defect in the anterior or anterolateral abdominal wall, often a result of a surgically created defect (incisional hernia) (see Fig. 16-52). Most occur through a defect in the linea alba (midline), but ventral hernias can occur anywhere the abdominal wall has been breached (including at laparoscopy ports). Properitoneal fat, omentum, and bowel often herniate through ventral wall defects.

Lumbar Hernia (Common)

Lumbar hernias most commonly occur after trauma or surgery disrupts the posterolateral abdominal wall musculature or fascia between the last rib and the iliac crest (Fig. 16-92). CT depicts not only the defect but the hernia contents (most often retroperitoneal fat, bowel, or kidney).

Spontaneous lumbar hernias can be divided into superior and inferior varieties. Superior lumbar hernias occur in areas of weakness in the superior lumbar triangle (Grynfeltt–Lesshaft triangle) immediately below the 12th rib. Inferior lumbar hernias occur in the smaller inferior lumbar triangle (Petit triangle) bordered inferiorly by the iliac crest.

Femoral Hernia (Uncommon)

Femoral hernias are considerably less common than ventral or inguinal hernias. Femoral hernias protrude into the femoral canal, medial to the femoral vessels and posterior to the inguinal ligament. They occur more often in women than men and are prone to complications of incarceration and strangulation.

Sciatic Hernia (Rare)

These hernias are rare, protruding through the greater sciatic foramen into the subgluteal region. Both small bowel and distal ureter can be included in the hernia sac.

Obturator Hernia (Rare)

Obturator hernias extend into the obturator canal in the superolateral aspect of the obturator foramen (Fig. 16-93). These hernias are most common in older women. They are best depicted on CT, which will reveal the hernia contents extending into the obturator canal, sometimes trapped between the pectineus and obturator externus muscles.

Perineal Hernia (Rare)

Perineal hernias usually afflict older women who have weakened pelvic floor musculature. Bowel can herniate through the urogenital diaphragm or the levator ani musculature.

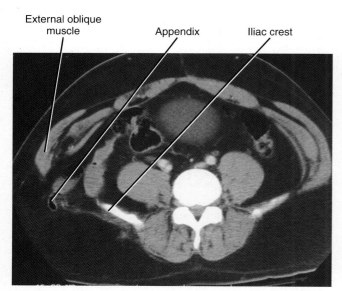

External oblique muscle   Appendix   Iliac crest

Figure 16-92 Axial image of the pelvis from a contrast-enhanced computed tomographic scan of a patient with a posttraumatic lumbar hernia.

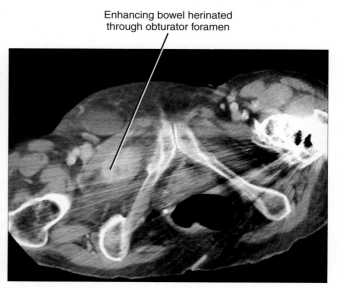

Enhancing bowel herinated through obturator foramen

Figure 16-93 Axial image of the lower pelvis from a contrast-enhanced computed tomographic scan of an elderly woman with small-bowel obstruction caused by an obturator hernia. (Courtesy Dr. William Chocallo).

Internal Hernias

Internal hernias are easy to miss, so one must be alert to subtle cues when evaluating patients with recurrent abdominal pain or episodic obstruction. Look for a "ball" or "glob" of small-bowel loops in an unusual location, sometimes with stasis and proximal bowel dilatation in addition to an abnormal course of adjacent mesenteric vasculature. Internal hernia should also be suspected when a cluster of dilated small bowel (possibly in a U shape) is identified against the abdominal wall in the absence of interposed omental fat. Internal hernias typically occur through acquired or congenital defects in the abdominal mesenteries.

Foramen of Winslow Hernia (Rare)

Foramen of Winslow hernias are characterized by small bowel or ascending colon slipping into the lesser sac via the epiploic foramen. Abdominal radiographs sometimes reveal gas-containing bowel loops high in the abdomen, posteromedial to the stomach. On CT, look for misplaced bowel tucked between the stomach, pancreas, and liver.

Paraduodenal Hernia (Rare)

Paraduodenal hernias are the most common type of internal hernia not related to a surgically created mesenteric defect. Herniation to the left is more common than to the right. Left paraduodenal hernias display a well-defined and fixed "ball" of jejunal loops lateral to the fourth portion of the duodenum. CT shows the "bag-of-bowel" situated between the pancreatic body and tail and the stomach, left of the ligament of Treitz. A fixed ball of jejunal loops inferolateral to the second portion of the duodenum is the hallmark of a right paraduodenal hernia.

Pericecal Hernia (Rare)

Pericecal hernias result from protrusion of distal ileum through cecal or appendiceal mesentery. Look for small bowel loops in the right paracolic gutter, dorsolateral to the cecum.

Transmesenteric and Transmesocolic Hernias (Uncommon)

Transmesenteric and transmesocolic hernias are internal hernias that can result from a surgical rent in a mesentery (adults) or from a congenital mesenteric defect (neonates). No sac encloses the herniated loops, but strangulation still can occur. CT will show typical signs of SBO plus converging mesenteric vessels at the hernia orifice. Transmesocolic hernias are a common complication of retrocolic gastric bypass, particularly when performed laparoscopically. Multiple dilated small-bowel loops adjacent to the stomach, and particularly dorsal to the stomach, should raise concern for herniation of jejunum through the mesocolon defect.

Suggested Readings

Aguirre D, Santosa AC, Casola G et al: Abdominal wall hernias: imaging features, complications, and diagnostic pitfalls at multi-detector row CT, *Radiographics* 25:1501-1520, 2005.

Balthazar EJ, Yen BC, Gordon RB: Ischemic colitis: CT evaluation of 54 cases, *Radiology* 211:381-388, 1999.

Ba-Ssalamah A, Prokop M, Uffmann M et al: Dedicated multidetector CT of the stomach: spectrum of diseases, *Radiographics* 23:625-644, 2003.

Bechtold RE, Chen MY, Stanton CA et al: Cystic changes in hepatic and peritoneal metastases from gastrointestinal stromal tumors treated with Gleevec, *Abdom Imaging* 28:808-814, 2003.

Bennett GL, Birnbaum BA, Balthazar EJ: CT of Meckel's diverticulitis in 11 patients, *AJR Am J Roentgenol* 182:625-629, 2004.

Berrocal T, Lamas M, Gutiérrez J et al: Congenital anomalies of the small intestine, colon, and rectum, *Radiographics* 19:1219-1236, 1999.

Blachar A, Federle MP, Dodson SF: Internal hernia: clinical and imaging findings in 17 patients with emphasis on CT criteria, *Radiology* 218:68-74, 2001.

Blachar A, Federle MP: Internal hernia: an increasingly common cause of small bowel obstruction, *Semin Ultrasound CT MR* 23:174-183, 2002.

Boudiaf M, Soyer P, Terem C et al: CT evaluation of small bowel obstruction, *Radiographics* 21:613-624, 2001.

Buckley JA, Fishman EK: CT evaluation of small bowel neoplasms: spectrum of disease, *Radiographics* 18:379-392, 1998.

Capps GW, Fulcher AS, Szucs RA et al: Imaging features of radiation-induced changes in the abdomen, *Radiographics* 17:1455-1473, 1997.

Catalano O: Computed tomographic appearance of sigmoid volvulus, *Abdom Imaging* 21:314-317, 1996.

Chintapalli KN, Chopra S, Ghiatas AA et al: Diverticulitis versus colon cancer: differentiation with helical CT findings, *Radiology* 210:429-435, 1999.

Chou CK, Mak CW, Huang MC et al: Differentiation of obstructive from non-obstructive small bowel dilatation on CT, *Eur J Radiol* 35:213-220, 2000.

Chou CK, Mak CW, Tzeng WS et al: CT of small bowel ischemia, *Abdom Imaging* 29:18-22, 2004.

Feczko PJ, Collins DD, Mezwa DG: Metastatic disease involving the gastrointestinal tract, *Radiol Clin North Am* 31:1359-1373, 1993.

Furukawa A, Yamasaki M, Takahashi M et al: CT diagnosis of small bowel obstruction: scanning technique, interpretation and role in the diagnosis, *Semin Ultrasound CT MR* 24:336-352, 2003.

Gore RM, Balthazar EJ, Ghahremani GG et al: CT features of ulcerative colitis and Crohn's disease, *AJR Am J Roentgenol* 167:3-15, 1996.

Gore RM, Levine MS: *Textbook of gastrointestinal radiology,* ed 3, Philadelphia, 2007, Elsevier Saunders.

Ha HK, Lee SH, Rha SE et al: Radiologic features of vasculitis involving the gastrointestinal tract, *Radiographics* 20:779-794, 2000.

Ha HK, Kim JS, Lee MS et al: Differentiation of simple and strangulated small-bowel obstructions: usefulness of known CT criteria, *Radiology* 204:507-512, 1997.

Halpert RD: Toxic dilatation of the colon, *Radiol Clin North Am* 25:147-155, 1987.

Hawn MT, Canon CL, Lockhart ME et al: Significance and outcome of CT diagnosis of pneumatosis of the gastrointestinal tract, *Am Surg* 70:19-23, 2004.

Ho LM, Paulson EK, Thompson WM: Pneumatosis intestinalis in the adult: benign to life-threatening causes, *AJR Am J Roentgenol* 188:1604-1613, 2007.

Horton KM, Corl FM, Fishman EK: CT evaluation of the colon: inflammatory disease, *Radiographics* 20:399-418, 2000.

Horton KM, Fishman EK: Current role of CT in imaging of the stomach, *Radiographics* 23:75-87, 2003.

Insko EK, Levine MS, Birnbaum BA et al: Benign and malignant lesions of the stomach: evaluation of CT criteria for differentiation, *Radiology* 228:166-171, 2003.

Jang HJ, Lim HK, Lee SJ et al: Acute diverticulitis of the cecum and ascending colon: the value of thin-section helical CT findings in excluding colonic carcinoma, *AJR Am J Roentgenol* 174:1397-1402, 2000.

Jayaraman MV, Mayo-Smith WW, Movson JS et al: CT of the duodenum: an overlooked segment gets its due, *Radiographics* 21:S147-S160, 2001.

Karahan OI, Dodd GD III, Chintapalli KN et al: Gastrointestinal wall thickening in patients with cirrhosis: frequency and patterns at contrast-enhanced CT, *Radiology* 215:103-107, 2000.

Kawamoto S, Horton KM, Fishman EK et al: Pseudomembranous colitis: spectrum of imaging findings with clinical and pathologic correlation, *Radiographics* 19:887-897, 1999.

Kernagis LY, Levine MS, Jacobs JE: Pneumatosis intestinalis in patients with ischemia: correlation of CT findings with viability of the bowel, *AJR Am J Roentgenol* 180:733-736, 2003.

Khurana B, Ledbetter S, McTavish J et al: Bowel obstruction revealed by multidetector CT, *AJR Am J Roentgenol* 178:1139-1144, 2002.

Laurent F, Drouillard J, Lecesne R et al: CT of small-bowel neoplasms, *Semin Ultrasound CT MR* 16:102-111, 1995.

Levine MS, Rubesin SE, Laufer I: *Double contrast gastrointestinal radiology,* ed 3, Philadelphia, 2000, Elsevier Saunders.

Levine MS, Rubesin SE, Laufer I et al: Diagnosis of colorectal neoplasms at double-contrast barium enema examination, *Radiology* 216:11-18, 2000.

Levy AD, Remotti HE, Thompson WM et al: Gastrointestinal stromal tumors: radiologic features with pathologic correlation, *Radiographics* 23:283-304, 2003.

Low RN, Chen SC, Barone R: Distinguishing benign from malignant bowel obstruction in patients with malignancy: findings at MR imaging, *Radiology* 228:157-165, 2003.

Lvoff N, Breiman RS, Coakley FV et al: Distinguishing features of self-limiting adult small-bowel intussusception identified at CT, *Radiology* 227:68-72, 2003.

Macari M, Megibow AJ, Balthazar EJ: A pattern approach to the abnormal small bowel: observations at MDCT and CT enterography, *AJR Am J Roentgenol* 188:1344-1355, 2007.

Maglinte DD: Small bowel imaging—a rapidly changing field and a challenge to radiology, *Eur Radiol* 16:967-971, 2006.

Maglinte DD, Sandrasegaran K, Lappas JC et al: CT enteroclysis, *Radiology* 245:661-671, 2007.

Mayo-Smith WW, Wittenberg J, Bennett GL et al: The CT small bowel feces sign: description and clinical significance, *Clin Radiol* 50:765-767, 1995.

Moore CJ, Corl FM, Fishman EK et al: CT of cecal volvulus: unraveling the image, *AJR Am J Roentgenol* 177:95-98, 2001.

Nagi B, Verma V, Vaiphei K et al: Primary small bowel tumors: a radiologic-pathologic correlation, *Abdom Imaging* 26:474-480, 2001.

Nevitt PC: The string of pearls sign, *Radiology* 214:157-158, 2000.

O'Malley ME, Wilson SR: US of gastrointestinal tract abnormalities with CT correlation, *Radiographics* 23:59-72, 2003.

Padidar AM, Jeffrey RB, Mindelzun RE et al: Differentiating sigmoid diverticulitis from carcinoma on CT scans: mesenteric inflammation suggests diverticulitis, *AJR Am J Roentgenol* 163:81-83, 1994.

Philpotts LE, Heiken JP, Westcott MA et al: Colitis: use of CT findings in differential diagnosis, *Radiology* 190:445-449, 1994.

Puylaert JB: Ultrasonography of the acute abdomen: gastrointestinal conditions, *Radiol Clin North Am* 41:1227-1242, 2003.

Rha SE, Ha HK, Lee SH et al: CT and MR imaging findings of bowel ischemia from various primary causes, *Radiographics* 20:29-42, 2000.

Saenz De Ormijana J, Aisa P, Añorbe E et al: Idiopathic enteroenteric intussusceptions in adults, *Abdom Imaging* 28:8-11, 2003.

Schmitt SL, Wexner SD: Bacterial, fungal, parasitic, and viral colitis, *Surg Clin North Am* 73:1055-1062, 1993.

Sebastià C, Quiroga S, Espin E et al: Portomesenteric vein gas: pathologic mechanisms, CT findings, and prognosis, *Radiographics* 20:1213-1224, 2000.

Segatto E, Mortelé KJ, Wiesner W et al: Acute small bowel ischemia: CT imaging findings, *Semin Ultrasound CT MR* 24:364-376, 2003.

Shadbolt CL, Heinze SB, Dietrich RB: Imaging of groin masses: inguinal anatomy and pathologic conditions revisited, *Radiographics* 21:S261-S271, 2001.

Shivanand G, Seema S, Srivastava DN et al: Gastric volvulus: acute and chronic presentation, *Clin Imaging* 27:265-268, 2003.

Takeyama N, Gokan T, Ohgiya Y et al: CT of internal hernias, *Radiographics* 25: 997-1015, 2005.

Warshauer DM, Lee JK: Adult intussusception detected at CT or MR imaging: clinical-imaging correlation, *Radiology* 212:853-860, 1999.

Wiesner W, Khurana B, Ji H et al: CT of acute bowel ischemia, *Radiology* 226:635-650, 2003.

Wiesner W, Mortelé KJ, Glickman JN et al: Pneumatosis intestinalis and portomesenteric venous gas in intestinal ischemia: correlation of CT findings with severity of ischemia and clinical outcome, *AJR Am J Roentgenol* 177: 1319-1323, 2001.

Zarvan NP, Lee FT, Yandow DR et al: Abdominal hernias: CT findings, *AJR Am J Roentgenol* 164:1391-1395, 1995.

CHAPTER **17**

Adrenal Glands

Neal C. Dalrymple

■ CLINICAL CONSIDERATIONS

Anatomy of the Adrenal Glands

Histologic Anatomy

Histologically, each adrenal gland is composed of two different types of tissue with different functions: the peripheral cortex and the central medulla. The adrenal cortex is derived embryologically from coelomic mesoderm that develops into three stratified zones of cortical tissue (zona glomerulosa, zona fasciculata, and zona reticularis) that are vital to fluid-electrolyte homeostasis. The adrenal medulla is derived from neural crest ectoderm and produces a variety of catecholamines that regulate hemodynamics and respond to stress. Table 17-1 provides a summary of the regional production of hormones.

Cross-Sectional Anatomy

The normal adrenal glands reside in a superior and anteromedial recess of the perirenal space, and adhere to the innermost layer of the perirenal fascia at this location. The right adrenal gland can usually be identified in a location superior to the right kidney with some tissue protruding between the posterior margin of the inferior vena cava and the medial portion of the right diaphragmatic crus. Often, the entire right adrenal gland is superior to the kidney, although a small portion may extend inferiorly anterior to the kidney. The short, right adrenal vein can be identified in most cases (Fig. 17-1). The adrenal vein is occasionally a useful landmark for identifying the adrenal gland when a mass distorts structures in the suprarenal region.

> *Pearl: Identification of the right adrenal vein can be useful in attempting to determine whether a large mass in the right upper quadrant arises from the adrenal gland or the adjacent kidney or liver.*

The left adrenal gland usually can be identified anterior and medial to the superior pole of the left kidney, and just lateral to the medial aspect of the left diaphragmatic crus. Vascular structures neighboring the left adrenal gland can sometimes cause confusion. For example, tortuous segments of the splenic artery and vein can course vertically adjacent to the left adrenal gland, simulating a nodule. For this reason, it is important to trace each adjacent structure before diagnosing an adrenal mass.

The cross-sectional appearance of the left adrenal gland often simulates an inverted "Y" shape, whereas the right more often simulates an inverted "V" shape. Because laparoscopic partial adrenalectomy can now be performed for functioning adenomas, it is sometimes helpful to provide a precise description for the location of small adrenal nodules. The anterior limb is usually described as the *body* of the gland. The posterior limbs are usually described as *medial* or *lateral*.

Note that the normal adrenal medulla has sufficient volume to result in fullness in the central part of the gland. A mildly rounded appearance of the adrenal gland at its center where the three limbs join is normal and should not be mistaken for a nodule.

Laboratory Findings Relevant to the Adrenal Gland

For some of us, the complexities of endocrinology exemplify the part of medicine we deliberately left behind when we chose to pursue radiology. Fear not! Only a rudimentary understanding of several laboratory values will be discussed to facilitate the radiologist as an intelligent investigator in imaging adrenal disease. We will divide the laboratory tests into those that assess cortical function and those that assess medullary function.

Laboratory Analysis of Adrenal Cortical Function

As mentioned previously, the adrenal cortex produces three main categories of substances: (1) *aldosterone* that regulates sodium absorption in the kidney and other organs, thus affecting electrolyte balance; (2) *cortisol* that regulates carbohydrate, protein, lipid, and nucleic acid metabolism; and (3) *androgens* (dehydroepiandrosterone [DHEA], dehydroepiandrosterone sulfate [DHEAS], and androstenedione) that play a role in the development of secondary sex characteristics in male individuals and virilization in female individuals (if excessive).

In addition to regulating fluid–electrolyte balance by promoting sodium retention, aldosterone also promotes renal potassium excretion. Therefore, hyperaldosteronism is suspected in the presence of hypertension, hypernatremia, and hypokalemia.

Table 17-1   Adrenal Endocrine Mediators by Location

Location	Product
Adrenal Cortex	
Zona glomerulosa	Aldosterone
Other zones	Cortisol Androgens (dehydroepiandrosterone, dehydroepiandrosterone sulfate, and androstenedione)
Adrenal Medulla	Epinephrine Small amounts of norepinephrine and dopamine

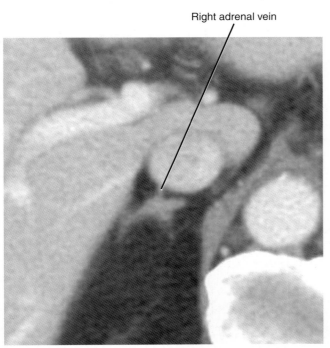

Right adrenal vein

Figure 17-1 Axial image from contrast-enhanced computed tomographic examination demonstrates the right adrenal vein as it bridges the body of the adrenal gland and posterior wall of the inferior vena cava.

Cortisol production in the adrenal cortex is regulated through a feedback mechanism to prevent overproduction. A *dexamethasone suppression test* introduces exogenous steroid that should suppress the normal adrenal cortex. Failure of suppression indicates unregulated cortisol production (Cushing syndrome).

17-Ketosteroids are found in the urine mainly as a breakdown product of androgens with a minor component coming from the breakdown of glucocorticoids. Increased levels of 17-ketosteroids in the urine usually indicate an adrenal causative agent for virilization in female individuals (carcinoma, hyperplasia) rather than an ovarian causative factor (arrhenoblastoma, polycystic ovarian syndrome).

Laboratory Analysis of Adrenal Medullary Function

A tumor of the chromaffin cells in the sympathetic nervous system is called *pheochromocytoma* if it arises within the adrenal medulla and *paraganglioma* when it arises in an extraadrenal location. Even when benign, these tumors can be lethal through the episodic release of catecholamines in the settings of stress, induction of anesthesia, voiding, pregnancy, biopsy, or manipulation. The rapid release of large amounts of catecholamines can result in headaches, palpitations, nausea, chest or abdominal pain, or hypertensive crisis.

The episodic nature of catecholamine release made the laboratory diagnosis of pheochromocytoma problematic in the past. Measurable levels of epinephrine and norepinephrine remain in the bloodstream for only a limited time; therefore, serum analysis is often unfruitful unless the sample is obtained immediately after or during a crisis. Because epinephrine and norepinephrine and their breakdown product *vanillylmandelic acid (VMA)* and *metanephrine* persist for a longer time in urine, urine assays have become the preferred method of diagnosis and are reported to have an accuracy rate as high as 95%. If immediate blood samples are available, assays may be able to determine whether epinephrine or norepinephrine is the predominant catecholamine. This can be useful in localizing tumors because the dominant catecholamine produced by the adrenal medulla is epinephrine, whereas extraadrenal paragangliomas produce mainly norepinephrine. Both epinephrine and norepinephrine are metabolized into VMA.

Pearl: Increased serum epinephrine level indicates the tumor is likely an adrenal pheochromocytoma, whereas elevated norepinephrine indicates an extraadrenal paraganglioma is more likely.

■ COMPARISON OF IMAGING MODALITIES

Table 17-2 presents a comparison of various imaging modalities for assessment of the adrenal glands.

■ CHARACTERIZING ADRENAL MASSES

First Things First: Is It Really the Adrenal Gland?

A number of normal and abnormal structures can mimic an adrenal mass. Adrenal mimics are much more common on the left side because of potential collateral venous pathways around the spleen and proximity of the left adrenal gland to the stomach and pancreas. Having a high index of suspicion is helpful in identifying subtle signs, such as traces of air in a gastric diverticulum, enhancement similar to nearby splenic tissue, or contiguity with adjacent vascular structures. Table 17-3 lists the most common mimics of adrenal masses.

Table 17-2   Imaging the Adrenal Glands: Relative Roles of Various Modalities

Modality	Role
Ultrasound	Detects some adrenal masses Limited role in characterization • Can distinguish cystic from solid lesions (Fig. 17-2) • Echogenic mass suggests myelolipoma or hemorrhage
CT	Sensitive for detection of adrenal masses Useful for staging primary adrenal neoplasms Useful for adrenal mass characterization • NCCT attenuation value < 10 HU highly specific for adenoma • Sensitive to small amounts of macroscopic fat (myelolipoma) • Relative washout of ≥40% or absolute washout of ≥60% highly specific for adenoma
MRI	Sensitive for detection of adrenal masses Useful for staging primary adrenal neoplasms Useful for adrenal mass characterization • Signal loss on opposed-phase gradient-echo images relative to in-phase images highly specific for adenoma • Sensitive for detection of blood products (hemorrhage) • Fat-suppression techniques useful for diagnosing myelolipoma
PET-CT	^{18}F-FDG is taken up in greater quantity by cells with more rapid metabolism (including cancer cells) Characterization of adrenal mass in a patient with history of malignancy • Most useful for lymphoma and lung cancer • Can be used with any tumor known to be FDG avid (Fig. 17-3) • Uptake of ^{18}F-FDG > liver suggests malignancy
MIBG	Diagnosis of pheochromocytoma Localization of extraadrenal paraganglioma Detect metastases from malignant pheochromocytoma (Fig. 17-4)

CT, Computed tomography; ^{18}*F-FDG*, F-18 fluorodeoxyglucose; *MIBG*, metaiodobenzylguanidine I123; *MRI*, magnetic resonance imaging; *NCCT*, noncontrast-enhanced computed tomography; *PET*, positron emission tomography.

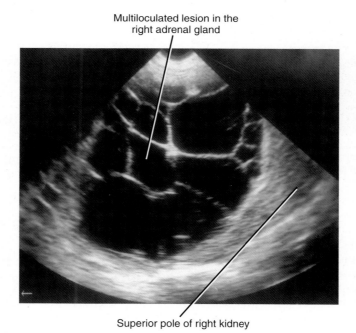

Multiloculated lesion in the
right adrenal gland

Superior pole of right kidney

Figure 17-2 Sagittal ultrasound image of the right adrenal gland demonstrates a multiloculated cystic lesion. This proved to be a hydatid cyst.

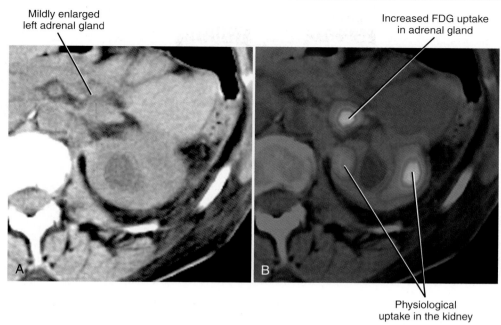

Mildly enlarged
left adrenal gland

Increased FDG uptake
in adrenal gland

Physiological
uptake in the kidney

Figure 17-3 Using positron emission tomography (PET) to characterize a small adrenal mass. **A,** Axial image from unenhanced computed tomography in a woman with known metastatic breast cancer demonstrates a small, soft-tissue attenuation mass in the left adrenal gland. **B,** The same image fused with fluoro-2-deoxy-D-glucose (FDG) PET image demonstrates increased uptake within the lesion (SUV = 3.6) compared with the background activity in the liver (SUV = 2.5, not shown). (Courtesy Kevin Banks, M.D.) *SUV,* Standardized uptake value.

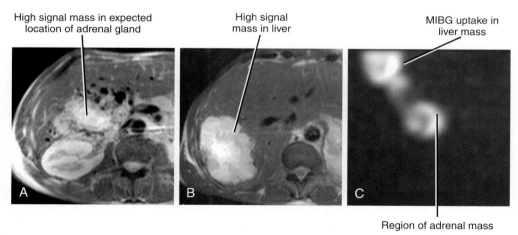

High signal mass in expected
location of adrenal gland

High signal
mass in liver

MIBG uptake in
liver mass

Region of adrenal mass

Figure 17-4 T2-weighted magnetic resonance images of a patient with metastatic pheochromocytoma shows **(A)** high signal in the primary adrenal lesion, as well as **(B)** high signal in a large liver metastasis. **C,** Coronal image from an I131-labeled (MIBG) study for this patient performed several days after the magnetic resonance imaging demonstrates intense uptake in both lesions.

Clinical Context

Associated imaging, physical examination, and laboratory findings are often essential to definitive characterization of an adrenal lesion. An adrenal mass in a patient with hypertension is likely to be an adenoma when associated with hypernatremia (Conn syndrome) or hirsutism and obesity (Cushing syndrome), but is more likely to be a pheochromocytoma if there is a history of episodic flushing. Each of these clinical syndromes is described in the section "Hyperfunctioning Lesions of the Adrenal Gland."

A known history of cancer increases the likelihood that a given adrenal mass is metastatic disease. More specific patterns of multiorgan involvement suggest syndrome-associated adrenal neoplasms, such as pheochromocytoma associated with neurofibromatosis,

Table 17-3   Mimics of Adrenal Mass

Mimics	Distinguishing Features
Plane-dependent pseudolesion on computed tomography (Fig. 17-5)	• Volume averaging of lateral limb of left adrenal gland • Present only on axial sections
Splenic varices (Fig. 17-6)	• Evidence of portal hypertension • Continuity with venous structures
Tortuous splenic artery	• Continuity with arterial structures
Gastric diverticulum	• Air–fluid or fluid–fluid level • Contiguous with stomach
Accessory spleen (Fig. 17-7)	• Enhancement pattern similar to spleen (computed tomography, magnetic resonance) • Uptake on technetium-99m–labeled, heat-damaged, red blood cell study or liver-spleen scan with single-photon emission computed tomography • Uptake of ferumoxides on magnetic resonance imaging
Pancreatic pseudocyst	• History or imaging evidence of pancreatitis
Tumors of the celiac ganglion (ganglioneuroma)	• Fat plane between mass and medial margin of the adrenal gland
Tumor of adjacent organ (e.g., kidney, stomach) or perirenal space (e.g., liposarcoma)	• Fat plane between mass and adrenal gland • "Claw sign" of adjacent organ or evidence of "divot" of adjacent kidney (angiomyolipoma)

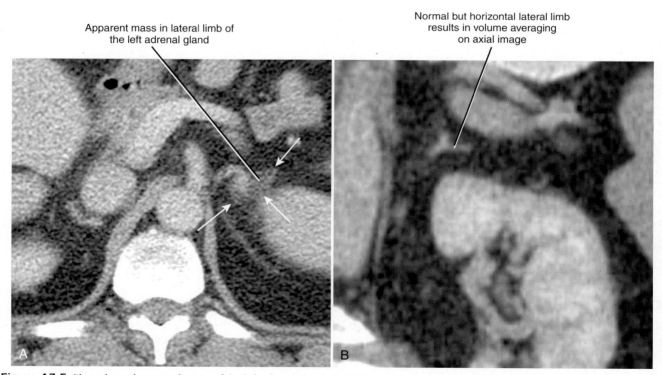

Figure 17-5 Plane-dependent pseudomass of the left adrenal gland. **A,** Axial image from a contrast-enhanced computed tomographic scan demonstrates a vague masslike appearance of the lateral limb caused by volume averaging (outlined by arrows). **B,** A coronal reformation demonstrates a horizontal configuration of the lateral limb with no mass.

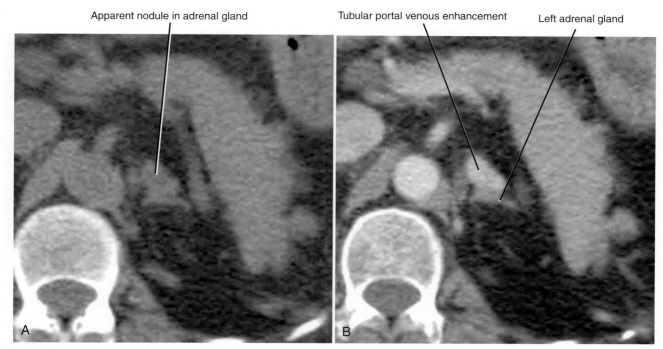

Apparent nodule in adrenal gland

Tubular portal venous enhancement   Left adrenal gland

A   B

Figure 17-6 Splenorenal varix as adrenal pseudomass. **A,** Axial unenhanced computed tomographic image demonstrates an apparent mass in the body of the left adrenal gland. **B,** On an axial image in the portal phase of enhancement, the lesion enhances uniformly compared with other portal structures and was found to be continuous with the splenic vein.

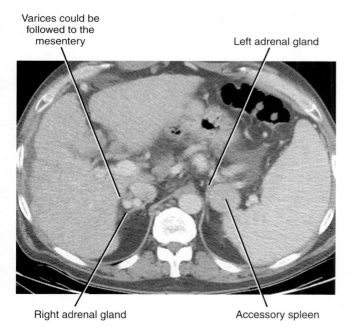

Varices could be followed to the mesentery

Left adrenal gland

Right adrenal gland   Accessory spleen

Figure 17-7 Axial image from a contrast-enhanced computed tomographic examination demonstrates bilateral adrenal pseudomass lesions. A patient with portal hypertension was referred for biopsy of left adrenal lesion. Notice the thin fat plane between the accessory spleen and left adrenal gland. Large varices cause an unusual pseudomass on the right side.

multiple endocrine neoplasia or von Hippel–Lindau syndrome (Fig. 17-8). A retroperitoneal mass in a young girl with hypertension and associated masses in the lung (pulmonary chondroma) or stomach (gastrointestinal stromal tumor) is suspicious for an extraadrenal paraganglioma in Carney's triad.

Mass Size, Shape, and Number

The size of an adrenal mass is a relatively strong discriminator between benign and malignant lesions. Most adrenal adenomas are small, averaging just larger than 2 cm in diameter in most series. At autopsy, only 2% of adrenal adenomas are larger than 4 cm and 0.03% are larger than 6 cm. Metastases, adrenal cortical carcinomas, and pheochromocytomas are often large at time of presentation (Fig. 17-9 and 17-10). Ninety-two percent of adrenal cortical carcinomas are larger than 6 cm at time of diagnosis. Thus, a small adrenal mass (<3 cm) with no suspicious imaging features in a patient without known risk for metastases can be followed with serial imaging unless an additional study (noncontrast computed tomography (CT), washout CT, or magnetic resonance imaging [MRI]) can characterize the mass definitively. A mass larger than 5 cm is suspicious for malignancy until proved otherwise.

As a rule of thumb, an adrenal limb thicker than 10 mm is considered to be enlarged. Unfortunately, adrenal shape is only occasionally helpful in characterizing adrenal gland enlargement. Diffuse bilateral enlargement of the adrenal glands usually indicates *adrenal hyperplasia* and can be either smooth or have a nodular

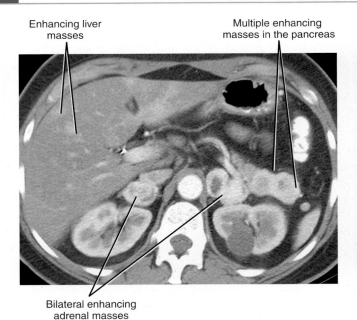

Enhancing liver masses

Multiple enhancing masses in the pancreas

Bilateral enhancing adrenal masses

Figure 17-8 Axial image from a contrast-enhanced computed tomographic examination demonstrates bilateral adrenal masses, as well as multiple masses in the pancreas and liver. The adrenal masses proved to be pheochromocytomas (metastatic to the liver), and the pancreatic masses islet cell tumors. This constellation of findings contributed to the ultimate diagnosis of von Hippel–Lindau disease.

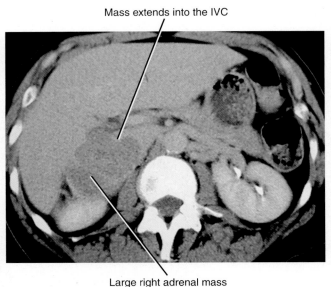

Mass extends into the IVC

Large right adrenal mass

Figure 17-10 Axial computed tomographic image of abdomen demonstrates a large right adrenal mass invading the inferior vena cava (IVC) in a patient with metastatic lung cancer. Caval extension is more common on the right side because of the short length of the right adrenal vein.

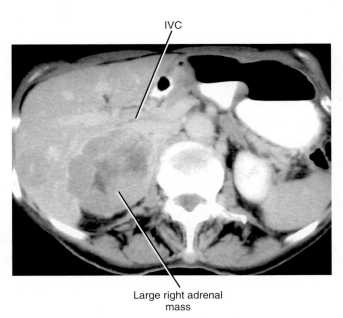

IVC

Large right adrenal mass

Figure 17-9 Axial image from a contrast-enhanced computed tomographic examination demonstrates a large right adrenal mass, partially displacing the inferior vena cava (IVC) anteriorly. This was surgically proved to be adrenal carcinoma.

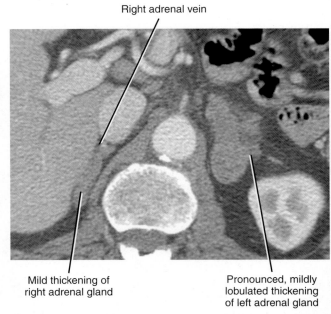

Right adrenal vein

Mild thickening of right adrenal gland

Pronounced, mildly lobulated thickening of left adrenal gland

Figure 17-11 Axial image of the adrenal glands from a contrast-enhanced computed tomographic examination demonstrates diffuse enlargement of both adrenal glands caused by adrenal hyperplasia.

contour (Fig. 17-11). Adrenal hyperplasia is associated with clinical findings of Conn or Cushing syndrome in adults and children, as well as virilization in infants. Uncommonly, adrenal metastases can cause diffuse enlargement of the gland (Fig. 17-12), although metastatic enlargement is usually less symmetric than that seen with hyperplasia.

The number of adrenal masses is a weak discriminator between benign and malignant lesions. Adrenal adenomas, carcinomas, metastases, lymphoma, and pheochromocytomas can all present as solitary or multiple

Gland retains adreniform
shape despite diffuse,
irregular enlargement

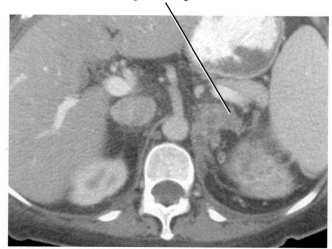

Figure 17-12 Axial contrast-enhanced computed tomographic image demonstrates diffuse enlargement of the left adrenal gland caused by metastatic renal cell carcinoma.

ROI placed over mass

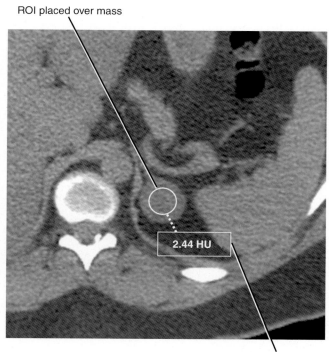

2.44 HU

Attenuation < 10 HU

Figure 17-13 Axial image from an unenhanced computed tomographic scan demonstrates a region-of-interest (ROI) attenuation measurement of a left adrenal mass. The mean attenuation of 2.44 HU is less than 10 HU and, therefore, highly specific for adenoma. Note that the ROI is placed to include most of the mass without extending beyond it.

adrenal masses. Nodular hyperplasia is easily mistaken for multiple metastatic nodules in a patient at risk for metastatic disease.

Attenuation Value or Signal Intensity within the Mass

Fluid

Fluid attenuation within an adrenal mass on CT (or fluid signal on MRI) is highly correlated with benignity, provided the lesion is homogeneous with smooth margins. In most cases, fluid attenuation results from averaging of intracellular lipid and soft-tissue components within an adenoma (Fig. 17-13). The attenuation value cutoff for diagnosing adenoma has been debated in the literature (some prefer the higher sensitivity for adenoma provided by a threshold of 15 HU), but currently, *most radiologists use 10 HU as the upper limit for diagnosis of adenoma* by attenuation value with noncontrast CT (NCCT). The use of this value provides a specificity of 98% for adrenal adenoma.

Necrotic malignant neoplasms can also demonstrate fluid attenuation centrally on NCCT (Fig. 17-14). However, these lesions are usually distinguished from adenoma by their size and enhancement characteristics. Some pheochromocytomas can appear predominately or nearly entirely cystic.

Pitfall: Water attenuation within an adrenal lesion does not automatically indicate a benign lesion. Necrosis within a malignant mass or lipid within a pheochromocytoma can also result in low attenuation on CT. In most cases, however, the malignant lesions will be large and will have irregular walls.

Adrenal cysts can be divided into endothelial cysts (simple cysts), pseudocysts (after hemorrhage or

Thick, irregular wall

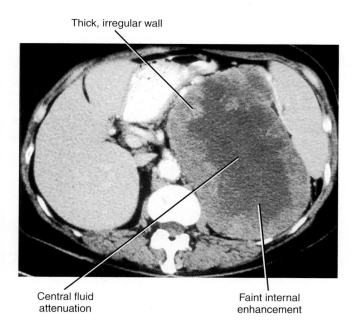

Central fluid
attenuation

Faint internal
enhancement

Figure 17-14 Axial image from a contrast-enhanced computed tomographic scan demonstrating fluid attenuation within central necrosis of adrenal cortical carcinoma. Despite the presence of fluid attenuation components, the presence of an irregular enhancing wall and large size suggest malignancy.

infection), hydatid cysts, and epithelial cysts. Because each of these is benign, there is little use in differentiating between them with imaging, with the exception of hydatid cysts that require treatment. Adrenal cysts typically measure water attenuation on CT and can appear identical to adenoma on unenhanced images unless a cyst wall is visible. CT demonstrates wall calcification in approximately 10% of endothelial cysts and 20% of pseudocysts (Figs. 17-15 and 17-16). With ultrasound, most adrenal cysts have characteristics similar to renal cysts (anechoic, enhanced through transmission),

whereas hydatid cysts are septated (see Fig. 17-2). MRI shows fluid signal intensity within adrenal cysts (high signal intensity on T2-weighted images and low signal intensity on T1-weighted images).

Fat/Lipid
MACROSCOPIC FAT

Macroscopic fat refers to the presence of adipocytes or deposits of extracellular fat in sufficient quantity to result in measured attenuation values lower than water (usually −30 to −90) by CT or detection by fat-suppression methods on MRI. Macroscopic fat within an adrenal gland is almost always a sign of myelolipoma, a benign hamartoma of the adrenal gland that consists of bone marrow elements. Because bone marrow contains variable amounts of fat, as well as red and white blood cell precursors, myelolipomas are often heterogeneous, containing both fat and soft-tissue elements on CT and MR images (Fig. 17-17). On MR images obtained with frequency-selective fat suppression, myelolipomas show loss of signal in regions of macroscopic fat (Fig. 17-18). No signal loss is expected centrally on opposed-phase imaging in areas of macroscopic fat, although signal loss will be present at fat–soft tissue interfaces. Small myelolipomas do not usually require treatment. Large myelolipomas can mimic retroperitoneal liposarcoma (Fig. 17-19). True lipomas of the adrenal gland also occur but are rare. Distinguishing between myelolipoma and lipoma on an imaging study is rarely important.

INTRACELLULAR LIPID

We describe tiny lipid droplets within the cytoplasm of cells as intracellular lipid. These are usually the endocrine products of adenomas, regardless of whether they are produced in quantities sufficient to produce symptoms or even to detect in the serum. Thus, all

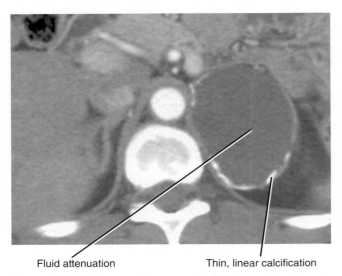

Fluid attenuation   Thin, linear calcification

Figure 17-15 Computed tomographic (CT) scan of an adrenal cyst. Axial image from a contrast-enhanced CT scan demonstrates thin wall calcification. Such calcification indicates endothelial cyst is likely, although similar calcification can be seen in adrenal pseudocysts.

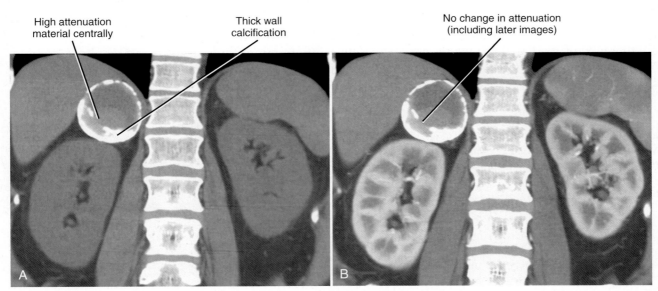

Figure 17-16 Coronal computed tomographic (CT) images of a calcified, cystic lesion of the right adrenal gland. Thick wall calcification is typical of adrenal pseudocyst, but appearance is confounded by internal high-attenuation material on unenhanced CT images (**A**). There is no enhancement after contrast administration (**B**) and the lesion remained stable in size for at least 6 years, consistent with benign disease.

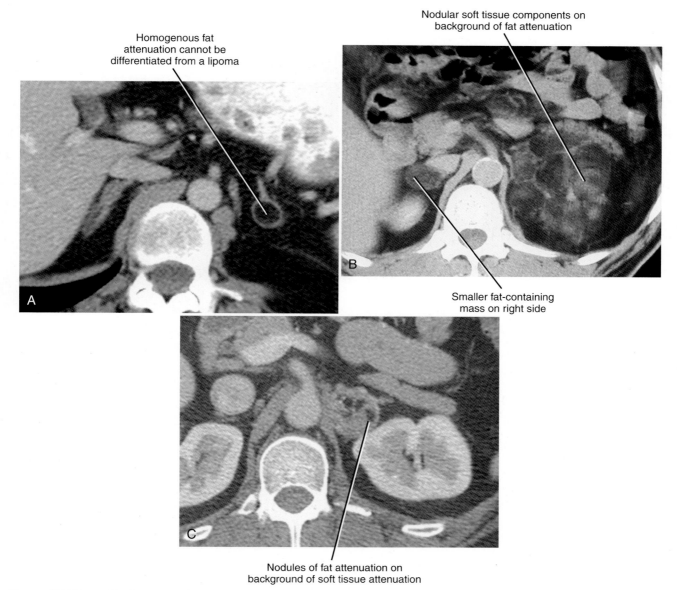

Homogenous fat attenuation cannot be differentiated from a lipoma

Nodular soft tissue components on background of fat attenuation

Smaller fat-containing mass on right side

Nodules of fat attenuation on background of soft tissue attenuation

Figure 17-17 Variable fat content of myelolipomas on axial computed tomographic images of different patients. **A,** Homogenous fat attenuation. **B,** Mix of fat and soft tissue in bilateral myelolipomas. **C,** Minimal fat content.

hyperfunctioning adenomas and most nonhyperfunctioning adenomas contain some amount of intracellular lipid. When intracellular lipid is interspersed with other tissue elements within an adrenal mass, the attenuation value on unenhanced CT approximates that of water.

With MRI, *chemical-shift imaging* (also called in- and opposed-phase imaging) provides specific evidence of intracellular lipid. To achieve this, technologists acquire T1-weighted gradient-echo images using specific variable echo-time settings that result in one image set with fat and water in phase, and another image set with fat and water out of phase. (Chapter 3 provides a more detailed explanation on chemical-shift imaging.) Tissues that contain sufficient intracellular lipid will lose signal intensity on opposed-phase images relative to in-phase images (Fig. 17-20).

Most adrenal adenomas consist of cells that contain enough intracellular lipid that the soft-tissue signal intensity seen on in-phase images decreases significantly on opposed-phase images. Unfortunately, some adrenal adenomas contain little intracellular lipid, and remain indeterminate on unenhanced CT and chemical-shift MRI. The differential diagnosis for a lesion that does not contain sufficient lipid to be characterized on unenhanced CT or chemical-shift MRI is broad, including lipid poor adenoma, metastasis, adrenal cortical carcinoma, pheochromocytoma, and lymphoma (Fig. 17-21).

Pitfall: *Lesions that do not lose signal on opposed-phase imaging are not necessarily malignant. Some adenomas lack sufficient intracellular lipid to cause signal loss with chemical-shift techniques.*

High signal on opposed phase
T1W image, consistent with
macroscopic fat

Signal loss with frequency
selective fat suppression

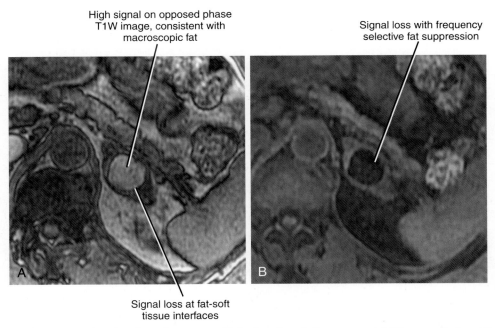

Signal loss at fat-soft
tissue interfaces

Figure 17-18 Magnetic resonance imaging shows fat content of left adrenal myelolipoma on axial **(A)** opposed-phase T1-weighted (T1W) and **(B)** fat-suppressed T1W images.

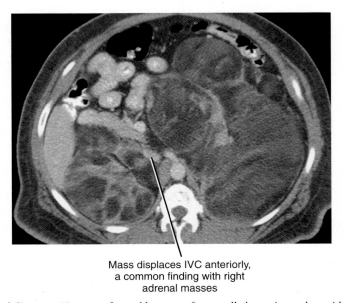

Mass displaces IVC anteriorly,
a common finding with right
adrenal masses

Figure 17-19 Large bilateral myelolipomas. Biopsy performed because of unusually large size and considerable organ displacement confirmed the diagnosis. *IVC,* Inferior vena cava.

The literature documents many attempts to quantify the diagnosis of intracellular lipid by MRI. Two commonly used methods—the signal intensity index and the adrenal-to-spleen ratio—are presented here.

Signal Intensity (SI) index =

$$\frac{(in\ phase\ SI) - (opposed\ phase\ SI)}{(in\ phase\ SI)} \times 100\%$$

The signal intensity index requires that identical imaging parameters are used for both in-phase and opposed-phase acquisitions. This is the case when both images are obtained as part of a dual-phase gradient-echo sequence widely available on newer MR systems. A signal intensity index value of more than 16.5% implies that an adrenal lesion is an adenoma.

When comparing in- and opposed-phase images that were not obtained as part of the same dual-echo

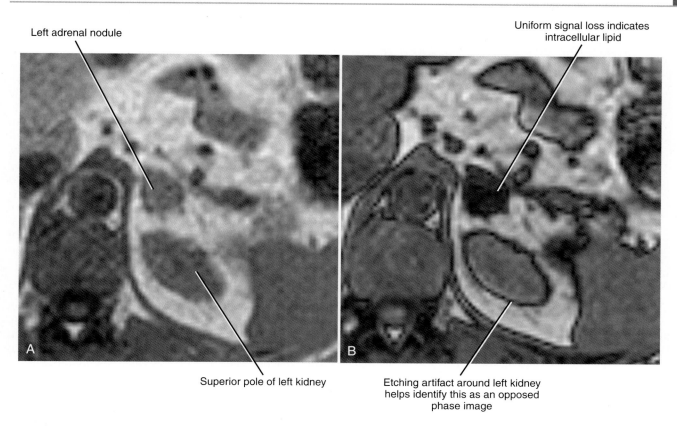

Left adrenal nodule

Uniform signal loss indicates
intracellular lipid

Superior pole of left kidney

Etching artifact around left kidney
helps identify this as an opposed
phase image

Figure 17-20 Chemical-shift imaging diagnosis of adrenal adenoma. **A,** Axial T1-weighted in-phase image of the left adrenal gland demonstrates intermediate signal in the adrenal gland. **B,** Axial image repeated out of phase demonstrates uniform signal loss, characteristic of an adenoma.

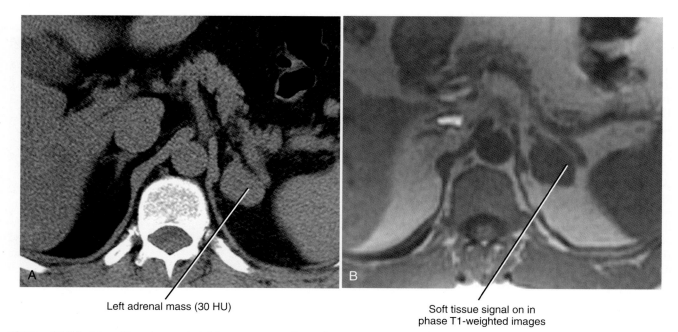

Left adrenal mass (30 HU)

Soft tissue signal on in
phase T1-weighted images

Figure 17-21 Adrenal lymphoma. **A,** Axial noncontrast-enhanced computed tomographic image demonstrates soft-tissue attenuation within a left adrenal mass. Axial T1-weighted magnetic resonance images performed **(B)** in phase and

Continued

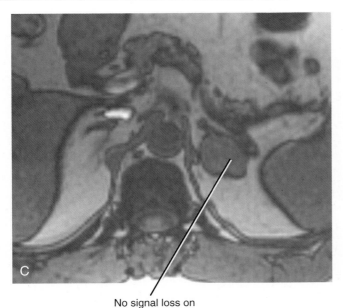

No signal loss on
opposed phase images

Figure 17-21, cont'd   (C) out of phase demonstrate no signal loss. Biopsy confirmed lymphoma in the adrenal gland.

sequence, a standard of reference is required. Because the spleen does not become steatotic and resides at the level of the adrenal glands, it provides a convenient reference for comparison.

Adrenal-to-spleen ratio =

$$\frac{(adrenal\ opposed\ phase\ SI)/(splenic\ opposed\ phase\ SI)}{(adrenal\ in\ phase\ SI)/(splenic\ in\ phase\ SI)}$$

Some use an adrenal-to-spleen ratio of 0.7 as a cutoff value, with a ratio less than 0.7 indicating adenoma. Similar ratios have been applied using renal or liver parenchyma and muscle, particularly if the patient has undergone splenectomy. Each has a different formula and threshold, but these are available in the literature. Those of us who avoid using a calculator whenever possible are fortunate that some literature suggests that qualitative assessment of signal loss is likely as accurate as quantitative analysis.

COMPUTED TOMOGRAPHY AND MAGNETIC
RESONANCE IMAGING FOR INTRACELLULAR LIPID:
ARE THEY COMPLEMENTARY OR REDUNDANT?
Because unenhanced CT and chemical-shift MRI both evaluate for the presence of intracellular lipid, some have suggested that lipid-poor adenomas that are indeterminate by NCCT criteria are likely to remain indeterminate with MRI. However, data have shown that a small but significant number of adrenal adenomas with an attenuation value that exceeds 10 HU on unenhanced CT can, in fact, be characterized as adenomas by chemical-shift MRI. Utility of MRI is greatest in those lesions with CT attenuation between 10 and 20 HU. If the CT attenuation measurement of a mass is greater than 30 HU, MRI

is unlikely to demonstrate intracellular lipid within the lesion.

MIMICS OF ADRENAL ADENOMA
Rarely, adrenal lesions other than adenoma can contain sufficient amounts of intracellular lipid to be detectable with NCCT or chemical-shift MRI. These include adrenal cortical carcinoma and metastases originating from lipid-rich primary tumors such as clear cell renal cell carcinoma and hepatocellular carcinoma. Fortunately, such lesions are exceedingly rare, and other imaging characteristics (e.g., size, margins, enhancement) often allow characterization as nonadenoma. Pheochromocytoma has also been reported as a potential CT mimic of adrenal adenoma both on unenhanced images and using washout criteria. For these reasons, one should not rely entirely on a single imaging characteristic when attempting to characterize an adrenal mass.

Calcification
Adrenal calcification is not uncommonly detected on CT examinations and has little significance in isolation. Calcification without an associated mass most often results from prior adrenal hemorrhage or granulomatous disease (Fig. 17-22). Because neonatal adrenal hemorrhage often goes undiagnosed, there is unlikely to be a history to corroborate this. Calcification is occasionally seen in adrenal adenoma, particularly when the adenoma is large.

Calcification can also be seen in some malignant adrenal masses (Fig. 17-23). Approximately 30% of adrenal cortical carcinomas and most neuroblastomas contain calcification on CT examinations. Metastases

Normal left adrenal gland

Trace calcification in right
adrenal gland

Figure 17-22   Computed tomographic scan performed for evaluation of potential renal donor shows trace calcification within an otherwise normal-appearing right adrenal gland. The patient has no known history of perinatal hemorrhage, although it is believed to be the most likely cause of this finding.

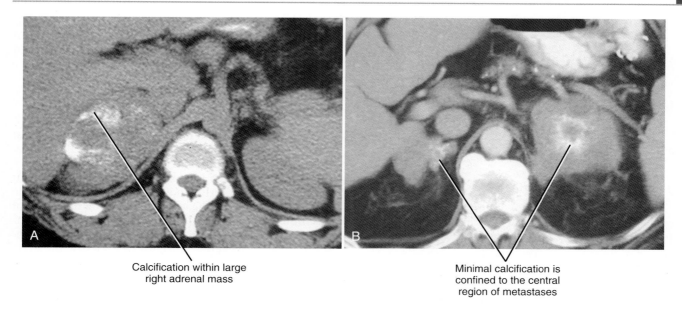

Calcification within large
right adrenal mass

Minimal calcification is
confined to the central
region of metastases

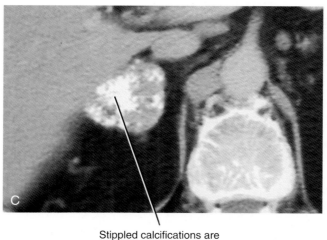

Stippled calcifications are
common in treated lymphoma

Figure 17-23 Calcification in malignant disease of the adrenal gland. **A,** Axial image from a noncontrast-enhanced computed tomographic (CT) examination demonstrates calcification in proven neuroblastoma. **B,** Axial image from a contrast-enhanced CT demonstrates calcification within bilateral adrenal metastases from colon cancer. **C,** Axial image from a contrast-enhanced CT scan demonstrate dense stippled calcifications from treated lymphoma.

from some types of adenocarcinoma (e.g., colon) are occasionally calcified as well. Lymphomatous involvement of the adrenal glands can result in calcification after therapy. Because calcified adrenal metastases and adrenal cortical carcinoma are uncommon, small calcified adrenal glands are more likely to be the sequelae of prior hemorrhage or granulomatous infection.

Calcification can also occur within the wall of a cystic adrenal mass. Mural calcification is reported to be uncommon and usually thin in endothelial cysts, and common and thick in pseudocysts (see Figs. 17-15 and 17-16). Cystic pheochromocytoma can also rarely contain mural calcification. In general, when mural calcification is present, lack of enhancing septa or other soft-tissue elements is a relatively good indicator of benign disease.

Hemorrhage

Adrenal hemorrhage occurs most often but not exclusively in neonates and victims of blunt abdominal trauma. Differentiating hematoma from other adrenal masses on enhanced CT can be challenging in adult trauma victims (Fig. 17-24). Although evidence of injury to nearby organs suggests hematoma, the presence of local trauma does not exclude other causative factors. Performing an unenhanced CT relatively soon after injury can demonstrate the increased attenuation of blood (usually 50-90 HU), although the attenuation value of a hematoma will decrease in the ensuing weeks after trauma.

MRI is also useful for characterizing suspected adrenal hemorrhage. Within the adrenal gland, the very high signal intensity typical of extracellular methemoglobin

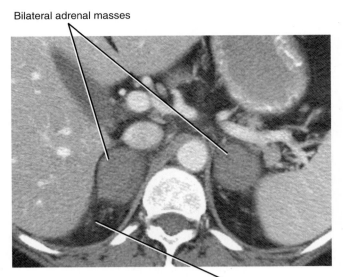

Bilateral adrenal masses

Mild fat stranding near
adrenal gland

Figure 17-24 Axial image from a contrast-enhanced computed to-mographic scan demonstrates bilateral adrenal hematomas in a patient who presented with acute abdominal pain and jaundice. There were no other significant findings. Percutaneous adrenal biopsy revealed only blood, and the lesions decreased in size on subsequent examinations.

hemorrhagic mass is being evaluated with MRI, it is important to include images obtained with and without fat suppression to aid in distinguishing between blood products and fat on T1-weighted images.

Enhancement of the Adrenal Gland

The presence of contrast enhancement within an adrenal lesion is not a reliable indicator of malignancy. Enhancement is expected within adrenal adenomas, some myelolipomas, and unusual lesions, such as cavernous hemangiomas of the adrenal gland (Fig. 17-25). Although the presence of contrast enhancement alone is not a useful discriminator, *patterns* of enhancement are more specific.

Because 10% to 40% of adrenal adenomas contain insufficient lipid to allow definitive characterization using unenhanced CT or MRI, multiple investigations have analyzed the patterns of enhancement and deenhancement or "washout" of adrenal masses in efforts to distinguish adrenal adenomas from malignant neoplasms.

Absolute Enhancement

Most adrenal adenomas enhance with IV contrast media, typically reaching peak enhancement during the arterial phase and rapidly decreasing in attenuation thereafter. During the portal venous phase, *most* adrenal adenomas have a mean attenuation value of 37 HU or less, whereas *most* metastases have an attenuation value of 45 HU or greater. Unfortunately, sufficient overlap exists between adenomas and metastases that the absolute attenuation measurement during the portal phase is not a reliable discriminator.

on T1-weighted images is uncommon except in cases of hemorrhage. Rare exceptions include some metastases from melanoma. Hemorrhage can occur secondary to a variety of adrenal tumors, such as myelolipoma, hemangioma, and pheochromocytoma. When a suspected

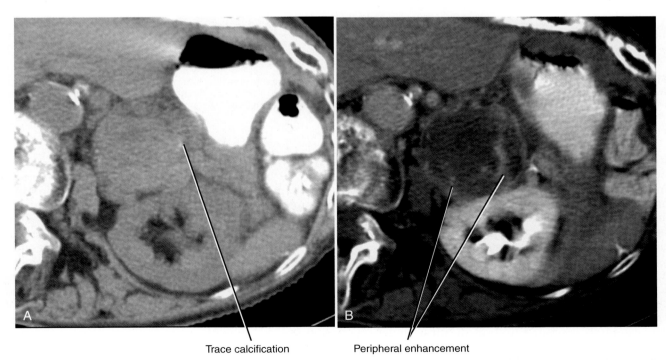

Trace calcification

Peripheral enhancement

Figure 17-25 Adrenal hemangioma on a computed tomographic scan including (A) precontrast and (B) delayed postcontrast images. Diagnosis was confirmed by biopsy, and the lesion has remained stable for 10 years. Progressive filling of the mass with contrast is typical of adrenal hemangiomas.

Adrenal Washout

Once intravenous contrast material has been administered for abdominal CT, adrenal adenomas demonstrate a reliable pattern of enhancement and deenhancement. After an early peak after contrast injection, both lipid-rich and lipid-poor adenomas decrease in attenuation rapidly, whereas most metastases and primary adrenal tumors retain contrast media for a prolonged period. "Washout" protocols based on these observations allow characterization of adrenal masses with high specificity.

ABSOLUTE WASHOUT

Studies performed for the specific purpose of characterizing an adrenal mass begin by obtaining unenhanced CT images. If the mean attenuation value of the adrenal mass is 10 HU or less, the lesion is characterized as an adenoma and no more imaging is performed. If the attenuation measurement is greater than 10 HU, intravenous contrast media is administered and enhanced images are obtained starting 65 seconds after start of injection. The adrenal glands are rescanned after an additional 15-minute delay. The absolute washout percentage is then calculated as follows:

Absolute washout =

$$\frac{Enhanced\ attenuation - Delayed\ attenuation}{Enhanced\ attenuation - Unenhanced\ attenuation} \times 100\%$$

Applying a threshold where a washout of 60% or greater is diagnosed as adenoma yields a specificity of 96% and sensitivity of 88% for adenoma.

RELATIVE WASHOUT

If an adrenal mass is detected after contrast-enhanced CT but before the patient leaves the department, and no precontrast images are available, all is not lost. Relative adrenal washout can be calculated using only initial enhancement images and 15-minute delayed images. The relative washout percentage is calculated as follows:

Relative washout =

$$\frac{Enhanced\ attenuation - Delayed\ attenuation}{Enhanced\ attenuation} \times 100\%$$

Applying a threshold of 40% or greater yields a specificity of 100% and sensitivity of 96% in the literature. Table 17-4 provides a summary of the imaging findings useful in characterizing adrenal masses discussed in the preceding section.

■ COLLISION TUMORS

The term *collision tumor* describes the presence of two or more abnormal tissue types within a single adrenal gland. The name applies regardless of whether the tissue types are all benign, all malignant, or a combination of benign and malignant. The diagnosis of collision tumor may be suggested when different

Table 17-4   Imaging Characteristics of Adrenal Masses on Computed Tomography

Finding	Most Likely Diagnosis
Diffuse enlargement	Favors adrenal hyperplasia
Mass < 4 cm	Probably adenoma unless known malignant neoplasm elsewhere
Mass > 4 cm	High probability of malignancy
Cystic with no enhancement	Adrenal cyst/pseudocyst
Cystic with enhancing components	Necrotic cortical carcinoma, metastasis, or cystic pheochromocytoma
Macroscopic fat	Myelolipoma
Intracellular lipid (<10 HU)	Adenoma
Calcification	Peripheral in cystic mass; calcified cyst or old hematoma Adreniform shape; granulomatous disease or old hemorrhage likely Large solid mass; carcinoma, metastatic adenocarcinoma, hemangioma
High attenuation (>50 HU)	Hematoma
Rapid washout	Adenoma (some pheochromocytomas)
Delayed persistent enhancement	Neoplasm other than adenoma

portions of an adrenal lesion, or two separate adrenal masses within the same gland, have different imaging characteristics on CT or MR images (Fig. 17-26). For example, if a clearly demarcated portion of an adrenal mass retains contrast on delayed enhanced CT or MR images whereas the remainder of the mass washes out, the possibility of a collision tumor should be suggested. Likewise, if a well-defined area within an adrenal mass fails to lose signal on opposed-phase MR images despite copious intracellular lipid in the remainder of the lesion, collision tumor should be suspected. Unfortunately, benign tumors such as adenomas and myelolipomas are not always homogeneous in imaging appearance, creating some overlap with collision tumors.

The coexistence of a malignant tumor with benign tissue such as adenoma can lead to sampling error during biopsy. Therefore, when performing percutaneous biopsy of an abnormal adrenal gland, it is critical to consult all relevant imaging studies in advance and to ensure that the most concerning area is sampled.

Pearl: When planning percutaneous biopsy of the adrenal gland, keep in mind that a heterogeneous adrenal mass may contain more than one tumor type. Biopsy of the most suspicious region or of each region with different imaging characteristics increases sensitivity of the biopsy.

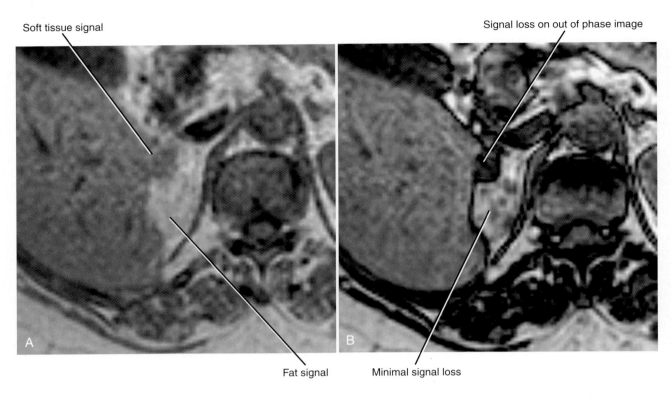

Soft tissue signal

Signal loss on out of phase image

Fat signal

Minimal signal loss

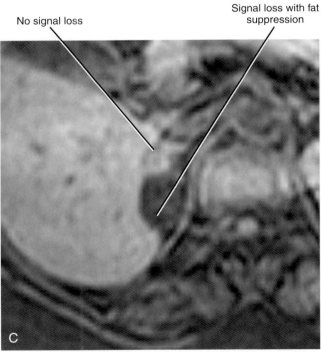

No signal loss

Signal loss with fat suppression

Figure 17-26 Presumed collision tumor on magnetic resonance imaging. Axial T1-weighted images of the right adrenal gland performed **(A)** in phase and **(B)** out of phase demonstrate a region of uniform signal loss within an adrenal mass on out-of-phase images typical of adenoma. **C,** Frequency-selective fat suppression proves fat within the larger component, typical of myelolipoma.

■ IMAGING EVALUATION FOR ABNORMAL ADRENAL FUNCTION

Although most adrenal lesions are asymptomatic, adrenal insufficiency or clinical evidence of excessive hormone production are occasional indications for adrenal imaging. Because the size and orientation of the adrenal glands is so variable, and because many of the disease process that alter function affect the glands diffusely, it is not surprising that cross-sectional imaging is often unfruitful. Occasionally, however, imaging findings play a significant role in management, particularly when unilateral adrenalectomy is contemplated.

Adrenal Insufficiency

Although some divide the causes of adrenal insufficiency into primary, secondary, and tertiary causes, it is probably more useful for the radiologist to consider both secondary and tertiary causes as a single group.

Primary Adrenal Insufficiency

Primary adrenal insufficiency, or *Addison's disease,* encompasses processes that directly damage adrenal tissue, resulting in decreased hormone production. Inflammatory and infectious disease processes that involve the adrenal glands are much more likely to result in adrenal insufficiency than metastatic disease. By the time infection results in a diagnosis of adrenal insufficiency, the most common imaging finding is adrenal calcification.

Autoimmune adrenalitis is probably the most common cause of Addison's disease in developed countries. Because of a gradual onset of vague clinical symptoms, it is rarely imaged in its early stages. More commonly, atrophic glands are identified only after irreparable damage has been done. Replacement hormone therapy is the only treatment. Calcification with or without nodularity suggests prior granulomatous infection or hemorrhage of the adrenal glands (Fig. 17-27).

Secondary Adrenal Insufficiency

Because adrenal gland function is regulated through multiple complex physiologic pathways, insufficiency can result from extraadrenal abnormalities. When this occurs it is called *secondary adrenal insufficiency.* Lesions that affect pituitary gland function (e.g., pituitary adenoma, craniopharyngioma, hemorrhage, infarction, or trauma) are among the most common causes of secondary adrenal insufficiency. Adrenal atrophy in response to long-term exogenous steroid use is another cause. In patients with secondary adrenal insufficiency, the adrenal glands may appear normal or atrophic on imaging examinations. Although the diagnosis of secondary adrenal insufficiency is usually made on the basis of a thorough endocrine evaluation, imaging plays a key role in detecting pituitary abnormalities.

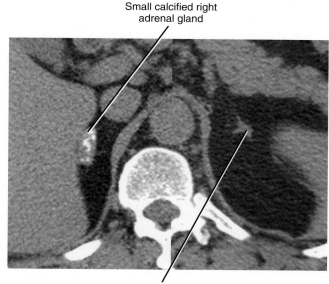

Small calcified right adrenal gland

Small left adrenal gland with no calcification

Figure 17-27 Axial noncontrast-enhanced computed tomographic image of the adrenal glands in a patient with idiopathic adrenal insufficiency. Although primary or secondary adrenal insufficiency can result in the diminutive appearance of the left gland, the calcifications on the right side suggest prior insult, such as from granulomatous disease.

Hyperfunctioning Lesions of the Adrenal Gland

Hyperfunctioning lesions of the adrenal gland can be divided into those arising from the adrenal cortex and those arising from the adrenal medulla. Hyperfunctioning masses usually present with a distinct clinical pattern, and imaging serves to identify the source of excess hormone production. Perhaps the most important point to remember is that hyperfunctioning adrenal masses are often small when detected, particularly aldosteronomas. In most cases, surgical resection of the offending lesion is curative.

Pearl: When searching for a hyperfunctioning adrenal mass, remember that they are often quite small. Identification of even a small nodule can facilitate curative resection.

Hyperfunctioning Lesions of the Adrenal Cortex

Hyperfunctioning lesions of the adrenal cortex produce aldosterone, glucocorticoids, or androgens. Primary hyperaldosteronism can result from a hyperfunctioning adrenal adenoma, adrenal hyperplasia (diffuse or nodular), or adrenal carcinoma. When caused by an adrenal adenoma, it is called *Conn syndrome;* otherwise, primary hyperaldosteronism is the preferred term. Because aldosterone promotes sodium resorption and potassium secretion, the combination of hypernatremia and hypokalemic alkalosis suggests hyperaldosteronism. Imaging is performed to look for an adrenal adenoma. These are often small nodules; lesions smaller than 1 cm may be clinically significant, so careful inspection of the gland is critical (Fig. 17-28). If a lesion cannot be identified, selective transcatheter sampling of the adrenal veins can be performed in the interventional suite to lateralize the source of excess aldosterone production.

Cushing syndrome describes a clinical presentation of central obesity, hypertension, hirsutism, amenorrhea, and abdominal striae caused by increased levels of cortisol. Causes include adrenal hyperplasia, adrenal adenoma, adrenal carcinoma, or administration of exogenous corticosteroids. When this syndrome is caused by adrenal hyperplasia, it is called *Cushing disease.* Imaging is performed to identify a potentially resectable lesion. Adenomas, when present, typically range in size from 2 to 5 cm and are readily identified by CT or MRI. More often, bilateral diffuse smooth or nodular hyperplasia of the adrenal glands is confirmed. Adrenalectomy is performed for focal lesions; therefore, differentiation between adenoma and the rare small adrenal cortical carcinoma is usually not important before surgery.

Excessive production of androgens by an adrenal mass is one cause of virilization in female individuals. Other causes include enzymatic defects resulting in adrenal hyperplasia and ovarian tumors. When an adrenal tumor is responsible, the mass is often malignant. Although there is little information available regarding these rare tumors, reported adenomas range from 2 to 6 cm in diameter, whereas carcinomas are typically much larger.

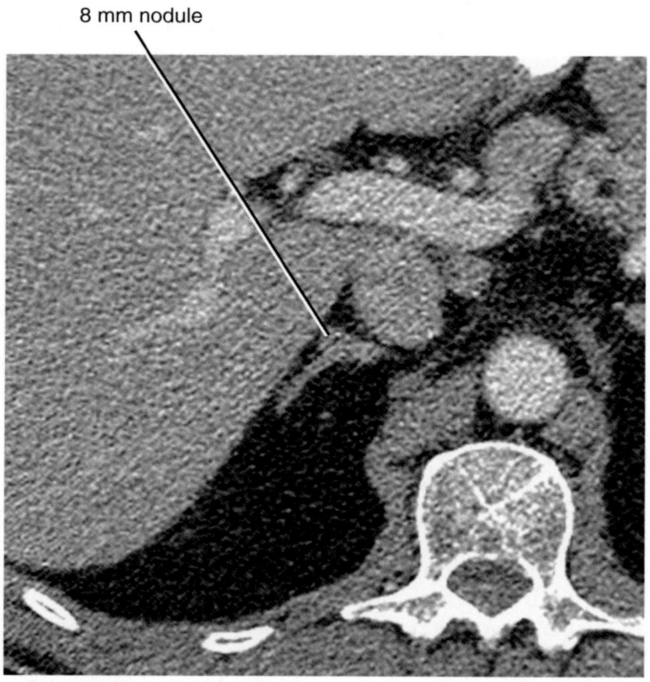

8 mm nodule

Figure 17-28 Axial image from a contrast-enhanced computed tomographic scan demonstrates a small right adrenal nodule in a patient with hyperaldosteronism. An aldosteronoma was removed surgically with clinical resolution.

Hyperfunctioning Lesions of the Adrenal Medulla: Pheochromocytoma

Pheochromocytomas are tumors of the adrenal medulla that produce an excess of catecholamines, predominantly epinephrine. If a similar tumor occurs outside the adrenal gland, it is called a *paraganglioma.* Patients usually present after experiencing episodes of headaches, palpitations, and excessive sweating that occur during each "crisis," or surge of catecholamine release. Additional symptoms include tremors, nausea and vomiting, chest or abdominal pain, and visual disturbances. Physical examination reveals hypertension and occasionally postural hypotension. A 24-hour urine sample demonstrates increased levels of VMA.

Approximately 10% of cases are extraadrenal paragangliomas, 10% are bilateral, and 25% are associated with hereditary syndromes. Although about 10% of adrenal pheochromocytomas are malignant, the number is greater with extraadrenal paragangliomas (40%). Notably, not all patients with pheochromocytoma are symptomatic. Therefore, pheochromocytoma should remain in the differential diagnosis for an incidentally discovered adrenal mass.

In symptomatic patients, the goal of imaging is to identify an adrenal or extraadrenal mass to confirm the diagnosis already suspected based on clinical and laboratory findings. Therefore, it is of great utility to be familiar with sites of extraadrenal paragangliomas to assist in diagnosis when an adrenal mass is absent. Nearly 98% of extraadrenal paragangliomas occur in the abdomen and pelvis, and the most common locations are listed in Box 17-1.

On CT, pheochromocytomas are usually 3 to 5 cm in diameter and frequently contain heterogeneous material, a combination of catecholamine, necrosis, and hemorrhage. Because of the low attenuation of lipid material within these tumors, attenuation values of less than 10 HU have been reported in 10% to 20% of cases (Fig. 17-29). Similar reports exist of rapid washout of enhancement with pheochromocytoma. Although these could result in misdiagnosis of a pheochromocytoma as an adenoma, combined infrequency of the tumor and high prevalence of clinical signs or symptoms in patients with pheochromocytoma make this a rare occurrence.

Pitfall: Because the catecholamines contained within pheochromocytomas are lipid, attenuation measurements of pheochromocytomas can overlap those of adenomas. Other associated imaging findings (thick wall) and clinical information are essential for accurate characterization.

BOX 17-1   Most Common Locations for Extraadrenal Paragangliomas

Urinary bladder (usually near the base)
Organ of Zuckerkandl (near aortic bifurcation)
Carotid and vagal bodies in the neck
Mediastinum including within the pericardium

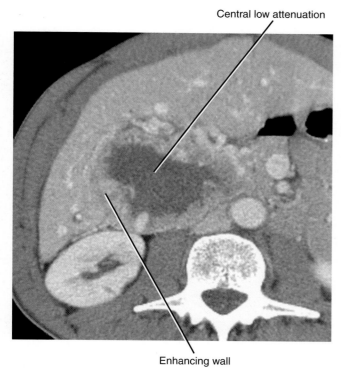

Central low attenuation

Enhancing wall

Figure 17-29 Axial image from a contrast-enhanced computed tomographic scan demonstrates low attenuation within a surgically proven pheochromocytoma. Despite fluid attenuation within the central region, overall lesion heterogeneity and large size are different from a typical adenoma.

Table 17-5 Hyperfunctioning Lesions of the Adrenal Gland

Clinical Syndrome	Adrenal Lesion (in Order of Incidence)	Size of Adrenal Nodule (When Present)
Cortex		
Primary Hyperaldosteronism		
Hypertension Hypernatremia Hypokalemia	Adenoma Hyperplasia Carcinoma	Small (<1 cm) when benign
Cushing Syndrome		2-5 cm
Hypertension Hirsutism Obesity	Hyperplasia Adenoma Carcinoma	
Virilization		Often >6 cm
Clitoromegaly Hirsutism	Carcinoma Adenoma	
Feminization		2-9 cm
Gynecomastia	Carcinoma Adenoma	
Medulla		
Pheochromocytoma		>3 cm
Hypertension Flushing	Benign (90%) Malignant (10%)	

The use of intravenous contrast media in patients with known or suspected pheochromocytoma merits mention. Sporadic increases in circulating catecholamines were reported using ionic contrast media several decades ago. As a result, some radiologists avoid iodinated contrast media in these patients and administer medications for adrenergic blockade when contrast administration is necessary for CT. More recently, a repeat of the study using nonionic contrast media demonstrated no measurable increase in catecholamines. Therefore, we do not currently avoid the intravenous use of nonionic contrast media in our patients with suspected pheochromocytoma.

The MRI appearance of pheochromocytoma is somewhat characteristic in approximately two-thirds of patients. Although the signal on T1-weighted images is variable, T2-weighted images usually show high signal intensity. Similar high signal intensity on T2-weighted images is often seen in extraadrenal paragangliomas and metastases (see Fig. 17-4). Although pheochromocytomas were originally described as classically "light-bulb" bright on T2-weighted MR images, we have not found this sign to be a highly specific discriminator when using state-of-the art MRI techniques.

Scintigraphy using metaiodobenzylguanidine (MIBG) is useful for characterization and localization of masses in patients suspected of having pheochromocytoma or extraadrenal paraganglioma (see Fig. 17-4). Marked uptake of the radiotracer is seen in approximately 90% of tumors. Because metastatic deposits from malignant pheochromocytoma share a similar avidity, MIBG is also useful for detecting areas of metastatic disease. Greater doses of I-131 MIBG can also be used to treat metastatic pheochromocytoma, with partial remissions reported in approximately 50% of patients. Table 17-5 summarizes the most common hyperfunctioning lesions of the adrenal gland.

Suggested Readings

Al-Hawary MM, Francis IR, Korobkin M: Non-invasive evaluation of the incidentally detected indeterminate adrenal mass, *Best Pract Res Clin Endocrinol Metab* 19(2):277-292, 2005.

Barzon L, Boscaro M: Diagnosis and management of adrenal incidentalomas, *J Urol* 163:398-407, 2000.

Blake MA, Kalra MK, Maher MM et al: Pheochromocytoma: an imaging chameleon, *Radiographics* 24:S87-S99, 2004.

Blake MA, Krishnamoorthy SK, Boland GW et al: Low-density pheochromocytoma on CT: a mimicker of adrenal adenoma, *Am J Roentgenol* 181(6):1663-1668, 2003.

Boland GWL, Lee MJ, Gazelle GS et al: Characterization of adrenal masses using unenhanced CT: an analysis of the CT literature, *Am J Roentgenol* 171:201-204, 1998.

Chong S, Lee KS, Kim HY et al: Integrated PET-CT for the characterization of adrenal gland lesions in cancer patients: diagnostic efficacy and interpretation pitfalls, *RadioGraphics* 26:1811-1826, 2006.

Dluhy RG: Pheochromocytoma—death of an axiom, *New Engl J Med* 346:1486-1488, 2002.

Dunnick NR, Korobkin M: Imaging of adrenal incidentalomas: current status, *Am J Roentgenol* 179:559-568, 2002.

Elsayes KM, Narra VR, Leyendecker JR et al: MRI of adrenal and extraadrenal pheochromocytoma, *Am J Roentgenol* 184:860-867, 2005.

Fujiyoshi F, Nakajo M, Fukukura Y et al: Characterization of adrenal tumors by chemical shift fast low-angle shot MR imaging: comparison of four methods of quantitative evaluation, *Am J Roentgenol* 180:1649-1657, 2003.

Haider MA, Ghai S, Jhaveri K et al: Chemical shift MR imaging of hyperattenuating (>10 HU) adrenal masses: does it still have a role? *Radiology* 231:711-716, 2004.

Israel GM, Korobkin M, Wang C et al: Comparison of unenhanced CT and chemical shift MRI in evaluating lipid-rich adrenal adenomas, *Am J Roentgenol* 183:215-219, 2004.

Kalra MK, Blake MA, Boland GW et al: CT features of adrenal pheochromocytomas: attenuation value and loss of contrast enhancement, *Radiology* 236(3):1112-1113, 2005.

McNicholas MMJ, Lee MJ, Mayo-Smith WW et al: An imaging algorithm for the differential diagnosis of adrenal adenomas and metastases, *Am J Roentgenol* 165:1453-1459, 1995.

Mitchell DG, Crovello M, Matteucci T et al: Benign adrenocortical masses: diagnosis with chemical shift MR imaging, *Radiology* 185:345-351, 1992.

Motta-Ramirez GA, Remer EM, Herts BR et al: Comparison of CT findings in symptomatic and incidentally discovered pheochromocytomas, *Am J Roentgenol* 185(3):684-688, 2005.

Mukherjee JJ, Peppercorn PD, Reznek RH et al: Pheochromocytoma: effect of nonionic contrast medium in CT on circulating catecholamine levels, *Radiology* 202(1):227-231, 1997.

Oelkers W: Adrenal insufficiency, *N Engl J Med* 335:1206-1212, 1996.

Park BK, Kim CK, Kim B et al: Comparison of delayed enhanced CT and chemical shift MR for evaluating hyperattenuating incidental adrenal masses, *Radiology* 243:760-765, 2007.

Paulsen SD, Nghiem HV, Korobkin M et al: Changing role of imaging-guided percutaneous biopsy of adrenal masses: evaluation of 50 adrenal biopsies, *Am J Roentgenol* 182:1033-1037, 2004.

Pena CS, Boland GW, Hahn PF et al: Characterization of indeterminate (lipid poor) adrenal masses: use of washout characteristics at contrast-enhanced CT, *Radiology* 217:798-802, 2000.

Pender SM, Boland GW, Lee MJ: The incidental nonhyperfunctioning adrenal mass: an imaging algorithm for characterization, *Clin Radiol* 53:796-804, 1998.

Raisanen J, Shapiro B, Glazer GM et al: Plasma catecholamines in pheochromocytoma: effect of urographic contrast media, *Am J Roentgenol* 143(1): 43-46, 1984.

Shapiro B, Copp JE, Sisson JC et al: Iodine-131 metaiodobenzylguanidine for the locating of suspected pheochromocytoma: experience in 400 cases, *J Nucl Med* 26(6):576-585, 1985.

Szolar DH, Korobkin M, Reittner P et al: Adrenocortical carcinomas and adrenal pheochromocytomas: mass and enhancement loss evaluation at delayed contrast-enhanced CT, *Radiology* 234(2):479-485, 2005.

Welch RJ, Sheedy PF, Stephens DH et al: Percutaneous adrenal biopsy: review of a 10-year experience, *Radiology* 193:341-344, 1994.

Yun M, Kim W, Alnafisi H et al: ^{18}F-FDG PET in characterizing adrenal lesions detected on CT or MRI, *J Nucl Med* 42:1795-1799, 2001.

CHAPTER 18

Kidneys

Neal C. Dalrymple

■ CLINICAL CONSIDERATIONS

The kidneys play a central role in homeostasis. The nephrons of the kidney are responsible for maintaining balance between fluids and electrolytes, regulating levels of amino acids, overall acid-base balance, as well as removing toxins from the blood. The kidney also has endocrine functions, helping to control blood pressure, bone mineralization, and erythrocyte production. Although each kidney is about the size of a fist, the approximately one million nephrons per kidney require nearly 20% of the total cardiac output to perform this multitude of functions.

Laboratory Assessment of Renal Function

Serum Creatinine

Despite the complexity of renal physiology, many attempt to assess renal function with a simple quantitative measure, the serum creatinine. Creatinine is a breakdown product of creatine, found within muscle. Most serum creatinine is excreted in the urine; therefore, if renal function is compromised, levels of creatinine in the serum increase.

Serum creatinine, however, is dependent not only on its disposal but also its production. Because production of creatinine is affected by sex, age, muscle mass, protein intake, and liver function, the serum creatinine can be an inaccurate predictor of renal function, particularly in those at the extremes of age and body weight.

Perhaps of even greater importance, serum creatinine is not a sensitive test for minor insults to the kidney in otherwise healthy individuals. A healthy individual who donates a kidney is likely to maintain a normal serum creatinine despite the loss of 50% of parenchymal tissue. However, this individual is more likely to show a decline in renal function from an additional insult. This illustrates the amount of reserve function that must be compromised before renal injury can be detected with a serum creatinine level. Thus, any upward trend in the serum creatinine value should be viewed with concern when considering the administration of potentially nephrotoxic or renally excreted intravenous contrast media.

Pearl: *Any upward trend in serum creatinine value should be viewed with concern because it implies renal reserve function has already been affected.*

Renal function is better evaluated by measured creatinine clearance, which takes into account not only the amount of creatinine in the blood but also the amount of creatinine within a specified volume of urine over a given period.

Estimated Creatinine Clearance and Glomerular Filtration Rate

Estimated creatinine clearance may be calculated using serum creatinine with adjustments made for sex, age, and body weight. Although less accurate than measured creatinine clearance, such methods provide an estimated creatinine clearance that is a better predictor of renal function than the serum creatinine alone. Several formulas are available for this calculation, and calculators and on-line sites are available to simplify the calculations. One of the most commonly used (and least complicated) equations is shown in Box 18-1.

The Modification of Diet in Renal Disease (MDRD) is another method for estimating renal function that yields a value often called *estimated glomerular filtration rate (eGFR)*. The MDRD calculation is more complicated than calculating creatinine clearance (taking into account body surface area, sex, and race) but is thought to be more accurate than estimated creatinine clearance, particularly among the elderly and obese. Many clinical laboratories now provide computer-generated calculations of estimated creatinine clearance or eGFR using patient data in the medical information system.

■ RENAL ANATOMY

Renal Parenchyma

The kidneys can be divided into three main regions from cranial to caudal. Each end of the kidney is commonly called a *pole*. The portion of the kidney between the poles is called the *interpolar region* and contains the renal hilum (Fig. 18-1).

On axial sections, the polar regions of the kidney typically form a closed circle or "donut" shape, with the "hole" formed by renal sinus fat. The anteromedial

BOX 18-1   Cockroft and Gault Equation for Calculating Estimated Creatinine Clearance

$$\text{Creatinine clearance} = \frac{(140 - \text{age}) \times \text{weight (kg)}}{72 \times \text{serum creatinine (mg/dL)}}$$

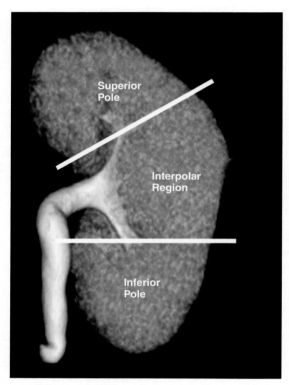

Figure 18-1 Annotated three-dimensional volume rendering of the left kidney acquired using a combined nephrographic phase and excretory phase during computed tomographic urography demonstrates regional anatomy of the kidney.

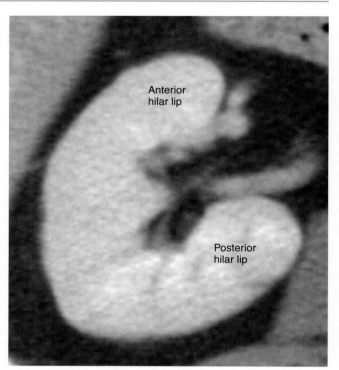

Figure 18-2 Annotated axial image of the right kidney from a contrast-enhanced computed tomographic scan demonstrates hilar anatomy of the kidney.

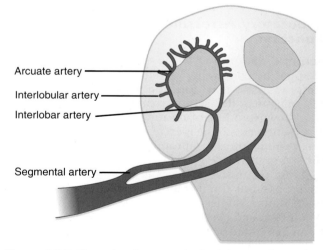

Figure 18-3 Illustration demonstrating basic intrarenal arterial anatomy.

aspect of the interpolar region is interrupted by the renal hilum to make a C shape. In this region, the anterior and posterior *hilar lip* is identified (Fig. 18-2). In most kidneys, the renal hilum faces more anteromedial in the upper half of the kidney and more directly medial in the lower half.

The solid renal parenchyma consists of the peripheral renal cortex and more central renal medulla. The nephrons within the cortex comprise some of the most highly perfused parenchymal tissue in the body. More tenuous vascular supply to the renal medulla makes it more susceptible to ischemia. Each segmental branch of the renal artery divides into multiple interlobar arteries that course along the periphery of the medullary pyramids and causes small interlobular branches (Fig. 18-3). Because the interlobular arteries form an arch overlying the pyramid, they are called the *arcuate arteries.* These terminal branches have no collateral circulation.

Renal Collecting System

Urine that is concentrated in the renal papilla is subsequently excreted into a lumen lined with transitional epithelium. The small portion of the lumen surrounding the papilla is called the *calyx.* The shape of the calyx is formed by the impression of the renal papilla. Increasing pressure within the lumen initially distends the fornices (acutely angled portions of the calyx along the sides of the papillae), whereas the central portion of the papillary

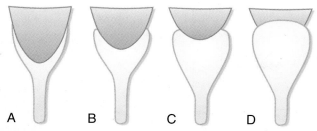

Figure 18-4 Illustration demonstrating the relation between the renal papilla and calyx. The normal appearance of the calyx is created by the impression of the renal papilla. **A,** Tips of the fornices are sharply defined. **B,** Mild hydronephrosis results in rounding of the fornices with mild shortening of the papillary impression. **C,** More severe hydronephrosis results in more pronounced shortening of the papilla. **D,** If pressure on the papilla persists, the ischemic papilla undergoes necrosis, allowing the calyx to protrude outward toward the cortex.

impression is preserved. Chronic obstruction, however, results in damage to the papilla, evident in the "clubbed" calyx of papillary necrosis (Fig. 18-4).

A *simple calyx* receives urine from a single papilla; a *compound calyx* receives urine from multiple papillae (Fig. 18-5). Urine from the calyces flows to the renal sinus via tributaries called *infundibula*. Occasionally, a papilla will communicate directly with an infundibulum or the renal pelvis and is considered to be an *aberrant papilla*. Unlike other filling defects within the renal collecting system (e.g., tumor, stone, clot), an aberrant papilla usually has a small fornix around it, seen as a halo on conventional urography (Fig. 18-6). However, sometimes ureteroscopy is required to confirm the diagnosis in patients with hematuria.

Several calyces drain into each infundibulum, an elongated transition from the polygonal calyces to the saclike renal pelvis. The renal pelvis then tapers like a funnel to join the ureter. The region where the renal pelvis joins the ureter is called the *ureteropelvic junction (UPJ)*.

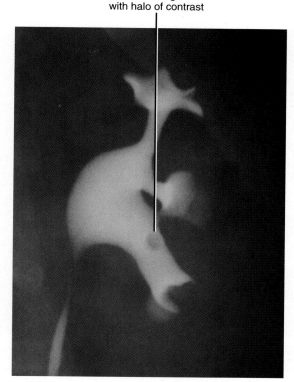

Rounded filling defect with halo of contrast

Figure 18-6 Frontal image of the left kidney from an intravenous urogram demonstrating an aberrant renal papilla in the lower pole infundibulum.

If the renal pelvis is entirely within the confines of the renal sinus, it is considered intrarenal. If the renal pelvis extends out of the renal sinus, it is considered to be an *extrarenal pelvis* (Fig. 18-7). Because an extrarenal pelvis is not confined by the renal parenchyma, there is a tendency for it to expand. Although this dilatation of the renal pelvis may occasionally mimic hydronephrosis, delicate and sharply defined calyces and thin infundibula can be used to differentiate an extrarenal pelvis from obstruction.

Pitfall: An extrarenal pelvis may be mistaken for hydronephrosis. The calyces, however, will have a normal appearance with an unobstructed extrarenal pelvis but will be dilated in cases of urinary obstruction.

Congenital Variants of Renal Anatomy

Abnormalities of Number

Unilateral *renal agenesis* occurs in approximately 1 in 1000 individuals with minimal impact on health, although it is sometimes associated with other congenital anomalies of the genitourinary tract and musculoskeletal system. Enlargement of a congenitally unilateral kidney is typical and presumed to be compensatory.

Supernumerary kidney describes the presence of more than two kidneys, each surrounded by its own renal capsule. In some cases, two separate kidneys drain into

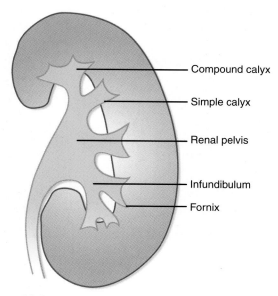

Compound calyx

Simple calyx

Renal pelvis

Infundibulum

Fornix

Figure 18-5 Illustration demonstrating the anatomy of the renal collecting system.

Sac-like renal pelvis is outside
the confines of the renal sinus

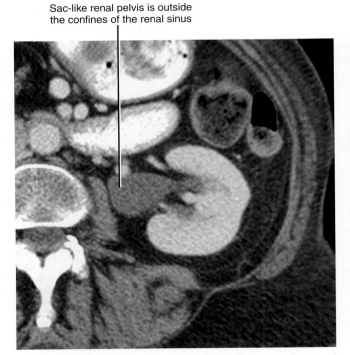

Figure 18-7 Axial image of the left kidney from a contrast-enhanced computed tomographic scan demonstrates an extrarenal pelvis. The ureter and calyces were not dilated (not shown), helping to differentiate this anatomic variant from obstruction.

Junctional cortical line

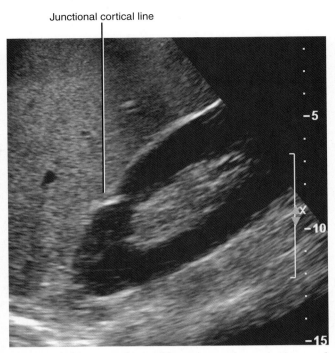

Figure 18-8 Junctional cortical line seen on a long-axis ultrasound image of the right kidney.

a bifid renal pelvis, ultimately drained by a common ureter. In other cases, each renal unit has its own ureter. Supernumerary kidneys are quite rare and have been associated with aortic coarctation, vaginal atresia, and urethral duplications.

Abnormalities of Lobation

As the lobules of metanephric blastema coalesce to form each kidney, they do not always result in a smooth, uniform band of cortex. A *junctional cortical line* is a common septum of capsule typically seen on ultrasound as an echogenic line at the site of fusion between the superior pole and middle third of the kidney (Fig. 18-8). When multiple clefts in the renal cortex are present throughout the kidney, it is described as *fetal lobulation*. Fetal lobulation is best differentiated from renal scars during the corticomedullary phase of enhancement on computed tomography (CT) or magnetic resonance imaging (MRI) because cortex can be followed into the indentation that occurs between calyces (Fig. 18-9). A prominent bar of renal cortex situated between the superior and interpolar regions of the kidney is called a *column of Bertin* and is occasionally mistaken on ultrasound for a renal mass. Normal parenchymal enhancement on CT or MRI allows definitive characterization.

Renal Ectopia

The upper pelvis is the most common ectopic location for the kidney; most cases are also associated with abnormalities of rotation. Extraaortic origin of the renal arteries and accessory renal arteries are common. When

Focal bulge could be mistaken
for a mass on sonography

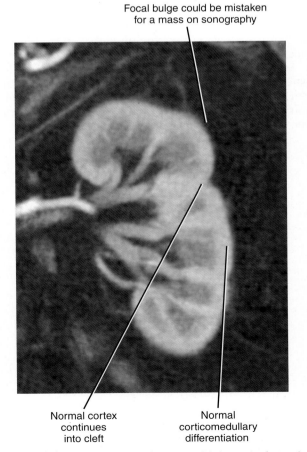

Normal cortex
continues
into cleft

Normal
corticomedullary
differentiation

Figure 18-9 Coronal computed tomographic image in the corticomedullary phase shows normal corticomedullary differentiation along the lobulated contour, consistent with fetal lobulation.

both kidneys are on the same side *crossed ectopia* is present, because the ureter from one kidney must cross the midline to insert into the bladder (Fig. 18-10). Crossed ectopia can be either fused or unfused. When fused, the condition is described as *crossed fused ectopia*. The fused kidneys can have a variety of orientations, including side by side, in-line, or perpendicular. Thoracic kidneys are the least common form of renal ectopia.

Abnormalities of Fusion

Horseshoe kidneys result from midline fusion of the kidneys, typically at the level of the origin of the inferior mesenteric artery. The isthmus connecting the kidneys is variable, ranging from normal renal cortex to a thin fibrous band. Blood supply is variable and often includes extraaortic and multiple vessel origins. The axes of the renal moeities are abnormal with the inferior "poles" angled medially. Prominent extrarenal pelves are typically positioned anteriorly (Fig. 18-11). *Pancake kidney* describes a more severe fusion anomaly with a single, flat kidney positioned low in the pelvis with an anterior collecting system drained by either one or two ureters.

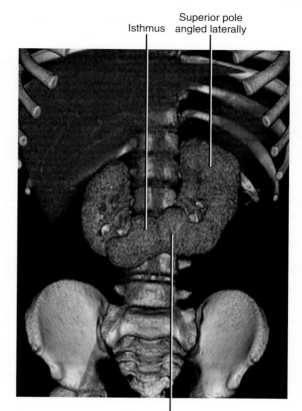

Isthmus
Superior pole
angled laterally

Inferior pole angled
medially toward isthmus

Figure 18-11 Three-dimensional volume rendering from contrast-enhanced multidetector computed tomography examination of the kidneys demonstrates typical orientation of a horseshoe kidney.

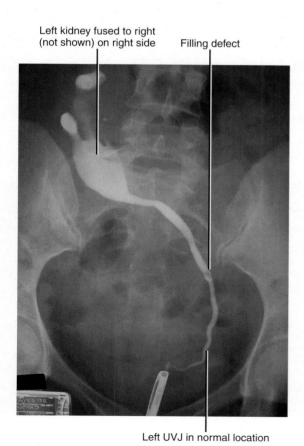

Left kidney fused to right
(not shown) on right side

Filling defect

Left UVJ in normal location

Figure 18-10 Crossed ectopia on intravenous pyelogram. The patient had right flank pain but had a solitary calcification in the left pelvis on plain radiograph (not shown). Retrograde urogram shows a calculus in the left ureter. Right-sided pain was related to crossed renal ectopia.

Ureteral Duplication

Duplication of the urinary tract is discussed in detail in Chapter 19. Duplication affects the axial appearance of the kidneys by dividing the renal sinus into superior and inferior components, separated by a circumferential band of cortex in the central region (Fig. 18-12).

Preprocedure Anatomic Considerations

Evaluation of the Living Renal Donor

Living renal donor allografts account for more than half of the transplanted kidneys in the United States. Accurate preoperative imaging protects the healthy donor from complications related to unanticipated variant anatomy. Literature supports the use of either multidetector computed tomography (MDCT) or MRI in donor evaluation. A potential benefit of MRI is the lack of exposure to ionizing radiation, although unenhanced CT would still be required to detect stones (the presence of stones increases the donor's risk for renal insufficiency later in life and could disqualify them as a donor candidate).

Imaging must provide detailed images of the renal parenchyma and a survey of arterial, venous, and ureteral anatomy. Table 18-1 provides a quick guide itemizing key imaging findings in the potential renal donor.

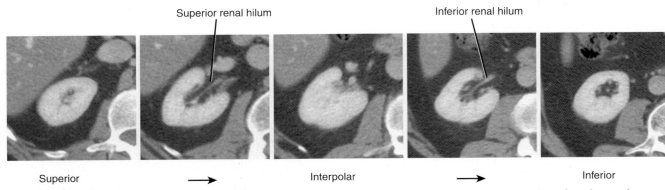

Superior renal hilum   Inferior renal hilum

Superior   →   Interpolar   →   Inferior

Figure 18-12 Axial sections of the right kidney from contrast-enhanced computed tomography demonstrate a bar of renal parenchyma separating renal hila in the superior and inferior poles, consistent with duplication.

Table 18-1   Imaging the Living Renal Donor

Inspected Areas	Comments
Stones	Always include unenhanced computed tomographic images to look for renal stones.
Renal arteries	Look carefully for accessory arteries at upper and lower poles (Fig. 18-13). Note diameter of arteries because small accessory arteries may be sacrificed in many cases. Note distance from origin to the first arterial division (Fig. 18-14). Identify abnormal course of main or accessory right renal artery anterior rather than posterior to inferior vena cava (Fig. 18-15).
Left renal vein	Look for retroaortic or circumaortic left renal vein. Note that retroaortic components are usually near the inferior poles (Fig. 18-16). Anterior components of circumaortic vein can be small. Note large lumbar veins (Fig. 18-17). Note multiple or large gonadal veins.
Right renal vein	Note number of veins by inspecting inferior vena cava along entire length of kidney.
Ureters	Look for duplication, large extrarenal pelvis.

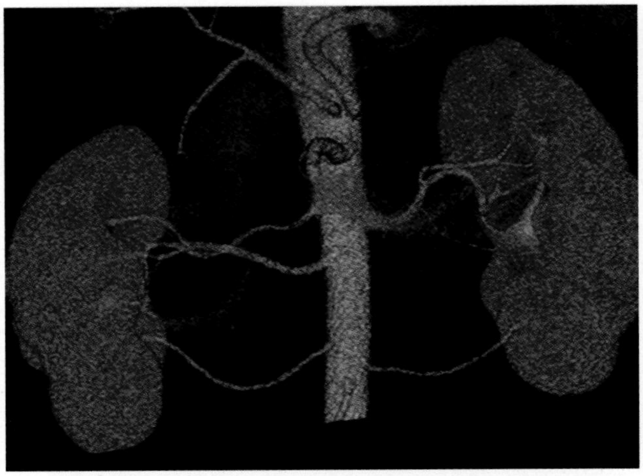

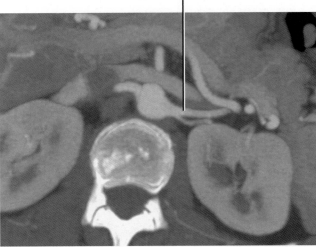

Figure 18-13 Volume rendering from a computed tomographic scan of the kidneys shows bilateral supernumerary renal arteries (three on right, two on left). Note origin of inferior accessories near inferior poles on each side.

First arterial branching
only 9 mm from aorta

Figure 18-14 Axial maximum intensity projection image from the arterial phase of a contrast-enhanced computed tomographic scan from a prospective renal donor demonstrates early prehilar branching of the left renal artery. In this case, the right kidney had more favorable anatomy for laparoscopic donor nephrectomy.

Crossing Vessels in Ureteropelvic Junction Obstruction

Conventional surgery for congenital UPJ obstruction involves an open pyeloplasty, in which some tissue is removed from the wall of the saclike renal pelvis to form a more tapered, efficient, funnel-shaped renal pelvis. Some forms of congenital UPJ obstruction are now treated with transureteroscopic endopyelotomy in which an incision is made from within the ureter using a ureteroscope. Because the fascia of the retroperitoneum prevents significant extravasation, the incision usually heals to form a larger lumen. If, however, a vessel crosses the UPJ at the level of obstruction, a blind incision made from the inside of the ureteral lumen can result in severe hemorrhage. Made

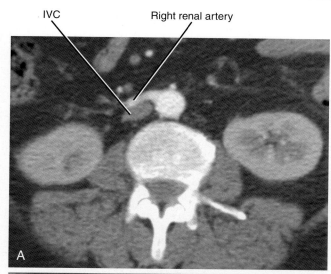

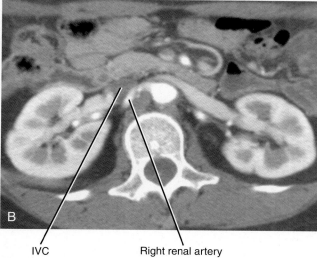

Figure 18-15 Relation between the right renal artery and the inferior vena cava (IVC). **A,** Axial image from contrast-enhanced computed tomography (CT) demonstrates an accessory right renal artery coursing anterior to the IVC. **B,** Axial CT image from a different patient demonstrates the more common location of the right renal artery posterior to the IVC.

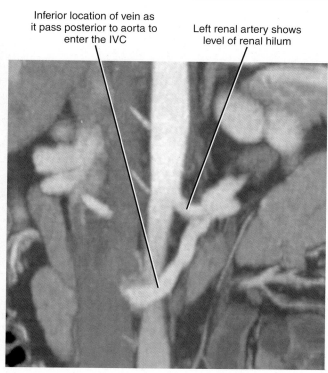

Figure 18-16 Coronal reformation from contrast-enhanced computed tomography performed for renal donation demonstrates a retroaortic left renal vein crossing the aorta well inferior to the level of the renal hila. *IVC,* Inferior vena cava.

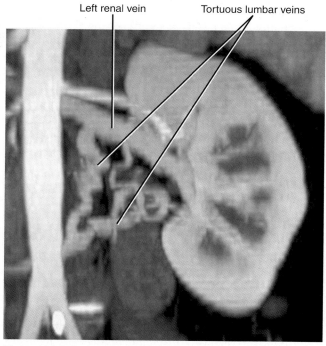

Figure 18-17 Coronal maximum intensity projection image from a contrast-enhanced computed tomographic scan demonstrates a dilated and tortuous lumbar veins joining the left renal vein.

aware of such a vessel, the urologist may choose to perform an alternate procedure to avoid hemorrhagic complications.

Recent advances in MDCT and MRI permit cross-sectional vascular studies to replace conventional angiography before UPJ repair (Fig. 18-18). Box 18-2 provides some tips regarding crossing vessels in UPJ obstruction.

■ NORMAL IMAGING APPEARANCE OF THE KIDNEYS

Ultrasound Appearance of the Kidneys

Ultrasound permits real-time optimization of imaging relative to the axis of each kidney. In most cases, the kidneys are situated with the inferior poles slightly

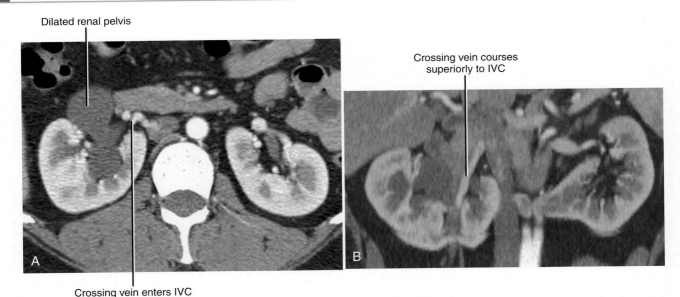

Dilated renal pelvis

Crossing vein courses
superiorly to IVC

A

B

Crossing vein enters IVC

Figure 18-18 Single-detector computed tomographic images from ureteropelvic junction deformity in the right side of a horseshoe kidney. **A,** Axial image demonstrates the dilated renal pelvis and crossing vessel. **B,** A curved planar reformation of the crossing vein demonstrates its course. Surgery was successful and the surgeon confirmed the anatomic survey was correct. *IVC,* Inferior vena cava.

BOX 18-2   Crossing Vessels in Ureteropelvic Junction Obstruction

1. Crossing vessels may be either *arterial* or *venous,* so remember to take a close look at both vascular phases.
2. The term *crossing vessel* does *not necessarily imply a causative relation.* In fact, some crossing vessels are near but not precisely at the level of obstruction. Any vessels adjacent to a site of potential endopyelotomy pose a potential hazard and should be reported.
3. Crossing vessels may be either *anterior* or *posterior* to the ureter, although anterior is more common.
4. The relation between the UPJ and vascular anatomy can be quite complex. *Best results are achieved if the radiologist can review the examination directly on a three-dimensional workstation.*

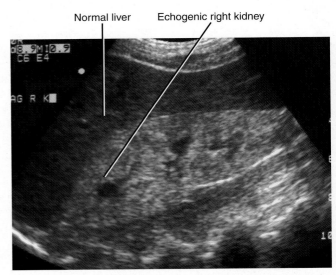

Normal liver   Echogenic right kidney

Figure 18-19 Sagittal ultrasound image of the right kidney demonstrates increased size and echogenicity of the kidney, findings typical of human immunodeficiency virus nephropathy. This kidney measured 14 cm in length. The left kidney (not shown) had a similar appearance.

---

more lateral and anterior than the superior poles. Each kidney should always be evaluated in long axis (coronal, sagittal, or both, depending on sonographic window) and axial to the kidney.

The cortex of a normal kidney is usually less echogenic than the adjacent normal liver. When the renal cortex is more echogenic than the adjacent liver, there is a high correlation with renal disease, although sensitivity is relatively low, according to Platt and colleagues (Fig. 18-19). When echogenicity of the renal cortex equals that of the liver, renal function is abnormal in approximately 38% of cases. In clinical practice, it is probably best to categorize the renal cortex as hypoechoic, isoechoic, or hyperechoic compared with

normal liver, and then state a correlative risk for associated renal parenchymal disease (Table 18-2).

Renal size can be measured in several ways. Calculation of the estimated renal volume is considered by some to be the most accurate assessment of renal size available with ultrasound, although renal length alone is more commonly reported. Most radiologists consider 10 to 12 cm to be an approximate reference range for renal length in adults, allowing for an additional 1 cm in either direction for patients at the extremes of height.

Table 18-2   Association between Renal Cortical Echogenicity and Renal Parenchymal Disease

Echogenicity of Renal Cortex*	Prevalence of Renal Disease
Hypoechoic	Low
Isoechoic	Moderate
Hyperechoic	High

*Echogenicity as compared with liver.

Size disparity greater than 1.5 cm between kidneys should raise suspicion that one kidney is abnormal.

Computed Tomographic Appearance of the Kidneys

The presence or absence of intravenous contrast media, as well as the phase of contrast enhancement, are key factors that determine the appearance of the renal parenchyma on CT (Table 18-3).

Table 18-3   Utility of Different Phases of Renal Contrast Enhancement

Phase of Enhancement	Timing	Appearance	Utility
Unenhanced	Before injection		Detect calcification Baseline HU for renal masses
Corticomedullary	25-40 seconds		Early enhancement of vascular masses and urothelial lesions Arterial anatomy Detect scars, infarcts
Nephrographic	70-90 seconds		Detect low-attenuation renal lesions Venous anatomy
Excretory	After 2 minutes Often 6-15 minutes for computed tomographic urography		Filling defects, obstruction

The *corticomedullary phase* is prolonged in the presence of ureteral or venous obstruction and can persist for days in cases of acute tubular necrosis (ATN; Fig. 18-20). The vascularity of some tumors may be most apparent during this phase (Fig. 18-21). However, small, low-attenuation lesions in the medulla are often obscured during this phase. The uniform high attenuation of the *nephrographic phase* provides an optimal background for detecting small, low-attenuation lesions in the renal parenchyma (Fig. 18-22).

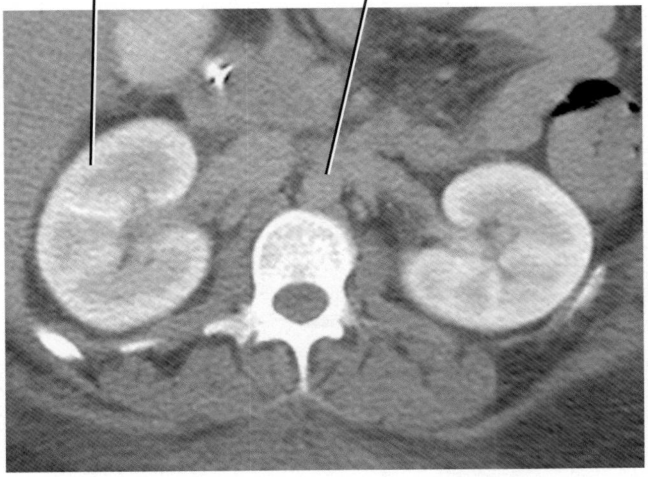

The visible contrast seen in the *excretory phase* has been concentrated many-fold. In fact, evaluation of the renal collecting system during the excretory phase often requires window and level settings approaching those used for evaluating the osseous structures (Fig. 18-23). Some centers use diuretics or fluid bolus, or both, during CT urography to dilute the excreted contrast to improve assessment of the urothelium.

Some divide the excretory phase into the *early excretory phase* (contrast mainly confined to the kidney) and *late excretory phase* (contrast in the ureters). The early excretory phase begins as early as 120 seconds after injection. Although ureteral contrast media is typically present before 3 minutes, longer delays provide more predictable opacification.

Magnetic Resonance Imaging

The renal cortex and medulla both have high signal intensity on T2-weighted images resulting in poor corticomedullary differentiation. However, T1-weighted images provide good corticomedullary differentiation. Calcifications and renal calculi are notoriously poorly demonstrated with MRI. The phases of nephrogram

Dense contrast in the renal cortex

No contrast in the aorta

Figure 18-20 Axial image from unenhanced computed tomography of the kidneys performed 2 days after an angiographic procedure demonstrates stasis of contrast in the renal cortex, resulting in a persistent corticomedullary phase of enhancement. Note that there is no contrast in the aorta.

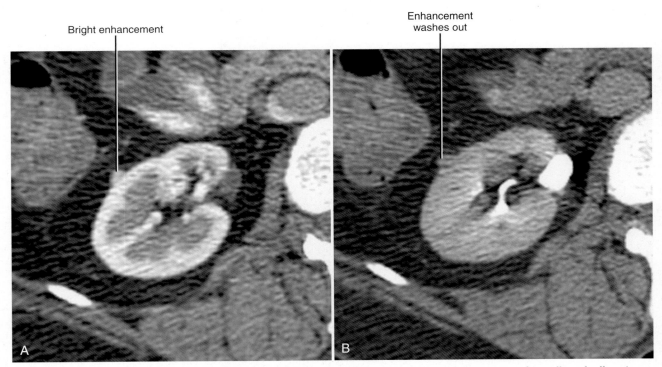

Bright enhancement

Enhancement washes out

Figure 18-21 Axial images from contrast-enhanced computed tomography demonstrate transient enhancement of a small renal cell carcinoma. **A,** Enhancement of the mass is conspicuous in the corticomedullary phase. **B,** Low-attenuation lesion in the late nephrographic/early excretory phase is less suspicious in appearance.

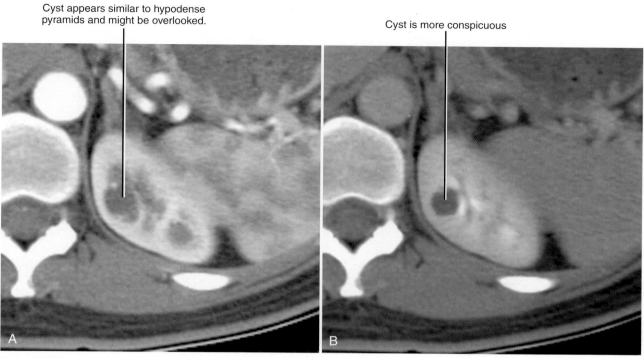

Cyst appears similar to hypodense pyramids and might be overlooked.

Cyst is more conspicuous

Figure 18-22 Axial images of the left kidney from a three-phase renal computed tomographic scan demonstrate improved conspicuity of low-attenuation lesions of the renal medulla during the nephrographic phase. **A,** A low-attenuation lesion is difficult to identify during the corticomedullary phase. **B,** The lesion becomes more conspicuous during the nephrographic phase.

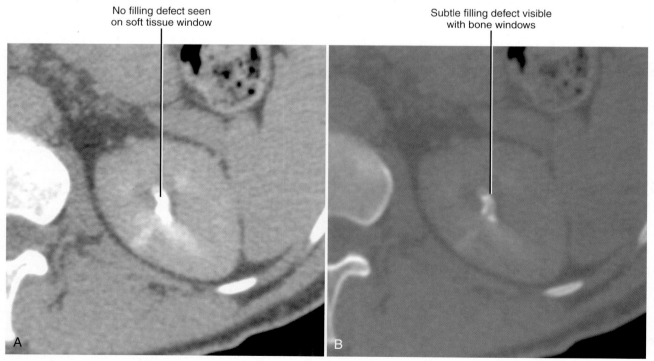

No filling defect seen on soft tissue window

Subtle filling defect visible with bone windows

Figure 18-23 Axial image of the left kidney obtained in the excretory phase of a computed tomographic urogram demonstrates the effects of window settings on visualizing structures near excreted contrast. **A,** Soft-tissue windows demonstrate no filling defect. **B,** A small calyceal defect is seen when the same image is viewed using bone windows. The defect proved to be blood clot from papillary necrosis.

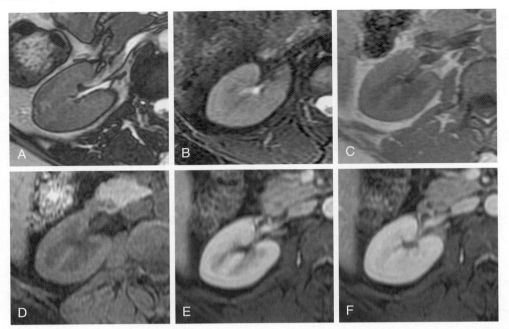

Figure 18-24 Normal magnetic resonance imaging appearance of the kidneys. **A,** Steady-state free precession, **(B)** T2-weighted with fat saturation, **(C)** T1-weighted, **(D)** T1-weighted with fat saturation, **(E)** postcontrast corticomedullary phase, and **(F)** postcontrast nephrographic phase.

development and contrast excretion parallel those seen on contrast-enhanced CT with one notable exception (Fig. 18-24). Unlike the excretory phase of enhanced CT, signal intensity within the renal collecting systems is reduced on T1- and T2-weighted MR images once excreted gadolinium-based contrast media becomes sufficiently concentrated. This phenomenon is due to T2-shortening and susceptibility (T2*) effects caused by concentrated gadolinium, and can potentially obscure filling defects and urothelial lesions.

◼ IMAGING EVALUATION FOR RENAL FAILURE

The goal of imaging patients with renal failure is to identify a correctable cause in an effort to recover or preserve renal function.

Types and Causes of Renal Failure

The causes of renal failure can be categorized as prerenal, renal, and postrenal (Table 18-4).

Ultrasound Evaluation for Renal Failure

Ultrasound is usually used in the initial evaluation of the patient with newly diagnosed renal failure. Even when there is another plausible explanation for decreased renal function (e.g., known prerenal causes), ultrasound offers the opportunity to rapidly and noninvasively identify a potentially correctible cause of renal failure. Table 18-5 summarizes a checklist approach to the ultrasound examination.

Table 18-4   Causes of Renal Failure

Category	Disease Process
Prerenal	Congestive heart failure, dehydration, diuretic use, burns, sepsis, hemorrhage, cirrhosis, diabetic keto-acidosis, renal artery stenosis*
Renal	Diabetes, hypertension, acute tubular necrosis,* chronic glomerulonephritis, autosomal dominant polycystic kidney disease,* multiple myeloma, interstitial nephritis, urate nephropathy, acute cortical necrosis, rhabdomyolysis
Postrenal	Ureteral obstruction,* bladder outlet obstruction,* neurogenic bladder*

*Entities for which sonography is most useful.

Table 18-5   Checklist Approach to Ultrasound for Renal Failure

Ultrasound Finding	Comments
Hydronephrosis	If present, obstruction is likely. Absence of hydronephrosis makes postrenal causes unlikely
Kidney size	Normal size: more likely acute. Cortical atrophy in one or both kidneys: suspect chronic or acute-on-chronic renal failure
Cortical echogenicity	Increased echogenicity has high association with parenchymal disease
Resistive index (RI)	Acute tubular necrosis usually results in an increased RI, whereas prerenal causes usually do not have an increased RI; postrenal causes often increase the RI, but hydronephrosis should be present in those cases
Bladder distension	If present, suspect neurogenic bladder or outlet obstruction

Increased Echogenicity

Increased cortical echogenicity is associated with many forms of chronic renal parenchymal disease and indicates a renal cause for renal failure. When abnormal echogenicity is detected, it is important to note whether it is unilateral or bilateral. Chronic glomerulonephritis usually causes bilateral increased renal echogenicity with smooth atrophy, whereas renal artery stenosis usually causes a similar but unilateral appearance (Fig. 18-25). Bilateral echogenic kidneys with renal hypertrophy can be seen associated with human immunodeficiency virus disease (see Fig. 18-19). The presence of contour irregularity usually indicates scarring, suggesting prior infection, reflux, or infarction. An acute change in renal cortical echogenicity is occasionally seen with pyelonehritis.

Hydronephrosis

Hydronephrosis is important to detect, because obstructive uropathy is often reversible if identified early. It is important to note, however, that the appearance of hydronephrosis does not necessarily indicate urinary obstruction (see Hydronephrosis and Its Mimics section later in this chapter).

For most people, obstruction of a single ureter does not induce renal failure. Obstruction can cause renal failure if it is bilateral (Box 18-3) or if there is preexisting disease in the unobstructed kidney. Ultrasound can often identify the cause in cases of bilateral obstruction (Fig. 18-26). In cases of unilateral obstruction with acute renal failure, sonographic evaluation may show evidence of chronic renal parenchymal disease in the unobstructed kidney.

BOX 18-3   Causes of Bilateral Hydronephrosis

Neurogenic bladder
Urethral stricture/valves
Bladder mass at trigone
Benign prostatic hyperplasia
Pelvic mass (cervical, rectal, uterine, prostate cancer)
Cystocele or uterine prolapse
Retroperitoneal fibrosis
Bilateral ureteral stones

Resistive Index

When hydronephrosis is absent, the causative factor for acute renal failure is almost certainly prerenal or renal. Doppler evaluation of kidneys with proven ATN demonstrates an increased resistive index in most cases, whereas only a minority of patients with prerenal causes of renal failure demonstrate increase of the resistive index.

Computed Tomographic Evaluation for Renal Failure

CT is occasionally used to evaluate patients with renal failure. In most cases, unenhanced CT is performed when the duration and cause of renal failure are unknown because exposure to iodinated contrast media could impair recovery of renal function. Unenhanced CT can identify hydronephrosis and hydroureter, urinary stones, and some masses. Renal size and cortical thickness can be assessed in a manner similar to ultrasound. CT angiography is occasionally performed when a vascular causative factor is suspected (renal artery stenosis or renal vein thrombosis) and MRI is contraindicated.

Magnetic Resonance Evaluation for Renal Failure

Unenhanced MRI can also be used to diagnose obstruction and identify the source (Fig. 18-27). MR angiography can be useful for the diagnosis of renal vascular abnormalities. Use of MR contrast agents in renal failure poses a lower risk than iodinated contrast material for exacerbating renal failure, but there is evidence that gadolinium-based MR contrast media pose some risk for systemic complications (nephrogenic systemic fibrosis) and should be used with caution in patients with severe or acute renal insufficiency. Static-fluid (T2-weighted) MR urography and phase-contrast MR angiography are useful techniques that do not require intravenous contrast material.

Nuclear Scintigraphy for Renal Failure

Renal scintigraphy can be performed with a variety of agents to provide assessment of either function or structure of the kidneys. Advantages of scintigraphy include accurate quantitative measurement of function

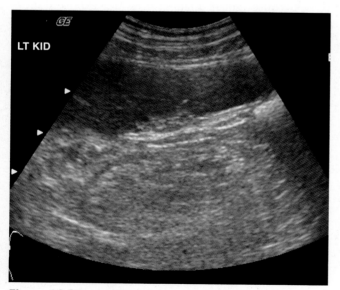

Figure 18-25 Sagittal ultrasound image of the left kidney demonstrates a unilateral small, smooth, echogenic kidney in a patient with renal artery stenosis. The right kidney has a normal appearance (not shown). The left kidney measured 7.8 cm, and the right kidney measured 10.9 cm. Arterial stenosis was confirmed by magnetic resonance angiography. If this appearance were present bilaterally, chronic renal disease such as chronic glomerulonephritis would be a more likely explanation.

Dilated upper pole calyx
and infundibulum   Dilated renal pelvis   Ureter

Soft tissue mass involving
posterior wall of bladder

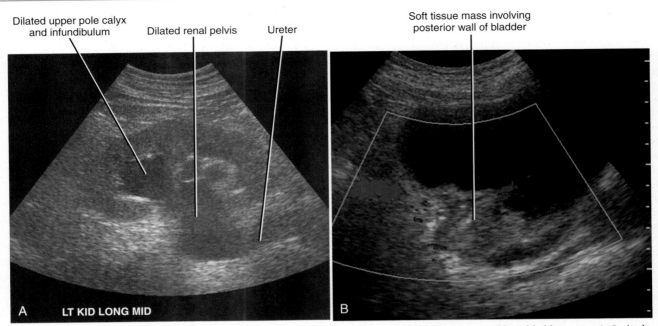

Figure 18-26 Ultrasound performed for acute renal failure demonstrates bilateral hydronephrosis caused by a bladder tumor. **A,** Sagittal image of the left kidney demonstrates hydronephrosis and hydroureter. The right kidney had a similar appearance (not shown). **B,** Transverse image of the bladder demonstrates a large bladder tumor in the region of the trigone.

Hydroureter   Hydronephrosis

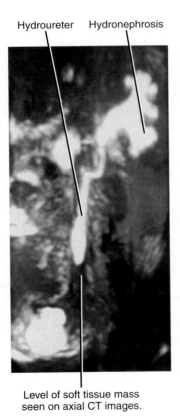

Level of soft tissue mass
seen on axial CT images.

Figure 18-27 T2-weighted maximum intensity projection image from a magnetic resonance urogram performed to evaluate urinary obstruction identified in a patient with an obstructing soft tissue mass in the pelvis on unenhanced computed tomography (CT). The patient had acute renal failure; therefore, contrast-enhanced CT was not performed.

and parenchymal mass without the risks for nephrotoxicity associated with iodinated contrast media or nephrogenic systemic fibrosis associated with gadolinium contrast agents.

Technetium 99m-mercaptoacetyltriglycin (MAG3) is excreted by the kidneys (mainly through secretion by proximal tubules) and provides evaluation of renal function, particularly in cases of suspected obstruction. Because repeat imaging does not expose the patient to additional radiation, multiple phases including delayed images may be obtained and allow the creation of quantitative curves that define the initial filling and then clearing of dilated collecting system structures. This method is the standard in evaluation of UPJ obstruction and often is used for other types of chronic obstruction. The dynamics of obstruction and quantification of relative renal function between the two kidneys may be important considerations in two general circumstances: (1) it is unclear whether obstruction is severe enough to warrant surgical intervention; or (2) significant parenchymal atrophy exists, and the relative merits of repair and nephrectomy are being compared. A furosemide challenge is often administered after initial excretion is observed to measure the impact of diuresis on the clearance of radiotracer from the renal pelvis.

Technetium 99m dimercaptosuccinic acid (DMSA) and glucoheptonate (GHA) are both used for evaluation of renal parenchyma. Despite different methods of accumulation, each is sequestered by the renal cortex, providing an opportunity to quantify the volume of renal parenchymal tissue in each kidney. The most common indication for cortical scintigraphy is to evaluate kidneys that have been injured by vesicoureteral reflux, chronic obstruction, or severe or repeated urinary infections. Poorly functioning kidneys with little residual parenchymal volume may be removed because preservation offers opportunities for future complications (infection, hypertension) without contributing significantly to renal function. The presence of significant renal parenchyma may justify surgical repair to maximize the functional contribution of that kidney.

■ DIFFUSE ABNORMALITIES OF THE KIDNEY

Size and Contour of Diffuse Renal Disease

Bilateral Small Smooth Kidneys

The bilateral small smooth kidney pattern describes most of what is often diagnosed on sonography as "medical renal disease," although the authors prefer the term *renal parenchymal disease*. These are chronic processes that lead to a loss of renal cortex gradually and uniformly. Small renal shadows may be seen on radiographs, and reniform shape is preserved on cross-sectional imaging. On ultrasound, the renal cortex is usually echogenic in this setting. Medullary cystic disease is encountered only rarely, and in addition to the echogenic atrophic cortex, the medullary pyramids are particularly hypoechoic. Table 18-6 lists the most common causes of bilateral smooth renal atrophy.

Unilateral Small Smooth Kidney

Global insult to one kidney may result in unilateral atrophy that is uniform and smooth. Table 18-7 lists causes of unilateral smooth renal atrophy. The most common cause is renal artery stenosis (see Fig. 18-25). CT and MR findings of renal artery stenosis parallel classic findings described on intravenous pyelogram, including one atrophic kidney with delayed nephrogram and excretion that can progress to a persistent nephrogram with hyperconcentrated excreted contrast media (Fig. 18-28). When the fine, weblike complex of ureteral arteries is recruited to contribute to collateral circulation, enlarged vessels are seen surrounding the proximal ureter, causing the classic "ureteral notching" seen on intravenous urogram (IVU).

Table 18-6   Causes of Bilateral Small Smooth Kidneys

Cause	Comments
Chronic glomerulonephritis	May have cortical nephrocalcinosis
Hypertensive nephrosclerosis	Longstanding hypertension
Bilateral renal artery stenosis	Often severe aortic disease or fibromuscular dysplasia
Analgesics	Papillary necrosis deforms calyces
Medullary cystic disease	Salt-wasting Cystic changes in medullary pyramids

Table 18-7   Causes of Unilateral Small Smooth Kidney

Cause	Comments
Renal artery stenosis	Delayed but increasingly dense nephrogram Delayed but hyperconcentrated contrast excretion Periureteral collaterals Ultrasound, computed tomography, or magnetic resonance evidence of renal artery narrowing
Postobstructive atrophy	Dilated, blunted collecting system
Chronic renal vein thrombosis	Enlargement of or calcification in renal vein
Radiation therapy	History of radiation
Renal hypoplasia	Decreased number of calyces (even unipapillary)
Page kidney	History of trauma Subcapsular fluid or calcification

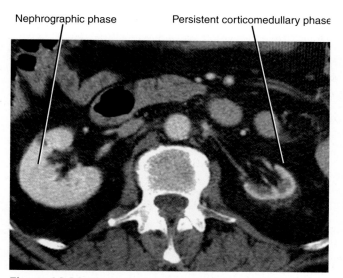

Nephrographic phase   Persistent corticomedullary phase

Figure 18-28 Contrast-enhanced computed tomography performed for trauma demonstrates evidence of renal artery stenosis. Findings include uniform atrophy with delayed progression of the nephrogram.

Although acute ureteral obstruction causes enlargement of the affected kidney, chronic obstruction leads to diffuse cortical loss. The overall size of the kidney depends on the level of residual collecting system distension. If the obstruction is relieved after atrophy has occurred, a small kidney with thin cortex and prominent calyces and renal pelvis is likely (Fig. 18-29). The degree of fluid replacement of the kidney and overall size of the kidney are likely related to the onset and duration of obstruction.

Unilateral Small Scarred Kidney

Loss of renal cortex in a nonuniform or irregular pattern can result from damage to the underlying papilla, infarction, or trauma. Although distortion of the renal contour caused by accidental or surgical trauma can

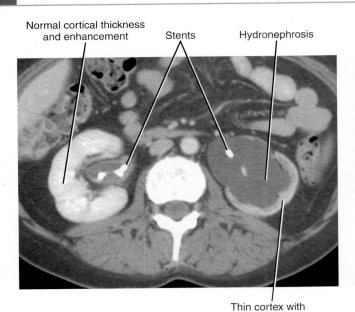

Normal cortical thickness and enhancement · Stents · Hydronephrosis

Thin cortex with poor enhancement

Figure 18-29 Axial image of the kidneys from a contrast-enhanced computed tomographic scan demonstrates unilateral cortical atrophy caused by chronic obstruction from cervical cancer. Bilateral ureteral stents are present.

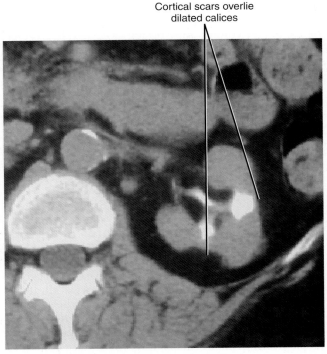

Cortical scars overlie dilated calices

Figure 18-31 Axial image of the left kidney in the excretory phase demonstrates parenchymal scars overlying calices, typical of processes that damage the renal papilla such as pyelonephritis, obstruction, and reflux. Defects caused by infarcts would be located between the calices.

affect any part of the kidney, scars resulting from injury to the papilla have an appearance that differs from those caused by infarcts (Figs. 18-30 and 18-31).

Note that multicystic dysplastic kidneys found in adults usually appear as a small, irregular calcified kidney as a result of congenital cysts and dysplasia of the renal cortex, not as a result of scarring.

Bilateral Small Scarred Kidneys
Vesicoureteral reflux is bilateral in more than 50% of cases diagnosed neonatally, with a smaller percentage diagnosed later in childhood or in adulthood. The pattern is identical to that seen with unilateral reflux, with parenchymal defects overlying dilated calyces in the upper and lower poles.

Renal infarcts from embolic disease and vasculitis are often bilateral (Fig. 18-32). Analgesic nephropathy or virtually any other cause of papillary necrosis can lead to damage to the cortex overlying affected papillae. Table 18-8 provides an overall summary of renal atrophy and its causes.

Bilateral Smooth Enlargement
Uniform enlargement of the kidneys can be difficult to detect. Smooth contours offer no indication that the kidneys are diseased. Variability in normal renal length, as well as the influences of variable renal axis

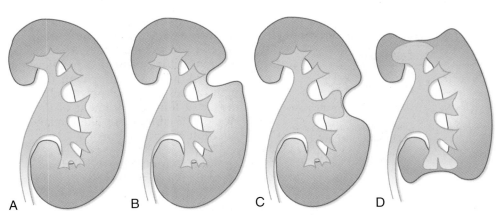

A   B   C   D

Figure 18-30 Location of renal scars related to diagnosis. **A,** Normal appearance. **B,** Defect between calyces caused by infarct. **C,** Defect overlying papilla from infection or obstruction. **D,** Polar parenchymal loss overlying calyces caused by reflux.

Table 18-8   Patterns of Diffuse Renal Atrophy: Summary

Pattern	Causes
Bilateral small smooth kidneys	Chronic glomerulonephritis Hypertensive nephrosclerosis Bilateral renal artery stenosis Analgesics Medullary cystic disease (salt wasting)
Unilateral small smooth kidneys	Renal artery stenosis Postobstructive atrophy Chronic renal vein thrombosis Radiation therapy Renal hypoplasia
Unilateral small scarred kidneys	Reflux nephropathy Pyelonephritis Prior surgery or percutaneous nephrostomy Prior trauma
Bilateral small scarred kidneys	Reflux nephropathy Infarcts Analgesic nephropathy

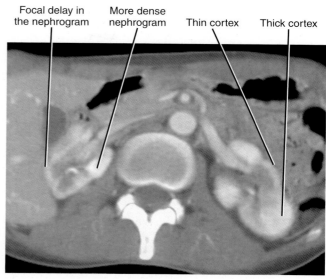

Focal delay in the nephrogram   More dense nephrogram   Thin cortex   Thick cortex

Figure 18-32 Axial image of the kidneys from contrast-enhanced computed tomography demonstrates bilateral irregular cortical volume loss caused by infarcts related to cocaine abuse. Regional differences in the nephrograms reflect regional differences in perfusion.

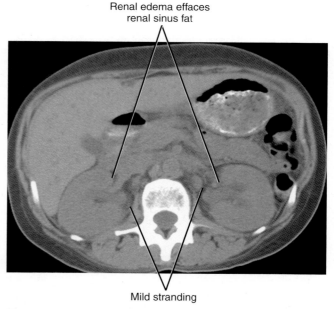

Renal edema effaces renal sinus fat

Mild stranding

Figure 18-33 Axial image of the kidneys from an unenhanced computed tomographic scan demonstrates diffuse bilateral smooth renal enlargement caused by lupus nephritis.

on measurements, confounds routine attempts to detect subtle abnormalities in kidney size. With imaging, most causes of renal enlargement result in obliteration of the renal sinus fat and perinephric fat stranding (Fig. 18-33). When bilateral enlargement is detected, the most common causative factors involve interstitial infiltration with neoplastic or inflammatory cells, or deposition of a substance. Table 18-9 lists some of the more common causes of renal enlargement.

Unilateral Smooth Enlargement

Because of the asymmetry, unilateral smooth renal enlargement is more conspicuous than bilateral enlargement. This is particularly true with the most common cause, ureteral obstruction, because hydronephrosis is usually present as well. Ureteral obstruction causes edema in the interstitium of the kidney that may enlarge the kidney out of proportion to the degree of hydronephrosis. Other causes of edema will also enlarge the involved kidney, including pyelonephritis, renal contusions, renal vein thrombosis, and acute renal arterial occlusion (Fig. 18-34). Infiltrating neoplasms, such

Table 18-9   Patterns of Diffuse Renal Enlargement

Pattern	Causes
Bilateral smooth enlargement	Diabetic nephropathy
	Acquired immune deficiency syndrome nephropathy
	Acute glomerulonephritis
	Collagen vascular disease and vasculitis
	Lymphoma and leukemia
	Amyloidosis
	Myeloma
	Additional rare causes
Unilateral smooth enlargement	Ureteral obstruction
	Compensatory hypertrophy
	Duplication
	Pyelonephritis including xanthogranulomatous pyelonephritis
	Renal vein thrombosis
	Urothelial carcinoma (previously transitional cell carcinoma)
	Medullary renal carcinoma
	Infiltrating renal cell carcinoma
	Collecting duct carcinoma
Bilateral irregular enlargement	Autosomal dominant polycystic kidney disease
	Acquired renal cystic disease
	Lymphoma
	Metastases
	Tuberous sclerosis
	Wilm's tumors

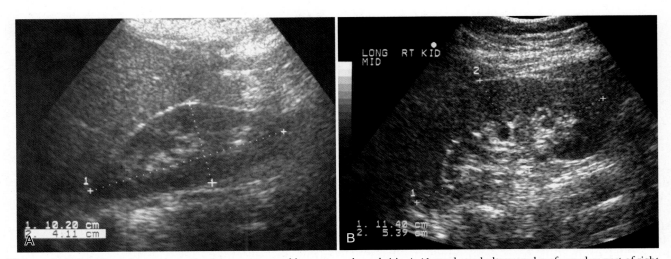

Figure 18-34 Unilateral smooth renal enlargement caused by acute pyelonephritis. **A,** Normal renal ultrasound performed as part of right upper quadrant sonogram. **B,** When the patient presented with acute pyelonephritis 1 month later, unilateral renal enlargement was noted with increase in size of more than 1 cm, as well as rounding of the poles.

as lymphoma, urothelial carcinoma, and medullary renal carcinoma, can also cause unilateral renal enlargement (Fig. 18-35).

Not all unilaterally enlarged kidneys are diseased. Renal hypertrophy commonly results in unilateral enlargement when the contralateral kidney is atrophic or absent. The normal reniform contour is preserved, and calyces appear normal. Urinary duplications contain parenchyma within the central region of the renal sinus, resulting in renal length that is larger than normal.

Enlarged Lobulated Kidneys

Irregular enlargement of the kidneys is usually the result of multiple bilateral masses. Autosomal dominant polycystic kidney disease (ADPKD) is the most common cause. In ADPKD, the kidneys contain numerous cysts that create irregular or lobulated contours on radiographs, cross-sectional imaging studies, or IVU (Fig. 18-36). Acquired renal cystic disease can cause enlargement but usually to a much lesser extent.

In tuberous sclerosis, the kidneys can be replaced with innumerable angiomyolipomas (AMLs). Unlike the sporadic form of AMLs, which appear as discrete masses, AMLs in tuberous sclerosis can be so numerous and large that it is often difficult to define specific lesions (Fig. 18-37).

When lymphoma results in multiple renal masses, the kidneys may be enlarged and irregular in contour. A similar appearance can occur with diffuse metastatic disease to the kidneys.

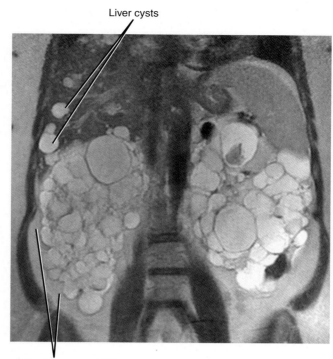

Liver cysts

Replacement of kidney with cysts results in lobulated contour

Figure 18-36 Coronal T2-weighted magnetic resonance image of the kidneys demonstrates bilateral renal enlargement with lobulated contours caused by autosomal dominant polycystic kidney disease.

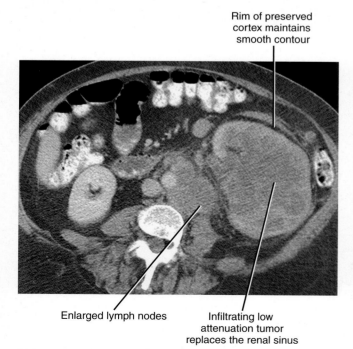

Rim of preserved cortex maintains smooth contour

Enlarged lymph nodes

Infiltrating low attenuation tumor replaces the renal sinus

Figure 18-35 Unilateral smooth renal enlargement caused by lymphoma. Reniform shape is preserved because soft-tissue infiltration expanded outward from the renal sinus. Medullary renal carcinoma and urothelial carcinoma can have a similar appearance.

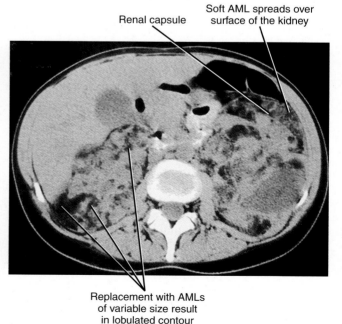

Renal capsule

Soft AML spreads over surface of the kidney

Replacement with AMLs of variable size result in lobulated contour

Figure 18-37 Axial image of the kidneys from an unenhanced computed tomographic scan demonstrates bilateral, lobulated renal enlargement from multiple angiomyolipomas (AMLs) in a patient with tuberous sclerosis.

Table 18-10 Diagnostic Implications of Abnormal Nephrograms

Pattern	Causes	
	Unilateral	**Bilateral**
Striated	Pyelonephritis Ureteral obstruction Renal vein thrombosis Contusion	Pyelonephritis Tubular obstruction (protein, crystals) Autosomal dominant polycystic kidney disease Hypotension
Delayed onset	Acute ureteral obstruction Renal artery stenosis Renal vein thrombosis	Tubular obstruction from deposition disease
Persistent	Acute ureteral obstruction Renal artery stenosis Renal vein thrombosis	Hypotension Acute tubular necrosis

Nephrograms

Patterns of nephrographic enhancement have been used by radiologists for years to identify and characterize categories of disease in the kidneys. It is easy to get complacent about nephrograms on cross-sectional images because there is so much other information available. However, the patterns of renal enhancement and transition can offer useful information about the physiologic state of the kidney and have the potential to augment the anatomic information on the examination. In general, nephrograms are evaluated in terms of uniformity of enhancement, rate of onset, and duration. Each category is discussed separately with an overall summary in Table 18-10.

Uniformity of Enhancement

Normal renal parenchyma appears homogeneous during the nephrographic phase of enhancement on IVU, CT, or MR images. One of the most common deviations from this normal pattern of enhancement is the *striated nephrogram*. The striated nephrogram appears as alternating bands of high and low attenuation or signal intensity, each several millimeters thick, perpendicular to the renal capsule (Fig. 18-38). Unilateral striated nephrograms are usually caused by acute ureteral obstruction, pyelonephritis, contusion or renal vein thrombosis. When bilateral, consider pyelonephritis, tubular obstruction (Tamm–Horsfall protein or rhabdomyolysis), hypotension, and ADPKD.

Global and *segmental absence of the nephrogram* are other forms of nonuniform enhancement. Failure to develop a nephrogram in all or part of a kidney indicates a perfusion abnormality (Fig. 18-39). These are usually segmental in nature, caused by an embolic infarct or trauma to a segmental branch of the renal artery. Less often, a hilar injury, large embolus, or renal extension of aortic dissection may prevent enhancement to the entire kidney. Depending on location of the thrombus and specific venous anatomy, renal vein thrombosis can result in either segmental or global absence of the nephrogram.

A *"flip-flop"* or reverse pattern of enhancement represents a region of hypoattenuation/diminished perfusion on early nephrographic images that becomes hyperattenuating in the same region on more delayed

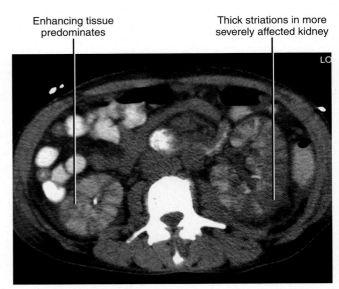

Enhancing tissue predominates

Thick striations in more severely affected kidney

Figure 18-38 Axial image of the kidneys from a contrast-enhanced computed tomographic (CT) scan demonstrates striated CT nephrograms in a patient with bacterial endocarditis, bilateral flank pain, and pyuria. Findings are consistent with bilateral pyelonephritis. Note that the right kidney was only mildly enlarged, and enhancing parenhyma predominates with thin lines of low attenuation. The left kidney is more enlarged and has larger bands of low attenuation, presumably because of higher pressure from interstitial edema.

images (Fig. 18-40). This can be seen with ischemia or infarction related to embolic disease, vasculitis, or trauma.

The *cortical rim sign* is perhaps the most specific sign of underperfusion to the kidney. A thin line of enhancement along the renal capsule indicates collateral circulation through peripelvic, capsular, and periureteral vessels (Fig. 18-41). Presence of a cortical rim sign usually indicates infarction but has also been reported in cases of ATN and renal vein thrombosis.

Delayed Development of Nephrogram

Once a common finding on IVU, the delayed development of a nephrogram is now seen as persistent corticomedullary phase of enhancement on CT or MRI

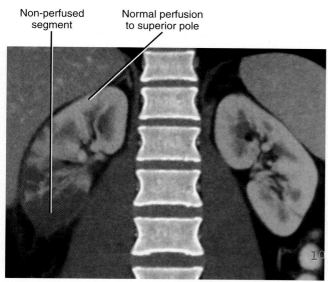

Non-perfused segment   Normal perfusion to superior pole

Figure 18-39 Coronal reformation from a contrast-enhanced computed tomographic scan performed for acute right flank pain in a patient with atrial fibrillation. A large segmental infarct is present in the inferior pole of the right kidney.

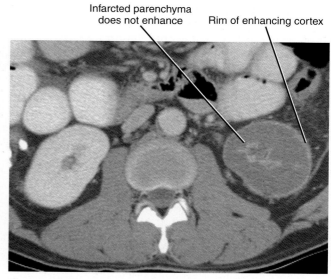

Infarcted parenchyma does not enhance   Rim of enhancing cortex

Figure 18-41 Cortical rim sign. Axial image of the kidneys from a contrast-enhanced computed tomographic scan performed 10 days after traumatic renal infarction demonstrates a thin rim of enhancement along the renal capsule. The acute appearance of this infarct is shown in Figure 9-23.

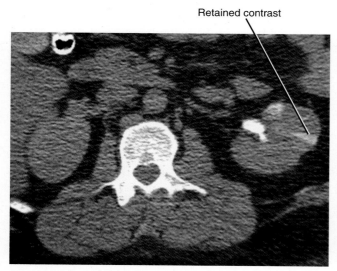

Retained contrast

Figure 18-40 "Flip-flop" enhancement of renal contusion. Axial image of the kidneys performed 2 hours after contrast injection demonstrates a wedge-shaped area of retained contrast in the same location as a low-attenuation defect on the initial scan (not shown). The delayed images were performed to exclude delayed hemorrhage from a splenic injury.

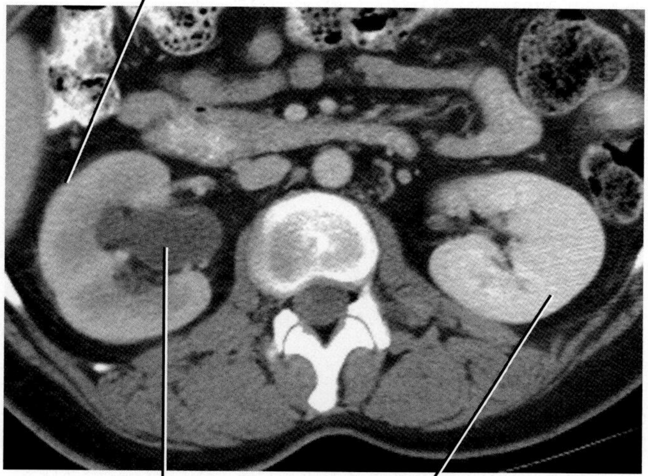

Persistent corticomedullary phase

Hydronephrosis   Uniform nephrogram with no corticomedullary differentiation

Figure 18-42 Axial image of the kidneys in the expected nephrographic phase (80 seconds after injection) of a contrast-enhanced computed tomographic scan demonstrates delayed cortical nephrogram on the right side because of distal ureteral obstruction from cervical cancer.

when the other kidney has progressed to a uniform nephrogram (Fig. 18-42). This occurs when there is a delay in either the delivery of contrast media to (arterial stenosis) or removal of (ureteral obstruction) contrast media from the kidney. Common causes include acute ureteral obstruction, renal artery stenosis, and renal vein thrombosis.

Persistently Dense Nephrogram

Although any of the processes that cause the delayed development of the nephrogram can also result in prolongation of the dense nephrogram once it develops, several other processes may have a brisk initial nephrogram followed by abnormal persistence. Hypotension (including systemic reactions to intravenous contrast media) causes stasis of urine and contrast within the tubules, resulting in a dense nephrogram that persists until normal perfusion resumes. If normotensive conditions are restored quickly, excretion usually begins and the nephrogram fades. If hypotension results in ATN or if ATN occurs for another reason, the nephrogram may persist longer (see Fig. 18-20).

Diffuse Signal Abnormalities of the Kidney on Magnetic Resonance Imaging

After the intravenous injection of gadolinium, MRI allows evaluation of the nephrogram pattern in a manner similar to CT. What might be overlooked is the impact of systemic disease on the signal intensity of the renal parenchyma before injection. Cortical nephrocalcinosis can decrease cortical signal on both T1- and T2-weighted images. Medullary nephrocalcinosis can accentuate the normal corticomedullary differentiation on T1-weighted images and can result in corticomedullary differentiation on T2-weighted images (usually absent). Iron deposition throughout the renal cortex can be seen in patients with paroxysmal nocturnal hemoglobinuria, sickle cell disease, and prosthetic heart valves related to intravascular hemolysis. When sufficient iron accumulates, it results in low-signal-intensity renal cortex with all pulse sequences (Fig. 18-43).

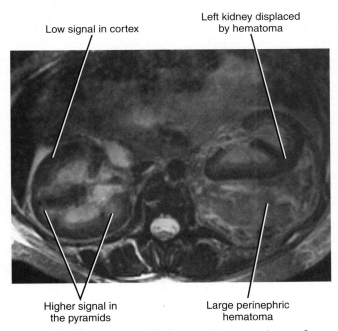

Low signal in cortex

Left kidney displaced by hematoma

Higher signal in the pyramids

Large perinephric hematoma

Figure 18-43 Axial T2-weighted magnetic resonance image of the kidneys in a patient with paroxysmal nocturnal hemoglobinuria demonstrates diffuse low signal throughout the renal cortex of both kidneys. Although the renal parenchyma usually has uniform high signal on T2-weighted images, iron deposition within the cortex results in differentiation from the underlying medullary pyramids. Imaging was performed to evaluate hemorrhage after renal biopsy on the left.

■ CHARACTERIZING FOCAL ABNORMALITIES OF THE KIDNEY

Characteristic imaging findings in the kidney allow a precise imaging diagnosis of many conditions, minimizing surgical removal of benign lesions in some cases and facilitating organ-sparing surgery in others. A methodical approach is helpful when analyzing renal lesions. We propose asking the following questions when confronted with a potential renal mass:

1. Could it be a normal variant or normal tissue surrounded by abnormal (scarred) kidney?
2. From where does it arise?
3. Does it have a characteristic shape?
4. What is it made of?
5. How does it enhance?

Renal Pseudotumor

Some normal anatomic structures or sequelae of remote renal injury result in masslike appearances within the kidney. We call these *pseudotumors* of the kidney.

The *hypertrophied column of Bertin* is recognized by its typical interpolar location and similarity to normal renal parenchyma on imaging studies. *Fetal lobulation* and *junctional cortical line* are discussed earlier in this chapter. The contour bulge of fetal lobulation can mimic a parenchymal mass on sonography but will demonstrate normal parenchymal enhancement with CT or MRI (see Fig. 18-9). The focus of increased echogenicity within a junctional cortical line can be confused with a small AML, but typical location should raise consideration of this anatomic variant, and linear shape of the abnormality is diagnostic (see Fig. 18-8). A prominent *diaphragmatic slip* can simulate the appearance of an exophytic renal mass (Fig. 18-44). This is easily clarified with CT.

Scarring from prior infection, reflux, or infarction can result in a bizarre renal contour. When a region of the kidney is spared from the causative insult, it can develop a masslike appearance. This can be confusing on ultrasound and even on nephrographic-phase CT scanning and MRI. Dynamic CT scanning or MRI will demonstrate normal corticomedullary differentiation in the spared parenchyma bordered by regions of cortical loss (Fig. 18-45). The spared masslike areas will also demonstrate normal uptake of radionuclide on renal scintigraphy.

Localizing Renal Abnormalities

Renal versus Perirenal Lesions

Localization is key to generating a differential diagnosis for abnormalities in and around the kidney. The first and most obvious question is, "Does the lesion come from the kidney or some other structure?" Although the origin is obvious in most cases, in some cases, determining the origin can be quite difficult. The classic quandary is the large mass in the right suprarenal region, distorting the superior pole of the right kidney

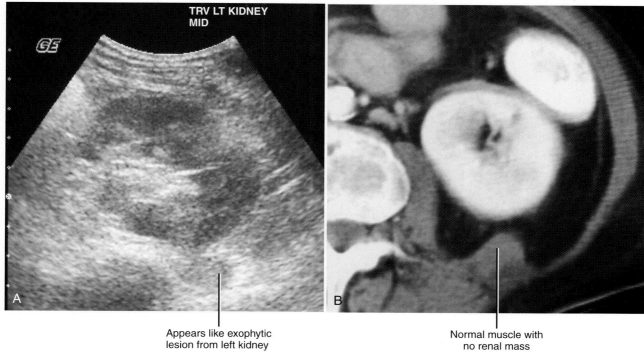

Appears like exophytic
lesion from left kidney

Normal muscle with
no renal mass

Figure 18-44 Diaphragmatic slip as a renal pseudomass. **A,** Transverse ultrasound image of the left kidney appears to show an exophytic mass posterior to the kidney. **B,** Transverse image from a contrast-enhanced computed tomographic scan performed the same day proves this to be a muscular slip of the diaphragm.

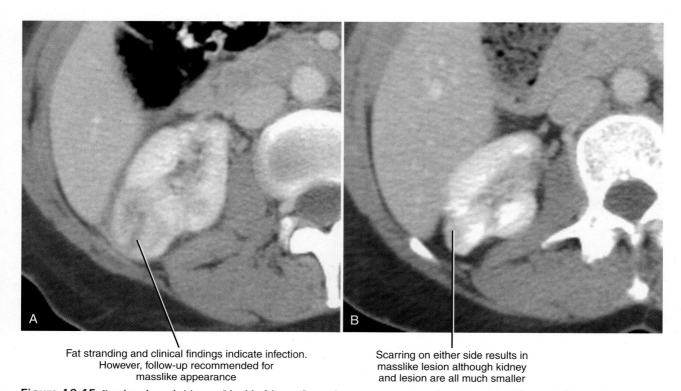

Fat stranding and clinical findings indicate infection.
However, follow-up recommended for
masslike appearance

Scarring on either side results in
masslike lesion although kidney
and lesion are all much smaller

Figure 18-45 Focal pyelonephritis as a "double fake-out" pseudotumor on computed tomography (CT). **A,** Axial image from contrast-enhanced CT performed at initial presentation with clinical signs of pyelonephritis demonstrates focal masslike bulge from the right kidney. **B,** Axial image from CT performed 6 weeks later to follow the bulge demonstrates scarring. Without the prior history and examination, scarring could be mistaken for an exophytic mass in the nephrographic phase.

Continued

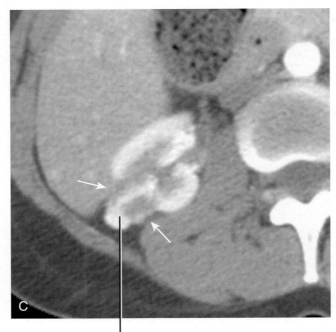

Bulge shows preserved cortex bordered
by areas of cortical loss (arrows)

Figure 18-45, cont'd C, Axial image in the corticomedullary phase of the same examination shows focal cortical defects *(arrows)* characteristic of scars.

and inferior margin of the liver and obscuring the adrenal gland. The *claw sign* is useful when present but not always best appreciated in the axial plane (Fig. 18-46). For masses centered in the suprarenal region, multiplanar imaging can be critical to determining the organ of origin.

Perirenal masses arise adjacent to but not from the kidney or any nearby organ (Fig. 18-47). A relatively narrow differential diagnosis exists for masses arising from within the perirenal space (Table 18-11).

The Renal Sinus

The renal sinus describes the space enveloped by renal parenchyma and normally contains fat, renal collecting system, renal vasculature, and lymphatics. Localizing an abnormality to the renal sinus limits a differential diagnosis considerably (Table 18-12). If a mass appears to arise from within the collecting system, considerations include transitional cell carcinoma, blood clot, and mycetoma. If a solid mass appears to arise outside of the collecting system but within the renal sinus, lymphoma is most common, although metastases also occur here. Fluid attenuation within the renal sinus on ultrasound, CT, or MRI could represent either renal sinus cysts or hydronephrosis. Several examples are shown in Figure 18-48.

Filling Defects within the Collecting System

Mucosal lesions (usually urothelial carcinoma but occasionally squamous cell carcinoma) are seen as dark filling defects against the bright background of excreted contrast on CT or T1-weighted MRI, and as nonmobile echogenic foci surrounded by anechoic

Cystic mass

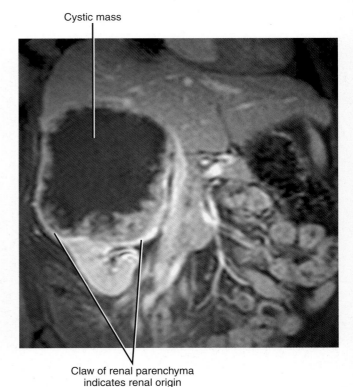

Claw of renal parenchyma
indicates renal origin

Figure 18-46 Claw sign. Coronal T1-weighted magnetic resonance image acquired after contrast administration shows a large, partially cystic renal cell carcinoma extending superiorly toward the liver. Compare this with the adrenal hematoma in Figure 9-28.

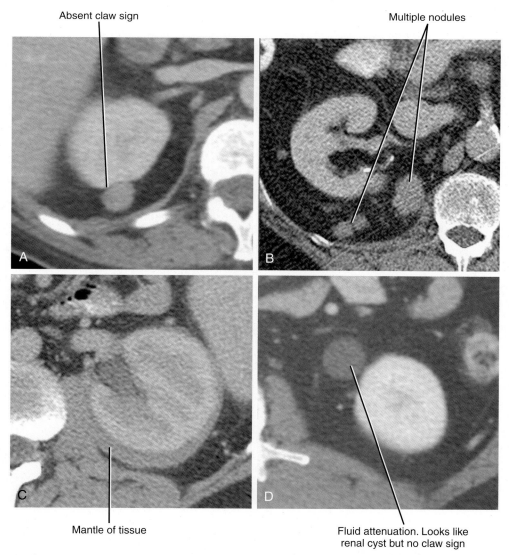

Absent claw sign

Multiple nodules

Mantle of tissue

Fluid attenuation. Looks like
renal cyst but no claw sign

Figure 18-47 Perirenal masses. **A,** Solitary perirenal mass is biopsy-proved metastatic lung cancer. **B,** Multiple perirenal masses in multiple myeloma. **C,** Mantle of perirenal soft tissue in Erdheim–Chester disease (this appearance is identical to perirenal lymphoma). **D,** Perirenal lymphangioma.

Table 18-11   Differential Diagnosis of Perirenal Masses

Diagnosis	Comments
Lymphoma	Most common perirenal soft-tissue mass Nodules or confluent mantle of tissue
Metastases	Multiple myeloma, melanoma, lung, breast
Lymphangioma	Fluid attenuation/signal intensity
Extramedullary hematopoiesis	Calcification and fat content
Hemorrhage	High attenuation on computed tomography (unless chronic) Heterogeneous with high-signal-intensity areas on T1-weighted magnetic resonance imaging
Abscess	Enhancing rim, gas
Erdheim–Chester disease	Rare form of non-Langerhans cell histiocytosis affecting retroperitoneum, mediastinum, or both Associated with sclerosis in long bones of the lower extremities and skin lesions

urine with sonography (Fig. 18-49). Table 18-13 describes common filling defects and some discriminating characteristics.

Shape of Focal Renal Masses

Defining the contour of a renal lesion can be helpful in narrowing the differential diagnosis. Most renal lesions can be described as spherical, mushroom shaped, or infiltrating (Table 18-14). Placing a lesion within one of these shape categories usually provides a more focused differential diagnosis, although most lesions must be further characterized based on additional features for definitive diagnosis.

Mass lesions that arise from the renal cortex tend to grow in a concentric fashion, resulting in a shape that is roughly *spherical*. Renal cortical cysts and renal cell carcinoma are the most common spherical lesions in the kidney and can, in most cases, be differentiated

Table 18-12   Abnormalities in the Renal Sinus

Diagnosis	Comments
Renal sinus cysts	Fluid attenuation Do not interconnect or collect excreted contrast Include both primary lymphatic cysts of the renal sinus (peripelvic cysts) and cortical cysts that herniate into the renal sinus (parapelvic cysts)
Hydronephrosis	Glovelike interconnection between the components Accumulates contrast material on delayed excretory images
Lymphoma	Smooth soft-tissue mass within sinus Often contiguous with retroperitoneal lymphadenopathy
Urothelial carcinoma	Expands renal collecting system (pelvis, calyces, or both) Usually enhances during arterial phase Filling defect on excretory-phase images
Sinus lipomatosis	Often present with obesity or advanced age, or both Thin collecting system on intravenous pyelogram, increased sinus fat on computed tomographic/magnetic resonance imaging Asymmetric lipomatosis with history of stones/inflammatory disease of the kidneys
Metastatic disease	Usually advanced cervical or testicular cancer with extensive lymphadenopathy in the retroperitoneum
Renal artery aneurysm	Round lesion with early arterial enhancement Calcification is common
Renal arteriovenous malformation	Tubular structures with early enhancement (see Fig. 18-66)

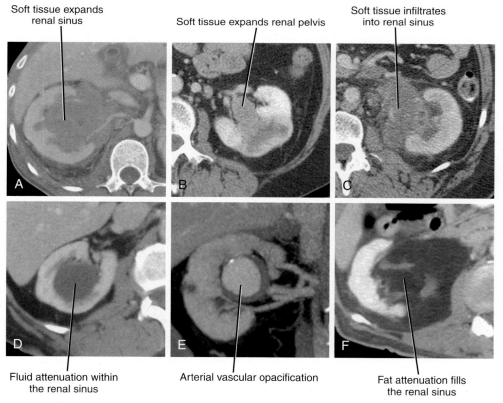

Figure 18-48 Examples of lesions in the renal sinus. **A,** Lymphoma. **B,** Urothelial carcinoma. **C,** Metastatic cervical carcinoma. **D,** Renal sinus cyst. **E,** Renal artery aneurysm. **F,** Renal sinus lipomatosis.

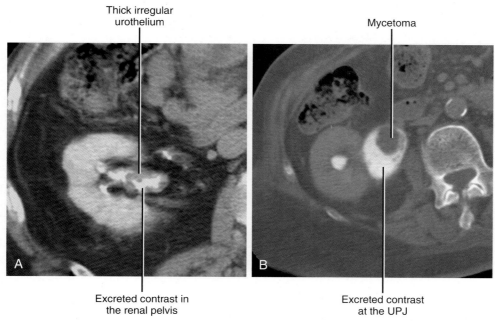

Thick irregular
urothelium

Mycetoma

Excreted contrast in
the renal pelvis

Excreted contrast
at the UPJ

A   B

Figure 18-49 Axial images of the right kidney in the excretory phase of contrast-enhanced computed tomographic examinations from two different patients demonstrate filling defects in the renal pelvis. **A,** Irregular mucosal thickening proved to be urothelial carcinoma. **B,** Mycetoma. *UPJ,* Ureteropelvic junction.

Table 18-13   Common Causes of Filling Defects in the Renal Collecting System

Causative Factor	Comments
Stone	Calcification on noncontrast-enhanced computed tomography
Blood clot	High attenuation on noncontrast-enhanced computed tomography High signal intensity on T1-weighted magnetic resonance imaging Mobile Castlike filling defect
Urothelial carcinoma	Soft tissue enhancement Irregular, papillary projections, expand renal pelvis
Sloughed papilla	Signs of papillary necrosis
Mycetoma	Immunocompromised patient, diabetes
Aberrant papilla	Halo of contrast in fornix around papilla

from one another on cross-sectional imaging based on attenuation and enhancement characteristics (Fig. 18-50). Metastases and renal abscesses also tend to be spherical. AMLs that are entirely intraparenchymal are often spherical.

A variant of spherical shape is the *mushroom shape,* typical of soft, pliable lesions of the renal cortex (Fig. 18-51). These lesions are exophytic with a visible "divot" in the renal parenchyma and often a somewhat flattened "crown." This is most commonly seen with small- to medium-size AMLs that extend beyond the renal cortex. Low-pressure cysts can have a similar appearance. Unfortunately, an occasional renal carcinoma will have this appearance; thus, the sign must be used with caution.

Inflammatory lesions of the kidney and masses that arise within the renal collecting system are more likely to maintain an approximation of the original renal contour as they expand the kidney. This *infiltrating appearance* is typical of pyelonephritis and urothelial carcinoma (Fig. 18-52) but can also be seen with lymphoma (see Fig. 18-35), infarcts (see Fig. 18-39), metastases, renal medullary carcinoma, and collecting duct carcinoma. Pyelonephritis is usually suspected on clinical grounds, whereas other infiltrating lesions may require transureteroscopic or percutaneous biopsy for diagnosis. Occasionally, an infiltrating form of renal cell carcinoma has a similar appearance.

Wedge-shaped abnormalities of the renal parenchyma usually have a vascular causative factor, with infarct most common (Fig. 18-53). Occasionally, focal pyelonephritis can mimic this appearance, likely because of regional hypoperfusion. Infiltrating transitional cell carcinomas occasionally have a similar impact on small vessels, resulting in wedge-shaped defects that are a combination of tumor and hypoperfusion.

Table 18-14   Using Shape to Characterize Focal Renal Abnormalities

Sphere	Mushroom	Infiltrating	Wedge
Cortical cyst*	AML*	Pyelonephritis*	Infarct*
RCC*	Cortical cyst*	Urothelial carcinoma*	Focal pyelonephritis
AML*	RCC (unusual)	Lymphoma	Infiltrating urothelial carcinoma
Abscess	Abscess	Metastasis	Vasculitis
Lymphoma	Defect from partial	RCC	Renal contusion
Oncocytoma	nephrectomy	Renal medullary carcinoma	
Calyceal diverticulum		Collecting duct carcinoma	

*More common lesions.
AML, Angiomyolipoma; *RCC*, renal cell carcinoma.

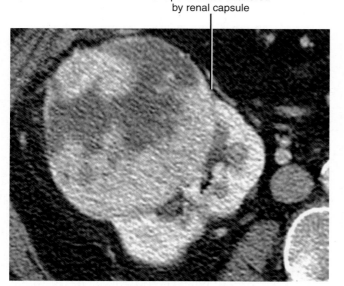

Shape of mass unaltered
by renal capsule

Figure 18-50 Axial image of the right kidney from a contrast-enhanced computed tomographic scan demonstrates a renal mass with a spherical shape typical of renal cell carcinoma.

Composition of Focal Renal Masses

Fat

AMLs consist of vascular, smooth muscle, and fatty elements to varying degrees. Although not all AMLs contain fat, the presence of fat in a renal mass indicates AML in almost all cases. In most cases, there is sufficient fat to allow detection with CT and MRI (Fig. 18-54). On sonography, AMLs appear echogenic (see Fig. 1-69) but may be difficult to distinguish from a hyperechoic RCC. Thin-section CT and chemical-shift imaging with MRI are helpful for identifying tiny amounts of fat within AMLs (Fig. 18-55).

One should be careful when using chemical-shift MRI to differentiate between AML and RCC. Macroscopic fat (common in AML but rare in RCC) will not suppress homogeneously on opposed-phase images. Rather, small amounts of macroscopic fat will demonstrate a peripheral low-signal-intensity ring caused by the fat–water interface. Intracellular lipid (common in RCC) will lose signal on opposed-phase images, without demonstrating a low-signal-intensity boundary artifact. Unlike macroscopic fat, intracellular lipid will not suppress significantly with chemically selective fat-saturation techniques.

RCC containing macroscopic fat is extremely rare. In most reported cases, calcification is also present. This is helpful because calcification is rarely present in AMLs. The rare reports of renal cell carcinoma containing fat but no calcification describe large renal masses (10 cm) that are presumed to have engulfed perirenal fat. Renal masses of such a size are almost always removed.

Surgeons often pack perinephric fat into sites of partial nephrectomy. These can have the appearance of a fatty mass on subsequent CT and MR images (Fig. 18-56). If history of surgery is not already provided, there is usually local postoperative distortion with focal thinning of the perinephric fat overlying the defect.

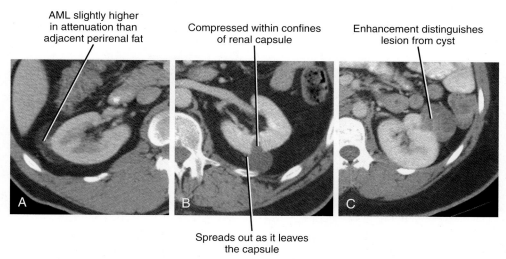

AML slightly higher
in attenuation than
adjacent perirenal fat

Compressed within confines
of renal capsule

Enhancement distinguishes
lesion from cyst

Spreads out as it leaves
the capsule

Figure 18-51 Mushroom-shaped lesions. **A,** Angiomyolipoma entirely spread out over the capsule. **B,** Simple cyst. **C,** Renal cell carcinoma (unusual case). *AML,* Angiomyolipoma.

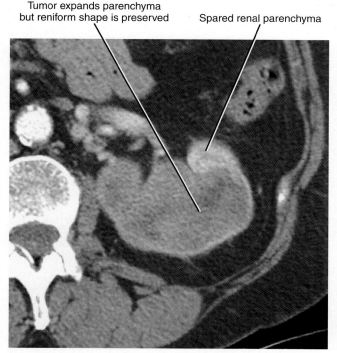

Tumor expands parenchyma
but reniform shape is preserved

Spared renal parenchyma

Figure 18-52 Axial image of the left kidney from a contrast-enhanced computed tomographic scan demonstrates the infiltrating appearance of intrarenal urothelial carcinoma.

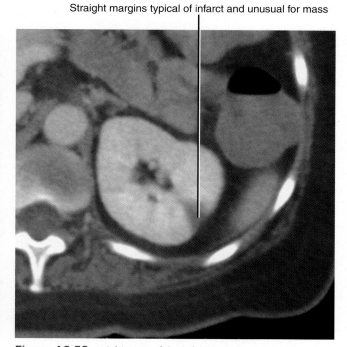

Straight margins typical of infarct and unusual for mass

Figure 18-53 Axial image of the left kidney from a contrast-enhanced computed tomographic scan demonstrates a wedge-shaped infarct in a patient with bacterial endocarditis.

Fluid

The presence of fluid within a renal lesion limits considerations to benign and malignant cysts, necrotic neoplasms, calyceal diverticula, or renal sinus cysts. On ultrasound, cystic lesions usually contain anechoic areas with enhanced through transmission. A lesion must have smooth walls and be completely anechoic to be characterized as a simple cyst by ultrasound. With CT, an attenuation threshold of 15 to 20 HU is often used to identify fluid, although the impact of image noise (particularly from beam hardening) limits attenuation measurement in small (<2 cm) lesions. Section thickness also impacts attenuation measurement in small lesions, because volume averaging will increase measured attenuation values. MRI can be more effective at characterizing small cystic lesions, because the fluid signal is less affected by lesion size.

The presence of fluid is less specific for lesion characterization than is the presence of fat. Rather, it is the

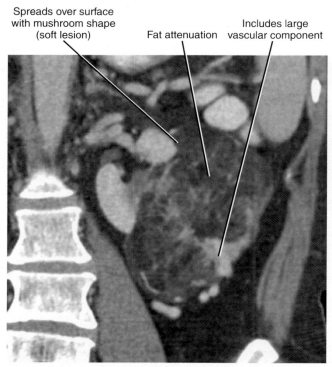

Spreads over surface with mushroom shape (soft lesion)

Fat attenuation

Includes large vascular component

Figure 18-54 Coronal reformation from a contrast-enhanced computed tomographic scan of the kidneys demonstrates a large fat-attenuation mass exophytic from the lateral aspect of inferior pole of the left kidney. This appearance is diagnostic of angiomyolipoma.

presence of nodules and septations that determine the likelihood of malignancy. Cystic renal carcinoma and multilocular cystic nephroma are leading considerations when there are enhancing septations within a predominantly cystic lesion. The presence of one or more enhancing nodules within a cystic mass is highly associated with malignant histology. The sonographic equivalent of enhancement in such cases is the demonstration of flow on color Doppler images.

Calyceal diverticula are urine-filled outpouchings from the intrarenal collecting system that can mimic other types of cystic lesions. The most common type arises from the fornix of a calyx and is called a *type I diverticulum* (Fig. 18-57). Type II diverticula arise from an infundibulum, and type III arise directly from the renal pelvis. Types I and II are located within the renal cortex. Type III diverticula are usually located within the renal sinus. All three usually appear cystic with cross-sectional imaging. Because they do not interface directly with a papilla, no urine is excreted directly into a calyceal diverticulum. Rather, they fill with urine via a thin communication to the normal collecting system. A postcontrast delay of 20 minutes or more may be necessary to demonstrate filling of a diverticulum with CT or MRI, depending on the size of the communication (Fig. 18-58).

Calyceal diverticula are prone to stasis and stone formation. When present, milk of calcium forms a fluid–calcium level within diverticula on upright radiographs (if suspected, allow several minutes for the sediment to

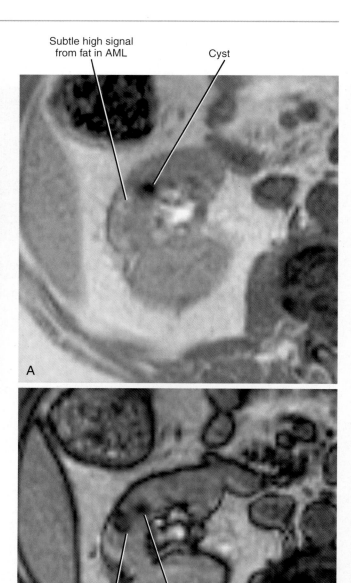

Subtle high signal from fat in AML

Cyst

A

India ink artifact around small AML

Cyst

B

Figure 18-55 Characterizing small angiomyolipomas (AMLs) with magnetic resonance imaging. **A,** Axial T1-weighted image performed in phase demonstrates a subtle high-attenuation lesion in the right kidney. **B,** Axial, out-of-phase, T1-weighted image shows India ink artifact around the lesion, indicating an interface between fat and fluid (renal cortex).

settle). A fluid–calcium level is often seen on CT without additional maneuvers, although if the diagnosis remains in doubt, prone positioning shows redistribution of the calcium. Rarely, carcinoma can arise within a calyceal diverticulum.

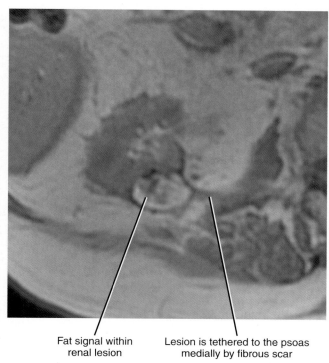

Fat signal within
renal lesion

Lesion is tethered to the psoas
medially by fibrous scar

Figure 18-56 Axial T1-weighted magnetic resonance image of the right kidney demonstrates a round, fat-containing lesion. This is a site of prior partial nephrectomy with perinephric fat packed into the site of resection.

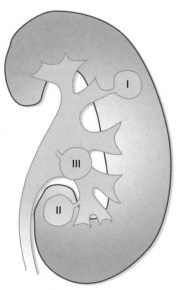

Figure 18-57 Illustration demonstrating variable origins of calyceal diverticula. *I*, From fornix (most common); *II*, from infundibulum; *III*, from renal pelvis.

Hemorrhage or Proteinaceous Debris

Occasionally, the contents of a benign cyst are not simple. That is to say, the cyst contains internal echoes with sonography, measures greater than 20 HU on CT, or does not follow the characteristic pattern of signal intensities of a simple cyst on MRI. The terms *complicated cyst* or *complex cyst* are often used to describe such lesions. Often, the contents of such cysts represent hemorrhagic or proteinaceous fluid. Lesions that are of uniform and very high attenuation on unenhanced CT (>70 HU) or uniform and very high signal intensity on unenhanced T1-weighted MR images are statistically likely to represent complicated cysts. However, we do not recommend relying solely on unenhanced CT or MRI to make a definitive diagnosis of benign cyst. Fortunately, definitive characterization can usually be accomplished with contrast-enhanced CT or MRI, as discussed in the next section.

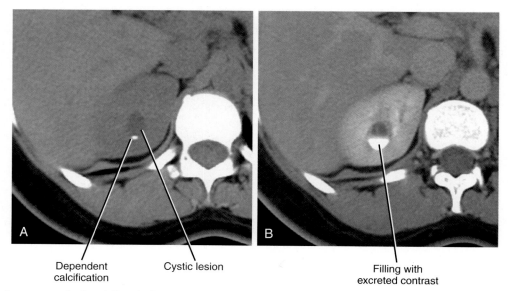

Dependent
calcification

Cystic lesion

Filling with
excreted contrast

Figure 18-58 Appearance of calyceal diverticulum on computed tomography (CT). **A,** Axial image of the right kidney from an unenhanced CT scan demonstrates minimal dependent calcium within a cystic lesion. **B,** Axial image at the same level during the excretory phase demonstrates excreted contrast filling the cyst indicating that it is a calyceal diverticulum.

Enhancement of Focal Renal Lesions

Regardless of echogenicity, attenuation, or signal intensity, benign simple renal cysts do not enhance after administration of intravenous contrast media and do not demonstrate blood flow with color Doppler imaging. Therefore, the presence of enhancement or flow within a lesion narrows the differential diagnosis to enhancing renal lesions. Depending on the lesion, enhancement on CT or MRI exams may be most apparent during either the corticomedullary or nephrographic phase (see Figs. 18-21 and 18-59).

Pearl: When CT or MRI is performed specifically to characterize a renal lesion, the examination should include unenhanced, corticomedullary-phase, and nephrographic-phase images.

Early literature suggested that any lesion with a measured increase in attenuation of 10 HU or more be considered enhancing. The fact is, small lesions (<2 cm) are susceptible not only to volume averaging (although less so with MDCT) but to beam hardening because of enhancement of the adjacent cortex. We recommend that small lesions with measured enhancement more than 10 HU be further imaged if not obviously malignant in appearance.

The most common solid enhancing renal mass by far is renal cell carcinoma. AMLs can enhance but usually contain fat. Unfortunately, AMLs with minimal fat and other benign but enhancing lesions, such as oncocytoma, cannot be reliably differentiated from malignancy. Thus, unless macroscopic fat is demonstrated, all enhancing renal masses are considered malignant until proved otherwise through biopsy or resection.

In most cases, it is not difficult to determine whether a lesion enhances on CT and MR images, provided a precontrast acquisition available. However, some renal lesions have baseline high attenuation on CT or high signal intensity on MRI, making subjective assessment of enhancement difficult. In such cases, subtraction images created by subtracting the precontrast data set from the postcontrast data set are helpful, because the baseline attenuation or signal is eliminated (Fig. 18-60). When subtraction is not possible, carefully placed ROIs can usually resolve the issue of enhancement.

Nonfatty renal masses that achieve a peak attenuation exceeding 100 HU after intravenous contrast administration are presumed to be renal carcinoma, with clear cell carcinoma the most likely subtype. Papillary renal cell carcinoma tends to enhance less avidly than clear cell carcinoma. This is important because papillary renal cell carcinoma can be mistaken for a benign cyst on nephrographic-phase CT or MR images if a careful assessment of lesion enhancement is not performed. AMLs with minimal fat can have a similar appearance to papillary renal cell carcinoma on enhanced CT and MR images. Although a "spoke wheel" pattern of vascularity has been described for oncocytomas angiographically, the distinction between renal cell carcinoma and oncocytoma cannot be reliably made based on CT and MRI enhancement patterns.

Because MRI does not expose patients to ionizing radiation, every MRI protocol should include unenhanced images. Unfortunately, many CT protocols do not include precontrast images in an effort to reduce radiation dose. Attempts have been made to distinguish between benign hyperdense cysts and renal cell carcinoma based on the attenuation change between the corticomedullary and nephrographic phases of enhancement on CT. Although a high-attenuation renal mass that changes less than 10 HU between these phases is likely benign, this finding does not entirely exclude renal cell carcinoma.

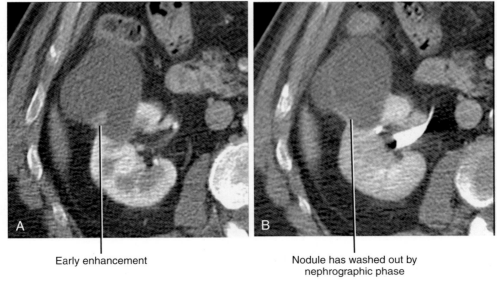

Early enhancement

Nodule has washed out by nephrographic phase

Figure 18-59 Value of multiphase examination for evaluation of cystic renal lesions. **A,** Axial computed tomographic image of the right kidney during the corticomedullary phase of enhancement demonstrates nodular enhancement within a cystic lesion. **B,** Enhancement is much less conspicuous during the nephrographic phase. A cystic renal cell carcinoma was removed surgically.

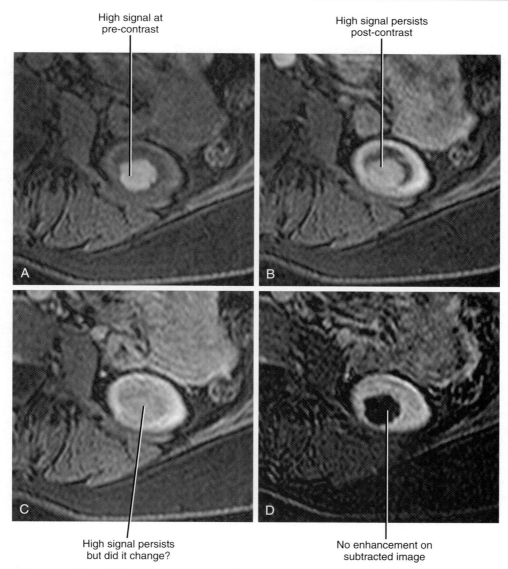

High signal at
pre-contrast

High signal persists
post-contrast

High signal persists
but did it change?

No enhancement on
subtracted image

Figure 18-60 Axial images of the left kidney demonstrate the utility of subtraction technique for hemorrhagic cysts on magnetic resonance imaging. **A,** T1-weighted baseline image, **(B)** corticomedullary phase after injection, **(C)** nephrographic phase, and **(D)** subtracted nephrographic-phase image. All series were performed with identical scan parameters including frequency-selective fat suppression.

■ DISTINGUISHING BENIGN FROM MALIGNANT RENAL LESIONS

Cystic Lesions

With ultrasound, benign simple renal cysts are round with a sharply defined far wall, are anechoic, and demonstrate acoustic enhancement. Although a thin septum of uniform thickness (no more than 1 mm thick) can be tolerated, any suggestion of thicker septa, mural or septal irregularity, internal echoes (other than layering milk of calcium), or mural nodularity precludes the diagnosis of simple cyst. Although some such lesions will be ultimately proved benign, further imaging evaluation is usually warranted. We rarely recommend treatment of a cystic-appearing renal mass on the basis of ultrasound alone.

In 1986, Morton Bosniak introduced a system for classifying renal cysts according to features seen with CT. Although the system has been modified several times since its introduction, it remains in widespread use today. The classification system uses several key imaging features, which are summarized in Table 18-15.

Although the Bosniak classification system is useful, a fair amount of subjectivity can be introduced. Discriminating between class IIf and III lesions is perhaps the most difficult distinction. Several useful principles exist in this regard. First, *benign septa should be quite thin*, even where they join together. If septa thicken where they meet each other or the wall, this suggests the class III category is appropriate (Fig. 18-61). Second, *any internal enhancement is suspicious*. Complex cystic lesions are best evaluated on both corticomedullary- and nephrographic-phase images, because the optimal time for visualizing enhancing components varies (see Fig. 18-59).

Table 18-15   Bosniak Classification of Cystic Renal Masses

Class	Imaging Features	Management
I	Simple cyst: water attenuation, no enhancement or septa	None
II	Mildly complicated cyst: few, thin septa or minimal thin-wall calcification	None
IIf	Indeterminate lesion with low malignant potential: high-attenuation cysts that are not exophytic, mildly irregular or increased number of septa	Imaging surveillance
III	Suspicious: many septa, coarse calcification, nodular wall components that do not enhance, heterogeneous attenuation	Surgical resection
IV	Highly suspicious: enhancing nodular wall components, irregular walls	Surgical resection

The Bosniak classification was originally developed for CT. However, studies have shown that the similar criteria can be applied to MR images. MRI using both fat suppression and subtraction is also effective for identifying subtle areas of enhancement and can be used effectively to further characterize problem lesions (Fig. 18-62). In thin patients with accessible lesions, ultrasound can also sometimes show internal cyst architecture not visible with CT. From a practical point of view, we divide lesions into three categories, as presented in Table 18-16.

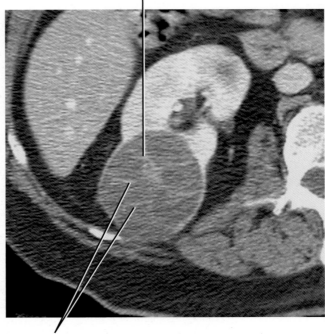

Nodular tissue at junction of septa

Multiple thin but enhancing septa

Figure 18-61 Axial image of the right kidney from a contrast-enhanced computed tomographic scan demonstrates a multiloculated cystic lesion proved to be renal cell carcinoma at surgery.

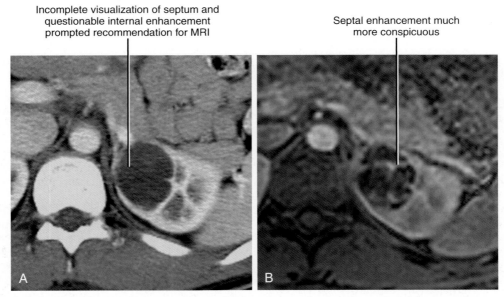

Incomplete visualization of septum and questionable internal enhancement prompted recommendation for MRI

Septal enhancement much more conspicuous

Figure 18-62 Value of subtracted magnetic resonance images for detecting septal enhancement. **A,** Axial computed tomographic image of the left kidney during the corticomedullary phase of enhancement demonstrates questionable faint attenuation abnormality that prompted a recommendation for magnetic resonance imaging (MRI). **B,** Subtracted postcontrast T1-weighted image demonstrates clear evidence of enhancement within the lesion, prompting resection of a cystic renal cell carcinoma.

Table 18-16   Simplified Approach to Renal Cysts

What to Do	Bosniak Class	Features
Leave it alone	I, II	Anechoic (US) Homogeneous water attenuation (CT) or SI (MR) Round with smooth, sharply defined margins Thin (≤1 mm) wall or septa (up to 2 septa) No more than thin mural or septal calcification No enhancement (CT/MR) or flow (Doppler US) Milk of calcium
Follow or further imaging	IIf	Low-level echoes (US) >2 thin septa Borderline attenuation change (10-20 HU) that is likely the result of beam hardening on CT Thick or nodular calcification
Intervene	III, IV	Thick, irregular, or nodular enhancing wall Unequivocal internal enhancement (CT/MR) or flow (Doppler US)

CT, Computed tomography; *MR,* magnetic resonance; *SI,* signal intensity; *US,* ultrasound.

Solid Lesions

In general, solid lesions discovered with sonography require further imaging with CT or MRI for definitive characterization. The only reliable discriminator between benign and malignant solid lesions on CT and MRI is the presence of macroscopic fat. When there is clear evidence of macroscopic fat within a solid mass on CT or MR images, a diagnosis of AML can usually be made. A solid renal mass that contains intracellular lipid detected with chemical-shift MRI in the absence of macroscopic fat should not be classified as an AML. Instead, intracellular lipid is a feature of the *clear cell subtype of renal cell carcinoma.*

Papillary renal cell carcinomas also have a characteristic MR appearance, often demonstrating low signal intensity on T2-weighted images, intermediate signal intensity on T1-weighted images, and only mild-to-moderate enhancement after intravenous administration of gadolinium-based contrast media. Unfortunately, AMLs with minimal or no fat can also have this appearance.

Occasionally, findings outside of the kidney can help confirm the malignant nature of a renal mass. For example, enhancing tissue within the renal vein or IVC suggests renal vein invasion by renal cell carcinoma. Unfortunately, even this sign is not entirely specific, because benign lesions such as AML have been reported to grow into the renal vein on rare occasions.

Infectious processes such as renal abscess or focal pyelonephritis can sometimes mimic a malignant neoplastic process (Fig. 18-63). In such cases, the clinical scenario is often the key to making the correct diagnosis. Short-term imaging follow-up after appropriate antibiotic therapy can also be helpful (see Fig. 18-45).

Percutaneous Biopsy of Focal Renal Lesions

Commonly accepted indications for percutaneous biopsy of focal renal lesions include distinguishing renal cell carcinoma from metastases or lymphoma in patients with a known malignancy, or from focal pyelonephritis or abscess when there are signs of infection.

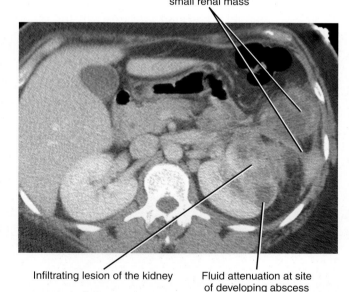

Stranding in perirenal fat and adjacent thickening of the colon more severe than expected for small renal mass

Infiltrating lesion of the kidney

Fluid attenuation at site of developing abscess

Figure 18-63 Axial image of the kidneys from a contrast-enhanced computed tomographic scan demonstrates masslike appearance in the kidney caused by focal pyelonephritis with abscess formation. Ample clinical signs of infection were present as well.

Biopsy is also indicated when tumor is unresectable so that a tissue diagnosis can be used to direct therapeutic decisions.

Recent literature supports an increasing role of percutaneous biopsy of small renal masses. This is due, in part, to the increased utilization of MDCT resulting in the incidental detection of an abundance of small enhancing renal masses. Although solid renal masses were once thought to be overwhelmingly malignant, recent series show a high number of benign lesions among small renal masses (nearly half of lesions less than 1 cm in diameter). Biopsy of small renal masses can be used to avoid surgery or ablation for benign lesions and to verify tissue type before ablation. The role of percutaneous biopsy in characterizing indeterminate cystic lesions of the kidney is more controversial.

Because of the renewed interest in renal biopsy, it is more important now than ever to distinguish primary vascular lesions of the kidney from other causes of renal mass.

Renal artery aneurysms are easily diagnosed with color Doppler ultrasound or enhanced CT and MRI (see Fig. 18-48E). Aneurysms follow the enhancement pattern of the aorta and renal artery, thus they tend to enhance more uniformly than renal carcinoma and wash out more quickly on CT and MRI. Often, a rim of mural thrombus or curvilinear wall calcification is evident. Maximum intensity projection or volume rendering may help map relations of the relevant vessels before embolization or surgery (Fig. 18-64).

Renal arteriovenous malformations and *fistulas* can be congenital (sometimes called *cirsoid malformations*) or acquired. Patients may have high-output heart failure, hypertension related to renal parenchymal hypoperfusion, or hematuria. On ultrasound, vascular structures are seen with high-velocity, low-resistance flow. There may be abnormal pulsatility in the renal vein (Fig. 18-65). On CT, large vessels are present within the renal sinus and hilum. With multiphase CT, the venous structures opacify almost as briskly as the arteries early in the arterial phase of enhancement (Fig. 18-66), a finding characteristic of arteriovenous communication. Findings are similar on MRI, although flow voids within the kidney can often suggest the diagnosis on unenhanced images.

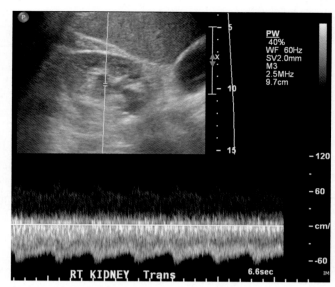

Figure 18-65 Spectral Doppler evaluation of a dilated structure in the renal sinus demonstrates pulsatility within the renal vein, commonly seen with arteriovenous communication.

Tubular structures enhance similar to aorta

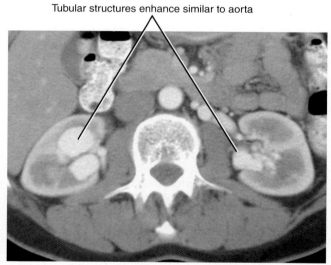

Figure 18-66 Bilateral renal arteriovenous malformations. Axial image of the kidneys from contrast-enhanced computed tomography performed in the arterial phase demonstrates arterial enhancement of dilated vessels in the renal sinus of each kidney.

■ NEPHROCALCINOSIS

Nephrocalcinosis refers to calcification of the renal parenchyma and is associated with a variety of conditions shown in Table 18-17. Medullary nephrocalcinosis is the most common type of nephrocalcinosis. This appears as punctuate or "smudgelike" calcifications within the renal papillae seen best on unenhanced CT (Fig. 18-67). Medullary nephrocalcinosis can be detected sonographically as echogenic renal pyramids. A Randall's plaque is a mild form of medullary nephrocalcinosis in which a concretion forms from the tip of the papilla, much like an icicle. Although Randall's plaques cannot pass into

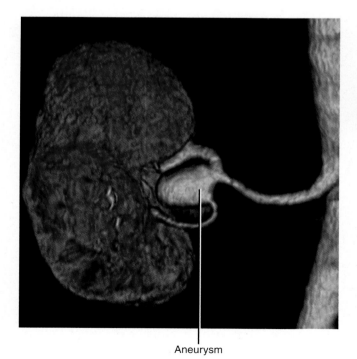

Aneurysm

Figure 18-64 Volume rendering from computed tomographic angiogram performed to plan a surgical approach to addressing this complex aneurysm at the initial division of the right renal artery.

Table 18-17   Causes of Nephrocalcinosis

Medullary	Hyperparathyroidism and other causes of hypercalcemia Medullary sponge kidney Renal tubular acidosis (type I) (Rarely, tuberculosis or furosemide use)
Cortical	Chronic glomerulonephritis Acute cortical necrosis (shock, toxic ingestion) Lithium toxicity (Rarely, Alport syndrome, chronic transplant rejection)
Both	Oxalosis (primary or secondary)

Larger, more central calcification is probably a calculus   Punctate calcifications in the renal medulla

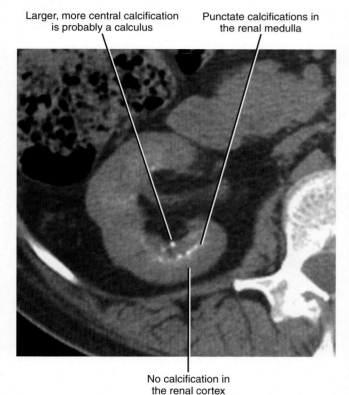

No calcification in the renal cortex

Figure 18-67 Axial image of the right kidney from an unenhanced computed tomographic scan in a patient with medullary sponge kidney demonstrates a typical appearance of medullary nephrocalcinosis.

Stippled calcification confined to the renal cortex

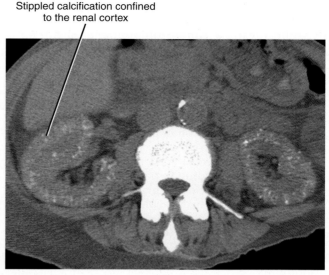

Figure 18-68 Axial image from an unenhanced computed tomographic scan demonstrates cortical nephrocalcinosis in a patient with lithium toxicity.

Small stone   No contrast in the aorta

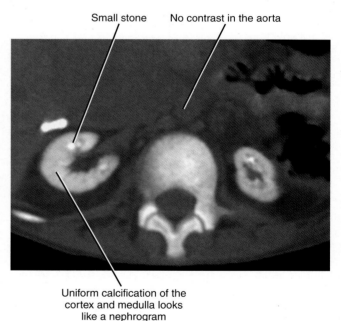

Uniform calcification of the cortex and medulla looks like a nephrogram

Figure 18-69 Axial image of the kidneys from an unenhanced computed tomographic scan demonstrates combined medullary and cortical nephrocalcinosis in a child who has undergone recent transplantation for primary hyperoxaluria (surgical drain anterior to right kidney).

the ureter while they are attached to the papilla, they may detach from the papilla and enlarge to form a calyceal stone.

Cortical nephrocalcinosis describes calcifications in the renal cortex and is much less common than medullary nephrocalcinosis. The calcifications can either be smooth, uniform, or tram-track–like calcifications, as usually seen with chronic glomerulonephritis or more patchy or striated calcifications associated with cortical necrosis or nephrotoxic medications (Fig. 18-68). Cortical nephrocalcinosis can occur in conjunction with medullary nephrocalcinosis in individuals with oxalosis (Fig. 18-69).

■ HYDRONEPHROSIS AND ITS MIMICS

Imaging Appearance of Hydronephrosis Related to Urinary Tract Obstruction

Suspected obstruction is one of the most common reasons to image the urinary tract. Despite their small size, the kidneys receive more than a liter of blood per minute and filter, on average, 180 L of fluid per day, of which 99% is reabsorbed. Needless to say, with such a dynamic organ, a simple plumbing problem turns quickly into a clinical crisis. As pressure builds in an obstructed urinary tract, the intrarenal collecting system distends. Note that although a preexisting extrarenal pelvis tends to dilate readily, a renal pelvis encased by solid parenchyma within the renal sinus is less distensible. Thus, the relative amount of pyelectasis and caliectasis is variable and dependent, in part, on anatomy. Prolonged high pressure within the calyx causes compression and decreased perfusion of the renal papillae, eventually leading to papillary necrosis.

On ultrasound, the dilated calyces, infundibula, and pelvis of obstructive hydronephrosis are easily demonstrated. It is important to be certain that the anechoic structures thought to represent hydronephrosis are truly the renal collecting system and not renal sinus cysts. In the setting of hydronephrosis, the dilated renal pelvis, infundibula, and calyces interconnect. Color Doppler can be useful to avoid confusing venous structures for dilated collecting system. Because hydronephrosis results in an increase in the interstitial pressure within the renal parenchyma, spectral Doppler evaluation may reveal an increase in resistive index (most studies use a threshold value of 0.70 or greater), although this finding is not specific.

Unenhanced CT is usually the first-line examination for suspected acute ureteral obstruction, particularly when stone disease is suspected. The presence of asymmetric fat stranding implies acute obstruction as the cause of hydronephrosis. Attenuation of the renal cortex of the obstructed kidney is often at least 5 HU less than the other kidney, a finding that is more specific than it is sensitive. As with ultrasound, renal sinus cysts are a common mimic of hydronephrosis on unenhanced CT.

On contrast-enhanced IVU, CT, and MRI examinations, the increased pressure caused by obstruction results in delayed onset of the nephrogram on the obstructed side. Eventually, the nephrogram becomes dense and striated (Fig. 18-70). Excretion is delayed compared with the contralateral side. On CT and MRI, delayed enhancement appears as a persistent corticomedullary phase (see Fig. 18-42). Because hydronephrosis acts like a sac of fluid, excreted contrast is dilute at first, accumulating slowly over time. Excreted contrast first makes crescents outlining the papillae, with subsequent puddling within dilated calyces. In complete obstruction, contrast excretion eventually ceases.

T2-weighted MRI is more sensitive than CT for detecting fluid around the kidney in the setting of acute obstruction, both within the fat and along the capsule (Fig. 18-71). Fat suppression improves conspicuity of fluid in the perirenal space. MRI is less sensitive than CT for detecting stones, however, and many calculi can be missed, particularly when not surrounded by urine.

Persistent urinary obstruction causes a transition from a state of high pressure to a state of normal pressure through declining renal function. Damage to the papillae and poor renal perfusion in the face of high interstitial pressure within the parenchyma eventually result in cortical atrophy (see Fig. 18-29). These effects are often seen in patients with congenital UPJ obstruction.

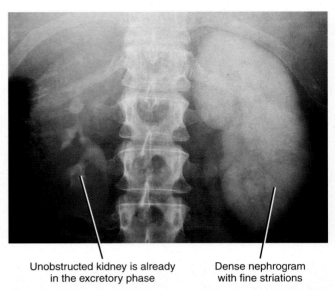

Unobstructed kidney is already in the excretory phase   Dense nephrogram with fine striations

Figure 18-70 Image from an intravenous urogram demonstrates a dense, striated left nephrogram in a patient with a left ureteral calculus.

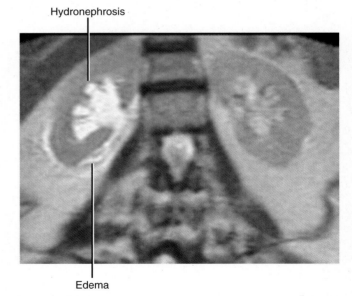

Hydronephrosis

Edema

Figure 18-71 Coronal T2-weighted image of the kidneys demonstrates right-sided hydronephrosis and perirenal edema in a patient with a right ureteral calculus.

Although UPJ obstruction is often identified in utero, severity and age at diagnosis are quite variable. Symptoms of UPJ obstruction can be exacerbated by diuresis (e.g., alcohol intake), and the fluid-filled renal sinus is vulnerable to rupture from trauma (Fig. 18-72).

Nuclear scintigraphy with MAG3 and diuretic augmentation is often used to evaluate patients with suspected UPJ obstruction. The normal kidney achieves maximum accumulation of radiotracer in about 5 minutes, with clearance of 50% of the tracer ($T_{1/2}$) within about 10 minutes. A $T_{1/2}$ exceeding 20 minutes is considered abnormal, indicating obstruction (Fig. 18-73). In UPJ obstruction, the degree of obstruction becomes worse

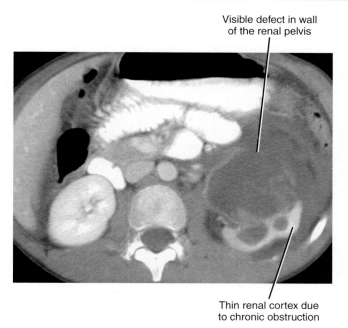

Visible defect in wall
of the renal pelvis

Thin renal cortex due
to chronic obstruction

Figure 18-72 Axial image of the kidneys from contrast-enhanced computed tomography performed after a low-speed motor vehicle collision demonstrates rupture of previously undiagnosed congenital ureteropelvic junction obstruction.

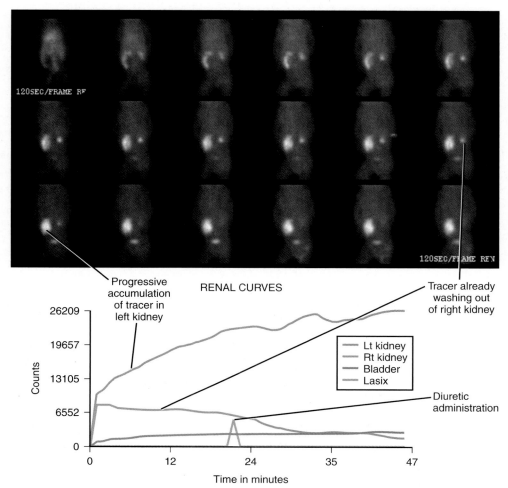

Progressive
accumulation
of tracer in
left kidney

RENAL CURVES

Tracer already
washing out
of right kidney

Diuretic
administration

— Lt kidney
— Rt kidney
— Bladder
— Lasix

Counts

Time in minutes

Figure 18-73 Posterior images from technetium 99m-mercaptoacetyltriglycin (MAG3) study performed with furosemide demonstrates abnormal clearing of urine from the left kidney as a result of congenital uteropelvic junction obstruction.

with further dilatation of the renal pelvis. Thus, low-grade UPJ obstruction subjected to diuresis (with either furosemide or beer) may become a high-grade obstruction.

Urinary obstruction usually occurs at the level of the ureter, because the long, thin tube is vulnerable to traveling stones, clots, and papillae, as well as a variety of tumors and even surgeons. Box 18-4 provides a list of the most common causes of ureteral obstruction. Bilateral hydronephrosis can be the result of abnormalities involving both ureters, the bladder, or the urethra, and causes of bilateral hydronephrosis are described in the section "Imaging Evaluation for Renal Failure" and summarized in Box 18-3.

Nonobstructive Mimics of Obstructive Hydronephrosis

Because urine can be difficult to distinguish from other types of simple fluid on grayscale ultrasound and unenhanced CT and MRI, many mimics of urinary tract obstruction exist for these examinations. Table 18-18 lists the most common nonobstructive conditions that can mimic urinary obstruction on imaging examinations.

BOX 18-4 Causes of Urinary Obstruction
Ureteral calculus
Blood clot/hematuria
Sloughed papilla
Cancer of the cervix and uterus
Prostatic hypertrophy
Bladder cancer
Ureteral cancer
Rectal cancer
Iatrogenic injury
Trauma
Neurogenic bladder
Urethral stricture
Radiation therapy

Table 18-18 Mimics of Urinary Obstruction

Mimic	Distinguishing Features and Comments
Renal sinus cysts (Figs. 18-74 through 18-76)	Do not contain contrast on excretory-phase images Are not confluent centrally (dilated calyces are confluent with the renal pelvis) Peripelvic cysts are primary lymphatic cysts of the renal sinus and are usually multiple Parapelvic cysts are exophytic cortical cyst that protrude into the renal sinus (Fig. 18-77)
Extrarenal pelvis (see Fig. 18-7)	Calyces are not dilated Ureter appears normal Often bilateral but may be asymmetric
Ureteral reflux (Fig. 18-78)	Suspect in infants and children with hydronephrosis and hydroureter Confirm with VCUG or bladder scintigraphy Consider reflux in adults with hydronephrosis and hydroureter but no evidence of obstruction on excretory-phase images by any technique Common finding with urinary diversions, less common with renal transplants
Hydronephrosis of pregnancy (Fig. 18-79)	Ureteral jet is usually present on color Doppler US and may be augmented by turning the patient away from the symptomatic side (relieves compression) No stone on low-dose NCCT or two-shot IVU A persistently dilated ureter below the common point of compression of the ureter between the gravid uterus and sacral promontory indicates distal ureteral obstruction rather than hydronephrosis of pregnancy
Bacterial pyelonephritis (Fig. 18-80)	US demonstrates ureteral jet and may show urothelial thickening With obstruction, attenuation of the renal parenchyma can be at least 5 HU lower on the symptomatic side because of infiltrating edema (fluid); this is not the case with cellular infiltration caused by pyelonephritis
Xanthogranulomatous pyelonephritis (Fig. 18-81)	Staghorn calculus typically present Excretory function is absent from all or part of the kidney Rounded structures are a combination of papillae infiltrated with lipid-laden macrophages and pus-filled calyces
Renal AVM (Fig. 18-82)	Dilated spaces fill with flow on color Doppler US or with contrast during contrast-enhanced CT or MRI
Autosomal dominant polycystic kidney disease (see Fig. 18-36)	Dilated spaces do not communicate with the renal pelvis on US and do not fill with contrast on excretory-phase images from contrast-enhanced CT or MRI
Megacalyces (Fig. 18-83)	With primary megacalycosis, calyces are often increased not only in size but in number (instead of 8-10 calyces, may have >20) Flat shape of the renal papillae results in "squaring" of the calyces Renal pelvis and the ureter are normal

AVM, Arteriovenous malformation; *CT,* computed tomography; *IVU,* intravenous urogram; *MRI,* magnetic resonance imaging; *NCCT,* noncontrast-enhanced computed tomography; *US,* ultrasound; *VCUG,* voiding cystourethrography.

Central cystic structures do not
connect to the renal pelvis

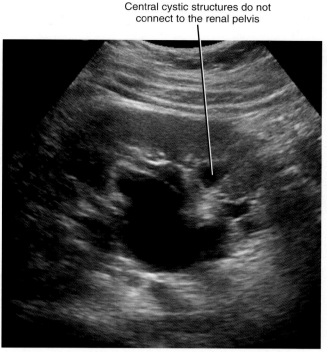

Figure 18-74 Differentiating renal sinus cysts from hydronephrosis on ultrasound. Diagnosis of renal sinus cyst was subsequently confirmed by a computed tomographic scan with delayed images.

Low attenuation structures
fill renal sinus

Peripelvic cysts remain unopacified

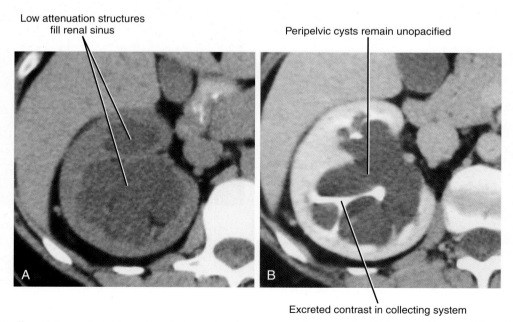

Excreted contrast in collecting system

Figure 18-75 Differentiating peripelvic cysts from hydronephrosis on computed tomography (CT). **A,** Axial image of the right kidney from enhanced CT has an appearance identical to hydronephrosis (although the ureter was normal more distally). **B,** Axial image of the same kidney in the excretory phase proves the cystic structures are not in continuity with the collecting system.

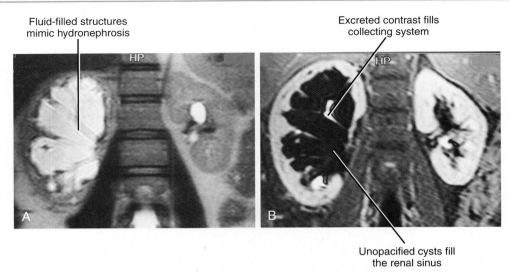

Fluid-filled structures
mimic hydronephrosis

Excreted contrast fills
collecting system

Unopacified cysts fill
the renal sinus

Figure 18-76 Differentiating renal sinus cysts from hydronephrosis on magnetic resonance imaging. **A,** Peripelvic cysts mimic hydronephrosis on coronal T2-weighted image. **B,** On excretory-phase, contrast-enhanced, T1-weighted images, thin collecting system structures become opacified; the cysts do not.

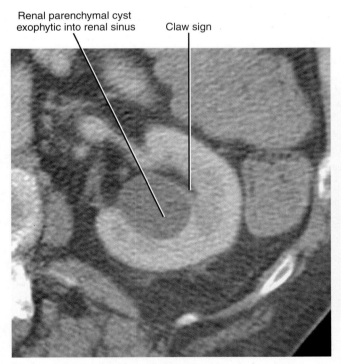

Renal parenchymal cyst
exophytic into renal sinus

Claw sign

Figure 18-77 Axial image of the left kidney from a contrast-enhanced computed tomographic scan demonstrates a rounded cortical cyst protruding into the renal sinus, characteristic of a parapelvic cyst. This type of spherical cystic lesion is occasionally confused with a dilated renal pelvis on sonography but should be accurately characterized because of the absence of caliectasis.

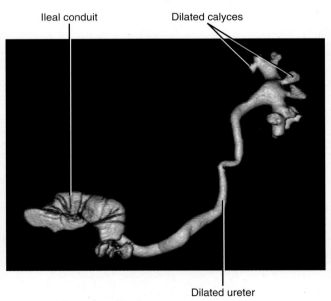

Ileal conduit

Dilated calyces

Dilated ureter

Figure 18-78 Three-dimensional volume rendering from a computed tomographic urogram performed for hematuria in a patient with ileal conduit because of cystectomy for bladder cancer. The appearance of hydroureteronephrosis on left side because of reflux is common with urinary diversions. The right kidney was replaced with recurrent urothelial carcinoma; thus, it did not opacify with contrast.

Bilateral
hydronephrosis

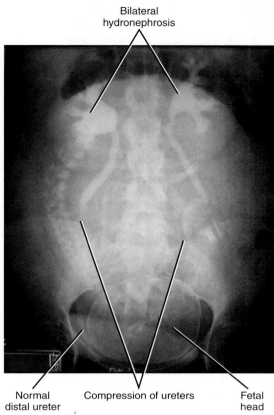

Normal   Compression of ureters   Fetal
distal ureter   head

Figure 18-79 Hydronephrosis of pregnancy. Image from an intravenous urogram demonstrates a third-trimester pregnancy compressing both ureters as they enter the pelvis, resulting in hydronephrosis and hydroureter. A short segment of normal distal ureter can be seen on the right side.

Dilated renal pelvis   Fat stranding

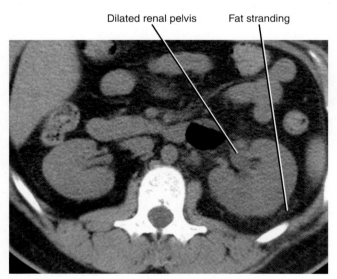

Figure 18-80 Axial image of the kidneys from unenhanced computed tomography performed for suspected ureterolithiasis demonstrates dilatation of the left renal pelvis associated with perinephric stranding. No calcifications were in the ureter, and the presence of pyuria and leukocytosis confirmed a diagnosis of pyelonephritis.

Areas of low attenuation
outlined by thin rim of cortex

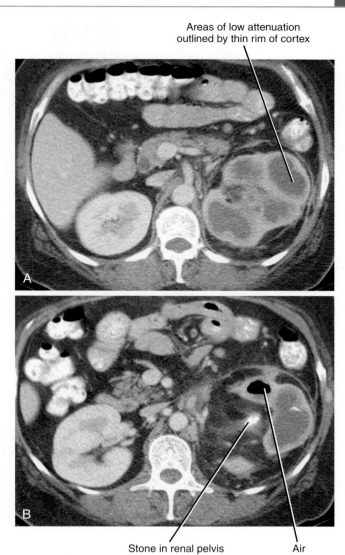

Stone in renal pelvis   Air

Figure 18-81 Xanthogranulomatous pyelonephritis (XGP) on computed tomography. **A,** Axial image of the kidneys from a contrast-enhanced computed tomographic scan of a patient with XGP demonstrates pronounced corticomedullary differentiation caused by foamy macrophages and pus-filled calyces in the medullary region. **B,** A more inferior image demonstrates an obstructing stone in the renal pelvis. Although unusual, air was also present in this patient who had symptoms of acute infection.

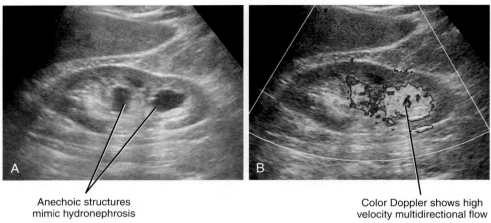

Anechoic structures
mimic hydronephrosis

Color Doppler shows high
velocity multidirectional flow

Figure 18-82 Renal arteriovenous malformation (AVM) as mimic of hydronephrosis. **A,** Sagittal image of the right kidney demonstrates a renal AVM that looks like hydronephrosis. **B,** Color Doppler imaging demonstrates pronounced flow within the anechoic structures.

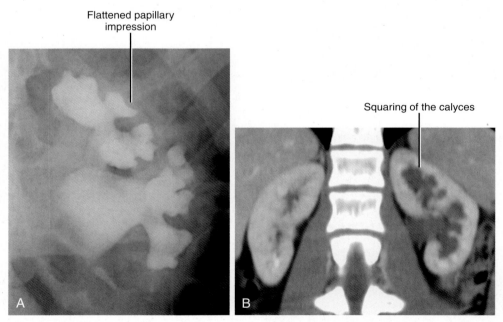

Flattened papillary
impression

Squaring of the calyces

Figure 18-83 Differentiating megacalycosis from hydronephrosis. **A,** Image from an intravenous urogram in a patient with megacalyces demonstrates the flattened appearance of the papillae. **B,** Coronal reformation from contrast-enhanced computed tomography of the same patient demonstrates squaring of the calyces, a result of the congenitally flat papillae.

Suggested Readings

Bachorzewska-Gajewska H, Jolanta M, Jacek SM et al: Undiagnosed renal impairment in patients with and without diabetes with normal serum creatinine undergoing percutaneous coronary intervention, *Nephrology* 11:549-554, 2006.

Biseglia M, Galliani CA, Senger C et al: Renal cystic diseases: a review, *Adv Anat Pathol* 13:26-56, 2006.

Carter AR, Horgan JG, Jennings TA et al: The junctional parenchymal defect: a sonographic variant of renal anatomy, *Radiology* 154:499-502, 1985.

Chang SL: Magnetic resonance imaging detected renal volume reduction in refluxing and nonrefluxing kidneys, *J Urol* 178:2550-2554, 2007.

Chow LC: Split-bolus MDCT urography with synchronous nephrographic and excretory phase enhancement, *Am J Roentgenol* 189:314-322, 2007.

D'Angelo PC, Gash JR, Horn AW et al: Fat in renal cell carcinoma that lacks calcification, *Am J Roentgenol* 178(4):931-932, 2002.

Gay SB, Armistead JP, Weber ME, Williamson BR: Left infrarenal region: anatomic variants, pathologic conditions, and diagnostic pitfalls, *Radiographics* 11:549-570, 1991.

Georgiades CS, Moore CJ, Smith DP: Differences of renal parenchymal attenuation for acutely obstructed and unobstructed kidneys on unenhanced helical CT: a useful secondary sign? *Am J Roentgenol* 176:965-968, 2001.

Hann L, Pfister RC: Renal subcortical rim sign: new etiologies and pathogenesis, *Am J Roentgenol* 138:51-54, 1982.

Johnson AJ, Levey AS, Coresh J et al: Clinical practice guidelines for chronic kidney disease in adults: part I. Definition, disease stages, evaluation, treatment and risk factors, *Am Fam Physician* 70(5):869-876, 2004.

Jonisch AI, Rubinowitz AN, Mutalik PG et al: Can high-attenuation renal cysts be differentiated from renal cell carcinoma at unenhanced CT? *Radiology* 243:445-450, 2007.

Kamel IR, Berkowitz JF: Assessment of the cortical rim sign in posttraumatic renal infarction, *J Comput Assist Tomogr* 20:5, 1996.

Kawamoto S, Lawler LP, Fishman E: Evaluation of the renal venous system on late arterial and venous phase images with MDCT angiography in potential living laparoscopic renal donors, *Am J Roentgenol* 184:539-545, 2005.

Laugharne M: Multidetector CT angiography in live donor renal transplantation: experience from 156 consecutive cases at a single centre, *Transplant Int* 20:156-166, 2007.

Lawler LP, Jarret TW, Corl FM et al: Adult ureteropelvic junction obstruction: insights with three-dimensional multi-detector row CT, *Radiographics* 25(1):121-134, 2005.

Lesavre A, Correas JM, Merran S et al: CT of papillary renal cell carcinomas with cholesterol necrosis mimicking angiomyolipomas, *Am J Roentgenol* 181:143-145, 2003.

Levy EM, Viscoli CM, Horwitz RI: The effect of acute renal failure on mortality: a cohort analysis, *JAMA* 275:1489-1494, 1996.

McCullough PA, Adam A, Becker CR et al: Risk prediction of contrast-induced nephropathy, *Am J Cardiol* 98(6A):27-36, 2006.

Mehran R, Aymong ED, Nkolsky E et al: A sample risk score for prediction of contrast-induced nephropathy after percutaneous coronary intervention, *J Am Coll Cardiol* 44(7):1393-1399, 2004.

Monil J, Pernas J, Montserat E et al: CT features of abdominal plasma cell neoplasms, *Eur Radiol* 15:1705-1712, 2005.

Namasivayam S, Kalra MK, Small WC et al: Multidetector row computed tomography evaluation of potential living laparoscopic renal donors: the story so far, *Curr Probl Diagn Radiol* 35:102-114, 2006.

O'Neill CW: Sonographic evaluation of renal failure, *Am J Kidney* 35(6):1021-1038, 2000.

Platt JF, Rubin JM, Ellis JH: Acute renal failure: possible role of duplex Doppler US in distinction between acute prerenal failure and acute tubular necrosis, *Radiology* 179:419-423, 1991.

Rudnick M: Contrast-induced nephropathy: what are the true clinical consequences? *Clin J Am Soc Nephrol* 3:263-272, 2008.

Sahani DV, Rastogi H, Greenfield AC et al: Multi-detector row CT in evaluation of 94 living renal donors by reader with varied experience, *Radiology* 235:905-910, 2005.

Saunders HS, Dyer RB, Shifrin RY et al: The CT nephrogram: implications for the evaluation of urinary tract disease, *Radiographics* 15:1069-1085, 1995.

Silverman SG, Gan YU, Mortele KJ et al: Renal masses in the adult patient: the role of percutaneous biopsy, *Radiology* 240:6-22, 2006.

Stanson AW, Friese JL, Johnson M et al: Polyarteritis nodosa: spectrum of angiographic findings, *Radiographics* 21:151-159, 2001.

Stevens LA, Coresh J, Greene T, Levey AS: Assessing kidney function—measured and estimated glomerular filtration rate, *N Engl J Med* 354:2473-2483, 2006.

Suh M, Coakley FV, Qayyum A et al: Distinction of renal cell carcinomas from high-attenuation renal cysts at portal venous phase contrast-enhanced CT, *Radiology* 228:330-334, 2003.

Suzer O, Shirkhoda A, Jafri SZ et al: CT features of renal infarction, *Eur J Radiol* 44:59-64, 2002.

Wile GE, Leyendecker JR, Krehbiel KA et al: CT and MR imaging after imaging-guided thermal ablation of renal neoplasms, *Radiographics* 27:325-339, 2007.

Wong WS, Moss AA, Federle MP et al: Renal infarction: CT diagnosis and correlation between CT findings and etiologies, *Radiology* 150:201-205, 1984.

Zagoria RJ, Gasser T, Leyendecker JR et al: Differentiation of renal neoplasms from high-density cysts: use of attenuation changes between the corticomedullary and nephrographic phases of computed tomography, *J Comput Assist Tomogr* 31:37-41, 2007.

CHAPTER 19

Ureters, Bladder, and Urethra

Neal C. Dalrymple

◼ ANATOMY OF THE URINARY TRACT

Anatomy of the Ureters

The ureters are muscular tubes with an internal lining of urothelium (previously called *transitional epithelium*). During development, each ureter begins as a ureteric bud arising from the mesonephric duct near the cloaca. The ureteric bud elongates in a cephalad direction until it reaches the metanephric blastema, which is induced to form a kidney.

Each ureter begins at a cone-shaped junction with the renal pelvis, the ureteropelvic junction (UPJ), then courses anterior to the psoas muscles in the retroperitoneum and enters the bladder at the trigone. The trigone is the triangular portion of bladder between the bladder neck and the two *ureteral orifices* (often called the *UO* by urologists). The ureters normally pass dorsal to the gonadal vessels and ventral to the iliac vessels. Organized antegrade peristaltic waves work in cooperation with gravity to facilitate passage of urine from each kidney to the bladder.

Anatomy of the Bladder

The urinary bladder is a highly distensible, muscular reservoir for urine that fills with continuous flow from the ureters and empties periodically through the urethra. Urothelium lines the lumen, and the detrusor muscle forms the bulk of the bladder wall. When empty (or nearly empty), the bladder is relatively flat in the craniocaudal direction. A layer of peritoneum rests over the dome of the bladder like a blanket. As it fills, the bladder becomes ellipsoid, lifting the peritoneum from the anterior abdominal wall (like peeking under the blanket). Therefore, the anterior bladder wall is in continuity with the extraperitoneal prevesical space (of Retzius). In women, the peritoneum drops behind the bladder before rising to encase the uterus, creating a peritoneal recess called the *vesicouterine pouch*. A similar peritoneal recess between the rectum and bladder in men is called the *rectovesical pouch*.

Early in development, the bladder empties through the umbilicus through a tube called the *urachus*. The urachus involutes in utero to form the median umbilical ligament, a long cord just superficial to the peritoneum that stretches from the bladder dome to the umbilicus. In the sagittal plane, the collapsed bladder dome is usually tented up anteriorly by its attachment to the median umbilical ligament (Fig. 19-1). A variety of abnormalities occur when obliteration of the lumen of the urachus is incomplete.

The interureteric ridge is a promontory on the posterior bladder wall between where the ureters enter the bladder. The uterovesical junction (UVJ) describes the short segment of ureter that courses through the muscular bladder wall, often protruding

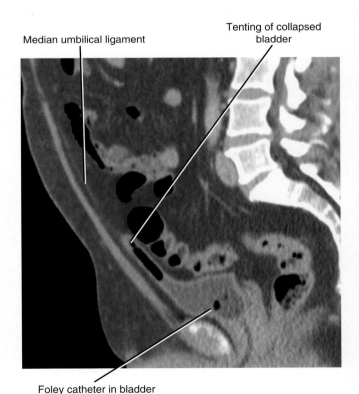

Median umbilical ligament

Tenting of collapsed bladder

Foley catheter in bladder accounts for air in lumen

Figure 19-1 Sagittal reformation from multidetector computed tomographic examination demonstrates tenting of the collapsed urinary bladder by the median umbilical ligament, a normal remnant of the urachus.

slightly into the bladder at the trigone (Fig. 19-2). These small normal protuberances of the UVJ are a helpful landmark when searching for ureteral jets by ultrasound.

Anatomy of the Female Urethra

The female urethra is a short tube (usually less than 4 cm) that provides an outlet from the cone-shaped bladder neck to the perineum. The urethra adheres firmly to the anterior wall of the vagina just posterior to the pubic symphysis. The urethral orifice opens within the vestibule just anterior to the vagina. The female urethra is lined along the proximal one-third with urothelium and along the distal two-thirds with stratified squamous epithelium. Several paraurethral glands near the meatus are known as *Skene's glands*. These are lined with columnar epithelium and secrete into the urethra via two Skene's ducts that may dilate to form palpable cysts. The secretions are similar to those made by the prostate, prompting some to hypothesize that Skene's glands are a prostate homologue. Some urologists even use the term *female prostatitis* to describe symptoms related to periurethral inflammation within the glands.

Anatomy of the Male Urethra

Male urethral anatomy is slightly more complex than that of the female urethra, although familiarity with several landmarks facilitates accurate identification of normal anatomic structures. From the bladder to meatus, the male urethra is divided into four main segments: prostatic, membranous, bulbous, and penile (Fig. 19-3). Combined, the prostatic urethra and membranous urethra make up the *posterior urethra*; the bulbous and penile comprise the *anterior urethra*.

The bladder narrows like a funnel into the bladder neck. Below the bladder neck, the *prostatic urethra* appears almost as an elongated teardrop with a posterior impression representing the verumontanum. The lumen of the prostatic urethra is lined with the same type of urothelium that lines the bladder, ureter, and renal pelvis. The verumontanum contains the urethral outlets for the ejaculatory ducts.

Just below the verumontanum, the urethra tapers for a segment about 1 cm in length, usually at or just below the inferior 1 cm or so of the pubic symphysis. This mildly narrowed segment is the *membranous urethra*. The membranous urethra opens into the long, curved *bulbous urethra*. The proximal bulbous urethra often has a mild hourglass impression from the *pars nuda muscle*, but the remainder of the bulbous urethra should have a larger diameter than any other part of the urethra. The bulbous urethra swings down then back up over the suspensory ligament to emerge from the scrotum as the *penile urethra*. The urothelium of the prostatic urethra progresses to stratified columnar epithelium in the bulbous and proximal penile urethra. As the penile urethra widens slightly at the *fossa navicularis* near the meatus, squamous epithelium predominates.

Two different types of glands make secretions that keep the urethral mucosa moist. A pair of *Cowper glands* is situated with one gland on each side of the membranous urethra. The secretions of each Cowper gland are delivered to the bulbar urethra through a thin Cowper duct. Multiple *glands of Littré* surround the penile urethra; each of these small glands secretes directly into the underlying mucosa through a short duct.

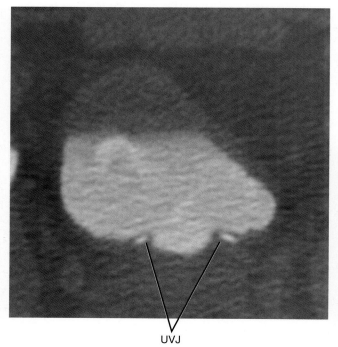

Figure 19-2 Axial image from computed tomographic urogram demonstrates normal appearance of the uterovesical junction *(UVJ)* on both sides.

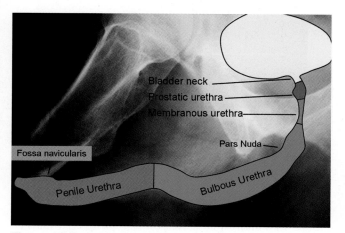

Figure 19-3 Illustration superimposed on a retrograde urethrogram demonstrates anatomic segments of the male urethra.

■ NORMAL IMAGING APPEARANCE OF THE URINARY TRACT

Normal Imaging Appearance of the Ureters

For decades, intravenous urography (IVU) and retrograde urography were the mainstays of ureteral imaging. Typically, a ureter exits each renal pelvis at approximately L2 to L3 and parallels the spine overlying the transverse processes. As the ureters enter the pelvis, they course first laterally, then curve toward the bladder trigone, entering at an angle that is variable but often approximates 45 degrees.

The ureters are usually divided into proximal, middle, and distal segments when describing abnormalities. Although radiologists often apply these terms loosely, a methodical system is commonly used by urologists when planning interventions. The *proximal ureter* refers to the segment from the UPJ to the superior margin of the sacrum, the *midureter* is the segment that overlies the sacrum (also referred to as the sacral ureter), and the *distal ureter* is the short segment between the inferior margin of the sacrum and the ureteral orifice (Fig. 19-4).

Often, radiologists prefer to localize lesions within the ureter, dividing each ureter into thirds of equal length. Because this may cause miscommunication between radiologists and urologists, it is best to use the terms *proximal third*, *middle third*, and *distal third* for clarification when using this geometric division of the ureter. Using anatomic landmarks (e.g., "at the level of the left L3 transverse process") also helps to avoid confusion.

Pitfall: Urologists divide the ureters into anatomic segments of unequal length based on anatomic landmarks. Failure to use the same system or to at least specify equal geometric division of the ureter by using the term third can lead to confusion.

Today, ureters are examined by computed tomography (CT) more often than with any other modality. Even without intravenous (IV) contrast, the course of the ureter can be followed from the renal pelvis to the bladder in most patients. At the level of the inferior margin of the renal hila, the ureters course lateral to the gonadal veins. Just inferior to the lower renal poles, each ureter typically crosses posterior to the ipsilateral gonadal veins from lateral to medial. Identifying the gonadal veins on each study prevents confusion between the vein and the ureters on more inferior images. This is particularly important because gonadal vein phleboliths can easily be confused with ureteral calculi.

Pearl: Following each gonadal vein and ureter to its cranial terminus helps avoid confusion between gonadal vein phleboliths and ureteral calculi, and facilitates identification of ureteral duplication.

It is sometimes difficult to continue following the ureters as they cross anterior to the iliac vessels, particularly if there is a paucity of fat in the retroperitoneum. One remedy is to identify where the ureters enter the bladder at an angle of approximately 45 degrees (Fig. 19-5). The ureters can then be followed back (a retrograde noncontrast-enhanced computed tomography [NCCT] study!) to the level of the iliac vessels. With practice, one may become as comfortable following each ureter retrograde as antegrade, allowing a stone protocol CT examination to be viewed in a "U" configuration, following one ureter from kidney to bladder and the other ureter from bladder to kidney.

On contrast-enhanced CT, the normal ureter may enhance slightly in the arterial and portal venous phases. Excretion of contrast into the ureters usually starts by

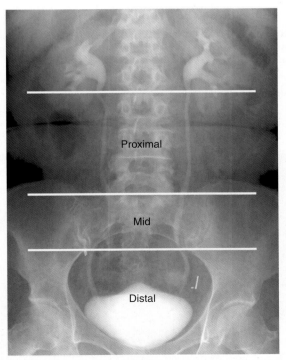

Figure 19-4 Image from an excretory urogram is used to illustrate convention used by urologists to divide the ureters into proximal, mid, and distal segments.

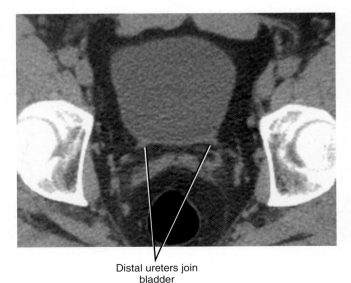

Distal ureters join bladder

Figure 19-5 Axial unenhanced computed tomographic image of the bladder demonstrates how the uterovesical junction can be used to identify the distal ureters.

about 2 minutes after injection. The high attenuation of excreted contrast defines the ureteral lumen well but can obscure the thin ureteral wall. Coronal images (often using thin-slab maximum intensity projection [MIP]) provide visualization of longer segments of the ureters, and even small abnormalities can be detected on coronal reformations using isotropic data. Using a thicker MIP technique allows longer segments to be viewed on fewer coronal sections but also limits detection of small filling defects.

On unenhanced magnetic resonance (MR) images, the ureters contain high-signal-intensity urine on T2-weighted images. On early excretory phase images after IV gadolinium-based contrast media administration, the urine within the ureteral lumen enhances on T1-weighted images. Unlike CT, the ureteral lumen does not become brighter as the excreted contrast agent becomes progressively more concentrated. Instead, T2* effects prevail at greater concentrations of gadolinium, causing loss of signal intensity. On T2-weighted images performed during the excretory phase of contrast-enhanced MRI, the ureters appear dark.

Administering a low dose of a diuretic such as furosemide (typically 5-10 mg) aids in ureteral distention and dilution of excreted contrast media. This reduces the negative effects that concentrated gadolinium has on signal intensity and permits contrast-enhanced excretory urography to be performed with MRI. Excretory-phase, gadolinium-enhanced, T1-weighted images can be acquired in the coronal plane to create an MR urogram (Fig. 19-6). Diuretic administration also benefits CT urography by distending the collecting systems and dispersing excreted contrast material more evenly.

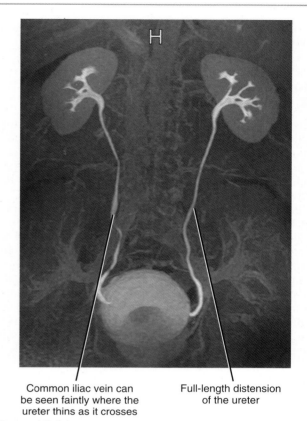

Common iliac vein can be seen faintly where the ureter thins as it crosses

Full-length distension of the ureter

Figure 19-6 Coronal thick-slab maximum intensity projection image from T1-weighted magnetic resonance urogram performed after the administration of intravenous (IV) contrast media. IV furosemide was administered to optimize ureteral opacification. (Reprinted from Leyendecker JR, Barnes CE, Zagoria RJ: MR urography: techniques and clinical applications, *Radiographics* 28:23-46, 2008, by permission.)

Normal Imaging Appearance of the Bladder

The bladder is often seen on a kidneys, ureter, and bladder radiograph (KUB) as a flattened ellipsoid (when empty) to elongated oval-shaped (when distended) soft-tissue density arising from the middle of the pelvic floor. In women, the uterus can often be seen faintly as it rests over the bladder dome. Looking for the normal bladder on each KUB helps with the detection of unsuspected bladder distension or bladder calcification.

On IVU and conventional cystography (including voiding cystourethrography [VCUG]), the empty bladder has a flattened configuration with multiple smooth bladder folds defining heaped up mucosa when the detrusor muscle is contracted. As the bladder becomes distended with opacified urine, the detrusor and mucosa are stretched smooth.

The appearance of the urinary bladder on CT depends on the phase of enhancement. On NCCT, differentiation between the low-attenuation urine and soft-tissue bladder wall is subtle but often can be defined. Each ureteral orifice often can be identified as an area of focal thickening of the posterior bladder wall approximately one third of the way up from the bladder neck. During the arterial phase of contrast administration, the mucosa often enhances slightly more than the muscle,

improving discrimination between bladder wall and the urine within. The detrusor muscle remains slightly dense during the portal venous phase. Although imaging with excreted contrast within the bladder improves the detection of filling defects, the contrast is often of such high attenuation that it causes beam-hardening artifact, which may obscure findings. This "blooming effect" can be minimized by windowing the images so that the dense contrast appears gray rather than bright white.

MRI provides excellent characterization of the bladder, even without contrast media. The urine is bright on T2-weighted images, providing excellent contrast with the mucosal surface. Similar to difficulties with very-high-attenuation contrast on CT, it is often helpful to window the urine to a gray level to avoid obscuring subtle features of the bladder wall on T2-weighted images. T1-weighted images performed after gadolinium-based contrast injection but before the excretory phase allows detection of subtle enhancement in the normal bladder wall, as well as brighter enhancement in mucosal lesions. Once the excreted contrast material fills the bladder, a stratified appearance is common, particularly on delayed images. This appearance is not related to true contrast layering, but rather results when thresholds in concentration are reached that result in relatively abrupt changes in signal intensity despite gradual changes in gadolinium concentration.

Normal Imaging Appearance of the Female Urethra

After filling the bladder with radiopaque contrast media, voiding demonstrates a slightly undulating, funnel-shaped structure that extends inferiorly from the bladder neck. This shape is often described as a "spinning top," and the undulations reflect impressions of the pelvic floor musculature.

Because of its short length, retrograde urethrography (RUG) of the female urethra is not a simple matter. A balloon within the lumen would occupy much of its length and contrast is likely to fill the bladder preferentially, leaving the urethra poorly distended. When necessary, these challenges can be overcome with a *double-balloon urethrogram*. This requires a bladder catheter designed specifically for this purpose (Fig. 19-7). Fortunately, the urethra usually can be imaged effectively with cross-sectional imaging. With careful inspection, urethral diverticula can be seen with CT, particularly if they contain stones (Fig. 19-8). Large masses can also be seen with CT if they enlarge the urethra or invade adjacent structures.

The female urethra is best demonstrated with MRI, particularly when an endovaginal coil is used to produce high-resolution images. On axial sections obtained with an external surface coil, the urethra is posterior to the pubic symphysis and anterior to the vagina, contained within an inverted cone-shaped space created by

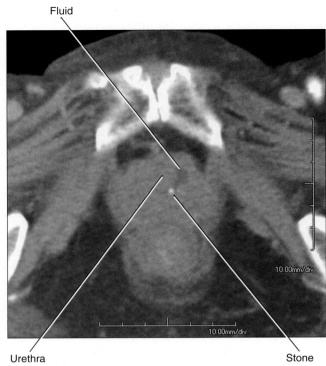

Figure 19-8 Axial image from a contrast-enhanced computed tomographic scan at the level of the urethra in a female patient demonstrates a small stone within a urethral diverticulum.

the puborectalis muscle. The anus is situated at the apex of that inverted cone (Fig. 19-9).

Ultrasound has been used effectively by some for evaluation of the female urethra. Transperineal, endovaginal, and endorectal techniques have all been described. Endourethral ultrasound can also be performed with a specialized transducer.

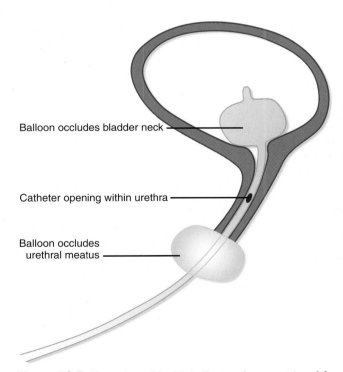

Figure 19-7 Illustration of double balloon catheter positioned for female retrograde urethrography.

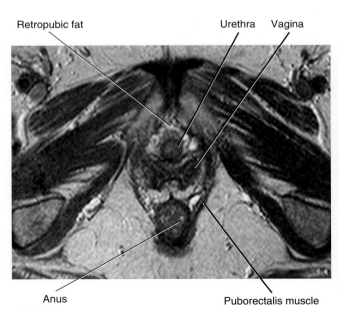

Figure 19-9 Axial T2-weighted magnetic resonance image of the female perineum demonstrates normal anatomic structures.

Normal Imaging Appearance of the Male Urethra

VCUG is the most commonly performed imaging technique for evaluation of the male urethra (Fig. 19-10). During voiding, the bladder neck opens, and the prostatic and membranous urethra widen. The bulbous and penile urethra usually become moderately distended and are typically of uniform caliber.

RUG is appropriate in the setting of trauma or suspected stricture. A Foley catheter is inserted into the urethra, and the balloon inflated with approximately 1 to 2 ml saline in the fossa navicularis. Alternatively, a catheter tip syringe can be inserted gently into the urethral meatus until snug. With the patient in an oblique position (providing relatively uniform body density throughout the length of the urethra by superimposing it over the thigh), water-soluble contrast is injected under fluoroscopy and images are obtained. The penile and bulbous segments are distended more with RUG than with VCUG (see Fig. 19-10). The posterior urethra, however, is generally less distended. A jet of contrast is often seen mixing with unopacified urine within the bladder and can have a bizarre appearance to the uninitiated.

■ CONGENITAL ABNORMALITIES

Duplication

During fetal development, part of the mesonephric duct forms a ureteral bud that migrates cranially. When the ureteric bud reaches the metanephric blastema, it branches into multiple divisions and induces development of the kidney around a branched collecting system. Early branching or complete duplication of the ureteric bud results in *duplication* of all or part of the affected renal collecting system and ureter. If the bud divides completely at its origin, duplication is complete (two ureteral orifices). Any division of the ureteric bud proximal to the bladder trigone leads to variable lengths of duplication between the renal pelvis and the bladder (Fig. 19-11). Some form of duplication is present in up to 4% of people, and although it is usually an incidental radiographic finding, it occasionally has significant health implications.

Partial duplications that unite to form a common ureter rarely cause symptoms (Fig. 19-12). However, it is useful to have knowledge of duplicated anatomy in the event of procedures that place the ureters at potential risk, such as donor nephrectomy, pelvic surgery, or radiofrequency ablation. On occasion, partial duplication of the ureters (probably paired with abnormalities of peristalsis) results in channeling of urine down one ureter and up the other, so-called yo-yo reflux.

Most cases of medically significant duplication are complete. With complete duplication, the ureter from the lower pole usually inserts into a normal location in the bladder trigone. The ureter from the superior pole is ectopic, usually entering the bladder inferior and medial to the expected location *(Weigert–Meyer rule)*. The most common location for the ectopic upper pole ureter is near or within the bladder neck. Even with complete duplication, if the ectopic ureteral orifice has normal morphology, it is not usually of clinical significance. However, when an ectopic ureter protrudes or herniates into the bladder lumen because of an abnormal angle of entry, it forms a ureterocele. Ectopic ureteroceles are prone to obstruction (Fig. 19-13). In addition, mass effect from a large ectopic ureterocele can distort the orifice of the orthotopic ureter, resulting in reflux to the lower pole.

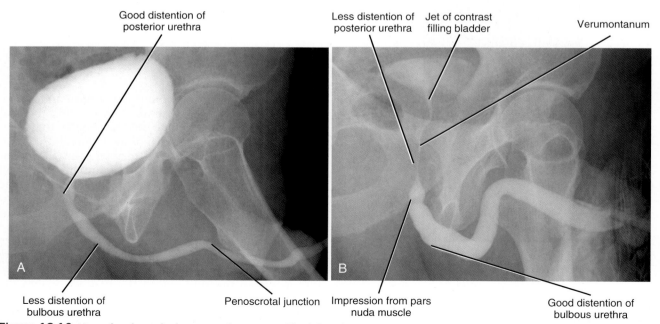

Good distension of posterior urethra

Less distension of posterior urethra   Jet of contrast filling bladder   Verumontanum

Less distension of bulbous urethra   Penoscrotal junction   Impression from pars nuda muscle   Good distension of bulbous urethra

Figure 19-10 Normal male urethral anatomy demonstrated by **(A)** voiding cystourethrography and by **(B)** retrograde urethrography.

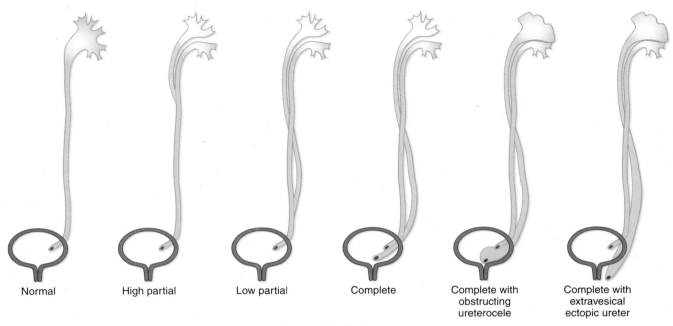

Figure 19-11 Illustration demonstrating the spectrum of ureteral duplication.

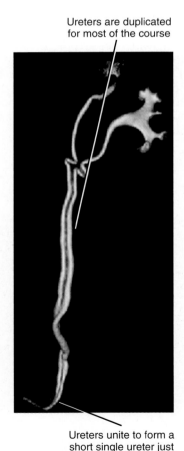

Figure 19-12 Volume-rendered three-dimensional image from computed tomographic urogram demonstrating low union of a partial ureteral duplication. *UVJ,* Ureterovesical junction.

The ectopic ureter from the upper pole can also insert into the urethra, vagina, prostate, or seminal vesicle. Female individuals with a ureteral orifice in the vagina or distal urethra suffer from incontinence. This leads to early diagnosis and favors preservation of some function in the upper pole moiety. Male individuals are more likely to have continent ectopia, with insertion into the prostate, seminal vesicle, or vas deferens. By the time many men are diagnosed with ectopic ureteral insertion, the upper pole moiety has severely compromised function because of obstructive uropathy.

Pearl: In female individuals, ectopic ureters often insert into the urethra or vagina and present with urinary incontinence at an early age. In male individuals, ectopic ureters often result in silent obstruction that may not be discovered until a later age.

Ureterocele

Simple ureteroceles occur without duplication and are located at the expected location of the normal ureteral orifice. Sometimes called *orthotopic ureteroceles,* these represent incomplete obliteration of the embryologic membrane between the ureter and bladder (Chwalla membrane). The flow of urine pushes the membrane, like wind filling a sail, causing the end of the ureter to push into the bladder. Simple ureteroceles are usually small and incidental (Fig. 19-14). Larger ureteroceles are prone to obstruction and stone formation (Fig. 19-15).

An *everting ureterocele* can occur when a ureterocele coexists with any cause of increased bladder pressure (usually benign prostatic hypertrophy). In such cases, the increased pressure within the bladder pushes the ureterocele back into the ureter, resulting in distal ureteral obstruction. On CT, an everting ureterocele results in the appearance of a membrane within the lumen of

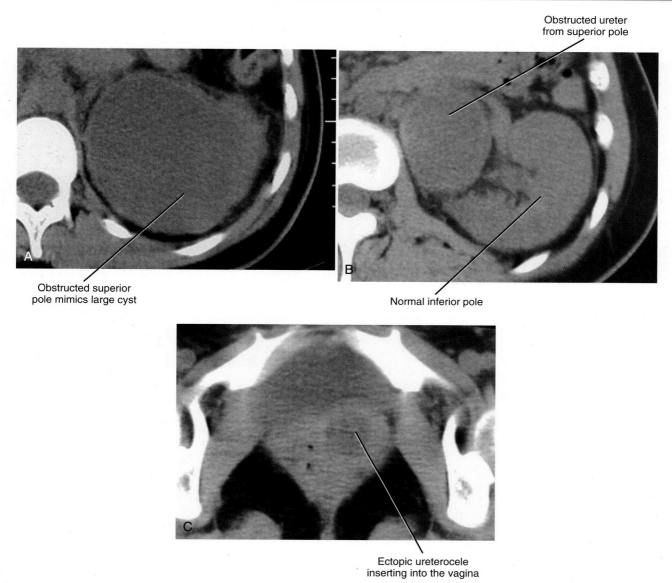

Figure 19-13 Axial images from noncontrast-enhanced computed tomography (CT) performed for suspected ureterolithiasis at the level of the superior pole **(A)**, at the level of the renal hilum **(B)**, and at the level of the perineum **(C)** demonstrate chronic obstruction of the upper pole from previously undiagnosed duplication. In this case, infection caused the symptoms that prompted evaluation with CT at age 20.

the ureter (Fig. 19-16). Because antegrade urography can push the ureterocele down into the bladder, combined antegrade urography and cystography may be required to confirm the diagnosis.

Ectopic Ureter

Just as ureteroceles can occur either with duplication or as an isolated abnormality, ectopic ureters can also occur without associated duplication. Isolated ureteral ectopia follows the same sex rules as duplication. Female individuals have a low insertion (bladder neck, urethra, or vagina) with associated incontinence and infections. In male individuals, ectopic ureters insert into the prostate, seminal vesicle, or vas deferens and can cause recurrent episodes of epididymoorchitis. In

up to 5% of ectopic ureters, no ureteral orifice is found and the ureter is assumed to be a blind-ending pouch. Most ectopic ureters cause obstruction. When the system is not duplicated, obstructive nephropathy damages the entire kidney. Because onset of the insult is in utero, kidneys can be dysplastic or hypoplastic when discovered (Fig. 19-17).

Circumcaval and Retrocaval Ureter

The portion of the inferior vena cava (IVC) below the renal vein usually develops from the supracardinal vein, which is posterior to the ureter. If, instead, the infrarenal IVC develops from the right subcardinal or postcardinal veins (these are anterior to the ureter), part of the ureter may become trapped behind the IVC. In the

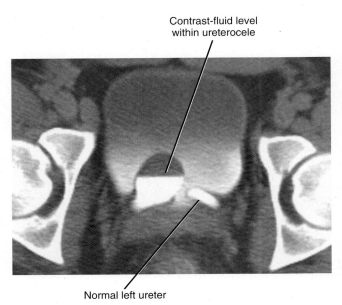

Contrast-fluid level
within ureterocele

Normal left ureter

Figure 19-14 Axial image from a contrast-enhanced computed tomographic scan of the bladder demonstrates a simple right uretero-cele on an examination performed for suspected acute appendicitis.

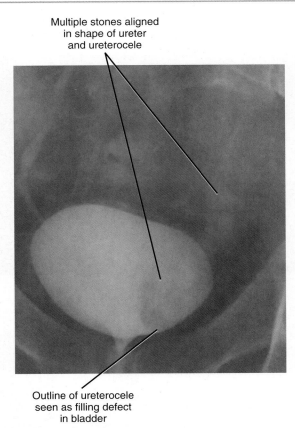

Multiple stones aligned
in shape of ureter
and ureterocele

Outline of ureterocele
seen as filling defect
in bladder

Figure 19-15 Images from an excretory urogram show multiple stones within a ureterocele and distal ureter.

most common form of this variant, the proximal right ureter courses posterior to the IVC at the L4 level, and loops around medial then anterior to the IVC before assuming a normal location for the distal segment. This loop around the IVC is cause for the name *circumcaval* ureter. This may give the illusion that the ureter is "hung up" on the L4 pedicle (Fig. 19-18). This anatomic variant often presents when a ureteral stone becomes obstructed in the circumcaval segment (Fig. 19-19). This can be confusing on unenhanced CT if a calculus is lodged posterior to the IVC. Following the ureters carefully from kidney to bladder on sequential axial images allows accurate diagnosis.

Rarely, the right ureter gets caught by a posterior branch from the IVC so that a segment courses posterior to the IVC. The ureter in such cases reemerges laterally and is called a *retrocaval ureter*.

Blind-Ending Ureteral Duplication

What happens if a ureteric bud never reaches the metanephric blastema? Without induction of the kidney, the bud never develops the familiar arborization of the intrarenal collecting system. Instead, it remains a blind-ending pouch. In an unduplicated system, the bud usually atrophies and the kidney never develops, accounting for some cases of renal agenesis. If, however, the bud had already divided into a potential duplication, refluxing urine maintains patency of the bud, which persists as a blind-ending ureteral duplication, sometimes called a *ureteral diverticulum*. In most cases, these are incidental findings on imaging examinations, although resection for infection and for pain have been reported.

Refluxing excreted contrast media can opacify a blind ending ureteral duplication during excretory urography,

but these anomalies are often better opacified on retrograde urography (Fig. 19-20). In some cases, expansion of the blind-ending ureter caused by reflux results in misdiagnosis as an ovarian cyst. Today, blind-ending ureters are more likely to be discovered with CT, although detection requires a methodical approach. Similar to identification of the ureter and gonadal vein on every examination, it is important to follow any dilated tubular structure in the retroperitoneum to confirm its beginning and end to avoid confusing a diverticulum with an obstructed ureter (Fig. 19-21).

Urachal Anomalies

The urachus is a tube that empties the bladder through the umbilicus during early fetal development. The urachus usually narrows and then closes late in development or at birth. The closed urachus becomes the *median umbilical ligament,* an extraperitoneal cord that extends from the bladder dome to the umbilicus between the transversalis fascia and parietal peritoneum. The median umbilical ligament can be seen on virtually every multidetector computed tomography examination of the pelvis. Minimal soft-tissue thickening, trace calcification, or both are commonly present in the bladder dome where the median umbilical ligament inserts (Fig. 19-22).

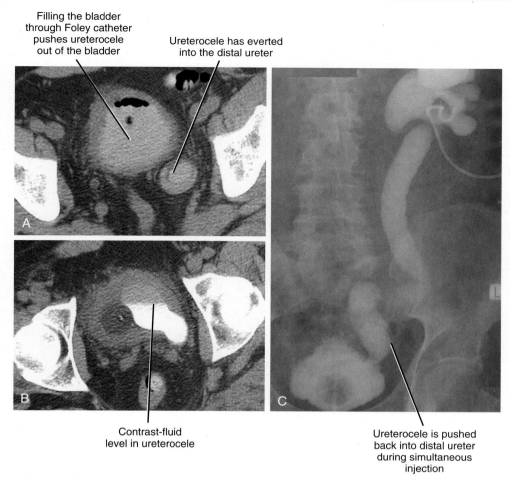

Filling the bladder
through Foley catheter
pushes ureterocele
out of the bladder

Ureterocele has everted
into the distal ureter

Contrast-fluid
level in ureterocele

Ureterocele is pushed
back into distal ureter
during simultaneous
injection

Figure 19-16 Axial images of the pelvis during (**A**) CT cystography and (**B**) during antegrade CT pyelography via nephrostomy tube demonstrate an everting ureterocele in a 52-year-man with urinary obstruction. **C,** Diagnosis was confirmed during simultaneous catheter injections under fluoroscopy.

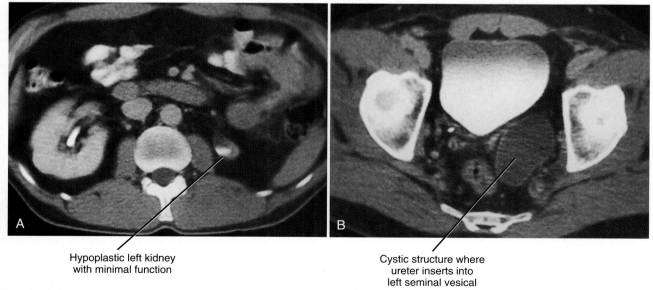

Hypoplastic left kidney
with minimal function

Cystic structure where
ureter inserts into
left seminal vesical

Figure 19-17 Simple ectopic ureter. **A,** Axial image from a contrast-enhanced computed tomographic (CT) scan at the level of the kidneys demonstrates hypoplasia of the left kidney caused by congenital partial obstruction. **B,** Axial image at the level of the bladder from the same CT examination demonstrates a cystic structure in the expected location of the distal left ureter. At surgery, ureteral insertion into the left seminal vesicle was confirmed.

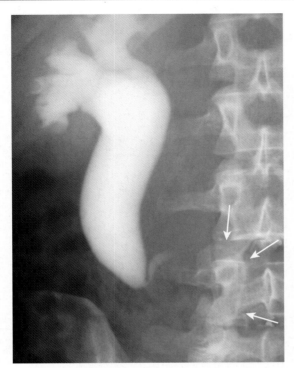

Figure 19-18 Image from an intravenous urogram demonstrates dilatation of the proximal ureter to the level of a circumcaval segment (*arrows*).

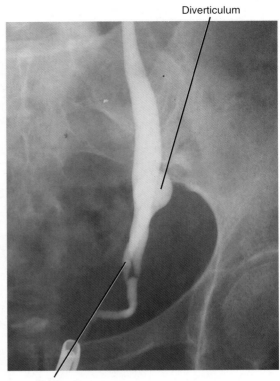

Figure 19-20 Blind-ending ureteral duplication demonstrated by retrograde urography. Because of saccular dilatation of the pouch, these are occasionally mistaken for adnexal cysts on ultrasound.

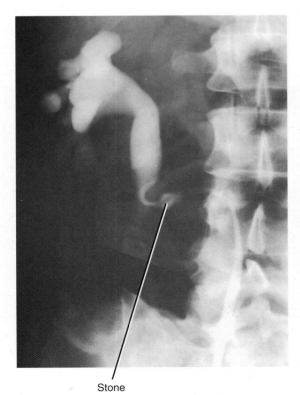

Figure 19-19 Retrograde urogram demonstrates a stone in a circumcaval segment of the ureter.

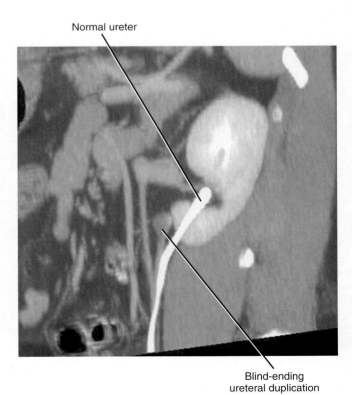

Figure 19-21 Sagittal-oblique reformatted image from excretory phase of computed tomography performed for nonurinary complaints demonstrates blind-ending ureteral duplication.

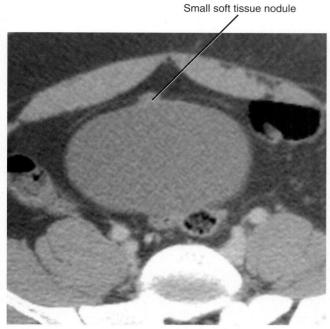

Small soft tissue nodule

Figure 19-22 Benign urachal remnant on computed tomography (CT). Axial image from a contrast-enhanced CT scan demonstrates a small soft-tissue nodule protruding slightly from the anterior bladder dome.

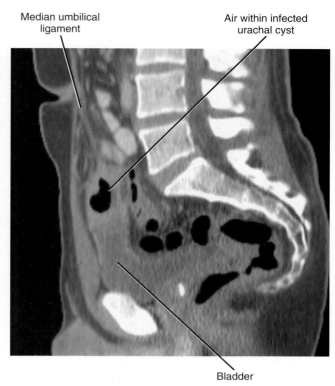

Median umbilical ligament

Air within infected urachal cyst

Bladder

Figure 19-24 Midline sagittal reformation of computed tomographic examination demonstrates an infected urachal cyst. The diagnosis was confirmed at surgery.

Failure of urachal closure may be complete *(patent urachus)*, may involve the bladder end *(urachal diverticulum)*, may involve the umbilical end *(urachal sinus)*, or may be sequestered in the middle *(urachal cyst)* (Fig. 19-23). A patent urachus presents with urine leaking from the umbilicus. Urachal diverticula often occur when urachal closure is impeded by bladder outlet obstruction. Urachal sinuses and cysts usually present when they become infected (Fig. 19-24).

Urachal carcinoma is the most dreaded consequence of persistent urachal tissue. Tumor can arise anywhere along the urachal remnant but most commonly occurs just anterior to the bladder dome. *Adenocarcinoma* accounts for 80% of cases, with urothelial and squamous cell carcinomas occurring considerably less often. Hematuria is absent when the tumor does not communicate with the bladder lumen. Because no vital structures are compressed by a mass in this region, urachal carcinomas are usually large at presentation (mean size, 8 cm), and initial symptoms may be related to a palpable anterior pelvic mass or metastatic disease. Masses range from solid to low attenuation on computed tomography, often with heterogeneous areas of contrast enhancement (Fig. 19-25). Dystrophic calcifications are common.

Pearl: When a mass is present in the midline near the bladder dome, think of processes related to a urachal remnant.

■ FILLING DEFECTS AND IMPRESSIONS

For the purposes of discussion, we define a filling defect as a space-occupying lesion that prevents contrast from completely filling the lumen of a hollow organ, thus altering its radiographic appearance (Fig. 19-26). We consider an impression to be a contour abnormality at

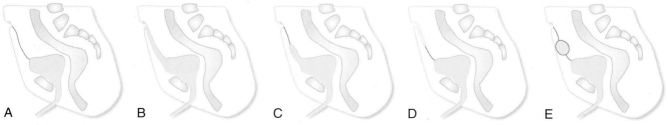

A   B   C   D   E

Figure 19-23 Illustrations demonstrating the spectrum of abnormalities related to closure of the urachus. **A,** Normal median umbilical ligament. **B,** Patent urachus. **C,** Urachal diverticulum. **D,** Urachal sinus. **E,** Urachal cyst.

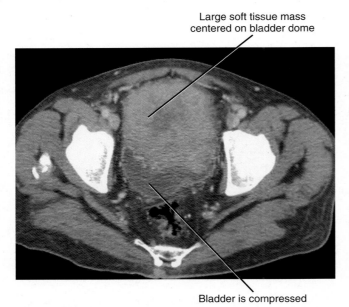

Large soft tissue mass
centered on bladder dome

Bladder is compressed

Figure 19-25 Axial image from a contrast-enhanced computed tomographic scan demonstrates a large, heterogeneously enhancing mass extending from the bladder dome toward the anterior abdominal wall. This was removed surgically and proved to be urachal carcinoma.

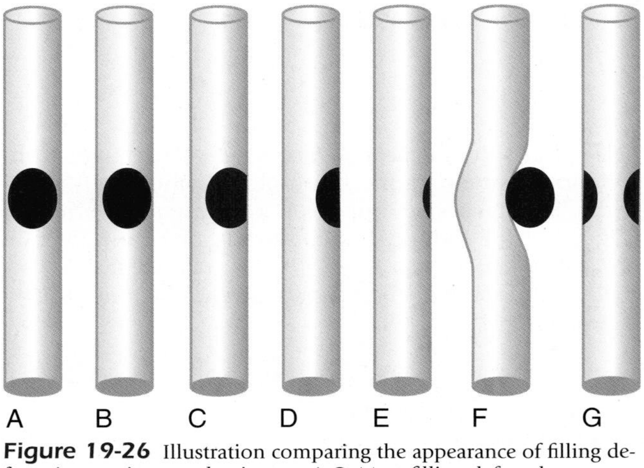

mind that some entities are neither filling defects nor impressions but can create a similar appearance (e.g., aberrant renal papilla).

Filling defects within the urinary tract are most often the result of material passing through the urinary tract (e.g., stone, blood clot) or polypoid mucosal lesions (e.g., urothelial carcinoma, polyp) (Figs. 19-27 and 19-28). Impressions usually result from normal anatomic structures (e.g., blood vessels, bowel, uterus, prostate) and adjacent mass or, in the case of bladder impressions, extrinsic fluid collections. Table 19-1 summarizes some common filling defects and impressions that involve the urinary tract.

Successfully characterizing a filling defect or impression often requires correlation of several different imaging studies or different phases from the same contrast-enhanced examination. Important features to evaluate include lesion morphology, composition, and enhancement.

Morphology is an important characteristic of a filling defect or impression. A blood clot usually forms a cast of the lumen that contains it. Stones within a ureter usually cause an acute inflammatory response, resulting in narrowing of the lumen distal to the stone. Tumors growing within the lumen of the ureter, on the other hand, fill the lumen gradually without much irritation to the

```
A    B    C    D    E    F    G
```

Figure 19-26 Illustration comparing the appearance of filling defects, impressions, and strictures. **A-C,** Most filling defects have contrast surrounding at least part of the lesion, resulting in acute angles with the wall. This indicates either a mucosal lesion or loose body within the lumen. **D,** A 90-degree interface with the wall could represent either a sessile filling defect or an impression from a submucosal lesion. **E, F,** Obtuse margins or deviation of the lumen usually indicates an impression from an extrinsic process. **G,** Circumferential narrowing is called a *stricture*.

the interface between intraluminal contrast and the wall of the lumen. Unlike filling defects that are surrounded by contrast, impressions bulge into fluid but are not engulfed by it. This appearance is often the result of superficial mucosal lesions, submucosal lesions, and extrinsic structures. This section includes filling defects and impressions together because the imaging appearance can overlap, and some entities (e.g., urothelial carcinoma) can have either appearance. Also keep in

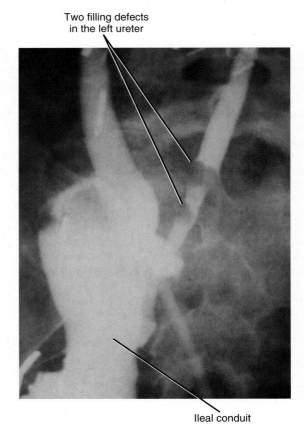

Two filling defects
in the left ureter

Ileal conduit

Figure 19-27 Loopogram performed in patient status post cystectomy and ileal conduit for bladder cancer. Filling defects seen within the left ureter were subsequently proved to be recurrent urothelial carcinoma.

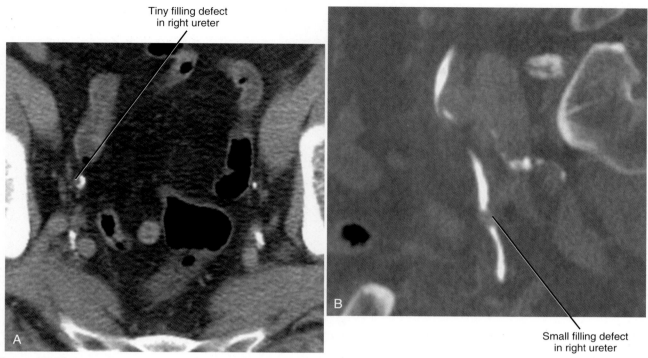

Tiny filling defect
in right ureter

Small filling defect
in right ureter

Figure 19-28 Small filling defect on computed tomographic urography. **A,** Axial excretory phase image of the pelvic ureters demonstrates a small filling defect outlined by excreted contrast within the right ureter. **B,** Sagittal maximum intensity projection image better demonstrates the lesion (urothelial carcinoma).

adjacent mucosal tissues. Instead of becoming narrowed, the ureter just distal to a urothelial cancer becomes mildly dilated. This appearance has been called the *goblet sign* (Fig. 19-29). A castlike defect within the ureter on antegrade urography and ball-valve obstruction of the ureter on retrograde urography is typical for a fibroepithelial polyp of the ureter (Fig. 19-30). Blood vessels that create an impression on the ureter are tubular structures. Normal vessels that commonly impress on the ureters include the gonadal and iliac vessels. Abnormal vascular impressions can result from anatomic variants, vascular occlusion (Fig. 19-31), or arteriovenous communication. *Ureteritis cystica* occurs in response to chronic urothelial irritation and consists of small, fluid-filled mucosal and submucosal cysts that create multiple round impressions in the ureter or renal pelvis, or both, on urographic images (Fig. 19-32). Although these cysts seen en face can appear as filling defects, those viewed in tangent can be seen to have obtuse or 90-degree angles with the ureteral wall. Ureteritis cystica usually occurs in response to the presence of a ureteral stent and usually affects the renal pelvis as well (pyeloureteritis cystic). Because the contours can sometimes appear irregular and overlap the appearance of superficial spreading urothelial carcinoma, clinical history and comparison with prior examinations is critical. In the appropriate clinical setting, the rounded impressions are characteristic and the lesions can be followed to resolution.

Pearl: Ureteral stones usually cause narrowing of the ureter just distal to impaction. Ureteral tumors usually cause dilatation just distal to the filling defect.

Lesion composition can also be helpful to characterize a filling defect or impression. Small lesions that consist entirely of calcified matrix represent stones. When visible, stones are hyperechoic with posterior acoustic shadowing and demonstrate "twinkle" artifact on color Doppler ultrasound. Sloughed papillae can calcify but typically are found in the setting of papillary necrosis. Small amounts of calcification can also be present within transitional cell carcinoma. Blood clots tend to be of higher attenuation than fluid (but much lower attenuation than calcium) on NCCT or high signal intensity on T1-weighted MRI. When CT shows mottled gas within a filling defect in the urinary tract, *mycetoma* is an important consideration, although mycetomas can also have a more bland appearance (Fig. 19-33).

The presence or absence of contrast enhancement is an important clue to the cause of a filling defect. Multiphase contrast-enhanced CT or MRI can demonstrate the vascularity of a urothelial tumor in the early phase of enhancement before it becomes obscured by excreted contrast media (Fig. 19-34). Vessels responsible for ureteral impressions enhance similar to vessels elsewhere. Blood clots, stones, sloughed papillae, fungus balls, and foreign bodies do not enhance after IV contrast administration.

The differential diagnosis of filling defects within the urethra differs from that for the ureters and bladder, because transients such as stones, clots, papillae, and mycetoma are seldom present in the urethra long enough to be included on imaging examinations. Fixed filling defects within the urethra include cancer, benign

Table 19-1   Filling Defects and Impressions of the Ureters and Bladder

Causative Factors	Distinguishing Features
Ureters and Bladder	
Stone	Calcified on NCCT Hyperechoic with shadowing or "twinkle" artifact on US Signal void on MRI No enhancement Inflammatory response with narrowing of ureter below Can change position
Blood clot	Castlike appearance conforms to urinary tract High attenuation on NCCT (usually 60–80 Hounsfield units) High signal intensity on T1W MRI Can change position or shape
Urothelial carcinoma	Irregular shape Goblet sign in ureter on urograms (IVU, CTU, or MRU) Often pedunculated in bladder Occasional faint calcification on NCCT Enhances Fixed shape and position
Squamous cell carcinoma	Sessile filling defect, ureteral stricture or bladder wall thickening Calcification in ureter, bladder wall, or on surface of tumor Associated with schistosomiasis, chronic irritation from indwelling catheters and bladder stones, chronic infections; greater incidence among paraplegics
Sloughed papilla	Other evidence of papillary necrosis Mobile May be calcified No enhancement
Ureters	
Blood vessels	Tubular impression on proximal ureter Venous impressions may efface with retrograde injection Enhancement comparable with other vessels on CT and MRI Ureteral notching seen with renal vein thrombosis, chronic arterial occlusion, and AVM
Ureteritis cystica	Often has history of recent ureteral stent Multiple round impressions, look like filling defects if viewed en face
Fibroepithelial polyp	Smooth, castlike filling defect on antegrade studies Ball-valve obstruction on retrograde studies
Bladder	
Adenocarcinoma	Primary urachal: large impression on bladder dome from urachal mass Primary nonurachal: diffuse bladder wall thickening Secondary: direct invasion from prostate, rectum, or colon; distant metastases from stomach, breast, or lung cancer; diffuse bladder wall thickening is common
Leiomyoma	Smooth impression with intact overlying mucosa Smoothly round or lentiform mural mass Similar attenuation (CT) or signal intensity (T1W MR) to muscle Low signal intensity on T2W MR images (such as leiomyomas elsewhere) Enhances after intravenous contrast administration
Lymphoma	Diffuse wall thickening or focal mass Lymphadenopathy on CT Enhances after intravenous contrast administration
Mycetoma	Immunocompromised patient Mottled gas Mobile No enhancement
Foreign body	History of foreign body insertion Characteristic shape No enhancement Potentially mobile but can be fixed in position

Table 19-1   Filling Defects and Impressions of the Ureters and Bladder—cont'd

Causative Factors	Distinguishing Features
Cystitis cystica and cystitis glandularis	Response to chronic irritation in the bladder Multiple nodular filling defects may have characteristic "cobblestone" appearance, although more focal lesions may mimic bladder cancer May be hypervascular on CT and MRI
Inflammatory pseudotumor	Also known as "pseudosarcomatous fibromyxoid tumor" Can mimic invasive malignant tumor Solitary bladder mass, often polypoid, spares trigone T2W MR images show high signal center with low signal in periphery Postcontrast T1W MR images show peripheral enhancement
Malakoplakia	Chronic granulomatous process More common in women and immunocompromised patients Varies appearance including diffuse wall thickening, multiple sessile or polypoid masses that may involve the distal ureters Usually enhances
Endometriosis	Premenopausal women Most bladder wall implants occur within the posterior wall (from the pouch of Douglas) or in the bladder dome High signal intensity on T1W MR images
Nephrogenic adenoma	Metaplasia of the urothelium caused by chronic irritation from infections, stones, and prior surgery Recurrence after resection common

AVM, Arteriovenous malformation; *CT*, computed tomography; *CTU*, computed tomographic urography; *MR*, magnetic resonance; *MRI*, magnetic resonance imaging; *MRU*, magnetic resonance urography; *NCCT*, noncontrast-enhanced computed tomography; *T1W*, T1-weighted; *T2W*, T2-weighted; *US*, ultrasound.

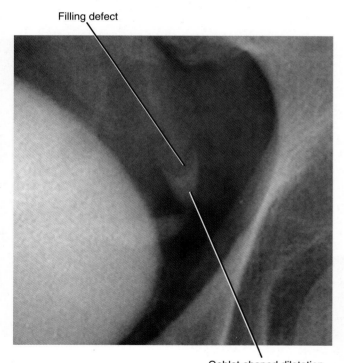

Figure 19-29 Image from excretory urogram demonstrates a filling defect in the distal left ureter with mild dilatation of the ureter beyond the defect. This "goblet" sign is commonly seen with urothelial carcinoma of the ureter.

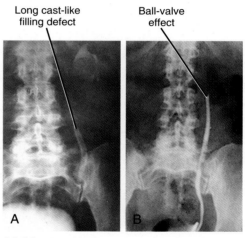

Figure 19-30 Fibroepithelial polyp of the ureter. **A,** Intravenous urogram demonstrates an elongated ureteral filling defect. **B,** Subsequent retrograde urogram demonstrates ball-valve obstruction. A fibroepithelial polyp of the ureter was removed surgically. (Courtesy Arthur Rosenfield, M.D.)

■ STRICTURES

Ureteral Strictures

Because the ureters are long, thin, delicate tubes, virtually any type of injury can result in a stricture. Indeed, the list of causative factors for ureteral stricture is long (Table 19-2). The most common cause of ureteral stricture is passage of a calculus or the instrumentation performed to achieve stone removal (Fig. 19-36). Because the passing of a ureteral stone seldom goes unnoticed, a history of stone passage is usually available. The risk for development of a stricture is increased with increased stone size and duration of obstruction.

fibroepithelial polyps, and condyloma (Fig. 19-35). Definitive diagnosis always requires endoscopic evaluation. Whereas carcinomas of the ureter and bladder most often appear as filling defects on radiographic studies, urethral carcinoma is more likely to appear as an irregular stricture.

Notching from
enlarged vessels

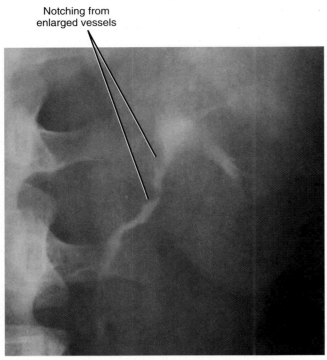

Figure 19-31 Image from an intravenous urogram demonstrates impressions on the proximal ureter and renal pelvis in a patient subsequently shown to have renal vein thrombosis. Ureteral notching is the result of enlarged collateral veins.

Although advancements in stone-removal techniques have greatly decreased the risk for stricture formation, evidence exists that silent urinary obstruction (without pain) develops in up to 3% of patients after ureteroscopic stone extraction. Thus, postprocedural imaging is sometimes performed to avoid damage to the kidney from delayed diagnosis of urinary obstruction.

Rounded impressions
seen in profile

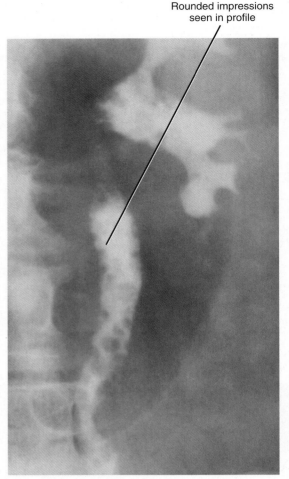

Figure 19-32 Pyeloureteritis cystica. Anteroposterior image of the left proximal ureter from a retrograde urogram demonstrates rounded filling defects and impressions. The spherical nature of the lesions and history of a recent ureteral stent suggest pyeloureteritis cystica.

Large filling defect
in bladder contains
mottled gas

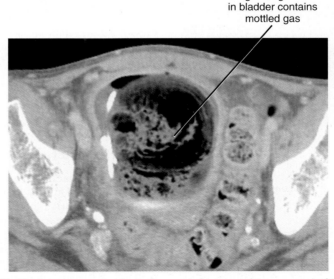

Figure 19-33 Axial image of the bladder from a contrast-enhanced computed tomographic scan acquired in the excretory phase demonstrates air within a large object filling most of the bladder. This appearance is typical for mycetoma (this one was removed), although air mixed with stool can have a similar appearance in cases of colovesical fistula.

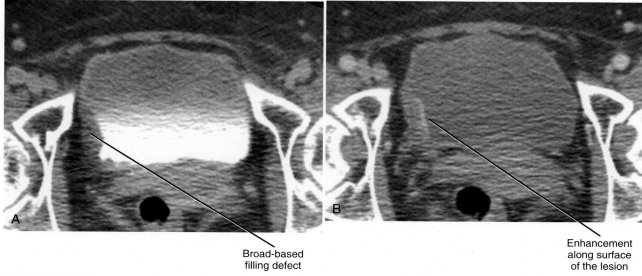

Broad-based
filling defect

Enhancement
along surface
of the lesion

Figure 19-34 Enhancement used to characterize filling defect in the bladder on computed tomography. **A,** Axial image of the bladder during the excretory phase demonstrates a sessile filling defect along the right wall of the bladder. **B,** Review of an image from the nephrographic phase demonstrates enhancement along the surface of the mass (urothelial carcinoma).

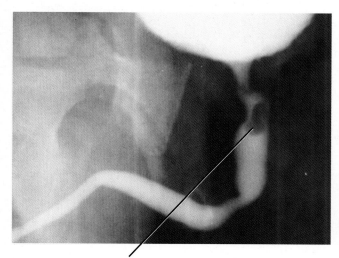

Fixed filling defect
with smooth margins

Figure 19-35 Filling defect on voiding cystourethrography. Smooth, fixed defect in the posterior urethra proved to be a benign fibroepithelial polyp.

Severe ureteral strictures are usually not difficult to diagnose. Hydronephrosis or flank pain prompts evaluation with some form of urography. Lesser degrees of narrowing are problematic, because normal peristalsis causes areas of apparent narrowing in the absence of stricture. On IVU, persistent narrowing on multiple views despite adequate distention elsewhere in the urinary tract should prompt evaluation by fluoroscopy (if the patient is still present) or retrograde urography. CT urography offers fewer opportunities to distinguish normal peristalsis from low-grade stricture. Although diuretics, fluid boluses, and/or compression improve ureteral distention, mild strictures can be easily missed

Table 19-2 Summary of Common Causes of Ureteral Stricture

Injury	Stone passage
	Instrumentation
	Penetrating trauma
	Blunt force trauma (near ureteropelvic junction most common)
	Radiation therapy
Malignant neoplasm	Urothelial carcinoma
	Cervical carcinoma
	Lymphoma
	Metastatic lymphadenopathy (most often pelvic primary)
Infection	Tuberculosis
	Schistosomiasis
Miscellaneous	Retroperitoneal fibrosis
	Endometriosis

on CT urograms when there is no associated mural thickening or mass. MR urography sequences are easily repeated, allowing better distinction between peristalsis and mild ureteral stricture.

Most benign strictures are short and smooth. The presence of mucosal irregularity, asymmetry, or focal wall thickening on imaging should raise concern for urothelial carcinoma (Fig. 19-37). Malignant strictures can also appear smooth, but in such cases, the transition is often abrupt with asymmetric shouldering (Fig. 19-38).

Retroperitoneal Fibrosis

Retroperitoneal fibrosis merits specific discussion because it is an unusual benign but often progressive disease that frequently first presents as ureteral obstruction. Retroperitoneal fibrosis is often idiopathic and

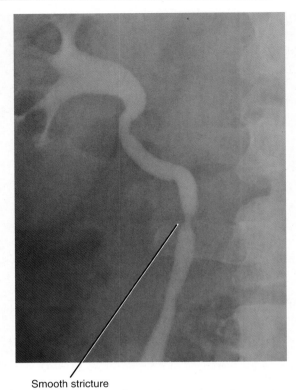

Smooth stricture

Figure 19-36 Intravenous urogram performed after passage of a ureteral calculus demonstrates a short stricture of the proximal ureter without associated obstruction.

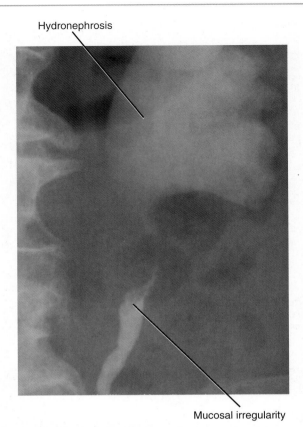

Hydronephrosis

Mucosal irregularity

Figure 19-37 Image from a retrograde urogram demonstrates an irregular stricture of the proximal left ureter caused by urothelial carcinoma.

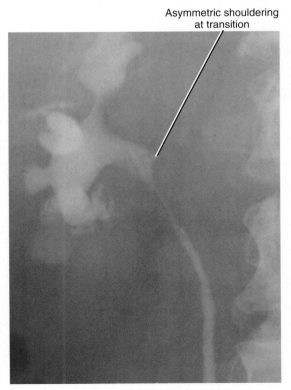

Asymmetric shouldering at transition

Figure 19-38 Asymmetric stricture in urothelial carcinoma. Retrograde urogram demonstrates an asymmetric ureteral stricture with abrupt shouldering at the margins. Urothelial carcinoma was resected surgically.

isolated, but it is sometimes associated with other conditions (Box 19-1).

With IVU, the most frequent findings include medial deviation of the middle third of both ureters with associated ureteral narrowing and proximal dilatation (Fig. 19-39). Deviation and obstruction are often asymmetric at presentation.

CT shows a smooth mantle of soft tissue surrounding the aorta, IVC, and ureters (Fig. 19-40). Although this bears some similarity to the appearance of retroperitoneal lymphadenopathy, the soft tissue in retroperitoneal fibrosis does not usually displace the aorta and IVC away from the spine, as is commonly seen with lymphoma (Fig. 19-41). Treatment for retroperitoneal fibrosis often involves initial placement of ureteral stents followed by ureterolysis, a surgical procedure that mobilizes the ureters into the peritoneal space. Imaging-guided percutaneous needle biopsy is

---

BOX 19-1   Conditions Associated with Retroperitoneal Fibrosis

Methysergide
Abdominal aortic aneurysm
Vascular graft/repair of the aorta
Autoimmune thyroid disease
Systemic lupus erythematosus
Vasculitis of small- and medium-size vessels
Rheumatoid arthritis
Ankylosing spondylitis
Fibrosing mediastinitis
Sclerosing mesenteritis
Inflammatory bowel disease
Sclerosing cholangitis
Primary biliary cirrhosis
Asbestos exposure

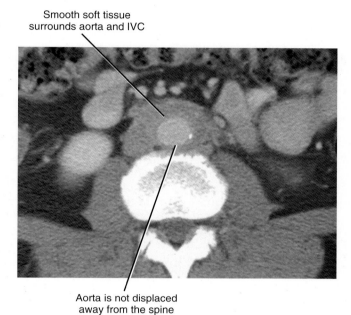

Smooth soft tissue surrounds aorta and IVC

Aorta is not displaced away from the spine

Figure 19-40 Computed tomography of retroperitoneal fibrosis. Axial image just below the kidneys demonstrates a smooth mantle of periaortic tissue. These images are from a different patient than those in Figure 19-39. *IVC,* Inferior vena cava.

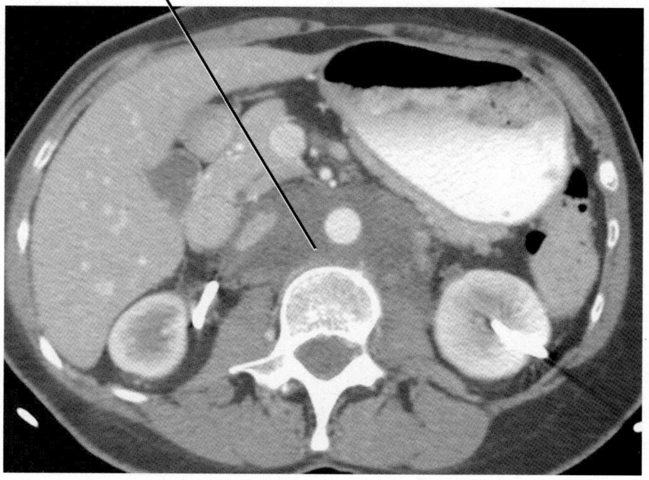

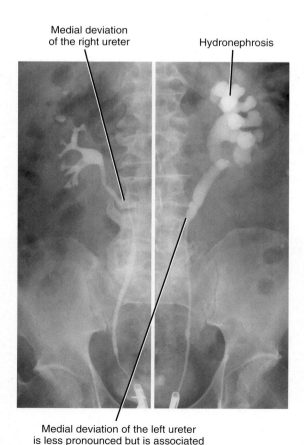

Medial deviation of the right ureter

Hydronephrosis

Medial deviation of the left ureter is less pronounced but is associated with narrowing

Figure 19-39 Juxtaposed images from right and left retrograde urograms in a patient with retroperitoneal fibrosis. Medial displacement is more pronounced with the right ureter, whereas narrowing is more severe on the left side, resulting in obstruction.

Soft tissue displaces the aorta away from the spine

Figure 19-41 Axial image from a contrast-enhanced computed tomographic scan in a patient with lymphoma demonstrates periaortic tissue that resembles retroperitoneal fibrosis, although the inferior vena cava and aorta are displaced away from the spine.

sometimes performed to exclude malignancy, but definitive diagnosis often requires open biopsy performed during ureterolysis.

Pearl: Periaortic lymphadenopathy associated with lymphoma tends to displace the aorta away from the spine, whereas the soft tissue associated with retroperitoneal fibrosis typically does not.

Urethral Strictures

Most urethral strictures are the result of prior infection or trauma. Urethritis is most often the result of infection with *Neisseria gonorrhoeae* or *Chlamydia trachomatis,* although a variety of other organisms are also associated. *Postinfectious strictures* preferentially affect the proximal bulbar urethra, likely because of stasis of residual urine in the dependent part of this segment, resulting in prolonged exposure of the glands of Littré to the pathogens (Fig. 19-42). Postinfectious urethral strictures are often irregular and multifocal, and can also involve the penile urethra (Fig. 19-43).

Posttraumatic strictures can occur anywhere along the urethra, but several locations are more common. Straddle injuries commonly affect the bulbar urethra where it is compressed against the symphysis pubis. Posttraumatic strictures are usually short, smooth, and solitary (Fig. 19-44). Blunt force trauma to the pelvis associated with pubic fractures or diastasis can result in fracture or even shattering of the prostate with subsequent stricture of the prostatic urethra. Injuries caused by instrumentation usually affect areas of transition, such as the penoscrotal junction and the membranous urethra.

Strictures associated with *urethral carcinoma* are usually solitary and can be either irregular or smooth (Fig. 19-45). Because the appearance of malignant and benign strictures overlap, most strictures are visualized with urethroscopy, and brushings/biopsies are obtained to verify the nature of the stricture.

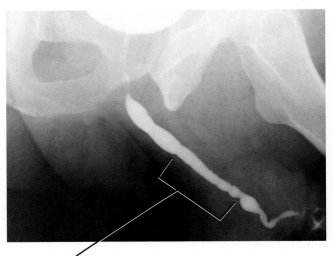

Narrowed segment

Figure 19-43 Voiding cystourethrography demonstrates a long segment of bulbous and penile urethra narrowed by multiple postinfectious strictures.

Because the length of the stricture influences the type of repair that is likely to be successful (buccal mucosa grafts are sometimes used to repair long strictures), ultrasound of the urethra can be performed during retrograde injection with saline to provide an accurate measurement without the magnification inherent to fluoroscopy (Fig. 19-46).

■ OUTPOUCHINGS FROM THE URINARY TRACT

Outpouchings can occur from virtually any part of the urinary tract. Some outpouchings are congenital, whereas others result from inflammation, infection, or abnormal pressures within the urinary tract. Table 19-3 lists a number of characteristic outpouchings from the urinary tract.

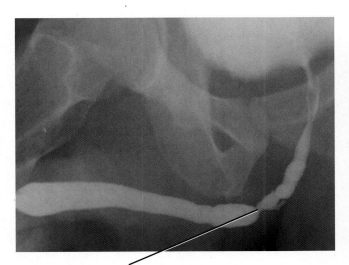

Dominant stricture in mid-bulbous urethra

Figure 19-42 Retrograde urethrogram performed after a history of urethritis demonstrates multifocal strictures in the bulbous urethra. Urethroscopy was performed and confirmed benign stricture.

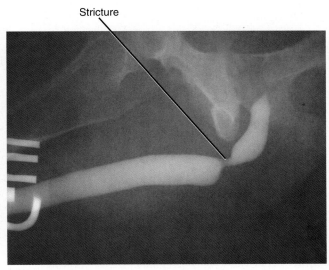

Stricture

Figure 19-44 Retrograde urethrography performed to follow straddle injury to the urethra shows a smooth, short stricture of the bulbous urethra.

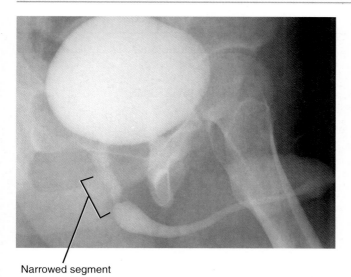

Narrowed segment

Figure 19-45 Voiding cystourethrography demonstrates smooth narrowing of the prostatic and membranous urethra. Urothelial carcinoma of the urethra was diagnosed at urethroscopy.

Outpouchings from the Ureter

Ureteral pseudodiverticulosis describes small outpouchings from the ureter, usually in the setting of chronic inflammation related to stone disease, ureteral stents, or both. The outpouchings are thought to result from a loosening of the subepithelial connective tissues, allowing hyperplastic urothelium to bulge out perpendicular to the lumen. The collections are small, less than 5 mm in diameter, and have a smooth appearance (Fig. 19-47). Interestingly, an association appears to exist between the presence of ureteral pseudodiverticulosis and urothelial carcinoma, although tumor does not necessarily arise within the outpouchings themselves. Evidence suggests

that as many as 50% of patients with ureteral pseudodiverticulosis either have a urothelial carcinoma or experience development of one within 2 to 10 years. More than 70% of patients with pseudodiverticulosis and a filling defect have a malignant urothelial tumor.

Blind-ending ureteral duplication (also called *ureteral diverticulum*) is a rare congenital outpouching from the ureter. Unlike the multiple small outpouchings of ureteral pseudodiverticulosis, a blind-ending duplication is a single tubular structure of variable length that results when a ureteric bud fails to induce the metanephron to form a kidney (see Figs. 19-20 and 19-21).

Outpouchings from the Bladder

Bladder Diverticula

Bladder diverticula are common, with increased incidence among older men. These are seen most often in the presence of high bladder pressure from outlet obstruction, usually related to prostatic hypertrophy. Areas of weakness between fibers of the detrusor muscle allow the mucosa to protrude through the muscle, resulting in a herniation of a thin layer of mucosa and serosa (technically, these are pseudodiverticula because the muscular component of the wall is absent, but these are commonly called *diverticula*). A natural separation occurs in muscle fibers at the trigone to allow each ureter to enter. This area of potential weakness is often the first site of bladder diverticulum formation (Fig. 19-48). These periureteral or *Hutch diverticula* can form even in low-pressure bladders. As described previously, diverticula can also form in the region of the urachus. These *urachal diverticula* arise from the midline of the bladder dome and are directed toward the umbilicus.

Because bladder diverticula are not surrounded by detrusor muscle, bladder contraction does not empty

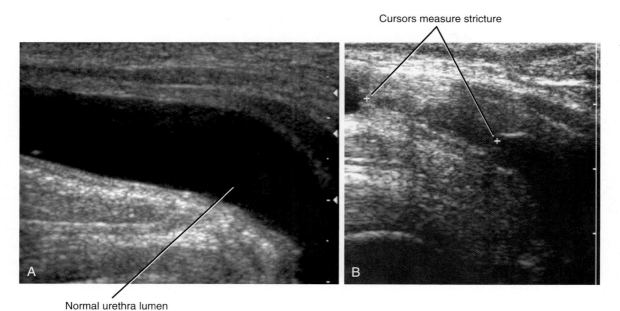

Cursors measure stricture

Normal urethra lumen

Figure 19-46 Urethral ultrasound in two patients. **A,** Sagittal ultrasonographic image obtained during regrade injection of saline demonstrates a normal segment of bulbous urethra. **B,** Sonographic measurement of bulbous urethral stricture shown in Figure 19-42. Because of the length of the stricture, a decision was made to use a buccal mucosal graft for repair.

Table 19-3   Outpouchings from the Urinary Tract

Diagnosis	Comments
URETERS	
Ureteral pseudodiverticulosis	Multiple small outpouchings from ureter Up to 50% develop urothelial carcinoma within 3 years (often in the bladder) Squamous cell carcinoma associated less commonly
Blind-ending ureteral duplication	Rare Blind-ending tube of variable length May become spherical or saclike
BLADDER	
Bladder diverticulum	Usually near ureteral orifice or midline bladder dome unless multiple (high-pressure bladder)
Cellules and saccules	Small outpouchings that protrude into but not beyond the detrusor muscle
Bladder within hernia	Inguinal or obturator hernia
URETHRA	
Urethral diverticulum	Fluid-filled periurethral sac Acquired in women; often present with postvoid dribbling Often congenital in male individuals; can present with outlet obstruction at birth
Urethral fistula or sinus	Prior infection or trauma
Cowper duct and gland	Paired ducts from bulbous urethra fill glands at level of membranous urethra
Glands of Littré	Associated with urethritis Strictures often present

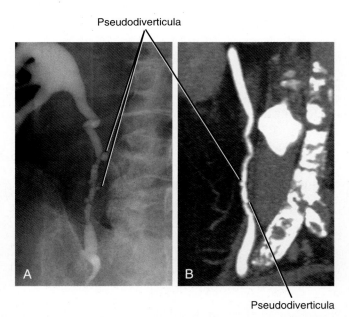

Figure 19-47 Ureteral pseudodiverticulosis. **A,** Image from retrograde urogram demonstrates multiple outpouchings typical of ureteral pseudodiverticulosis. **B,** Coronal maximum intensity projection image from computed tomographic urogram in a different patient with ureteral pseudodiverticulosis.

them. In fact, if a diverticulum develops as a result of bladder outlet obstruction, detrusor contraction can result in only a small amount of voided urine with preferential filling of the diverticulum (Fig. 19-49). In this case, the urine shifts from the bladder to the

diverticulum, then refills the bladder after the detrusor muscle relaxes (so-called yo-yo voiding).

A distended diverticulum can mimic the bladder, not only on fluoroscopy but occasionally on CT or MRI. The true bladder can be correctly identified if the ureters are

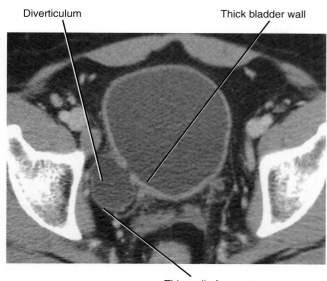

Diverticulum   Thick bladder wall

Thin wall of
diverticulum

Figure 19-48 Axial image of the bladder from contrast-enhanced computed tomographic scan demonstrates a periureteral bladder diverticulum. Compare the thickness of the wall of the diverticulum with the remainder of the bladder wall.

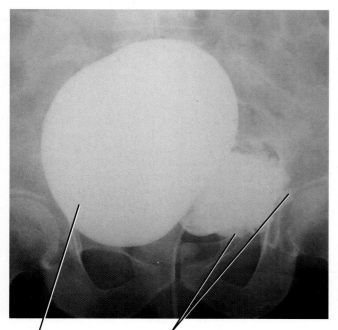

Smooth wall
of diverticulum

Cellules within
trabeculated bladder wall

Figure 19-49 Anteroposterior image from a cystogram shows two rounded structures: Which one is the diverticulum? The catheter courses left into the trabeculated bladder. The larger, smooth structure is the diverticulum, which expands when the patient tries to void.

seen entering the trigone or the bladder neck, and the urethra can be identified during voiding or in the presence of a catheter. Patients with bladder diverticula often have a trabeculated bladder, whereas a diverticulum has a smooth, thin wall.

Pearl: Large bladder diverticula are usually smooth, whereas the adjacent bladder is often trabeculated.

In cases of chronically increased bladder pressures (prostatic hypertrophy, urethral strictures, spastic type neurogenic bladder), innumerable outpouchings from the urinary bladder occur, ranging from marked trabeculation to frank diverticula. Small protrusions of mucosa into but not beyond the detrusor muscle are called *cellules* and are usually multiple (see Fig. 19-49). Because these become slightly larger, some call the outpouching *saccules*, although discrimination between cellules and saccules is arbitrary. When the lumen herniates beyond the outer margin of the detrusor muscle, it is called a *bladder diverticulum.*

It is important to inspect any bladder diverticula closely for mucosal irregularity or filling defects. Stasis within a diverticulum increases the risk for stone formation, infection, and urothelial carcinoma. Because the wall of a bladder diverticulum lacks the muscular layer, bladder cancers arising within diverticula are more likely to invade through the wall early, and small tumors can be associated with nodal and distant metastatic disease (Fig. 19-50).

Occasionally, the bladder will be pulled into hernias of the pelvic wall, particularly inguinal and obturator hernias. This can create the appearance of an elongated bladder diverticulum (Fig. 19-51). If initially identified on IV urography or cystography, a radiopaque instrument may be used to analyze the relation of the outpouching with other anatomic landmarks, such as the inguinal ligament. On CT, the diagnosis is less elusive, although when the connection between the two bladder components is long and thin, it may require an attentive observer to note.

Outpouchings of the Urethra

Urethral Diverticula
The term *urethral diverticulum* has been used to describe several different entities. *Acquired diverticula* usually develop after infection and occur more often in women.

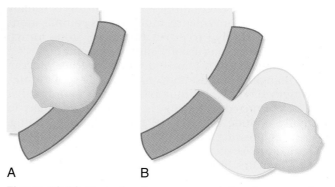

A   B

Figure 19-50 Illustration demonstrates early invasive nature of bladder cancer arising within a diverticulum. **A,** Tumors that arise from the mucosa within the bladder lumen must invade through the detrusor muscle to extend beyond the bladder. **B,** Because bladder diverticula lack a muscular component, the same tumor invades the perivesical fat earlier if it arises within a diverticulum.

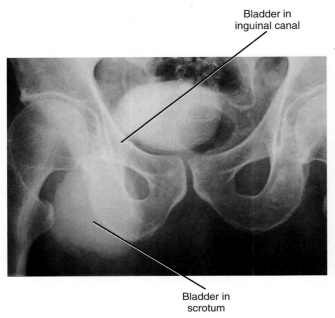

Bladder in
inguinal canal

Bladder in
scrotum

Double density of the
urethra containing and
surrounded by contrast

Diverticulum wraps
around urethra

Figure 19-51 Anteroposterior image from an intravenous urogram demonstrates an elongated outpouching of the urinary bladder as it is pulled into a right inguinal hernia.

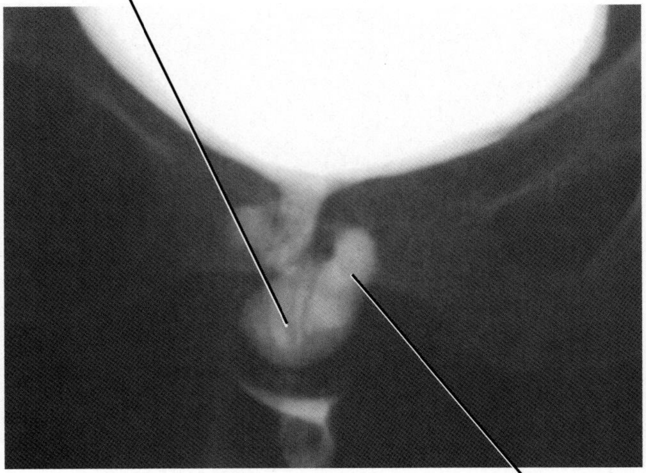

Figure 19-52 Anteroposterior image from a voiding cystoure-thrography in a woman with a urethral diverticulum.

Congenital diverticula are sometimes found as a cause of urethral obstruction in male infants. Some consider acquired diverticula to be "pseudodiverticula" because they are enclosed by postinflammatory fibrosis rather than an epithelial lining. However, this differentiation is rarely important to the radiologist, and often is neglected in medical dictionaries and pathology texts.

DIVERTICULA OF THE FEMALE URETHRA

The most common urethral diverticulum is the acquired type that occurs in up to 6% of adult women. Thought to occur when an infected periurethral gland bursts into the urethra and maintains communication, these diverticula are confined by the fascial planes of the periurethral space. Because they can fill during voiding, women with diverticula may experience postvoid dribbling when the diverticulum later empties. Although this is usually only a social inconvenience, more serious complications can occur, including recurrent infections, stone formation, and carcinoma (usually adenocarcinoma).

The diagnosis of a female urethral diverticulum can be challenging. Because they may fill only sporadically, sensitivity of VCUG is limited. If VCUG is performed, it can be optimized by having the woman use a finger to partially occlude the urethral meatus during voiding, increasing pressure within the urethra. If it does fill, the diverticulum is seen to wrap around the urethra and usually remains filled after voiding (Fig. 19-52). RUG is more effective than VCUG but requires a double-balloon catheter, as described previously.

MRI has become the preferred technique for evaluating women with suspected urethral diverticulum. Because the outpouching rarely empties completely, T2-weighted images demonstrate a fluid-containing

sac adjacent to or partially surrounding the urethra. Knowledge of female perineal anatomy is key to interpretation, and the diverticulum is often seen wrapping around the urethra on axial images (Fig. 19-53). The actual connection between the diverticulum and the urethra is sometimes visualized by MRI, particularly when an endovaginal coil is used. When evaluating a urethral diverticulum with MRI, contrast enhancement with gadolinium-based contrast media can be helpful to assess for infection or tumor. Urethral diverticula can usually be easily differentiated from Gartner's duct cysts, which are more posterior or lateral, within the wall of the vagina, and Bartholin gland cysts, which are near the vestibule and do not wrap around the urethra.

DIVERTICULA OF THE MALE URETHRA

Acquired diverticula also occur in men as the result of trauma, prolonged catheterization, or periurethral infection, although they are much less common than in women (Fig. 19-54). These are not difficult to identify by RUG but could be overlooked on routine cross-sectional imaging. As in women, symptoms often include infection and postvoid dribbling, although the latter symptom is not unusual to a lesser degree in men without diverticula.

Some also apply the term *urethral diverticulum* to a congenital abnormality that can cause bladder outlet obstruction in male infants. Others consider these to be anterior urethral valves, whereas still others describe subtle differences between what they consider to be congenital anterior urethral diverticula and anterior urethral valves. In any case, these are a wide-mouthed protrusion that distends with urine, compressing the adjacent urethral lumen.

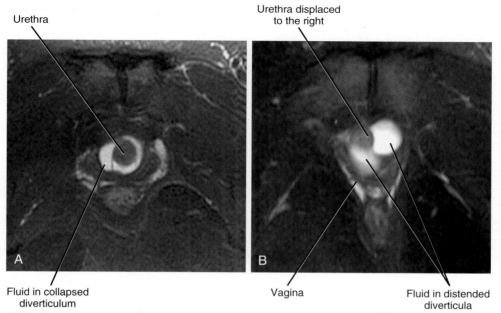

Urethra

Urethra displaced to the right

Fluid in collapsed diverticulum

Vagina

Fluid in distended diverticula

Figure 19-53 Axial, fat-suppressed, T2-weighted images of urethral diverticula in two separate female patients. **A,** Collapsed diverticulum appears as a thin, fluid-filled sac surrounding the urethra. **B,** In a different patient, two distended diverticula exert mass effect on the urethra and vagina.

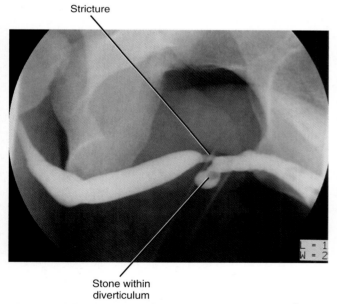

Stricture

Stone within diverticulum

Figure 19-54 Retrograde urethrography demonstrates an acquired male urethral diverticulum after prolonged bladder catheterization. The diverticulum is adjacent to a stricture at the penoscrotal junction. A small filling defect proved to be a stone.

Urethral Fistula and Sinus

A urethral fistula is a linear outpouching of the urethra that reaches the skin surface or another hollow viscous (bladder or bowel). A tract that ends in a blind pouch is called a *urethral sinus.* Both urethral fistulae and sinuses can result from poor urethral healing after trauma; breakdown of tissues because of inflammation, surgery, or radiation; or primary tumor of the urethra (Box 19-2)

BOX 19-2   Causes of Urethral Fistulae

Trauma
Surgery to adjacent structures
Radiation therapy
Tuberculous urethritis
Other chronic urethritis
Malignant tumor
Penile prosthesis

Diagnosis is usually made with VCUG, RUG, or both. In each case, a curvilinear tract is identified leading away from the urethra.

If a sinus or fistula leads to other structures in the pelvis or perineum, some benefit may exist to imaging with CT. Depending on the circumstances, dilute contrast media may be injected into the urethra or bladder, and the patient may be asked to void before imaging (Fig. 19-55).

Cowper Ducts and Glands

Cowper glands are paired periurethral glands in men and are situated on either side of the membranous urethra, embedded within the tissues of the genitourinary diaphragm. A duct drains each gland by running a course parallel to the urethra until it empties into the bulbous urethra through a small orifice. Generally, these glands are of no clinical significance. They can become infected, but this is difficult to diagnose at the time because they are rarely imaged and symptoms are that of urethritis. If obstructed, they can become dilated (some call this *Cowper syringocele*) and can compress or burst into the adjacent urethra. The main significance of the Cowper glands

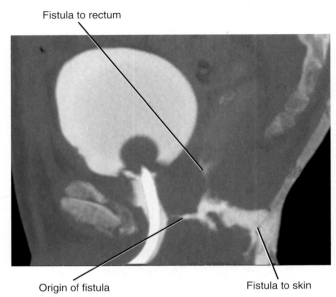

Figure 19-55 Sagittal maximum intensity projection image from a computed tomographic cystogram performed several weeks after traumatic injury to the prostatic urethra demonstrates a fistulous communication from the urethra to the skin and to the rectum.

and ducts to the radiologist is the occasional filling during retrograde examination (Fig. 19-56). Retrograde filling through a mildly patulous orifice has no clinical significance but could be confused with a sinus tract or acquired diverticulum.

Glands of Littré

Multiple small mucinous glands help lubricate the penile urethra. These glands of Littré can unwittingly become the host of infection during episodes of urethritis. As the

glands swell with bacteria, the openings to the urethra become patulous, allowing reflux of contrast during RUG (Fig. 19-57). Because the glands may never return to normal, reflux does not necessarily imply active urethritis and is often associated with urethral strictures. This glandular tissue is also believed to be the origin of rare cases of urethral adenocarcinoma.

■ WALL THICKENING

Ureteral Wall Thickening

Thickening of the ureter can be diffuse or focal. Diffuse thickening is often the result of inflammation from a stent or pyelonephritis (Fig. 19-58). Atypical infections such as tuberculosis and schistosomiasis or neoplastic processes such as lymphoma can also thicken the wall of the ureter. Superficial spreading urothelial carcinoma is an unusual cause of wall thickening in the ureter and usually results in marked mucosal irregularity on excretory phase images.

Urothelial carcinoma is the most common cause of focal thickening in the ureter. In most cases, malignant thickening also demonstrates increased contrast enhancement, although urothelial enhancement is also common in inflammatory processes. For this reason, it is helpful to include nephrographic phase images of the ureters and bladder routinely on enhanced CT and MR examinations. When obstructive, urothelial carcinoma can delay or prevent urinary excretion of contrast; therefore, mucosal masses are often best seen as enhancing masses or focal thickening outlined by a background of low-attenuation or low-signal-intensity urine (Fig. 19-59).

Bladder Wall Thickening

Diffuse thickening of the bladder wall on cross-sectional imaging is usually the result of trabeculation in response to chronic bladder outlet obstruction. For

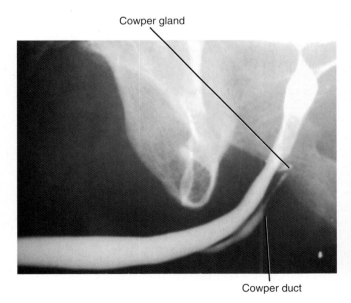

Figure 19-56 Retrograde urethrography demonstrates filling of a Cowper duct and gland. This is considered to be a normal finding, although filling is more common in patients with a history of urethritis.

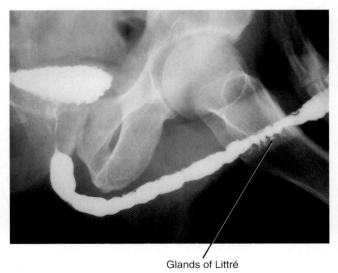

Figure 19-57 Retrograde urethrography performed in a patient with recurrent urethritis demonstrates filling of enlarged glands of Littré. Multifocal strictures are present in the penile and bulbous urethra.

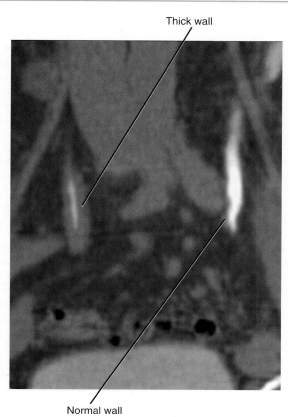

Thick wall

Normal wall

Figure 19-58 Coronal multiplanar reformation from the excretory phase of a computed tomographic urogram demonstrates diffuse thickening of the right ureter. A stent had been removed several weeks before the study, but because of severe thickening, brushings were performed revealing inflammation with no malignant cells.

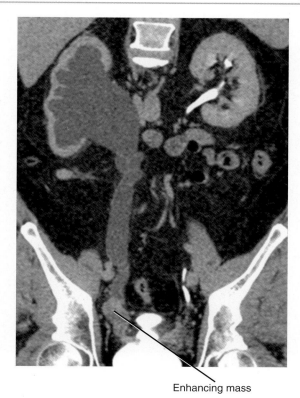

Enhancing mass

Figure 19-59 Curved planar reformation of the right ureter from a computed tomographic urogram. An enhancing mass in the obstructed distal right ureter is seen against a background of low-attenuation urine. Note normal excretion on the left side.

this reason, diffuse bladder wall thickening is a common finding in older men who have prostatic hyperplasia (Fig. 19-60). However, outlet obstruction from any cause, including prostate cancer and benign or malignant urethral stricture, or spastic-type of neurogenic bladder can also cause diffuse bladder wall thickening (Fig. 19-61). Bladder diverticula are commonly seen when thickening is due to outlet obstruction.

The term *cystitis* is used to describe a wide variety of inflammatory disorders in the bladder. The most common form of cystitis is due to bacterial infection (commonly referred to as *urinary tract infection [UTI]*). Inflammatory cystitis can also result from medications (cyclophosphamide is the classic example), radiation, or atypical infections such as tuberculosis and schistosomiasis. Changes from cystitis range from mild, diffuse wall thickening to irregular nodular wall thickening (Fig. 19-62). Hemorrhagic cystitis refers to bleeding from hyperemic mucosa and can be associated with any form of acute cystitis or from rapid decompression of an obstructed bladder. In hemorrhagic cystitis, wall thickening is accompanied by blood clots in the lumen (they often fill the lumen). Interstitial cystitis is an idiopathic form that appears to be immune mediated, and can cause wall thickening and decreased bladder capacity. The bladder wall can also become secondarily involved by extravesical inflammatory processes such

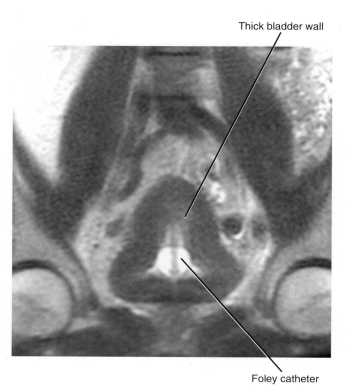

Thick bladder wall

Foley catheter

Figure 19-60 Coronal T2-weighted magnetic resonance image of the pelvis demonstrates a severely thickened bladder wall after catheter decompression of bladder outlet obstruction caused by benign prostatic hyperplasia.

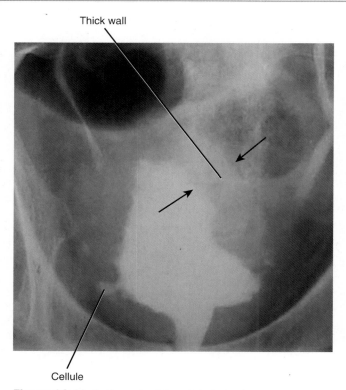

Thick wall

Cellule

Figure 19-61 Radiograph of the pelvis during intravenous urography demonstrates diffuse bladder wall thickening and trabeculation caused by neurogenic bladder. *Arrows* identify the inner and outer margins of the bladder wall.

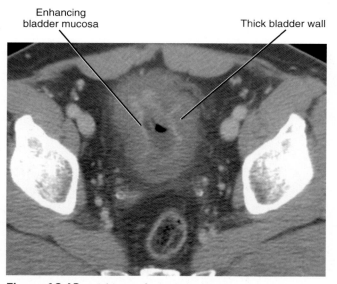

Enhancing bladder mucosa

Thick bladder wall

Figure 19-62 Axial image from a contrast-enhanced computed tomographic scan in a patient with interstitial cystitis demonstrates diffuse thickening of the bladder wall. Air is in the lumen of the bladder because of recent catheterization. Note subtle mucosal enhancement defining the inner margin of the bladder wall.

as diverticulitis and Crohn disease. Table 19-4 summarizes benign causes of bladder wall thickening.

When diffuse bladder wall thickening is irregular, it should raise concern for malignancy. Although a variety of benign entities can result in nodular bladder

changes, irregular thickening is more often seen with urothelial carcinoma or involvement with lymphoma (Figs. 19-63). When lymphoma is the cause of bladder wall thickening, usually evidence of disease exists elsewhere, although isolated bladder lymphoma can occur. Because considerable overlap exists in the appearance of benign and malignant disease in cases of irregular bladder wall thickening, cystoscopy is required for diagnosis.

Focal bladder wall thickening is usually the result of malignant disease (see Fig. 19-34). The most common cause is urothelial carcinoma; therefore, identification of focal bladder wall thickening should prompt a search for invasion into the perivesical fat and adjacent organs, as well as for enlarged lymph nodes along the pelvic and paraaortic chains. When focal thickening is located at the bladder dome, urachal carcinoma is a consideration. Percutaneous biopsy may be required for diagnosis urachal carcinoma if the mass does not extend through the bladder mucosa.

Leiomyoma of the bladder wall is a rare cause of focal wall thickening that appears smooth and well defined on imaging. Although the submucosal nature of the mass is occasionally apparent on imaging (Fig. 19-64), cystoscopy is usually required for diagnosis.

Eosinophilic cystitis is a rare inflammatory process of the bladder that may present as focal bladder wall thickening or bladder mass, indistinguishable from urothelial carcinoma (Fig. 19-65). Biopsy is required for diagnosis, demonstrating eosinophilic infiltration and fibrosis. Most cases respond to therapy with antiinflammatory medications and resection of masses, although some cases progress to chronic fibrosis.

Urethral Wall Thickening

Whereas the male urethra is only rarely examined with cross-sectional imaging, the female urethra is commonly included on axial CT and MR sections through the perineum. The predictable anatomy of the region already discussed allows identification of masses that affect the female urethra. Iatrogenic thickening of the female urethra can be seen when *collagen* has been injected in an effort to treat stress urinary incontinence (Fig. 19-66). When injections have been performed, thickening is usually uniform with no evidence of enhancement on MR.

Carcinoma of the female urethra can result in symmetric or asymmetric enlargement of the urethra on cross-sectional images (Fig. 19-67). Squamous cell carcinoma is the most common type of urethral cancer, followed by urothelial carcinoma. When malignancy arises within a urethral diverticulum, adenocarcinoma is the most common subtype. Each of these tumors is best demonstrated with MRI, showing distortion of the normal anatomy on T2-weighted images and heterogeneous contrast enhancement on postcontrast T1-weighted images. Benign *leiomyomas* of the female urethra are less common than carcinoma, often appear more focal, and tend to have more uniform contrast enhancement on MRI.

Table 19-4   Benign Causes of Bladder Wall Thickening

Diagnosis	Clinical and Imaging Characteristics
Bacterial cystitis	Associated with pyuria Thick bladder wall with or without stranding of the perivesical fat May have air within bladder lumen
Bladder outlet obstruction	More common in male individuals Enlarged prostate or posterior urethra (stricture or valves) Trabeculated bladder with cellules and diverticula
Neurogenic bladder	Spinal cord injury and other central nervous system disorders Multiple types, but those with bladder wall thickening typically have small bladder volume
Interstitial cystitis	Clinical syndrome of urinary frequency, urgency, nocturia, and pelvic pain with sterile urine cultures Imaging is usually normal, especially in early stages In late phases, bladder volume is small
Radiation cystitis	History of pelvic irradiation Variable imaging appearance, but usually small volume with thick wall May see radiation-related changes in adjacent pelvic organs or bones Calcifications or fistulae may be present
Hemorrhagic cystitis	History of rapid decompression of obstructed bladder or radiation to the pelvis Magnetic resonance imaging shows variable signal in bladder wall depending on the stage of blood products
Schistosomiasis	Most common in Africa No distinguishing features in acute phase In chronic phase, see small bladder with thick wall that contains curvilinear calcification Distal ureter may be calcified Increased risk for squamous cell carcinoma
Tuberculosis	Consider in patients with cystitis refractory to therapy with sterile urine cultures More common in immunocompromised patients Acute infection: imaging shows thick wall with no distinguishing features Chronic infection: sinus tracts and fistulae may be present.
Malacoplakia	More common in women and individuals with diabetes Associated with urinary tract infections, especially with *Escherichia coli* May have multiple masslike lesions or diffuse wall thickening Mass lesions may invade adjacent pelvic structures, mimicking cancer
Emphysematous cystitis	Patients with diabetes Air in the bladder wall with or without air within the bladder lumen
Cystitis cystica and cystitis glandularis	Nodular reaction to chronic irritation/infection resulting in small, fluid-filled submucosal cysts or larger nodules of glandular hyperplasia that often coexist on imaging and at cystoscopy Even with extensive changes, the muscular layer of the bladder remains intact on imaging
Nephrogenic adenoma	Result of chronic bladder irritation from stones, infection, or surgery May develop after bladder biopsy Polypoid or sessile masses at imaging, often multiple
Eosinophilic cystitis	Rare eosinophilic infiltrate of bladder wall Reported associations with parasitic infections and allergies Diffuse or masslike thickening of bladder wall Irregularity of the mucosal surface and stranding of the perivesical fat are common findings
Endometriosis	Focal areas of wall thickening Focal areas of high signal on T1-weighted magnetic resonance (MR) images within region of bladder wall thickening
Amyloidosis of bladder wall	Diffuse wall thickening on computed tomography Low signal on T2-weighted MR images with corresponding lack of enhancement
Lupus cystitis	Symptoms and imaging appearance usually similar to interstitial cystitis but occurs in patients with systemic lupus erythematosus. Caused by vasculitis and deposition of immune complexes within the bladder wall Cases of hemorrhagic cystitis have been reported

Enhancing mass fills most of the bladder lumen

Residual bladder lumen

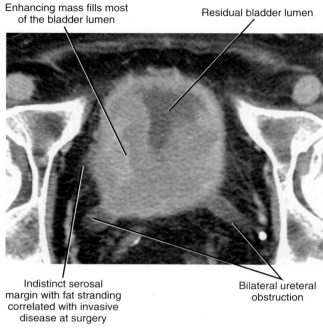

Indistinct serosal margin with fat stranding correlated with invasive disease at surgery

Bilateral ureteral obstruction

Figure 19-63 Axial image from a contrast-enhanced computed tomographic scan of the pelvis demonstrates diffuse bladder involvement with urothelial carcinoma. Local extravesical invasion along the right margin was confirmed at surgery.

Focal bladder wall thickening

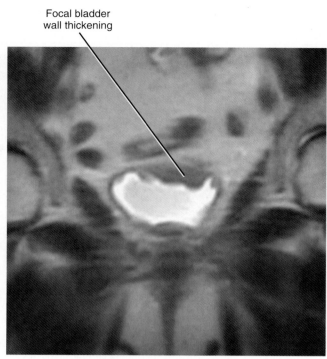

Figure 19-65 Coronal T2-weighted magnetic resonance image of a woman being evaluated for a cystocele who was incidentally found to have focal bladder wall thickening. This was thought to represent urothelial carcinoma on imaging, but biopsy revealed eosinophilic cystitis.

Overlying mucosa is intact

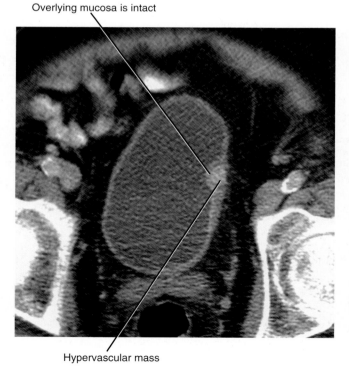

Hypervascular mass

Figure 19-64 Axial image from a contrast-enhanced computed tomographic scan demonstrates an enhancing submucosal lesion confirmed to be a leiomyoma of the bladder wall after excision.

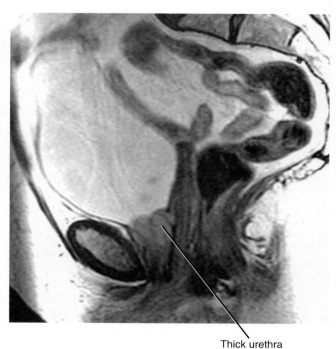

Thick urethra

Figure 19-66 Sagittal midline T2-weighted magnetic resonance image of the pelvis in a woman treated for stress urinary incontinence using periurethral collagen injections. Uniform thickening of the urethra is present.

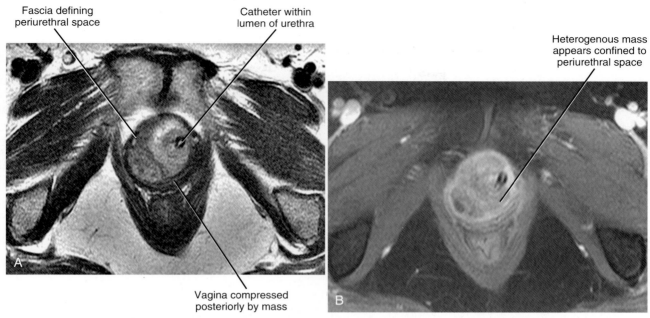

Fascia defining periurethral space

Catheter within lumen of urethra

Heterogenous mass appears confined to periurethral space

Vagina compressed posteriorly by mass

Figure 19-67 Magnetic resonance imaging demonstrating urethral thickening in papillary urothelial carcinoma of the female urethra. **A,** Axial T2-weighted imaging with a Foley catheter in place demonstrates asymmetric wall thickening in the urethral space. **B,** Postcontrast injection T1-weighted imaging with fat suppression demonstrates heterogeneous enhancement of the mass.

Carcinoma of the male urethra is seen more often as a stricture than wall thickening because urethrography is used more commonly than cross-sectional imaging. The bulbous and membranous urethra are the most common location, followed by the penile urethra and, rarely, the prostatic urethra. Squamous cell carcinoma is the most common subtype of male urethral cancer, although urothelial carcinoma is more common in the prostatic urethra. Adenocarcinoma occasionally arises within the glands of Littré or Cowper gland.

■ CALCIFICATIONS

Noncontrast-enhanced CT has largely replaced plain radiography for the diagnosis of ureteral stone disease. Not surprisingly, CT also allows detection of stones within the bladder and urethra. In each case, describing the size and precise location of the stone(s) provides the urologist with potentially valuable information regarding appropriate management. The use of NCCT for the diagnosis of ureteral calculi presenting as flank pain is discussed in Chapter 8.

Several types of bladder stones have a characteristic imaging appearance. Stones that consist mainly of calcium oxalate dihydrate often form spicules at the periphery, similar to a toy jack (hence the name *jack stones*) (Fig. 19-68). Because calcium oxalate dehydrate stones are relatively fragile, this appearance predicts a greater rate of success for extracorporeal shockwave lithotripsy.

Uric acid stones are often considered radiolucent, although some large uric acid stones are faintly seen on plain films. Because uric acid stones have an appearance similar to any other urinary calculus on NCCT, the presence of a moderate-to-large stone on CT that is not seen on a good-quality plain film suggests it is composed of uric acid.

Occasionally, foreign bodies within the urinary tract become encrusted with mineral deposits. This usually occurs within the bladder because foreign bodies elsewhere in the urinary tract are more likely to cause

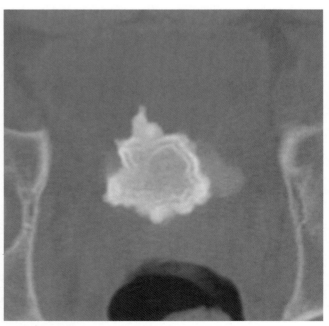

Figure 19-68 Axial image from noncontrast-enhanced computed tomography of the pelvis demonstrates the typical appearance of a jack stone in the urinary bladder. The spiculated appearance is common when the stone is composed of calcium oxalate dihydrate.

obstruction and require immediate therapy. Sometimes the foreign body is a stent or other device placed intentionally. Stent encrustation resulting from delayed stent removal or exchange can result in severe patient morbidity and present a serious challenge to the urologist. Because the calcification is so dense that it can obscure subtle details when CT is viewed in soft-tissue windows, it is important to use bone windows to allow better appreciation of the components within the mineral/foreign body complex (Fig. 19-69).

Pitfall: *Soft-tissue windows often do not allow differentiation between calcification around ureteral stents and the stent material. Use of bone windows facilitates*

discrimination between the stent and the surrounding encrustation.

Pearl: *Accurate identification of stent encrustation allows the urologist to prepare for a complicated stent removal procedure.*

Calcification within the walls of the urinary tract usually signifies the presence of a chronic disease process or exposure. Calcification occurs most commonly in the bladder, probably because the thickness of the bladder wall allows accumulation of detectable mineral, and stasis of urine prolongs exposure to many of the causative agents (Fig. 19-70). Box 19-3 lists most of the causes of bladder wall calcification. Although rare in the

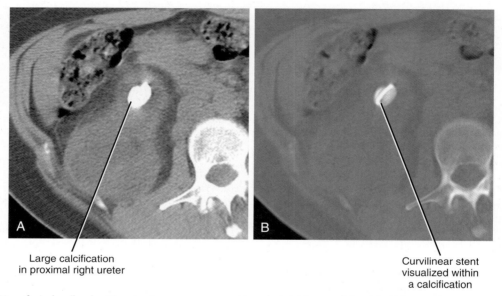

Large calcification
in proximal right ureter

Curvilinear stent
visualized within
a calcification

Figure 19-69 Use of window/level settings to detect stent encrustation. **A,** Axial image of the right kidney and proximal ureter from noncontrast-enhanced computed tomography viewed in a standard soft-tissue setting demonstrates a large calcification in the proximal right ureter. **B,** The same image viewed in bone windows allows differentiation between calcification and the stent. Encrustation resulted in a nonfunctioning stent with chronic obstruction of the right kidney.

Thickened region
of bladder wall
contains calcification

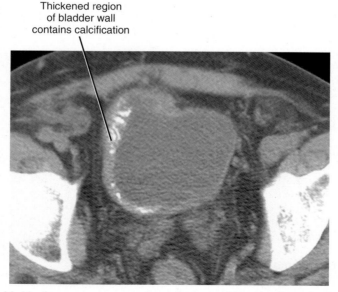

Figure 19-70 Axial image of the bladder from a noncontrast-enhanced computed tomography scan in a patient with biopsy-proven amyloid deposition in the bladder.

BOX 19-3   Causes of Bladder Wall Calcification

Schistosomiasis
Urothelial carcinoma
Tuberculosis
Radiation cystitis
Cytoxan cystitis
Interstitial cystitis
Amyloidosis

United States, schistosomiasis remains the most common cause of bladder calcification worldwide. In the United States, urothelial carcinoma is a more common cause of bladder wall calcification on CT (Fig. 19-71).

■ GAS AND CHYLE
IN THE URINARY TRACT

Gas

Gas in the urinary tract is often an incidental finding in patients who have a catheter in the bladder or have had recent catheterization. However, air in the bladder without a history of instrumentation can be a sign of urinary tract infection or fistulous communication with bowel (Figs. 19-72 and 19-73).

Mucosal or submucosal air within the urinary bladder almost always signals *emphysematous cystitis*, a severe form of bladder infection. Although it is usually not difficult to localize air to within the bladder wall on CT

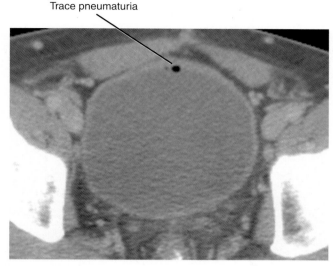

Trace pneumaturia

Figure 19-72 Axial image of the bladder from a contrast-enhanced computed tomographic scan from a patient who presented with fever and abdominal pain demonstrates a trace amount of intraluminal gas. The patient had not undergone bladder catheterization. Pyuria was found at urinalysis, leading to the diagnosis of urinary tract infection.

(Fig. 19-74), findings may be more subtle on plain films. Gas in the bladder wall can easily be mistaken for gas in the rectum, although rectal gas mixed with stool usually has a mottled appearance, whereas gas within the bladder wall often appears curvilinear on plain films (Fig. 19-75).

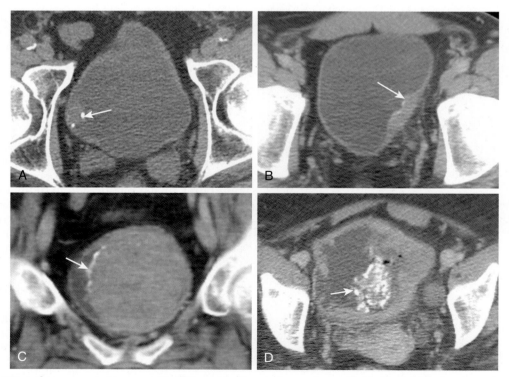

Figure 19-71 Images from computed tomographic (CT) examinations in four patients with bladder calcification *(arrows)* associated with urothelial carcinoma. **A,** Punctate calcifications, **(B)** subtle smooth surface calcification, **(C)** more pronounced surface calcification (coronal image from CT urogram), and **(D)** mottled focal calcification in the papillary portion of a diffuse bladder tumor.

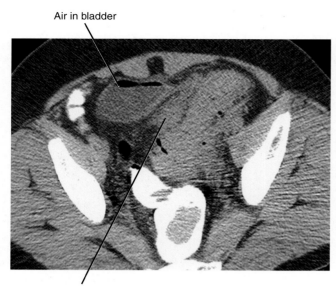

Air in bladder

Stranding bridges
the sigmoid colon
and bladder

Figure 19-73 Axial image from computed tomography performed to evaluate diverticulitis. Patient had no history of bladder catheterization, and air within the bladder proved to be due to a colovesical fistula. The bladder is displaced to the right by inflamed sigmoid colon.

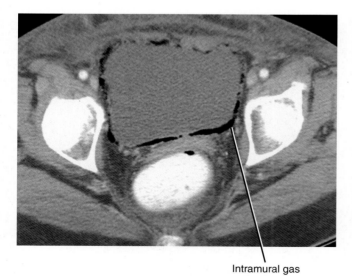

Intramural gas

Figure 19-74 Axial image of the bladder from a contrast-enhanced computed tomographic scan demonstrates gas in the wall of the bladder indicating emphysematous cystitis.

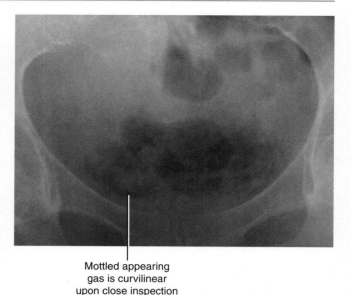

Mottled appearing
gas is curvilinear
upon close inspection

Figure 19-75 Magnified view of the pelvis from an abdominal radiograph performed in the intensive care unit for a patient with urosepsis. Mottled and curvilinear gas in the pelvis was shown to represent emphysematous cystitis on the computed tomography scan performed in Figure 19-74.

Pearl: Curvilinear dependent collections of gas usually indicate that they are located within the bladder wall, signaling infection more severe than seen with pneumaturia (gas in the bladder lumen) alone.

Gas within the ureters is rare and most often results from reflux of air introduced into the bladder or kidney iatrogenically. As with the bladder, the possibility of infection should always be considered. Gas-producing infection within the lumen of the upper urinary tract is called *emphysematous pyelitis* (an entity distinct from emphysematous pyelonephritis) and is discussed in Chapter 18.

Chyluria

Fat attenuation or signal within the bladder usually indicates the presence of chyle caused by a connection between lymphatic system and urinary tract. Chyluria was originally described in association with filariasis infiltrating the lymphatic system of the kidney but can also be seen in association with urinary obstruction, renal abscess, tumors of the kidney or prostate, and tuberculosis. Recently, chyluria has been described in association with partial nephrectomy, and postsurgical chyluria is likely the most common cause encountered in the United States. Chyluria also occurs occasionally after radiofrequency ablation of renal tumors. Although usually asymptomatic, prolonged loss of chyle in the urine can result in hypoproteinemia and subsequent immunocompromise. Detection of a fat–fluid level on CT is usually the first indication of chyluria, but appropriate windowing is necessary to differentiate fat from air (Fig. 19-76). Chyluria often resolves spontaneously but may require surgical ligation of lymphatics in some cases.

Fat-fluid level
in the bladder

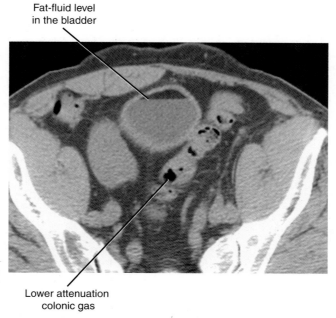

Lower attenuation
colonic gas

Figure 19-76 Axial image of the pelvis from an unenhanced computed tomographic scan of a patient after partial nephrectomy demonstrates fat attenuation in the nondependent portion of the bladder. Mistaking this finding for gas could prompt incorrect diagnosis of infection or colovesical fistula, but appropriate windowing shows the attenuation to be higher than that of colonic gas.

Suggested Readings

Ashley RA, Inman BA, Leibovich BC et al: Urachal carcinoma: clinicopathologic features and long-term outcomes of an aggressive malignancy, *Cancer* 107:712-720, 2006.

Barry KA, Jafri SZ: Eosinophilic cystitis: CT findings, *Abdom Imaging* 19:272-273, 1994.

Capps GW, Fulcher AS, Szucs RA et al: Imaging features of radiation-induced changes in the abdomen, *Radiographics* 17:1455-1473, 1997.

Chow LC, Kwan SW, Olcott EW et al: Split-bolus MDCT urography with synchronous nephrographic and excretory phase enhancement, *Am J Roentgenol* 189:314-322, 2007.

Dillman JR, Caoili EM, Cohan RH: Multi-detector CT urography: a one-stop renal and urinary tract imaging modality, *Abdom Imaging* 32:519-529, 2007.

Gittes RF: Female prostatitis, *Urol Clin* 29:613-616, 2002.

Herndon CD, McKenna PH: Antenatally detected proximal ureteral diverticulum, *Urology* 55(5):774, 2000.

Kawashima A: Imaging of urethral disease: a pictorial review, *Radiographics* 24(suppl 1):S195-S216, 2004.

Kottra JJ, Dunick NR: Retroperitoneal fibrosis, *Radiol Clin North Am* 34:1259-1275, 1996.

Krishnan A: The anatomy and embryology of posterior urethral valves, *J Urol* 175:1214-1220, 2006.

Leyendecker JR, Barnes CE, Zagoria RJ: MR urography: techniques and clinical applications, *Radiographics* 28:23-46, 2008.

Miller FH, Keppke AL, Yaghmi V et al: CT diagnosis of chyluria after partial nephrectomy, *Am J Roentgenol* 188:25-28, 2007.

Parker B, Patel B, Coffield KS: Ureteritis cystica presenting as a retractile ureteral polyp, *J Urol* 168:195-196, 2002.

Prasad SR, Menias CO, Narra VR: Cross-sectional imaging of the female urethra: technique and results, *Radiographics* 25:749-761, 2005.

Roberts WW: Ureteral stricture formation after removal of impacted calculi, *J Urol* 159:723-726, 1998.

Socher SA, Dewolf WC, Morgentaler A: Ureteral pseudodiverticulosis: the case for the retrograde urogram, *Urology* 47:924-927, 1996.

Thali-Schwab CM: Computed tomographic appearance of urachal adenocarcinomas: review of 25 cases, *Eur Radiol* 15:79-84, 2005.

Thomas AA, Lane BR, Thomas AZ et al: Emphysematous cystitis: a review of 135 cases, *BJU Int* 100:17-20, 2007.

Uibu T, Oska P, Auvinen A: Asbestos exposure as a risk factor for retroperitoneal fibrosis, *Lancet* 363:1422-1426, 2004.

Vaglio A, Salvarani C, Buzio C: Retroperitoneal fibrosis, *Lancet* 367:241-251, 2006.

Wasserman NF, Zhang G, Posalaky IP et al: Ureteral pseudodiverticula: frequent association with uroepithelial malignancy, *Am J Roentgenol* 157:69-72, 1991.

Wasserman NF: Inflammatory disease of the ureter, *Radiol Clin North Am* 34:1131-1156, 1996.

Weizer AZ: Routine postoperative imaging is important after ureteroscopic stone manipulation, *J Urol* 168:46-50, 2002.

Wong-You-Cheong JJ, Woodward PJ, Manning MA et al: Inflammatory and non-neoplastic bladder masses: radiologic-pathologic correlation, *Radiographics* 26:1847-1868, 2006.

Wong-You-Cheong JJ, Woodward PJ, Manning MA et al: Neoplasms of the urinary bladder: radiologic-pathologic correlation, *Radiographics* 26:553-580, 2006.

Yu JS: Urachal remnant diseases: spectrum of CT and US findings, *Radiographics* 21:451-461, 2001.

CHAPTER 20

Male Reproductive System

Anthony I. Zarka, Adam J. Jung, and Neal C. Dalrymple

■ ANATOMY OF THE MALE REPRODUCTIVE SYSTEM

Testis and Epididymis

The testes develop in the retroperitoneum during early fetal development. Each testis is attached to the inferior scrotal wall by the *gubernaculum testis,* which does not grow significantly in length as the rest of the fetus develops. As a result, the testes are tethered to the scrotum. As the torso grows, the spermatic cord stretches in length, maintaining the vascular supply in the form of the testicular artery and vein, and maintaining the reproductive pathway through the vas deferens. Thus, although this process is often described as the testes "descending" into the scrotum during the second month of gestation, it may be more accurate to say the fetal abdomen grows away from the testis. In adulthood, the gubernaculum remains as a part of the mesentery-like structure that maintains appropriate orientation of the testis within the scrotum. Redundancy of this mesorchium results in the *"bell-clapper"* deformity that increases the risk for testicular torsion. If there is more complete failure of scrotal attachment, the result is an "undescended testis," which is more appropriately termed *cryptorchidism.*

A portion of the peritoneal space is trapped by the testis and gubernaculum. This pocket of peritoneum is called the *processus vaginalis* and typically obliterates late in development. Persistent communication of the processus vaginalis with the peritoneal space provides a pathway for peritoneal fluid and disease to descend into the scrotum. Discontinuous areas that fail to obliterate result in noncommunicating hydrocele.

Each testis receives arterial supply from a testicular artery that arises from the abdominal aorta. The *pampiniform plexus* is a network of veins that provide venous outflow along the spermatic cord, ultimately uniting to form a single testicular vein on each side. The left testicular vein courses along the retroperitoneum from the inguinal canal to the left renal vein. The right testicular vein usually joins the inferior vena cava at the level of the inferior pole of the right kidney, although it does occasionally join the right renal vein.

Testicular parenchyma consists primarily of *seminiferous tubules* where spermatogenesis takes place. These are soft, convoluted tubular structures that resemble strands of spaghetti several microns in diameter. The tubules are compacted together and are encapsulated within the tunica albuginea, giving the testis its ovoid shape (Fig. 20-1). A small incision or laceration in the tunica allows the seminiferous parenchyma to spill out like spaghetti from a plastic bag. The mediastinum testis is a septum that runs within the testicular parenchyma, providing a lattice for the vascular structures and efferent ductules that carry sperm from the seminiferous tubules to the epididymis.

Sperm travels through the mediastinum testis to the head of the epididymis, which also consists of multiple tubular structures. These tubules begin to coalesce into more organized, straightened tubules in the epididymal tail until they finally channel into a single tube, the *vas deferens.* The vas deferens courses along the spermatic cord to the internal inguinal ring. Once inside the pelvis, it deviates away from the gonadal vessels, and travels inferior and medial to insert into the ejaculatory ducts near the ostium of the ipsilateral seminal vesicle.

Prostate and Seminal Vesicles

The prostate has an inverted cone shape. As such, the base of the prostate is cranial and the apex is caudal. The bladder sits atop the prostatic base, with the seminal vesicles situated between the posteroinferior bladder wall and rectum. The urogenital diaphragm delineates the caudal-most border of the prostatic apex. The prostate gland is separated from the rectum posteriorly by *Denonvilliers (rectovesical) fascia.* Santorini's plexus of veins (a venous plexus that surrounds the ventral and lateral prostate gland) and the pubic symphysis border the prostate anteriorly. The levator ani complex borders the lateral walls of the prostate caudally; the obturator internis muscles abut the lateral margin more cranially.

The prostate gland can be divided into one-third nonglandular and two-thirds glandular elements. The nonglandular components of the gland consist primarily of the anterior *fibromuscular stroma* and *prostatic urethra.* The fibromuscular stroma is located directly anterior to the urethra and includes the majority of the anterior lobe of the prostate (Fig. 20-2).

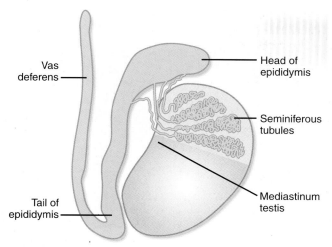

Figure 20-1 Schematic illustration of anatomy of the testis and epididymis.

The bladder neck enters the base of the prostate centrally to join the proximal prostatic urethra. The ejaculatory ducts enter the prostatic urethra at a posterior mound called the *verumontanum*, defining the beginning of the distal prostatic urethra.

The glandular components of the prostate consist of the *peripheral zone, central zone, transitional zone,* and *periurethral glandular tissues.* The peripheral zone is localized around the posterior periphery of the gland and extends anterolaterally toward the anterior fibromuscular stroma but does not surround it. It contains and surrounds the entire posterolateral aspect of the gland, similar to a baseball mitt holding a baseball. In young men, the peripheral zone comprises approximately 70% of the prostate and envelops the entire central gland, which consists of the transitional zone, central zone, and periurethral glandular tissue. The transitional and central zones comprise approximately 5% and 25% of the gland, respectively, in the young male individual. As men age, this ratio inverts with the transitional zone taking up the majority of the central glandular tissue as it undergoes significant proliferative changes resulting in benign prostatic hyperplasia

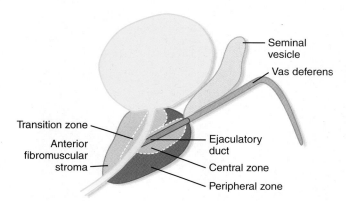

Figure 20-2 Schematic illustration of prostatic anatomy in the sagittal plane.

(BPH). Hyperplastic changes in the transitional zone and periurethral glandular tissues compress the central zone against the surrounding peripheral zone into a thin rim resulting in the surgical pseudocapsule. This pseudocapsule is separate and different from the true fibrous capsule, which is a 2- to 3-mm fibromuscular layer that encapsulates the external surface of the prostate. The surgical pseudocapsule serves as the surgical plane for transurethral prostatectomy often used for treatment of BPH.

■ NORMAL IMAGING APPEARANCE OF THE MALE REPRODUCTIVE SYSTEM

Scrotal Contents

Not only does the design of the scrotum provide a climate conducive to spermatogenesis, but it also places the testes and paratesticular tissues in a location convenient to physical inspection and evaluation by ultrasound (US). Because of wide availability of high-resolution transducers with excellent near-field resolution and color, spectral, and power Doppler, nearly all scrotal imaging is performed by sonography. Because no ionizing radiation is involved, serial examinations can be performed to evaluate disease progression or regression without concern for patient safety.

By US, each testis is an ovoid structure that is homogenous and mildly hypoechoic compared with the sparse adjacent soft tissues (Fig. 20-3). Because it is not possible to compare the echogenicity of the testes with other organs, it may be difficult to identify diffuse bilateral abnormalities of echogenicity. Fortunately, most testicular disease processes result in focal, multifocal, or diffuse unilateral abnormalities.

An echogenic line (the *mediastinum testis*) can usually be identified with US, bisecting the testis along its long axis asymmetrically (Fig. 20-4). A mediastinal artery is visible about 50% of the time and can mimic a small cyst or mass when viewed in cross section. Elongating the vessel and use of color Doppler imaging confirm the vascular nature of this finding (Fig. 20-5). Capsular arteries underlie the tunica albuginea and give rise to centripetal branches that radiate inward. Spectral Doppler demonstrates a low-resistance arterial waveform, with resistive indices typically between 0.50 and 0.75.

The head of the *epididymis* is seen on sagittal US images as a triangular, solid structure adjacent to the superior pole of the testis. Although the epididymal head is usually mildly echogenic compared with the testis, the tubules become more organized in the tail, which can render the tail hypoechoic. This can result in a "two-toned" appearance at the junction of the epididymal head and body (Fig. 20-6).

Prostate and Seminal Vesicles

Typical appearance of the prostate on CT is an ovular soft-tissue density, often difficult to separate from the surrounding fascia and musculature. Large BPH nodules

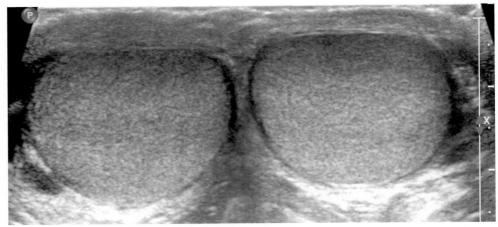

Figure 20-3 Normal "buddy shot." Transverse ultrasound image includes both testes, allowing comparison of echogenicity between the two.

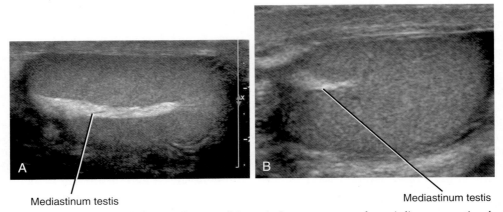

Mediastinum testis

Mediastinum testis

Figure 20-4 Mediastinum testis. **A,** Sagittal ultrasound image of the testis demonstrates an echogenic line representing the fibrofatty tissue of the mediastinum testis. **B,** Transverse image demonstrates a typical eccentric location. This example is slightly more pronounced than typical but is not abnormal.

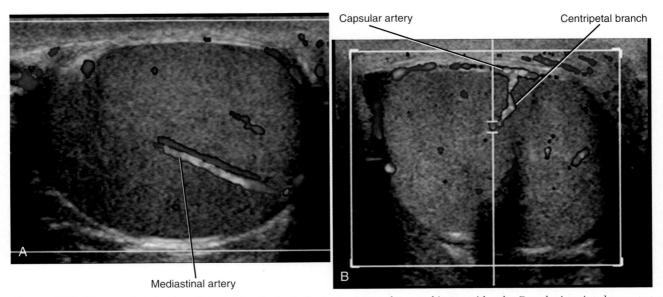

Capsular artery   Centripetal branch

Mediastinal artery

Figure 20-5 Ultrasound evaluation of arterial flow in the testis. **A,** Transverse ultrasound image with color Doppler imaging demonstrates mediastinal artery and vein. **B,** Color Doppler imaging demonstrates capsular artery and centripetal branch.

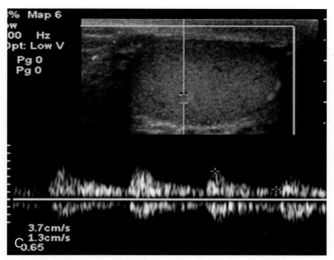

Figure 20-5, cont'd C, Spectral Doppler imaging demonstrates a normal low-resistance waveform.

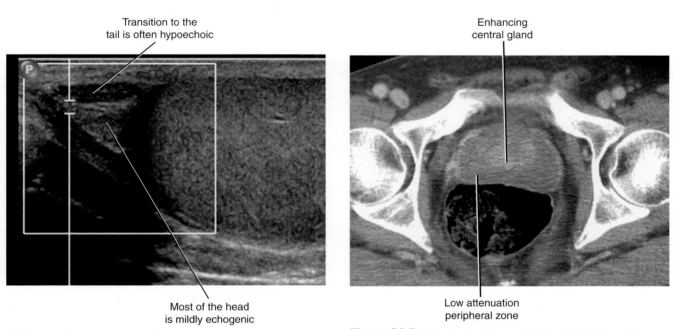

Transition to the
tail is often hypoechoic

Enhancing
central gland

Most of the head
is mildly echogenic

Low attenuation
peripheral zone

Figure 20-6 Sagittal ultrasound image demonstrates the head of the epididymis. This "two-toned" appearance from a mildly echogenic head to a hypoechoic tail is a normal finding and should not be mistaken for a mass.

Figure 20-7 Enhanced axial computed tomography in a 42-year-old man demonstrates some limited zonal anatomy.

and global prostatic enlargement are sometimes evident as irregular soft-tissue nodules seen encroaching into the bladder base, often with associated bladder wall thickening. Crude zonal anatomy can be appreciated on contrast-enhanced images in patients with BPH, as the central gland enhances heterogeneously, delineating it from the surrounding hypovascular peripheral zone (Fig. 20-7). Calcification within the prostate gland is common and usually asymptomatic, although it is more common in men with recurrent prostatitis, BPH, and a variety of metabolic disorders. Calcification of the seminal vesicles and vas deferens are also common and are associated with diabetes mellitus.

MRI provides exquisite anatomic detail of the prostate. Multicoil imaging using the body coil for excitation, and combined endorectal and external surface phased array coils for signal reception have been well established in the literature for 1.5 Tesla (1.5T) systems. However, the optimal technique for 3T imaging of the prostate is still evolving. The theoretical twofold increase in the signal-to-noise ratio achieved on 3T systems relative to 1.5T systems can be utilized to increase spatial resolution, increase temporal resolution for dynamic contrast-enhanced studies, or diminish overall scan time. Now that endorectal coils are commercially available for 3T imaging of the prostate, this technique will likely begin to replace imaging at 1.5T.

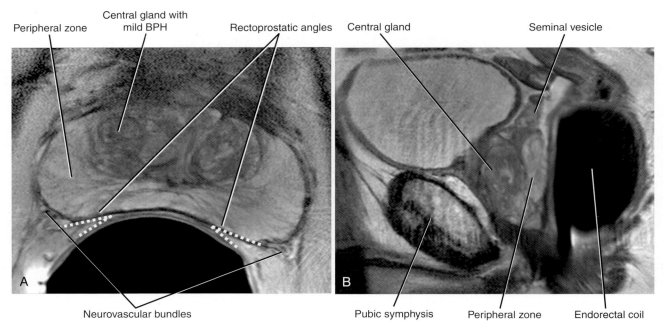

Figure 20-8 Normal zonal anatomy of the adult prostate on high-resolution T2-weighted magnetic resonance images obtained with an endorectal coil in the **(A)** axial and **(B)** sagittal planes. Images were obtained on a 3-Tesla magnet. On magnetic resonance images, the transitional zone and central zone are considered together as one region called the *central gland*. *BPH*, Benign prostatic hyperplasia.

T2-weighted MR images provide improved definition of multiplanar prostatic zonal anatomy compared with other imaging modalities (Fig. 20-8). The peripheral zone consists of glandular tissue high in water content, giving it a bright appearance on T2-weighted images. The transitional and central zones of the central gland are difficult to delineate as separate structures in the young male individual, but together appear as intermediate signal intensity on T2-weighted imaging. As the patient ages, the transitional zone and periurethral glandular tissues enlarge, compressing the central zone and creating the surgical pseudocapsule between the hyperplastic transitional zone and the surrounding peripheral zone.

The seminal vesicles can be best visualized on coronal and axial images as clusters of high-T2 signal-intensity tubules just cranial to the posterior prostatic base (Fig. 20-9). The course of the urethra through the prostate is best depicted on sagittal images.

The *neurovascular bundles* can be appreciated on T1- and T2-weighted axial images as small clustered foci of low signal in the rectoprostatic angles, which are the two acute angles formed by the outer rim of the posterior peripheral zone and anterior rectal wall. The site where each neurovascular bundle penetrates the true prostatic capsule provides an avenue for extracapsular spread of prostate cancer; thus, familiarity with this region is critical to MR staging. The true prostatic capsule appears as a region of low signal intensity 1 to 2 mm thick surrounding the exterior surface of the gland on T2-weighted images.

Pearl: Inspection of the neurovascular bundle within each rectoprostatic angle is key to detecting extracapsular extension of prostate cancer on MRI.

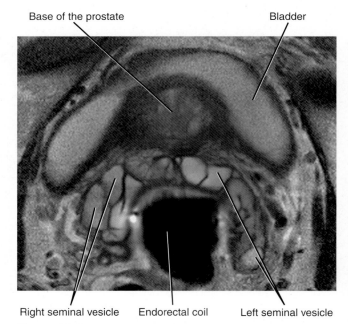

Figure 20-9 Normal appearance of the seminal vesicles on magnetic resonance imaging. Axial T2-weighted image at the level of the prostate base demonstrates the midportion of both seminal vesicles.

■ SCROTAL PAIN

Differential Diagnosis and Triage of Patients with Scrotal Pain

The main goal of imaging for acute scrotal pain is to identify those disease processes that require urgent surgical therapy. Sonographic evaluation usually allows effective triage of patients into one of three categories as shown in Table 20-1.

Although these processes can be usually differentiated from one another using US, correct diagnosis often requires "hands-on" sonographic evaluation because correlating physical examination findings such as tenderness with sonographic findings can improve specificity. Because many of these disease processes have helpful clinical discriminators, it can be useful to ask the patient questions regarding onset, location, and duration of pain while scanning. Table 20-2 lists additional clinical discriminators.

Torsion or Infection?

Time is a critical factor in the diagnosis and treatment of testicular torsion. Surgical correction within **6 hours** of the onset of pain is associated with salvage rates of greater than 90%, but the likelihood of testicular salvage declines rapidly thereafter. Because physical examination findings cannot always reliably distinguish between epididymitis and testicular torsion, patients with epididymitis are often sent for sonographic evaluation to exclude torsion before initiating medical therapy.

Fortunately, the imaging findings of infection and torsion are also usually quite disparate (Table 20-3).

Table 20-1   Triage of Patients with Scrotal Pain According to Ultrasound Findings

Management	Ultrasound Diagnosis
No treatment necessary	No abnormal findings Epididymal cyst Torsion of appendix testis or appendix epididymis Scrotal pearl Idiopathic hydrocele Small varicocele Segmental infarction Testicular cyst Tubular ectasia of the rete testis
Medical therapy usually sufficient	Epididymitis Orchitis
Surgical intervention should be considered	Testicular mass Paratesticular mass Large varicocele (transvenous intervention also available) Testicular abscess or pyocele Inguinal hernia
Urgent surgical intervention required	Testicular torsion Fournier gangrene

Table 20-2   Differentiating Common Causes of Scrotal Pain

Diagnosis	Clinical Discriminators	Ultrasound Discriminators
Epididymitis	Gradual onset Focal tenderness over epididymis Positive Prehn sign: lifting testis relieves pain Cremasteric reflex present Fever, pyuria, dysuria may be present	Enlargement or thickening of the epididymis Increased vascularity in epididymis with color Doppler imaging
Orchitis	Gradual onset Usually progression from epididymitis Mumps orchitis may be bilateral	Increased vascularity to testis with color Doppler imaging Testis hypoechoic or heterogeneous
Testicular torsion	Sudden onset Negative Prehn sign: lifting testis does not relieve pain Cremasteric reflex absent Horizontal, superior position	Absent/decreased flow to affected testis with color and spectral Doppler imaging Loss of diastolic flow and venous flow on spectral Doppler imaging Diffuse enlargement Heterogeneity "Spiral" appearance of spermatic cord on color Doppler imaging
Segmental infarction of the testis	History of sickle cell disease, vasculitis, polycythemia vera, torsion/detorsion	Regional distribution of hypoperfusion on color Doppler imaging May be hypoechoic Abnormal region becomes smaller on subsequent examinations as it progresses to fibrosis
Varicocele	Palpable enlargement on physical examination that increases with Valsalva maneuver or standing	Dilated venous structures that enlarge with Valsalva maneuver Increased flow on color Doppler with Valsalva maneuver
Torsion of testicular or epididymal appendage	Focal tenderness "Blue dot" visible through skin at site of tenderness	Avascular nodule corresponds to site of focal tenderness Appendages > 5 mm are likely torsed
Hernia	Bowel sounds in scrotal mass Associated bowel obstruction Often reducible	Peristalsis of bowel or movement of fat with Valsalva maneuver
Fournier gangrene	Marked skin discoloration Crepitus	Echogenic foci of soft-tissue gas

Table 20-3 Ultrasound Findings in Epididymitis and Testicular Torsion

Characteristics	Epididymitis	Epididymoorchitis	Testicular Torsion
Epididymis size	Enlarged	Enlarged	Enlarged
Testis size	Normal	Enlarged	Enlarged
Flow to epididymis	Increased	Increased	Decreased
Flow to testis	Normal	Increased	Decreased
Spiral cord sign	Absent	Absent	Present

Typical sonographic features of epididymitis include an enlarged epididymis with increased blood flow on color Doppler (Fig. 20-10). In epididymoorchitis, there is also increased blood flow to the testis, which is often enlarged and mildly hypoechoic (Fig. 20-11). Although the testis and epididymis are typically enlarged and hypoechoic with torsion as well, blood flow is decreased or absent (Fig. 20-12). When evaluating blood flow for possible torsion, it is essential to keep in mind that there is often hyperemia surrounding an ischemic or infarcted testicle, so flow within the testicular parenchyma must be present to exclude torsion (Fig. 20-13). A spiral appearance of the spermatic cord vessels has also been described as a sign of torsion. Spectral Doppler evaluation usually demonstrates a low-resistance arterial waveform in orchitis and a high-resistance arterial waveform with decreased, absent, or reversed diastolic flow in testicular torsion. With torsion, loss of venous flow may precede loss of arterial flow on spectral Doppler imaging.

Imaging findings may be confusing, however, when the patient has undergone torsion followed by detorsion. In this scenario, considerable hyperemia to the testis and epididymis can exist, similar to the appearance seen in epididymoorchitis. The clinical history, however, is usually different because torsion/detorsion typically results in marked and abrupt fluctuation in symptoms, unlike the gradual progression usually seen with infectious processes of the scrotum.

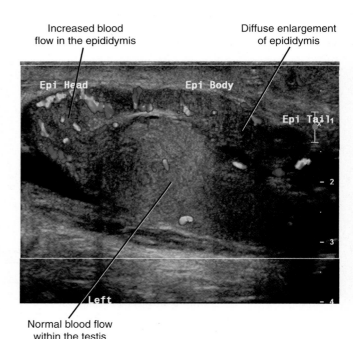

Increased blood flow in the epididymis

Diffuse enlargement of epididymis

Normal blood flow within the testis

Figure 20-10 Ultrasound findings of epididymitis. Sagittal ultrasound image with color Doppler demonstrates diffuse enlargement and increased vascularity of the epididymis.

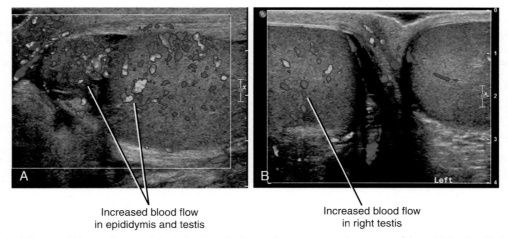

Increased blood flow in epididymis and testis

Increased blood flow in right testis

Figure 20-11 Epididymoorchitis on ultrasound. **A,** Color Doppler image demonstrates enlargement of the epididymis with increased blood flow to both the epididymis and testis. **B,** Transverse midline color Doppler image of both testes allows direct comparison of vascularity, increased on the patient's right side in this case.

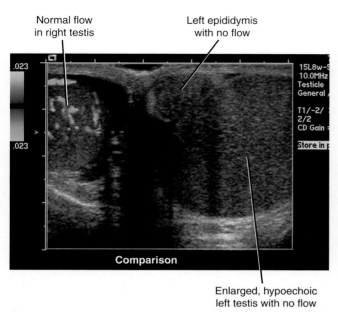

Normal flow
in right testis

Left epididymis
with no flow

Comparison

Enlarged, hypoechoic
left testis with no flow

Figure 20-12 Ultrasound findings in testicular torsion. Transverse midline color Doppler ultrasound image in a patient with severe left scrotal pain demonstrates enlargement of the left testis and epididymis compared with the right side. No flow is detected within the left testis, whereas normal flow is demonstrated on the right side.

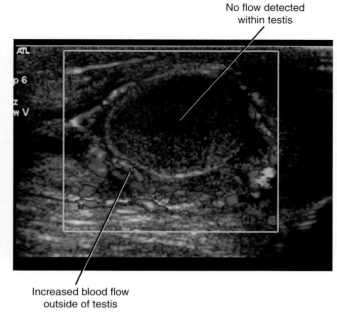

No flow detected
within testis

Increased blood flow
outside of testis

Figure 20-13 Peripheral hyperemia in testicular torsion. Color Doppler ultrasound image demonstrates increased blood flow surrounding an infarcted testis, but no flow within the testis itself. The presence of peripheral flow does not exclude torsion.

Pitfall: Intermittent episodes of torsion and detorsion can result in color and spectral Doppler findings similar to epididymoorchitis. A history of abrupt onset and relief of symptoms can be a key clinical discriminator suggesting torsion-detorsion syndrome.

A Few Words About Appendages

The appendix epididymis and appendix testis are small (usually ≤5 mm), nodular appendages of benign soft tissue that are often seen protruding from the respective structure. They are usually obscured by adjacent soft tissues during sonography but become more conspicuous when a hydrocele is present (Fig. 20-14). Rarely, one of these appendages may undergo torsion independent of the other scrotal structures, resulting in pain but no risk to the testis. This is more common in boys aged 7 to 14 years but can occur in adults as well. If sonography demonstrates no evidence of infection or torsion, and pain can be directly correlated to an appendix of the testis or epididymis, a diagnosis of appendiceal torsion can be made, resulting in appropriate conservative management.

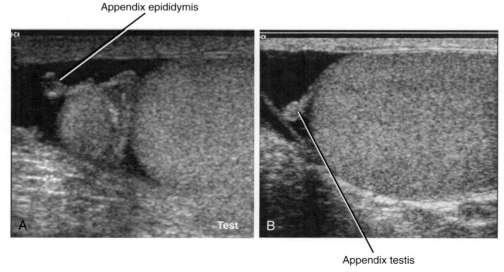

Appendix epididymis

Appendix testis

Figure 20-14 Appendices in the scrotum. **A,** Sagittal ultrasound (US) image of the epididymal head demonstrates a small appendix epididymis. **B,** Sagittal US image of the testis in a different patient demonstrates an appendix testis. In both cases, a small amount of hydrocele facilitated visualization.

Complications of Inflammatory Disease in the Scrotum

Several complications can occur when epididymitis, orchitis, or both go untreated or are incompletely treated. The most common of these complications is development of an infected hydrocele called a *pyocele*. A pyocele consists of infected fluid between the layers of the tunica vaginalis. Unlike simple hydroceles that develop in response to local inflammation, pyocele are usually septated and contain internal echoes (Fig. 20-15).

Epididymoorchitis can progress to form an *intratesticular abscess*. The pressure created by an expanding abscess within the confines of the tunica albuginea usually causes severe pain. Increased interstitial pressure can also decrease perfusion to the remainder of the testis, eventually resulting in global or segmental infarction. On US, abscesses are usually hypoechoic compared with adjacent testicular parenchyma, although internal echoes may be sufficient to make the abscess nearly isoechoic. Color Doppler imaging can be useful, demonstrating absent flow within the abscess cavity (Fig. 20-16).

Pitfall: Testicular abscess can be nearly isoechoic to adjacent testicular parenchyma. A focal area of absent testicular perfusion within a background of hyperemia on color Doppler imaging should prompt suspicion of abscess.

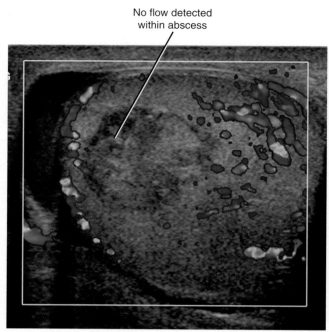

No flow detected within abscess

Figure 20-16 Testicular abscess. Color Doppler ultrasound performed for severe testicular pain demonstrates a focal heterogeneous lesion with absent color flow. Enterobacter abscess was confirmed surgically. The absence of color flow within the lesion and clinical presentation help differentiate this lesion from testicular cancer.

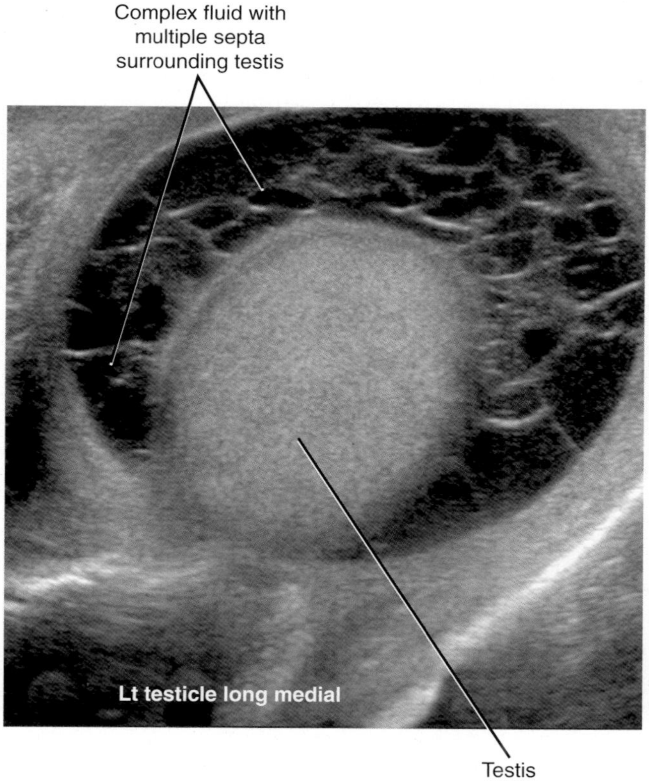

Complex fluid with multiple septa surrounding testis

Testis

Lt testicle long medial

Figure 20-15 Ultrasound of the scrotum performed after 1 week of swelling and pain demonstrates a pyocele that was subsequently debrided surgically.

Surgical debridement is usually performed for pyocele, and orchiectomy is standard treatment for testicular abscess. If pain and other symptoms of infection are sufficiently mild, intensive antibiotic therapy may be attempted with serial US examinations to look for signs of response or progression.

Fournier Gangrene

The scrotum and perineum are also prone to cellulitis. Left untreated, a life-threatening fasciitis can develop. The gas-producing organisms of Fournier gangrene visibly progress in a matter of hours, and rapid surgical debridement followed by aggressive antibiotic therapy is key to escaping the persistently high mortality rate (30-50%).

Two schools of thought exist regarding the use of imaging in the diagnosis and surgical planning of patients suspected of having Fournier gangrene: (1) Don't image—just get them to the operating room; and (2) scan quickly with CT to define the expected extent of debridement necessary. If imaging is requested, speed of performance and interpretation are of the utmost importance. Key findings include gas and fat stranding in the subcutaneous soft tissues (Fig. 20-17). Because successful debridement is defined not only by width of resection but also by depth, try to identify areas of gas in adjacent muscles or other deep soft tissues.

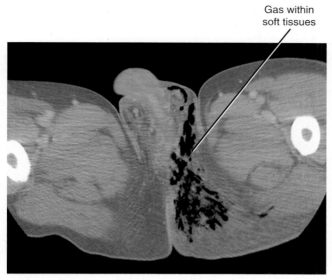

Gas within
soft tissues

Figure 20-17 Axial image from contrast-enhanced computed tomography performed in search of an abscess in a case of severe cellulitis of the perineum. Extensive gas within the soft tissues indicates this is Fournier gangrene, requiring immediate surgical debridement.

■ FOCAL TESTICULAR LESIONS

Benign or Malignant?

Sonography is the imaging modality of choice when characterizing an intratesticular mass and is nearly 100% sensitive for detection of testicular tumors. Once US has confirmed the presence of a clinically suspected testicular tumor, the next step is differentiating the more common malignant lesions from less common benign ones.

Confident diagnosis of a benign intratesticular lesion can prevent unnecessary orchiectomy. The benign lesions that are easiest to characterize are cystic. These include cysts of the tunica albuginea, simple testicular cysts, and tubular ectasia of the rete testis. A key difference between these benign conditions and a cystic malignant neoplasm is that a solid component is absent in the former conditions. Diagnosis of an intratesticular varicocele can also be made with confidence in most cases using Doppler sonography.

Diagnosis of other benign intratesticular lesions demands more caution. Examples include epidermoid cyst, abscess, hematoma, focal infarction, and granulomatous orchitis. In many cases, the appearances of these lesions overlap that of malignancy; therefore, clinical factors (e.g., a history of trauma or fever) may be crucial in determining initial management. Table 20-4 summarizes US findings that favor a benign diagnosis.

Testicular Cysts

Cysts of the tunica albuginea are usually found in men older than 40 years. They are located at the periphery of the testis, usually at the upper anterior or lateral margins. At grayscale US, they are usually biconvex or lentiform in shape and meet all the criteria of a simple cyst (Fig. 20-18). The cysts are typically unilocular but can be multilocular. Simple intratesticular cysts are similar in appearance to those of the tunica but can be located anywhere in the testis and can be solitary or multiple.

Germ cell tumors that undergo necrosis and teratomas with cystic components also can have a cystic appearance. However, cystic malignant lesions have a complex appearance with solid components or thick septations, or both, that distinguish them from simple cysts (Fig. 20-19).

Ectasia of the Rete Testis

The normal rete testis is a group of small tubules located within the mediastinum testis that serves as a pathway for spermatozoa to travel from the seminiferous tubules of the testicular parenchyma to the epididymis. Enlargement of these tubules is often idiopathic but can also result from epididymitis or vasectomy. Tubular ectasia of the rete testis is often bilateral and is more common in men older than 55 years.

Mild-to-moderate tubular ectasia could be confused with a testicular mass on older US units, but newer technology usually reveals the fine tubular nature of the

Table 20-4   Focal Testicular Lesions: Ultrasound Findings That Favor Benign Disease

Finding	Comments
Anechoic with smooth margins	Cyst of tunica albuginea or true intratesticular cyst depending on location
Absence of flow on color Doppler	Rare in malignancy Common in most benign lesions except for intratesticular varicocele
Enlargement of epididymis or thickening of the scrotum	Common with infection or inflammation including granulomatous orchitis
Tubular shape	Small tubes: rete testis Large tubes: intratesticular varicocele
Concentric rings (laminated)	Epidermoid cyst
Straight margins or wedge shape	Focal testicular infarct
Pronounced mediastinal adenopathy with small testicular lesions	Consider sarcoidosis

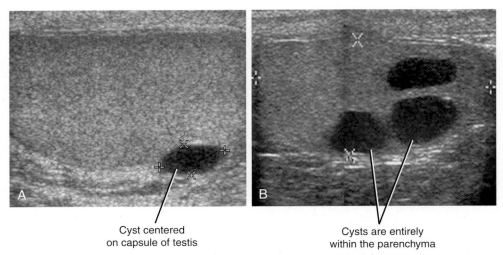

Cyst centered
on capsule of testis

Cysts are entirely
within the parenchyma

Figure 20-18 Benign testicular cysts. **A,** Sagittal ultrasound image demonstrates an oval-shaped simple cyst centered on the tunica albuginea. Note that it results in a slight bulge in contour, making it palpable. **B,** Sagittal image of multiple intratesticular cysts. Although some are adjacent to the tunica, not all of them are. These were not palpable.

Wall nodules

Solid nodules

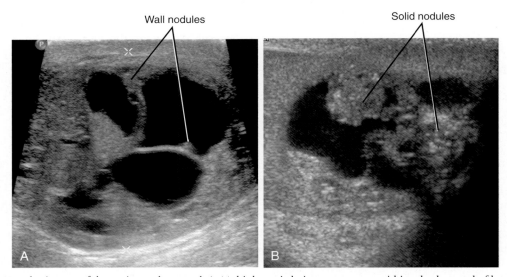

Figure 20-19 Neoplastic cysts of the testis on ultrasound. **A,** Multiple cystic lesions are present within a background of heterogeneous soft tissue in this mixed germ cell tumor. **B,** Larger soft-tissue nodules protrude into cystic regions in this immature teratoma. Neither lesion should be mistaken for a simple cyst.

abnormality on US (Fig. 20-20). More pronounced cases may appear grossly cystic (Fig. 20-21). If there is any doubt, MRI can be performed, demonstrating high signal intensity on T2-weighted images (as opposed to low signal intensity typical of most solid testicular neoplasms) (Fig. 20-22).

Pearl: Ectasia of the rete testis can be diagnosed confidently with high-resolution US when fine tubular structures conform to the shape of the mediastinum testis.

Intratesticular Varicocele

Intratesticular varicoceles can occur in isolation or in combination with extratesticular varicoceles. At grayscale US, multiple anechoic, serpentine tubular struc-

tures demonstrate venous flow that is accentuated with the Valsalva maneuver (Fig. 20-23). Although most varicoceles occur spontaneously, they occasionally occur because of compression of the testicular vein by a retroperitoneal mass.

Epidermoid Cysts

Epidermoid cysts, although true cysts, appear solid because of their keratinous contents. Although they are typically removed surgically, testis-preserving enucleation of the lesion can be performed in place of orchiectomy.

On US, most epidermoid cysts are round, circumscribed, laminated, or "onion skinned" in appearance,

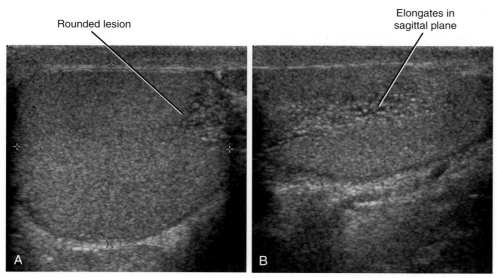

Figure 20-20 Tubular ectasia of the rete testis. **A,** Transverse ultrasound image demonstrates a heterogeneous round lesion seen in the periphery of the testis. A fine cystic/tubular echotexture makes tubular ectasia likely. **B,** Long-axis view proves the lesion to elongate, conforming to the mediastinum testis, confirming the diagnosis.

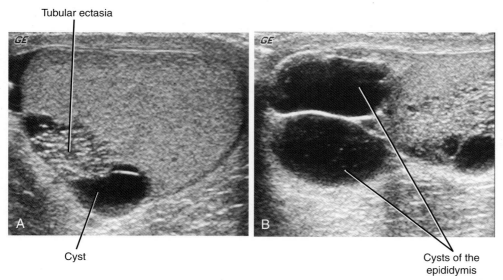

Figure 20-21 Cystic ectasia of the rete testis. **A,** Transverse ultrasound image of the testis shows a combination of fine tubular structures and larger cysts within the mediastinum testis. **B,** Long-axis view demonstrates multiple cysts within the head of the epididymis.

and color flow is absent (Fig. 20-24). In some cases, the echogenic and hypoechoic material is less organized, resulting in heterogeneous mass without lamellations, although color flow is still absent. Less organized lesions usually have a well-defined rim at the margin of the lesion, although the rim can be either hypoechoic or hyperechoic.

Pearl: On US, epidermoid cysts are usually round, circumscribed masses with a lamellated appearance and no internal flow on color Doppler imaging.

MRI can be performed in problematic cases. Epidermoid cysts are typically heterogeneous with areas of high signal intensity on T2-weighted images, predominantly low signal intensity on T1-weighted images, and absent internal enhancement after injection of intravenous gadolinium-based contrast media. This is in contrast with germ cell tumors, which are usually low signal intensity on T2-weighted images with demonstrable enhancement. Any uncertainty in the imaging characteristics must raise the possibility of an intratesticular malignancy.

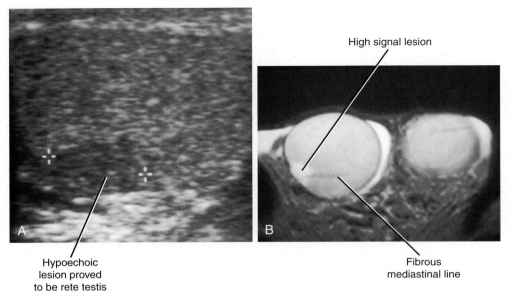

Figure 20-22 Rete testis on magnetic resonance (MR) imaging. **A,** Admittedly old sonogram demonstrated an indeterminate lesion in the testis. Location suggested rete testis, but echotexture was indeterminate. **B,** Axial T2-weighted MR image of the same patient demonstrates high signal intensity within the testicular lesion, characteristic of tubular ectasia.

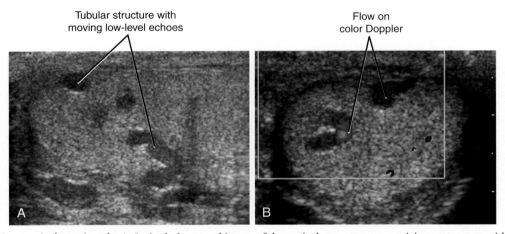

Figure 20-23 Intratesticular varicocele. **A,** Sagittal ultrasound image of the testis demonstrates a serpiginous structure within the testis. During scanning, low-level echoes could be seen to move. **B,** Transverse color Doppler image demonstrates flow within the varicocele.

Testicular Abscess

As mentioned earlier, intratesticular abscesses are a complication of epididymoorchitis. By US, abscesses are hypoechoic with low-level internal echoes, demonstrate no internal color flow, and often have hypervascular margins (see Fig. 20-16). Clinical presentation and sonographic findings of epididymoorchitis are important features because seminomas can rarely become necrotic and simulate an abscess.

Testicular Hematoma

Intratesticular hematoma usually results from blunt scrotal trauma, although it can also occur spontaneously in the setting of vasculitis. Although the grayscale appearance can vary greatly depending on the acuity of the injury, a consistent feature is the lack of internal vascularity (Fig. 20-25). Because hematomas can compress the adjacent testicular parenchyma, resulting in ischemia or infarction, they are usually removed surgically unless quite small.

Notably, testicular neoplasms can be found serendipitously in men with scrotal trauma. Although the lack of blood flow usually allows discrimination from a germ cell tumor, small hematomas treated conservatively should be followed with repeat US in 1 to 2 weeks to demonstrate resolution and differentiate from a rare hypovascular mass. Hematomas can be indistinguishable from abscess on US, although the clinical presentations are usually quite different.

Lamellae

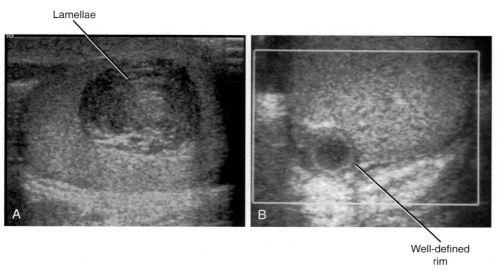

Well-defined
rim

Figure 20-24 Ultrasound appearance of two surgically-proven epidermoid inclusion cysts of the testis. **A,** Classic "onion-skin" appearance of lamellae within a testicular lesion. No flow was detected on color Doppler. **B,** Ringlike margin defines lesion without internal color flow.

No detectable flow
within hematoma

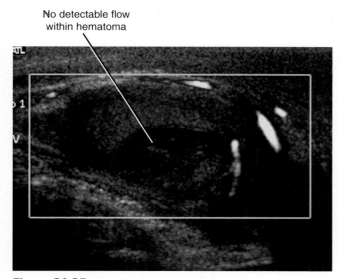

Figure 20-25 Ultrasound performed for scrotal pain and swelling after a motor vehicle collision demonstrates a heterogeneous, predominantly hypoechoic lesion within the testis. No flow is shown within the lesion on power Doppler imaging. A hematoma was evacuated surgically.

Segmental Infarction of the Testis

In recent years, reports of infarction involving only a portion of a testicle have increased. As yet, this remains a poorly understood phenomenon. Although many reports describe an association with sickle cell disease or vasculitis, segmental infarction has also been described in association with surgical injury to the spermatic cord (usually during hernia or varicocele repair) and in the absence of risk factors.

Grayscale US typically shows a hypoechoic, wedge-shaped lesion at the periphery of the testis (Fig. 20-26). Although the appearance can be confused with a germ cell tumor, straight margins and lack of blood flow

allow correct diagnosis in most cases. If MRI is performed, straight margins are usually appreciated demarcating the enhancing and nonenhancing portions of the testis. A rim of contrast enhancement has been reported to occur in acute and subacute cases.

Granulomatous Orchitis

Granulomatous orchitis can be seen in sarcoidosis or infections such as brucellosis, tuberculosis, coccidioidomycosis, leprosy, and syphilis. Both the epididymis and testis are involved in most cases. In fact, several series have shown enlargement of the epididymis and thickening of the scrotum and tunica albuginea to be good predictors of benign, inflammatory disease.

Sarcoidosis is usually a systemic disease, although scrotal symptoms are occasionally the presenting complaint. The incidence of sarcoidosis is much greater among young black men. In most cases of testicular involvement, multiple bilateral hypoechoic nodules are present within the testes, usually with some degree of epididymal enlargement (Fig. 20-27). Whereas multiple bilateral testicular lesions in the appropriate clinical setting may prompt open biopsy, solitary lesions of sarcoidosis cannot be reliably distinguished from germ cell neoplasms with imaging and usually result in orchiectomy.

Pearl: Testicular sarcoidosis usually results in multiple bilateral hypoechoic testicular lesions with mild enlargement of the epididymis.

Interestingly, some reports describe an association between sarcoidosis and development of germ cell tumors. In one series, white men with sarcoidosis were 100 times more likely to experience development of germ cell tumors than those without it. This has two main implications. First, the presence of isolated mediastinal lymphadenopathy in association with testicular cancer should raise the possibility of coexisting cancer

Preserved tissue

Infarcted tissue

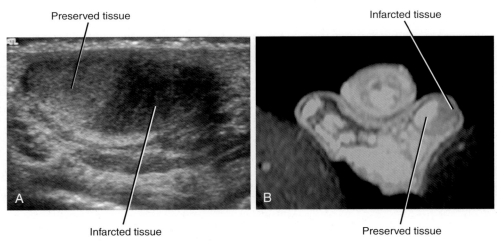

Infarcted tissue

Preserved tissue

Figure 20-26 Presumed segmental infarction of the testis. **A,** Sagittal ultrasound (US) image of the left testis demonstrates a linear demarcation between normal echogenicity and a hypoechoic region. **B,** Axial T1-weighted magnetic resonance image performed after contrast injection demonstrates a similar well-defined transition. The patient reported a remote history of trauma. No change was found on serial follow-up US examinations.

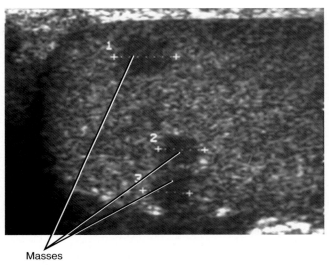

Masses

Figure 20-27 Sarcoidosis of the testis. Sagittal ultrasound image of the testis demonstrates multiple hypoechoic masses within the testis. Similar findings were present in the other testis. Diagnosis was confirmed with open biopsy.

and sarcoidosis. Second, this observation has led some to advocate for orchiectomy over observation for testicular sarcoidosis to prevent future development of testicular cancer.

Germ Cell Tumors of the Testis

Testicular tumors are classified as germ cell and non–germ cell neoplasms. Ninety-five percent of testicular tumors are germ cell neoplasms arising from spermatogenic cells. Non–germ cell tumors of the testis include primary neoplasms of the sex cords and stroma, of which 10% are malignant, and nonprimary neoplasms such as lymphoma, leukemia, and metastases.

Germ cell neoplasms of the testis are further characterized as seminoma or nonseminomatous (NSGCT). NSGCTs include embryonal carcinoma, yolk sac tumor, choriocarcinoma, and teratoma. These latter neoplasms rarely occur in their pure form, and any combination of these form a mixed germ cell tumor. Mixed germ cell tumors are considered NSGCTs, even when they contain a seminomatous component. The average age of a patient with a classic seminoma is approximately 40 years. Mixed germ cell tumors occur in younger men, typically in their 30s.

The grayscale appearance of seminoma ranges from complete replacement of the testis to a small, well-defined lesion (Fig. 20-28). Most tumors are uniformly hypoechoic, although larger tumors are often heterogeneous and sometimes partially cystic or necrotic in appearance. They are often lobulated and rarely infiltrating, multifocal, or bilateral (Fig. 20-29). Color and power Doppler US usually demonstrate increased vascularity.

In contrast, NSGCTs (including mixed variety) are usually more heterogenous in appearance than seminoma (Fig. 20-30). US findings include heterogeneous solid components, occasional cystic regions, and in some cases, echogenic foci caused by calcification, cartilage, or immature bone. The latter features indicate components of teratoma that are seen in more than 50% of mixed germ cell tumors.

A "burned-out" or regressed germ cell tumor is diagnosed when a patient has documented dissemination of germ cell tumor but only a small remnant tumor is found in the testis at orchiectomy. It is believed that the primary tumor outgrows its blood supply, then undergoes necrosis followed by fibrosis and calcification. The sonographic appearance is variable, but typically a small heterogeneous and potentially calcified mass is identified in a patient with evidence of metastatic disease. Pathologic evaluation may reveal some residual malignant cells within the testicular lesion.

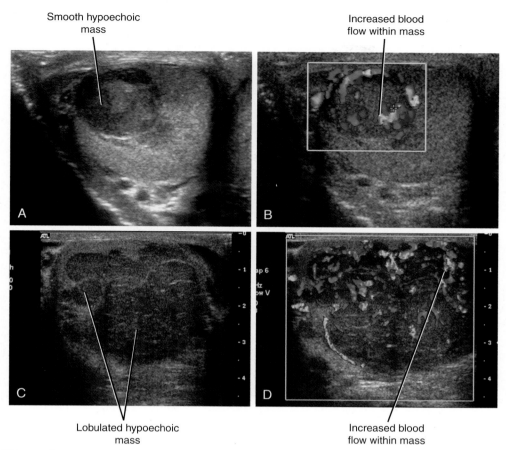

Smooth hypoechoic
mass

Increased blood
flow within mass

Lobulated hypoechoic
mass

Increased blood
flow within mass

Figure 20-28 Ultrasound appearance of seminoma in two patients. **A,** Well-defined hypoechoic lesion. **B,** Color Doppler imaging demonstrates increased internal blood flow in same lesion as **(A),** a feature absent with an epidermoid cyst, hematoma, or abscess. **C,** A hypoechoic mass with lobulated margins nearly replaces the testis in another patient. **D,** Color Doppler imaging demonstrates hypervascularity within this lesion as well.

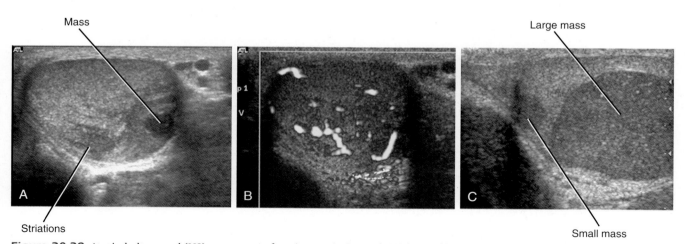

Mass

Large mass

Striations

Small mass

Figure 20-29 Atypical ultrasound (US) appearance of seminoma. **A,** Grayscale US image demonstrates a small hypoechoic mass with adjacent striations within the parenchyma. **B,** Power Doppler image demonstrates increased blood flow within the striations. The striations correlated with an infiltrative pattern of tumor at pathology. **C,** In a different patient, US demonstrates multiple separate testicular masses found to represent multifocal seminoma at pathology.

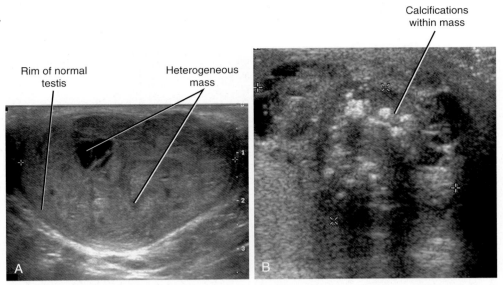

Figure 20-30 Ultrasound (US) appearance of nonseminomatous germ cell tumor. **A,** Sagittal US image of the testis demonstrates heterogeneous soft tissue within a proven mixed germ cell tumor. **B,** US image of a high-grade immature teratoma in a different patient demonstrates a heterogenous mass with calcifications.

Pearl: Most seminomas are uniformly hypoechoic (US) or hypointense (MRI) relative to the normal testis, whereas NSGCTs are more likely to be heterogeneous, cystic, or calcified.

Stromal Tumors of the Testis

Approximately 5% of primary testicular neoplasms arise from the testicular stroma rather than from germ cells. These include *Leydig cell* and *Sertoli cell* tumors. Both types of tumors are benign in approximately 90%

of cases. About one in three stromal tumors has enough hormonal activity to present with endocrine symptoms (precocious puberty, gynecomastia, impotence). These hormone-secreting tumors are more likely to be small at time of diagnosis (Fig. 20-31). Thus, the presence of a small testicular mass in a patient with hormonal abnormalities suggests the diagnosis of a stromal tumor. Tumors that are not hormonally active present as an enlarging mass that cannot be distinguished from a germ cell tumor by imaging.

Pearl: Hormonally active testicular stromal tumors may be quite small at the time of diagnosis.

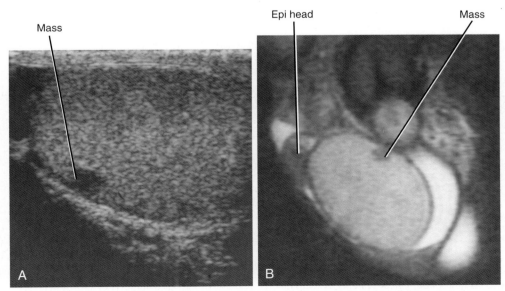

Figure 20-31 Small Leydig cell tumor in a 41-year-old man with gynecomastia. **A,** Sagittal ultrasound image demonstrates a small hypoechoic mass. **B,** T2-weighted imaging sagittal to the testis demonstrates a low-signal-intensity lesion. Leydig cell tumor was found at pathology. *Epi,* Epididymis.

Large cell calcifying Sertoli cell tumor is an unusual type of stromal tumor that typically calcifies, resulting in an unusual echogenic appearance on US (Fig. 20-32). This large cell variant of the Sertoli cell tumor is usually benign and is associated with Carney's complex (cardiac myxoma, skin pigmentation, pituitary adenoma, fibroadenoma of the breast) and Peutz–Jeghers syndrome (gastrointestinal polyposis and mucocutaneous pigmentation).

Testicular Lymphoma

Testicular involvement with lymphoma usually occurs in the setting of systemic disease, although primary testicular lymphoma can occur. US typically shows masslike enlargement of a hypoechoic testis (Fig. 20-33). Blood flow is preserved within the affected region, although not usually increased. Although masslike enlargement of the testis from lymphoma is indistinguishable from diffuse germ cell tumor, bilateral involvement is much more common with lymphoma, occurring in up to 40%

of patients. Age is a discriminator, because testicular masses in men older than 60 are more likely to be lymphoma than germ cell tumor. Because of poor delivery of chemotherapeutic agents to the testis, testicular disease may persist or recur after otherwise successful systemic therapy.

Pearl: A testicular mass in a man older than 60 is more likely to be lymphoma than a germ cell tumor.

Leukemia in the Testis

Although primary leukemia of the testis is rare, the testis is a common site of recurrence. As with lymphoma, recurrence is thought to be caused by poor vascular delivery of chemotherapeutic medications to the testes. The sonographic appearance of leukemia in the testes is variable, including solitary and multiple hypoechoic mass lesions, diffuse infiltration of the parenchyma resulting in heterogeneity, and either unilateral or bilateral disease.

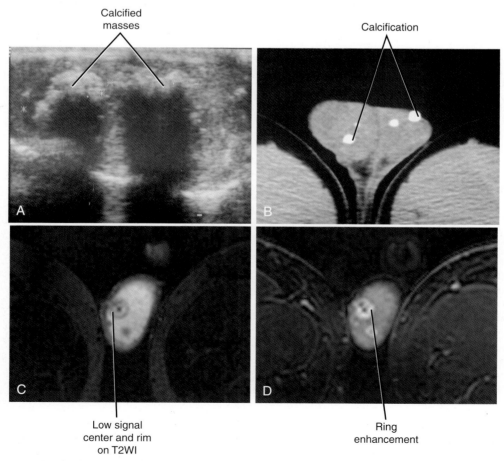

Figure 20-32 Large-cell calcifying Sertoli tumor of the testis. **A,** Sagittal ultrasound image demonstrates multiple calcified masses in the testis. **B,** Axial image of the scrotum from contrast-enhanced computed tomographic scan demonstrates testicular calcifications. **C,** T2-weighted magnetic resonance image (T2WI) demonstrates target lesions with low-signal-intensity rim and signal void (calcification) at the center. **D,** Dynamic T1-weighted image after administration of contrast demonstrates enhancing rings around the calcifications.

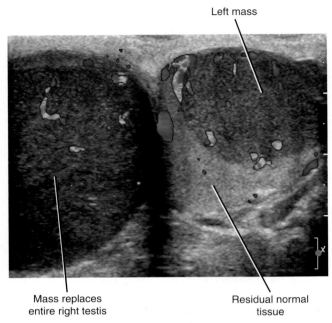

Left mass

Mass replaces entire right testis

Residual normal tissue

Figure 20-33 Transverse midline color Doppler ultrasound image of the testes in a 46-year-old man with scrotal enlargement demonstrates a focal hypoechoic mass in the left testis and complete replacement of the right testis with tumor. Biopsy of the right testis yielded a diagnosis of acute lymphoblastic type B-cell lymphoma.

Other Rare Testicular Lesions

Adrenal rests are a benign proliferation of adrenal tissue within the testis, usually in infants with congenital adrenal hyperplasia. These rests are rarely found in adults with Cushing syndrome, and are typically less than 5 mm in diameter, multiple, and bilateral. Correct diagnosis and treatment with glucocorticoids usually results in regression of the masses, avoiding unnecessary orchiectomy. Testicular vein sampling has been successful in problematic cases because the presence of increased glucocorticoids is diagnostic.

Metastases to the testes are unusual. When encountered, the most common primary tumors include carcinoma of the prostate, lung, or gastrointestinal tract, renal cell carcinoma, rhabdomyosarcoma, and melanoma. Lesions are most often multiple and bilateral, although solitary, unilateral testicular metastases have been reported.

Carcinoid tumors of the testis have been reported and can be primary or metastatic. A primary testicular carcinoid tumor cannot be distinguished from germ cell tumor based on imaging findings.

■ DIFFUSE TESTICULAR LESIONS

Approach to Diffusely Abnormal Testicular Echogenicity

Prior or current infection, torsion, or malignant infiltration can all result in diffusely abnormal testicular echogenicity (Table 20-5). Differentiating among these is

Table 20-5 Causes of Diffusely Abnormal Testicular Echogenicity

Diagnosis	Comments
Epididymoorchitis	Enlarged epididymis Increased blood flow on color Doppler imaging
Testicular torsion	Absent or high-impedance blood flow to testis Peripheral hyperemia in torsion-detorsion syndrome
Prior epididymoorchitis or torsion	Atrophic testis Striated appearance of the testicular parenchyma on ultrasound
Diffuse germ cell tumor	Enlarged testis Thin rim of compressed residual parenchyma visible with ultrasound
Lymphoma or leukemia	Enlarged testis(es) Bilateral involvement common

crucial to avoid unnecessary orchiectomy or a missed opportunity for treatment.

Testicular atrophy can be seen in association with varicocele, medications (including anabolic steroids), cryptorchidism, or prior insult to the testis from infection or ischemia. Orchitis can result in diffuse parenchymal damage, followed by fibrosis and atrophy (Fig. 20-34). In many cases, linear striations of perivascular fibrosis are seen sonographically. However, it is important to listen to the patient because germ cell tumors can arise within testes that have been injured in the past (likely at

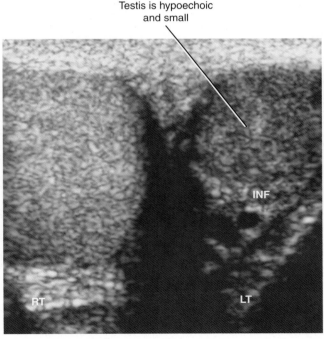

Testis is hypoechoic and small

INF

RT

LT

Figure 20-34 Transverse ultrasound of both testes in a man who reported a prior history of mumps orchitis on the left side. The left testis *(LT)* is much smaller and diffusely hypoechoic compared with the right. *INF,* Inferior.

the same rate as in the normal testis, despite anecdotal reports of an increased incidence). A small testis that is shown to increase in size on serial US examinations is concerning for malignancy.

An enlarged, diffusely abnormal testis can result from acute infection, torsion, or malignant infiltration. A combination of clinical factors and imaging findings can reliable differentiate among these in most cases. Viral orchitis caused by mumps occurs in prepubertal boys. If US is performed acutely, the testis is enlarged with increased flow on color Doppler and minimal or no associated findings in the epididymis. Although unusual, severe cases of bilateral mumps orchitis can result in infertility.

Bacterial orchitis is usually the result of sexually transmitted infection and is almost always accompanied by epididymitis. US shows evidence of epididymal enlargement, often accompanied by reactive hydrocele and scrotal thickening (Fig. 20-35). Color Doppler shows increased blood flow to both the testis and epididymis (see Fig. 20-11). Often, laboratory evidence of sexually transmitted disease (e.g., chlamydia) or pyuria exists. Infectious orchitis of any cause can occur bilaterally. Mumps orchitis is the one cause of orchitis that commonly spares the epididymis (Fig. 20-36).

Pearl: With the exception of mumps orchitis, infectious and inflammatory disorders of the testis also involve the epididymis. Malignant neoplasms of the testis usually spare the epididymis.

Testicular torsion is almost always unilateral and tends to affect boys in childhood or adolescence. A history describing an abrupt onset of pain usually prompts the diagnosis even before imaging. On US, blood flow is usually absent or diminished with high impedance

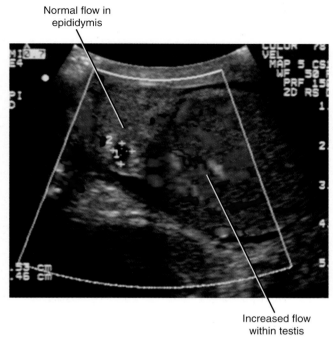

Normal flow in epididymis

Increased flow within testis

Figure 20-36 Color Doppler ultrasound image of a patient with mumps orchitis demonstrates increased blood flow to the testis but not to the epididymis.

within the enlarged testis, although there may be reactive hyperemia in the surrounding soft tissues.

Malignant replacement of the testis can occur with germ cell tumors, lymphoma, or leukemia. As described earlier, lymphoma usually occurs in men older than 50. Leukemic infiltration of the testis is most often seen after chemotherapy for systemic disease. Testicular involvement with germ cell tumors is usually unilateral; with myeloproliferative neoplasms, it is more often bilateral. Malignant replacement almost always results in testicular enlargement and normal to increased blood flow. A thin rim of preserved testicular parenchyma is often sonographically visible compressed against the tunica albuginea by the tumor, forming a thick pseudocapsule (Fig. 20-37). No such rim of spared tissue occurs with orchitis.

Pearl: Replacement of the testis with tumor is rarely complete and usually results in a rim of preserved tissue in the periphery. Because this is not always obvious, detection may require a directed search.

Testicular Microlithiasis

Testicular microlithiasis, an uncommon and usually incidental entity, has a characteristic, often striking appearance. At US, microlithiasis appears as multiple punctate (2-3 mm) echogenic foci within the testicular parenchyma that do not produce shadowing (Fig. 20-38). The finding is usually bilateral, and five or more foci per transducer field is a widely used threshold to make the diagnosis. Although an association between testicular microlithiasis and testicular germ cell tumors has been

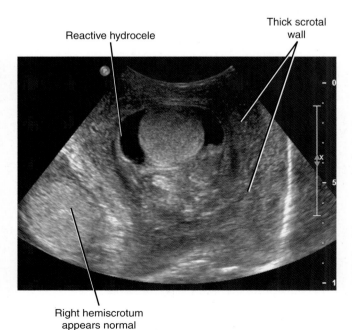

Reactive hydrocele

Thick scrotal wall

Right hemiscrotum appears normal

Figure 20-35 Ultrasound of the left testis in a patient with severe epididymitis demonstrates severe scrotal wall thickening, an uncommon finding with germ cell tumors of the testis.

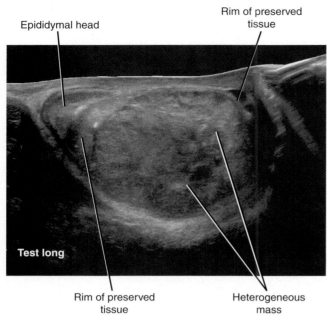

Epididymal head

Rim of preserved tissue

Rim of preserved tissue

Heterogeneous mass

Test long

Figure 20-37 Transverse ultrasound image of a testis that is almost completely replaced with mixed germ cell tumor, demonstrating the rim of preserved tissue commonly seen with large neoplasms of the testis. Additional imaging findings that favor malignancy over infection include the normal epididymis and lack of scrotal wall edema.

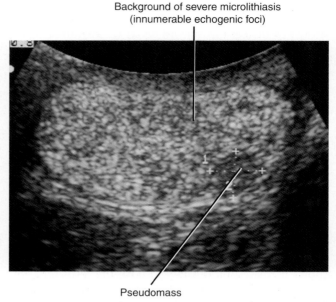

Background of severe microlithiasis (innumerable echogenic foci)

Pseudomass

Figure 20-39 Pseudomass from focal sparing in testicular microlithiasis. Operative biopsy performed using ultrasound guidance showed no evidence of malignancy.

reported, determining the precise risk or causal relation has been more elusive. Nonetheless, many advocate surveillance for testicular cancer once the diagnosis of microlithiasis has been made.

The distribution of microlithiasis within the testis is often not uniform. In cases of severe microlithiasis, regions of sparing can mimic a mass (Fig. 20-39). Because most germ cell tumors have defined margins, the lack of such a margin raises the possibility of a pseudomass

related to sparing in microlithiasis. In some cases, biopsy is required for diagnosis.

■ EXTRATESTICULAR SCROTAL MASS

In addition to the testis, scrotal masses can arise from the epididymis, spermatic cord, and scrotal soft tissues, or enter the scrotum through a patent processus vaginalis.

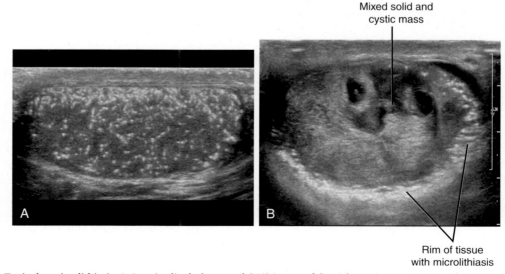

Mixed solid and cystic mass

Rim of tissue with microlithiasis

A

B

Figure 20-38 Testicular microlithiasis. **A,** Longitudinal ultrasound (US) image of the right testis in a patient with testicular microlithiasis. Nonshadowing echogenic foci are scattered diffusely throughout the testis. **B,** Longitudinal US image of the left testis demonstrates a nonseminomatous germ cell tumor within a background of microlithiasis. Note the rim of preserved testicular tissue in the periphery (echogenic because of compressed microlithiasis).

Fluid-Containing Paratesticular Lesions

Epididymal Cyst and Spermatocele

Cysts of the epididymis are extremely common. Most epididymal cysts are asymptomatic, and they are more common in older men and after vasectomy. Anechoic lesions are described as simple cysts with sonography (Fig. 20-40). The presence of low-level echoes or a sedimentation level suggests a spermatocele (Fig. 20-41). In either case, these lesions are benign and are treated only when significantly symptomatic.

Papillary cystadenomas are cystic or solid lesions that arise within the epididymis in approximately 60% of male individuals with von Hippel–Lindau disease (vHL). When predominantly cystic, they usually have papillary projections or septations that separate them from simple epididymal cysts. In other cases, they appear predominantly solid with small internal cystic spaces. Small epidymal masses in patients with vHL are often followed by serial ultrasound examination and removed only if they increase in size.

Hydrocele

Usually a trace amount of fluid is present within the scrotum between the layers of the processes vaginalis. When there is more than a trace amount of fluid, it is called a *hydrocele.* Hydroceles can be classified as communicating or noncommunicating, depending on patency of the processes vaginalis resulting in communication with the peritoneal cavity. In most cases, the fluid is simple, idiopathic, and asymptomatic. With the high-resolution US transducers currently available, it is common to see low-level echoes within idiopathic hydroceles (Fig. 20-42).

A "reactive hydrocele" occurs in response to infection, torsion, or trauma (Fig. 20-43). More complex fluid adjacent to an infected epididymis or testis, or both, is likely to contain bacteria and is called a *pyocele* (see Fig. 20-15).

A *communicating hydrocele* may be the result of generalized ascites extending into the scrotum. Knowledge of

Cysts

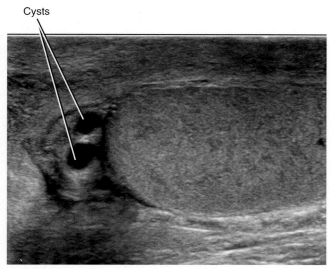

Figure 20-40 Sagittal ultrasound image of the epididymal head demonstrates two incidental simple cysts.

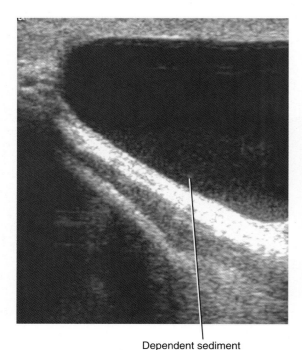

Dependent sediment

Figure 20-41 Sagittal ultrasound image of the epididymis demonstrates a large cystic structure with a sediment layer of low-level echoes. These findings are consistent with a spermatocele.

Echoes within hydrocele   Appendix epididymis

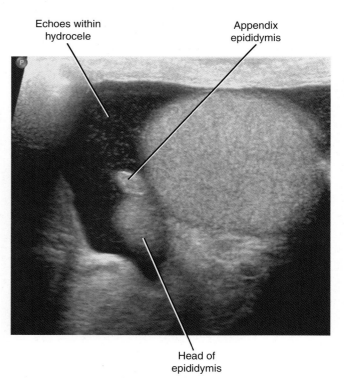

Head of epididymis

Figure 20-42 Sagittal ultrasound image of the scrotum demonstrates an idiopathic and painless hydrocele containing low-level echoes. This is a common finding not to be confused with a spermatocele, which is a contained cystic structure with a sedimentation level within the epididymis.

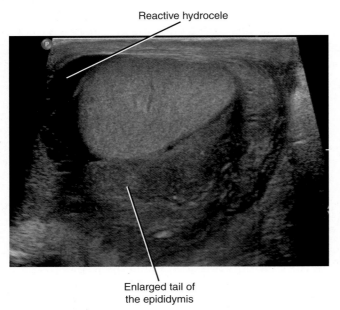

Reactive hydrocele

Enlarged tail of
the epididymis

Figure 20-43 Reactive hydrocele in a patient with severe epididymoorchitis. Transverse ultrasound image demonstrates fluid within the scrotum and a massively enlarged epididymis.

this pathway is useful when peritoneal malignancy presents initially as a scrotal mass (Fig. 20-44). Unusual extratesticular masses detected on physical examination or ultrasound should prompt performance of CT examination of the abdomen and pelvis to evaluate for spread of an abdominal malignancy. Occasionally, inflammatory processes of the abdomen, such as pancreatitis, can extend into the scrotum via extraperitoneal pathways.

Pearl: *Because there is potential communication between the scrotum and the peritoneal space, CT of the*

abdomen and pelvis should be considered to evaluate unusual extratesticular masses that remain incompletely characterized by ultrasound.

Solid Paratesticular Masses

Solid paratesticular masses are uncommon, and most are benign. The most common solid extratesticular scrotal mass is *adenomatoid tumor*. These are benign tumors most often found in the tail of the epididymis but that can arise elsewhere in the epididymis or from the tunica albuginea of the testis or spermatic cord. The appearance is highly variable, ranging from a solid lesion isoechoic to the testis (common) to cystic (uncommon) (Fig. 20-45).

Sperm granuloma is another uncommon, solid-appearing benign intrascrotal extratesticular mass that arises from the epididymis. Thought to be a granulomatous reaction to extravasated spermatozoa, these masses are more common after vasectomy but can be idiopathic or associated with prior infection or trauma. On ultrasound, a sperm granuloma is usually hypoechoic with no demonstrable blood flow with Doppler interrogation. A similar appearance can be seen with fibrous pseudotumor, a nonneoplastic fibrous mass arising from the epididymis or tunica albuginea.

Rare solid paratesticular masses include lesions of the spermatic cord, including benign *lipomas* and *leiomyomata* (Fig. 20-46) and *soft-tissue sarcomas* (rhabdomyosarcoma, liposarcoma). *Epidermal inclusion cysts* can occur outside the testis, usually in the midline near the median raphe. Diagnosis is usually easy when subcutaneous, but an intrascrotal, extratesticular epidermal inclusion cyst results in an unusual solid paratesticular mass (Fig. 20-47). *Polyorchidism* can create the appearance of a paratesticular tumor.

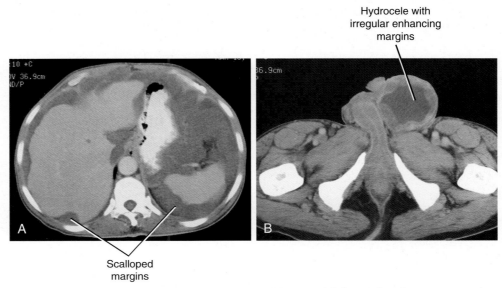

Hydrocele with
irregular enhancing
margins

Scalloped
margins

Figure 20-44 Scrotal presentation of peritoneal neoplasm in a 63-year-old man with left scrotal swelling. A computed tomographic (CT) examination was recommended when complex fluid and irregular scrotal wall thickening were found by US (not shown). **A,** Axial CT image of the upper abdomen demonstrates fluid attenuation scalloping the liver and spleen consistent with mucinous peritoneal tumor. **B,** Axial section through the perineum demonstrates similar material within the scrotum. Mucinous adenocarcinoma of the appendix was found at surgery.

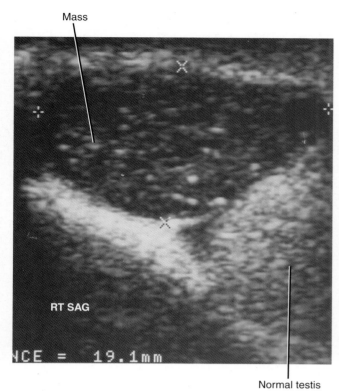

Mass

RT SAG

NCE = 19.1mm

Normal testis

Figure 20-45 Adenomatoid tumor. Sagittal ultrasound image of the testis identified a solid lesion in the head of the epididymis that accounted for the palpable abnormality that was the presenting complaint. This was surgically removed and found to be an adenomatoid tumor of the testis. Although it is more common for adenomatoid tumors to be isoechoic compared with the adjacent testis, some are hypoechoic, as in this case.

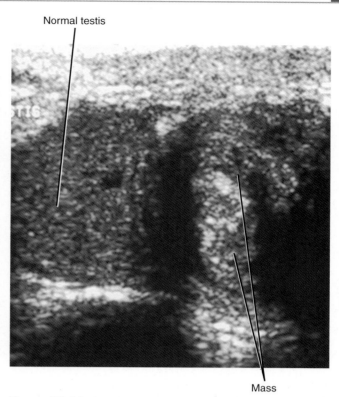

Normal testis

Mass

Figure 20-46 Sagittal ultrasound image of the right testis demonstrates a normal testis that is displaced superiorly in the scrotum by a mass that was subsequently shown to be a leiomyoma of the spermatic cord.

Paratesticular Masses That Change with Valsalva Maneuver

Varicocele

Varicoceles consist of dilated venous structures adjacent to (less commonly within) the testis. These are a common finding with scrotal sonography, occurring in up to 20% of asymptomatic male individuals. They are found in up to 40% of men with infertility and are thus thought to have an adverse effect on spermatogenesis. On US images, serpiginous venous structures are visible adjacent to the testis. With Valsalva maneuver, increased color flow occurs within the varicocele and the veins often increase in diameter (Fig. 20-48). Varicoceles are more common on the left side and usually arise spontaneously, although they occasionally occur as a result of obstruction of the testicular vein by a retroperitoneal mass.

Inguinal Hernia

Up to 5% of men will have a documented inguinal hernia during their lifetime. A hernia that enters the scrotum can present as a scrotal mass. Differentiation from other scrotal masses with US is usually simple; hernias can often be seen moving through the inguinal canal and into the scrotal sac with Valsalva maneuver. When bowel is present within the hernia sac, identification of peristalsis is diagnostic. If there is any doubt about the diagnosis, CT can be helpful, particularly when performed at rest and during Valsalva maneuver.

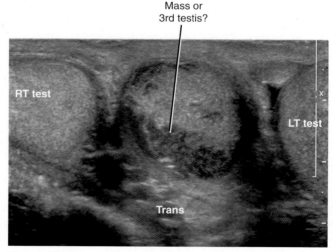

Mass or 3rd testis?

RT test

LT test

Trans

Figure 20-47 Solid extratesticular mass. Transverse midline ultrasound image demonstrates a heterogeneous, solid, soft-tissue mass between the two testes. The mass was removed and found to be an extratesticular epidermal inclusion cyst. *LT test,* Left testis; *RT test,* right testis.

Paratesticular Calcifications

Scrotal pearls are small, calcified, loose bodies within the scrotum (Fig. 20-49). These are thought to represent appendages of the testis and epididymis that have undergone torsion and become detached. They may be palpable but are otherwise asymptomatic and have no clinical significance.

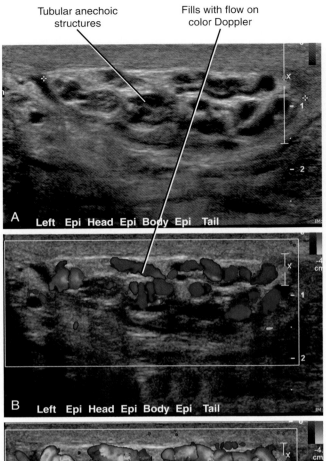

Tubular anechoic
structures

Fills with flow on
color Doppler

A   Left Epi Head Epi Body Epi Tail

B   Left Epi Head Epi Body Epi Tail

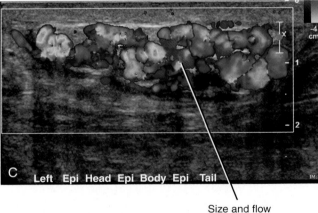

C   Left Epi Head Epi Body Epi Tail

Size and flow
increase with Valsalva

Figure 20-48 Appearance of varicocele on ultrasound. **A,** Grayscale image shows a group of serpiginous hypoechoic structures near the epididymis *(Epi).* **B,** Color Doppler image demonstrates flow within the structures. **C,** When the patient performs a Valsalva maneuver, the vessels become larger with increased blood flow.

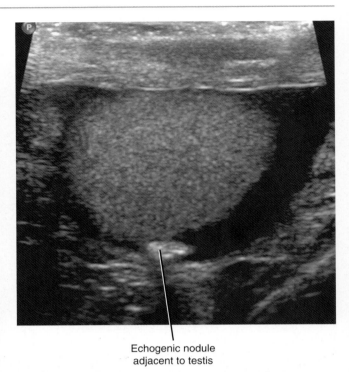

Echogenic nodule
adjacent to testis

Figure 20-49 Scrotal pearl on ultrasound (US). A shadowing echogenic nodule is present deep to the testis on the transverse US image. This could be moved manually.

■ STAGING TESTICULAR CANCER

As mentioned in Chapter 10, imaging plays little role in the preoperative staging of testicular cancer because orchiectomy is almost always performed immediately once a testicular mass is identified. Knowledge of the patterns of disease spread, however, can be useful in optimizing postoperative imaging for metastatic disease. In addition, familiarity with typical patterns of nodal spread allows the radiologist to recommend testicular examination when unsuspected disease is present.

The most common mode of spread for testicular cancer is along the lymphatic drainage that parallels the gonadal veins. In patients with known testicular cancer, it is helpful to follow the gonadal vein from the inguinal canal through the retroperitoneum to its termination near the level of the renal hila. On the right side, the vein usually enters the IVC just inferior or anterior to the right renal vein (Fig. 20-50). On the left side, the gonadal vein usually joins the left renal vein (Fig. 20-51). In many cases of testicular cancer, the only signs of nodal disease are found in the retroperitoneum, at or just below the level of the renal hila. Clusters of small lymph nodes along the gonadal vein may be sampled with retroperitoneal lymph-node dissection or followed by imaging, depending on tumor type and at the discretion of the urologist and oncologist.

Occasionally, this pattern of lymphadenopathy is found in men with acute abdominal pain. Identification of retroperitoneal lymph nodes at the level of the renal hila in a man without a history of lymphoma should prompt physical examination and sonographic evaluation of the testes (Fig. 20-52).

Pearl: Retroperitoneal lymphadenopathy isolated to the level of the renal hila in a man should prompt scrotal evaluation with physical examination and ultrasound in search of a testicular mass.

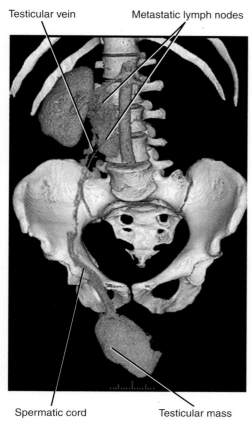

Figure 20-50 Three-dimensional volume rendering from multi-detector computed tomographic examination performed in a patient with right testicular germ cell tumor and retroperitoneal lymph nodes. The lymph nodes are located near the termination of the testicular vein as it enters the inferior vena cava.

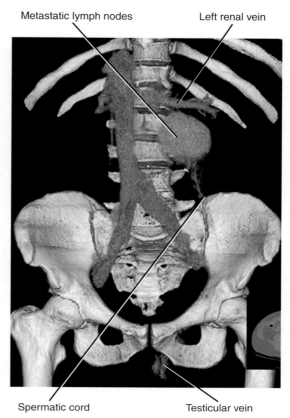

Figure 20-51 Three-dimensional volume rendering from a multi-detector computed tomographic scan performed in a patient with a germ cell tumor of the left testis metastatic to the retroperitoneum. This illustrates the typical pattern of spread to lymph nodes near the termination of the left testicular vein near the left renal vein.

■ ABNORMALITIES OF THE PROSTATE

Cystic Lesions of the Prostate and Seminal Vesicles

Cystic lesions of the prostate and seminal vesicles are reported to occur in up to 7.6% of asymptomatic men. Utricle cysts and müllerian duct cysts are believed to be embryologically different but have similar imaging appearances. Both appear as midline or paramedian cystic structures best seen on MRI or transrectal US (Fig. 20-53). They are both typically high signal intensity on T2-weighted images and variable signal intensity on T1-weighted images, because they may contain blood or proteinaceous fluid.

Utricle cysts typically arise from the verumontanum, are usually small in size (8-10 mm), communicate with the posterior urethra, and are confined to the base of the prostate without extraprostatic extension. Utricle cysts can be associated with genital anomalies including cryptorchidism, ipsilateral renal agenesis, and/or hypospadias. *Müllerian duct cysts* are typically larger and extend superior to the base of the prostate without a urethral communication. They typically reside in the rectovesicular space and can be associated with ipsilateral renal agenesis. Both utricle cysts and müllerian duct

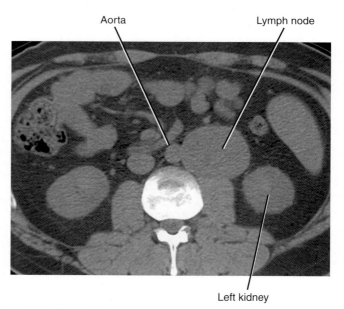

Figure 20-52 Axial image from an initial noncontrast-enhanced computed tomographic examination performed in a patient from Figure 20-51. When the large left paraaortic lymph node was identified on axial sections, the radiologist recommended a testicular ultrasound (US) over the objections of the emergency department physician. The US examination revealed a testicular mass subsequently proved to be a mixed germ cell tumor.

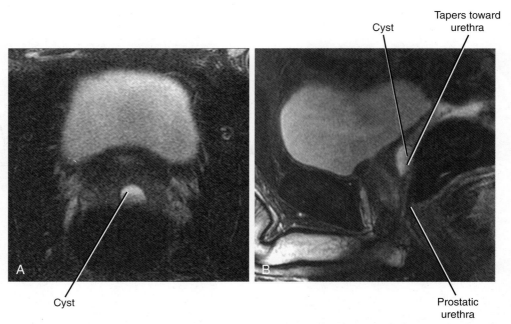

Figure 20-53 Utricle cyst of the prostate. **A,** Axial and **(B)** sagittal midline T2-weighted imaging of the prostate demonstrate a fluid-signal cystic lesion posterior to and communicating with the prostatic urethra.

cysts are associated with hematospermia, hematuria, urinary frequency, urinary urgency, dysuria, urinary obstruction, infertility, and pelvic pain.

Retention cysts of the prostate are common and are a result of glandular dilatation of the acini caused by obstruction of the ductule. They typically appear as 1- to 2-cm unilocular low-attenuation structures on CT, and have high signal intensity on T2-weighted and variable signal intensity on T1-weighted MR images. Retention cysts are identical in appearance to common prostatic cystic changes seen with BPH, with the exception that retention cysts can occur anywhere in the prostate.

Cysts of the seminal vesicles, ejaculatory ducts, and vas deferens are also rarely seen on imaging studies, typically as incidental findings. Ejaculatory duct cysts are intraprostatic and typically midline or paramedian. They result from ejaculatory duct obstruction and dilatation, and often contain stones. Seminal vesicle and vas deferens cysts are extraprostatic and lateral in location. Congenital seminal vesicle cysts are often associated with ipsilateral renal agenesis, dysplasia, or hypoplasia. Sinner syndrome refers to renal agenesis or dysgenesis with the presence of ipsilateral seminal vesicle cysts.

Prostatic abscess is an unusual complication of prostatitis. Abscesses are more common in immunocompromised patients; patients with comorbid conditions such as renal failure, cirrhosis, or diabetes; and patients who require chronic urethral catheterization. Abscesses can involve any portion of the gland but are most often seen in the transitional zone. Prostatic abscesses can be diagnosed and drained using transrectal ultrasound (TRUS). Prostatic abscess typically appears sonographically as a hypoechoic collection with internal echoes and possible septations. MRI and CT can demonstrate a rim-enhancing fluid collection, possibly with septations (Fig. 20-54). Prostate abscesses can extend outside the prostate and involve the seminal vesicles. Imaging should include the entire pelvis and kidneys if extraprostatic spread or urethral obstruction is clinically suspected.

Benign Prostatic Hyperplasia

BPH is present in more than half of all men by age 60, and moderate-to-severe lower urinary tract symptoms develop in more than half of men with BPH. Although some still use the term benign prostatic *hypertrophy,* it is a misnomer because the histologic changes are those of hyperplasia. The percentage of male individuals with BPH further increases to more than 90% by the age of 85. As such, recognition of the characteristic appearance of BPH-related changes on imaging studies is important.

BPH is associated with obstruction of the prostatic urethra, increased prostatic smooth muscle tone, and decreased prostatic compliance caused by altered collagen deposition. Hyperplasia occurs largely in the transitional zone and periurethral glandular tissue (>95%), although a minority of BPH nodules occur in the peripheral zone (<5%). Because the latter can present as a palpable mass on digital rectal examination, accurate imaging diagnosis can prevent unnecessary biopsies.

On MRI, T2-weighted images demonstrate multifocal heterogeneous nodules within the transitional zone with associated global enlargement of the prostate gland. Signal characteristics on T2-weighted imaging are based largely on the composition of the BPH nodules. Predominantly stromal and collagen-filled nodules are hypointense, whereas highly glandular BPH nodules are hyperintense compared with adjacent prostate parenchyma. A low-signal-intensity envelope surrounds many of these BPH nodules on T2-weighted images, and the lack of this dark rim has

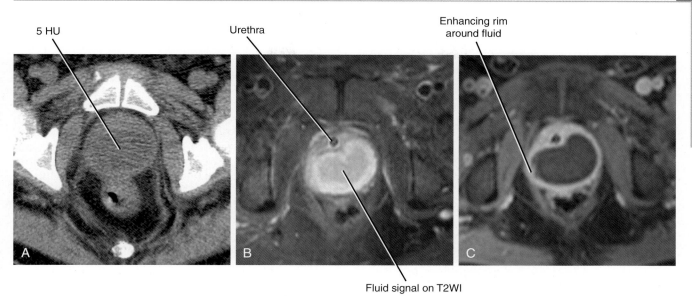

Figure 20-54 Prostate abscess on computed tomography and magnetic resonance imaging. Fifty-year-old man with pelvic pain and fever. **A,** Axial image from noncontrast-enhanced computed tomography shows fluid attenuation in the prostate but little anatomic detail. **B,** Axial T2-weighted imaging (T2WI) and **(C)** axial postcontrast T1-weighted imaging demonstrate a large fluid collection within the prostate with no extraprostatic extension. Transrectal drainage was performed.

been associated with transitional zone prostate cancers. Large BPH nodules often cause deviation of the prostatic urethra to one side, causing obstructive lower urinary tract symptoms (Fig. 20-55). Large BPH nodules in the base of the prostate are often seen extending cranially into the inferior bladder wall (Fig. 20-56).

Transitional zone hypertrophy can also cause compression of the central zone against the peripheral zone, result-ing in the appearance of the thin surgical pseudocapsule (Fig. 20-57). The peripheral zone may also become compressed and thinned, however to a much lesser extent. Differentiation of BPH from prostate cancer can usually be made based on zonal location and characteristic heterogeneous appearance of BPH.

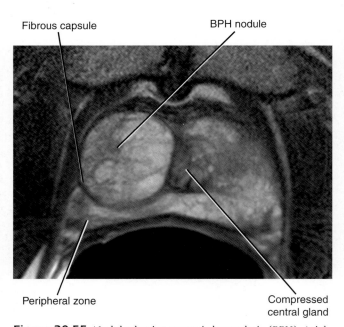

Figure 20-55 Nodular benign prostatic hyperplasia (BPH). Axial T2-weighted magnetic resonance image of the prostate demonstrates a large nodule of glandular BPH (high signal intensity) expanding the central gland on the right side and displacing the other central glandular tissue (and the urethra) toward the left side.

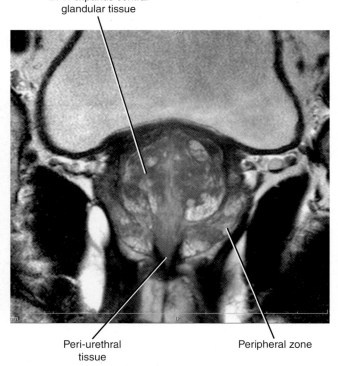

Figure 20-56 Coronal T2-weighted magnetic resonance image demonstrates enlargement of the central glandular tissue, displacing the bladder base superiorly. In this case, benign prostatic hyperplasia (BPH) is predominantly stromal, with mixed but predominantly low signal intensity on T2-weighted imaging (T2WI) (compare with Fig. 20-55).

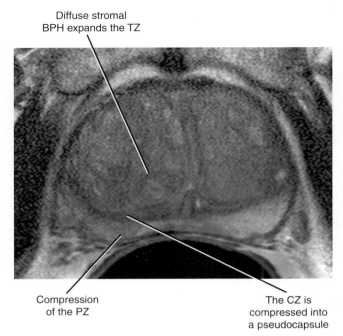

Diffuse stromal
BPH expands the TZ

Compression
of the PZ

The CZ is
compressed into
a pseudocapsule

Figure 20-57 Surgical pseudocapsule from benign prostatic hyperplasia. Axial T2-weighted magnetic resonance image demonstrates diffuse stromal expansion of the transitional zone (TZ), compressing the central zone (CZ) into a low-signal-intensity band just anterior to the peripheral zone (PZ). The PZ is also compressed, but to a lesser degree.

Prostate Cancer

Prostate cancer remains the second most common malignant neoplasm in men (skin cancer is the most common), with approximately 218,890 new cases and 27,050 deaths in the United States in 2007, as estimated by the American Cancer Society. MRI performed with an endorectal coil (erMRI) was developed specifically to evaluate prostate cancer in an attempt to give clinicians information regarding tumor location, stage, and treatment response.

Greater than 95% of prostate cancers are adenocarcinomas, of which more than 70% occur within the peripheral zone. erMRI has focused primarily on evaluation of peripheral zone cancers because currently there is significant variability and lack of standardized imaging criteria for the detection of central and transitional zone cancers. For this reason, this section primarily focuses on peripheral zone cancers.

Magnetic Resonance Imaging of Prostate Cancer

Commercially available coils and software now make high-spatial-resolution multiparametric erMRI of the prostate more available than ever. Many centers are adopting a multiparametric approach, with high-resolution T2-weighted anatomic imaging of the prostate in three planes, large field-of-view (FOV) T1-weighted axial anatomic imaging for nodal disease, high temporal resolution dynamic contrast-enhanced imaging, diffusion-weighted imaging (DWI), and MR spectroscopy. However,

the incremental benefit of each of these components of a comprehensive MR examination of the prostate remains an area of active investigation.

ANATOMIC IMAGING

High-spatial-resolution, small FOV, multiplanar, T2-weighted images focused on the prostate are used to delineate focal areas of decreased T2 signal intensity in the otherwise "bright" peripheral zone (Fig. 20-58). These low-signal regions are indicative of prostate cancer. However, decreased signal intensity in the peripheral zone on T2-weighted images is not specific for prostate cancer and can be seen in chronic prostatitis, postbiopsy hemorrhage, prostatic intraepithelial neoplasia, trauma, fibrosis, and normal peripheral-zone stroma. These entities can mimic prostate cancer and limit the specificity of T2-weighted MRI. The literature also reports significant interobserver variability of MRI interpretation for prostate cancer staging and localization based largely on reader experience.

Large FOV T1-weighted images are used primarily for the depiction of postbiopsy hemorrhage and assessment of lymph-node and bone involvement. The T1-weighted sequence is planned to cover from the pubic symphysis to the aortic bifurcation. Postbiopsy hemorrhage usually causes high signal intensity on T1-weighted images, although the signal intensity of blood products is variable. Therefore, it is recommended that erMRI examinations be performed at least 6 to 8 weeks after biopsy to minimize false positive results. Longer waiting periods may be required for more extensive 12-core or saturation-type biopsies.

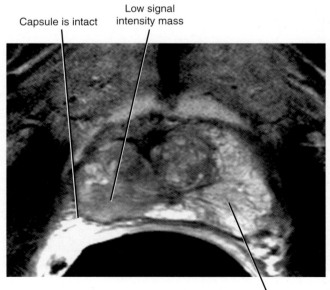

Capsule is intact

Low signal
intensity mass

Normal PZ on left side

Figure 20-58 Typical appearance of prostate cancer on magnetic resonance imaging. Axial T2-weighted imaging demonstrates a low-signal-intensity mass replacing much of the peripheral zone (PZ) on the right side. Organ-confined tumor was confirmed at surgery.

Prognosis, management, and treatment options for prostate cancer are greatly affected by cancer stage. Specifically, cancers with extracapsular extension, denoted as T3 or greater disease, have worse prognosis and are more likely to recur after prostatectomy or radiation therapy than tumors confined to the gland. Standardized axial T2-weighted imaging criteria for extracapsular extension are listed in Box 20-1, and examples are shown in Figure 20-59. Overt seminal vesicle invasion of cancer is often best seen on coronal T2-weighted images. Multiplanar correlation can help increase overall accuracy for tumor detection and localization.

Because of the limited specificity and considerable interobserver variability associated with T2-weighted MRI, multiparametric imaging is often performed. In addition to traditional anatomic imaging, adding MR spectroscopic imaging (MRSI), DWI, and/or dynamic perfusion imaging helps to improve specificity of the examination.

MAGNETIC RESONANCE SPECTROSCOPY, DIFFUSION-WEIGHTED IMAGING, AND DYNAMIC CONTRAST ENHANCEMENT

Certain metabolic changes have been shown to be typical of prostate cancer in both ex vivo and in vivo studies. MRSI delineates this metabolic fingerprint for prostate cancer. Voxels containing prostate cancer demonstrate increased levels of choline and decreased levels of citrate and polyamines.

Similarly, prostate cancer has been shown to demonstrate decreased apparent diffusion coefficient values in DWI when compared with benign prostatic tissue. As with T2-weighted imaging, success has been greatest in the peripheral zone. Several studies report using b values of 0 and 500 sec/mm^2 for DWI in the peripheral zone. Other studies report some success in identifying tumor within the transitional zone using greater b values (1000 sec/mm^2), although there is still overlap between benign and malignant tissues.

High-temporal-resolution, dynamic, contrast-enhanced imaging has the potential to further increase specificity for detecting prostate cancers. Aggressive cancers have been shown to demonstrate increases in total uptake, rate of uptake, and relative rate of washout of contrast on dynamic imaging. However, cancer-related tumor angiogenesis and associated changes in contrast uptake pharmacokinetics are often difficult to differentiate from inflammation seen in prostatitis.

BOX 20-1 Signs of Extracapsular Extension of Prostate Cancer on Axial T2-Weighted Magnetic Resonance Images

- Obliteration of the rectoprostatic angle
- Asymmetry of neurovascular bundle
- Interruption of the low-signal-intensity capsule of the prostate
- Bulging of the prostatic contour
- Tumor signal intensity within periprostatic fat
- Low signal intensity within the normally bright seminal vesicle

---

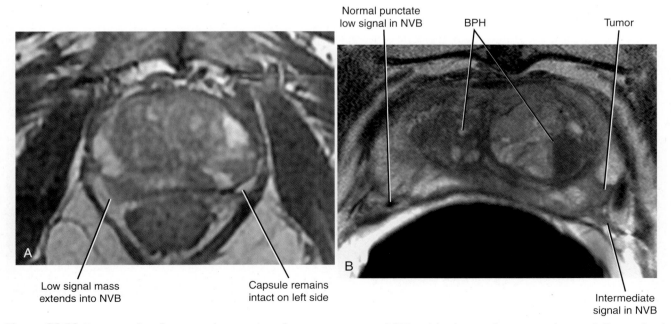

Normal punctate low signal in NVB   BPH   Tumor

Low signal mass extends into NVB   Capsule remains intact on left side

Intermediate signal in NVB

Figure 20-59 Two examples of extracapsular extension of prostate cancer on axial T2-weighted magnetic resonance images. **A,** Tumor signal extends beyond the capsule, into the fat in the expected location of the right neurovascular bundle (NVB). **B,** Abnormal signal within the left NVB in a different patient. Extracapsular extension was proved at surgery. *BPH,* Benign prostatic hyperplasia.

Ultrasound Evaluation of Prostate Cancer

High-frequency TRUS allows differentiation of zonal anatomy and detection of typical hypoechoic peripheral zone prostate cancers. However, greater than 40% of prostate cancers are isoechoic to adjacent prostate tissue, and sensitivity of TRUS remains low for cancer detection. Ultrasound does, however, provide an effective imaging method for guiding biopsies of the prostate.

Metastatic Prostate Cancer

Prostate cancer typically spreads along the obturator, internal/external/common iliac, and presacral lymph-node chains. Because the average size of positive lymph nodes at dissection is 7 mm, standard size criteria are not sensitive for early lymph-node involvement. Bone metastases likely occur through hematogenous spread of cancer cells from the periprostatic veins lateral to the prostate, to the internal iliac veins, to the presacral venous plexus, to the veins of the spine.

Although prostate cancer is sometimes apparent on CT as a region of increased contrast enhancement in the peripheral zone, sensitivity and specificity remain limited. CT has thus been limited to the assessment of lymph nodes, metastatic disease to bone, and radiation treatment planning. Prostate cancer causes predominantly osteoblastic metastases to the axial skeleton, which are evident on CT imaging. Unfortunately, lymph-node morphology, attenuation, enhancement, and size on CT images do not reliably distinguish normal lymph nodes from those involved with tumor. Preliminary results using ultrasmall superparamagnetic iron oxide particle–based agents to detect metastases in normal-size lymph nodes with MR imaging have been promising, but no such agents are approved for use in the United States.

◼ PENILE IMAGING

Erectile Dysfunction

Erectile dysfunction has three main types: too much (priapism), too little (impotence or flaccid erectile dysfunction), or the wrong direction (Peyronie disease).

Imaging is used to a variable amount in the diagnosis and treatment of erectile dysfunction, largely based on local expertise.

Priapism

These days, priapism (a sustained, often painful erection) is most often caused by medications. These include medications intended to induce erection, as well as a variety of antidepressants and psychotropic medications. Imaging plays no role in the diagnosis or treatment of these patients. Imaging can be helpful, however, in high-flow priapism induced by trauma.

Because each corpus cavernosum has a centrally located cavernosal artery surrounded by venous sinuses, traumatic injury can result in development of an arteriovenous fistula or pseudoaneurysm, or both. Increased arterial inflow with normal-to-decreased venous outflow (if damaged) results in a sustained, painful erection. Ultrasound with color Doppler helps identify the location and nature of the vascular defect (Fig. 20-60). Accurate preoperative characterization can minimize the amount of exploration necessary and optimize vascular repair or placement of a shunt for decompression.

Doppler Evaluation for Flaccid Erectile Dysfunction

Spectral Doppler US can be useful in the evaluation of patients who are unable to achieve an erection by screening for arterial insufficiency or venous leak. Serial interrogation of the cavernosal arteries is performed before and after the intracavernosal injection of prostaglandin. The presence of a tardus parvus waveform or a lack of change after injection, or both, suggest arterial insufficiency, in which case transcatheter intervention may be helpful in improving arterial inflow. More commonly, there is ineffective closure of the venous outflow, called a *venous leak*. With normal venous closure, loss of diastolic flow indicating high-resistance arterial flow occurs. With venous leak, only minimal decrease in diastolic flow 30 minutes after prostaglandin injection occurs.

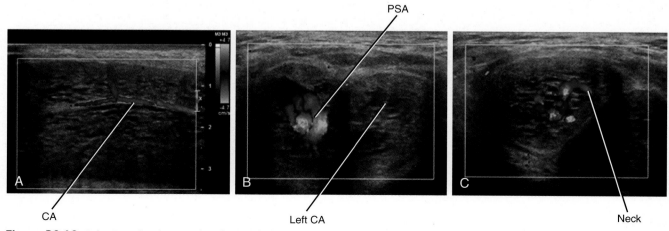

Figure 20-60 Color Doppler ultrasound performed for posttraumatic high-flow priapism. **A,** Slightly enlarged but otherwise normal-appearing right cavernosal artery (CA) near the base of the penis. **B,** While following each cavernosal artery, a pseudoaneurysm (PSA) was discovered on the right side. **C,** Identification of the precise location of the pseudoaneurysm neck by color Doppler ultrasound facilitated vascular repair.

Peyronie Disease

Peyronie disease describes the development of fibrous plaques in the corpora cavernosa, altering the uniformity of erection and ultimately resulting in a bent shape during erection. Causes include prior trauma, autoimmune connective tissue disease, and use of β-blocker medications. In most cases, diagnosis is made on clinical grounds. On occasion, a physician seeks imaging to confirm the diagnosis. Calcified plaques are sometimes visible on plain radiographs and CT, but Peyronie disease is more precisely characterized with US (Fig. 20-61).

Penile Cancer

Penile cancer describes lesions that arise from the soft tissues of the penis excluding the urethra, usually within the skin or subcutaneous soft tissues. Squamous cell carcinoma is the most common tumor type and is usually slow growing. About 4% of penile cancers are a more aggressive sarcomatoid type of tumor. When performed, imaging is usually used to identify nodal disease, which spreads first to inguinal lymph nodes and then into the pelvic lymph nodes.

Traditional surgical treatment is total penectomy, leaving a urethral meatus in the perineum for voiding. A recent preference for partial penectomy or stepwise excision (Mohs surgery) makes imaging useful on occasion. MRI provides excellent anatomic detail and is useful for determining the presence and extent of cavernosal invasion, presence of invasion into the corpus spongiosa and urethra, and the presence of nodal disease (Fig. 20-62). When performing MRI, consider using an extremity coil and small FOV to achieve the highest spatial resolution possible. On T2-weighted images, the low signal of the tunica albuginea divides

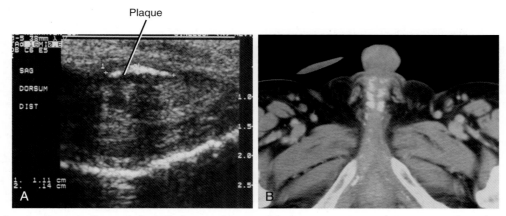

Figure 20-61   Imaging Peyronie disease. **A,** Sagittal ultrasound image of the corpus cavernosum demonstrates echogenic, mildly shadowing plaque in the near field. **B,** Axial computed tomographic image of the same patient demonstrates calcified plaques in both cavernosa.

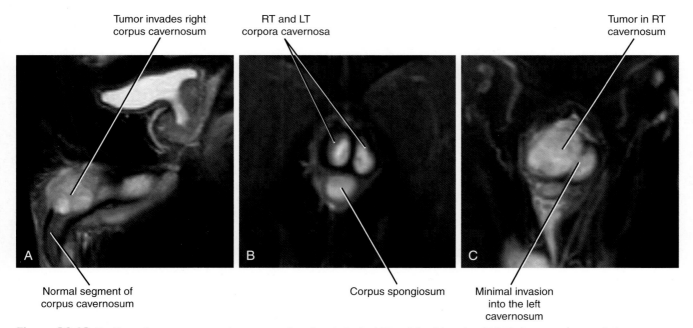

Figure 20-62   Penile carcinoma on magnetic resonance imaging. **A,** Sagittal T2-weighted imaging (T2WI) demonstrates a soft-tissue mass within the subcutaneous tissues and right corpus cavernosum. **B,** Axial T2WI distal to the mass demonstrates the zonal anatomy of the penis with dark bands defining the tunica albuginea surrounding the corpora cavernosa. **C,** Axial T2WI at the level of the mass demonstrates tumor extending from the right (RT) into the left (LT) corpus cavernosum. This was confirmed at surgery.

the right and left corpora cavernosa from each other and from the corpus spongiosum. Images orthogonal to the axis of the penis are most helpful. Postcontrast T1-weighted images can be useful if performed early, but enhancement of the cavernosa is typically so intense that discrimination between vascular tumors and normal tissue is virtually impossible by 1 minute.

Suggested Readings

Akbar SA, Sayyed TA, Jafri SZ et al: Multimodality imaging of paratesticular neoplasms and their rare mimics, Radiographics 23:1461-1476, 2003.

Cho JH, Chang JC, Park BH et al: Sonographic and MR imaging findings of testicular epidermoid cysts, Am J Roentgenol 178:743-748, 2002.

Coakley FV, Hricak HH: Radiologic anatomy of the prostate gland: a clinical approach, Radiol Clin North Am 38(1):15-29, 2000.

Dogra VS, Gottlieb RH, Oka M, Rubens DJ: Sonography of the scrotum, Radiology 227:18-36, 2003.

Dogra VS, Gottlieb RH, Rubens DJ, Liao L: Benign intratesticular cystic lesions: US features, Radiographics 21:S273-S281, 2001.

Dogra VS, Gottlieb RH, Rubens DJ et al: Testicular epidermoid cysts: sonographic features with histopathologic correlation, J Clin Ultrasound 29:192-196, 2001.

Fernandez-Perez GC, Tardaguila FM, Velasco M et al: Radiologic findings of segmental testicular infarction, Am J Roentgenol 184:1587-1593, 2005.

Grossman GD, Coakley FV: Benign prostatic hyperplasia: clinical overview and value of imaging, Radiol Clin North Am 38(1):15-29, 2000.

Ishikawa M, Okabe H, Oya T et al: Midline prostatic cysts in healthy men: incidence and transabdominal sonographic findings, Am J Roentgenol 181:1669-1672, 2003.

Jung JA, Coakley FV, Vigneron DB et al: Prostate depiction at endorectal MR spectroscopic imaging: investigation of a standardized evaluation system, Radiology 233:701-708, 2004.

Kim CK, Park BK: Update of prostate magnetic resonance imaging at 3 T, J Comp Assist Tomogr 32:163-172, 2008.

Lin EP, Bhatt S, Rubens DJ et al: Testicular torsion: twists and turns, Semin Ultrasound CT MRI 28:317-328, 2007.

Madaan S, Joniau S, Klockaerts K et al: Segmental testicular infarction: conservative management is feasible and safe, Eur Urol 53:441-445, 2008.

Massarweh NN, Bhalani VK, Shaw KK et al: Testicular presentation of sarcoidosis and organ preservation: case report and review of management strategies, Urology 67:200, 2006.

McDermott VG, Meakem TJ 3rd, Stolpen AH, Schnall MD: Prostatic and periprostatic cysts: findings on MR imaging, Am J Roentgenol 164:123-127, 1995.

McNeal JE: The prostate gland: morphology and pathobiology, Monogr Urol 9:36-54, 1998.

McNeil JE: Normal and pathologic anatomy of the prostate, Urology 17:11-16, 1981.

Miedler JD, MacLennan GT: Primary testicular lymphoma, J Urol 178:2645, 2007.

Ocak I, Bernardo M, Metzger G et al: Dynamic contrast-enhanced MRI of prostate cancer at 3 T: a study of pharmacokinetic parameters, Am J Roentgenol 189:849, 2007.

Parsons RB, Fisher AM, Bar-Chama N, Mitty HA: MR imaging in male infertility, Radiographics 17:627-637, 1997.

Rayson D, Burch PA, Richardson RL: Sarcoidosis and testicular carcinoma, Cancer 83:337-343, 1998.

Salmeron I, Ramirez-Escobar MA, Puertas F et al: Granulomatous epididymo-orchitis: sonographic features and clinical outcome in brucellosis, tuberculosis and idiopathic granulomatous epididymo-orchitis, J Urol 159:1954-1957, 1998.

Shin SL, Outwater EK: Benign large cell calcifying Sertoli cell tumor of the testis in a prepubescent patient, Am J Roentgenol 189:W65-W66, 2007.

Shoskes DA, Lee CT, Murphy D et al: Incidence and significance of prostatic stones in men with chronic prostatitis/chronic pelvic pain syndrome, Urology 70:235-238, 2007.

Tynski Z, MacLennan GT: "Burnt-out" testicular germ cell tumors, J Urol 174:2013, 2005.

van Veen RN, van Wessem KJ, Halm JA et al: Patent processus vaginalis in the adult as a risk factor for the occurrence of indirect inguinal hernia, Surg Endosc 21:202-205, 2007.

Wang L, Mullerad M, Chen HN et al: Prostate cancer: incremental value of endorectal MR imaging findings for prediction of extracapsular extension, Radiology 232(1):133-139, 2004.

Woodward PJ, Sohaey R, O'Donoghue MJ et al: Tumors and tumorlike lesions of the testis: radiologic-pathologic correlation, Radiographics 22:189-216, 2002.

CHAPTER 21

Female Reproductive System

David Childs and Neal C. Dalrymple

■ CLINICAL CONSIDERATIONS

There are a wide variety of indications for imaging the female pelvis. From acute pelvic pain and abnormal uterine bleeding (AUB) to identifying and characterizing pelvic masses or potential causes of infertility, imaging plays a crucial role in diagnosis and management. However, imaging studies obtained to evaluate pelvic pathology can often be difficult to interpret in isolation. The pelvis contains elements of the gastrointestinal and urinary tracts, as well as the reproductive system, all of which can be affected by congenital, inflammatory, and neoplastic processes. The dissemination of pelvic inflammation or neoplasm via the peritoneal cavity or extraperitoneal spaces can make the organ of origin difficult or impossible to determine with imaging alone. Furthermore, the pelvic structures and organs lie in close proximity to one another, and intervening fat planes can be subtle or absent on imaging studies, particularly in thin patients. This explains the difficulty often encountered in distinguishing between pelvic inflammatory disease and appendicitis. Therefore, radiologists must rely on accurate clinical information to improve specificity and ensure appropriate management.

Certain clinical data should be sought by the radiologist when interpreting imaging studies of the female pelvis. Appropriate questions to ask are included in Table 21-1.

The differential diagnosis of acute pelvic pain is discussed in Chapter 8. Therefore, after a brief discussion of female pelvic anatomy, this chapter focuses primarily on nonacute abnormalities of the female pelvis.

Anatomy of the Female Reproductive System

Uterus

The uterus is a muscular pouch that forms from paired müllerian ducts. The ducts first fuse; then some of the intervening tissue resorbs to form the fallopian tubes, uterus, and upper one-third of the vagina (Fig. 21-1). Most congenital anomalies of the uterus and vagina result from either failure of the ducts to fuse or failure of the intervening tissue to resorb. The mucosal lining of the uterus is called the *endometrium*. The muscular wall is the myometrium. The uterine fundus protrudes into the peritoneal space, encased by a blanket of peritoneum that forms the broad ligament on either side.

Ovaries

The egg-producing ovaries are themselves egg shaped, each approximately 3 cm in length in adults. Ovarian cortex makes up the bulk of each ovary, consisting predominantly of ova-containing follicles with some intervening stroma. The central medulla does not contain ova. The ovary is under the control of follicle-stimulating hormone and luteinizing hormone produced by the pituitary gland. Together, these hormones promote maturation of an ovarian follicle (usually only one) each menstrual cycle until it bursts, releasing an ovum into the peritoneal cavity and fallopian tube. After ovulation, the "empty" follicle is called the *corpus luteum*.

Fallopian Tubes

The fallopian tubes are a continuation of the müllerian ducts that form the uterus and provide communication between the peritoneal cavity and the outside world. It is necessary, of course, for the two worlds to meet for fertilization to occur. The fallopian tube averages 10 cm in length and can be subdivided into four segments (Fig. 21-2).

Broad Ligaments

The uterus, fallopian tubes, ovaries, and some blood vessels are "shrink-wrapped" in the peritoneal lining that also covers the floor of the peritoneal cavity. The folded peritoneum that extends from each side of the uterus toward each pelvic sidewall is called the *broad ligament*. The broad ligament helps maintain a predictable relation between the infundibulum of each fallopian tube and the adjacent ovary, and is one of several structures that provide support to the uterus. The broad ligament also facilitates bidirectional extraperitoneal spread of inflammation and neoplasm between the uterus and ovaries and other pelvic structures.

Pelvic Floor

The bony pelvis is basically shaped like a large ring. The pelvic organs are supported by a complex set of fascial, ligamentous, and muscular structures, which are attached to each other and to the bony framework of the pelvis, to counter the effects of gravity (and Valsalva).

Table 21-1   Appropriate Inquiries When Interpreting Female Pelvic Imaging Studies

Inquiry	Significance
Clinical History	
Are symptoms acute or chronic?	Ovarian cyst rupture/hemorrhage and torsion of ovary or fibroid often present with sudden onset of symptoms
Is the patient premenopausal or postmenopausal?	Affects normal measurements such as endometrial thickness
Is the patient on hormone replacement?	Affects appearance of endometrium
Could the patient be pregnant?	Affects appearance of endometrium and likelihood of ectopic pregnancy
Is the patient sexually active?	Affects likelihood of ectopic pregnancy and PID
Any vaginal discharge, dysfunctional uterine bleeding?	Helps localize origin of symptoms to the reproductive tract
Any fever or chills?	Helps distinguish between infectious and neoplastic processes
Has the patient had an appendectomy, hysterectomy, oophorectomy, or other pelvic surgery?	Helps eliminate diseases of these organs from the differential diagnosis and may explain altered anatomy
Physical Findings	
Any vaginal discharge or cervical motion tenderness?	Increases likelihood of PID
Any point tenderness?	Helps direct search
Any peritoneal signs?	Helps distinguish infectious or inflammatory ascites from malignant ascites
Laboratory Data	
Urinalysis	Helps localize disease process to the urinary tract
White blood cell count	Helps distinguish between infectious and noninfectious processes
Pregnancy test or β-hCG	Helps establish likelihood of intrauterine pregnancy, ectopic pregnancy, or gestational trophoblastic disease; the level of β-hCG should double every 48 hours during the early stages of pregnancy
CA-125	Commonly expressed by ovarian carcinoma Increase (most use > 30 units/mL) has high association with ovarian cancer in postmenopausal women, less straightforward in premenopausal women when normal levels are more variable

β-hCG, β-Human chorionic gonadotropin; *PID,* pelvic inflammatory disease.

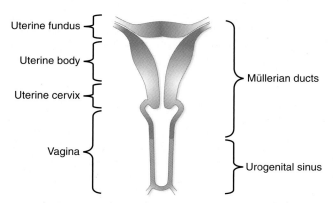

Figure 21-1 Illustration demonstrating origin of the uterus and vagina.

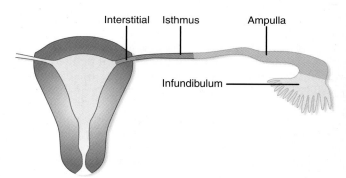

Figure 21-2 Illustration demonstrating the anatomic segments of the fallopian tube.

The *levator ani complex* is a key element of this slinglike support system and has multiple components, including the *puborectalis* and *iliococcygeus* muscles. The puborectalis provides anterior support, attached to either side of the pubic bone near the symphysis, and makes a sling around the anus, keeping the anus, vagina, and urethra bound to the pubis (Fig. 21-3). The iliococcygeus provides posterior and lateral support through multiple interdependent osseous and fascial attachments. The

levator plate is a posterior midline condensation of the ileococcygeus best seen as a linear attachment to the coccyx on sagittal magnetic resonance (MR) images (Fig. 21-4).

Perineum
The urethra, vagina, and rectum pass through the U-shaped levator hiatus. The urethra is most anterior and often has a target-like appearance on T2-weighted MR images. Just posterior to the urethra is the vagina, which

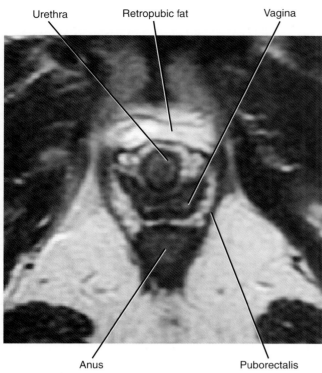

Urethra   Retropubic fat   Vagina

Anus   Puborectalis

Figure 21-3 Axial T2-weighted magnetic resonance image demonstrates normal axial anatomy of the female perineum. Familiarity with these normal structures is critical to diagnosis of abnormalities of the urethra and vagina.

typically has an H or butterfly shape. The anus is posterior to the vagina. The urethra and vagina end in the external urethral meatus and vaginal introitus, respectively, both of which lie in the vestibule between the labia minora. *Skene's glands* adjacent to the urethra

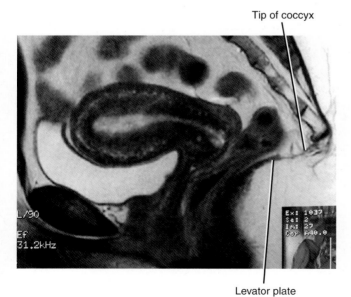

Tip of coccyx

Levator plate

Figure 21-4 Sagittal T2-weighted magnetic resonance (MR) image in the midline demonstrates the levator plate, a posterior condensation of fascia extending from the levator ani complex to the coccyx. This is a key anatomic landmark in the dynamic MR evaluation of pelvic floor laxity.

produce mucus that lubricates the mucosal surface. Embedded within the posterior aspect of the labia minora are the paired *Bartholin glands,* with ducts that drain on either side of the vaginal introitus.

■ NORMAL IMAGING APPEARANCE OF THE FEMALE PELVIS

Ultrasound

Ultrasound (US) is the first-line modality for most applications in the female pelvis. Transvaginal ultrasound *(TVUS)* provides high-resolution images of the uterus. With the transducer only millimeters away, US provides excellent detail of the endometrium and myometrium in most patients. The orientation of TVUS images can be disorienting. To the uninitiated, it sometimes helps to rotate images of the uterus clockwise 90 degrees (Fig. 21-5).

Transabdominal scanning provides less-detailed information regarding the uterus and ovaries in most cases, but remains useful by providing perspective regarding the orientations and relations of the pelvic organs, particularly if a large mass is present. Occasionally, ovaries not visible with transvaginal sonography become visible with a transabdominal approach.

Hormonal influences on the endometrium result in a variable appearance of the endometrial stripe *(EMS)* on TVUS during the alternating proliferative and secretory phases of each menstrual cycle (Fig. 21-6). A hypoechoic layer of functional myometrium is usually seen surrounding the echogenic apposed endometrial mucosa; it is important that this dark line be omitted from the EMS measurement. During the proliferative phase, the hypoechoic line of the inner myometrium is outside all three echogenic endometrial lines. In premenopausal women, the EMS typically measures up to 8 mm during the proliferative phase and up to 14 mm during the secretory phase. After menses, the EMS becomes thin (2-3 mm). Because of variability, absolute EMS thickness is less important than uniformity in premenopausal women.

The postmenopausal endometrium becomes atrophic, usually measuring 2 to 3 mm in thickness with uniformly increased echogenicity (Fig. 21-7). A cutoff for EMS measurement of *5 mm or less* is used to effectively exclude malignancy with a sensitivity of 96% (this is discussed in greater detail later in the Imaging Evaluation for Abnormal Uterine Bleeding section). Little data have been reported regarding the significance of an EMS measurement of greater than 5 mm found incidentally in an asymptomatic postmenopausal woman.

Despite variable location of the ovaries, they can be identified with transvaginal sonography in nearly all premenopausal women. The ovaries can be more challenging to identify after menopause but are still identified in the majority of women. The normal ovary contains multiple small anechoic follicles, typically ranging from 1.0 to 2.5 cm (Fig. 21-8). Most consider a cystic structure in the ovary that exceeds 2.5 cm in diameter to be a cyst, and most of these are functional cysts that

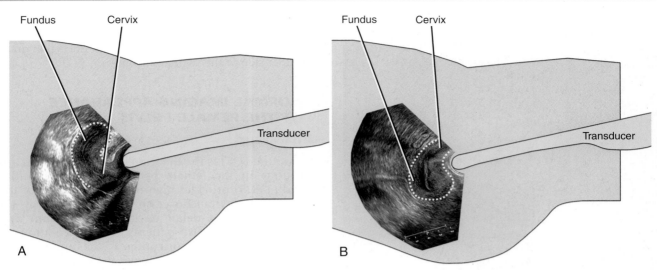

Fundus   Cervix

Transducer

Fundus   Cervix

Transducer

A

B

Figure 21-5 Schematic illustration demonstrating the sagittal perspective of the uterus with transvaginal ultrasound. **A,** Sagittal relation between the transducer and an anteverted uterus. Tilting your head toward the right provides the usual imaging perspective. **B,** Sagittal relation between the transducer and a retroverted uterus.

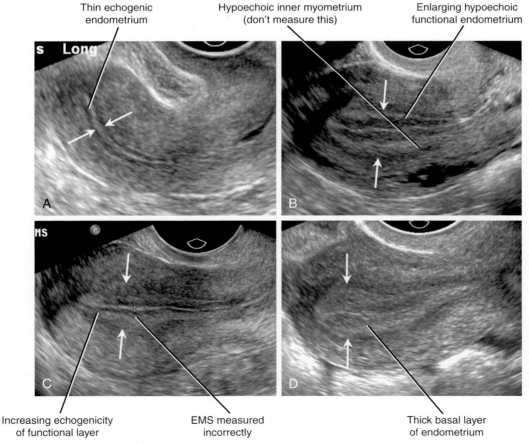

Thin echogenic endometrium

Hypoechoic inner myometrium (don't measure this)

Enlarging hypoechoic functional endometrium

Increasing echogenicity of functional layer

EMS measured incorrectly

Thick basal layer of endometrium

Figure 21-6 Cycle-related changes in the appearance of the endometrial stripe (EMS) on transvaginal ultrasound. **A,** Early proliferative endometrium. **B,** Late proliferative endometrium. **C,** Early secretory endometrium. **D,** Late secretory endometrium. *Opposing arrows* on each image demonstrate correct cursor placement to measure thickness of the EMS.

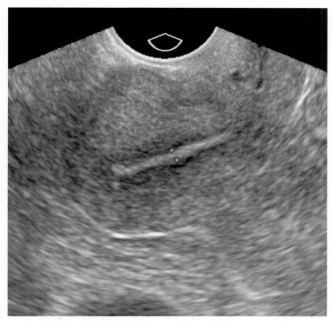

Figure 21-7   Sagittal transvaginal ultrasound image of a post-menopausal woman with abnormal bleeding. This thin (4-mm), uniformly echogenic stripe is normal and effectively excludes the presence of endometrial carcinoma or polyps.

will resolve over time. Depending on the phase of the ovulatory cycle, a *corpus luteum* may be present. With US, the corpus luteum typically has an irregular, thick wall that demonstrates increased flow on color Doppler. This appearance has prompted use of the term *ring of fire*.

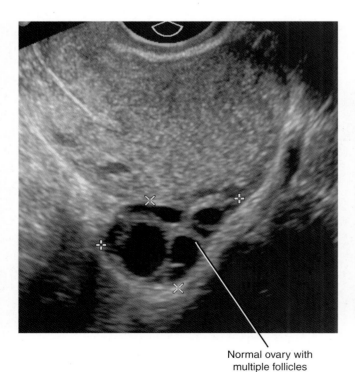

Normal ovary with
multiple follicles

Figure 21-8   Sagittal transvaginal ultrasound image demonstrates a normal ovary posterior to the retroverted uterus.

Computed Tomography

Computed tomography (CT) is used to image women with pelvic symptoms when US is negative or inconclusive. It is also used for staging and following neoplastic disease. CT provides broader perspective of anatomy and pathology compared with US and is less operator dependent. With newer multidetector computed tomography (MDCT) scanners, routine multiplanar reformations help better define pelvic anatomy, although soft-tissue contrast remains limited.

The uterus usually appears as an oblong soft-tissue structure near the midline on CT images, situated posterior to the bladder and anterior to the rectum. CT appearance of the EMS varies considerably, inapparent in some cases and low attenuation in others.

More rapid scan acquisition with MDCT often results in an earlier phase of uterine enhancement compared with single-detector CT. Although the impact of hormonal cyclic changes on the US appearance is well-recognized, few consider that the vascular changes that contribute to transitions from proliferative to secretory phases result in different patterns of uterine enhancement on CT. Heterogeneous uterine enhancement on MDCT is usually a normal finding (Fig. 21-9). The normal endometrium appears hypoattenuating relative to the myometrium on unenhanced CT images, and this relation persists through the portal phase of imaging after administration of intravenous contrast material. This appearance is often confused with endometrial fluid by inexperienced CT readers.

The ovaries can be found by CT in virtually all cases. On axial sections, note the region where the uterus

Heterogeneous
myometrium

Low attenuation
endometrium

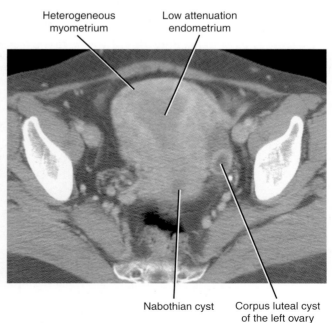

Nabothian cyst

Corpus luteal cyst
of the left ovary

Figure 21-9   Axial image from multidetector computed tomographic examination performed with intravenous contrast demonstrates heterogenous enhancement of the normal myometrium.

changes from oval shaped to tapered as the contour becomes defined by the broad ligament. In most cases, this tapering causes the uterus to "point" toward each ovary, or at least to a thin band of broad ligament that can be followed to the ovary. The *ovarian veins* are readily identified in most cases, and following each ovarian vein inferiorly should demonstrate where it joins the suspensory ligament of the ovary, usually between the ovary and iliac vessels. CT reveals less detail regarding the normal ovary compared with US. Often, individual follicles cannot be discerned, or only the dominant follicle is seen by CT.

Magnetic Resonance Imaging

MRI is used to image the female pelvis when US and CT are inconclusive. MR is also the most accurate imaging modality for characterizing congenital uterine anomalies and for staging most gynecologic malignancies. Cinematic MRI can be useful for the evaluation of pelvic floor laxity. When performing MRI of the pelvis, it can be helpful to have the patient fast or to administer glucagon to reduce artifact from bowel peristalsis. For evaluation of the uterus, imaging planes should be chosen relative to the uterine axes rather than relative to the pelvis (Fig. 21-10).

On T2-weighted MR images, the uterus can be divided into three distinct layers: the central high-signal-intensity endometrium, the low-signal-intensity junctional zone, and the outer intermediate-signal-intensity myometrium (Fig. 21-11). Thickness of the endometrium varies throughout the menstrual cycle in premenopausal women, with a width of up to 14 mm considered normal during the secretory stage of the menstrual cycle. In postmenopausal women, an endometrial thickness of 5 mm or less is considered normal.

The *junctional zone*, regarded as a distinct stratum by MRI, is actually the basal layer of the myometrium. This layer is easy to identify on T2-weighted images because it appears as a smooth, dark band between the

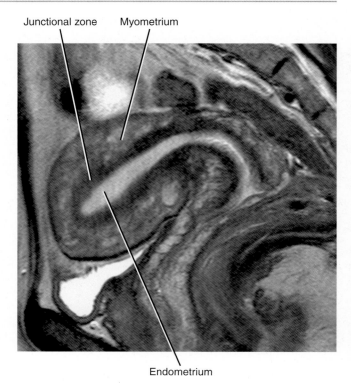

Junctional zone   Myometrium

Endometrium

Figure 21-11 Sagittal T2-weighted magnetic resonance image through the uterine corpus demonstrates the zonal anatomy of the uterus. The low-signal junctional zone can clearly be seen as a smooth uniform band separating the hyperintense endometrium from the intermediate-signal outer myometrium.

hyperintense endometrium and the intermediate signal myometrium. The junctional zone should appear smooth, and a thickness of less than 8 mm is considered normal. Zonal anatomy often becomes less distinct in postmenopausal women (Fig. 21-12).

Uterine zonal anatomy cannot be distinguished on unenhanced T1-weighted images. After contrast administration, the myometrium enhances briskly, whereas

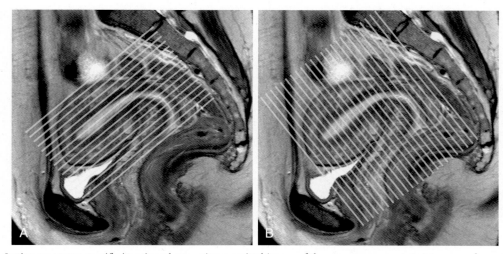

Figure 21-10 Setting up uterus-specific imaging planes using a sagittal image of the uterus as a scout. **A,** Images performed coronal to the uterine fundus optimize visualization of the outer fundal contour, critical in characterizing müllerian anomalies. **B,** Images performed axial to the uterine fundus facilitate assessment of endometrial masses and their invasion into the myometrium.

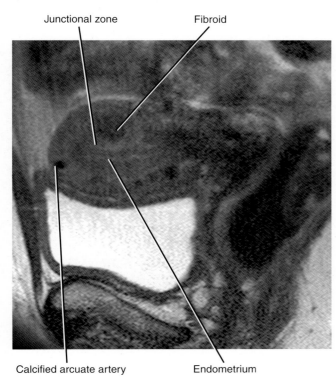

Junctional zone   Fibroid

Calcified arcuate artery   Endometrium

Figure 21-12 Sagittal T2-weighted magnetic resonance image of a postmenopausal uterus. Zonal anatomy is much less distinct than in Figure 21-11.

the endometrium undergoes more delayed progressive contrast enhancement, eventually becoming isointense or hyperintense to myometrium. In postmenopausal women, a zone of normal *subendometrial enhancement* on postcontrast T1-weighted images is often more helpful in demarcating the transition from endometrium to myometrium than is the often inapparent junctional zone on T2-weighted images (Fig. 21-13).

The zonal anatomy of the cervix is best appreciated on T2-weighted imaging sequences. From central to peripheral, the three anatomic zones include the *endocervix*, the *inner fibromuscular stroma* (FMS), and the *outer FMS* (Fig. 21-14). The endocervical mucosa, secretions, and plicae palmatae (mucosal folds) appear as increased signal intensity centrally within the cervix on T2-weighted images. The inner FMS has low signal intensity, likely the result of a densely packed zone of fibroblasts and smooth muscle cells. The outer FMS, composed of more loosely packed tissue, is low-to-intermediate signal intensity on T2-weighted images.

The ovary also has an identifiable zonal anatomy on T2-weighted imaging with a low-signal cortex peripherally, an intermediate-signal medulla centrally, and high signal intensity cysts and follicles (Fig. 21-15). In normal premenopausal women, the appearance of the ovaries varies with the menstrual cycle. Normal follicles range in size from several millimeters up to 2.5 cm, and should appear of homogenously low signal intensity on T1-weighted images and high signal intensity on

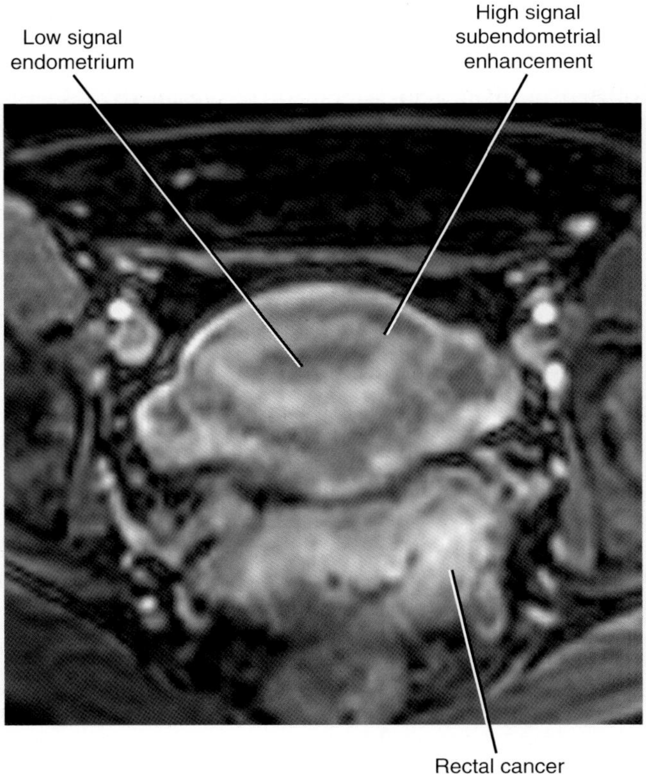

Low signal endometrium   High signal subendometrial enhancement

Rectal cancer

Figure 21-13 Subendometrial enhancement defining zonal anatomy during early phases of dynamic contrast-enhanced T1-weighted magnetic resonance imaging of the postmenopausal uterus. In this case, axial sections were obtained in the evaluation of rectal cancer.

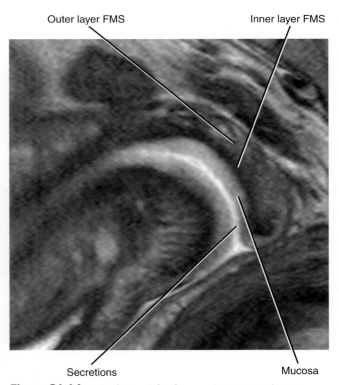

Outer layer FMS   Inner layer FMS

Secretions   Mucosa

Figure 21-14 Sagittal T2-weighted magnetic resonance image through the cervix demonstrates the normal zonal anatomy. The endocervix is comprised of very high signal intensity secretions and slightly lower signal intensity mucosa. The fibromuscular stroma (FMS) is divided into a low-signal inner layer and an intermediate-signal outer layer. Signal within the FMS layers is determined by cell density.

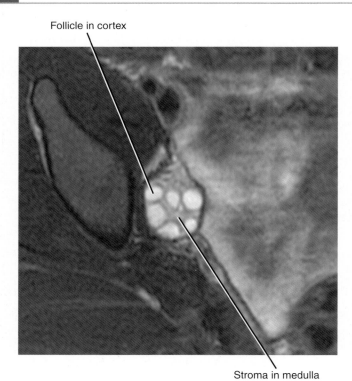

Follicle in cortex

Stroma in medulla

Figure 21-15 Axial T2-weighted magnetic resonance image of the normal right ovary.

Hysterosalpingography

Hysterosalpingography (HSG) is the only imaging modality to reliably demonstrate the normal fallopian tubes. Through opacification of the endometrial canal and fallopian tubes, HSG can identify and characterize most abnormalities associated with female infertility. Although mildly invasive, risk to the patient is low and the diagnostic yield is high.

Injection into the cervix opacifies a funnel-shaped endometrial canal that should have a smooth appearance without filling defects (Fig. 21-16). The fallopian tubes opacify next and should be thin and gracile proximally, then gradually widening until contrast spills from the ampullary portion into the peritoneal space.

■ IMAGING EVALUATION FOR ABNORMAL UTERINE BLEEDING

Abnormal uterine bleeding (AUB) is the most common indication for US among postmenopausal women. The most common cause of postmenopausal bleeding is endometrial atrophy, reported to be responsible in 75% of cases. Other causes of AUB include endometrial polyps, submucosal fibroids, endometrial hyperplasia, and estrogen withdrawal. Although endometrial carcinoma accounts for only 10% of cases of postmenopausal bleeding, AUB is the most common presentation for endometrial carcinoma.

TVUS is the initial imaging modality of choice in this patient population, given its relative low cost, high accuracy in depicting the endometrium, and near-universal availability. An EMS measurement of 5 mm or less is considered normal. A measurement of greater than 5 mm should be considered abnormal in the presence of abnormal bleeding, a cutoff that detects 96% of endometrial carcinoma cases. Some prefer to use a threshold of 4 mm to increase sensitivity, but this is accompanied by an increase in the number of false-positive examinations.

T2-weighted images. Dominant follicles become corpus lutea in the secretory phase of the menstrual cycle, often displaying smooth, thick walls that enhance avidly after intravenous contrast administration. The corpus luteum involutes if pregnancy does not occur, and imaging at this stage reveals a convoluted cyst contour. In postmenopausal women, the ovaries progressively decrease in size over time and appear as oval structures of low signal intensity. Dormant follicular cysts can be seen in normal postmenopausal ovaries as small, simple cysts.

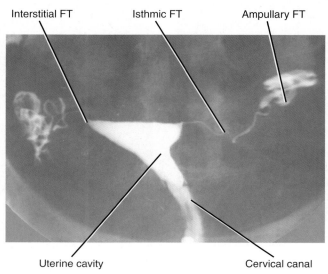

Interstitial FT   Isthmic FT   Ampullary FT

Uterine cavity   Cervical canal

Figure 21-16 Image from a hysterosalpingogram (HSG) demonstrating normal anatomy of the female reproductive system. *FT,* Fallopian tube.

Although TVUS is sensitive for detecting endometrial abnormalities, it is often unable to definitively distinguish between benign and malignant processes. Cases of abnormally thickened endometrium should, therefore, be investigated further with sonohysterography, endometrial biopsy, or hysteroscopy. Hysteroscopy is considered by many to be the gold standard for endometrial evaluation, but it is costly and invasive. Current techniques of pipette endometrial biopsy can be performed during an office visit but provide only a small, blind sample of endometrium. This is effective for diffuse abnormalities of the endometrium but is less sensitive for focal abnormalities.

Saline infusion sonohysterography (TVUS with saline infusion) is a minimally invasive procedure that provides a more detailed evaluation of the endometrium. Infusion of saline allows evaluation of the endometrium as a single layer, rather than the opposed layers that comprise the usual EMS. This improves differentiation between focal and diffuse disease, and improves characterization of subendometrial lesions (Fig. 21-17). For the procedure, a speculum is used to visualize the cervical os, which is then cannulated with a small catheter. Catheters in use range from simple pediatric feeding tubes to HSG catheters with retention balloons. The speculum is then withdrawn, and the endovaginal US probe is inserted parallel to the catheter. The endometrial cavity is then filled with sterile saline (usually 5-10 mL). In a study comparing sonohysterographic findings with subsequent hysteroscopy and pathology, the imaging results were found to be congruent with the pathology results in 92.6% of the 122 patients studied.

Pearl: When performing sonohysterography with an HSG catheter, inflate the balloon using saline rather than air to minimize acoustic shadowing. Continued

scanning while deflating the balloon at the end of the examination improves visualization of the lower uterine segment.

■ CHARACTERIZING UTERINE MASSES

Endometrial Masses

Types of Endometrial Masses
The most common causes of abnormal thickening of the EMS include endometrial hyperplasia, endometrial polyps, submucosal fibroids, and endometrial carcinoma.

ENDOMETRIAL HYPERPLASIA
Endometrial hyperplasia is excessive proliferation of the endometrial glands, focal or diffuse, and is thought to result from unopposed estrogen stimulation. Such stimulation is commonly seen in the setting of *tamoxifen* therapy in patients with breast carcinoma. Cellular atypia can be present, in which case the risk for development of endometrial carcinoma is increased. Hyperplasia usually appears as enlargement of the EMS on TVUS or MRI, a nonspecific finding. In some cases, cystic dilatation of the endometrial glands results in anechoic spaces on TVUS (Fig. 21-18). Cystic endometrial hyperplasia is particularly common with tamoxifen use. On MRI, these cystic spaces appear as small foci of increased signal intensity on T2-weighted images, which do not enhance after contrast administration.

ENDOMETRIAL POLYPS
Endometrial polyps can be considered as a more focal form of endometrial hyperplasia. Although they can be multifocal, most are sessile or pedunculated solitary

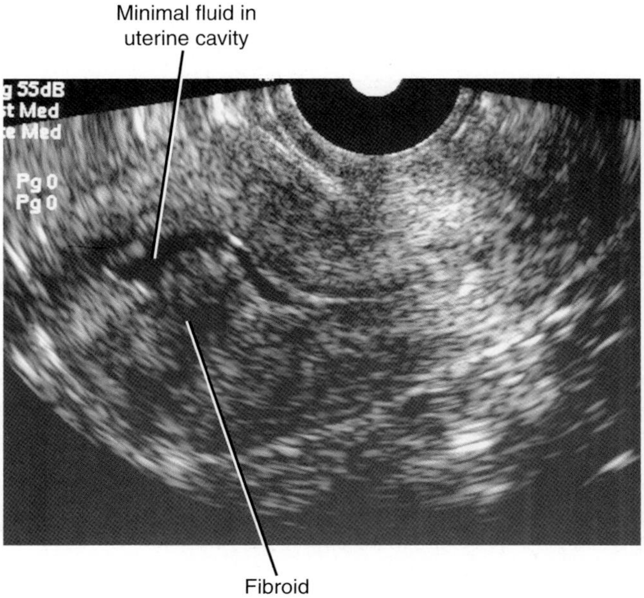

Minimal fluid in uterine cavity

Fibroid

Figure 21-17 Submucosal fibroid characterized by sonohysterography. Sagittal transvaginal ultrasound image of the uterus after saline infusion demonstrates a smooth, spherical mass protruding into the lumen of the endometrial canal. This was found to be nearly pedunculated at hysteroscopic resection.

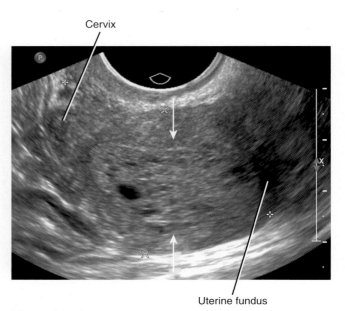

Cervix

Uterine fundus

Figure 21-18 Sagittal midline transvaginal ultrasound image of a retroverted uterus in a patient receiving tamoxifen. The endometrial stripe (between *arrows*) is enlarged (19 mm) with small areas of cystic change. Biopsy confirmed benign endometrial hyperplasia.

lesions. Polyps typically appear as diffuse or focal echogenic thickening of the endometrium on TVUS, and most occur in the uterine fundus and cornua (Fig. 21-19). Polyps tend to be nearly isoechoic to endometrium and can have a frondlike appearance on sonohysterography. When fluid is present in the endometrial canal, the margins of the polyp might be defined and a stalk identified in some cases.

The MR signal characteristics of polyps are variable. Polyps are often hypointense relative to the adjacent endometrium on T2-weighted images but can be isointense (Fig. 21-20). Both solid and cystic components are often visible. Polyps demonstrate variable enhancement on postcontrast images, often enhancing more than adjacent endometrium on early dynamic images but less than the endometrium on delayed images. Although only occasionally visible on MRI, identification of a stalk strongly suggests the diagnosis. Whereas subtle discriminators may allow differentiation of polyps from endometrial cancer in some cases (fibrous core, intratumoral cysts, endometrial cysts, and lack of muscular invasion), overlap is present in the appearances of benign polyps and early endometrial carcinoma.

SUBMUCOSAL FIBROIDS

Submucosal fibroids are a common cause of AUB. In some cases, a large fibroid is predominantly myometrial, with only a small submucosal component. In others, a

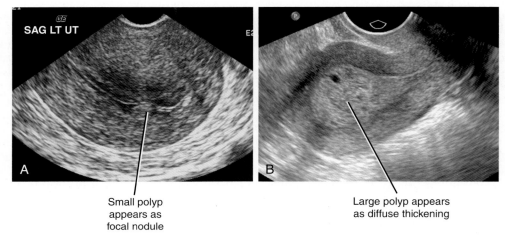

Small polyp appears as focal nodule

Large polyp appears as diffuse thickening

Figure 21-19 Transvaginal ultrasound appearance of benign endometrial polyps in two different patients. **A,** Sagittal image of a retroverted uterus demonstrates a rounded area of focal thickening of the endometrial stripe (EMS). **B,** Sagittal image demonstrates diffuse thickening of the EMS with a small cystic area. No features distinguish this from hyperplasia or endometrial carcinoma.

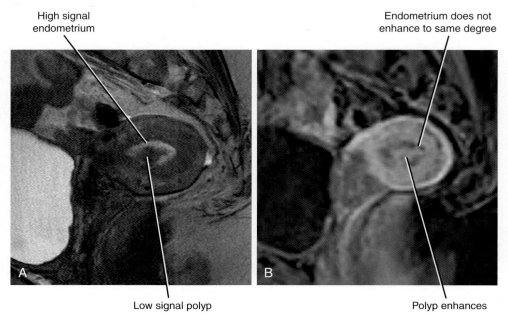

High signal endometrium

Endometrium does not enhance to same degree

Low signal polyp

Polyp enhances

Figure 21-20 Endometrial polyp on magnetic resonance imaging. **A,** Sagittal T2-weighted image demonstrates a focal lesion within the endometrial canal that has a signal lower than the adjacent endometrium. **B,** Sagittal early postcontrast T1-weighted image demonstrates enhancement within the lesion.

pedunculated submucosal fibroid mimics the appearance of an endometrial polyp. In such cases, US or MR aids in the diagnosis.

On TVUS, submucosal fibroids usually appear as a spherical hypoechoic mass that distorts the EMS (Fig. 21-21). Acoustic shadowing is common but not always present. MRI demonstrates similar distortion of the endometrial canal (Fig. 21-22). Fibroids usually have decreased signal intensity compared with polyps on T2-weighted images.

ENDOMETRIAL CARCINOMA

Endometrial cancer is the most common invasive gynecologic malignancy in the United States, with a peak incidence in the sixth and seventh decades. Risk is increased in women treated with tamoxifen. Adenocarcinoma accounts for 60% of endometrial carcinoma. Other types include adenosquamous, clear cell, and a spectrum of sarcomatous tumors. Thickening of the EMS is the most common imaging finding, but in many cases, cancer cannot be distinguished from benign causes of EMS thickening. For this reason, endometrial biopsy is typically performed for unexplained endometrial thickening.

Staging Endometrial Carcinoma

Endometrial carcinoma staging is performed according to surgical and pathologic criteria defined by the International Federation of Gynecology and Obstetrics *(FIGO)*. Corresponding TNM staging corresponds to FIGO criteria. Tables 10-8 and 10-9 outline both staging systems. In most centers, hysterectomy is performed in all cases of endometrial carcinoma, unless there is evidence of advanced metastatic disease. Pretreatment imaging has played little role. Recently, considerable literature has demonstrated accuracy of pretreatment imaging with MRI, and this has become more common in large cancer centers.

Endometrium   Fibroid

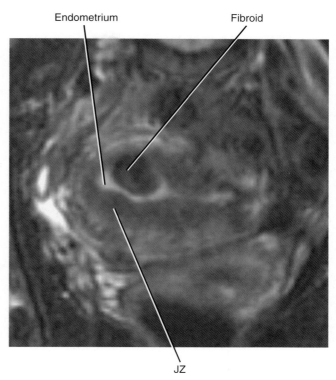

JZ

Figure 21-22 Submucosal fibroid on magnetic resonance imaging. T2-weighted imaging acquired axial to the uterine fundus demonstrates an oval-shaped, smooth, low-signal-intensity mass protruding into the high-signal-intensity endometrial canal. Signal intensity in the mass is even lower than in the adjacent junctional zone *(JZ)*.

Two key points should be kept in mind regarding the role of imaging in staging endometrial carcinoma once a diagnosis is made. First, identification of myometrial involvement is important, because there is increasing use of minimally invasive approaches in women who wish to maintain fertility or who are poor surgical candidates. Second, precise delineation of the depth of myometrial invasion is paramount, because superficial myometrial invasion *(<50%, stage IB)* is treated with simple hysterectomy, whereas deep invasion *(>50%, stage IC)* also requires lymphadenectomy because of an increased incidence of nodal metastases.

At many centers in the United States, MRI is the preferred imaging modality for preoperative staging of endometrial carcinoma. Stage IA disease (confined to the endometrium) can be suggested when an endometrial mass fails to extend into the junctional zone on T2-weighted images (Fig. 21-23) or the zone of subendometrial enhancement on dynamic contrast-enhanced T1-weighted images (helpful in postmenopausal women with poor zonal anatomy on T2-weighted images).

Interruption of the normally dark continuous junctional zone by higher signal intensity tumor is considered a sign of myometrial invasion (Fig. 21-24). Determining the depth of myometrial invasion (greater or less than 50%) is best achieved with images obtained axial and/or sagittal with respect to the uterus (Fig. 21-25). T1-weighted imaging after administration of gadolinium chelates is complementary and perhaps most useful when the junctional zone is indistinct. Endometrial

EMS

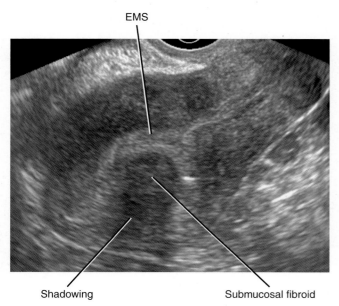

Shadowing   Submucosal fibroid

Figure 21-21 Submucosal fibroid on transvaginal ultrasound. Sagittal image of the uterus demonstrates a spherical hypoechoic mass that distorts the endometrial stripe *(EMS)*. Acoustic shadowing is more common with fibroids than with other endometrial masses.

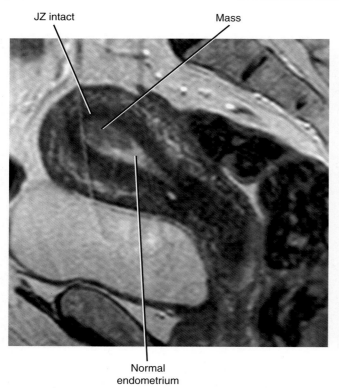

JZ intact   Mass

Normal
endometrium

Figure 21-23 Stage IA endometrial carcinoma on magnetic resonance imaging. Sagittal T2-weighted image of the uterus demonstrates a low-signal-intensity mass with irregular margins within the high-signal endometrial canal. The junctional zone (*JZ*) is intact in this premenopausal patient.

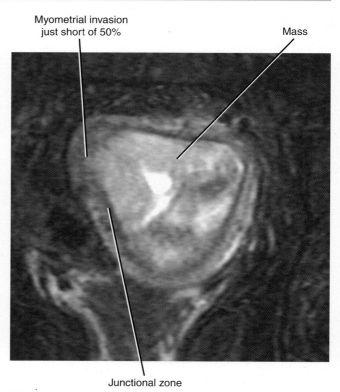

Myometrial invasion
just short of 50%   Mass

Junctional zone

Figure 21-24 Findings of stage IB endometrial carcinoma on magnetic resonance imaging. Coronal T2-weighted imaging of the uterus demonstrates a heterogeneous signal mass replacing most of the endometrial canal. A segment of the junctional zone is interrupted with invasion of just less than 50% thickness of the myometrium.

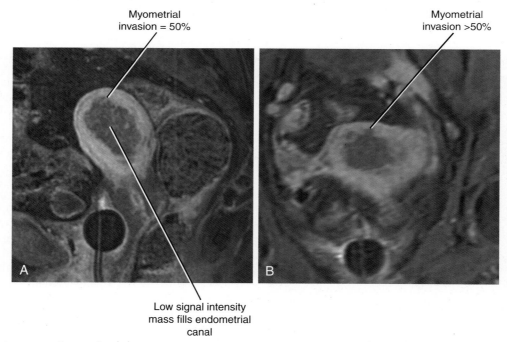

Myometrial
invasion = 50%   Myometrial
invasion >50%

Low signal intensity
mass fills endometrial
canal

Figure 21-25 Stage IC endometrial carcinoma on magnetic resonance imaging. Because the junctional zone was indistinct in this postmenopausal woman, postcontrast T1-weighted imaging was the key to staging. **A,** Sagittal postcontrast image demonstrates poorly enhancing endometrial mass invading the myometrium by approximately 50%. **B,** Postcontrast image axial to uterine fundus identifies invasion exceeding 50%. In view of this finding, lymph node dissection is indicated. (Courtesy Chad Rabinowitz, MD.)

carcinoma typically enhances in a delayed manner relative to myometrium (similar to normal endometrial enhancement). Therefore, invasive endometrial carcinoma will appear hypointense relative to the enhancing myometrium (see Fig. 21-25). Factors that may confound evaluation of myometrial invasion by MRI include an abnormal junctional zone caused by adenomyosis, distortion of the endometrial canal and myometrium because of fibroids, and thinning of the uterine wall because of large tumors.

> *Pearl: Interruption of the junctional zone by tumor signal is a sign of myometrial invasion. Interruption of the zone of subendometrial enhancement on early dynamic contrast-enhanced MR images has the same significance and is of particular value when the junctional zone is indistinct.*

When tumor extends into the cervix, stage II disease is diagnosed. Extension beyond the uterus denotes stage III disease if contained in the true pelvis (Fig. 21-26), and stage IV disease if extending beyond the true pelvis or invading the bladder or rectum.

CT is useful for identifying nodal disease and signs of local spread in the pelvis. It is also useful to survey large anatomic areas for metastatic disease. CT is not accurate for determining depth of myometrial invasion and is less accurate than high-quality MRI for identifying subtle signs of bladder or rectal invasion.

Myometrial Masses

Fibroids

The most common lesion found within the uterus is the leiomyoma, or fibroid, which is a benign neoplasm composed of smooth muscle cells. Fibroids (easier than saying "leiomyomata") occur in greater than 25% of women older than 35 years and are classified according to their location (Fig. 21-27). Classification is helpful in determining whether a given fibroid is likely to account for the patient's symptoms and what type of therapy (if any) may be appropriate.

Intramural fibroids are the most common type of fibroids and are contained within myometrium. Because they do not affect the endometrium or serosa, they are the least likely to cause symptoms. If a portion of a fibroid protrudes into the endometrial canal, it is considered a *submucosal fibroid*. AUB and infertility (including a history of spontaneous abortions) are the most common symptoms associated with submucosal fibroids. In some cases, submucosal fibroids become pedunculated within the endometrial canal and can even pass into the endocervical canal or vagina.

When a fibroid displaces the uterine serosa outward, it is considered to be *subserosal*. The appearance of subserosal fibroids ranges from a bulge in the uterine contour to an entirely *pedunculated* mass that can mimic an adnexal tumor (Fig. 21-28). Fibroids can also be found within the broad ligament, appearing completely detached from the uterus. Visualizing the connection of the mass to the uterus helps differentiate a pedunculated subserosal fibroid from an ovarian mass. Fibroids arise from the uterus and, therefore, are typically supplied by branches of the uterine artery. The *bridging vascular sign* refers to visualization of a vascular pedicle extending from the uterus to the fibroid on US or MR images. Ovarian tumors are typically supplied and drained by the ovarian vessels, although ovarian artery supply is occasionally seen with fibroids.

Fibroids vary in sonographic appearance. Most fibroids are heterogenous but predominately hypoechoic

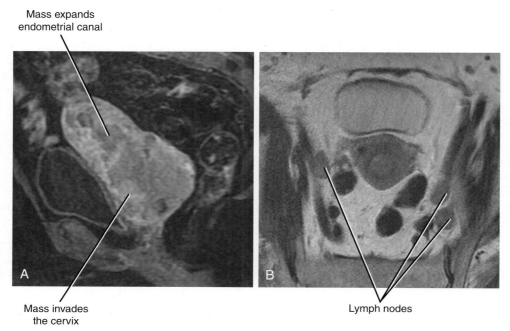

Mass expands
endometrial canal

Mass invades
the cervix

Lymph nodes

Figure 21-26 Stage IIIC endometrial carcinoma on magnetic resonance imaging. **A,** Sagittal postcontrast T1-weighted imaging demonstrates expansion of the endometrial canal with extensive invasion of the cervix (mimics cervical cancer). **B,** Axial T2-weighted imaging with small field of view identifies enlarged lymph nodes in the pelvis, increasing the stage from IIB to IIIC.

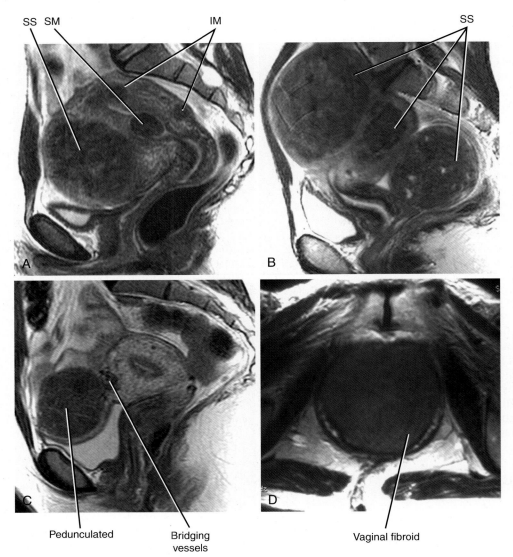

SS SM IM SS

Pedunculated   Bridging vessels   Vaginal fibroid

Figure 21-27 Classifying fibroids according to location on T2-weighted magnetic resonance images. **A,** Sagittal image demonstrates submucosal (SM), subserosal (SS), and intramural (IM) fibroids. **B,** Sagittal image with multiple subserosal fibroids. **C,** Sagittal image demonstrates a pedunculated subserosal fibroid with bridging vascular sign. **D,** Axial image of perineum demonstrates a vaginal fibroid.

in appearance. Acoustic shadowing is common. Often, a discrete mass is difficult to define, and distortion of the uterine contour with posterior shadowing is the clue to the presence of fibroids. Small, diffuse tumors can cause the uterus to appear enlarged and heterogeneous. When present, calcifications can be seen as echogenic foci or a hyperechoic peripheral rim. Cystic spaces can be seen with necrosis.

With MRI, smaller solitary fibroids are usually well-defined and demonstrate characteristically low signal on T2-weighted images compared with the myometrium. A peripheral halo of increased T2 signal has also been described and attributed to perilesional edema, dilated veins, or dilated lymphatics. Fibroids are often cellular, enhancing as much as the myometrium on CT or MRI (Fig. 21-29).

As fibroids grow larger than 3 to 5 cm, they commonly undergo *degeneration* and necrosis as they outgrow their blood supply. Areas of hemorrhage (bright on T1-weighted MR images), cystic change (nonenhancing bright areas on T2-weighted MR images or decreased echogenicity on US), or hyalinization (also bright on

T2-weighted MR images) are commonly present in large fibroids (Fig. 21-30). Characterizing the type of degeneration is not usually important except in the case of acute hemorrhage. Fat can rarely be present in a uterine fibroid (lipoleiomyoma). Sarcomas of the uterine wall are quite rare and cannot be reliably distinguished from benign fibroids unless invasion of adjacent organs is present.

Although histologically benign, uterine fibroids are not clinically insignificant. Aside from uterine bleeding and abdominal discomfort, fibroids can cause a host of other problems. Multiple fibroids can be associated with an increased risk for pregnancy loss. A lower uterine or cervical fibroid can narrow the pelvic outlet, complicating attempts at vaginal delivery. This is compounded by the fact that many (but not all) fibroids increase in size during pregnancy. Pedunculated fibroids can undergo torsion, resulting in severe pain.

When interpreting imaging examinations performed specifically to evaluate fibroids for potential uterine artery embolization, it is important to mention fibroid location and blood supply. Subserosal fibroids are more

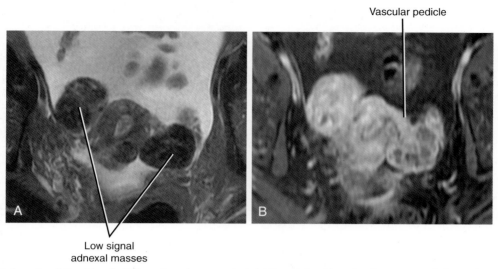

Figure 21-28 Pedunculated fibroids mimicking adnexal masses. **A,** Axial T2-weighted imaging demonstrates bilateral low-signal masses in both adnexal regions. Notice an intermediate-signal stalk connecting the left mass to the uterus. **B,** Axial fat-suppressed T1-weighted imaging demonstrates enhancement within both lesions. An enhancing stalk extends from the uterus to the left mass (vascular pedicle) consistent with an exophytic fibroid.

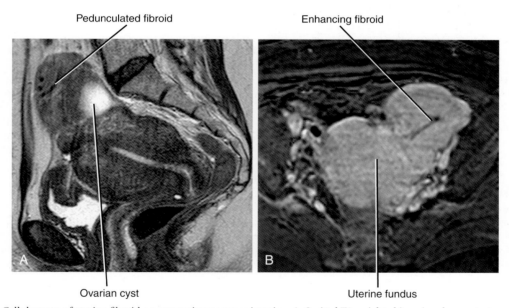

Figure 21-29 Cellular type of uterine fibroid on magnetic resonance imaging. **A,** Sagittal T2-weighted imaging demonstrates an exophytic mass from the uterine fundus that has similar signal intensity to the myometrium. An area of high signal is due to an adjacent ovarian cyst. **B,** Axial postcontrast T1-weighted imaging demonstrates diffuse enhancement of the mass. This was removed and proved to be a benign leiomyoma.

likely to parasitize regional nonuterine blood flow, rendering them less susceptible to embolization. Likewise, fibroids with significant ovarian artery supply are unlikely to respond to embolization of the uterine artery alone. Submucosal fibroids can slough into the endometrial canal after embolization, whereas treated subserosal fibroids can detach from the uterus and become free within the peritoneal cavity.

A potential mimic of the fibroid is a *myometrial contraction,* also referred to as uterine peristalsis. Although most commonly seen in the gravid uterus with grayscale sonography, contractions are occasionally imaged in the nongravid uterus with MRI, particularly in the week before menstruation. They appear as transient low-signal-intensity distortions of the myometrium on T2-weighted MR images. The contraction distorts the underlying endometrium but not the external contour. The main distinguishing feature separating uterine peristalsis from leiomyoma is the transient nature of the entity. Adenomyosis is another potential mimic of uterine fibroids and is discussed in the following section.

Adenomyosis

Adenomyosis is a condition in which ectopic endometrial glands and stroma are embedded within the myometrium. Women usually present with dysmenorrhea,

Cystic degeneration   Large fibroid   Endometrial stripe is faintly seen

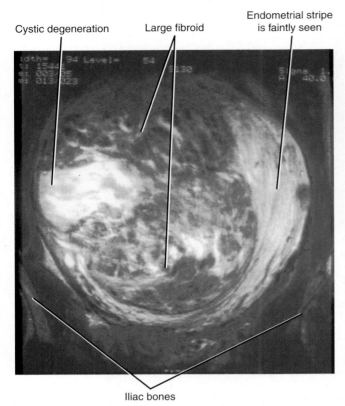

Iliac bones

Figure 21-30 Coronal T2-weighted magnetic resonance image of the pelvis demonstrates a 20-cm heterogeneous mass arising from the wall of the uterus. Areas of high signal are consistent with cystic degeneration. This was removed out of concern that it could be a sarcoma, but no malignant tissue was found.

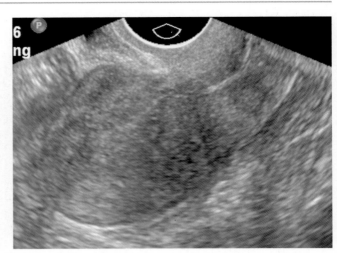

Figure 21-31 Adenomyosis on transvaginal ultrasound (US) performed for pain and abnormal bleeding. Sagittal image of the uterus demonstrates heterogeneous echotexture within the fundus without distinct mass. A diagnosis of adenomyosis was suggested based on the US findings and confirmed after hysterectomy performed to treat intractable symptoms.

menorrhagia, or both. A spectrum of tissue distribution, ranging from focal areas to diffuse uterine infiltration, is present.

On US, adenomyosis appears as heterogeneous uterine enlargement (Fig. 21-31). Additional sonographic findings have been reported, including tiny cysts adjacent to the endometrium and linear echogenic striations extending from the endometrium to the myometrium.

Adenomyosis can be diagnosed definitively on T2-weighted MR images as focal or diffuse widening of the junctional zone. The junctional zone is considered definitely widened if 12 mm or more in thickness (Fig. 21-32). A junctional zone of 8 mm or less is considered normal. A thickness of 9 to 11 mm is indeterminate, in which case ancillary findings are important, including poorly defined margins of the junctional zone, high-signal foci on T1- or T2-weighted sequences, and linear hyperintense striations radiating from the endometrium into the myometrium on T2-weighted images. The high-signal foci have been variously explained as ectopic endometrium, cystically dilated endometrial glands, and areas of hemorrhage.

Adenomyoma is a term used to describe focal adenomyosis, an entity that can be confused with a leiomyoma. Both entities demonstrate decreased signal intensity on T2-weighted sequences. Features that favor adenomyoma over leiomyoma include ill-defined margins, elliptical

shape with orientation along the endometrium, and the ancillary findings discussed earlier. In addition, adenomyosis typically does not distort the serosal or endometrial contours of the uterus. Rarely, adenomyoma can be polypoid or predominately cystic, potentially creating confusion with other entities.

Adenomyosis is occasionally seen on HSG performed in evaluation of infertility. Small, discrete, contrast-filled outpouchings seen extending from the endometrial cavity are diagnostic (Fig. 21-33).

Uterine Lymphoma

Lymphoma is an unusual cause of uterine enlargement. In most cases, uterine involvement is part of widespread disease, although primary lymphoma of the uterine fundus and uterine cervix can rarely occur. Whether primary or secondary, the most common imaging finding is diffuse uterine enlargement, evident on any cross-sectional imaging modality. Because the disease usually infiltrates the myometrium, the endometrium usually appears normal, allowing differentiation from endometrial carcinoma. With MRI, diffuse enlargement of the myometrium with an intact junctional zone and normal endometrium is characteristic.

Cervical Masses

The external cervical os can be visualized directly during physical examination. However, masses entirely within the endocervical canal or within the muscular wall of the cervix can be missed by examination. Therefore, imaging plays a limited, but nonetheless important role in evaluating the cervix. Fortunately, the differential diagnosis of cervical masses is relatively short, and many cervical abnormalities have distinctive imaging characteristics (Table 21-2).

Focus of high signal

Focal adenomyosis

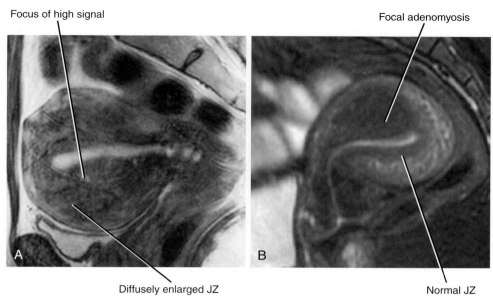

A

B

Diffusely enlarged JZ

Normal JZ

Figure 21-32 Adenomyosis on magnetic resonance imaging. **A,** Sagittal T2-weighted imaging demonstrates diffuse thickening of the junctional zone (JZ). When thickening is this severe, it may be mistaken for abnormal myometrial signal. **B,** Sagittal T2-weighted imaging of a retroflexed uterus demonstrates focal thickening of the JZ in the anterior fundus.

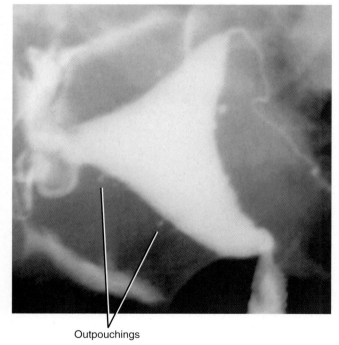

Outpouchings

Figure 21-33 Appearance of adenomyosis on hysterosalpingography (HSG). Small outpouchings from the endometrial cavity are a characteristic finding in adenomyosis.

Nabothian Cysts

Nabothian cysts are retention cysts of the cervical mucosa and are the most common mass of the uterine cervix. They are more common in multiparous women, and are readily identified on TVUS and MRI (Fig. 21-34). They are typically superficial but can be located deep within the muscular wall on occasion. TVUS reveals

internal debris caused by hemorrhage in some cases, although most have the appearance of a simple cyst. On T2-weighted sequences, they appear as hyperintense lesions within the normally hypointense FMS of the cervix. Intermediate to slightly high signal intensity can be seen on T1-weighted images, depending on the content of mucin or blood products. No enhancement should be present on postcontrast imaging.

Occasionally, a variant consisting of complex multicystic dilation of the endocervical glands can occur, known as a *tunnel cluster.* Although this conglomerate of small cystic glands is a benign entity, its imaging appearance can overlap that of a rare malignant lesion known as *adenoma malignum,* which is a subtype of mucinous adenocarcinoma associated with watery vaginal discharge. In this case, the presence of any interposed solid components, particularly those showing enhancement, would favor a diagnosis of adenoma malignum rather than tunnel cluster.

Cervical Fibroid

Fibroids are much more common in the uterine corpus but do occur in the cervix. As in the myometrium, they typically demonstrate low signal intensity on T2-weighted MR images. Various types of degeneration can occur, resulting in highly variable signal characteristics that can potentially mimic carcinoma. Most cervical fibroids arise within the wall of the cervix. Rarely, a pedunculated submucosal fibroid of the uterine corpus prolapses into the endocervical canal or vagina (Fig. 21-35).

Cervical Cancer

Cervical carcinoma is the third most common gynecologic malignancy and a major cause of mortality and morbidity among women worldwide. It is associated with human papilloma virus infection. A vaccine is now

Table 21-2   Cervical Masses

Diagnosis	Discriminators
Nabothian cysts	Small, simple cysts along endocervical canal on US or MR May have internal debris on transvaginal US MR: bright on T2WI, variable on T1WI No enhancement with contrast or flow on color Doppler
Cervical carcinoma	Soft-tissue mass expands endocervical canal Enhances with intravenous contrast on CT or MR May extend superiorly into uterine fundus or to adjacent organs Can be associated with adenopathy
Adenoma malignum	Extremely rare complex cystic lesion May have solid components Associated with Peutz–Jeghers syndrome in some patients (hamartomatous polyps, skin lesions) Associated with mucinous ovarian tumors
Cervical fibroid	Can arise primarily in wall of cervix or prolapse into cervix/vagina from uterine corpus Usually low signal on T2WI, but degeneration causes variable signal in larger fibroids
Cervical polyp	Mass within endocervical canal (looks like stage I cancer) May protrude into the vagina on imaging or physical examination
Cervical pregnancy	Serum β-hCG positive Gestational sac within cervical canal Decidual reaction thickens endometrial stripe Fetal cardiac activity
Lymphoma	Usually one component of widespread disease Rarely occurs as primary cervical lymphoma Infiltrative appearance of the wall, sparing the mucosa

β-hCG, β-Human chorionic gonadotropin; *CT*, computed tomography; *MR*, magnetic resonance; *T2WI*, T2-weighted imaging; *US*, ultrasound.

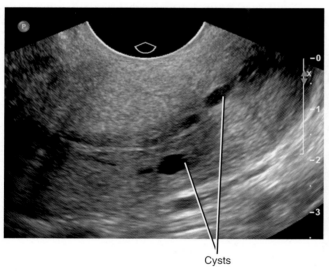

Cysts

Figure 21-34 Sagittal transvaginal ultrasound image of an anteverted uterus demonstrates several small nabothian cysts within the cervix.

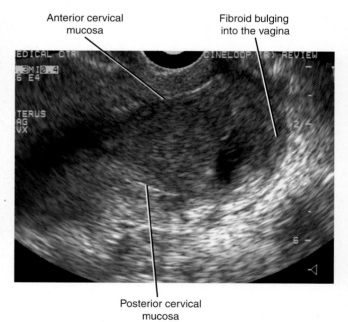

Anterior cervical mucosa

Fibroid bulging into the vagina

Posterior cervical mucosa

Figure 21-35 Cervical fibroid. Sagittal transvaginal ultrasound image of the cervix demonstrates a cone-shaped mass widening the endocervical canal. This was removed and found to be a pedunculated submucosal fibroid passing through the cervix into the vagina.

available that may eventually decrease incidence of the disease. Early disease is usually asymptomatic. More advanced disease results in vaginal bleeding and a palpable mass. Widespread screening with the Pap smear has decreased the percentage of cervical carcinomas in the invasive stages at presentation.

When cervical cancer is seen by TVUS, it usually appears as a soft-tissue mass expanding the endocervical canal (Fig. 21-36). US can also be used to define the extent of involvement or obstruction of the uterine fundus,

or both. Although some centers use US to characterize depth of involvement and local spread of disease, it is used less commonly for staging than CT and MRI.

When cervical carcinoma is visible on CT, it is usually a large soft-tissue mass. Hematometros (blood within a

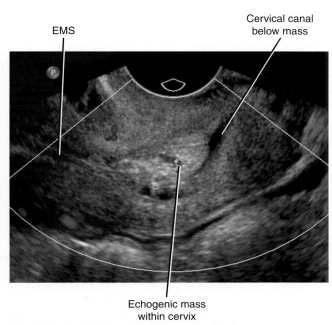

Figure 21-36 Sagittal transvaginal ultrasound image of the cervix and lower uterine segment demonstrates a soft-tissue mass within the endocervical canal. This cervical cancer was not visible on speculum examination. *EMS*, endometrial stripe.

the mass itself and is unable to accurately define depth of invasion within the cervix with low stage disease.

The sensitivity of MRI for detecting parametrial invasion is advantageous to making patient management decisions. The most important transition in staging is distinguishing early disease (stages I and IIA) from advanced disease (stage IIB and higher). When a tumor breaches the FMS and extends into the parametrium, it reaches at least stage IIB status, and optimal management changes from surgical resection to radiation alone or combined with chemotherapy. Extension to the lower one third of the vagina (stage IIIA) or pelvic sidewall (stage IIIB), or invasion of adjacent organs (stage IV) such as the bladder or rectal mucosa renders the tumor nonoperable (Fig. 21-38).

Cervical carcinoma is usually hyperintense on T2-weighted images, which provides high lesion conspicuity in comparison with the low-signal-intensity FMS. On dynamic contrast-enhanced MRI, smaller tumors enhance homogenously and earlier than normal cervical stroma. Large tumors are often necrotic and have variable degrees of central enhancement, but usually have an enhancing rim. Perhaps the most important finding on T2-weighted images is the preservation of an intact hypointense stromal ring, which has been shown to be highly accurate in excluding parametrial extension, particularly in the case of small tumors. With larger tumors, however, edema altering signal of the

dilated endometrial cavity) is more commonly seen than the mass itself on CT (Fig. 21-37). CT is commonly used for staging extracervical disease. CT can identify nodal disease, distant metastases, as well as severe cases of extension into adjacent organs (see Table 10-10 for staging). Urinary obstruction, when present, indicates disease involving the ureter at the pelvic sidewall (stage IIIb). However, CT allows only limited visualization of

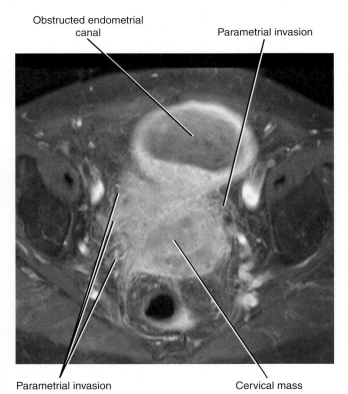

Figure 21-38 Cervical cancer with parametrial invasion on magnetic resonance imaging. Axial T1-weighted imaging with fat suppression after contrast administration demonstrates a cervical mass with a dilated endometrial canal. Soft tissue with indistinct margins extends into the parametrial tissues, reaching the pelvic sidewall on the right side, consistent with stage IIIB disease.

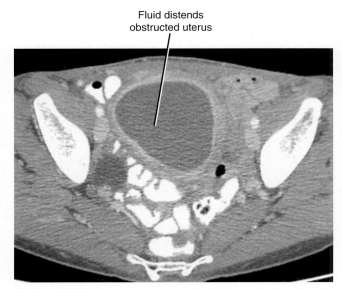

Figure 21-37 Computed tomographic (CT) presentation of cervical carcinoma. Axial CT image of the pelvis demonstrates hematometros caused by malignant obstruction of the endocervical canal. This appearance is found more often by CT than is the cervical mass itself.

ring can lead to false-positive results; therefore, caution must be used and tumor morphology must be taken into consideration.

Parametrial spread is also suggested by visualization of an irregular peripheral margin or abutment and/or encasement of periuterine vessels. In the case of a lesion involving the upper one third of the vagina, disruption of the vaginal wall indicates parametrial extension. Vaginal involvement is diagnosed by observing disruption of the normally low signal wall of the H-shaped vagina on T2-weighted images. Hydronephrosis, pelvic sidewall involvement, or both are considered stage IIIB disease. Local findings suggestive of pelvic sidewall involvement include tumor within 3 mm of or abutting the obturator internus, levator ani, and pyriformis muscles, as well as the iliac vessels. Loss of parametrial signal and increased pelvic muscular signal have also been described on T2-weighted images in stage IIIB disease.

MRI has been shown to be helpful in the assessment of bladder invasion (stage IV). Criteria used for bladder invasive disease include focal obliteration of the normally hypointense bladder wall on T2-weighted images and distinct nodular masses extending into the bladder lumen. Preservation of the hypointense bladder wall and intervening perivesicle fat exclude bladder involvement. Rectal involvement presents as segmental thickening and disruption of the anterior rectal wall.

■ CHARACTERIZING ADNEXAL MASSES

The differential diagnosis for adnexal masses is long and varied. A methodical approach helps the radiologist to narrow the differential diagnosis in most cases. The majority of adnexal masses can be characterized effectively by asking the following questions:

1. Does it arise from the ovary?
2. What does it consist of?
3. If it does not come from the ovary, where does it come from?

Does It Arise from the Ovary?

The differential diagnosis for an adnexal lesion depends on its structure of origin; that is, is it ovarian or extraovarian? Begin by identifying both ovaries if possible; the presence of two separate normal ovaries excludes a mass of ovarian origin. If the ovaries are not immediately apparent, it is often useful to follow the round ligament away from the tapered cornual region of the uterus because this often points toward the ovary on US, CT, and MRI. Some advocate identifying the suspensory ligament of the ovary near the common or external iliac vessels and tracing it medially to the ovary, although it is often difficult to find. If ovarian follicles are not visible, or if an abnormality is so large as to distort normal anatomy, tracing the ovarian veins from the inferior vena cava (right) or left renal vein (left) down into the pelvis is often effective.

Pearl: *Following the gonadal vessels from the inferior vena cava (right side) or left renal vein (left side) is helpful in finding atrophic ovaries or determining whether a large mass arises from the ovary.*

As with other organs, the *claw sign* is useful in determining whether a mass originates from the ovary or the uterus (Fig. 21-39). Pedunculated lesions from the uterus (usually a fibroid) should have a vascular pedicle extending from the uterus to the mass that can usually be found with imaging. This can be identified on US by finding an imaging plane that includes *vascular bridging* between the uterus and the mass (Fig. 21-40). On MRI, demonstration

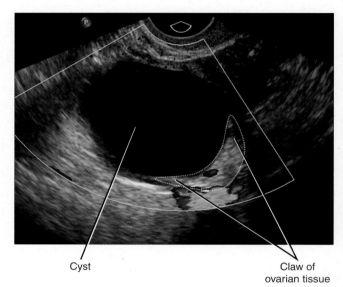

Cyst   Claw of
                                        ovarian tissue

Figure 21-39 Transvaginal ultrasound of the pelvis demonstrates a simple cyst within the right adnexal region. A "claw" of ovarian parenchyma around the cyst (outlined) indicates this is an ovarian rather than paraovarian cyst.

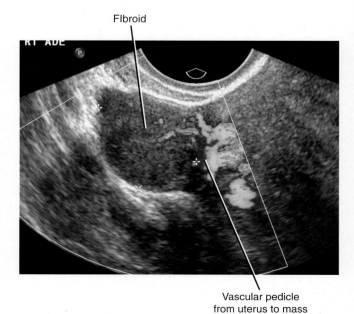

Fibroid

Vascular pedicle
from uterus to mass

Figure 21-40 Vascular pedicle from uterus to pedunculated fibroid identified by transvaginal ultrasound using power Doppler.

of the vascular pedicle is facilitated by prescribing an imaging plane between the mass and the adjacent uterine cornu, a task that requires radiologist participation or a technologist with considerable experience in performing pelvic MRI (or luck!) (see Fig. 21-27C).

A history of bilateral oophorectomy does not necessarily exclude a mass of ovarian origin. Occasionally, a portion of the ovary is inadvertently left behind during oophorectomy. This tends to occur in the setting of prior pelvic inflammation, resulting in adhesions. The residual ovarian tissue can continue to function and result in a complex cystic mass that can become symptomatic (*ovarian remnant syndrome*).

What Does It Consist of?

Ovarian lesions are first characterized by their composition. The simplest approach categorizes lesions as predominantly cystic or predominantly solid. This provides a useful framework for further refinement of the differential diagnosis.

Predominantly Cystic Ovarian Lesions

SIMPLE FLUID (UNILOCULAR CYSTS)

Simple-appearing unilocular cysts lack septa and mural nodularity, lack enhancing features (CT and MRI) or internal flow with color Doppler, and are anechoic (US), low attenuation (CT), or follow the signal intensity of simple fluid on MR. Unilocular cysts can be normal or worrisome, depending on size and patient age. For simple cysts less than 2.5 cm in diameter in premenopausal women, many prefer the term *follicle* and consider this to be a normal finding that requires no follow-up. Others use 3.0 cm as a threshold for follow-up. Simple-appearing unilocular cysts smaller than 5 cm in premenopausal women usually represent functional cysts and are followed conservatively. Unilocular cysts 5 to 10 cm are also usually benign but cannot be distinguished from neoplastic cysts such as serous cystadenoma. Although some advocate removal of all cysts larger than 5 cm, many centers now opt for follow-up sonography performed in approximately 6 weeks. An increase in size raises suspicion for neoplasm and usually prompts surgical excision. Cysts larger than 10 cm should be considered neoplastic in any adult age group.

In postmenopausal women, simple asymptomatic unilocular cysts up to 5 cm can be followed with US. If 5 cm or greater, or if symptomatic, a significant risk for neoplasia exists necessitating more aggressive gynecologic evaluation. Increased CA-125 levels also increase clinical concern for malignancy in postmenopausal patients with unilocular cystic lesions. Increased CA-125 in the serum is less specific in premenopausal women.

CYSTIC AND SOLID TISSUE

In the evaluation of predominantly cystic lesions that are not unilocular, suspicion for malignancy should increase as the number of complicating features increases (Fig. 21-41). Note that these morphologic features can be well demonstrated on US, CT, or MRI. Features suggesting malignancy are included in Box 21-1. Applying these criteria to MRI, Hricak and

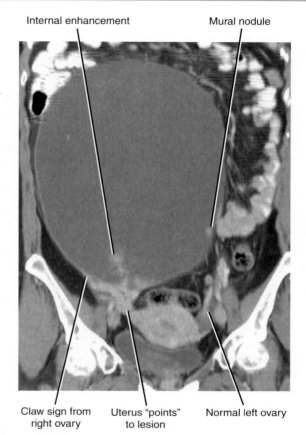

Internal enhancement   Mural nodule

Claw sign from   Uterus "points"   Normal left ovary
right ovary   to lesion

Figure 21-41 Coronal reformation from contrast-enhanced computed tomography demonstrates a large cystic mass (ovarian carcinoma) arising from the right ovary (a relation that was less clear on axial images). An area of solid enhancing tissue within this large but otherwise simple-appearing cystic lesion is present.

BOX 21-1   Imaging Features That Suggest Ovarian Malignancy

Primary Features

A solid mass or large solid component

Wall thickness greater than 3 mm

Septal thickness greater than 3 mm and/or vegetations or nodularity

Necrosis

Size larger than 5 cm*

Secondary Features

Involvement of pelvic organs or the side wall

Peritoneal, mesenteric, or omental disease

Ascites

Lymphadenopathy

*Hricak and colleagues used a size of larger than 4 cm as a primary feature of malignancy, although many authors advocate increased suspicion with cystic lesions greater than 5 cm, and some studies advocate a cutoff as high as 10 cm. Most cystic ovarian carcinomas are larger than 7.5 cm at time of diagnosis.

colleagues noted an accuracy rate of 93% in the diagnosis of ovarian malignancy when either two primary or one primary and one secondary feature was present. The features presented in Box 21-1 are not specific for primary ovarian neoplasms and can be seen in metastatic lesions.

Some investigators have advocated the use of the pulsatility index (PI) and resistive index (RI) obtained from the ovarian arteries with Doppler US to distinguish between benign and malignant ovarian masses. Although evidence suggests that, in general, the PI and RI are lower in malignant ovarian masses than in benign lesions, significant overlap exists between the two. Furthermore, an established threshold is lacking, and the use of these indices must take into account the phase of the menstrual cycle, because low resistance flow in the ovarian artery is common during the luteal phase. It is recommended, therefore, that ovarian artery Doppler findings be interpreted in the context of lesion morphology and correlated with the phase of the menstrual cycle.

FAT

The presence fat within an adnexal mass almost always indicates that it is a mature cystic teratoma of the ovary, also called a *dermoid cyst*. Note that there are other types of teratomas (immature teratomas and monodermal teratomas such as struma ovarii, which is filled with thyroidal colloid), so use of the full term is preferred. Mature cystic teratomas are benign germ cell tumors and the most common ovarian neoplasm. Mature cystic teratomas are bilateral in 10% to 25% of cases; therefore, finding one should prompt a search for a second lesion. Fat content within a mature cystic teratoma can be identified by US as an echogenic region with shadowing, the so-called iceberg sign (Fig. 21-42). This can be confused with bowel or omental fat, so it is helpful

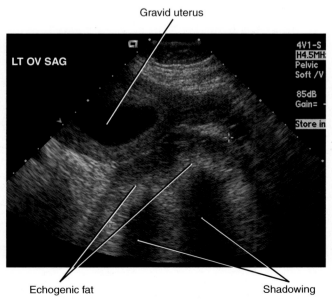

Gravid uterus

LT OV SAG

4V1-S
H4.5MH:
Pelvic
Soft /V

85dB
Gain=

Store in

Echogenic fat

Shadowing

Figure 21-42 Ultrasound appearance of shadowing fat ("iceberg sign") in a proven mature cystic teratoma of the left ovary. This presented as an adnexal mass during the first trimester of pregnancy.

to confirm the diagnosis by CT or MR (Fig. 21-43). On CT, characteristic fat attenuation can be readily identified, often layering with fluid. Nodular calcifications are also common.

With MR, high signal intensity is seen on T1- and T2-weighted images performed without fat suppression. With frequency-selective fat suppression, fat will become dark (Fig. 21-44). Caution should be used with short tau inversion recovery (STIR) sequences, which provide nonfrequency-selective fat suppression, because decreased signal can be seen with both fat (mature cystic teratoma) and blood (endometrioma). Most mature cystic teratomas also show chemical-shift artifact, which can aid in diagnosis when fat-suppressed images are not provided. Laparoscopic removal is usually performed after diagnosis, because these lesions predispose the ovary to undergo torsion.

Pitfall: STIR images can decrease the signal of both fat and blood products. Therefore, frequency-selective fat suppression should be used instead of STIR for the evaluation of adnexal masses.

The amount of fat within mature cystic teratomas varies. Lesions can be nearly entirely fatty or completely devoid of detectible fat. Tiny amounts of fat within a suspected teratoma are often best demonstrated with thin-section CT or chemical-shift MRI.

BLOOD

The presence of blood products within a cystic adnexal mass has less specificity than the presence of fat, but it is still a useful finding. The presence of blood products in the absence of features associated with malignancy usually indicates either *endometrioma* or *hemorrhagic cyst*. Ovarian carcinoma occasionally contains areas of hemorrhagic fluid; therefore, irregular enhancing walls, mural nodules, or thick, enhancing septa are suspicious for malignancy regardless of the fluid composition. With endometriosis, cysts are often multiple and of various shapes and sizes, but intervening septa are thin and uniform. Like dermoid cysts, endometriomas are commonly bilateral.

On US images, hemorrhagic cyst contents often appear as low-level echoes (Fig. 21-45). If the blood is more organized, there may be a lacy or weblike pattern within the cyst. Occasionally, a retracting clot can be seen as an echogenic mass, with absent flow with color Doppler imaging, adherent to the wall. By CT, blood products can produce a sedimentation layer or may appear uniformly dense. Administration of intravenous contrast results in no internal enhancement on CT and MRI.

On MRI, the methoglobin that accumulates within endometriomas because of repeated hemorrhage results in characteristically high signal on T1-weighted images, high signal that persists with frequency-specific fat suppression (Fig. 21-46). Although signal intensity on T2-weighted images is also higher than that of soft tissue, it is lower than that of water, an appearance often described as "T2 shading." To some, the term *shading* refers to the gradation in signal intensity within an endometrioma that can occur because of the gradation in concentration of blood contents from the nondependent to the dependent

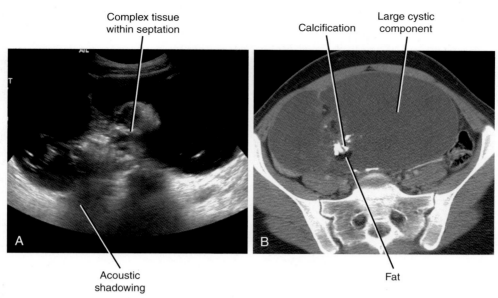

Complex tissue
within septation

Calcification

Large cystic
component

Acoustic
shadowing

Fat

Figure 21-43 Mature cystic teratoma of the ovary demonstrated by ultrasound (US) and computed tomography (CT). **A,** Transverse US image demonstrates a predominantly cystic lesion with complex soft tissue contained within septations. Areas of shadowing could represent fat or calcification. **B,** Transverse CT image of the same patient reveals fat adjacent to coarse calcifications. No enhancement of the soft-tissue components is present. A benign cystic teratoma was removed.

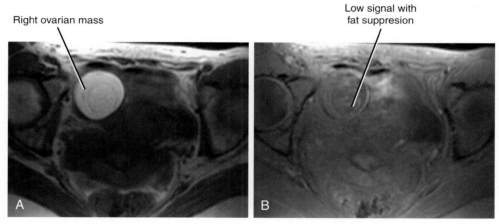

Right ovarian mass

Low signal with
fat suppresion

Figure 21-44 Mature cystic teratoma of the ovary on axial magnetic resonance images. **A,** Axial T1-weighted imaging (T1WI) demonstrates a high-signal-intensity mass in the right ovary. **B,** Axial T1WI with frequency-selective fat suppression demonstrates signal loss within the right ovarian lesion, consistent with fat content.

portion of the lesion. However, this graded appearance is not always present within an endometrioma on T2-weighted images, and we prefer the former definition.

In contrast with endometriomas, the signal within hemorrhagic functional ovarian cysts is more variable on MR, depending on the age of blood products. Because most hemorrhagic functional cysts are imaged in the acute phase, signal is usually low on T1-weighted images but often intermediate on T1-weighted images with frequency-specific fat suppression. When high signal intensity is present on T1-weighted images, it is often seen as a peripheral rim. Signal on T2-weighted images is also variable, although most have heterogeneous signal with at least one focus of high signal.

Hemorrhagic cysts tend to be solitary rather than multicentric, and in contradistinction to endometrial cysts, typically regress within 2 months.

CALCIFICATION
Large, coarse foci of well-defined calcification are common in mature cystic teratomas of the ovary. Notice how many qualifiers were used at the beginning of that sentence? The calcified ectodermal component of a mature cystic teratoma is toothlike and should be large and well-defined (see Fig. 21-43). Beware of fine, indistinct, or powder-like calcifications because they can be found within malignant ovarian neoplasm, as well as in their metastatic deposits in the peritoneal cavity (Fig. 21-47).

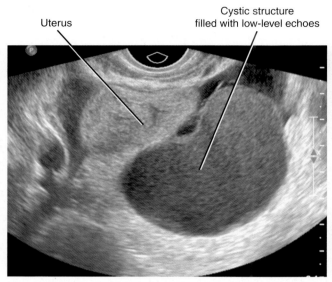

Uterus   Cystic structure filled with low-level echoes

Figure 21-45 Transvaginal ultrasound of the pelvis demonstrates a 7-cm cystic structure in the left adnexa with low-level echoes. There was no flow with color Doppler (not shown). This failed to resolve and pain persisted. An endometrioma was removed surgically.

Pitfall: Although the presence of fat is a reliable sign of a mature cystic teratoma, the presence of calcium is less specific and can also be seen in ovarian cancer.

GAS

Gas is occasionally found with an adnexal mass. This is a reliable sign of infection and is most commonly found within tuboovarian abscess. Gas can also be found within an infected cystic mass such as mature cystic teratoma (Fig. 21-48).

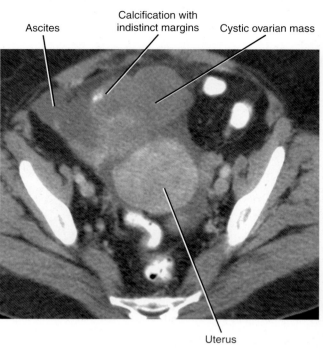

Ascites   Calcification with indistinct margins   Cystic ovarian mass

Uterus

Figure 21-47 Malignant ovarian calcifications. Axial computed tomographic image of the pelvis demonstrates calcification with indistinct margins within a complex right ovarian lesion. Enhancing soft tissue within the lesion and adjacent ascites also support the proven diagnosis of ovarian carcinoma. Compare this appearance with the well-defined ectodermal calcification within the mature cystic teratoma in Figure 21-43.

Predominantly Solid Ovarian Lesions

Predominantly solid ovarian masses can be benign or malignant, primary or secondary. Although epithelial neoplasms are more often cystic, they can be entirely solid. *Metastases* to the ovary are often predominantly

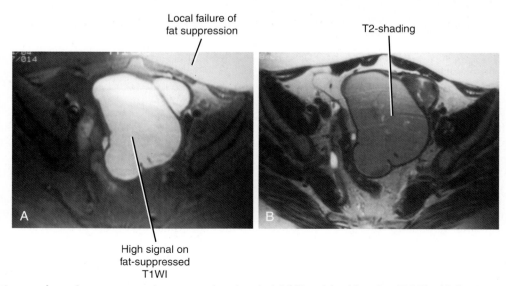

Local failure of fat suppression

T2-shading

High signal on fat-suppressed T1WI

Figure 21-46 Large endometrioma on magnetic resonance imaging. **A,** Axial T1-weighted imaging (T1WI) with frequency-selective fat suppression demonstrates a cystic lesion with very high signal within the pelvis. **B,** Axial T2WI without fat suppression demonstrates "shading"—that is, signal intensity that is higher than that of soft tissue but lower than that of water.

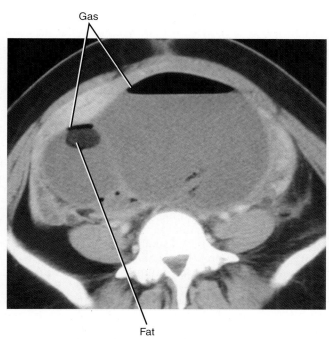

Gas

Fat

Figure 21-48 Axial image from contrast-enhanced computed tomography demonstrates nondependent gas within a large cystic mass in the pelvis. The presence of fat (shown) and calcification (not shown) supported the diagnosis of an infected mature cystic teratoma. The diagnosis was confirmed at surgery.

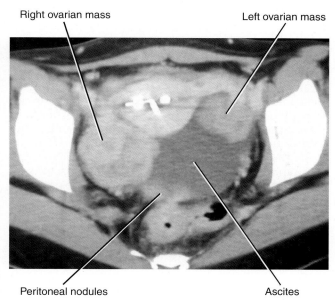

Right ovarian mass   Left ovarian mass

Peritoneal nodules   Ascites

Figure 21-49 Metastases to the ovaries on computed tomography (CT). Axial image from contrast-enhanced CT examination performed in a woman with known gastric cancer. Predominantly solid masses are present in both ovaries. The presence of ascites facilitates visualization of additional peritoneal metastases in the cul-de-sac. An intrauterine contraceptive device is present within the uterus.

solid but can show a mixture of solid and cystic elements. Other ovarian neoplasms that can appear predominately solid on imaging studies include Brenner tumor, dysgerminoma, yolk sac tumor, and a variety of sex cord-stromal tumors. *Brenner tumors* are associated with other cystic ovarian neoplasms, such as mucinous cystadenoma or cystic teratoma in 30% of cases. *Dysgerminomas* are malignant germ cell tumors that are histologically similar to testicular seminoma. They occur most often in women younger than 30 years.

Although it can be difficult, differentiating between primary and metastatic lesions is important because therapy and prognosis differs. Although the majority of primary ovarian carcinomas are unilateral, metastases tend to be bilateral. A known primary tumor (especially stomach, colon, or breast) favors metastatic disease (Fig. 21-49). Unfortunately, MRI is not much better than US or CT for distinguishing between primary and metastatic ovarian neoplasms. On T2-weighted imaging, metastatic tumors can have hypointense solid components corresponding to areas of collagenous stroma produced by the ovary against the metastatic disease. As mentioned later, low T2-weighted signal intensity is commonly found in solid primary ovarian tumors.

Although the sonographic appearance of solid ovarian masses is nonspecific, one particular neoplasm has a somewhat characteristic appearance. The typical appearance of a fibroma/fibrothecoma/thecoma is that of a uniformly hypoechoic mass with posterior acoustic attenuation (because of dense fibrous tissue). When a mass of this appearance is associated with ascites and pleural effusion, a diagnosis of *Meigs syndrome* should be considered. The differential diagnosis for *ovarian fibrothecoma* (as we will call this group of lesions subsequently) includes Brenner tumor and leiomyoma.

The same histologic feature (i.e., fibrous tissue) that gives the fibrothecoma its characteristic appearance on US images also creates a characteristic MRI appearance. These lesions tend to be hypointense on T2-weighted MR images because of varying degrees of fibrous tissue. As with US, the differential diagnosis includes Brenner tumors and fibroids. Signal intensity is intermediate to low on T1-weighted images. Although theca cells are highly vascular, connective tissue is not. Enhancement is, therefore, variable depending on the ratio of these two tissues within the lesion. Typically, both fibrothecomas and Brenner tumors are only modestly enhancing after administration of intravenous gadolinium chelates and can rarely be definitively distinguished with imaging.

Pearl: The primary differential diagnosis for a solid adnexal mass that appears uniformly hypoechoic on US (with posterior acoustic attenuation) and uniformly low in signal intensity on T2-weighted MR images (with modest enhancement after gadolinium chelate administration) is fibrothecoma, Brenner tumor, or pedunculated or broad ligament leiomyoma.

If It Does Not Come from the Ovary, Where Does It Come From?

Nonovarian adnexal masses are common and easily confused with ovarian lesions. As mentioned earlier, the presence of two normal ovaries separate from an adnexal lesion excludes primary ovarian origin. Once the ovaries are excluded, a variety of other adnexal processes should be considered.

Broad Ligament

Several types of masses may arise within the broad ligament. The most common are paraovarian cysts. *Paraovarian cysts* (also called *paratubal cysts*) are adnexal cysts that arise from the mesonephric (wolffian) structures, paramesonephric (müllerian) structures, or mesothelial inclusions. These extraovarian lesions are common, estimated to represent up to 10% of adnexal masses. Most paraovarian cysts are close to the round ligament and uterus, and often adjacent to but separate from the ovary (hence the name). Uncomplicated paraovarian cysts can appear similar to functional cysts. Just as ovarian cysts predispose the ovary to torsion, large paraovarian cysts can also result in torsion.

Peritoneal inclusions cysts and intraligamentous fibroids can also arise within the broad ligament. Because each can present as an adnexal mass even when arising from outside the broad ligament, these entities are discussed separately in the following subsections.

Peritoneum

A variety of peritoneal abnormalities can present as adnexal masses. *Peritoneal inclusion cysts* form as loculated collections (unilocular or multilocular) of ascitic fluid secondary to peritoneal adhesions. An imaging clue to their extraovarian location is a peculiar shape, which conforms to the adjacent pelvic organs, bowel, and side wall. These are more common in women who have a history of pelvic inflammatory disease or pelvic surgery.

As mentioned earlier, endometriosis consists of small peritoneal deposits seen only with direct visualization that can develop into *endometriomas* (sometimes called *endometriotic cysts*) containing blood products. These cysts can arise either within or separate from the ovaries.

Metastases to the peritoneum can result in masses in the adnexa. Gastric, colorectal, appendiceal, and pancreatic carcinoma are the primary extraovarian malignancies most commonly associated with peritoneal carcinomatosis. Primary peritoneal carcinoma is less common but has a pattern of disease spread similar to ovarian carcinoma.

Peritoneal metastases to the adnexa are commonly bilateral and are usually associated with ascites. Metastatic deposits may attach to the ovary, the broad ligament, or the uterus. History of a known primary malignancy and/or the presence of ascites and masses in other peritoneal recesses should prompt suspicion of the diagnosis.

Fallopian Tube

Hydrosalpinx is another common extraovarian adnexal mass. Although distended fallopian tubes usually contain simple fluid (hydrosalpinx), they can also contain blood (hematosalpinx) or pus (pyosalpinx). On TVUS, tubular anechoic or hypoechoic structures are seen in the adnexa (Fig. 21-50). The appearance of adjacent tubular structures may mimic septations of a complex cystic mass. Low-attenuation structures with similar shapes are seen on CT, usually located between the uterus and ovary. On MR, signal characteristics vary with the contents, but more importantly, the morphology of the lesion should allow accurate diagnosis. Hydrosalpinx usually appears as a C- or S-shaped structure. Identification of longitudinal mucosal folds (plicae) is considered specific. If there is extensive folding of the tube, the appearance can simulate a multilocular cystic mass, with a more "cog-wheel" appearance. In this case, evaluation in multiple planes may be helpful, as well as recognition of incomplete septa that would suggest a tubular morphology. When pyosalpinx progresses to form a thick-walled complex cystic mass, it is called a *tuboovarian abscess* (Fig. 21-51). *Fallopian tube carcinoma* is a rare cause of adnexal mass (<1% of gynecologic malignancies) but should be considered if soft tissue is seen within hydrosalpinx on US or MRI.

Because *ectopic pregnancy* usually presents with pain, it is discussed in Chapter 8. However, it is also discussed briefly here because ectopic pregnancy should always be considered in the differential diagnosis of a complex adnexal mass in a premenopausal female patient. The sonographic appearance in the adnexa is usually an echogenic ring with a sonolucent center (see Figure 8-52). In

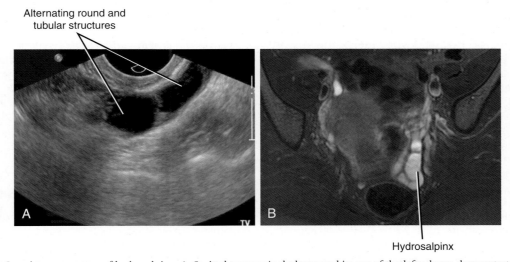

Alternating round and tubular structures

Hydrosalpinx

Figure 21-50 Imaging appearance of hydrosalpinx. **A,** Sagittal transvaginal ultrasound image of the left adnexa demonstrates adjacent round and tubular anechoic structures. **B,** Axial T2-weighted magnetic resonance image in the same patient better demonstrates the tubular nature of the structure.

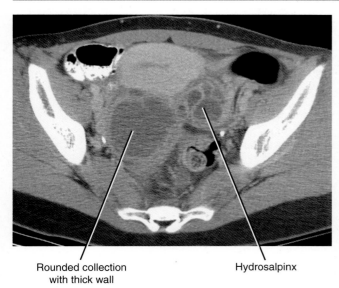

Figure 21-51 Axial computed tomographic image in a 24-year-old woman with pelvic pain and fever demonstrates hydrosalpinx on the left side and a more rounded, thick-walled collection on the right side. Bilateral tuboovarian abscesses were found at laparoscopy.

Rounded collection with thick wall

Hydrosalpinx

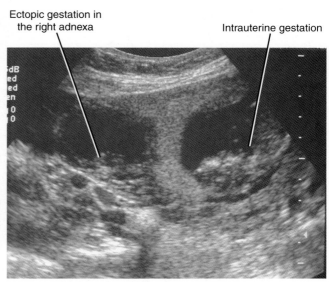

Ectopic gestation in the right adnexa

Intrauterine gestation

Figure 21-52 Concurrent intrauterine and ectopic pregnancy. Transverse ultrasound image of the uterus demonstrates gestational sacs in both the uterine cavity and within the right adnexa. Cardiac activity was demonstrated in both locations (not shown).

most cases, the ring is more echogenic than the adjacent ovary, and usually demonstrates increased vascularity around the periphery of the lesion on color Doppler imaging. Vascularity may be decreased with spontaneous termination of the pregnancy or after treatment with methotrexate. In some cases, presentation is late enough in pregnancy to allow visualization of a fetal pole. Hemoperitoneum is often present.

Identification of an intrauterine gestation makes ectopic pregnancy unlikely but does not exclude the diagnosis completely. The incidence of concurrent intrauterine and ectopic pregnancy has increased in recent years, likely related to fertility treatments. Characteristic findings of ectopic pregnancy in the adnexa should raise concern even in the presence of an intrauterine gestation (Fig. 21-52). Remember also that although most ectopic pregnancies occur within the extrauterine segments of the fallopian tube, additional locations include the interstitial segment of the fallopian tube, the cervix, as well as within the peritoneal cavity.

Uterus

Pedunculated fibroid (leiomyoma) is a common non-ovarian adnexal mass. Whether protruding between the peritoneal layers of the broad ligament (intraligamentous fibroid) or a freely mobile mass resting along the adnexa (pedunculated subserosal fibroid), the key distinguishing imaging feature of a pedunculated fibroid is the bridging vascular sign that results from the uterine blood supply extending to the mass. A pedicle of bridging vessels can be found by US, CT, or MRI (see Figs. 21-27, 21-28, and 21-40). Imaging of uterine fibroids is discussed in greater detail earlier in this chapter (see the Myometrial Masses section).

As discussed in the section on congenital uterine anomalies, although only one fully formed uterine horn comprises the unicornuate uterus, a *rudimentary horn* is often present. This tissue from the hypoplastic second horn is often solid but may be cystic if there is functioning endometrium within an obstructed horn. A rudimentary horn is a rare cause of a solid or cystic adnexal mass.

Bowel

Because of the proximity of the colon, appendix, and small bowel loops to the adnexa, abnormalities of the gastrointestinal tract can uncommonly mimic an adnexal mass. *Carcinoma of the colon, appendix,* and *small bowel* can present initially as an adnexal mass. Identification of the ovary separate from the mass and continuity of an intestinal loop with the mass are key image features. *Duplication cysts* of intestinal loops in the pelvis can mimic a cystic adnexal mass.

Appendicitis can mimic a tuboovarian abscess or cystic ovarian mass if a fluid-filled appendix happens to be located in the adnexal region. *Appendiceal abscess* and *mucocele* of the appendix can also present as cystic structures in the adnexa. *Diverticular abscess* can also be confused with an adnexal mass.

Lymphatics

Lymphoceles often develop after lymph-node dissection and should be considered when simple cysts (often large) occur in the adnexa along the pelvic sidewalls after pelvic surgery. They are usually lateral to the ovary, adjacent to the iliac vessels, and surgical clips are often found in the vicinity.

Urinary Tract

Although the origin of a *bladder diverticulum* is usually obvious, it can occasionally be mistaken for a cystic mass in the pelvis when the diverticulum is large and the bladder is collapsed. In rare cases, *ureteral diverticula* arising from the distal ureter have been mistaken for an adnexal mass with sonography (Table 21-3).

Table 21-3   Summary of Adnexal Masses

Morphology	Diagnosis	Imaging and Clinical Features (variably present)
Unilocular Cyst	Simple cyst	Simple fluid Thin wall <5 cm* No enhancement or Doppler flow
	Paraovarian cyst or peritoneal inclusion cyst	Separate from ovary
	Hemorrhagic cyst	Low-level echoes on US Blood products on MRI Resolves on follow-up
	Endometrioma	Low-level echoes on US Blood products on MRI with shading on T2-weighted images Does not resolve on follow-up
	Ovarian cystadenoma	Size > 5 cm Slight wall thickening is common
	Ovarian carcinoma	Postmenopausal patient with increased CA-125
Complex Cyst	Functional cyst	Few thin septa No nodularity or enhancement/flow
	Hemorrhagic cyst	Weblike fibrin strands or dependent clot with no enhancement/flow Blood products on MRI
	Hydrosalpinx or pyosalpinx	Tubular shape Incomplete septa Fever or adnexal tenderness (pyosalpinx)
	Benign or malignant ovarian neoplasm	Thick septa (>3 mm) Nodularity of wall or septa Internal enhancement
	Mature cystic teratoma	Contains fat attenuation/signal Calcification
Cyst with Thick, Hypervascular Wall	Corpus luteum	Premenopausal, midcycle Thick, crenulated wall Wall less echogenic than endometrium (unlike ectopic pregnancy) Resolves Resistive index usually between 0.39 and 0.70
	Ectopic pregnancy	Premenopausal Positive β-hCG Thick wall that is often as echogenic as endometrial stripe Resistive index < 0.39 or > 0.70
	Ovarian neoplasm	Increases in size Postmenopausal with increased CA-125 Ascites
Solid Mass	Fibroma/fibrothecoma/thecoma	Solid, often large hypoechoic mass with sound attenuation on US Low signal on T2-weighted MRI May be associated with pleural effusion
	Pedunculated or broad ligament fibroid	Bridging vascular sign Low signal on T2-weighted MRI
	Ovarian torsion	Acute pain Flow decreased/absent Peripheral follicles ("string of pearls" sign)
	Metastases	Known malignancy Often bilateral Ascites is common
	Sex-cord stromal tumor	Clinical findings related to hormonal activity Often small at time of diagnosis
	Dysgerminoma	Large, multilobulated mass Enhancing fibrovascular septa
	Granulosa cell tumor	Secrete estrogen Usually predominantly solid but may have cystic component

Table 21-3   Summary of Adnexal Masses—cont'd

Morphology	Diagnosis	Imaging and Clinical Features
	Brenner tumor	Often bilateral
		Small solid tumors but often associated with benign cystic neoplasms
		Low signal on T2-weighted MRI
		Calcification in 50%

*Functional cysts and benign serous inclusion cysts are less common in postmenopausal women but still more common than malignancy. Some advocate surveillance with ultrasound in this population of ovarian cysts > 1 cm.
β-*hCG*, β-Human chorionic gonadotropin; *MRI*, magnetic resonance imaging; *US*, ultrasound.

■ ABNORMALITIES OF THE LOWER PELVIS AND PERINEUM

Benign Perineal Lesions

Several common lesions of the central regions of the lower pelvis and perineum that are seen in close association with the urethra and vagina are discussed here.

Urethral Diverticula

Urethral diverticula are discussed in detail in Chapter 19. In brief, they appear as cystic masses in close association with the midurethra, usually seen wrapping around the posterolateral wall on TVUS and on axial CT and MR images. Water attenuation/signal is usually noted. Real-time transvaginal sonography facilitates identification of the connection with the urethra. Stones can form within diverticula and have typical characteristics of calcification on all imaging modalities. Tumors have been reported within diverticula, including adenocarcinoma and squamous cell carcinoma.

Paraurethral Cysts

Multiple small glands secrete mucus into the female urethra and are variably called *paraurethral, periurethral,* or *Skene's glands* in the literature. These glands are believed by some to be the female analogue to the prostate gland and likely account for a minority of urethral cancers in women. Cysts may arise from a Skene's gland or its short duct that empties into the urethra. Such paraurethral cysts or Skene's duct cysts are rare, more common in infants,

but can be seen at virtually any age. On imaging, paraurethral cysts occur in a location similar to urethral diverticula, but are more likely to be large and spherical and less likely to wrap around the urethra. In addition, communication with the urethra is not evident by imaging.

Gartner Duct Cysts

Gartner duct cysts typically arise in the anterolateral aspect of the upper vaginal wall and are usually seen as small (<2 cm) fluid-attenuation structures in the region of the upper vagina on axial CT images (Fig. 21-53). MR demonstrates a similar appearance with fluid signal on T1- and T2-weighted sequences. These cysts represent remnants of the mesonephric (Wolffian) ducts and are sometimes associated with other developmental anomalies of the genitourinary system.

Bartholin Gland Cysts

In contradistinction to Gartner duct cysts, which occur in the upper vagina, Bartholin gland cysts occur in the lower vagina. These cysts represent obstructed vestibular glands of the vagina and are located in the posterolateral aspect of the vagina behind the labia minora. These are seen most often as labial cysts on CT performed for other reasons (see Fig. 21-53). When seen on MRI, internal signal intensity is often high on T2-weighted images and variable on T1-weighted images depending on mucoid content. These are seldom seen by sonography unless directed sonography of the

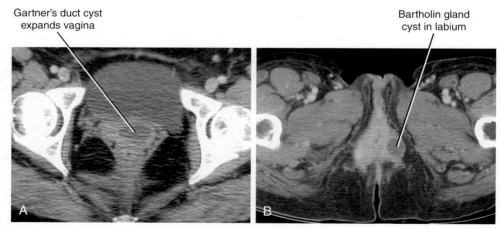

Gartner's duct cyst expands vagina

Bartholin gland cyst in labium

Figure 21-53 Vaginal cysts on computed tomography (CT). **A,** Axial image from a contrast-enhanced CT scan demonstrates a low-attenuation lesion in the region of the upper vagina (compare with anatomy shown in Fig. 21-3). This is too cephalad to be a urethral diverticulum (bladder still in view) and is a typical location for a Gartner's duct cyst. **B,** Axial image from CT of a different patient demonstrates a low-attenuation lesion in the posterior left labium. This infected Bartholin gland cyst was excised.

perineum is performed with a high-resolution linear transducer.

Malignancy in the Perineum

Perineal malignancies are occasionally imaged for staging, preoperative planning, or both. Primary vulvar and vaginal malignancies occur infrequently and are usually squamous cell carcinoma. Both entities are associated with human papillomavirus. Although diagnosis is almost always made clinically, imaging is useful for determining the extent of disease.

CT is often performed, mainly to identify abnormal lymph nodes. In most cases, CT does not provide sufficient soft-tissue discrimination to allow accurate local staging of the tumor.

MR defines location and extent of disease better than CT. *Primary squamous cell carcinoma of the vagina* usually arises from the posterior wall in the upper third of the vagina. T2-weighted images demonstrate a vaginal mass with signal that is increased compared with the low signal seen in the normal vagina. Distortion of the H-shaped vaginal contour can be seen on axial images. High-resolution, small field-of-view images optimize definition of local disease spread, whereas inclusion of a larger field of view axial acquisition of the entire pelvis (often T1 weighted) permits lymph-node staging. Crucial findings to report include the tumor size, local extent, and presence of adenopathy.

Pearl: Primary vaginal carcinoma is most often of squamous cell type and usually arises from the posterior wall of the upper vagina.

Adenocarcinoma of the vagina is less common and usually arises from the anterior wall of the upper vagina. The signal intensity of adenocarcinoma on T2-weighted images is typically higher than that seen with squamous cell carcinoma. *Primary vaginal melanoma* can occur anywhere in the vagina but occurs more commonly in the lower vagina. The MRI appearance of primary vaginal melanoma is quite variable, depending on the content of melanin and/or hemorrhage within the tumor. Signal intensity on T1-weighted images is more likely to be high or intermediate than with other vaginal tumors.

Most tumors (80-90%) that affect the vagina actually are due to extension from primary bladder, vulvar, cervical, or rectal tumors. Discontinuous vaginal metastases have been reported from known genital tract malignancies.

Dynamic Pelvic Floor Imaging

The pelvic floor is supported by a complex network of muscles and ligaments that form a sort of hammock to hold the bladder, uterus (if present), rectum, and peritoneal contents within expected confines of the pelvis. Damage to the supporting structures can alter the usual mechanics that control voiding and defecation. Childbirth and hysterectomy provide the insults most commonly held responsible for laxity, although multiple other disorders that affect the connective tissues or increase abdominal pressure are believed to contribute as well. Some estimate that up to 50% of

women who have given birth have some degree of prolapse in their perineum. Although a detailed discussion of the imaging evaluation of pelvic floor laxity is beyond the scope of this textbook, we chose to mention some imaging findings that might be discovered incidentally and warrant further assessment as clinically indicated.

From an imaging standpoint, pelvic floor laxity is most often encountered incidentally on CT examinations performed for other reasons (Fig. 21-54). Axial CT or MR images at the level of the pubic symphysis should include the urethra, vagina, and anus contained by the sling of the puborectalis muscle. Abnormal descent of pelvic structures into the perineum indicates pelvic floor prolapse. The type of prolapsed is named according to descending structure to include *cystocele* (bladder), *uterine prolapse* (uterus), *enterocele* (small bowel), and *rectocele* (rectum).

In addition to discomfort and incontinence, pelvic floor laxity can result in obstructive symptoms in the urinary and gastrointestinal tracts. Cystocele predisposes to urinary stasis leading to infection and stone formation (Fig. 21-55). Occasionally, the distal ureters prolapse with the bladder trigone, resulting in partial ureteral obstruction. Rectocele can result in constipation or obstipation, often seen as an increase in the amount of fecal material in the colon on CT.

Multiple types of prolapse often coexist, but it may be difficult to characterize each by physical examination alone. Because a number of different surgical approaches can be used depending on the structures involved, many surgeons seek preoperative imaging. Fluoroscopy was the mainstay for imaging the pelvic floor for many

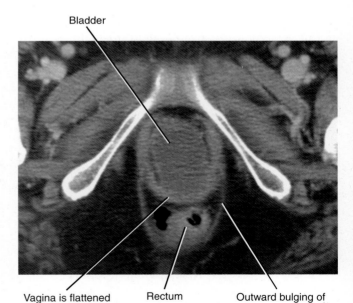

Bladder

Vagina is flattened and stretched by bladder

Rectum

Outward bulging of puborectalis muscle

Figure 21-54 Pelvic floor laxity as unexpected finding on computed tomography (CT). Axial image at the level of the pubic symphysis from contrast-enhanced CT performed for abdominal pain includes the bladder (indicating cystocele) and rectum (indicating rectocele). Compare this with normal axial perineal anatomy shown in Figure 21-3.

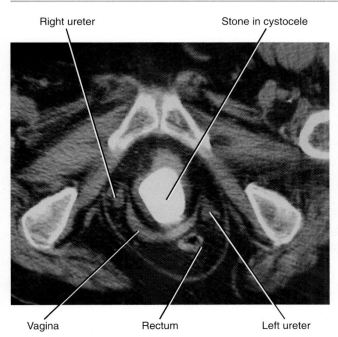

Figure 21-55 Axial image at the level of the pubic symphysis from an unenhanced computed tomographic (CT) scan demonstrates a large bladder stone within a cystocele. The examination was performed without contrast because the patient had renal failure. Bilateral hydronephrosis was also present on more superior images (not shown).

years, using contrast instilled into the bladder and rectum (sometimes using oral contrast for small-bowel visualization as well) to allow visualization of these structures during voiding and defecation.

Dynamic MRI of the pelvic floor is becoming a more common examination. Although techniques vary, MR is less dependent on inserting contrast media into the structures and provides visualization not only of the lumen of each structure but also of the supporting muscular elements. Dynamic information is obtained by acquiring a series of repeated midline sagittal T2-weighted images obtained at rest and during Valsalva (Fig. 21-56).

■ IMAGING EVALUATION FOR INFERTILITY

Infertility is generally defined as at least 1 year of unprotected sexual intercourse that does not result in pregnancy. The initial workup involves a battery of diagnostic tests for both the male and female partner. In addition to laboratory tests used to assess hormonal factors, imaging is often used to evaluate the female partner for patency and structure of the reproductive system.

Evaluation for Tubal and Endometrial Patency

Tubal patency can be evaluated with HSG, laparoscopic hydrotubation, or sonohysterography. The laparoscopic technique is invasive and expensive, and some have questioned any benefit over HSG. In addition to diagnostic information, HSG also provides access for recanalization of a proximally obstructed fallopian tube by various catheterization techniques. HSG also remains the most accurate method for diagnosing abnormalities of the fallopian tube such as *salpingitis isthmica nodosa* and provides more detail regarding endometrial scarring than does MRI (Fig. 21-57).

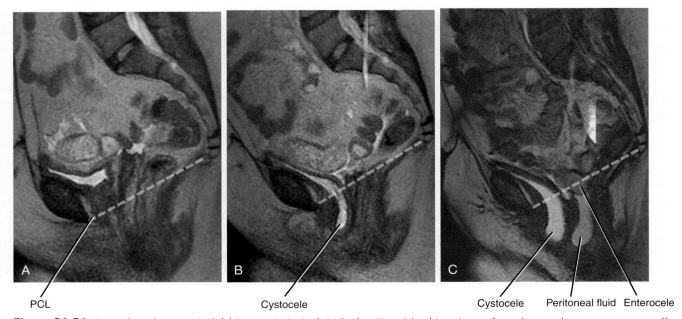

Figure 21-56 Cystocele and rectovaginal dehiscence. A, Sagittal single-shot T2-weighted imaging performed at rest demonstrates a normally positioned bladder base. The pubococcygeal line (PCL) is shown. B, With Valsalva, the bladder base descends well below the pubic symphysis, diagnostic of cystocele. C, Sagittal dynamic CINE FIESTA at maximal stress not only shows the cystocele but also wide separation of the vagina from the rectum (which fills with physiologic free fluid), diagnostic of rectovaginal fascial dehiscence. There is minimal descent of small bowel compatible with a small enterocele.

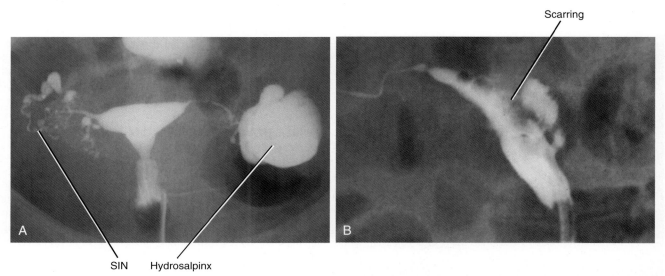

Figure 21-57 Hysterosalpingography appearance in two cases of acquired infertility. **A,** Outpouchings from the right fallopian tube caused by salpingitis isthmica nodosa (SIN). Hydrosalpinx is present on the left side. **B,** Scarring of the endometrial canal (synechiae) characteristic of Asherman syndrome related to prior instrumentation.

Saline infusion sonohysterosalpingography (sono-HSG) has emerged as an alternative method to evaluate tubal patency and the endometrial cavity. Saline is infused after cervical cannulation, followed by endovaginal sonographic evaluation of the uterus and tubes. Although the technique has proved accurate for assessment of tubal patency, it has also been shown to be superior to HSG for the detection of certain uterine anomalies and characterization of uterine lesions such as fibroids and polyps.

A study comparing the relative accuracies of HSG, endovaginal sonography (EVS), and MRI for diagnosis of uterine müllerian anomalies found both EVS and MRI to be clearly superior to HSG. MRI does have some advantages over EVS, however, including its noninvasive nature, limitless multiplanar capability, and precise delineation of the external uterine contour.

Structural Anomalies of the Uterus and Vagina

Evaluation for congenital (müllerian duct) anomalies is a crucial component of the infertility workup, because approximately 25% of women with uterine anomalies suffer from subfertility. Although uterine anomalies are often imaged with HSG, US, or CT, MRI provides the most precise characterization in most cases. Because surgical treatment is beneficial for some anomalies but unnecessary in others, MRI is often used to provide a definitive diagnosis.

Uterine anomalies arise when the müllerian ducts fail to fuse or the intervening tissue fails to resorb after fusion. As noted earlier, the distal müllerian ducts form the fallopian tubes, uterine corpus, cervix, and upper two thirds of the vagina (see Fig. 21-1). Müllerian anomalies are frequently associated with renal anomalies; therefore, the kidneys should be routinely imaged when evaluating a patient with a suspected müllerian anomaly.

Pearl: Müllerian duct anomalies are commonly associated with renal anomalies such as agenesis. It is useful to include the kidneys when imaging for suspected müllerian duct anomalies.

Müllerian duct anomalies are classified by the American Society of Reproductive medicine into seven classes. Class 1 anomalies include varying degrees of *uterine hypoplasia,* as well as complete *uterine agenesis,* which can include the upper two thirds of the vagina (Mayer–Rokitansky–Küster–Hauser syndrome) (Fig. 21-58). The ovaries are present, helping to distinguish this entity from androgen insensitivity.

Class 2 anomalies are defined as hypoplasia or agenesis of one of the two müllerian ducts, commonly referred to as a *unicornuate uterus.* The uterus appears elongated, curved, off the midline, and has been referred to as "banana shaped." In the case of agenesis, only one uterine horn is present. In the case of hypoplasia, there is one fully formed horn and a *rudimentary horn* that may or may not communicate with the endometrial canal (Fig. 21-59). Unicornuate uterus is associated with ipsilateral renal anomalies in up to 40% of cases.

Class 3 anomalies represent complete failure of müllerian duct fusion, a condition known as *uterus didelphys.* No communication occurs between two endometrial canals, resulting in widely divergent separate uterine horns, vertical septation of the vagina, and separate cervices. The uterine horns are often located in different spatial planes, making it difficult to achieve a classic coronal view (Fig. 21-60). Each uterine horn demonstrates normal zonal anatomy.

Class 4 and 5 anomalies are perhaps the most important from a perspective of infertility. A class 4 anomaly results from incomplete fusion of the uterine horns, a condition known as *bicornuate uterus.* The horns are symmetric with an intervening cleft, resulting in two divergent horns (Fig. 21-61). The cleft not only separates

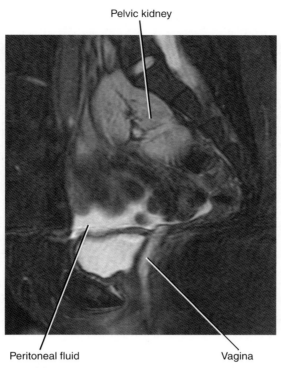

Pelvic kidney

Peritoneal fluid   Vagina

Figure 21-58 Uterine agenesis (class I anomaly) on magnetic resonance imaging. Sagittal T2-weighted imaging demonstrates the presence of a vagina but no uterus. Ovaries were present (not shown) and likely account for the peritoneal fluid. A pelvic kidney is present, a reminder that müllerian anomalies are commonly associated with other genitourinary and musculoskeletal anomalies.

the two horns but results in a concavity of the external fundal contour greater than 1 cm in depth. The two endometrial canals may or may not communicate at their caudal margins. However, unlike didelphys, the cervical portion shares common muscular stroma.

Class 5 anomalies, representing 55% of all müllerian duct anomalies, result from failed resorption of the medial septum after fusion of the two ducts. Class 5 anomalies are

also known as *septate uterus*. The imaging appearance can be similar to a bicornuate uterus, but the distinction is critical, because the septate uterus has a higher association with infertility, and the surgical correction for each is different.

Septate uterus can be treated with hysteroscopic metroplasty (resection of the septum from the inside) in an attempt to improve fertility. In the rare case that repair

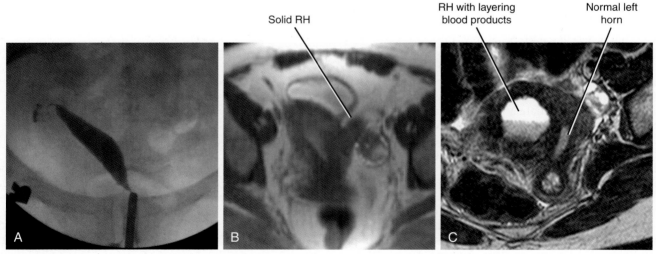

Solid RH   RH with layering   Normal left
                            blood products   horn

A   B   C

Figure 21-59 Unicornuate uterus. **A,** Hysterosalpingography demonstrates a thin "banana-shaped" endometrial canal with a single fallopian tube coming from the apex. **B,** T2-weighted imaging (T2WI) coronal to the uterine fundus in the same patient shows a normal-appearing right uterine horn with a small solid rudimentary horn (RH) on the left. **C,** Axial T2WI in a different patient shows a normal left horn with an obstructed right RH.

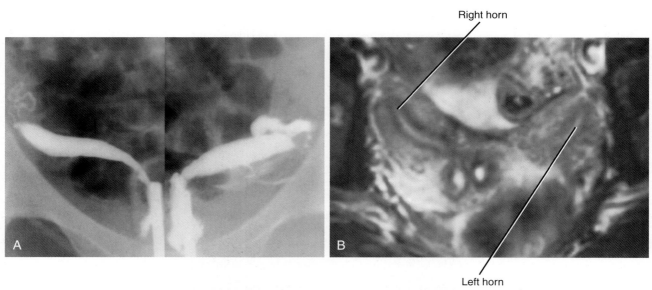

Figure 21-60   Uterus didelphys. **A,** Fused image from injection of two separate cervices demonstrates widely diverging uterine horns. Note that individually, each horn has the appearance of a unicornuate uterus. **B,** T2-weighted magnetic resonance image coronal to the uterus in the same patient demonstrates widely divergent horns (it was difficult to obtain a plane that included the fundus of both sides, a common situation with uterus didelphys).

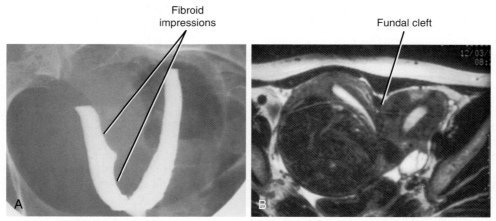

Figure 21-61   Bicornuate uterus with fibroids. **A,** Hysterosalpingography image demonstrates diverging horns with less angulation than seen in Figure 21-60. Note the impression made by large fibroids. **B,** T2-weighted magnetic resonance image coronal to the uterine fundus demonstrates two endometrial canals with a pronounced cleft in the fundus, definitive evidence that this is *not* a septate uterus.

of a bicornuate uterus is considered appropriate, an open surgical approach is used. The key for differentiation between bicornuate and septate uterus is the external contour of the fundus. The contour can be convex, flat, or minimally concave with a septate uterus, but any cleft in the uterine fundus measures less than 10 mm in depth (Fig. 21-62). A cleft of 10 mm or greater indicates a bicornuate uterus. Occasionally, it is difficult to identify the outer contour of the fundus on T2-weighted imaging. In such cases, a T1-weighted image without fat suppression coronal to the uterine fundus can improve definition. In the case of septate uterus, it is helpful for purposes of resection to note whether the septum is predominantly muscular or fibrous.

Pearl: When two endometrial canals are identified, it is critical to evaluate the outer fundal contour on images performed coronal to the uterus. The absence of a cleft indicates it is a septate uterus. The presence of a cleft indicates bicornuate or didelphys uterus. MR signal of the tissue between two endometrial canals has no impact on the diagnosis of septate versus bicornuate uterus.

A class 6 uterus, commonly referred to as an *arcuate uterus,* results from near-complete resorption of the medial septum. This causes a flattening of the fundal contour and broad smooth indentation of the endometrium superiorly (Fig. 21-63). Some choose to disregard this as a diagnosis because it has no proven impact on fertility and can be quite subjective.

A class 7 uterus can be seen in women whose mothers were treated with diethylstilbestrol during pregnancy. This results in a T-shaped hypoplastic uterus with

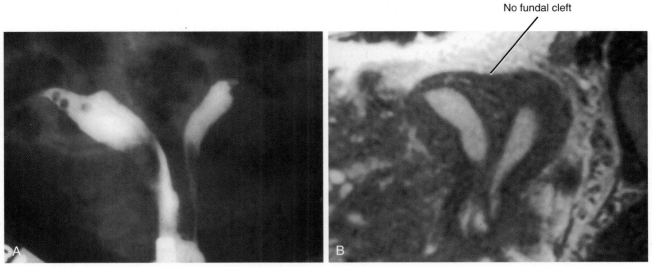

Figure 21-62 Septate uterus. **A,** Hysterosalpingography demonstrates two uterine canals. The angle is consistent with either septate or bicornuate uterus. **B,** T2-weighted magnetic resonance image coronal to the uterine fundus demonstrates a smooth outer contour to the fundus, diagnostic of a septate rather than bicornuate uterus. Note that the signal of the intervening septum is identical to that of the myometrium elsewhere in the uterus (muscular septum).

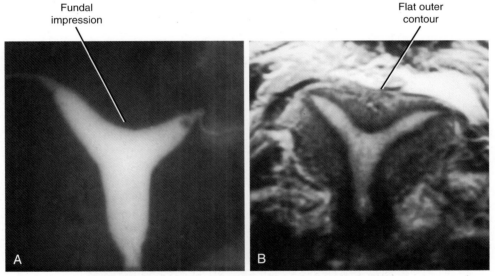

Figure 21-63 Arcuate uterus. **A,** Hysterosalpingography demonstrates a shallow impression into the fundal region of the endometrial cavity. **B,** T2-weighted magnetic resonance image coronal to the uterine fundus demonstrates a flat outer fundal contour and similar shallow impression on the endometrial cavity.

irregularly narrowed vertical and horizontal segments of the endometrial cavity (Fig. 21-64).

Incomplete or failed resorption of tissue in the vagina can lead to obstruction because of vaginal atresia or a vaginal septum. This is usually diagnosed in adolescence, as the onset of menstruation results in distension of the uterus and vagina with blood (hematometrocolpos) (Fig. 21-65). The level of obstruction can be as low as an imperforate hymen, and sometimes attempts at surgical repair are made without imaging. On occasion, however, imaging is performed to identify the level of a higher vaginal septum or vaginal atresia when initial attempts at surgery become more complex than anticipated. Occasionally, a vaginal septum is present on one side of a uterus didelphys. In such cases, renal agenesis is sometimes seen on the same side as the septum.

Uterine Fibroids

Submucosal fibroids have been implicated as a contributing cause to subfertility, with improved fertility rates demonstrated after myomectomy. Large submucosal fibroids that distort the uterine cavity are associated with pregnancy loss. Intramural fibroids in the cornual regions can obstruct the interstitial tube, and large subserosal lesions extending into the broad ligament can exert mass effect on the fallopian tubes. Mechanical effects

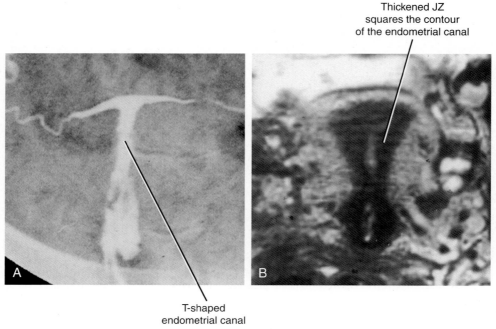

Thickened JZ
squares the contour
of the endometrial canal

T-shaped
endometrial canal

Figure 21-64 Diethylstilbestrol-related uterine hypoplasia. **A,** Hysterosalpingography demonstrates the characteristic T-shape of the endometrial canal. **B,** T2-weighted magnetic resonance image coronal to the uterine fundus demonstrates squaring of the junctional zone (JZ) that defines the shape of the endometrial canal.

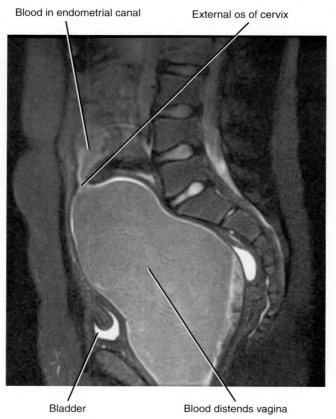

Blood in endometrial canal   External os of cervix

Bladder   Blood distends vagina

Figure 21-65 Sagittal T2-weighted magnetic resonance image demonstrates hematometrocolpos in a 12-year-old girl with pelvic pain and delayed menarche. A vaginal septum (not included on this image) was resected.

on the endometrial cavity have also been described, particularly with large (>5 cm) submucosal fibroids. This effect has been associated with fetal malpresentation and an increased rate of Cesarean deliveries related to obstruction of the birth canal by bulky lesions in the lower uterine segment. Large tumors greater than 5 cm are also at increased risk for degeneration that can result in significant pain.

Suggested Readings

Alborzi S, Dehbashi S, Khodaee R: Sonohysterosalpingographic screening for infertile patients, *Int J Gynaecol Obstet* 82(1):57-62, 2003.

American Fertility Society: The American Fertility Society classifications of adnexal adhesions, distal tubal obstruction, tubal occlusion secondary to tubal ligation, tubal pregnancies, Müllerian anomalies and intrauterine adhesions, *Fertil Steril* 49:944-955, 1988.

Ascher SM: MR imaging of the female pelvis: the time has come, *Radiographics* 18:931-945, 1998.

Atri M: Ectopic pregnancy versus corpus luteum cyst revisited: best Doppler predictors, *J Ultrasound Med* 22:1181-1184, 2003.

Bipat S, Glas AS, van der Velden J, et al: Computed tomography and magnetic resonance imaging in staging of uterine cervical carcinoma: a systematic review, *Gynecol Oncol* 91(1):59-66, 2003.

Brown DL: A practical approach to the ultrasound characterization of adnexal masses, *Ultrasound Q* 23:87-105, 2007.

Chang SD: Imaging of the vagina and vulva, *Radiol Clin North Am* 40(3):637-658, 2002.

Chaudhry S, Reinhold C, Guermazi A et al: Benign and malignant diseases of the endometrium, *Top Magn Reson Imaging* 14:339-357, 2003.

Chung HH, Kang SB, Cho JY et al: Accuracy of MR imaging for the prediction of myometrial invasion of endometrial carcinoma, *Gynecol Oncol* 104:654-659, 2007.

Condous G, Kirk E, Lu C et al: Diagnostic accuracy of varying discriminatory zones for the prediction of ectopic pregnancy in women with a pregnancy of unknown location, *Ultrasound Obstet Gynecol* 26:770-775, 2005.

Crosignani PG, Rubin BL: Optimal use of infertility diagnostic tests and treatments. The ESHRE Capri Workshop Group, *Hum Reprod* 15(3):723-732, 2000.

Dwyer PL, Rosamilia A: Congenital urogenital anomalies that are associated with the persistence of Gartner's duct: a review, *Am J Obstet Gynecol* 195:354-359, 2006.

Eilber KS, Raz S: Benign cystic lesions of the vagina: a literature review, *J Urol* 170:717-722, 2003.

Erdem M, Bilgin U, Bozkurt N, Erdem A: Comparison of transvaginal ultrasonography and saline infusion sonohysterography in evaluating the endometrial cavity in pre- and postmenopausal women with abnormal uterine bleeding, *Menopause* 14(5):846-852, 2007.

Fielding JR: Practical MR imaging of female pelvic floor weakness, *Radiographics* 22:295-304, 2002.

Foshager MC, Walsh JW: CT anatomy of the female pelvis: a second look, *Radiographics* 14:51-66, 1994.

Fung MFK, Reid A, Faught W et al: Prospective longitudinal study of ultrasound screening for endometrial abnormalities in women with breast cancer receiving tamoxifen, *Gynecol Oncol* 91:154-159, 2003.

Garcia CR, Tureck RW: Submucosal leiomyomas and infertility, *Fertil Steril* 42:16-19, 1984.

Goldstein RB, Bree RL, Benacerraf BR et al: Evaluation of the woman with post-menopausal bleeding: Society of Radiologists in Ultrasound-Sponsored Consensus Conference Statement, *J Ultrasound Med* 20:1025-1036, 2001.

Green GE, Mortele KJ, Glickman JN et al: Brenner tumors of the ovary: sonographic and computed tomographic imaging features, *J Ultrasound Med* 25:1245-1251; quiz 1252-1244, 2006.

Hashimoto M, Okane K, Hirano H, Watari J: Pictorial review: subperitoneal spaces of the broad ligament and sigmoid mesocolon—imaging findings, *Clin Radiol* 53:875-881, 1998.

Hricak H, Chen M, Coakley FV et al: Complex adnexal masses: detection and characterization with MR imaging—multivariate analysis, *Radiology* 214:39-46, 2000.

Hricak H, Gatsonis C, Coakley FV et al: Early invasive cervical cancer: CT and MR Imaging in Preoperative Evaluation ACRIN/GOG Comparative Study of Diagnostic Performance and Interobserver Variability. *Radiology* 245(2):491-498, 2007.

Hricak H, Lacey CG, Sandles LG et al: Invasive cervical carcinoma: comparison of MR imaging and surgical findings, *Radiology* 166:623-631, 1998.

Hricak H, Yu KK: Radiology in invasive cervical cancer, *Am J Roentgenol* 167:1101-1196, 1996.

Imaoka I, Akihiko W, Michimasa M et al: MR imaging of disorders associated with female infertility: use in diagnosis, treatment, and management, *Radiographics* 23:1401-1421, 2003.

Jung SE, Lee JM, Rha SE et al: CT and MR imaging of ovarian tumors with emphasis on differential diagnosis, *Radiographics* 22:1305-1325, 2002.

Kanso HN, Hachem K, Aoun NJ et al: Variable MR findings in ovarian functional hemorrhagic cysts, *J Magn Reson Imaging* 24:356-361, 2006.

Kaur H, Silverman PM, Iyer RB et al: Diagnosis, staging, and surveillance of cervical carcinoma, *Am J Roentgenol* 180:1621-1631, 2003.

Kim YS: MR imaging of primary uterine lymphoma, *Abdom Imaging* 22:441-444, 1997.

Kim SH, Han MC: Invasion of the urinary bladder by uterine cervical carcinoma: evaluation with MR imaging, *Am J Roentgenol* 168:393-397, 1997.

Kinkel K: Pitfalls in staging uterine neoplasm with imaging: a review, *Abdom Imaging* 31:164-173, 2006.

Macura KJ: Magnetic resonance imaging of pelvic floor defects in women, *Top Magn Reson Imaging* 17:417-426, 2006.

Manfredi R: Endometrial cancer: magnetic resonance imaging, *Abdom Imaging* 30:626-636, 2005.

Murase E, Siegelman ES, Outwater EK et al: Uterine leiomyomas: histopathologic features, MR imaging findings, differential diagnosis, and treatment, *Radiographics* 19(5):1179-1197, 1999.

Nalaboff KM, Pellerito JS, Ben-Levi E: Imaging the endometrium: disease and normal variants, *Radiographics* 21(6):1409-1424, 2001.

Okamoto Y, Tanaka YO, Nishida M: MR imaging of the uterine cervix: imaging-pathologic correlation, *Radiographics* 23:425-445, 2003.

Outwater EK, Siegelman ES, Hunt JL: Ovarian teratomas: tumor types and imaging characteristics, *Radiographics* 21:475-490, 2001.

Ouyang DW, Economy KE, Norwitz ER: Obstetric complications of fibroids, *Obstet Gynecol Clin North Am* 33(1):153-169, 2006.

Parikh JH, Barton DPJ, Ind TEJ et al: MR imaging features of vaginal malignancies, *Radiographics* 28:49-63; quiz 322, 2008.

Patel MD: Practical approach to the adnexal mass, *Radiol Clin North Am* 44:879-899, 2006.

Pellerito JS, McCarthy SM, Doyle MB et al: Diagnosis of uterine anomalies: relative accuracy of MR imaging, endovaginal sonography, and hysterosalpingography, *Radiology* 183(3):795-800, 1992.

Saksouk FA, Johnson SC: Recognition of the ovaries and ovarian origin of pelvic masses with CT, *Radiographics* 24:S133-S146, 2004.

Siegelman ES, Outwater EK: Tissue characterization in the female pelvis by means of MR imaging, *Radiology* 212:5-18, 1999.

Smith-Bindman R, Kerlikowske K, Feldstein VA et al: Endovaginal ultrasound to exclude endometrial cancer and other endometrial abnormalities, *JAMA* 280:1510-1517, 1998.

Smith-Bindman R, Weiss E, Feldstein V: How thick is too thick? When endometrial thickness should prompt biopsy in postmenopausal women without vaginal bleeding, *Ultrasound Obstet Gynecol* 24:558-565, 2004.

Stein MW, Ricci ZJ, Novack L et al: Sonographic comparison of the tubal ring of ectopic pregnancy with the corpus luteum, *J Ultrasound Med* 23:57-62, 2004.

Sugiyama K, Takehara Y: MR findings of pseudoneoplastic lesions in the uterine cervix mimicking adenoma malignum, *Br J Radiol* 80:878-883, 2007.

Tamai K, Koyama T, Umeoka S et al: Spectrum of MR features of adenomyosis, *Best Pract Res Clin Ostet Gynaecol* 20:583-602, 2006.

Thurmond AS, Machan LS, Maubon AJ et al: A review of selective salpingography and fallopian tube catheterization, *Radiographics* 20:1759-1768, 2000.

Togashi K, Morikawa K, Kataoka LM, Konishi J: Cervical cancer, *J Magn Reson Imaging* 8:391-397, 1998.

Torricelli P, Ferraresi S, Fiocchi F et al: 3-T MRI in the preoperative evaluation of depth of myometrial infiltration in endometrial cancer, *Am J Roentgenol* 190:489-495, 2008.

Wolfman DJ, Ascher SM: Magnetic resonance imaging of benign uterine pathology, *Top Magn Reson Imaging* 17(6):399-407, 2006.

Yang A, Mostwin JL, Rosenshein NB, Zerhouni EA: Pelvic floor descent in women: dynamic evaluation with fast MR imaging and cinematic display, *Radiology* 179(1):25-33, 1991.

PROBLEM SOLVING: INTERVENTIONS

Percutaneous Biopsy and Drainage

John R. Leyendecker and Matthew Blurton

Before the 1980s, open surgery was considered to be the best option for sampling an indeterminate mass or evacuating an infected or symptomatic fluid collection within the abdomen or pelvis. Since then, the development and refinement of percutaneous image-guided techniques have allowed for far less invasive means of accomplishing these objectives. With the proper selection of potential candidates, guidance modality, and approach, image-guided percutaneous techniques have proved safe, efficient, and effective. This chapter discusses some of the considerations and decisions involving percutaneous biopsy and fluid drainage procedures.

■ PERCUTANEOUS INTERVENTIONS: FOUR STEPS TO SUCCESS

The successful performance of a percutaneous intervention involves several steps beyond the physical act of placing a catheter or needle in a patient: (1) Determine necessity and risk; (2) choose target and approach; (3) choose a modality; and (4) assess efficacy.

Determine Necessity and Risk

Most image-guided interventions begin with an initial referral from a clinician who does not routinely perform percutaneous procedures. Therefore, one cannot expect the referring physician to be familiar with all of the details regarding the indications, contraindications, techniques, expected outcomes, and complications associated with the requested procedure. Regardless of the opinion or expertise of the referring physician, the radiologist has a responsibility to assess each potential case independently to determine whether the procedure can be performed safely, whether percutaneous access is the preferred approach, and whether the patient is likely to benefit from the procedure (Fig. 22-1). Rare is the referring physician who will stand by your side in court, taking responsibility for the poor outcome of a nonindicated procedure that you performed at their request. In addition, thorough knowledge of the case at hand projects a sense of competence and confidence to the patient, who will appreciate that you took the time to familiarize yourself with their situation. One should only consider percutaneous biopsy of a mass or organ when patient management or treatment decisions depend on definitive characterization of an abnormality that cannot reasonably be characterized noninvasively. Generally accepted indications for percutaneous fluid drainage include suspected infection, need for fluid characterization, or relief of symptoms. Abscess drainage in the setting of cholecystitis, perforated appendicitis, diverticulitis, or Crohn disease may be indicated as a temporizing rather than curative measure.

Pearl: The radiologist has a responsibility to assess each potential case independently to determine whether the procedure can be performed safely, whether percutaneous access is the preferred approach, and whether the patient is likely to benefit from the procedure.

Choose Target and Approach

Before performing any biopsy or drainage, one should review all available relevant imaging studies to choose an appropriate target (mass or fluid collection), determine the safest approach to the lesion, and anticipate complications. The most appropriate target for biopsy may not be the lesion initially selected by the referring clinician (Fig. 22-2). Some referring clinicians review diagnostic imaging examinations without ever consulting a radiologist or an official interpretation. Such individuals may refer a patient for biopsy of a particular lesion, unaware that a far more favorable target exists elsewhere in the body. By carefully studying the imaging data in advance, the radiologist can also plan the safest and most direct access to the lesion in question, potentially saving time and consternation during the procedure. Once the access site is chosen, one can estimate the likelihood of certain complications, such as pneumothorax, and appropriately inform the patient.

Pearl: The most appropriate target for biopsy may not be the lesion initially selected by the referring clinician.

Choose a Modality

The choice of an appropriate guidance modality (computed tomography [CT], sonography, fluoroscopy, magnetic resonance imaging [MRI]) is important to the success of any percutaneous intervention. When

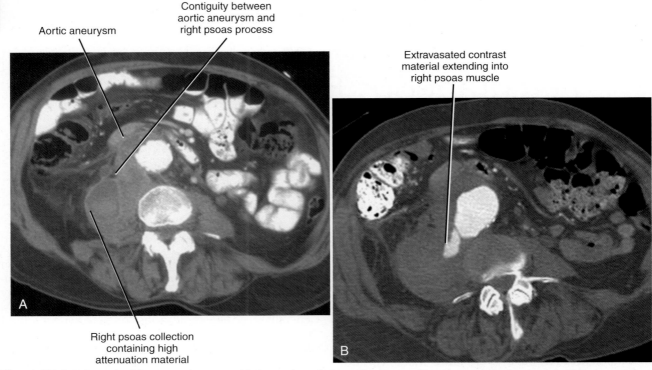

Figure 22-1 Enhanced axial computed tomographic image through the midabdomen of a patient with back pain and mildly increased white blood cell count (**A**) and repeat examination (**B**) performed within 24 hours of initial study. The referring surgeon insisted on percutaneous drainage of possible right psoas abscess after initial study (**A**). The radiologist refused, citing concern for ruptured aortic aneurysm. The repeat study (**B**) confirmed the radiologist's suspicions, and the patient underwent immediate surgery.

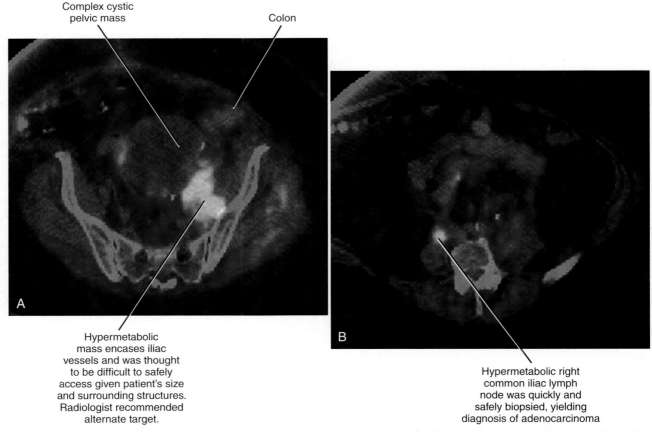

Figure 22-2 Axial fused data set from positron emission tomographic/computed tomographic study through the pelvis (**A**) and lower abdomen (**B**) of a patient with a complex pelvic mass. The referring gynecologist requested biopsy of the hypermetabolic pelvic sidewall component in **A**. This was noted to surround the iliac vessels by the radiologist, who recommended biopsy of the easier-to-access hypermetabolic right common iliac artery lymph node in **B**. Biopsy of the lymph node recommended by radiologist yielded the diagnosis of adenocarcinoma.

choosing a modality, one must consider such factors as lesion visibility and location, proximity and visibility of surrounding structures, modality availability, and operator experience.

Assess Efficacy

In the case of percutaneous biopsy, assessing efficacy refers to evaluating the adequacy of the tissue obtained. Unless the radiologist is skilled at reviewing cytology preparations under a microscope, this can best be accomplished by having a cytologist or cytotechnologist review the specimen(s) at the time of tissue sampling. In the case of percutaneous abscess drainage, efficacy can be assessed by imaging the area of interest after catheter placement or fluid aspiration. When a large residual collection persists despite attempts at complete aspiration, repositioning or "upsizing" the needle or catheter may be necessary. In addition to assessing appropriate catheter position and function, repeat imaging allows early detection of procedure-related complications.

■ SELECTING A MODALITY

Fluoroscopy

Fluoroscopy is rarely used to primarily access a soft-tissue mass or fluid collection within the abdomen or pelvis. However, fluoroscopy may be useful for guiding musculoskeletal procedures based on bony landmarks and may occasionally be utilized to access a superficial air-containing collection requiring drainage. Fluoroscopy greatly facilitates drainage tube manipulations and procedures that require catheter exchanges over a guidewire. Contrast material injected under fluoroscopy can be used to check drainage tube patency and residual abscess cavity size, as well as to delineate fistulous tracts and demonstrate communications between fluid collections. Fluoroscopy may also be a useful adjunct to sonography.

Ultrasound

Ultrasound is a popular guidance modality for percutaneous biopsy and abscess drainage (Figs. 22-3 and 22-4). The high temporal resolution of ultrasound facilitates both accuracy and efficiency without subjecting the patient and operator to ionizing radiation. Ultrasound also allows for an unlimited number of imaging planes from which the operator can select the safest projected path. Color Doppler imaging is effective at demonstrating intervening vascular structures, and system portability permits procedures to be performed at the patient's bedside. Ultrasound is also easy to combine with fluoroscopy. One unique feature of ultrasound is the ability to use it to displace structures such as bowel that lie along the projected needle path. This is accomplished by applying gentle but firm

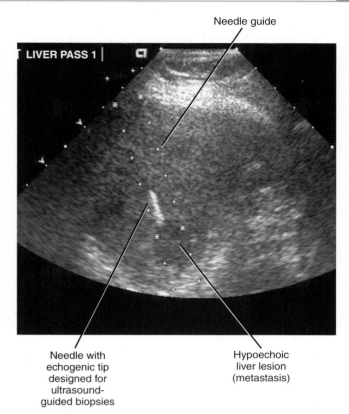

Figure 22-3   Ultrasound-guided liver biopsy with a needle designed with an echogenic tip for ultrasound-guided procedures.

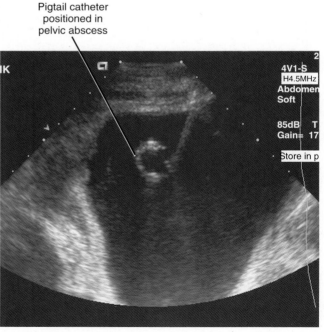

Figure 22-4   Pigtail drainage catheter successfully positioned in pelvic abscess using ultrasound guidance. Catheter visibility is excellent due to superficial location and hypoechoic nature of collection.

continuous pressure with the transducer over the bi-opsy site until bowel is displaced to the side. This technique has the added benefit of decreasing the distance from the skin to the target, improving accuracy and target visibility. Unfortunately, the many benefits of sonography are counterbalanced by limited tissue penetration, limited field of view, and the need for an adequate sonographic window. Depending on the background echogenicity, standard needles and catheters may occasionally be difficult to visualize with ultrasound (Fig. 22-5). Visualization of deep structures may be limited in obese patients and in patients with air-filled bowel overlying the region of interest. Air within an abscess cavity may also obscure visualization (Fig. 22-6). The use of tools such as needle guides and echogenic needles designed specifically for ultrasound-guided procedures may improve operator confidence (see Fig. 22-3). If using an adjustable-angle needle guide, one must be certain that the adjustment on the guide matches the angle setting on the ultrasound machine.

Computed Tomography

CT provides excellent spatial resolution, field of view, and depth of penetration. However, vascular structures may be difficult to differentiate from surrounding soft tissues on noncontrast CT images, and conventional CT

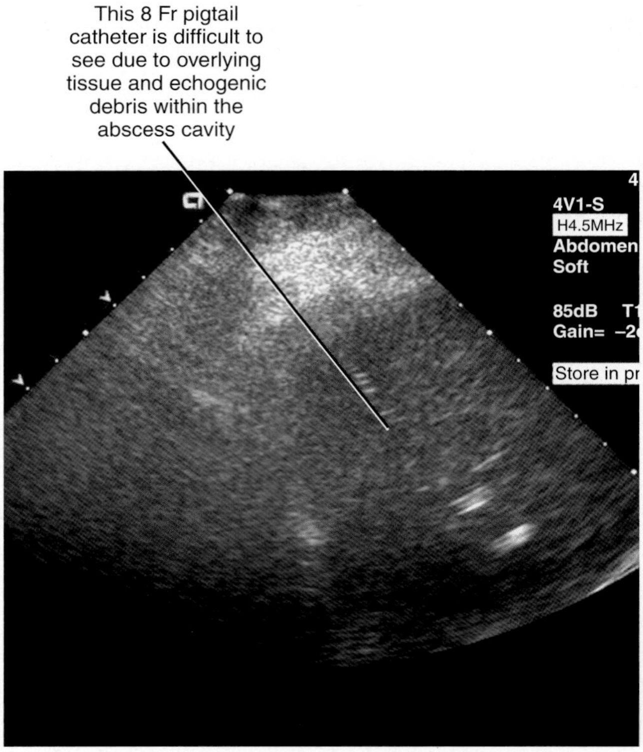

Figure 22-5 Abdominal abscess drained under ultrasound guidance. Note that drainage catheter is difficult to see because of the echogenic nature of the fluid and deeper location of the collection. *Fr,* French.

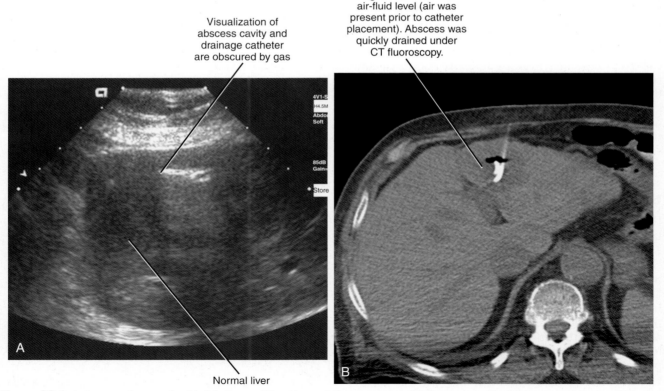

Figure 22-6 Attempt at ultrasound-guided drainage of liver abscess **(A)** was unsuccessful due to poor visualization caused by gas within the collection. The abscess subsequently drained successfully by computed tomographic (CT) fluoroscopy **(B).**

guidance offers relatively poor temporal resolution. Intermittent imaging can be cumbersome for the operator attempting to access a mobile target, and one must rely on estimated trajectories when attempting to avoid nearby structures (Fig. 22-7). Conventional CT imaging is limited to the axial or oblique axial plane (with gantry angulation), lacks portability, and exposes the patient to ionizing radiation.

The lack of real-time imaging capability has been perceived as a profound weakness of conventional CT guidance. CT-fluoroscopy units, which became available in the 1990s, improved on conventional CT techniques by providing operator-controlled near–real-time imaging capability. Table and scanner controls, as well as image display, are available in the scanner room to allow efficient operation. Therefore, the operator is exposed to ionizing radiation during CT-fluoroscopy procedures and requires shielding such as a lead apron. Radiation exposure to the operator results from scatter, as well as direct irradiation when the operator's hands are directly within the beam during needle manipulations. Needle holders have been specifically designed to minimize this latter problem, although traditional surgical instruments may also serve to alleviate exposure of the operator's hands. In most situations, intermittent monitoring with hands outside the radiation beam is sufficient for needle guidance. Improved efficiency still results from close proximity of the operator to the patient and rapid image acquisition and reconstruction. Because of the potential of CT-fluoroscopy to result in unacceptably high radiation doses to patients and operators, care must be taken to reduce patient exposure (e.g., through modification of tube current and exposure times) and operator exposure (e.g., through appropriate shielding and efficient technique). In addition to improving procedure efficiency, CT fluoroscopy has the potential to improve needle positioning and diagnostic yield of difficult percutaneous biopsies (mobile or small targets), and facilitate safe placement of needles around obstacles such as ribs, bowel, and blood vessels (Figs. 22-8 and 22-9).

Magnetic Resonance Imaging

MRI offers excellent spatial and contrast resolution in addition to a multiplanar capability that has the potential to greatly expand the number of access routes. MRI can take advantage of the intrinsic tissue properties of a lesion to improve conspicuity without requiring intravenous contrast injection. This latter benefit has particular implications for the monitoring of percutaneous ablation therapies. Despite these advantages, the expense and limited availability of MR scanners, as well as the need for MR-compatible equipment and appropriately trained individuals, have limited widespread performance of MRI-guided interventions.

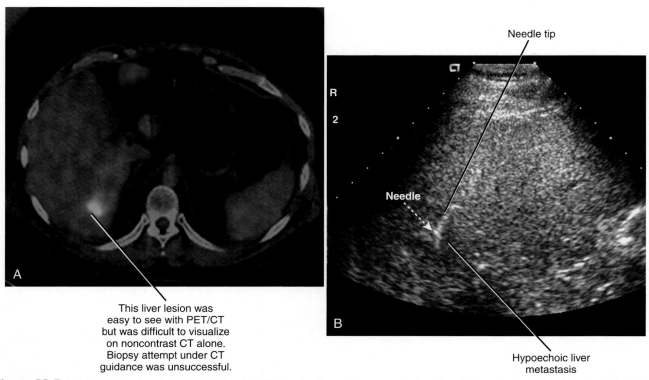

Needle tip

Needle

This liver lesion was easy to see with PET/CT but was difficult to visualize on noncontrast CT alone. Biopsy attempt under CT guidance was unsuccessful.

Hypoechoic liver metastasis

Figure 22-7 Axial positron emission tomographic (PET)/computed tomographic (CT) image **(A)** shows hypermetabolic liver metastasis in the right lobe of the liver. Biopsy attempt was unsuccessful under CT guidance because of respiratory motion and poor visibility but was quickly accomplished under ultrasound guidance **(B)**.

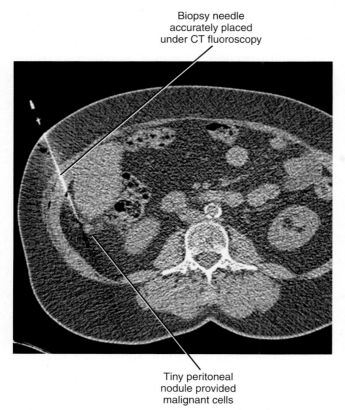

Biopsy needle
accurately placed
under CT fluoroscopy

Tiny peritoneal
nodule provided
malignant cells

Figure 22-8 A biopsy was successfully performed on tiny peritoneal metastasis using computed tomographic fluoroscopy.

■ ACCESS CONSIDERATIONS

Preprocedure Access Questions

When planning a percutaneous biopsy or abscess drainage, one must choose among the various potential paths by which the lesion can be accessed. When planning access, one should resist the urge to "wing it" when the patient is on the table and should consider the following questions in advance:

1. *How can or should the patient be positioned?* Prone imaging may not be an option for a patient with an open abdominal wound. A patient with severe back problems may not tolerate supine positioning for extended periods.

2. *What is the most direct path to the lesion?* Even a slight deviation in needle angle will result in inaccurate needle placement when covering a large distance. Also, thin needles are difficult to control over long distances.

3. *Are there any critical structures that must be avoided?* Some critical structures (such as the inferior epigastric arteries) are small but nonetheless important.

4. *Can the target lesion be approached along its long access?* This facilitates a longer throw or needle pass in the case of biopsies, and easier wire and catheter manipulation in the case of drainage procedures (Fig. 22-10).

5. *Will the patient be able to sleep or sit with a catheter in place? Will the proposed access site facilitate easy self-catheter care?*

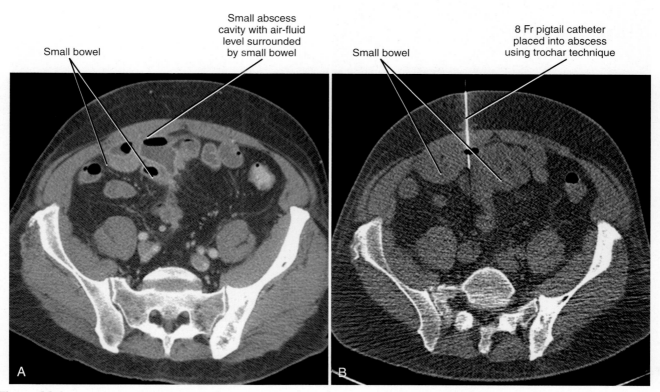

Small bowel

Small abscess
cavity with air-fluid
level surrounded
by small bowel

Small bowel

8 Fr pigtail catheter
placed into abscess
using trochar technique

A

B

Figure 22-9 Enhanced axial computed tomographic (CT) image **(A)** shows a small anterior abdominal abscess with air–fluid level surrounded by small bowel loops. The abscess was quickly drained under CT fluoroscopic guidance **(B)**. *Fr,* French.

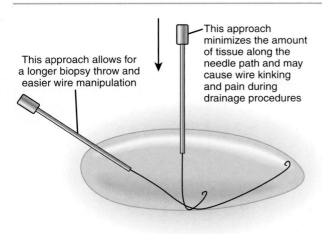

Figure 22-10 Illustration showing the potential benefit of approaching a fluid collection along its long axis.

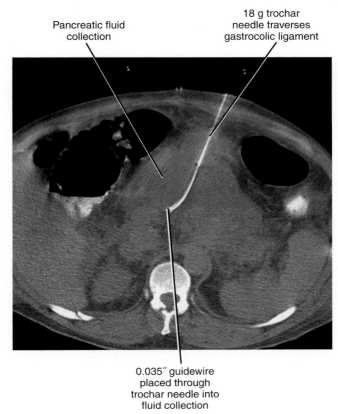

Figure 22-11 Axial noncontrast computed tomographic image shows anterior transperitoneal approach to acute pancreatic fluid collection. *18 g*, 18-gauge.

6. *Have all potential access strategies been considered?* Would the patient be better served by a less conventional approach (e.g., transrectal, transvaginal, endoscopic)?
7. *For which complications should I be prepared?* Surprises are best reserved for birthday parties and scary movies.

Potential Approaches

When planning access to an abnormality, many options can be considered. These can be organized into anterior or posterior, transperitoneal or extraperitoneal, percutaneous or endoluminal, and transvisceral or nontransvisceral approaches. When considering a transvisceral approach, one should make every attempt to avoid transgressing the pancreas, spleen, gallbladder, colon, uterus, ovaries, and prostate gland, unless the target lesion lies within one of those organs. Some of the more common approaches are discussed in more detail in the following subsections. When planning the approach to a tumor or fluid collection, be sure to look for small but important structures that should be avoided (e.g., the ureters).

Anterior Transperitoneal (Transabdominal) Approach

The anterior transperitoneal (transabdominal) approach (Fig. 22-11) allows for comfortable supine positioning of the patient. Peritoneal mesenteries and ligaments (e.g., gastrocolic ligament) are transgressed without difficulty. In thin patients, retroperitoneal structures can be approached in this manner. Bowel creates the greatest impediment to this approach. An effort should be made to avoid the inferior epigastric vessels that run deep to the rectus muscles. Avoiding the rectus muscles by puncturing through an aponeurosis may prevent rectus sheath hematoma. Traversing the peritoneum can be painful for the patient, so care must be taken to provide adequate anesthesia.

Anterior Extraperitoneal Approach

Patients may be positioned supine or lateral decubitus for the anterior extraperitoneal approach (Fig. 22-12), which is useful for biopsy of pelvic lymph nodes and pelvic sidewall lesions, as well as drainage of iliopsoas abscesses. The ureters, external iliac vessels, and deep circumflex iliac arteries are the main structures to avoid with this approach.

Posterior Extraperitoneal (Retroperitoneal) Approach

The posterior extraperitoneal (retroperitoneal) approach (Fig. 22-13) usually requires prone or decubitus positioning of the patient but has the advantage of avoiding the intraperitoneal organs. The anterior pararenal approach allows access to many pancreatic fluid collections. A catheter placed in this manner can serve as a guide for a subsequent retroperitoneal surgical approach to the pancreas.

Transgluteal (Transsciatic) Approach

Deep pelvic structures can be approached through the sciatic foramen (Fig. 22-14). Patients are positioned prone or lateral decubitus for this approach. The gluteal vessels and sciatic nerve/sacral plexus are avoided by staying close to the sacrum and below the level of the piriformis muscle. The main limitations of this

White arrow shows
anterior extraperitoneal
approach to fluid collection

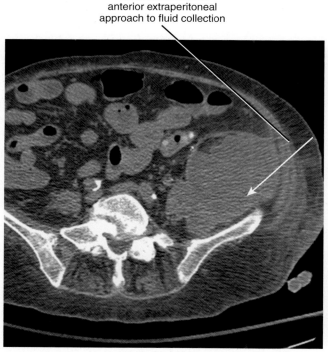

Figure 22-12 Unenhanced axial computed tomographic image through the upper pelvis demonstrating anterior extraperitoneal approach to abscess collection.

Rim enhancing
fluid collection
posterior to uterus

Urinary bladder

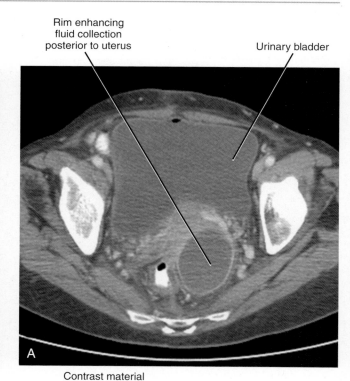

A

Anterior pararenal
fluid collection

Drainage catheter
placed over 11th rib
into anterior pararenal
fluid collection

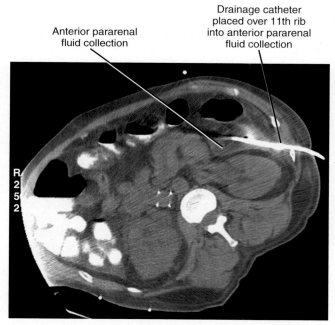

Figure 22-13 Unenhanced axial computed tomographic image demonstrates posterior extraperitoneal approach to pancreatic fluid collection.

Contrast material
within urinary
bladder

Drainage catheter

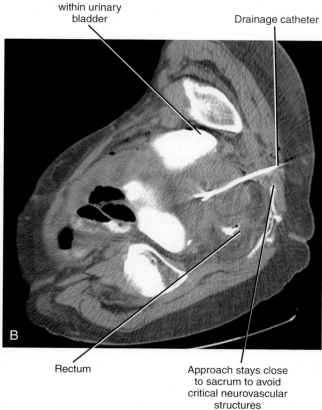

B

Rectum

Approach stays close
to sacrum to avoid
critical neurovascular
structures

Figure 22-14 Enhanced axial computed tomographic image of a deep pelvic abscess (**A**) inaccessible from an anterior approach. The abscess was successfully drained from a transgluteal approach (**B**). Access was facilitated by lateral decubitus positioning of the patient.

approach are patient discomfort and limited patient access to the skin entry site for self-care.

Pearl: The gluteal vessels and sciatic nerve/sacral plexus are avoided during a transsciatic approach by staying close to the sacrum and below the level of the piriformis muscle.

Transhepatic Approach

The liver can be safely traversed when necessary to access fluid collections or biopsy targets within the right adrenal gland, kidney, mesentery, and pancreatic region (Fig. 22-15). An attempt should be made to avoid major hepatic vessels, the gallbladder, and major bile ducts. When placing a transhepatic catheter into an extrahepatic collection, one should try to ensure that no catheter side holes remain within the hepatic parenchyma.

Transenteric Approach

Transgastric access is often necessary to perform a biopsy or drain abnormalities of the pancreas, peripancreatic region, and lesser sac. Percutaneous drainage of pancreatic pseudocysts can be safely accomplished through the stomach, but the resulting tract between the pseudocyst and the stomach cannot be expected to persist for long once the catheter is removed. Rarely, it may be necessary to traverse small bowel to perform a biopsy on otherwise inaccessible lesions of the abdomen and pelvis. This can usually be safely and successfully performed with a 22-gauge needle. Interloop abscess aspiration may be attempted through the small bowel, but catheter placement is typically not performed in such circumstances.

Transrectal and Transvaginal Approaches

Transrectal and transvaginal approaches are used to access collections low in the pelvis or to perform a biopsy on low pelvic structures such as the prostate. Ultrasound guidance is typically preferred, and specially designed needle guides are helpful. A variety of patient positions can be utilized. The vaginal wall can be difficult and painful to puncture and dilate, and over-the-wire techniques may be challenging from a transrectal or transvaginal approach. Adequate anesthesia is important, and preprocedure antibiotics may be beneficial.

Other Approaches

A variety of alternative biopsy approaches has been described for particularly challenging lesions. These include transrenal, transcystic (through the bladder), and transosseous (through bone) approaches, among others. As with all interventional procedures, an analysis of the potential risks and benefits should be performed before embarking on a difficult procedure. One must also keep in mind that the best approach may be offered by an alternative service with a different set of tools and skills. For example, a transjugular approach to the liver may be preferred in a patient with coagulopathy. Endoscopic techniques excel at pancreatic pseudocyst drainage and pancreatic mass biopsy. Finally, some lesions are best accessed using laparoscopic or open surgical techniques.

Tricks for Improving Percutaneous Access

When a tumor or fluid collection appears inaccessible via the approaches described in the previous subsections, one should consider some additional ways to improve access (Box 22-1). Sometimes changes in patient position or respirations may be beneficial. This is particularly true for abnormalities within or behind mobile structures such as the liver and kidneys. Decubitus positioning and expiratory breath holding may be beneficial when traversing the pleural space (Fig. 22-16). The CT scanner gantry angle can be altered to circumvent ribs or the pleural space when necessary.

Hydrodissection refers to the displacement of nontarget structures away from a target with an injection of sterile water or saline (Fig. 22-17). Saline should be avoided when performing radiofrequency ablation because it is conductive.

When ultrasound guidance is used to guide a procedure, bowel loops can also be displaced by applying firm, continuous pressure over the access site with the transducer. The tip of a 22-gauge biopsy needle can be

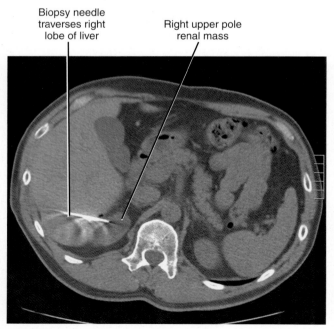

Biopsy needle traverses right lobe of liver

Right upper pole renal mass

Figure 22-15 Transhepatic biopsy of right upper pole renal mass under computed tomographic guidance.

BOX 22-1   Alternative Ways to Improve Access to Lesions of the Abdomen and Pelvis

Change patient position.
Alter patient respirations.
Inject sterile saline or water (hydrodissection).
Apply pressure with the ultrasound transducer.
Use a curved needle (through a straight guide).
Catheterize the bladder.
Angle the CT scanner gantry.

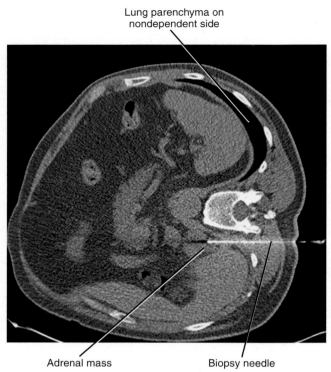

Lung parenchyma on
nondependent side

Adrenal mass   Biopsy needle

Figure 22-16 Unenhanced axial computed tomographic (CT) image from CT-guided biopsy of right adrenal mass. Right lateral decubitus positioning helps avoid visceral pleura of the lung, although the needle crosses the pleural space.

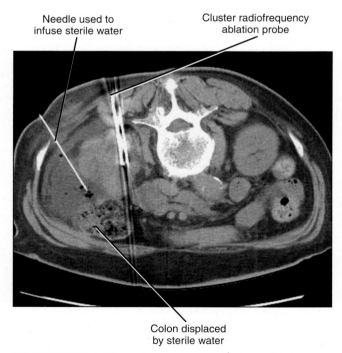

Needle used to   Cluster radiofrequency
infuse sterile water   ablation probe

Colon displaced
by sterile water

Figure 22-17 Axial unenhanced computed tomographic image through the kidneys shows use of hydrodissection to displace the colon away from the kidney during radiofrequency ablation of a renal tumor.

bent with a hemostat into a gentle curve to maneuver around critical structures. When placed through a guide needle, this smaller caliber curved needle emerges at an angle from the guide.

A full bladder can obscure lesions of the pelvis and may simulate a pathologic fluid collection. Therefore, placement of a bladder catheter helps facilitate access to lesions deep within the pelvis (Fig. 22-18).

What to Do When You Cannot See the Lesion

Occasionally, an attempt may be made to perform a biopsy on a lesion that is visible on a preprocedure imaging study but not during the actual procedure. When this occurs, first make certain that all imaging parameters have been optimized. This is particularly important for ultrasound-guided procedures. Adjustments in the focal zone, gain settings, transducer frequency, or imaging plane may reveal the lesion. The next step when ultrasound is being used is to reposition the patient or alter respirations. Turning the patient on his or her side or having the patient take a deep breath may move the lesion to a more favorable location. If CT guidance is being used, consider using anatomic landmarks to guide tissue sampling. Useful landmarks include nearby vessels, calcifications, ducts, surgical clips, or surface contour deformities. Occasionally, intravenous contrast administration may be necessary. Unfortunately, the benefits of contrast enhancement may be fleeting, so consider positioning the needle near the expected location of the lesion before contrast administration. When a lesion is difficult to visualize, always consider alternative imaging modalities.

Pearl: When injecting contrast to better define a target lesion during CT-guided biopsy, consider positioning the needle near the expected location of the lesion before contrast administration, because the benefits of contrast enhancement may be fleeting.

■ MAXIMIZING SUCCESS

Percutaneous Biopsy

In our opinion, three criteria define a successful percutaneous biopsy (ignoring the financial compensation aspect for a moment): (1) Sufficient tissue is obtained to establish a diagnosis; (2) the information obtained makes a meaningful contribution to the patient's care; and (3) the patient does not suffer serious irreparable damage. In general, one should expect a successful outcome in at least 80% of abdominal and pelvic percutaneous biopsy procedures. Assuming one can successfully navigate the gauntlet of intervening organs and vessels to arrive at the target lesion, the adequacy of tissue obtained is controlled by the needle type, needle size, and sampling technique. We cannot provide a complete and detailed dissertation on needle selection in a text of this scope, but a few points warrant further consideration. In many cases, the choice of needle depends on user experience and preference.

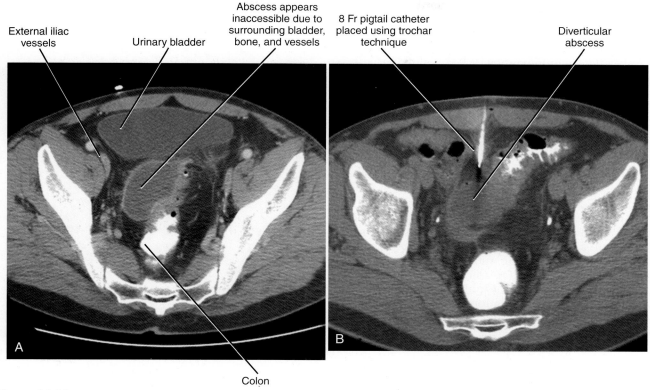

Figure 22-18 Enhanced axial computed tomographic image (**A**) through the pelvis of a patient with a diverticular abscess. After emptying the urinary bladder, the abscess was accessible from an anterior approach (**B**). *Fr,* French.

Fine Needle Aspiration Needles

Fine needle aspiration (FNA) needles usually have a removable stylet and a tip with one or more sharp points. FNA needles are used to obtain tissue via aspiration or capillary action. Most FNAs are performed with needles ranging from 25 to 20 gauge. FNA technique is typically used to sample focal mass lesions. Although a thinner needle creates smaller holes in tissue, thinner is not always better. Thinner needles are harder to control because of their tendency to bend and deviate from the projected path. To improve needle tracking and permit multiple biopsy passes without the need for repeat needle positioning, a larger-caliber guide needle (usually 20 to 18 gauge) can be positioned at the leading edge of a mass. Repeat samples can be subsequently obtained with a 20-gauge or thinner needle placed coaxially through the guide needle. When FNA is performed, we recommend having a cytopathologist or technologist evaluate the specimen for adequacy.

Core Biopsy Needles

Core biopsy needles typically consist of an outer sheath and an inner needle with a chamber that stores the tissue sample. Core biopsy needles can be manually activated or are available as spring-loaded "guns." Core biopsies are often performed when larger tissue samples are desired, when attempts at FNA are unsuccessful, or when tissue architecture must be preserved (e.g., for staging hepatitis). Before performing a core needle biopsy, it is important to understand the design of the needle with particular attention to the additional excursion that the needle tip will make once fired. One should make certain that the projected needle excursion does not extend into vital structures. Some core biopsy guns come with adjustable throws. It is important to be certain that the proper setting is selected before inserting the needle. When a core biopsy is obtained, a "touch-prep" can be performed to evaluate the specimen, although some pathologists discourage this practice. It may be helpful to consult with your pathologists as to the type and amount of sample they prefer for analysis before performing a biopsy.

Pitfall: Before performing a core biopsy with a spring-loaded needle, ensure that critical structures are not in the line of fire.

Biopsy Technique

When using an FNA needle, tissue is obtained by making multiple quick needle excursions of 1 to 2 cm through the target lesion. The outer guide needle may be used to gently redirect the biopsy needle to different parts of the lesion (to a minor degree). One can often rely on capillary action to obtain cells. Once blood is seen in the needle hub, further excursions are usually not helpful with the capillary FNA technique. When removing the needle, it helps to place a finger over the needle hub to minimize tissue loss to vacuum effect. One should avoid prolonged sampling because this may allow the specimen to clot in the needle. Preparation of the slides should commence immediately after sampling for the same reason. Some individuals prefer to actively apply suction with a syringe during FNA, although we only rarely have found this necessary. Use of a short connecting tube between the syringe and needle may facilitate manipulations. When aspirating with a syringe, relieving suction when withdrawing the needle helps to avoid sampling nontarget tissues and aspirating the specimen into the syringe.

When performing a biopsy, avoid sampling the center of a necrotic mass because this will likely result in inadequate cells for characterization. When performing a core biopsy, it may be helpful to include a small margin of normal organ in the sample. This can be confirmed by the presence of a visible zone of transition in the specimen. Repeated biopsies of the same area within a mass often result in sampling the area of hemorrhage created by the first pass. Multiple regions can be sampled within a large mass by first sampling the far side of the mass and performing subsequent biopsies more proximally. When sampling a firm but mobile mass, it may be necessary to use a more abrupt stabbing motion during FNA to prevent deviation of the mass away from the needle. A core biopsy gun may also be helpful in such a setting.

Pitfall: Repeated biopsies of the same area within a mass often result in sampling the area of hemorrhage created by the first pass.

Maximizing Success During Percutaneous Fluid Drainage

We consider a successful percutaneous fluid drainage to be one with the following results: (1) permanent elimination of an infected fluid collection; (2) significant relief of patient symptoms; (3) stabilization of a patient until a more definitive procedure can be performed; or (4) simplification of subsequent surgery or patient management. In general, one should be successful in at least 80% of percutaneous drainage procedures. A lower success rate may result from patient selection, as well as technique. Fluid collections should not be drained simply because they are present on an imaging study, and one should always be aware of abscess mimics that should not be drained, including necrotic or vascular neoplasm (Fig. 22-19), pseudoaneurysm, surgical packing material, bowel, and implanted devices (Fig. 22-20).

It may be difficult to establish the infected nature of a fluid collection based solely on imaging characteristics. Although laboratory analysis of aspirated fluid is the most definitive way to establish the infected nature of a fluid collection, some imaging findings increase the likelihood that a fluid collection is infected (Box 22-2). Unfortunately, any one of the findings listed in Box 22-2 can occur in the absence of infection. Nuclear scintigraphy with gallium-67– or indium-111–labeled leukocytes may be helpful to establish the infected nature of a fluid collection noninvasively, but these tests are rarely performed before fluid aspiration.

Pitfall: Many imaging findings in abdominal and pelvic abscesses may also be present in sterile hematomas and necrotic or cystic neoplasms. Surgically placed

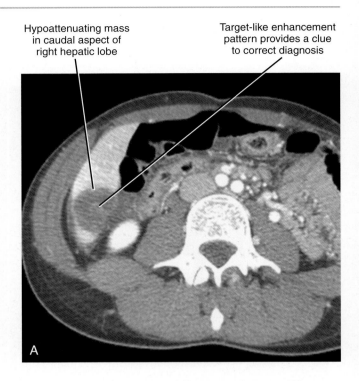

Hypoattenuating mass in caudal aspect of right hepatic lobe

Target-like enhancement pattern provides a clue to correct diagnosis

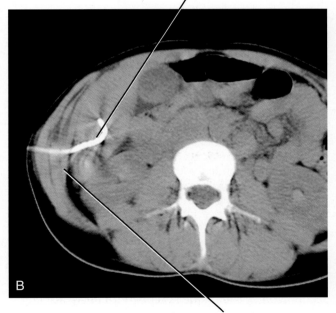

Tip of pigtail catheter failed to form due to lack of fluid-filled cavity. Aspiration yielded no fluid.

Pigtail catheter placed using trochar technique

Figure 22-19 Enhanced axial computed tomographic image (**A**) through caudal right hepatic lobe in a patient with fever and increased white blood cell count shows a hypoattenuating lesion thought to represent hepatic abscess. Attempt to percutaneously drain lesion was unsuccessful (**B**), and biopsies performed during same procedure were inconclusive. Epithelioid hemangioendothelioma was subsequently found at surgery.

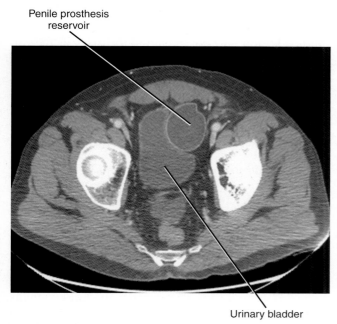

Penile prosthesis
reservoir

Urinary bladder

Figure 22-20 Enhanced axial computed tomographic scan through the pelvis of a patient with penile prosthesis. Note the reservoir in the left lower quadrant. Attempts at percutaneous drainage of such devices have resulted in litigation.

BOX 22-2   Imaging Findings That May Be Present in Infected Fluid Collections

Gas
Rim enhancement
Debris
Septa
Surrounding fat stranding

---

packing or hemostatic material may closely mimic the appearance of a postoperative abscess.

A sterile fluid collection often can be managed by complete aspiration through a 20- to 18-gauge needle at the time of sampling. Small abscesses (<5 cm in diameter) often can be successfully managed by antibiotics combined with complete aspiration at the time of diagnosis. Successful needle aspiration of infected fluid usually can be accomplished with an 18-gauge trochar needle or 5 French (Fr) needle sheath system. A specifically designed needle with multiple side holes may facilitate aspiration of thicker fluid. Aspiration alone is unlikely to succeed if the collection communicates with the biliary tract, pancreatic duct, or bowel. Pancreatic pseudocysts rarely resolve completely after aspiration alone.

Although some individuals advocate management of larger (e.g., >5 cm) infected or symptomatic fluid collections by aspiration alone, most practitioners prefer catheter drainage for collections of this size. A daunting variety of catheters is available for image-guided percutaneous abscess drainage. The various catheter designs are distinguished, in part, by material composition,

inner lumen diameter, distal tip design, locking mechanism, and side hole location, size, and number. Some designs (sump catheters) have multiple lumens. In our experience, sump catheters are rarely necessary for routine abscess drainage. In most cases, the choice of catheter design does not significantly affect outcome and should be at the discretion of the individual radiologist.

Catheter diameter may be a more important determinant of success than catheter design. Two major schools of thought exist regarding the choice of catheter diameter: (1) use the smallest catheter that will accomplish the task, or (2) use the largest catheter that can be placed safely. Smaller catheters are better tolerated by patients, and in our experience, many abscesses can be successfully drained with an 8 to 8.5 Fr catheter. However, smaller catheters may become blocked with debris and are more prone to kinking. Larger catheters are less likely to become obstructed or kink but are more cumbersome to place and may be less comfortable for the patient.

As with catheter design, placement technique varies with operator preference. Some practitioners prefer an over-the-wire technique. This method has the advantage of initially puncturing with a needle that is considerably thinner than the catheter. This may reduce the risk for complications such as bowel injury related to inaccurate placement. Over-the-wire technique also allows fluid sampling before catheter placement without the need for an additional puncture. The access needle can also be used to deliver local anesthetic to the deep tissues along the needle tract. Over-the-wire technique requires several exchanges of equipment and risks loss of access because of wire dislodgment or kinking. This technique works best when the cavity size allows for sufficient wire to coil within it and is unsuitable for small collections. An over-the-wire technique may be beneficial in the setting of a loculated fluid collection because the guide wire can serve to break up septa and create communications between loculations.

Catheters can also be placed using a trochar technique, which involves primary placement of the catheter in the fluid collection using a sharp inner trochar to dissect through the tissues. This technique has the advantage of speed, although one must be careful not to deviate from the projected path to avoid serious injury to surrounding structures. One must also be certain that the catheter tip is well within the fluid collection before deployment, or an extracavitary tube placement will result (Fig. 22-21). Larger catheters can be difficult to place using this technique, and one should use only catheters designed for this purpose.

Final catheter position can be important to the success of a percutaneous drainage procedure. In general, drainage will be more effective when working with gravity. When draining a fluid collection, it is important to provide sufficient catheter length to allow for catheter movement with respiration and changes in patient position. A catheter that travels through a large mobile pannus can become dislodged when the patient rolls from side to side or sits upright. When draining a large collection, be sure to place enough catheter length within the

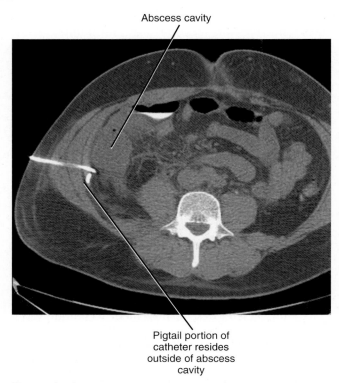

Abscess cavity

Pigtail portion of catheter resides outside of abscess cavity

Figure 22-21 Axial computed tomographic (CT) image through the abdomen performed immediately after an attempt at CT-guided abscess drainage using the trochar technique. Note that the catheter was deployed prematurely, resulting in extracavitary placement.

cavity to allow for cavity shrinkage (Fig. 22-22). A catheter positioned in the most superficial part of a large fluid collection may not remain in the cavity as the volume of fluid decreases and the catheter withdraws with patient movement and catheter maintenance (Fig. 22-23). Catheters that cross ascites before entering a collection have a tendency to pull back into the peritoneal space with respirations and patient motion (Fig. 22-24).

Pearl: When draining a fluid collection, be sure to provide sufficient catheter length within the collection to allow for catheter movement at the skin and cavity collapse.

Once a catheter has been placed within a fluid cavity, limited imaging should be performed to verify satisfactory position. We recommend verifying catheter position before complete aspiration of the cavity contents. It is often easier to determine that a catheter is satisfactorily positioned and that no bowel loops have been transgressed when the cavity is not completely collapsed around the catheter. Once the fluid contents have been aspirated to the extent desired, a collection device (either a drainage bag or suction bulb) is attached to the catheter. Usually, fluid is sent to the laboratory for analysis. To avoid seeding the bloodstream with bacteria, we do not routinely flush an abscess cavity with saline immediately after catheter placement. An appropriately positioned drainage catheter is generally left in place until output declines to less than 10 to 15 ml/day.

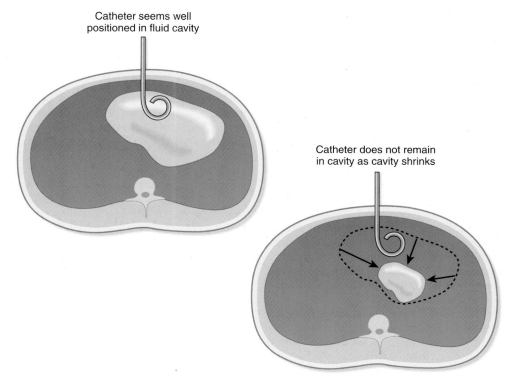

Catheter seems well positioned in fluid cavity

Catheter does not remain in cavity as cavity shrinks

Figure 22-22 The problem with insufficient catheter length within a fluid collection.

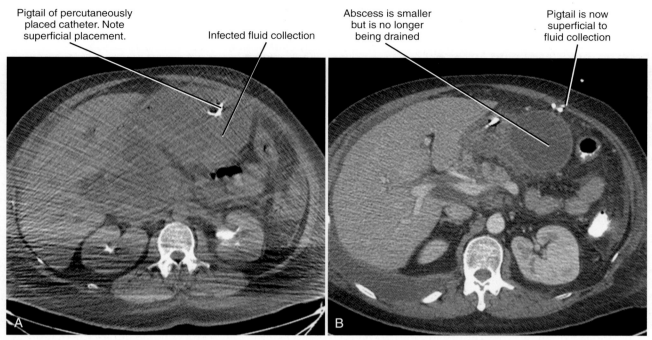

Pigtail of percutaneously placed catheter. Note superficial placement.

Infected fluid collection

Abscess is smaller but is no longer being drained

Pigtail is now superficial to fluid collection

Figure 22-23   Axial computed tomographic scans performed immediately after percutaneous drainage of an anterior abdominal abscess (**A**), and several days later after fever recurred and catheter drainage ceased (**B**). Note that the catheter position was too superficial in **A**, resulting in eventual extracavitary position in **B**.

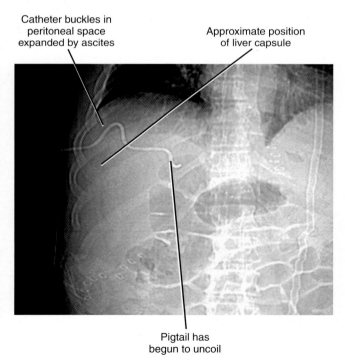

Catheter buckles in peritoneal space expanded by ascites

Approximate position of liver capsule

Pigtail has begun to uncoil

Figure 22-24   Scanogram from a computed tomographic scan performed after a drainage catheter was placed through ascites into a hepatic abscess. Despite the precarious catheter position, the abscess was treated successfully.

Special Fluid Drainage Circumstances

Infected Pancreatic Necrosis
Some patients with infected pancreatic necrosis may be managed successfully with percutaneous drainage. Drainage of infected pancreatic necrosis represents a significant commitment of time and effort by the radiologist. Multiple large-bore catheters (with diameters often exceeding the 8-14 Fr catheters typically placed by radiologists), suction, intermittent catheter manipulations, frequent irrigation, and additional efforts at debridement are usually necessary to remove solid debris.

Highly Viscous Collection
Collections that resist drainage despite satisfactory placement of a relatively large-bore catheter may occasionally be managed successfully by the transcatheter introduction of fibrinolytic agents.

Bowel Perforation
Patients with overt signs of uncontained bowel perforation into the peritoneal cavity (free air, peritoneal signs, enteric contrast leakage) are usually better served by surgical intervention.

Tumor Abscess
Infected, cavitated tumors that cannot be surgically resected occasionally can be managed with catheter drainage. However, the patient and referring physician should be informed that such an infection is unlikely to be cured with catheter drainage alone, and that drainage

may be necessary for the duration of the patient's remaining life.

Abscesses Associated with Lower Likelihood of Success

Collections that communicate with bowel, are multiple or highly loculated, contain a large amount of necrotic debris, or have deep gas bubbles may be more difficult to eradicate completely via catheter drainage (Fig. 22-25). However, percutaneous drainage should be considered in such cases when other options, such as surgery, are not viable.

Troubleshooting Catheters

Sometimes, despite seemingly flawless placement, a percutaneous drain fails to accomplish its intended goal. Generally, there are two reasons for persistent cavity despite adequate catheter position: (1) insufficient removal of fluid via the catheter, or (2) excessive fluid production. Table 22-1 addresses the former situation.

When high catheter output persists despite antibiotics and prolonged drainage, one should attempt to determine whether the fluid cavity communicates with bowel, bile duct, renal collecting system, or pancreatic duct. In such cases, additional procedures such as biliary or urinary diversion may be necessary to allow the communication to close. In the case of a pancreatic duct communication, the administration of octreotide may decrease pancreatic secretions and improve outcome, provided the pancreatic duct is not obstructed. Communication with the pancreatic or bile duct, bowel, or ureter can be documented by gently injecting sterile water-soluble contrast media through the drainage catheter during fluoroscopic observation.

Table 22-1   No Catheter Output Despite Residual Fluid Cavity

Potential Cause	Potential Solution
Fluid too viscous	Upsize catheter, consider fibrinolytics
Catheter in suboptimal position	Reposition or replace catheter
Catheter obstructed	Attempt to unblock or exchange catheter over wire
Catheter kinked at skin	Remove dressing and resecure catheter
Loculated fluid	Consider additional catheters or fibrinolytics

■ MINIMIZING COMPLICATIONS

Despite careful planning and meticulous technique, complications cannot be completely eradicated from one's interventional practice. The typical practice can expect a major complication rate related to percutaneous abdominal and pelvic interventions of about 10% or less. One's own rate will depend on the definition of complication, as well as the difficulty of cases referred. Box 22-3 lists the most common complications to be potentially encountered during a percutaneous intervention in the abdomen and pelvis.

Careful attention to details before beginning a percutaneous procedure can help minimize risk to the patient. Laboratory values (e.g., platelet level, international normalized ratio) should be assessed for evidence of coagulopathy, and the patient's medications should be reviewed to identify any that can predispose to bleeding complications (e.g., anticoagulants or antiplatelet agents). A review of the patient's allergies may reveal

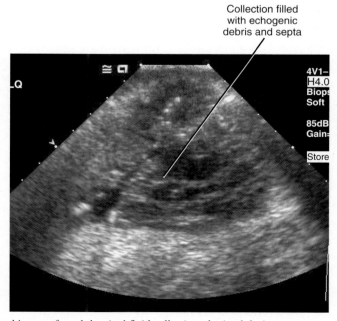

Collection filled with echogenic debris and septa

Figure 22-25 Grayscale ultrasound image of an abdominal fluid collection obtained during an attempt at ultrasound-guided drainage. Despite successful catheter placement, this collection did not respond to percutaneous drainage because of the complex nature of its contents.

BOX 22-3   Most Common Abdominal and Pelvic Interventional Complications

Bleeding
Arteriovenous fistula or pseudoaneurysm
Infection
Pneumothorax (subphrenic procedures)
Empyema (subphrenic drainage procedures)
Bowel perforation
Other nontarget organ injury

Table 22-2   Small but Important Vessels to Avoid During Procedures

Vessel	Location
Intercostal arteries	These travel along the underside of the ribs and may be injured during intercostals procedures (Fig. 22-26).
Inferior epigastric arteries	These travel just deep to the rectus muscles. These arteries gradually transit from lateral to medial as they course from the pelvis toward the umbilicus (Fig. 22-27).
Gluteal arteries	These structures are at risk during transgluteal/transsciatic procedures. They travel through the sciatic foramen close to the ischium. They are best avoided by staying as medial as possible during a transsciatic approach (close to the sacrum).
Deep circumflex iliac artery	This artery runs along the anteromedial surface of the iliacus muscle and may be injured when using an anterior extraperitoneal approach (see Fig. 22-27).

allergies to such things as latex or local anesthetics. It is important to ensure that pheochromocytoma has been excluded through appropriate laboratory studies before adrenal biopsy.

Although one can never eliminate the possibility of a complication, attention to certain details will help minimize the severity of a complication once it occurs. Patients should have reliable intravenous access and be connected to monitoring equipment (e.g., pulse oximeter, sphygmomanometer) before beginning a procedure. Oxygen, suction, and relevant emergency medications should be readily available if needed. Every major abdominal intervention should be followed by a period of close observation (generally between 1 and 4 hours depending on the procedure). Antibiotics are typically administered before drainage of an infected fluid collection. When using imaging guidance to perform an intervention, one should always survey the area around the target lesion to account for all nearby critical structures. If the exact location of a nearby organ is not known in advance, it may be difficult to avoid.

Pearl: During an imaging-guided intervention, if you do not know where a nearby nontarget structure or organ is, you cannot be certain you will avoid it.

Bleeding

Procedure-related hemorrhage is the most common complication related to percutaneous interventional procedures outside of the thorax. Because of the nature of most procedures (i.e., jabbing the patient with a sharp object), some degree of hemorrhage is expected after a biopsy or drainage procedure. For this reason, preexisting coagulopathy or thrombocytopenia should be corrected before proceeding with most interventions. Hemorrhage requiring surgical intervention, blood transfusion, or other urgent management often results from injury of a medium-sized or larger vessel and can be minimized by careful selection of the needle tract and appropriate use of imaging guidance. Table 22-2 lists some frequently injured vascular structures.

Critical vessels can be avoided during CT-guided procedures through careful needle tract planning. Real-time imaging with color Doppler ultrasound is especially helpful in avoiding vascular structures (Fig. 22-28). The use of a needle guide also helps to ensure a safe needle passage. When using a needle guide, choose a needle path that does not intersect any major vascular structure.

Bleeding also can result from transgression of an organ capsule during an intervention. One should attempt to minimize trauma to the capsule by limiting patient motion and respirations during the time that the capsule is breached. When a patient cannot or will not cooperate, one should carefully consider additional means of ensuring cooperation (e.g., improved communication, pain management, or sedation) or alternative means of obtaining tissue. The use of a coaxial needle system during biopsy minimizes the number of times an organ capsule is traversed and can be helpful when multiple samples are anticipated. This potential benefit is somewhat offset by the requirement for larger gauge access. When a patient is breathing freely with the outer guide needle in place, it is important to prevent constraining the free motion of the needle to prevent capsular laceration.

When sampling liver lesions, we recommend leaving at least 1 cm of normal parenchyma between the lesion and the liver capsule along the needle path. Although we acknowledge that this is not always possible when sampling subcapsular lesions, it does help to tamponade bleeding (Fig. 22-29). When ascites is present, we try to minimize amount of ascites between the liver and the abdominal wall, acknowledging that the issue of whether the presence of ascites increases the risk for peritoneal hemorrhage from percutaneous biopsy remains a controversial one. Additional situations that may be associated with an increased risk for a bleeding complication during a percutaneous biopsy include use of large-gauge needles, the presence of cirrhosis, a hypervascular or malignant target lesion, and underlying coagulopathy or thrombocytopenia.

Infection

The risk for introducing infection during a percutaneous intervention is low and can be minimized through careful attention to sterile technique. The greatest risk for introducing infection into a patient probably exists

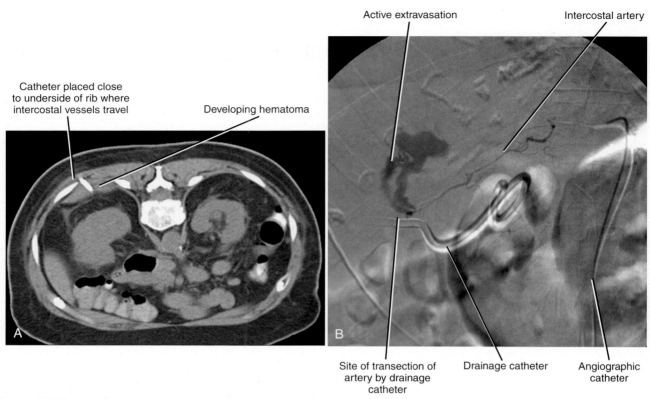

Catheter placed close to underside of rib where intercostal vessels travel

Developing hematoma

Active extravasation

Intercostal artery

Site of transection of artery by drainage catheter

Drainage catheter

Angiographic catheter

A

B

Figure 22-26 Axial computed tomographic scan (**A**) performed after intercostal placement of a drainage catheter into an abdominal fluid collection (collection visible on different slice) and subsequent digital subtraction arteriogram (**B**) performed after patient became hemodynamically unstable. Transected intercostal artery was embolized.

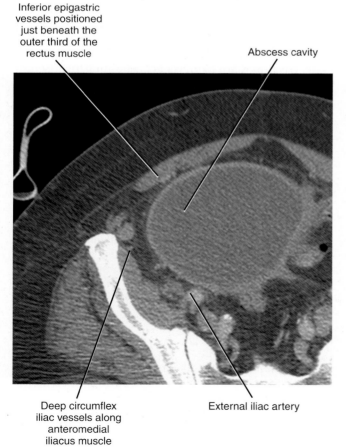

Inferior epigastric vessels positioned just beneath the outer third of the rectus muscle

Abscess cavity

Deep circumflex iliac vessels along anteromedial iliacus muscle

External iliac artery

Figure 22-27 Unenhanced axial computed tomographic image through the pelvis of a patient with an abscess shows the position of some critical vessels to be avoided.

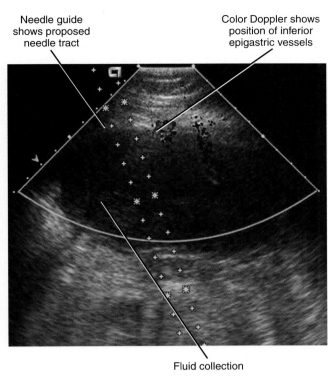

Needle guide shows proposed needle tract

Color Doppler shows position of inferior epigastric vessels

Fluid collection

Figure 22-28 Use of color Doppler and needle guide to avoid inferior epigastric vessels during US-guided fluid aspiration.

for drainage of sterile fluid collections. One should be particularly leery of leaving drainage catheters in sterile collections that are in continuity with implanted surgical devices because infection in this setting can have severe consequences. The risk for introducing infection into a previously sterile collection leads many interventionalists to sample fluid before placing a catheter. If clear fluid is obtained, many individuals prefer to aspirate the collection as completely as possible before removing the needle. When the sterility of a collection is in question, a stat Gram stain can be useful to help determine whether catheter placement is indicated.

Postprocedure sepsis can complicate percutaneous abscess drainage and can have serious consequences. Clinical manifestations may include fever, chills, rigors, and hypotension. Sepsis presumably results from the introduction of bacteria directly into the bloodstream during catheter placement and manipulation. Preprocedure antibiotics may help reduce the risk for postprocedure sepsis, although even patients receiving antibiotics are at risk. To further reduce the risk for sepsis, we recommend minimizing guidewire and catheter manipulation during and after placement into an infected fluid collection. We do not advocate routinely flushing an abscess cavity with saline immediately after catheter placement.

Nontarget Injury

Structures other than blood vessels are at risk for injury during percutaneous intervention. The likelihood of injuring a structure or organ relates directly to its proximity

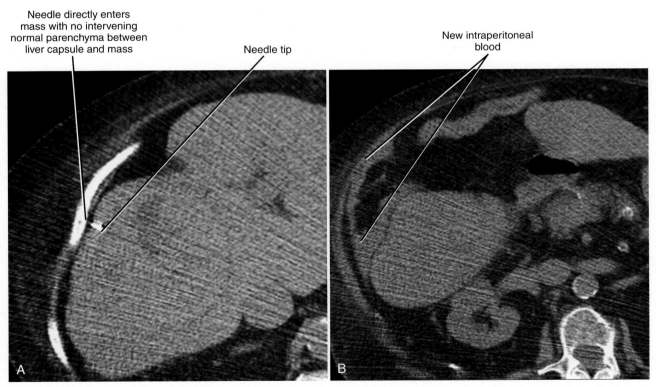

Needle directly enters mass with no intervening normal parenchyma between liver capsule and mass

Needle tip

New intraperitoneal blood

A   B

Figure 22-29 Axial computed tomographic (CT) images during (**A**) and after (**B**) CT-guided fine needle aspiration of hepatocellular carcinoma. The biopsy needle did not cross normal parenchyma before entering the mass. The postprocedure CT scan (**B**) was performed when the patient began reporting severe abdominal pain.

to the target. Before any intervention, one should always ensure that enough of the region around the target lesion is visualized. A few moments should be dedicated to identifying normal anatomic structures around the region of interest that are to be avoided.

The gallbladder is occasionally inadvertently entered during percutaneous biopsy or aspiration in or near the liver. If this occurs, we recommend aspirating the contents of the gallbladder as completely as possible to avoid bile leakage and subsequent bile peritonitis.

The bowel can be inadvertently crossed or entered during a variety of procedures. When a relatively thin needle (e.g., 20 gauge or thinner) is used, it can usually be withdrawn without adverse consequences. When larger needles inadvertently transgress bowel, the patient should be monitored for evidence of peritonitis. Puncture of the colon is generally considered more significant than puncture of small bowel. Prophylactic antibiotic coverage may be considered when the bowel is transgressed. When a drainage catheter is inadvertently placed within bowel, it can be left in place for approximately 2 weeks to allow a mature tract to form. Enteric contrast material administered before a CT-guided procedure is helpful for distinguishing between bowel and abnormal fluid collections. When performing an ultrasound-guided intervention, one should always look for evidence of peristalsis or other typical features of bowel before proceeding. When performing an ultrasound-guided pelvic intervention, the introduction of water per rectum can sometimes be helpful in delineating the rectum and sigmoid colon. Preprocedure placement of a bladder catheter may help reduce the risk for bladder injury during pelvic interventions.

The pleura can be avoided during upper abdominal interventions by choosing the most anterior and caudal approach feasible. The intercostal route often results in transgression of the pleural space and increased risk for pneumothorax, empyema, and pleural fistula (Fig. 22-30). The patient and referring physician should be made aware of the significant possibility of these complications when the parietal pleura cannot be avoided. Every effort should be made to avoid the lung during an abdominal intervention. If a new pleural effusion is noted on chest radiography performed after a subphrenic drainage procedure, one should consider the possibility of hemothorax, empyema, or abdominopleural fistula. Some practitioners intentionally collapse the lung before an intervention near the diaphragm to avoid injuring the lung during the procedure. The lung is reexpanded on successful complete of the intervention.

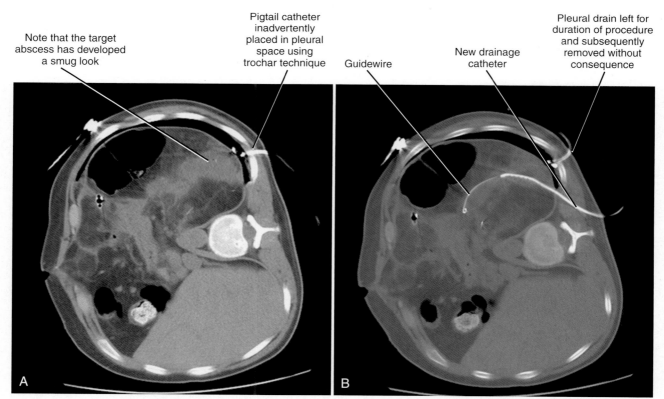

Figure 22-30 Axial computed tomographic scans performed after an initial attempt at catheter placement into abdominal fluid collection using trochar technique (**A**) and after reattempt (**B**) because of inadvertent placement of first catheter in pleural space.

Suggested Readings

Arellano RS, Maher M, Gervais DA et al: The difficult biopsy: let's make it easier, *Curr Probl Diagn Radiol* 32:218-226, 2003.

Bakal CW, Sacks D, Burke DR et al: Quality improvement guidelines for adult percutaneous abscess and fluid drainage, *J Vasc Interv Radiol* 14:S223-S225, 2003.

Cardella JF, Bakal CW, Bertino RE et al: Quality improvement guidelines for image-guided percutaneous biopsy in adults, *J Vasc Interv Radiol* 14:S227-S230, 2003.

Cinat ME, Wilson SE, Din AM: Determinants for successful percutaneous image-guided drainage of intra-abdominal abscess, *Arch Surg* 137:845-849, 2002.

Feld RI: Ultrasound-guided biopsies: tricks, needle tips, and other fine points, *Ultrasound Q* 20:91-99, 2004.

Froelich JJ, Wagner HJ: CT fluoroscopy: tool or gimmick? *Cardiovasc Intervent Radiol* 24:297-305, 2001.

Gervais DA, Ho C, O'Neill MJ et al: Recurrent abdominal and pelvic abscesses: incidence, results of repeated percutaneous drainage, and underlying causes in 956 drainages, *Am J Roentgenol* 182:463-466, 2004.

Gobien RP, Stanley JH, Schabel SI et al: The effect of drainage tube size on adequacy of percutaneous abscess drainage, *Cardiovasc Intervent Radiol* 8:100-102, 1985.

Gupta S, Nguyen HL, Morello FA et al: Various approaches for CT-guided percutaneous biopsy of deep pelvic lesions: anatomic and technical considerations, *Radiographics* 24:175-189, 2004.

Hui GC, Amaral J, Stephens D et al: Gas distribution in intraabdominal and pelvic abscesses on CT is associated with drainability, *Am J Roentgenol* 184:915-919, 2005.

Jaffe TA, Nelson RC, Delong DM et al: Practice patterns in percutaneous image-guided intraabdominal abscess drainage: survey of academic and private practice centers, *Radiology* 233:750-756, 2004.

Liermann D, Kickuth R: CT fluoroscopy-guided abdominal interventions, *Abdom Imaging* 28:129-134, 2003.

Maher MM, Gervais DA, Kalra MK et al: The inaccessible or undrainable abscess: how to drain it, *Radiographics* 24:717-735, 2004.

Mehta RP, Johnson MS: Update on anticoagulant medications for the interventional radiologist, *J Vasc Interv Radiol* 17:597-612, 2006.

Men S, Akhan O, Koroglu M: Percutaneous drainage of abdominal abscess, *Eur J Radiol* 43:204-218, 2002.

Mueller PR, Simeone JF, Butch RJ et al: Percutaneous drainage of subphrenic abscess: a review of 62 patients, *Am J Roentgenol* 147:1237-1240, 1986.

Nawfel RD, Judy PF, Silverman SG et al: Patient and personnel exposure during CT fluoroscopy-guided interventional procedures, *Radiology* 216:180-184, 2000.

Otto R: Interventional ultrasound, *Eur Radiol* 12:283-287, 2002.

Park JK, Kraus FC, Haaga JR: Fluid flow during percutaneous drainage procedures: an in vitro study of the effects of fluid viscosity, catheter size, and adjunctive urokinase, *Am J Roentgenol* 160:165-169, 1993.

Shankar S, vanSonnenberg E, Silverman S et al: Imaging and percutaneous management of acute complicated pancreatitis, *Cardiovasc Intervent Radiol* 27:567-580, 2004.

Sudakoff GS, Lundeen SJ, Otterson MF: Transrectal and transvaginal sonographic intervention of infected pelvic fluid collections: a complete approach, *Ultrasound Q* 21:175-185, 2005.

Thomas J, Turner SR, Nelson RC et al: Postprocedure sepsis in imaging-guided percutaneous hepatic abscess drainage: how often does it occur? *Am J Roentgenol* 186:1419-1422, 2006.

Wagner LK: CT fluoroscopy: another advancement with additional challenges in radiation management, *Radiology* 216:9-10, 2000.

Yu SC: The utility of a drainage needle for percutaneous abscess drainage, *Am J Roentgenol* 185:58-63, 2005.

Index

Note: "b" following an entry indicates a box, "f" indicates a figure, "t" indicates a table, and "CD" indicates material discussed in the bonus CD chapters.